2017
Twentieth Edition

The Complete Learning Disabilities Directory

Associations • Products • Resources
Conferences • Services • Web Sites

A SEDGWICK PRESS Book

Grey House
Publishing

PUBLISHER: Leslie Mackenzie
EDITORIAL DIRECTOR: Laura Mars

PRODUCTION MANAGER & COMPOSITION: Kristen Thatcher
ASSOCIATE EDITORS: Daniella D'souza, Venessa Weedmark
MARKETING DIRECTOR: Jessica Moody

A Sedgewick Press Book
Grey House Publishing, Inc.
4919 Route 22
Amenia, NY 12501
518.789.8700
FAX 845.373.6390
www.greyhouse.com
e-mail: books@greyhouse.com

Table of Contents

Table of Contents

Introduction

The Complete Learning Disabilities Directory has been a comprehensive and sought-after resource for professionals, families and individuals with learning disabilities since 1992. This twentieth edition is the most comprehensive and current source of resources for the LD community available today. This title is a consistent National Health Information Awards Winner for providing "...the Nation's Best Consumer Health Infomation Programs and Materials in the category of Health Promotion/Disease and Injury Prevention Information."

Praise for previous editions:

> ***Tremendous Asset . . .*** *"this title would be a tremendous asset to any professional, parent, or student who seeks to deepen their knowledge about challenges and rewards of recognizing different learning styles and behaviours which may one day not be seen as a 'disability.'"*
>
> —Pinnacle Health System

> ***Highly Recommended . . .*** *"By virtue of its size, comprehensiveness, and frequency of updates, this directory stands out as a singularly important resource for academic and public libraries. It is highly recommended."*
>
> —ARBA

> ***Five-Star Review . . .*** *"This is a must-have resource for individuals who work with people with different types of learning disabilities. . . . any professional, parent, or student wanting to learn more. This is by far the best of all the resources available for learning disabled individuals. No need to search the Internet to find this information; this book provides it all at your fingertips!"*
>
> —Doody's Review Service

According to James Wendorf, Executive Director of The National Center for Learning Disabilities (NCLD), "Stigma, underachievement and misunderstanding of LD continue to be stubborn barriers for parents and children to overcome. [2014 data indicates] that, left unaddressed, as many as 60 million individuals risk being left behind, burdened by low self- esteem, subjected to low expectations, and diminished in their ability to pursue their dreams."

Facts from the NCLD:
- 2.4 million American public school students (approximately 5%) are identified with LD
- Two-thirds of students identified with LD are male
- More students with LD live in poverty than children from the general population
- Many people attribute LD, inaccurately, to: excessive TV watching; poor diet; and childhood vaccinations
- In the past decade, the number of students with LD receiving regular HS diplomas has risen from 57 to 68%

The Complete Learning Disabilities Directory supports the LD population, from those with a learning disability to their support network, in a number of ways. Following this Introduction is an in-depth Glossary from *LD Online*, a leading web site about learning disabilities and ADHD. This Glossary provides more than 200 clear, detailed definitions of acronyms and specialized terms frequently used in books, articles, medical offices and educational environments that are devoted to individuals with learning disabilities and their network of family, friends, and professionals.

The Complete Learning Disabilities Directory, with 4,622 listings, provides a comprehensive look at the variety of resources available for the many different types of learning disabilities, from those that occur in spoken language, to those that affect organizational skills. It includes a wide array of testing resources, crucial for early diagnosis, and is arranged in subject-specific chapters for quick, effective research.

The Table of Contents is your guide to this database in print form. *The Complete Learning Disabilities Directory's* listings are arranged into 21 major chapters and 100 subchapters, making it easy to pinpoint the exact type of desired reference, including Associations, National/State Programs, Publications, Audio/Video, Web Sites, Products, Conferences, Schools, Learning/Testing Centers, and Summer Programs. Listings provide thousands of valuable contact points, including 10,363 key executives, web sites, fax numbers, descriptions, founding year, designed-for age for products, and size of LD population for schools.

The Complete Learning Disabilities Directory provides comprehensive and far-reaching coverage not only for individuals with LD, but for parents, teachers and professionals. Users will find answers to legal and advocacy questions, as well as specially designed computer software and a full range of assistive devices.

As information overload distracts to immobility, *The Complete Learning Disabilities Directory* gives you the confidence that this one resource with important LD information is all you need. It assures those in the LD community that this crucial information is readily available at every school and library across the country, not just at state or district level special education resource centers. Now, every special education teacher, student, and parent can have, right at their fingertips, a wealth of information on the critical resources that are available to help individuals achieve in school and in their community.

This valuable resource includes three indexes: Geographic, Entry Name & Publisher and Subject.

This data in *The Complete Learning Disabilities Directory* is also available for subscription on G.O.L.D. – Grey House OnLine Databases. Subscribers to G.O.L.D. can access their subscription via the Internet and do customized searches that make finding information quicker and easier. Visit http://gold.greyhouse.com for more information.

Glossary

The education field is so full of acronyms and specialized words that it can seem like a confusing alphabet soup! Find out what AYP, IEP, 504, and many other abbreviations and words mean in this glossary of frequently used terms.

Academic Achievement Standards

Academic achievement standards refer to the expected performance of students on measures of academic achievement; for instance, "all students will score at least 76% correct on the district-developed performance-based assessment." Also known as performance standards. See also **academic content standards**.

Academic Content Standards

Academic content standards are developed by state departments of education to demonstrate what they expect all students to know and be able to do in the core **content areas**. According to **NCLB**, **ELL** students "will meet the same challenging State academic content and student academic achievement standards as all children are expected to meet." See also **academic achievement standards**.

Academic English

The English language ability required for academic achievement in context-reduced situations, such as classroom lectures and textbook reading assignments. This is sometimes referred to as Cognitive/Academic Language Proficiency (CALP).

Accommodation (For English Language Learners)

Adapting language (spoken or written) to make it more understandable to second language learners. In assessment, accommodations may be made to the presentation, response method, setting, or timing/scheduling of the assessment (Baker, 2000; Rivera & Stansfield, 2000).

Accommodation (For Students With Disabilities)

Techniques and materials that allow individuals with LD to complete school or work tasks with greater ease and effectiveness. Examples include spellcheckers, tape recorders, and expanded time for completing assignments.

Accuracy

The ability to recognize words correctly.

Adequate Yearly Progress (AYP)

An individual state's measure of yearly progress toward achieving state academic standards. "Adequate Yearly Progress" is the minimum level of improvement that states, school districts and schools must achieve each year.

Affective Filter

The affective filter is a metaphor that describes a learner's attitudes that affect the relative success of second language acquisition. Negative feelings such as lack of motivation, lack of self-confidence and learning anxiety act as filters that hinder and obstruct language learning. This term is associated with linguist Stephen Krashen's **Monitor Model** of second language learning.

Affix

Part of word that is "fixed to" either the beginnings of words (prefixes) or the endings of words (suffixes). The word *disrespectful* has two affixes, a prefix (*dis-*) and a suffix (*-ful*).

Age Equivalent Score

In a norm-referenced assessment, individual student's scores are reported relative to those of the norming population. This can be done in a variety of ways, but one way is to report the average age of people who received the same score as the individual child. Thus, an individual child's score is described as being the same as students that are younger, the same age, or older than that student (e.g. a 9 year old student my receive the same score that an average 13 year old student does, suggesting that this student is quite advanced).

Alphabetic Principle

The basic idea that written language is a code in which letters represent the sounds in spoken words.

Americans With Disabilities Act (ADA)

A federal law that gives civil rights protections to individuals with disabilities similar to those provided to individuals on the basis of race, color, sex, national origin, age, and religion. It guarantees equal opportunity for individuals with disabilities in public accommodations, employment, transportation, state and local government services, and telecommunications.

Analogy-Based Phonics

In this approach, students are taught to use parts of words they have already learned to read and decode words they don't know. They apply this strategy when the words share similar parts in their spellings, for example, reading screen by analogy to green. Students may be taught a large set of key words for use in reading new words.

Analytic Phonics

In this approach, students learn to analyze letter-sound relationships in previously learned words. They do not pronounce sounds in isolation.

Annual Measurable Achievement Objectives (AMAO)

Within Title III of NCLB, each state is required to determine Annual Measurable Achievement Objectives (AMAOs). AMAOs indicate how much English language proficiency (reading, writing, speaking, listening, and comprehension) children served with Title III funds are expected to gain each year. See also AYP, for similar content area requirements

The AMAO requirements include reporting on these three things:

1. Annual increases in the number or percentage of children making progress in learning English.

2. Annual increases in number or percentage of children attaining English proficiency.

3. ELL children making AYP.

Aphasia

see Developmental Aphasia

Assessment

Assessment is a broad term used to describe the gathering of information about student performance in a particular area. See also formative assessment and summative assessment.

Assistive Technology

Equipment that enhances the ability of students and employees to be more efficient and successful. For more information, go to **"LD Topics: Technology."**

Attention Deficit / Hyperactivity Disorder (ADHD)

Any of a range of behavioral disorders in children characterized by symptoms that include poor concentration, an inability to focus on tasks, difficulty in paying attention, and impulsivity. A person can be predominantly inattentive (often referred to as ADD), predominantly hyperactive-impulsive, or a combination of these two.

Attention Deficit Disorder (ADD)

see ADHD

Auditory Discrimination

Ability to detect differences in sounds; may be gross ability, such as detecting the differences between the noises made by a cat and dog, or fine ability, such as detecting the differences made by the sounds of letters "m" and "n."

Auditory Figure-Ground

Ability to attend to one sound against a background of sound (e.g., hearing the teacher's voice against classroom noise).

Auditory Memory

Ability to retain information which has been presented orally; may be short term memory, such as recalling information presented several seconds before; long term memory, such as recalling information presented more than a minute before; or sequential memory, such as recalling a series of information in proper order.

Auditory Processing Disorder (APD)

An inability to accurately process and interpret sound information. Students with APD often do not recognize subtle differences between sounds in words.

Authentic Assessment

Authentic assessment uses multiple forms of evaluation that reflect student learning, achievement, motivation, and attitudes on classroom activities. Examples of authentic assessment include performance assessment, portfolios, and student self-assessment.

Automaticity

Automaticity is a general term that refers to any skilled and complex behavior that can be performed rather easily with little attention, effort, or conscious awareness. These skills become automatic after extended periods of training. With practice and good instruction, students become automatic at word recognition, that is, retrieving words from memory, and are able to focus attention on constructing meaning from the text, rather than decoding.

Base Words

Words from which many other words are formed. For example, many words can be formed from the base word *migrate*: *migration, migrant, immigration, immigrant, migrating, migratory*.

Basic Interpersonal Communication Skills (BICS)

Basic Interpersonal Communication Skills (BICS) is often referred to as "playground English" or "survival English." It is the basic language ability required for face-to-face communication where linguistic interactions are embedded in a situational context called **context-embedded language**. BICS is part of a theory of language proficiency developed by **Jim Cummins**, which distinguishes this conversational form of language from **CALP** (Cognitive Academic Language Proficiency).

BICS, which is highly contextualized and often accompanied by gestures, is cognitively undemanding and relies on context to aid understanding. BICS is much more easily and quickly acquired than CALP, but is not sufficient to meet the cognitive and linguistic demands of an academic classroom .

Behavior Intervention Plan (BIP)

A plan that includes positive strategies, program modifications, and supplementary aids and supports that address a student's disruptive behaviors and allows the child to be educated in the least restrictive environment (LRE).

Bicultural

Identifying with the cultures of two different ethnic, national, or language groups. To be bicultural is not necessarily the same as being bilingual. In fact, you can even identify with two different language groups without being bilingual, as is the case with many Latinos in the U.S.

Bilingual Education

An educational program in which two languages are used to provide content matter instruction. Bilingual education programs vary in their length of time, and in the amount each language is used.

Bilingual Education, Transitional

An educational program in which two languages are used to provide content matter instruction. Over time, the use of the native language is decreased and the use of English is increased until only English is used.

Bilingualism

Bilingualism is the ability to use two languages. However, defining bilingualism can be problematic since there may be variation in proficiency across the four language dimensions (listening, speaking, reading and writing) and differences in proficiency between the two languages. People may become bilingual either by acquiring two languages at the same time in childhood or by learning a second language sometime after acquiring their first language.

Biliteracy

Biliteracy is the ability to effectively communicate or understand written thoughts and ideas through the grammatical systems, vocabularies, and written symbols of two different languages.

Blend

A consonant sequence before or after a vowel within a syllable, such as *cl, br,* or *st*; it is the written language equivalent of consonant cluster.

California English Language Development Test (CELDT)

CELDT is a language proficiency test developed for the California Department of Education. Progress on language proficiency assessments like the CELDT is a requirement for ELLs under the **No Child Left Behind Act** .

Center For Applied Linguistics (CAL)

CAL is a private, non-profit organization consisting of a group of scholars and educators who use the findings of linguistics to identify and address language-related problems. CAL carries out a wide range of activities including research, teacher education, analysis and dissemination of information, design and development of instructional materials, technical assistance, conference planning, program evaluation, and policy analysis. Visit the **CAL website**.

Central Auditory Processing Disorder (CAPD)

A disorder that occurs when the ear and the brain do not coordinate fully. A CAPD is a physical hearing impairment, but one which does not show up as a hearing loss on routine screenings or an audiogram. Instead, it affects the hearing system beyond the ear, whose job it is to separate a meaningful message from non-essential background sound and deliver that information with good clarity to the intellectual centers of the brain (the central nervous system).

Cloze Passage

A cloze passage is a reading comprehension exercise in which words have been omitted in a systematic fashion. Students fill in the blanks, and their responses are counted correct if they are exact matches for the missing words. Cloze exercises assess comprehension and background knowledge, and they are also excellent indicators of whether the reading level and language level of the text are appropriate for a given student.

Cognates

Words in different languages related to the same root, e.g. *education* (English) and *educación* (Spanish).

Cognitive/Academic Language Proficiency (CALP)

Cognitive/Academic Language Proficiency (CALP) is the language ability required for academic achievement in a context-reduced environment. Examples of context-reduced environments include classroom lectures and textbook reading assignments, where there are few environmental cues (facial expressions, gestures) that help students understand the content. CALP is part of a theory of language developed by Jim Cummins, and is distinguished from Basic Interpersonal Communication Skills **(BICS)**.

Collaborative Writing

Collaborative writing is an instructional approach in which students work together to plan, draft, revise, and edit compositions.

Comprehension Strategies

Techiniques to teach reading comprehension, including summarization, prediction, and inferring word meanings from context.

Comprehension Strategy Instruction

The explicit teaching of techniques that are particularly effective for comprehending text. The steps of explicit instruction include direct explanation, teacher modeling ("think aloud"), guided practice, and application. Some strategies include *direct explanation* (the teacher explains to students why the strategy helps comprehension and when to apply the strategy), *modeling* (the teacher models, or demonstrates, how to apply the strategy, usually by "thinking aloud" while reading the text that the students are using), *guided practice* (the teacher guides and assists students as they learn how and when to apply the strategy) and *application* (the teacher helps students practice the strategy until they can apply it independently).

Connected Instruction

A way of teaching systematically in which the teacher continually shows and discusses with the students the relationship between what has been learned, what is being learned, and what will be learned.

Content Area

Content areas are academic subjects like math, science, English/language arts, reading, and social sciences. Language proficiency may affect these areas, but is not included as a content area. Assessments of language proficiency differ from those of language arts.

Context Clues

Sources of information outside of words that readers may use to predict the identities and meanings of unknown words. Context clues may be drawn from the immediate sentence containing the word, from text already read, from pictures accompanying the text, or from definitions, restatements, examples, or descriptions in the text.

Context-Embedded Language

Context-embedded language refers to communication that occurs in a context of shared understanding, where there are cues or signals that help to reveal the meaning (e.g. visual clues, gestures, expressions, specific location).

Context-Reduced Language

Context-reduced language refers to communication where there are few clues about the meaning of the communication apart from the words themselves. The language is likely to be abstract and academic. Examples: textbook reading, classroom lecture.

Continuous Assessment

An element of responsive instruction in which the teacher regularly monitors student performance to determine how closely it matches the instructional goal.

Cooperative Learning

A teaching model involving students working together as partners or in small groups on clearly defined tasks. It has been used successfully to teach comprehension strategies in content-area subjects.

Criterion-Referenced Test

Criterion-referenced tests are designed to determine whether students have mastered specific content, and allow comparisons with other students taking the same assessment. They are nationally and locally available.

Curriculum-Based Assessment

A type of informal assessment in which the procedures directly assess student performance in learning-targeted content in order to make decisions about how to better address a student's instructional needs.

Decoding

The ability to translate a word from print to speech, usually by employing knowledge of sound-symbol correspondences. It is also the act of deciphering a new word by sounding it out.

Developmental Aphasia

A severe language disorder that is presumed to be due to brain injury rather than because of a developmental delay in the normal acquisition of language.

Developmental Spelling

The use of letter-sound relationship information to attempt to write words (also called *invented spelling*)

Dialogue Journal

A type of writing in which students make entries in a notebook on topics of their choice, to which the teacher responds, modeling effective language but not overtly correcting the student's language (O'Malley & Valdez-Pierce, 1996, p.238).

Differentiated Instruction

An approach to teaching that includes planning out and executing various approaches to content, process, and product. Differentiated instruction is used to meet the needs of student differences in readiness, interests, and learning needs.

Digital Literacy

Digital literacy is the ability to effectively navigate, evaluate, and generate information using digital technology (e.g. computers, software, digital devices, and the Internet).

Direct Instruction

An instructional approach to academic subjects that emphasizes the use of carefully sequenced steps that include demonstration, modeling, guided practice, and independent application.

Direct Vocabulary Learning

Explicit instruction in both the meanings of individual words and word-learning strategies. Direct vocabulary instruction aids reading comprehension.

Domain-Specific Words And Phrases*

Vocabulary specific to a particular field of study (domain), such as the human body (CCSS, p. 33); in the Standards, domain-specific words and phrases are analogous to Tier Three words (Language, p. 33).

Dominant Language

The dominant language is the language with which a bilingual or multilingual speaker has greatest proficiency and/or uses more often. See **primary language**.

Dual Language Program/Dual Immersion

Also known as two-way immersion or two-way bilingual education, these programs are designed to serve both language minority and language majority students concurrently. Two language groups are put together and instruction is delivered through both languages. For example, in the U.S., native English-speakers might learn Spanish as a foreign language while continuing to develop their English literacy skills and Spanish-speaking ELLs learn English while developing literacy in Spanish. The goals of the program are for both groups to become biliterate, succeed academically, and develop cross-cultural understanding. See the ERIC **Two-way Online Resource Guide** or the NCELA publication, **Biliteracy for a Global Society**.

Dyscalculia

A severe difficulty in understanding and using symbols or functions needed for success in mathematics.

Dysgraphia

A severe difficulty in producing handwriting that is legible and written at an age-appropriate speed.

Dyslexia

A language-based disability that affects both oral and written language. It may also be referred to as reading disability, reading difference, or reading disorder.

Dysnomia

A marked difficulty in remembering names or recalling words needed for oral or written language.

Dyspraxia

A severe difficulty in performing drawing, writing, buttoning, and other tasks requiring fine motor skill, or in sequencing the necessary movements.

Early Childhood English Language Learner (ECELL)

An ECELL is a child who is between the ages of zero and five (early stages of development) and who is in the process of learning English as a second language.

Editing*

A part of writing and preparing presentations concerned chiefly with improving the clarity, organization, concision, and correctness of expression relative to task, purpose, and audience; compared to revising, a smaller-scale activity often associated with surface aspects of a text; see also **revising**, **rewriting**.

ELD

English language development (ELD) means instruction designed specifically for English language learners to develop their listening, speaking, reading, and writing skills in English. This type of instruction is also known as "English as a second language" (**ESL**), "teaching English to speakers of other languages" (**TESOL**), or "English for speakers of other languages" (**ESOL**). ELD, ESL, TESOL or ESOL are versions of English language arts standards that have been crafted to address the specific developmental stages of students learning English.

Embedded Phonics

In this approach, students learn vocabulary through explicit instruction on the letter-sound relationships during the reading of connected text, usually when the teacher notices that a student is struggling to read a particular word. Letter-sound relationships are taught as part of sight word reading. If the sequence of letter-sounds is not prescribed and sequenced, but is determined by whatever words are encountered in text, then the program is not systematic or explicit.

Emergent Literacy

The view that literacy learning begins at birth and is encouraged through participation with adults in meaningful reading and writing activities.

Emergent Reader Texts*

Texts consisting of short sentences comprised of learned sight words and CVC words; may also include rebuses to represent words that cannot yet be decoded or recognized; see also **rebus**.

English As A Second Language

English as a Second Language (ESL) is an educational approach in which English language learners are instructed in the use of the English language. Their instruction is based on a special curriculum that typically involves little or no use of the native language, focuses on language (as opposed to content) and is usually taught during specific school periods. For the rest of the school day, students may be placed in mainstream classrooms, an immersion program, or a bilingual education program. Every bilingual education program has an ESL component (U.S. General Accounting Office, 1994). See also **ELD**, **pull-out ESL**, **ESOL**.

English Language Learner (ELL)

Students whose first language is not English and who are in the process of learning English.

Entry Criteria

Entry criteria are a set of guidelines that designate students as English language learners and help place them appropriately in bilingual education, ESL, or other language support services. Criteria usually include a home language survey and performance on an English language proficiency test.

ESL

See English As A Second Language

ESOL

ESOL stands for 'English for speakers of other languages' (see **ESL**).

Evidence*

Facts, figures, details, quotations, or other sources of data and information that provide support for claims or an analysis and that can be evaluated by others; should appear in a form and be derived from a source widely accepted as appropriate to a particular discipline, as in details or quotations from a text in the study of literature and experimental results in the study of science.

Exceptional Students Education (ESE)

Refers to special education services to students who qualify.

Executive Function

The ability to organize cognitive processes. This includes the ability to plan ahead, prioritize, stop and start activities, shift from one activity to another activity, and to monitor one's own behavior.

Exit Criteria

Exit criteria are a set of guidelines for ending special services for English language learners and placing them in mainstream, English-only classes as fluent English speakers. This is usually based on a combination of performance on an English language proficiency test, grades, standardized test scores, and teacher recommendations. In some cases, this redesignation of students may be based on the amount of time they have been in special programs.

Experimental Writing

Efforts by young children to experiment with writing by creating pretend and real letters and by organizing scribbles and marks on paper.

Expressive Language

The aspect of spoken langauge that includes speaking and the aspect of written language that includes composing or writing.

Family Educational Right To Privacy Act (FERPA)

A federal law that protects the privacy of student education records.

Fluency

The ability to read a text accurately, quickly, and with proper expression and comprehension. Because fluent readers do not have to concentrate on decoding words, they can focus their attention on what the text means.

Focused Question*

A query narrowly tailored to task, purpose, and audience, as in a research query that is sufficiently precise to allow a student to achieve adequate specificity and depth within the time and format constraints.

Formal Assessment

The process of gathering information using standardized, published tests or instruments in conjunction with specific administration and interpretation procedures, and used to make general instructional decisions.

Formal English

See **Standard English**.

Formative Assessment

Formative assessments are designed to evaluate students on a frequent basis so that adjustments can be made in instruction to help them reach target achievement goals.

Free Appropriate Public Education (FAPE)

A requirement of IDEA; all disabled children must receive special education services and related services at no cost.

Functional Behavioral Assessment (FBA)

A problem-solving process for addressing student problem behavior that uses techniques to identify what triggers a given behavior(s) and to select interventions that directly address them.

General Academic Words And Phrases*

Vocabulary common to written texts but not commonly a part of speech; in the Standards, general academic words and phrases are analogous to Tier Two words and phrases (Language, p. 33).

Grade Equivalent Scores

In a norm-referenced assessment, individual student's scores are reported relative to those of the norming population. This can be done in a variety of ways, but one way is to report the average grade of students who received the same score as the individual child. Thus, an individual child's score is described as being the same as students that are in higher, the same, or lower grades than that student (e.g. a student in 2nd grade my earn the same score that an average forth grade student does, suggesting that this student is quite advanced).

Grapheme

A letter or letter combination that spells a single phoneme. In English, a grapheme may be one, two, three, or four letters, such as *e*, *ei*, *igh*, or *eigh*.

Graphic Organizers

Text, diagram or other pictorial device that summarizes and illustrates interrelationships among concepts in a text. Graphic organizers are often known as maps, webs, graphs, charts, frames, or clusters.

Independent Educational Evaluation (IEE)

An evaluation conducted by a qualified examiner, who is not employed by the school district at the public's expense.

Independent School District (ISD)

ISD is a commonly-used acronym in education plans to refer to the school system the child attends.

Independent(Ly)*

A student performance done without scaffolding from a teacher, other adult, or peer; in the Standards, often paired with proficient(ly) to suggest a successful student performance done without scaffolding; in the Reading standards, the act of reading a text without scaffolding, as in an assessment; see also proficient(ly), scaffolding.

Indirect Vocabulary Learning

Vocabulary learning that occurs when students hear or see words used in many different contexts — for example, through conversations with adults, being read to, and reading extensively on their own.

Individualized Education Program (IEP)

A plan outlining special education and related services specifically designed to meet the unique educational needs of a student with a disability.

Individualized Transition Plan (ITP)

A plan developed by the IEP team to help accomplish the student's goals for the transition from high school into adulthood.

Individuals With Disabilities Education Act (IDEA)

The Individuals with Disabilities Education Act is the law that guarantees all children with disabilities access to a free and appropriate public education.

Informal Assessment

The process of collecting information to make specific instructional decisions, using procedures largely designed by teachers and based on the current instructional situation.

Information Gap

'Information gap' is an oral language activity in which a student is rated on his or her success in verbally describing visual information that is hidden from a partner, such as a picture, map, or object (O'Malley & Valdez-Pierce, 1996).

Instructional Conversations

[D]iscussion-based lessons geared toward creating opportunities for students' conceptual and linguistic development. They focus on an idea or a student. The teacher encourages expression of students' own ideas, builds upon information students provide and experiences they have had, and guides students to increasingly sophisticated levels of understanding (Goldenberg, 1991).

Intelligence Quotient (IQ)

A measure of someone's intelligence as indicated by an intelligence test, where an average score is 100. An IQ score is the ratio of a person's mental age to his chronological age multiplied by 100.

Language Learning Disability (LLD)

A language learning disability is a disorder that may affect the comprehension and use of spoken or written language as well as nonverbal language, such as eye contact and tone of speech, in both adults and children.

Language Majority

Language majority refers to a person or language community that is associated with the dominant language of the country.

Language Minority (LM)

Language minority refers to a person from a home where a language other than the dominant, or societal, language is spoken. So, that person may (1) be fully bilingual, (2) speak only the home language, (3) speak only English, or (4) speak mostly the home language but have limited English proficiency.

Language Proficiency

To be proficient in a second language means to effectively communicate or understand thoughts or ideas through the language's grammatical system and its vocabulary, using its sounds or written symbols. Language proficiency is composed of oral (listening and speaking) and written (reading and writing) components as well as academic and non-academic language (Hargett, 1998).

Lau Remedies

Lau Remedies are policy guidelines for the education of English language learners, based on the ruling in the **Lau vs. Nichols** suit, mandating school districts' compliance with the civil rights requirements of Title VI (Lyons, 1992).

Lau V. Nichols

'Lau vs. Nichols' is a lawsuit filed by Chinese parents in San Francisco in 1974, which led to a landmark Supreme Court ruling that identical education does not constitute equal education under the Civil Rights Act. School districts must take "affirmative steps" to overcome educational barriers faced by non-English speakers (Lyons, 1992).

Learning Disability (LD)

A disorder that affects people's ability to either interpret what they see and hear or to link information from different parts of the brain. It may also be referred to as a learning disorder or a learning difference.

Least Restrictive Environment (LRE)

A learning plan that provides the most possible time in the regular classroom setting.

LEP

See Limited English Proficient.

Limited English Proficient (LEP)

Limited English proficient is the term used by the federal government, most states, and local school districts to identify those students who have insufficient English to succeed in English-only classrooms. Increasingly, English language learner (ELL) or English learner (EL) are used in place of LEP.

Linguistically And Culturally Diverse (LCD)

The term 'linguistically and culturally diverse' is commonly used to identify communities where English is not the primary language of communication, although some individuals within the community may be bilingual or monolingual English speakers.

Listening Comprehension

Understanding speech. Listening comprehension, as with reading comprehension, can be described in "levels" – lower levels of listening comprehension would include understanding only the facts explicitly stated in a spoken passage that has very simple syntax and uncomplicated vocabulary. Advanced levels of listening comprehension would include implicit understanding and drawing inferences from spoken passages that feature more complicated syntax and more advanced vocabulary.

Literacy

Reading, writing, and the creative and analytical acts involved in producing and comprehending texts.

Literacy Coach

A reading coach or a literacy coach is a reading specialist who focuses on providing professional development for teachers by providing them with the additional support needed to implement various instructional programs and practices. They provide essential leadership for the school's entire literacy program by helping create and supervise a long-term staff development process that supports both the development and implementation of the literacy program over months and years.

Local Education Agency (LEA)

A public board of education or other public authority within a state that maintains administrative control of public elementary or secondary schools in a city, county, township, school district or other political subdivision of a state.

Mainstream

"Mainstream" is a term that refers to the ordinary classroom that almost all children attend. Accommodations may be made for children with disabilities or who are English language learners, as part of the general educational program.

Metacognition

Metacognition is the process of "thinking about thinking." For example, good readers use metacognition before reading when they clarify their purpose for reading and preview the text.

Monitor Model

In the monitor model, linguist Stephen Krashen proposes that language learning is accomplished either through learning (formal, conscious learning about language) or through acquisition (informal, subconscious learning through experience with language). He suggests that there is an internal "monitor," which is developed through formal learning which is a part of the conscious process of error correction in when speaking a new language. The monitor plays only a minor role in developing fluency, compared to the role of acquisition. This model later became part of Krashen and Terrell's Natural Approach to language teaching (Krashen & Terrell, 1983).

Monitoring Comprehension

Readers who monitor their comprehension know when they understand what they read and when they do not. Students are able to use appropriate "fix-up" strategies to resolve problems in comprehension.

More Sustained Research Project*

An investigation intended to address a relatively expansive query using several sources over an extended period of time, as in a few weeks of instructional time.

Morpheme

The smallest meaningful unit of language. A morpheme can be one syllable (*book*) or more than one syllable (*seventeen*). It can be a whole word or a part of a word such as a prefix or suffix. For example, the word *ungrateful* contains three morphemes: *un*, *grate*, and *ful*.

Morphemic Relationship

The morphemic relationship is the relationship between one morpheme and another. In the word books, book is a free morpheme (it has meaning by itself) and -s is a bound morpheme (it has meaning only when attached to a free morpheme).

Morphology

The study of how the aspects of language structure are related to the ways words are formed from prefixes, roots, and suffixes (e.g., *mis-spell-ing*), and how words are related to each other.

Morphophonology

Using a word's letter patterns to help determine, in part, the meaning and pronunciation of a word. For example, the morpheme *vis* in words such as *vision* and *visible* is from the Latin root word that means *to see*; and the *ay* in *stay* is pronounced the same in the words *gray* and *play*.

Mother Tongue

This term variably means (a) the language learned from the mother, (b) the first language learned, (c) the native language of an area or country, (d) the stronger (or dominant) language at any time of life, (e) the language used most by a person, (f) the language toward which the person has the more positive attitude and affection (Baker, 2000). See also **native language**.

Multiple Intelligences

A theory that suggests that the traditional notion of intelligence, based on IQ testing, is far too limited. Instead, it proposes eight different intelligences to account for a broader range of human potential in children and adults. These intelligences are: linguistic, logical-mathematical, spatial, bodily-kinesthetic, musical, interpersonal, intrapersonal, naturalist.

Multiple Literacies

Multiple literacies reach beyond a traditional 'reading and writing' definition of literacy to include the ability to process and interpret information presented through various media.

Multisensory Structured Language Education

An educational approach that uses visual, auditory, and kinesthetic-tactile cues simultaneously to enhance memory and learning. Links are consistently made between the visual (what we see), auditory (what we hear), and kinesthetic-tactile (what we feel) pathways in learning to read and spell.

Naming Speed

The rate at which a child can recite "overlearned" stimuli such as letters and single-digit numbers.

Native Language

The first language a person acquires in life, or identifies with as a member of an ethnic group (Baker, 2000). See also **mother tongue**.

Natural Approach

The Natural Approach is a methodology for second language learning which focuses on communicative skills, both oral and written. It is based on linguist Stephen Krashen's theory of language acquisition, which assumes that speech emerges in four stages: (1) preproduction (listening and gestures), (2) early production (short phrases), (3) speech emergence (long phrases and sentences), and (4) intermediate fluency (conversation). This approach was developed by Krashen and teacher Tracy Terrell (1983) (Lessow-Hurley, 1991).

Newcomer Program

A newcomer program addresses the needs of recent immigrant students, most often at the middle and high school level, especially those with limited or interrupted schooling in their home countries. Major goals of newcomer programs are to acquire beginning English language skills along with core academic skills and to acculturate to the U.S. school system. Some newcomer programs also include primary language development and an orientation to the student's new community (Genesee, et al, 1999).

No Child Left Behind (NCLB)

The No Child Left Behind Act of 2001 is the most recent reauthorization of the Elementary and Secondary Education act of 1965. The act contains President George W. Bush's four basic education reform principles: stronger accountability for results, increased flexibility and local control, expanded options for parents, and an emphasis on teaching methods based on scientifically-based research.

Nonverbal Learning Disability

A neurological disorder which originates in the right hemisphere of the brain. Reception of nonverbal or performance-based information governed by this hemisphere is impaired in varying degrees, causing problems with visual-spatial, intuitive, organizational, evaluative, and holistic processing functions. For more information, go to **Nonverbal LD**.

Norm-Referenced Assessment

A type of assessment that compares an individual child's score against the scores of other children who have previously taken the same assessment. With a norm-referenced assessment, the child's raw score can be converted into a comparative score such as a percentile rank or a stanine.

Norm-Referenced Test

Norm-referenced tests (NRTs) are designed to discriminate among groups of students, and allow comparisons across years, grade levels, schools, and other variables. They are nationally, commercially available.

Occupational Therapy (OT)

A rehabilitative service to people with mental, physical, emotional, or developmental impairments. Services can include helping a student with pencil grip, physical exercises that may be used to increase strength and dexterity, or exercises to improve hand-eye coordination.

Office For Civil Rights (OCR)

A branch of the U.S. Department of Education that investigates allegations of civil rights violations in schools. It also initiates investigations of compliance with federal civil rights laws in schools that serve special student populations, including language-minority students. The office has developed several policies with regard to measuring compliance with the **Lau v. Nichols** decision. OCR is also responsible for enforcing Title VI of the Civil Rights Act of 1964. For more information, see the **OCR resources about ELLs** and **OCR Disability Discrimination: Overview of the Laws**.

Office Of Special Education Programs (OSEP)

An office of the U.S. Department of Education whose goal is to improve results for children with disabilities (ages birth through 21) by providing leadership and financial support to assist states and local districts.

Onset

The initial consonant sound(s) in a monosyllabic word. This unit is smaller than a syllable but may be larger than a phoneme (the onset of *bag* is *b-*; of *swim* is *sw-*).

Onset And Rime

Onsets and rimes are parts of monosyllabic words in spoken language. These units are smaller than syllables but may be larger than phonemes. An onset is the initial consonant sound of a syllable (the onset of bag is b-; of swim is sw-).

The rime is the part of a syllable that contains the vowel and all that follows it (the rime of bag is -ag; of swim is -im).

Onset-Rime Phonics Instruction

In this approach, students learn to break monosyllabic words into their onsets (consonants preceding the vowel) and rimes (vowel and following consonants). They read each part separately and then blend the parts to say the whole word.

Onset-Rime Segmentation

Onset-rime segmentation is separating a word into the onset, the consonant(s) at the start of a syllable, and the rime, the remainder of the syllable. For example, in swift, sw is the onset and ift is the rime.

Oral Language Difficulties

A person with oral language difficulties may exhibit poor vocabulary, listening comprehension, or grammatical abilities for his or her age.

Orthographic Knowledge

The understanding that the sounds in a language are represented by written or printed symbols.

Orton-Gillingham

A multisensory approach to remediating dyslexia created by Dr. Samuel Orton, a neuropsychiatrist and pathologist, and Anna Gillingham, an educator and psychologist.

Other Health Impairments (OHI)

A category of special education services for students with limited strength, vitality or alertness, due to chronic or acute health problems (such as asthma, ADHD, diabetes, or a heart condition).

Paraprofessional Educator

Also known as instructional aides and teachers' aides, these individuals provide assistance to teachers in the classroom. They do not provide primary direct instruction, but may help clarify material to students through home language or other supports. In classrooms funded through Title I, instructional paraprofessionals must have at least an Associates' degree or its equivalent, or have passed a test.

Pervasive Developmental Disorder (PDD)

The category of special education services for students with delays or deviance in their social/language/motor and/or cognitive development.

Phoneme

The smallest unit of speech that serves to distinguish one utterance from another in a language.

Phonemic Awareness

The ability to notice, think about, and work with the individual sounds in spoken words. An example of how beginning readers show us they have phonemic awareness is combining or blending the separate sounds of a word to say the word (/c/ /a/ /t/ – cat.)

Phonics

Phonics is a form of instruction to cultivate the understanding and use of the alphabetic principle. It emphasizes the predictable relationship between phonemes (the sounds in spoken language) and graphemes (the letters that represent those sounds in written language) and shows how this information can be used to read or decode words.

See also: Analogy-based phonics, Analytic phonics, Embedded phonics, Onset-rime phonics instruction, Phonics through spelling, Synthetic phonics, Systematic and explicit phonics instruction.

Phonological Awareness

A range of understandings related to the sounds of words and word parts, including identifying and manipulating larger parts of spoken language such as words, syllables, and onset and rime. It also includes phonemic awareness as well as other aspects of spoken language such as rhyming and syllabication.

Physical Therapy (PT)

Instructional support and treatment of physical disabilities, under a doctor's prescription, that helps a person improve the use of bones, muscles, joints and nerves.

Point Of View*

Chiefly in literary texts, the narrative point of view (as in first- or third-person narration); more broadly, the position or perspective conveyed or represented by an author, narrator, speaker, or character.

Portfolio Assessment

A portfolio assessment is a systematic collection of student work that is analyzed to show progress over time with regard to instructional objectives (Valencia 1991, cited in O' Malley & Valdez-Pierce, 1996). Student portfolios may include responses to readings, samples of writing, drawings, or other work.

Pre-Reading

Prereading activities are activities used with students before they interact with reading material. They're designed to provide students with needed background knowledge about a topic, or to help students identify their purpose for reading.

Prefix

A prefix is a word part added to the beginning of a root or base word to create a new meaning. The most common prefixes include dis- (as in disagree), in- (as invaluable), re- (as in repeat), and -un (as in unfriendly).

Prewriting

Prewriting is any activity designed to help students generate or organize their ideas before writing.

Primary Language

The primary language is the language in which bilingual/multilingual speakers are most fluent, or which they prefer to use. This is not necessarily the language first learned in life. See also **dominant language**.

Print Awareness

Basic knowledge about print and how it is typically organized on a page. For example, print conveys meaning, print is read left to right, and words are separated by spaces.

Print Or Digital (Texts, Sources)*

Sometimes added for emphasis to stress that a given standard is particularly likely to be applied to electronic as well as traditional texts; the Standards are generally assumed to apply to both.

Proficient(Ly)*

A student performance that meets the criterion established in the Standards as measured by a teacher or assessment; in the Standards, often paired with independent(ly) to suggest a successful student performance done without scaffolding; in the Reading standards, the act of reading a text with comprehension; see also independent(ly), scaffolding.

Pull-Out ESL

Pull-out ESL is a program in which **LEP** students are "pulled out" of regular, mainstream classrooms for special instruction in English as a second language.

Push-In ESL

In contrast with pull-out ESL instruction, a certified ESL teacher provides ELLs with instruction in a mainstream or content-area classroom.

Readability

Readability refers to the level of difficulty in a written passage. This depends on factors such as length of words, length of sentences, grammatical complexity and word frequency.

Reading Coach

See Literacy Coach.

Reading Comprehension

See text comprehension.

Reading Disability

Another term for dyslexia, sometimes referred to as reading disorder or reading difference.

Reading First

Reading First is a federal program that focuses on putting proven methods of early reading instruction in classrooms. Through Reading First, states and districts receive support to apply scientifically based reading research and the proven instructional and assessment tools consistent with this research to ensure that all children learn to read well by the end of third grade.

Rebus*

A mode of expressing words and phrases by using pictures of objects whose names resemble those words.

Receptive Language

The aspect of spoken language that includes listening, and the aspect of written language that includes reading.

Reciprocal Teaching

Reciprocal teaching is a multiple-strategy instructional approach for teaching comprehension skills to students. Teachers teach students four strategies: asking questions about the text they are reading; summarizing parts of the text; clarifying words and sentences they don't understand; and predicting what might occur next in the text.

Repeated And Monitored Oral Reading

In this instructional activity, students read and reread a text a certain number of times or until a certain level of fluency is reached. This technique has been shown to improve reading fluency and overall reading achievement. Four re-readings are usually sufficient for most students. Students may also practice reading orally through the use of audiotapes, tutors, peer guidance, or other means.

Response To Intervention (RTI)

Response to Intervention is a process whereby local education agencies (LEAs) document a child's response to scientific, research-based intervention using a tiered approach. In contrast to the discrepancy criterion model, RTI provides early intervention for students experiencing difficulty learning to read. RTI was authorized for use in December 2004 as part of the Individuals with Disabilities Education Act (IDEA).

Responsive Instruction

A way of making teaching decisions in which a student's reaction to instruction directly shapes how future instruction is provided.

Revising*

A part of writing and preparing presentations concerned chiefly with a reconsideration and reworking of the content of a text relative to task, purpose, and audience; compared to editing, a larger-scale activity often associated with the overall content and structure of a text; see also **editing**, **rewriting**.

Rewriting*

A part of writing and preparing presentations that involves largely or wholly replacing a previous, unsatisfactory effort with a new effort, better aligned to task, purpose, and audience, on the same or a similar topic or theme; compared to revising, a larger-scale activity more akin to replacement than refinement; see also **editing**, **revising**.

Rime

The vowel and all that follows it in a monosyllabic word (the rime of *bag* is *-ag*; of *swim* is *-im*).

Root Word

Words from other languages that are the origin of many English words. About 60 percent of all English words have Latin or Greek origins.

Scaffolding

A way of teaching in which the teacher provides support in the form of modeling, prompts, direct explanations, and targeted questions — offering a teacher-guided approach at first. As students begin to acquire mastery of targeted objectives, direct supports are reduced and the learning becomes more student-guided. The teacher provides contextual supports for meaning during instruction or assessment, such as visual displays, classified lists, or tables or graphs (O' Malley & Valdez-Pierce, 1996, p.240).

Scaffolding*

Temporary guidance or assistance provided to a student by a teacher, another adult, or a more capable peer, enabling the student to perform a task he or she otherwise would not be able to do alone, with the goal of fostering the student's capacity to perform the task on his or her own later on.

Self-Advocacy

The development of specific skills and understandings that enable children and adults to explain their specific learning disabilities to others and cope positively with the attitudes of peers, parents, teachers, and employers.

Self-Monitoring

The ability to observe yourself and know when you are doing an activity act according to a standard. For example, knowing if you do or do not understand what you are reading. Or whether your voice tone is appropriate for the circumstances or too loud or too soft.

Semantic Maps

A semantic map is a strategy for graphically representing concepts. As a strategy, semantic maps involve expanding a student's vocabulary by encouraging new links to familiar concepts. Instructionally, semantic maps can be used as a prereading activity for charting what is known about a concept, theme, or individual word. They can also be used during reading as a way to assimilate new information learned from the text.

Semantic Organizers

Graphic organizers that look somewhat like a spider web where lines connect a central concept to a variety of related ideas and events.

Sentence Combining

Sentence combining is an instructional approach that involves teaching students to combine two or more simple sentences to form a more complex or sophisticated sentence.

Short Research Project*

An investigation intended to address a narrowly tailored query in a brief period of time, as in a few class periods or a week of instructional time.

Sight Words

Words that a reader recognizes without having to sound them out. Some sight words are "irregular," or have letter-sound relationships that are uncommon. Some examples of sight words are *you*, *are*, *have* and *said*.

Small Learning Communities

Small learning communities are an increasingly popular approach for teaching adolescents. This approach uses personalized classroom environments where teachers know each individual student and can tailor instruction to meet their academic and social/emotional needs. The goal is to increase students' sense of belonging, participation, and commitment to school.

Social English

Often referred to as "playground English" or "survival English", this is the basic language ability required for face-to-face communication, often accompanied by gestures and relying on context to aid understanding. Social English is much more easily and quickly acquired than academic English, but is not sufficient to meet the cognitive and linguistic demands of an academic classroom. Also referred to as Basic Interpersonal Communication Skills (BICS).

Source*

A text used largely for informational purposes, as in research.

Special Education (SPED)
Services offered to children who possess one or more of the following disabilities: specific learning disabilities, speech or language impairments, mental retardation, emotional disturbance, multiple disabilities, hearing impairments, orthopedic impairments, visual impairments, autism, combined deafness and blindness, traumatic brain injury, and other health impairments.

Specific Learning Disability (SLD)
The official term used in federal legislation to refer to difficulty in certain areas of learning, rather than in all areas of learning. Synonymous with learning disabilities.

Speech Impaired (SI)
A category of special education services for students who have difficulty with speech sounds in their native language.

Speech Language Pathologist (SLP)
An expert who can help children and adolescents who have language disorders to understand and give directions, ask and answer questions, convey ideas, and improve the language skills that lead to better academic performance. An SLP can also counsel individuals and families to understand and deal with speech and language disorders.

Standard English*
In the Standards, the most widely accepted and understood form of expression in English in the United States; used in the Standards to refer to formal English writing and speaking; the particular focus of Language standards 1 and 2 (CCSS, pp. 26, 28, 52, 54).

State Education Agency (SEA)
A state education agency is the agency primarily responsible for the state supervision of public elementary and secondary schools.

Story Structure
In story structure, a reader sees the way the content and events of a story are organized into a plot. Students learn to identify the categories of content (setting, characters, initiating events, internal reactions, goals, attempts, and outcomes). Often students recognize the way the story is organized by developing a story map. This strategy improves students' comprehension and memory of story content and meaning.

Strategic Instructional Model (SIM)
SIM promotes effective teaching and learning of critical content in schools. SIM strives to help teachers make decisions about what is of greatest importance, what we can teach students to help them to learn, and how to teach them well.

Striving Readers Act
Striving Readers is aimed at improving the reading skills of middle school- and high school-aged students who are reading below grade level. Striving Readers supports the implementation and evaluation of research-based reading interventions for struggling middle and high school readers in Title I eligible schools that are at risk of not meeting or are not meeting adequate yearly progress (AYP) requirements under the No Child Left Behind Act, or that have significant percentages or number of students reading below grade level, or both.

Striving Readers Legislation

Striving Readers is a government program designed to improve the reading skills of middle and high school students who read below grade level. Authorized in 2005 as part of the No Child Left Behind Act, this program supports initiatives to improve literacy instruction across the curriculum and works to build a scientific research base for strategies that improve literacy skills for adolescents.

Suffix

"A suffix is a word part that is added to the end of a root word. The four most frequent suffixes account for 97 percent of suffixed words in printed school English. These include -ing, -ed, -ly, and -es."

Summarizing

Summarizing is a process in which a reader synthesizes the important ideas in a text. Teaching students to summarize helps them generate main ideas, connect central ideas, eliminate redundant and unnecessary information, and remember what they read.

Summative Assessment

Summative assessment is generally carried out at the end of a course or project. In an educational setting, summative assessments are typically used to assign students a course grade.

Supplemental Services

Services offered to students from low-income families who are attending schools that have been identified as in need of improvement for two consecutive years. Parents can choose the appropriate services (tutoring, academic assistance, etc.) from a list of approved providers, which are paid for by the school district.

Syllabication

The act of breaking words into syllables.

Syllable

A part of a word that contains a vowel or, in spoken language, a vowel sound (*e-vent*, *news-pa-per*).

Synthetic Phonics

In this instructional approach, students learn how to convert letters or letter combinations into a sequence of sounds, and then how to blend the sounds together to form recognizable words.

Systematic And Explicit Phonics Instruction

The most effective way to teach phonics. A program is systematic if the plan of instruction includes a carefully selected set of letter-sound relationships that are organized into a logical sequence. Explicit means the programs provide teachers with precise directions for the teaching of these relationships.

Teachers Of English To Speakers Of Other Languages (TESOL)

TESOL is a professional association of teachers, administrators, researchers and others concerned with promoting and strengthening instruction and research in the teaching of English to speakers of other languages.

Technical Subjects*

A course devoted to a practical study, such as engineering, technology, design, business, or other workforce-related subject; a technical aspect of a wider field of study, such as art or music.

Text Complexity Band*

A range of text difficulty corresponding to grade spans within the Standards; specifically, the spans from grades 2–3, grades 4–5, grades 6–8, grades 9–10, and grades 11–CCR (college and career readiness).

Text Complexity*

The inherent difficulty of reading and comprehending a text combined with consideration of reader and task variables; in the Standards, a three-part assessment of text difficulty that pairs qualitative and quantitative measures with reader-task considerations (CCSS, pp. 31, 57; Reading, pp. 4–16).

Text Comprehension

The reason for reading: understanding what is read by reading actively (making sense from text) and with purpose (for learning, understanding, or enjoyment).

Textual Evidence

See evidence.

Total Physical Response (TPR)

Total Physical Response is a language-learning approach based on the relationship between language and its physical representation or execution. TPR emphasizes the use of physical activity for increasing meaningful learning opportunities and language retention. A TPR lesson involves a detailed series of consecutive actions accompanied by a series of commands or instructions given by the teacher. Students respond by listening and performing the appropriate actions.

Transition

Commonly used to refer to the change from secondary school to postsecondary programs, work, and independent living typical of young adults. Also used to describe other periods of major change such as from early childhood to school or from more specialized to mainstreamed settings.

Transitional Bilingual Education

An educational program in which two languages are used to provide content matter instruction. Over time, the use of the native language is decreased and the use of English is increased until only English is used.

Unified School District (USD)

USD is a common acronym used in education plans to refer to the elementary, middle, and high schools within the school district.

Universal Design For Learning (UDL)

UDL provides a framework for creating flexible goals, methods, materials, and assessments that accommodate learner differences.

Vocabulary

Vocabulary refers to the words a reader knows. Listening vocabulary refers to the words a person knows when hearing them in oral speech. Speaking vocabulary refers to the words we use when we speak. Reading vocabulary refers to the words a person knows when seeing them in print. Writing vocabulary refers to the words we use in writing.

With Prompting And Support/With (Some) Guidance And Support

See scaffolding.

Word Attack

Word attack is an aspect of reading instruction that includes intentional strategies for learning to decode, sight read, and recognize written words.

Word Parts

Word parts include affixes (prefixes and suffixes), base words, and word roots.

Word Roots

Word roots are words from other languages that are the origin of many English words. About 60 percent of all English words have Latin or Greek origins.

Working Memory

The ability to store and manage information in one's mind for a short period of time. In one test of working memory a person listens to random numbers and then repeats them. The average adult can hold 7 numbers in their working memory. Working memory is sometimes called Short-term memory

These terms and definitions were collected from the following sources: Dr. Jean Lokerson, ERIC Digest; Southwest Educational Laboratory (SEDL); Dr. Linda Wilmshurst and Dr. Alan Brue, A Parent's Guide to Special Education, American Management Association, 2005; The Partnership for Reading; Learning Disabilities Council; Dr. Don Deshler, University of Kansas.

*Source: Common Core State Standards. National Governors Association Center for Best Practices, Council of Chief State School Officers, 2010.

http://www.ldonline.org/glossary?theme=print

User Guide

Descriptive listings in *The Complete Learning Disabilities Directory (LDD)* are organized into 21 chapters and 84 subchapters. You will find the following types of listings throughout the book:

- National Agencies & Associations
- State Agencies & Associations
- Camps & Summer Programs
- Exchange Programs
- Classroom & Computer Resources
- Print & Electronic Media
- Schools & Learning Centers
- Testing & Training Resources
- Conferences & Workshops

Below is a sample listing illustrating the kind of information that is or might be included in an entry. Each numbered item of information is described in the paragraphs on the following page.

↦ 1234

2 → **Association for Children and Youth with Disabilities**

3 → **1704 L Street NW**

Washington, DC 20036

4 → **075-785-0000**

5 → **FAX: 075-785-0001**

6 → **800-075-0002**

7 → **TDY: 075-785-0002**

8 → **info@AGC.com**

9 → **www.AGC.com**

10 → Peter Rancho, Director
Nancy Williams, Information Specialist
Tanya Fitzgerald, Marketing Director
William Alexander, Editor

11 → Advocacy organization that ensures children and youth with learning disabilities receive the best possible education. Services include speaking with an informed specialist, free publications, database searches, and referrals to other organizations.

12 → *$6.99*

13 → *204 pages*

14 → *Paperback*

User Key

1 ➤ **Record Number:** Entries are listed alphabetically within each category and numbered sequentially. The entry numbers, rather than page numbers, are used in the indexes to refer to listings.

2 ➤ **Organization Name:** Formal name of organization. Where organization names are completely capitalized, the listing will appear at the beginning of the alphabetized section. In the case of publications, the title of the publication will appear first, followed by the publisher.

3 ➤ **Address:** Location or permanent address of the organization.

4 ➤ **Phone Number:** The listed phone number is usually for the main office of the organization, but may also be for sales, marketing, or public relations as provided by the organization.

5 ➤ **Fax Number:** This is listed when provided by the organization.

6 ➤ **Toll-Free Number:** This is listed when provided by the organization.

7 ➤ **TDY:** This is listed when provided by the organization. It refers to Telephone Device for the Deaf.

8 ➤ **E-Mail:** This is listed when provided by the organization and is generally the main office e-mail.

9 ➤ **Web Site:** This is listed when provided by the organization and is also referred to as an URL address. These web sites are accessed through the Internet by typing http:// before the URL address.

10 ➤ **Key Personnel:** Name and title of key executives within the organization.

11 ➤ **Organization Description:** This paragraph contains a brief description of the organization and their services.

The following apply if the listing is a publication:

12 ➤ **Price:** The cost of each issue or subscription, often with frequency information. If the listing is a school or program, you will see information on age group served and enrollment size.

13 ➤ **Number of Pages:** Total number of pages for publication.

14 ➤ **Paperback:** The available format of the publication: paperback; hardcover; spiral bound.

National

1 AVKO Educational Research Foundation

3084 Willard Rd
Birch Run, MI 48415-9404

810-686-9283
866-285-6612
Fax: 810-686-1101
www.avko.org
webmaster@avko.org

Don McCabe, President
Linda Heck, Vice-President
Michael Lane, Treasurer
AVKO is a non-profit membership organization that focuses on the development and production of materials and techniques to help students with learning disabilities achieve literacy. Resource subjects focus on reading and spelling, handwriting (manuscript and cursive) and key boarding.

2 America's Health Insurance Plans

601 Pennsylvania Ave. NW
South Building, Ste 500
Washington, DC 20004-2601

202-778-3200
Fax: 202-331-7487
www.ahip.org
info@ahip.org

Marilyn Tavenner, President & CEO
Jeanette Thornton, SVP Health Plan Operations
Mark Hamelburg, SVP Federal Programs
Purpose is to represent the interests of members on legislative and regulatory issues at the federal and state levels, and with the media, consumers, and employers. Provides information and services such as newsletters, publications, a magazine and on-line services. Conducts education, research, and quality assurance programs and engages in a host of other activities to assist members.

3 American Association of Collegiate Registrars and Admissions Officers

One Dupont Circle NW
Ste 520
Washington, DC 20036-1148

202-293-9161
Fax: 202-872-8857
www.aacrao.org
corporateinfo@aacrao.org

Michael Reilly, Executive Director
Janie Barnett, Associate Executive Director
Saira Burki, Associate Director, Marketing
Provides professional development, guidelines and voluntary standards to be used by higher education officials regarding the best practices in records management, admissions, enrollment management, administrative information technology and student services. It also provides a forum for discussion regarding policy initiation and development, interpretation and implementation at the institutional level and in the global educational community.
9,500 members

4 American Bar Association Center on Children and the Law

321 N Clark St
Chicago, IL 60654

312-988-5000
800-285-2221
www.americanbar.org/groups
ctrchildlaw@abanet.org

Prudence Beidler Carr, Director
Claire Chiamulera, Communications
Niya Davis, Administration
Aims to improve children's lives through advances in law, justice, knowledge, practice and public policy.
400,000 members

5 American Camp Association

5000 State Rd 67 N
Martinsville, IN 46151-7902

765-342-8456
800-428-2267
Fax: 765-342-2065
www.acacamps.org
contactus@acacamps.org

Tisha Bolger, President
Rue Mapp, Vice President
Craig Whiting, Treasurer
The American Camp Association brings together camping professionals dedicated to ensuring the quality of camp programs, and providing children with the unique enjoyment of camp experiences.
9,000+ members

6 American College Testing

500 Act Dr
Iowa City, IA 52243-0168

319-337-1000
Fax: 319-339-3021
www.act.org

Martin Roorda, Chief Executive Officer
Richard Patz, Chief Measurement Officer
Paul Weeks, SVP Client Relations
An independent, not-for-profit organization that provides more than a hundred assessment, research, information, and program management services in the broad areas of education and workforce development.

7 American Counseling Association

6101 Stevenson Ave
Alexandria, VA 22304-3304

703-823-9800
800-347-6647
Fax: 703-823-0252
www.counseling.org
membership@counseling.org

Catherine Roland, President
Richard Yep, ACA CEO
The ACA is a non-profit organization working towards the growth and enhancement of the counseling profession.

8 American Dance Therapy Association (ADTA)

10632 Little Patuxent Pkwy
Ste 108
Columbia, MD 21044-3263

410-997-4040
Fax: 410-997-4048
www.adta.org
info@adta.org

Jody Wager, MS, BC-DMT, Board President
Margaret Migliorati, Vice President
Leslie Armeniox, Secretary
Works to establish and maintain high standards of professional education and competence in the field of dance/movement therapy. ADTA stimulates communication among dance/movement therapists and members of allied professions through publication of the ADTA Newsletter, the American Journal of Dance Therapy, monographs, bibliographies, and conference proceedings.

9 American Dyslexia Association

442 S. Tamiami Trail
Osprey, FL 34229

www.american-dyslexia-association.com
office@american-dyslexia-association.com
The American Dyselxia Association Inc. is a non-profit organization, providing information and teaching aids for dyslexic and dyscalculic people with free information and teaching aids.

10 American Occupational Therapy Association

4720 Montgomery Ln
Ste 200
Bethesda, MD 20814-3449

301-652-6611
800-729-2682
Fax: 301-652-7711
www.aota.org
praota@aota.org

Founded to represent the interests and concerns of occupational therapy practitioners and students of occupational therapy and to improve the quality of occupational therapy services. Advances the quality, availability, use, and support of occupational therapy through standard-setting, advocacy, education and research on behalf of its members and the public.
56,000 members

11   American Psychological Association
750 First St. NE
Washington, DC 20002-4242

202-336-5500
800-374-2721
Fax: 202-336-5518
TDD: 202-336-6123
www.apa.org
psycinfo@apa.org

Susan McDaniel, President
Jaime Diaz-Granados, Executive Director
Ian King, Executive Director, Membership
Its objectives are to advance psychology as a science and profession and as a means of promoting health, education and human welfare.
117,500 members

12   American Public Human Services Association (APHSA)
1133-19th St. NW
Ste 400
Washington, DC 20036-3623

202-682-0100
Fax: 202-289-6555
www.aphsa.org
carolyn.marshall@aphsa.org

Tracy Wareing Evans, Executive Director
Evelyn Hunt-Williams, Human Resources Director
Donna Jarvis-Miller, Director of Membership
A nonprofit, bipartisan organization of state and local human service agencies and individuals who work in or are interested in public human service programs. Mission is to develop and promote policies and practices that improve the health and well-being of families, children, and adults

13   American Red Cross (National Headquarters)
2025 E Street NW
Washington, DC 20006

202-303-4498
800-733-2767
www.redcross.org
info@usa.redcross.org

Gail J. McGovern, President & CEO
Bonnie McElveen Hunter, Chairman of the Board
Brian J. Rhoa, Chief Financial Officer
A humanitarian organization led by volunteers, guided by its Congressional Charter and the fundamental principles of the International Red Cross Movement to provide relief to victims of disasters and help people prevent, prepare for, and respond to emergencies.

14   American Rehabilitation Counseling Association (ARCA)
5999 Stevenson Ave
Alexandria, VA 22304-3304

703-823-9800
800-347-6647
Fax: 703-461-9260
TDD: 937-775-3153
www.arcaweb.org

Quiteya D. Walker, President
Henry McCarthy, President-Elect
Ruth Mercado-Cruz, Treasurer
An organization of rehabilitation counseling practitioners, educators, and students who are concerned with improving the lives of people with disabilities. The mission is to enhance the lives of people with disabilities and to promote excellence in the rehabilitation counseling profession.

15   American Speech-Language-Hearing Association (ASHA)
2200 Research Blvd
Rockville, MD 20850-3289

301-296-5700
800-498-2071
Fax: 301-296-8580
TTY: 301-296-5650
www.asha.org
nsslha@asha.org

Jaynee A. Handelsman, President
Arlene A. Pietranton, Chief Executive Officer
Edie R. Hapner, Vice President for Planning
Promotes the interests of and provide the highest quality services for professionals in audiology, speech-language pathology, and speech and hearing science, and to advocate for people with communication disabilities.
186,000 members 1958

16   Association of Educational Therapists
7044 S. 13th St.
Oak Creek, WI 53154

414-908-4949
www.aetonline.org
customercare@AETOnline.org

Alice Pulliam, President
Susan Grama, Treasurer
Kaye Ragland, Secretary
A national professional organization dedicated to establishing ethical professional standards, defining the roles and responsibilities of the educational therapist, providing opportunities for professional growth, and to studying techniques and technologies, philosophies and research related to the practice of educational therapy.

17   Association on Higher Education and Disability (AHEAD)
107 Commerce Centre Dr
Ste 204
Huntersville, NC 28078

704-947-7779
Fax: 704-948-7779
www.ahead.org

Jamie Axelrod, President
Michael Johnson, Treasurer
Stephan Hamlin-Smith, Executive Director
Membership for professionals invloved in the development of policy and the provision of quality services to meet the needs of persons with disabiities in all aspects of higher education.

18   Attention Deficit Disorder Association
15000 Commerce Pkwy
Ste C
Mount Laurel, NJ 08054-2212

856-439-9099
800-939-1019
www.add.org
mail@add.org

Duane Gordon, President
Michelle Frank, Vice President
Melissa Reskof, Secretary
The National Attention Deficit Disorder Association is an organization focused on the needs of adults and young adults with ADD/ADHD, offering resources and research to help children, families, and professionals.

19   Autism Research Institute
4182 Adams Ave
San Diego, CA 92116

619-281-7165
866-366-3361
Fax: 619-563-6840
www.autism.com
matt@autism.com

Stephen Edelson, Ph.D., Executive Director
Jane Johnson, Managing Director
Valerie Paradiz, Ph.D., Director
Founded to conduct and foster scientific research designed to improve methods of diagnosing, treating and preventing autism. ARI also disseminates research findings to parents and others worldwide seeking help.

20 Autism Society
4340 East-West Hwy
Ste 350
Bethesda, MD 20814   301-657-0881
                                   800-328-8476
                              Fax: 301-657-0869
                         www.autism-society.org
                        info@autism-society.org
Scott Badesch, President & CEO
John Dabrowski, Chief Financial Officer
Tonia Ferguson, Vice President, Public Policy
Works to increase public awareness about the day-to-day issues faced by those on the autism spectrum. Offers a national contact center, local chapters throughout the country, a quarterly magazine and an annual conference.

21 Autism Treatment Center of America
2080 S Undermountain Rd
Sheffield, MA 01257-9643   413-229-2100
                                    877-766-7473
                               Fax: 413-229-3202
                         www.autismtreatmentcenter.org
Barry Kaufman, Founder & CEO
Samahria Lyte Kaufman, Co-Founder
Bryn Hogan, Executive Director
Provides innovative training programs for parents and professionals caring for children challenged by Autism, Autism Spectrum Disorders, Pervasive Developmental Disorder (PDD) and other developmental difficulties. The Son-Rise Program teaches a specific yet comprehensive system of treatment and education designed to help families and caregivers enable their children to dramatically improve in all areas of learning.

22 Best Buddies International
100 Southeast Second St
Ste 2200
Miami, FL 33131   305-374-2233
                                    800-892-8339
                               Fax: 305-374-5305
                            www.bestbuddies.org
                           info@bestbuddies.org
Anthony K. Shriver, Founder & Chairman
J.R. Fry, VP State Development
Mark Lewis, Vice President, Marketing
A non-profit organization dedicated to enhancing the lives of people with intellectual disabilities by providing opportunities for one-to-one friendships and integrated employment. Best Buddies is an international community that reaches students in middle schools, high schools and college campuses across the country and abroad.

23 Birth Defect Research for Children (BDRC)
976 Lake Baldwin Lane
Ste 104
Orlando, FL 32814   407-895-0802
                               Fax: 407-566-8341
                            www.birthdefects.org
                          staff@birthdefects.org
Betty Mekdeci, Founder
Mike Mekdeci, Co-Founder
A non-profit organization that provides parents and expectant parents with information about birth defects and support services for children. BDRC also has a parent-matching program that links families who have children with similar birth defects.

24 Boy Scouts of America
1325 West Walnut Hill Lane
Irving, TX 75015-2079   972-580-2000
                               Fax: 972-580-2502
                              www.scouting.org
                        BSA.Legal@scouting.org
Robert Mazzuca, CEO
Provides an educational program for boys and young adults to build character, to train in the responsibilities of participating citizenship, and to develop personal fitness.
1910

25 Brain Injury Association of America
1608 Spring Hill Rd
Ste 110
Vienna, VA 22182-2241   703-761-0750
                                    800-444-6443
                               Fax: 703-761-0755
                                www.biausa.org
                               info@biausa.org
Bud Elkind, Chairman of the Board
Douglas L. Brewer, Vice Chairman
Susan H. Connors, President & CEO
A national organization serving and representing individuals, families and professionals who are touched by a life-altering traumatic brain injury.

26 CASANA
416 Lincoln Avenue
2nd Fl.
Pittsburgh, PA 15209   412-343-7102
                            www.apraxia-kids.org
Sharon Gretz, M.Ed, Executive Director
David Hammer, M.A.; CCC-sLP, Director of Speech Services
Kathy Hennessy, Education Director
The Childhood Apraxia of Speech Association is a 501 (C) (3) nonprofit publicly funded charity whose mission is to strengthen the support systems in the lives of children with apraxia so that each child is afforded their best opportunity to develop speech and communication.

27 Career Education Colleges and Universities (CECU)
1101 Connecticut Ave NW
Ste 900
Washington, DC 20036   202-336-6700
                                    866-711-8574
                               Fax: 202-336-6828
                                www.career.org
                         membership@career.org
Steve Gunderson, President & CEO
Michael Dakduk, Executive Vice President
Kelley Blanchard, VP, Professional Development
Formerly APSCU, CECU provides education, advocacy, and training for professionals in postsecondary and higher education.

28 Center for Adult English Language Acquisition (CAELA)
Center for Applied Linguistics
4646 - 40th Street NW
Ste 200
Washington, DC 20016-1859   202-362-0700
                               Fax: 202-362-3740
                              www.cal.org/caela
                               info@cal.org
Joy Peyton, Director
Grace Burkart, Director, Language & Literacy
Carolyn Temple Adger, Director, Language in Society
A national center focusing on literacy education for adults and out-of-school youth learning English as a second language.

29 Center for Applied Linguistics
4646 - 40th St NW
Washington, DC 20016-1867   202-362-0700
                               Fax: 202-362-3740
                                 www.cal.org
                                info@cal.org
Donna Christian, President
Joy Peyton, Vice President
A private, non-profit organization working to improve communication through better understanding of language and culture. Dedicated to providing a comprehensive range of research-based language tools and resources related to language and culture.

30 Center for Applied Special Technology (CAST)
40 Harvard Mills Square
Ste 3
Wakefield, MA 01880-3233   781-245-2212
                                 Fax: 978-531-0192
                                       www.cast.org
                                       cast@cast.org
Anne Meyer, Co-Founder
David H. Rose, Co-Founder
Ada Sullivan, Interim Chief Executive Officer
CAST has earned international recognition for innovative, technology-based educational resources and strategies based on the principals of Universal Design for Learning (UDL). The mission is to expand opportunities for all individuals, especially those with disabilities, through the research and development of innovative, technology-based educational resources and strategies.

31 Center for Parent Information & Resources
Formerly NICHCY
c/o Statewide Parent Advocacy Ntwk
35 Halsey St., 4th Fl
Newark, NJ 07102
                             www.parentcenterhub.org
                                      malizo@spannj.org
Myriam Alizo, Project Assistant
Formerly housing the National Dissemination Center for Children with Disabilities, CPIR is a website that now houses NICHCY's legacy resources, in addition to resources of their own, continuuing to offer informational assistance to parents of children with disabilities.

32 Closing the Gap
Computer Technology in Special Education & Rehab.
526 Main St
P.O. Box 68
Henderson, MN 56044-0068   507-248-3294
                                 Fax: 507-248-3810
                                  www.closingthegap.com
                                  info@closingthegap.com
Dolores Hagen, Founder
Budd Hagan, Co-Founder
Connie Kneip, VP/General Manager
An organization that focuses on computer technology for people with special needs through its bi-monthly newsletter, annual international conference and other professional development resources.

33 Commission on the Accreditation of Rehabilitation Facilities (CARF)
6951 East Southpoint Rd
Tucson, AZ 85756-9407   520-325-1044
                                     888-281-6531
                                 Fax: 520-318-1129
                                 TDD: 520-495-7077
                                       www.carf.org
                                  feedback@carf.org
Brian J. Boon, President & CEO
Cindy L. Johnson, Strategic Development Officer
Leslie Ellis-Lang, Managing Director
An independent, non-profit accreditor of human service providers in the areas of aging services, behavioral health, child and youth services, DMEPOS, employment and medical rehabilitation.

34 Council for Exceptional Children (CEC)
2900 Crystal Dr
Ste 1000
Arlington, VA 22202-3557   703-243-0446
                                     888-232-7733
                                 Fax: 703-264-9494
                                 TTY: 866-915-5000
                                    www.cec.sped.org
                                  service@cec.sped.org
Antonis Katsiyannis, President
Diane Shinn, Director, Marketing
Deborah Ziegler, Director, Policy & Advocacy

An international professional organization dedicated to improving educational outcomes for individuals with exceptionalities, students with disabilities, and/or the gifted. Advocates for appropriate governmental policies, sets professional standards, provides continual professional development, advocates for underserved individuals with exceptionalities, and helps professionals obtain resources necessary for effective professional practice.

35 Council for Learning Disabilities
11184 Antioch Rd
Box 405
Overland Park, KS 66210   913-491-1011
                                 Fax: 913-491-1012
            http://council-for-learning-disabilities.org
                                  lneaseCLD@aol.com
Diane Bryant, President
Deborah Reed, Vice President
Linda Nease, Executive Director
An international organization concerned about issues related to students with learning disabilities. Working to build a better future for students with LD has been the primary goal of CLD for more than 20 years. Involvement in CLD helps members stay abreast of current issues that are shaping the field, affecting the lives of students, and influencing professional careers.

36 Council on Rehabilitation Education (CORE)
1699 East Woodfield Rd
Ste 300
Schaumburg, IL 60173-2088   847-944-1345
                                 Fax: 847-944-1346
                                    www.core-rehab.org
                                  kandre@core-rehab.org
Patricia Nunez, President
Frank Lane, Ph.D., CRC, LCPC, Chief Executive Officer
Kristie Andre, Administrative Assistant
Seeks to provide effective delivery of rehabilitation services to individuals with disabilities by stimulating and fostering continuing review and improvement of master's degree-level rehabilitation counselor education programs.

37 Department of VSA and Accessibility
Kennedy Center for the Performing Arts
2700 F St, NW
Washington, DC 20566   202-467-4600
                                     800-444-1324
                                 Fax: 202-429-0868
                                 TTY: 202-416-8524
                                  www.kennedy-center.org
David M. Rubenstein, Chairman
Deborah F. Rutter, President
Christoph Eschenbach, Music Director, NSO
An international, non-profit organization founded to create a society where all people with disabilities learn through, participate in and enjoy the arts.

38 Disability Rights Education & Defense Fund (DREDF)
3075 Adeline St
Ste 210
Berkeley, CA 94703   510-644-2555
                                     800-348-4232
                                 Fax: 510-841-8645
                                 TTY: 510-644-2555
                                       www.dredf.org
                                       info@dredf.org
Susan Henderson, Executive Director
Arlene B. Mayerson, Directing Attorney
Mary Lou Breslin, Senior Policy Advisor
A national civil rights law and policy center directed by individuals with disabilities and parents who have children with disabilities. Advances the civil and human rights of people with disabilities through legal advocacy, training, education, and public policy and legislative development.

39 **Distance Education Accrediting Commission (DEAC)**
Formerly DETC
1101 - 17th St NW
Ste 808
Washington, DC 20036 202-234-5100
Fax: 202-332-1386
www.deac.org
info@deac.org
Leah Matthews, Executive Director
Nan Ridgeway, Director, Accreditation
Robert Chalifoux, Director, Media and Events
A non-profit educational association founded to promote
sound educational standards and ethical business practices
within the correspondence and distance education fields.

40 **Division for Communicative Disabilities and Deafness
(DCDD)**
Council for Exceptional Children
1110 North Glebe Rd
Ste 300
Arlington, VA 22201-5704 703-243-0446
888-232-7733
Fax: 703-264-9494
TTY: 866-915-5000
http://community.cec.sped.org/dcdd/home
info@dcdd.us
Rebecca Jackson, President
The DCDD is concerned with the well-being, development,
and education of infants, toddlers, children, and youth with
communication and learning disorders, ranging from mild to
profound, and/or who are deaf or hard of hearing. Aims to
provide information to families regarding the development
of communicationa and learning disabilities.

41 **Division for Culturally & Linguistically Diverse Excep-
tional Learners**
Council for Exceptional Children
1110 North Glebe Rd
Ste 300
Arlington, VA 22201-5704 888-232-7733
Fax: 703-264-9494
TTY: 866-915-5000
http://community.cec.sped.org/ddel
sgreen34@csu.edu
Kelly M. Carrero, President
Ya-Yu Lo, Secretary
Diana Baker, Treasurer
The official division of the Council for Exceptional Children
that promotes the advancement and improvement of educa-
tional opportunities for culturally and linguistically diverse
learners with disabilities and/or gifts and talents, their fami-
lies, and the professionals who serve them.

42 **Division for Early Childhood of CEC**
Council for Exceptional Children
3415 South Sepulveda Blvd
Ste 1100
Los Angeles, CA 90034 310-428-7209
Fax: 855-678-1989
www.dec-sped.org/
dec@dec-sped.org
Peggy Kemp, Executive Director
Ben Rogers, Assistant Director
Sharon Walsh, Government Relations
An international membership association that aims to assist
those those who work with or on behalf of children with disabilities from birth through age eight and their families, promoting and advocating for policies that hope to ensure the
best outcomes for child development.
1973

43 **Division of Research**
Council for Exceptional Children
1110 N Glebe Rd
Ste 300
Arlington, VA 22202-3557 703-620-3660
888-232-7733
Fax: 703-264-9494
TTY: 866-915-5000
www.cecdr.org
info@cec.sped.org
Kristen McMaster, President
John Hosp, President Elect
David Lee, Vice President
Devoted to the advancement of research related to the educa-
tion of individuals with disabilities and/or who are gifted.
The goals of CEC-DR include the promotion of equal part-
nership with practitioners in designing, conducting and in-
terpreting research in special education.

44 **Division on Career Development & Transition (DCDT)**
Council for Exceptional Children
1110 North Glebe Rd
Ste 300
Arlington, VA 22201-5704 703-620-3660
888-232-7733
Fax: 703-264-9494
TTY: 866-915-5000
http://community.cec.sped.org/dcdt/home
jrazeghi@gmu.edu
Darlene Unger, President
Valerie Mazzotti, Vice President
Jane Razeghi, Executive Director
Promotes national and international efforts to improve the
quality of and access to career, vocational and transition ser-
vices. Works to influence policies affecting career develop-
ment and transition services for persons with disabilities.

45 **Division on Visual Impairments and Deafblindness**
Council for Exceptional Children
2900 Crystal Dr
Ste 1000
Arlington, VA 22202 703-245-3660
888-232-7733
Fax: 703-264-9494
TTY: 866-915-5000
http://commuity.cec.sped.org/dvi/home
service@cec.sped.org
Tiffany Wild, President
Nicole Johnson, Secretary
Mackenzie Savaiano, Director
Division offering support and resources to further the educa-
tion of visually impaired individuals, and assist the CEC in
its efforts to improve educational accessibility for persons
who are gifted and exceptional.

46 **Dyscalculia International Consortium (DIC)**
7420 Calhoun St
Dearborn, MI 48126 313-300-1901
Fax: 888-710-0951
www.dyscalculia.org
help@dyscalculia.org
Renee Hamilton-Newman, President
Samira Guyot, Chief Attorney - Education Law
Molly Simpson, Administrative Assistant
A non-profit educational organization dedicated to advancing understanding and treatment of specific learning disabilities in mathematics AKA dyscaculia. Aims to provide free
information to the public about math learning disability and
the best practices for diagnosis and treatment.

47 **Easter Seals**
233 South Wacker Dr
Ste 2400
Chicago, IL 60606 312-726-6200
800-221-6827
Fax: 312-726-1494
www.easterseals.com
info@easterseals.com

Richard W. Davidson, Chairman
Joseph Kern, 1st Vice Chairman
Eileen Howard Boone, 2nd Vice Chairman
Easter Seals' mission is to create solutions that change lives for children and adults with disabilities, their families, and their communities, by identifying the needs of people with disabilities and providing appropriate developmental and rehabilitation services. Easter Seals operates 550 web sites that provide services to children and adults with disabilities and their families.

48   Eden Autism Services
2 Merwick Rd
Princeton, NJ 08540   609-987-0099
                                              Fax: 609-987-0243
                                         http://edenautism.org
                                         info@edenservices.org
Peter H. Bell, President & CEO
Jennifer Bizub, Chief Operating Officer
John Inzilla, Chief Financial Officer
Provides year round educational services, early intervention, parent training, respite care, outreach services, community based residential services and employment opportunities for individuals with autism.

49   Educational Equity Center
FHI360
71 Fifth Ave
Fl 6
New York, NY 10003-6903   212-243-1110
                                              Fax: 212-627-0407
                                              TTY: 212-243-1110
                                              www.edequity.org
                                              lcolon@fhi360.org
Merle Froschl, Co-Founder/Director
Barbara Sprung, Co-Founder/Co-Director
Linda Colon, Senior Program Manager
A national not-for-profit organization that promotes bias-free learning through innovative programs and materials. The mission is to decrease discrimination based on gender, race/ethnicity, disability, and level of family income

50   Families and Advocates Partnership for Education (FAPE)
PACER Center
8161 Normandale Blvd
Minneapolis, MN 55437   952-838-9000
                                              888-248-0822
                                              Fax: 952-838-0199
                                              TTY: 952-838-0190
                                              www.fape.org
                                              pacer@pacer.org
Paula Goldberg, Executive Director
The FAPE project is a strong partnership that aims to improve the educational outcomes for children with disabilities. FAPE links families, advocates, and self-advocates to information about the Individuals with Disabilities Education Act (IDEA). The project represents the needs of seven million children with disabilities.

51   Federation for Children with Special Needs
529 Main St
Ste 1M3
Boston, MA 02129   617-236-7210
                                              800-331-0688
                                              Fax: 617-241-0330
                                              TDD: 617-236-7210
                                              www.fcsn.org
                                              fcsninfo@fcsn.org
Richard Robison, Executive Director
John Sullivan, Associate Executive Director
Maureen Jerz, Director, Development
The mission of the Federation is to provide information, support and assistance to parents of children with disabilities, their professional partners and their communities. Major services include information and referral and parent and professional training.

52   Friends-In-Art
4317 Vermont Court
Columbia, MO 65203   573-445-5564
                                              www.friendsinart.com
                                              lwb6c9@mizzou.edu
Lynn Hedl, President
Dwayne Estes, Vice President
Lisa Altschul, Corresponding Secretary
Aims to expand the art experience of blind people, encourages blind people to visit museums, galleries, concerts, the theater and other enjoyable public places, offers consultation to program planners establishing accessible art and museum exhibits and presents Performing Arts Showcases at the American Council of the Blind's national convention.

53   Higher Education for Learning Problems (HELP)
Marshall University
Myers Hall
520 - 18th St
Huntington, WV 25703-1530   304-696-6252
                                              Fax: 304-696-3231
                                              www.marshall.edu/help
                                              help@marshall.edu
Debbie Painter, Director
Missi Fisher, Assistant Director
K. Renna Moore, Administrative Assistant
Provides educational support, remediation, and mentoring to individuals diagnosed with a learning disability and/or ADD/ADHD. Comprise of Community H.E.L.P., College H.E.L.P., Medical/Law H.E.L.P., and Diagnostic H.E.L.P.

54   Independent Living Research Utilization Program
TIRR Memorial Hermann
1333 Moursund
Houston, TX 77030   713-520-0232
                                              Fax: 713-520-5785
                                              TTY: 713-520-0232
                                              www.ilru.org
                                              ilru@ilru.org
Lex Frieden, Director
Richard Petty, Co-Director
Darrell Jones, Program Director
A national center for information, training, research, and technical assistance in independent living. Its goal is to expand the body of knowledge in independent living and to improve utilization of results of research programs and demonstration projects in this field.

55   Institute for Educational Leadership
4301 Connecticut Ave., NW
Ste 100
Washington, DC 20008   202-822-8405
                                              Fax: 202-872-4050
                                              www.iel.org
                                              iel@iel.org
Martin J Blank, President & CEO
Maame Appiah, Director, Operations
S. Kwesi Rollins, Director, Leadership Programs
The Institute aims to improve education and the lives of children and their families through positive and visionary change.

56   Institute for Human Centered Design (IHCD)
Formerly Adaptive Environments
200 Portland St
Boston, MA 02114   617-695-1225
                                              800-949-4232
                                              Fax: 617-482-8099
                                              TTY: 617-695-1225
                                         http://adaptiveenvironments.org
                                              info@HCDesign.org
Ralph Jackson, FAIA, President
Valerie Fletcher, Executive Director
Gabriela Bonome-Sims, Director, Administration
The IHCD seeks to improve accessibility standards for disabled people through improvement and innovation in design. The institute offers information on both legal standards and best practices for universal design.

57 Institutes for the Achievement of Human Potential (IAHP)
8801 Stenton Ave
Wyndmoor, PA 19038-8397
215-233-2050
800 736 4663
Fax: 215-233-9312
www.iahp.org
institutes@iahp.org
Janet Doman, Founder & Director
Douglas Doman, Vice-Director
Dr. Leland Green, Medical Director
Nonprofit educational organization that serves children by introducing parents to the field of child brain development. Parents learn how to enhance significantly the development of their children physically, intellectually and socially.

58 International Dyslexia Association
40 York Rd
4th Fl
Baltimore, MD 21204
410-296-0232
Fax: 410-321-5069
www.dyslexiaida.org
info@ydslexiaida.org
Rick Smith, Chief Executive Officer
Elisabeth Liptak, Director, Professional Dev.
Cyndi Powers, Director, Special Projects
The International Dyslexia Association is an international organization that concerns itself with the complex issues of dyslexia. The IDA membership consist of a variety of professionals in partnership with people with dyslexia and their families and all others interested in The Association's mission.

59 International Literacy Association (ILA)
Formerly International Reading Association
800 Barksdale Rd
P.O. Box 8139
Newark, DE 19714-8139
302-731-1600
800-336-7323
Fax: 302-731-1057
www.literacyworldwide.org
customerservice@reading.org
William Teale, President
Marcie Craig Post, Executive Director
Stephen Sye, Associate Executive Director
The mission of the International Reading Association is to promote reading by continuously advancing the quality of literacy instruction and research worldwide.

60 LD OnLine
2775 South Quincy St
Arlington, VA 22206
FAX 703-998-2060
www.ldonline.org
Noel Gunther, Executive Director
Christian Lindstrom, Director, Learning Media
Rachel Walker, Outreach Consultant
Provides information and referrals to both parents and educators dealing with children that are diagnosed with learning disabilities.

61 Landmark School Outreach Program
Landmark School
429 Hale St
P.O. Box 227
Prides Crossing, MA 01965
978-236-3216
Fax: 978-927-7268
www.landmarkoutreach.org
outreach@landmarkschool.org
Dan Ahearn, Director of Outreach
Patricia Newhall, Associate Director, Outreach
Kaia Cunningham, Assistant Director
Offers strategies, research, and professional development to help educators improve learning for children with language-based learning disabilities.

62 Learning Ally: National Headquarters
20 Roszel Rd
Princeton, NJ 08540
609-452-0606
800-221-4792
www.lcarningally.org
princetonstudio@learningally.org
Andrew Friedman, President & CEO
Connie Murphy, Executive Vice President
Cynthia Hamburger, Chief Operating Officer
National, non-profit organization working to provide better access to learning aids that can assist children with reading-related disabilities. Offers informational resources for educators, parents, and professionals intended to help connect them with access to these learning aids and guides on implementing them at home or in the classroom.

63 Learning Disabilities Association of America (LDAA)
4156 Library Rd
Pittsburgh, PA 15234-1349
412-341-1515
Fax: 412-344-0224
www.ldaamerica.org
info@ldaamerica.org
Mary-Clare Reynolds, Executive Director
Maureen Swanson, Director
Myrna Mandlawitz, Policy Director
LDA is a grassroots, membership organization seeking to improve policy and accessibility for individuals with learning disabilities.

64 Learning Resource Network
P.O.Box 9
River Falls, WI 54022-0009
715-426-9777
800-678-5376
Fax: 888-234-8633
www.lern.org
info@lern.org
William A. Draves, President
Julie Coates, SVP Information Services
Greg Marsello, SVP Development
Organization dedicated to offering informational resources and consultative expertise on continuing education and life-long learning. Disseminates publications, newsletters, webinars, and conferences that provide strategies and methodologies for professionals in educational institutions.

65 Matrix Parent Network & Resource Center
94 Galli Dr
Ste C
Novato, CA 94949-5739
415-884-3535
800-578-2592
Fax: 415-884-3555
www.matrixparents.org
info@matrixparents.org
Denise LaBuda, Board President
Nora Thompson, Executive Director
Sandi Strang, Director, Parent Services
Providing families who have children with disabilities and other special needs with the tools they need to effectively advocate for themselves.

66 McRel International Formerly Edvantia Inc.
4601 DTC Blvd
Ste 500
Denver, CO 80237-2596
303-337-0990
800-858-6830
www.mcrel.org
info@mcrel.org
Patrick Woods, Chair
Bryan Goodwin, President & CEO
Robin Jarvis, Chief Program Officer
Organization offering educational services through evaluation, analysis, and research in order to assist schools with providing optimal learning outcomes.

67 **Menninger Clinic**
12301 S. Main St.
Houston, TX 77035-6207   713-275-5000
                                 800-351-9058
                            Fax: 713-275-5107
                       www.menningerclinic.com
                          epoa@menninger.edu
C. Edward Coffey, President & CEO
Avni Cirpili, Chief Nursing Officer
Edward Poa, Chief Inpatient Services
The mission of Menninger is to be a national resource providing psychiatric care and treatment of the highest standard, searching for better understanding of mental illness and human behavior, disseminating their findings, and applying this knowledge in useful ways to promote individual growth and better mental health.

68 **NASDSE**
225 Reinekers Lane
Ste 420
Alexandria, VA 22314   703-519-3800
                          Fax: 703-519-3808
                             www.nasdse.org
Fred Balcolm, President
Bill East, Executive Director
Nancy Reder, Deputy Executive Director
The National Association of State Directors of Special Education provides leadership focused on the improvement of educational services and positive outcomes for children and youth with disabilities throughout the United States.

69 **NASP**
4340 East West Highway
Ste 402
Bethesda, MD 20814   301-657-0270
                             866-331-6277
                        Fax: 301-657-0275
                       http://nasponline.org
Susan Gorin, Executive Director
Lauren Blackwell, Manager, Membership Marketing
Katherine Cowan, Director, Communications
The National Association of School Psychologists empowers school psychologists by advancing effective practices to improve students' learning, behavior, and mental health.

70 **National ARD/IEP Advocates**
4510 Redstart
Houston, TX 77035   281-265-1506
                        Fax: 253-295-9954
                           www.narda.org
                          louis@narda.org
Louis H. Geigerman, Founder & President
Sidney A. Wohlman, Child Advocate
Barbara Kluchin, Professional Advocate
National ARD Advocates is dedicated to obtaining the appropriate educational services for children with special needs.

71 **National Adult Education Professional Development Consortium (NAEPDC)**
444 North Capitol St., NW
Ste 422
Washington, DC 20001   202-624-5250
                          Fax: 202-624-1497
                             www.naepdc.org
                          jcarter@naepdc.org
Beverly Smith, Chair
Jeff Carter, Executive Director
Dr. Gene Sofer, Director, Government Relations
An organization dedicated to enhancing adult education through professional development and dissemination of information and assistive resources.

72 **National Association for Adults with Special Learning Needs (NAASLN)**
P.O.Box 716
Bryn Mawr, PA 19010   888-562-2756
                          Fax: 614-392-1559
                             www.naasln.org
Richard Cooper, President
Joan Hudson-Miller, President
Frances A. Holthaus, Vice President
An association for those who serve adults with special learning needs. Members include educators, trainers, employers and human service providers

73 **National Association for Child Development (NACD)**
549 - 25th St
Ogden, UT 84504-2422   801-621-8606
                          Fax: 801-621-8389
                               www.nacd.org
Robert J. Doman Jr, Founder & Director
Laird Doman, COO & Family Liason
Ellen R. Doman, Educational Director
Provides neurodevelopmental evaluations and individualized programs for children and adults, updated on a quarterly basis. Stresses parent training and parent implementation of the program.

74 **National Association for Community Mediation (NAFCM)**
P.O.Box 5246
Louisville, KY 40255   602-633-4213
                             www.nafcm.org
                          info@nafcm.org
D.G. Mawn, Associate Director
Brennan Frazier, Membership Coordinator
Supports the maintenance and growth of community-based mediation programs and processes; acts as a resource for mediation information; locates a center to help individuals and groups resolve disputes.

75 **National Association for Gifted Children (NAGC)**
1331 H St, NW
Ste 1001
Washington, DC 20005   202-785-4268
                          Fax: 202-785-4248
                               www.nagc.org
                             nagc@nagc.org
George Betts, President
M. René Islas, Executive Director
Adrian Wiles, Manager, Member Services
An organization of parents, teachers, educators, other professionals, and community leaders who unite to address the unique needs of children and youth with demonstrated gifts and talents as well as those children who may be able to develop their talent potential with appropriate educational experiences.

76 **National Association for the Education of Young Children (NAEYC)**
1313 L St NW
Ste 500
Washington, DC 20005-4110   202-232-8777
                                    800-424-2460
                               Fax: 202-328-1846
                                  www.naeyc.org
                                naeyc@naeyc.org
Deb Cassidy, President
Rhian Evans Allvin, Executive Director
Stephanie Morris, Deputy Executive Director
Dedicated to improving the well-being of all children, with particular focus on the quality of educational and developmental services for children from birth through age 8. Also the largest organization working on behalf of young adults with nearly 100,000 members, a national network of over 300 local, state and regional affiliates, and a growing global alliance of like-minded organizations.

77 National Association of Councils on Developmental Disabilities (NACDD)
1825 K. St, NW
Ste 600
Washington, DC 20006   202-506-5813
                                                   Fax: 202-506-5846
                                                      www.nacdd.org
                                                    infos@nacdd.org
Donna A. Meltzer, Chief Executive Officer
Robin Troutman, Deputy Director, Operations
Cindy Smith, Director, Public Policy
A national member-driven organization consisting of 55 State and Territorial Councils. Places high value on meaningful participation and contribution by Council members and staff of all Member Councils, and continually working towards positive system change on behalf of individuals with developmental disabilities and their families.

78 National Association of Parents with Children in Special Education (NAPCSE)
3642 E Sunnydale Dr
Chandler Heights, AZ 85142   800-754-4421
                                                   Fax: 800-424-0371
                                                      www.napcse.org
                                                  contact@napcse.org
Dr. George Giuliani, President
A national membership organization dedicated to rendering all possible support and assistance to parents whose children receive special education services, both in and outside of school. NAPCSE was founded to promote a sense of community and provide a national forum for ideas.

79 National Association of Private Special Education Centers (NAPSEC)
601 Pennsylvania Ave NW
Ste 900 - South Building
Washington, DC 20004   202-434-8225
                                                   Fax: 202-434-8224
                                                      www.napsec.org
                                                    napsec@aol.com
Sherry Kolbe, Executive Director
A non-profit association whose mission is to ensure access for individuals to private special education as a vital component of the continuum of appropriate placement and services in American education. The association consists solely of private special education programs that serve both both privately and publicly placed individuals of all ages with disabilities.

80 National Association of Special Education Teachers (NASET)
1250 Connecticut Ave NW
Ste 200
Washington, DC 20036-2643   202-296-7739
                                                       800-754-4221
                                                   Fax: 800-754-4221
                                                      www.naset.org
                                                  contactus@naset.org
Dr. Roger Pierangelo, Executive Director
Dr. George Giuliani, Executive Director
A national membership organization dedicated to providing all possible support and assistance to those preparing for or teaching in the field of special education.

81 National Association of the Education of African American Children with Learning Disabilities
P.O. Box 09521
Columbus, OH 43209   614-237-6021
                                                   Fax: 614-238-0929
                                                       www.aacld.org
                                                    info@aacld.org
The NAEAACLD links information and resources provided by an established network of individuals and organizations experienced in minority research and special education with parents, educators and others responsible for providing an appropriate education for African American students.

82 National Autism Association
One Park Avenue
Ste 1
Portsmouth, RI 02871   401-293-5551
                                                       877-622-2884
                                                   Fax: 401-293-5342
                                  http://nationalautismassociation.org
                                              naa@nationalautism.org
Lori McIlwain, Co-Founder/Board Chairperson
Wendy Fournier, President/Founding Board Member
Kelly Vanicek, Executive Director
The mission of the National Autism Association is to respond to themost urgent needs of the autism community, providing real help and hope so that all affected can reach their full potential.

83 National Business and Disability Council at The Viscardi Center
201 I.U. Willets Rd
Albertson, NY 11507   516-465-1400
                                                   Fax: 516-465-1591
                                   www.viscardicenter.org/services/nbdc
                                              info@viscardicenter.org
Brandon M. Macsata, General Consultant
Beatrice Schmidt, Corporate Services Specialist
Gary Karp, Training Consultant
A leading resource for employers seeking to integrate people with disabilities into the workplace and companies seeking to reach them in the consumer marketplace. The NBDC has played a major role in helping businesses create accessible work conditions for employees and accessible products and services for consumers.

84 National Center for Families Literacy (NCFL)
325 W Main St
Ste 300
Louisville, KY 40202   502-584-1133
                                                       877-326-5481
                                                   Fax: 502-584-0172
                                                 www.familieslearning.com
                                             notify@familieslearning.org
Sharon Darling, President & Founder
Mission is to create a literate nation by leveraging the power of family. Family literacy is an intergenerational approach based on the indisputable evidence that low literacy is an unfortunate and debilitating family tradition.

85 National Center for Learning Disabilities (NCLD)
32 Laight St
2nd Fl
New York, NY 10013   212-545-7510
                                                       888-575-7373
                                                   Fax: 212-545-9665
                                                       www.ncld.org
                                                      help@ncld.org
Frederic M. Poses, Chairman of the Board
Mimi Corcoran, President & CEO
Rashonda Ambrose, Marketing Director
Works to ensure that the nation's 15 million children, adolescents and adults with learning disabilities have every opportunity for succees in school, work and life. NCLD also provides essential information to parents, professionals and individuals with learning disabilities, promotes research and programs to foster effective learning and advocates for policies to protect and strengthen educational rights and opportunities.

86 National Center for Youth Law
405 14th St
15th Fl
Oakland, CA 94612   510-835-8098
                                                   Fax: 510-835-8099
                                                      www.youthlaw.org
                                                   info@youthlaw.org
Peter B. Edelman, President
Jesse Hahnel, Executive Director
Hannah Benton, Staff Attorney

Uses the law to improve the lives of low-income children. Also works to ensure that low-income children have the resources, support, and opportunities they need for a healthy and productive future. Much of NCYL's work is focused on poor children who are additionally challenged by abuse and neglect, disability, or other disadvantage.

87   National Council of Juvenile and Family Court Judges (NCJFCJ)

P.O. Box 8970
Reno, NV 89507 775-507-4777
Fax: 775-507-4848
www.ncjfcj.org
contactus@ncjfcj.org

Judge Katherine Tennyson, President
Joey Orduna Hastings, Chief Executive Officer
Michael Noyes, Chief Program Officer
The vision of the NCJFCJ is that every child and young person be reared in a safe, permanent, and nurturing family, where love, self-control, concern for others, and responsibility for the consequences of one's actions are experienced and taught as fundamental values for a successful life. Also advocates that every family in need of judicial oversight has access to fair, effective and timely justice.

88   National Council on Rehabilitation Education (NCRE)

1099 E. Champlain Dr, Ste A
PMB # 137
Fresno, CA 93720 559-906-0787
Fax: 559-412-2550
www.ncre.org
info@ncre.org

Noel Estrada-Hernández, President
Michael Accordino, 1st Vice-President
Denise Catalano, 2nd Vice-President
A professional organization of educators dedicated to quality services for persons with disabilities through education and research. NCRE advocates-up-to-date education and training and the maintenance of professional standards in the field of rehabilitation

89   National Disabilities Rights Network (NDRN)

820 1st St NE
Ste 740
Washington, DC 20002 202-408-9514
Fax: 202-408-9520
TTY: 202-408-9521
www.ndrn.org
info@ndrn.org

Kim Moody, President
Curtis L. Decker, Executive Director
Non-profit membership organization for the federally mandated Protection and Advocacy (P&A) Systems and Client Assistance Programs (CAP) for individuals with disabilities. Serves a wide range of individuals with disabilities including, but not limited to, those with cognitive, mental, sensory, and physical disabilities. Services include guarding against abuse; advocating for basic rights; and ensuring accountability in health care, education, employment, housing, and transportation.

90   National Education Association (NEA)

1201 - 16th St NW
Washington, DC 20036-3290 202-833-4000
Fax: 202-822-7974
www.nea.org

Lily Eskelsen García, President
Becky Pringle, Vice President
John C. Stocks, Executive Director
The National Education Association, along with it's state-wide affiliates, seeks to advance public education, working with professionals and members at every educational level - from pre-school to university.

91   National Federation of the Blind

200 E. Wells St.
at Jernigan Place
Baltimore, MD 21230 410-659-9314
Fax: 410-685-5653
www.nfb.org
nfb@nfb.org

Mark A. Riccobono, President
The largest and most influential membership organization of blind people in the United States. The NFB improves the lives of the blind through advocacy, education, research, technology, and programs encouraging independence and self-confidence. It is also the leading force in the blindness field today and the voice of the nation's blind.

92   National Institute for Learning Development

801 Greenbrier Parkway
Chesapeake, VA 23320 757-423-8646
877-661-6453
Fax: 757-451-0970
http://nild.org

Kristin Barbour, Executive Director
Allison Jenson, Program Development Manager
Susie Hartung, Program Coordinator
NILD is a global institute offering services to parents, students, and educators in areas of accreditation, professional development, and educational therapy.

93   National Institute of Art and Disabilities Art Center

551 - 23rd St
Richmond, CA 94804-1626 510-620-0290
Fax: 510-620-0326
www.niadart.org
admin@niadart.org

Deborah Dyer, Executive Director
Tim Buckwalter, Director
Belinda Sifford, Director of Client Services
An innovative visual arts center assisting adults with developmental and other physical disabilities. Provides an art program that promotes creativity, independence, dignity, and community integration for people with developmental and other disabilities.

94   National Joint Committee on Learning Disabilities

2775 S Quincy St
Arlington, VA 22206 301-296-5707
Fax: 703-998-2060
www.ldonline.org/njcld
mbklotz@naspweb.com

Elsa Cardenas-Hagan, NJCLD Chair
Stan Dublinske, NJCLD Secretary & Treasurer
Mary Beth Klotz, NJCLD Website Contact
A partner of LD OnLine, the NJCLD's mission is to provide multi-organizational leadership and resources to optimize outcomes for individuals with learning disabilities. LD Online serves as the official website for the NJCLD.

95   National Organization for Rare Disorders (NORD)

55 Kenosia Ave
Danbury, CT 06810 203-744-0100
800-999-6673
Fax: 203-263-9938
www.rarediseases.org
orphan@rarediseases.org

Marshall Summar, Board Chairman
Peter Saltonstall, President & CEO
Martha L. Rinker, VP, Public Policy
A unique federation of voluntary health organizations dedicated to helping people with rare diseases and assisting the organizations that serve them. Committed to the identification, treatment, and cure of rare disorders through programs of education, advocacy, research, and service.

96 **National Organization on Disability (NOD)**
77 Water St
Ste 204
New York, NY 10005 646-505-1191
Fax: 646-505-1184
www.nod.org
info@nod.org

Gov. Tom Ridge, Board Chairman
Carol Glazer, President
Miranda Pax, Director, External Affairs
The mission of the National Organization on Disability is to expand the participataion and contribution of America's 54 million men, women and children with disabilities in all aspects of life.

97 **National Rehabilitation Association**
P.O. Box 150235
Alexandria, VA 22315 703-836-0850
888-258-4295
Fax: 703-836-0848
www.nationalrehab.org
info@nationalrehab.org

Eleanor Williams, President
Dr. Fredric Schroeder, Executive Director
Tanya Griffey, Membership Coordinator
A membership organization that promotes ethical and state of the art practice in rehabilitation with the goal of the personal and economic independence of persons with disabilities. Members include rehabilitation counselors, physical, speech and occupational therapists, job trainers, consultants, independent living instructors, students in rehabilitation programs, and other professionals involved in the advocacy of programs and services for people with disabilities.

98 **National Rehabilitation Information Center (NARIC)**
8400 Corporate Dr
Ste 500
Landover, MD 20785 301-459-5900
800-346-2742
Fax: 301-459-4263
TTY: 301-459-5984
www.naric.com
naricinfo@heitechservices.com

Mark X Odum, Project Director
Jessica H. Chaiken, Media & Info Services Manager
Natalie J. Collier, Library and Acquisitions Manager
The mission of the Center is to collect and disseminate the results of research funded by the National Institute on Disability, Independent Living and Rehabilitation Research (NIDLRR).

99 **Non Verbal Learning Disorders Association (NLDA)**
507 Hopmeadow St
Simsbury, CT 06070 860-658-5522
Fax: 860-658-6688
www.nlda.org
info@nlda.org

Patricia Carrin, Founder/ President
Marcia Rubinstein, Founder/Executive Liaison
A non-profit organizaion dedicated to research, education, and advocacy for nonverbal learning disorders.

100 **Parent Advocacy Coalition for Educational Rights (PACER)**
8161 Normandale Blvd
Bloomington, MN 55437 952-838-9000
800-537-2237
Fax: 952-838-0199
TTY: 952-838-0190
www.pacer.org
pacer@pacer.org

Alison Bakken, Board President
Jeff Betchwars, Board Vice-President
Paula F. Goldberg, Executive Director

The mission of PACER is to expand opportunities and enhance the quality of life of children and young adults with disabilities and their families, based on the concept of parents helping parents.

101 **Parent Educational Advocacy Training Center (PEATC)**
8003 Forbes Place
Ste 310
Springfield, VA 22151 703-923-0010
800-869-6782
Fax: 800-693-3514
TTY: 703-923-0010
partners@peatc.org

Suzanne Bowers, Executive Director
Nichole Drummond, Deputy Director
Heather Arbeen, Senior Information Specialist
A non-profit that believes children with disabilities reach their full potential when families and professionals enjoy an equal, respectful partnership. PEATC also provides support education, and training to families, schools and other professionals committed to helping children with disabilities.

102 **Parents Helping Parents**
Sabrato Center for Nonprofits-San Jose
1400 Parkmoor Ave
Ste 100
San Jose, CA 95126 408-727-5775
855-727-5775
Fax: 408-286-1116
www.php.com
info@php.com

Maria Daane, Executive Director
Jane Floethe Ford, Director, Education Services
Nancy O'Rourke, Chief Development Officer
Helping children with special needs receive the resources, love, hope, respect, health care, education and other services they need to achieve their full potential by helping to create strong families and dedicated professionals.

103 **Rehabilitation Engineering and Assistive Technology Society of North America (RESNA)**
1700 N Moore St
Ste 1540
Arlington, VA 22209 703-524-6686
Fax: 703-524-6630
TTY: 703-524-6639
www.resna.org
membership@resna.org

Roger O. Smith, President
Michael J. Brogioli, Executive Director
An interdisciplinary association of people with a common interest in technology and disability. The purpose is to use technology to improve the potential of people with disabilities and enable them to achieve their goals.

104 **Rehabilitation International (RI Global)**
866 United Nations Plaza
Office 422
New York, NY 10017 212-420-1500
Fax: 212-505-0871
www.riglobal.org
info@riglobal.org

Jan A. Monsbakken, President
Venus Ilagan, Secretary General
A global network of people with disabilities, service providers, researchers, government agencies and advocates promoting and implementing the rights and inclusion of people with disabilities.

105 **Sertoma Inc.**
1912 East Meyer Blvd
Kansas City, MO 64132-1141 816-333-8300
Fax: 816-333-4320
www.sertoma.org
infosertoma@sertomahq.org

Don Bartelmay, President
Cheryl Cherny, President Elect
Edwin Dlugopolski, Senior Vice-President
Activities focus on helping people with speech and hearing problems, but also have programs in the areas of youth, national heritage, drug awareness and community services.

106   Smart Kids with Learning Disabilities
38 Kings Highway North
Westport, CT 06880   203-226-6831
                                        Fax: 203-226-6708
                                http://smartkidswithld.org
Smart Kids with Learning Disabilities is a non-profit organization dedicated to empowering the parents of children with learning disabilites (LD) and attention-deficit disorder (ADHD) by providing resources to help understand and evaluate their child's capabilities.

107   Son-Rise Program
Autism Treatment Center of America
2080 Undermountain Rd
Sheffield, MA 01257-9643   413-229-2100
                                             877-766-7473
                                        Fax: 413-229-3202
                             www.autismtreatmentcenter.org
                                      autism@option.org
Barry Kaufman, Founder
Raun Kaufman, Director of Global Education
Since 1983, the Autism Treatment Center of America has provided innovative training programs and workshops for parents and professionals caring for children challenged by Autism, Autism Spectrum Disorders, Pervasive Developmental Disorder (PDD) and other developmental difficulties.

108   Stuttering Foundation of America
P.O. Box 11749
Memphis, TN 38111-0749   901-761-0343
                                             800-992-9392
                                        Fax: 901-761-0484
                                    www.stutteringhelp.org
                                  info@stutteringhelp.org
Jane H. Fraser, President
Founded with the goal to provide the best and most up-to-date information and help available for the prevention of stuttering in young children and the most effective treatment available for teenagers and adults.

109   Team of Advocates for Special Kids (TASK)
100 West Cerritos Ave
Anaheim, CA 92805   714-533-8275
                                             866-828-8275
                                        Fax: 714-533-2533
                                           www.taskca.org
                                       task@.taskca.org
Marta Anchondo, Executive Director
TASK's mission is to enable children with disabilities to reach their maximum potential by providing them, their families and the professionals who serve them, with training, support information resources and referrals, and by providing community awareness programs. TASK's TECH Center is a place for children, parents, adult consumers, and professionals to learn about assistive technology by providing hands-on access to computer hardware, software and adaptive equipment.

110   Technology and Media Division
Council for Exceptional Children
2900 Crystal Dr
Ste 1000
Arlington, VA 22202-3557   703-245-3660
                                             888-232-7733
                                        Fax: 703-264-9494
                                     TTY: 866-915-5000
                                           www.tamcec.org
                                   contactus@tamcec.org
Antonis Katsiyannis, President

TAM works to promote the availability and effective use of technology and media for children, birth to 21, with disabilities and/or who are gifted.

111   The American Printing House for the Blind, Inc.
1839 Frankfort Ave
P.O. Box 6085
Louisville, KY 40206-0085   502-895-2405
                                             800-223-1839
                                        Fax: 502-899-2284
                                              www.aph.org
                                            info@aph.org
The world's largest non-profit organization creating educational, work place, and independent living products and services for people who are visually impaired.

112   The College Board
250 Vesey St
New York, NY 10281   212-713-8000
                                        Fax: 866-360-0114
                                      TTY: 609-882-4118
                                      www.collegeboard.org
                             ssd@info.collegeboard.org
David Coleman, President & CEO
Jeremy Singer, Chief Operating Officer
Jack Buckley, Senior Vice President, Research
Founded in 1900. Offers testing accommodations that minimize the effect of disabilities on test performance. The SAT Program tests eligible students with documented visual, physical, hearing, or learning disabilities who require testing accommodations for SAT.

113   US Autism & Asperger Association
12180 S. 300 E.
Ste 532
Draper, UT 84020-0532   888-928-8476
                                     http://usautism.org
Lawrence Kaplan, Chairman/CEO
Phillip DeMio, Chief Medical Officer
US Autism & Asperger Association (USAAA) is a 501 (c) (3) nonprofit organization for Autism and Asperger education, support, and solutions.

114   US Department of Education: Office for Civil Rights
400 Maryland Ave, SW
Washington, DC 20202-1100   202-453-6100
                                             800-421-3481
                                        Fax: 202-453-6012
                                      TTY: 800-877-8339
                                              www.ed.gov
                                            ocr@ed.gov
Catherine E. Lhamon, Assistant Secretary
James Ferg-Cadima, Dep. Assistant Secretary, Policy
The mission of the Office for Civil Rights is to ensure equal access to education and to promote educational excellence throughout the nation through vigorous enforcement of civil rights.

115   Washington PAVE: Specialized Training of Military Parents (STOMP)
6316 South 12th St
Tacoma, WA 98465-1900   253-565-2266
                                             800-572-7368
                                        Fax: 253-566-8052
                                      TTY: 800-573-7368
                                           www.wapave.org
                                       pave@wapave.org
Tracy Kahlo, Executive Director
Heather Hebdon, STOMP Program Director
Elma Rounds, CFO / Office Manager
STOMP is a parent-directed project that exists to empower military parents, individuals with disabilities, and service providers with knowledge, skills and resources so that they might access services to create a collaborative environment for a family and professional partnerships without regard to geographic location.

116 World Institute on Disability (WID)
3075 Adeline St
Ste 155
Berkeley, CA 94703 510-225-6400
Fax: 510-225-0477
TTY: 510-225-0478
www.wid.org
wid@wid.org
Carol J. Bradley, Chair
Anita Shafer Aaron, Executive Director
Thomas Foley, Deputy Director
A non-profit public policy center dedicated to promoting independence and full societal inclusion of people with disabilities.

117 YACHAD/National Jewish Council for Disabilities
11 Broadway
13th Fl
New York, NY 10004 212-613-8229
Fax: 212-613-0796
www.yachad.org
njcd@ou.org
Dr. Jeffrey Lichtman, International Director
Elizabeth Fishel, Director, National Yachad
Joe Goldfarb, Director, Summer Programs
Yachad/NJCD is dedicated to addressing the needs of all individuals with disabilities and including them in the Jewish community. Summer Programs include a variety of summer experiences for youth and adults with developmental disabilities.

118 YAI Network
460 West 34th St
11th Fl
New York, NY 10001-2382 212-273-6100
www.yai.org
staff@yai.org
Matthew Sturiale, Chief Executive Officer
Sanjay Dutt, Chief Financial Officer
Roberta G. Koenigsberg, Chief Compliance Officer
A national leader in the provision of services, education and training in the field of developmental and learning disabilities.

Alabama

119 Easter Seals - Alabama
5960 E Shirley Ln
Montgomery, AL 36117 334-395-4489
800-388-7325
Fax: 334-395-4492
www.easterseals.com/alabama
info@al.easterseals.com
John Ives, Chairman
Randy Thomas, Chairman Elect
Lynne Stokley, Chief Executive Officer
Easter Seals provides services to children and adults with disabilities and other special needs, and support to their families.

120 Easter Seals - Birmingham Area
2717 3rd Avenue S
Birmingham, AL 35233 205-942-6277
Fax: 205-945-4906
www.eastersealsbham.org
Shaun Cosby, Chairperson
Paul Ebert, Vice Chairperson
David Higgins, Executive Director
Easter Seals has been helping individuals with disabilities and special needs, and their families, live better lices for more than 80 years. From child development centers to physical rehabilitation and job training for people with disabilities, Easter Seals offers a variety of services to help people with disabilities address life's challenges and achieve personal goals.

121 Easter Seals - Central Alabama
2125 E South Blvd
Montgomery, AL 36116 334-288-0240
Fax: 334-288-7171
www.eastersealsca.org
info@eastersealsca.org
Debbie Lynn, Executive Director
Ed Collier, Director, Programs
Amy Berry, Speech Therapy/Referrals
Provides quality life enhancing programs and services to meet the needs of children and adults with disabilities.

122 Easter Seals - West Alabama
1110 Dr. Edward Hillard Dr
Tuscaloosa, AL 35401 205-759-1211
800-726-1216
Fax: 205-349-1162
www.eastersealswestal.org
eswa@eswaweb.org
Ronny Johnston, Director
Alvin Hawthorne, Director, Finance
Holly Hillard, Director, Development
Serves children and adults with disabilities while maintaining a reputation for quality, and comprehensive services.

123 International Dyslexia Association of Alabama
280 Marwood Drive
Birmingham, AL 35244 256-551-1442
855-247-1381
Fax: 205-942-2688
www.idaalabama.org
info@idaalabama.org
Linda Brady, President
Denise Gibbs, Vice President
Diane McTamney, Secretary
ALIDA will provide dyslexic individuals in Alabama with a unified voice to represent their interests to the public, to the educational community, to the legislature, and to others. ALIDA will also serve as a vehicle to increase awareness and understanding of dyslexia in Alabama.

124 Learning Disabilities Association of Alabama
PO Box 244023
Montgomery, AL 36124-4023 334-277-9151
Fax: 334-284-9357
www.ldaal.org
Tamara Massey-Garrett, President
Linda Hames, First Vice President
Pat Morrow, Second Vice President
A non-profit grassroots organization whose members are individuals with learning disabilities, their families, and the professionals who work with them. LDAA is dedicated to identifying causes and promoting prevention of learning disabilities and to enhance the quality of life for all individuals with learning disabilities and their families by encouraging effective identification and intervention, fostering research, and protecting their rights inder the law.

Alaska

125 Center for Human Development (CHD)
University of Alaska Anchorage
2702 Gambell St
Ste 103
Anchorage, AK 99503-2836 907-272-8270
800-243-2199
Fax: 907-274-4802
TTY: 907-264-6206
www.alaskachd.org
info@alaskachd.org
Karen Ward, Director
Jenny Miller, LEND Training Director
Ken Hamrick, AWP Program Director
One of 61 University Centers located in every state and territoyr, which attempts to bring together the resources of the university and the community in support of individuals with developmental disabilities.

126 **Easter Seals - Alaska**
670 W Fireweed Ln
Ste 105
Anchorage, AK 99503-2562   907-277-7325
                                    Fax: 907-272-7325
                              www.alaska.easterseals.com
Vilma Gutierrez-Osborne, CEO
Easter Seals assists more than one million children and
adults with disabilities and their families annually through a
nationwide network of more than 450 service sites.

Arizona

127 **Arizona Center for Disability Law**
5025 E Washington St
Ste 202
Phoenix, AZ 85034   602-274-6287
                                          800-927-2260
                                    Fax: 602-274-6779
                                    TTY: 602-274-6287
                                        www.acdl.com
                              center@azdisabilitylaw.org
Anthony DiRienzi, President
Art Gode, Vice President
John Chalmers, Treasurer
Advocates for the legal rights of persons with disabilities to
be free from abuse, neglect and discrimination; and to have
access to education, healthcare, housing and jobs, and other
services in order to maximize independence and achieve
equality.

128 **Center for Applied Studies in Education Learning
(CASE)**
ASU/SSFD
2801 S University Ave
Ste 209, Education Bldg.
Little Rock, AZ 72204   501-569-3423
                                    Fax: 501-569-8238
                                    rhbradley@ualr.edu
Bob Bradley, Professor
Improves the quality of education and human services in Arkansas and globally through a number of inter-related activities: conducting research on the effectiveness of programs
and practices in education and human services; providing
technical assistance in statistics, research design, measurement methodologies, data management, and program evaluation to students, faculty, and external groups and agencies;
providing formal and informal consultation, technical
assistance and instruction.

129 **Institute for Human Development: Northern Arizona
University**
PO Box 5630
Ste 27A, 912 Riordan Rd.
Flagstaff, AZ 86011-5630   928-523-4791
                                    Fax: 928-523-9127
                                    TTY: 928-523-1695
                                        www.nau.edu
                                        ihd@nau.edu
Richard Carroll, Executive Director
The Institute values and supports the independence, produc-
tivity and inclusion of Arizona's citizens with disabilities.
Based on the values and beliefs, the Institute conducts train-
ing, research and services that further these goal.

130 **International Dyslexia Association of Arizona**
985 W Silver Spring Place
Oro Valley, AZ 85755-6548   480-941-0308
                                  www.dyslexia-az.org
                              arizona.ida@gmail.com
Meredith Puls, President
Yvonne Gill, Vice President
Melissa A.L. Pallister, Treasurer

The Arizona Branch of The International Dyslexia Association (AIDA) is a 501 (c) (3) non-profit, scientific organization dedicated to educating the public about the learning
disability, dyslexia. The Arizona Branch has four objectives: to increase awareness in the dyslexic and general community; to network with other learning disability groups and
legislators in education; to increase membership; to raise
funds for future projects that will make a difference in our
community.

131 **Parent Information Network**
Arizona Department of Education
2384 N Steves Blvd
Flagstaff, AZ 86004-6105   928-679-8106
                                          800-352-4558
                                    Fax: 928-679-8124
                                        www.ade.az.gov
                                        pins@azed.gov
Becky Raabe, Director
Provides free training and information to parents on federal
and state laws and regulations for special education, parental
rights and responsibilities, parent involvement, advocacy,
behavior, standards and disability related resources. Provides a clearinghouse of information targeted to parents of
children with disabilities. Also assists schools in promoting
positive parent/professional/ regional partnerships.

Arkansas

132 **Easter Seals - Arkansas**
3920 Woodland Heights Rd
Little Rock, AR 72212-2495   501-227-3600
                                    Fax: 501-227-4021
                              www.eastersealsar.com
Rick Fleetwood, Chairman
Angela Harrison-King, Vice Chairman
Elaine Eubank, President & CEO
Easter Seals' mission is to provide exceptional services to
ensure that all people with disabilities or special needs have
equal opportunities to live, learn, work and play in their
communities.

133 **Learning Disabilities Association of Arkansas (LDAA)**
P.O. Box 23514
Little Rock, AR 72221   501-666-8777
                                    Fax: 501-666-4070
                                  www.ldaarkansas.org
                        ldaarkansas@yahoo.com
Nathan Green, President
Rebecca Walker, Vice President
Becca Green, Treasurer
A nonprofit, volunteer organization of parents and profes-
sionals. LDAA is devoted to defining and finding solutions
to the broad spectrum of learning disabilities.

California

134 **Berkeley Policy Associates**
440 Grand Ave
Ste 500
Oakland, CA 94610-5085   510-465-7884
                                    Fax: 510-465-7885
                                    TDD: 510-465-4493
                                    www.impaqint.com
                                  info@bpacal.com
Sharon R. Benus, Chief Executive Officer
Avi Benus, President
Davis Baker, Chief Program Officer
Conducts social policy research and program evaluations in
various topic areas, including disability policy. Although
the research typically does not focus on specific disabilities,
the reports or other deliverables deriving from the projects
may include specific information relating to particular disabilities, and are available for purchase.

135 California Association of Private Special Education Schools
520 Capitol Mall
Ste 280
Sacramento, CA 95814   916-447-7061
                                Fax: 916-447-1320
                                www.capses.com
                                director@capses.com
Suzy Fitch, President
Rebecca Foo, Secretary, Past President
Dan Maydeck, Treasurer
Dedicated to preserving and enhancing the leadership role of the private sector in offering quality alternative services to students with disabilities.
191 members 1973

136 Community Alliance for Special Education (CASE)
Hamm's Bldg., 1550 Bryant St
Ste 735
San Francisco, CA 94103   415-431-2285
                                Fax: 415-431-2289
                                www.caseadvocacy.org
                                info@caseadvocacy.org
Joseph Feldman, Director
Provides special education advocacy, representation at individual education program (IEP) meetings and due process proceedings, free technical assistance consultations and training throughout the San Francisco Bay area.
1979

137 Dyslexia Awareness and Resource Center
928 Carpinteria St
Ste 2
Santa Barbara, CA 93103-3477   805-963-7339
                                Fax: 805-963-6581
                                www.dyslexiacenter.org
                                info@dyslexiacenter.org
Joan Esposito, Program Director
Leslie V Esposito, Executive Director
Provides it services, free of charge, to help educate, advocate, support and raise the awareness of the public about dyslexia, attention deficit disorder and other learning differences and the means to learn about and rise above these differences.
1990

138 Easter Seals - Bay Area, Lakeport
1950 Parallel Dr
Lakeport, CA 95453-4811   707-263-3949
                                877-263-3994
                                Fax: 707-263-3985
                                http://noca.easterseals.com
                                bbonnett@noca.easterseals.com
Bonnie Bonnett, Site Manager
Susan Armiger, CEO
Pat Straub, Administrative Assistant
Easter Seals provides services to children and adults with disabilities and other special needs and support to their families.

139 Easter Seals - Camp Heron
16403 Hwy 9
Boulder Creek, CA 95006-9696   831-338-3383
                                Fax: 831-338-0200
                                www.campharmon.org
                                campharmon@es-cc.org
Scott Webb, Director
Cynthia Carman, Camp Registrar
Ruth Hutchison, Board Chair
Camp Harmon offers camping opporunities to people with disabilities. Offers sessions designed for a specific age group and specific to developmental and/or physical disabilities.

140 Easter Seals - Central California, Aptos
9010 Soquel Dr
Aptos, CA 95003-4002   831-684-2166
                                800-400-0671
                                Fax: 831-684-1018
                                www.centralcal.easterseals.com
                                info@es-cc.org
Tom Conway, Chief Executive Officer
June Stockbridge, Director of Human Resources
Stella Lauerman, Director of Program Services
Create solutions that change lives of children and adults with disabilities or other special needs and their families.

141 Easter Seals - Central California, Fresno
2505 W Shaw Ave
Ste 2
Fresno, CA 93711   559-241-7233
                                Fax: 559-228-9200
                                www.centralcal.easterseals.com
June Stockbridge, CEO
Create solutions that change lives of children and adults with disabilities or other special needs and their families.

142 Easter Seals - Nothern California, Novato
20 Pimentel Ct
Ste A1
Novato, CA 94949-5656   415-382-7450
                                Fax: 415-382-6052
                                http://noca.easterseals.com
                                pstraub@noca.easterseals.com
Pat Straub, Exec. Asst.
Craig C. King, CEO
Easter Seals provides services to children and adults with disabilities and other special needs and support to their families.

143 Easter Seals - Southern California
1570 E 17th St
Santa Ana, CA 92705-4770   714-834-1111
                                Fax: 714-834-1128
                                http://southerncal.easterseals.com
Kimberly Michel, Chair
Andre Filip, First Vice Chair
Kimberly Striegl, Second Vice Chair
Provides excpetional services to ensure that all peopel with disabilities or other special needs and their families have equal opportunities to live, learn, work and play in their communities.

144 International Dyslexia Association of Los Angeles
PO Box 8943
Calabasas, CA 91372-0808   818-506-8866
                                Fax: 818-222-9260
                                http://dyslexiala.org
                                info@dyslexiala.org
Elizabeth Lutsky, MA, ET/P, President
Jennifer Kalan, MA, ET/P, Vice President
Sarae Shenkin, MA, BCET, Treasurer
The Los Angeles County Branch of The International Dyslexia Association believes that all individuals have the right to realize their potential, that individual learning abilities can be strengthened, and that language and reading skills can be achieved.

145 International Dyslexia Association of Northern California (NCBIDA)
PO Box 5010
San Mateo, CA 94402-0010   650-328-7667
                                Fax: 650-375-8504
                                www.dyslexia-ncbida.org
                                office@dyslexia-ncbida.org
Frances Dickson, MA, President
Andrea Shuel, MA, Vice-President
Sherry Sachar, Secretary
Formed to increase public awareness of dyslexia in Northern California and Northern Nevada. Have been serving individuals with dyslexia, their families and professionals in the field in this community for 30 years.

146   International Dyslexia Association of San Diego
12285 Oak Knoll Rd.
Poway, CA 92064   619-295-3722
                                         800-657-0381
                                     Fax: 619-295-3722
                                     www.dyslexiasd.org
                                     sdidainfo@gmail.com
Christine Wyeth, MA, LEP, President
Debra Cohen, MEd, Vice President
Megan V. Cohen, MEd, Past President
A nonprofit scientific and educational organization dedicated to the study and treatment of the learning disability. This branch was informed to increase public awareness of dyslexia.

147   Learning Ally: Menlo Park Recording Studio
431 Burgess Dr
Ste 120
Menlo Park, CA 94025   650-493-3717
                                     www.learningally.org
                                     hhall@learningally.org
Harry Hall, Studio Leader
To create opportunities for individuals, from Kindergarten through Graduate Level, who cannot read standard print because of a visual impairment, learning disability or other physical disability, to succeed in school by providing accessible educational materials.

148   Learning Disabilities Association of California
PO Box 1114
Claremont, CA 91711   909-621-1494
                                         866-532-6322
                                     www.ldaca.org
                                     contact@ldaca.org
Arline Krieger, President
Pam Hamilton, 1st Vice-President
EunMi Cho, 3rd Vice-President
A non-profit volunteer organization of parents, professionals and adults with learning disabilities. Its purpose is to promote and support the education and general welfare of children and adults of potentially normal intelligence who manifest learning, perceptual, and/or behavioral handicaps.

149   Legal Services for Children
1254 Market St
3rd Fl
San Francisco, CA 94102-4816   415-863-3762
                                     Fax: 415-863-7708
                                     www.lsc-sf.org
                                     zabrina@lsc-sf.org
Shella Brenner, Director of Finance & Operations
Ron Gutierrez, Clinical Director
Abigail Trillin, Executive Director
Nonprofit law firm for children and youth. Legal Services for Children provides free legal and social services to children and youth under 18 years old in the San Francisco Bay area.
1975

150   Lutheran Braille Workers
13471 California St.
P.O. Box 5000
Yucaipa, CA 92399-1450   909-795-8977
                                         800-925-6092
                                     Fax: 909-795-8970
                                     www.lbwinc.org
                                     lbw@lbwinc.org
Phillip Pledger, Executive Director
The mission of Lutheran Braille Workers is to provide the message of salvation, through faith in Jesus Christ, to individuals who are blind or visually impaired throughout the world.
1943

151   Orange County Learning Disabilities Association
PO Box 25772
Santa Ana, CA 92799-5772   949-646-0133
                                     www.oclda.org
                                     info@oclda.org
Joyce Riley, President
A private, self-help, volunteer, non-profit, charitable organization of parents and professionals who are concerned with the welfare of children and adults who have learning disabilities.
1960

Colorado

152   Easter Seals - Colorado Camp Rocky Mountain Village
PO Box 115
Empire, CO 80438   303-569-2333
                                     Fax: 303-569-3857
                              www.co.easterseals.com
                          campinfo@easterealscolorado.org
Lynn Robinson, President
Nancy Hanson, VP, Human Resources
Krasimir Koev, Primary Contact
Provides services to children and adults with disabilities and other special needs, and support to their families.

153   Learning Ally: Denver Recording Studio
1355 S Colorado Blvd
Ste 801, Bldg C
Denver, CO 80222-3305   303-757-0787
                                     www.learningally.org
                                     asantos@learningally.org
Audrey Santos, Studio Leader
Produces the textbooks that students and professionals with print impairments need for the academic and career success that lead to lifelong self-sufficiency and self-fulfillment. Also provide and educational outreach program to schools to help them use and understand the program and our services.

154   Learning Disabilities Association of Colorado
55 Madison St
Ste 750
Denver, CO 80206   303-894-0992
                                     Fax: 303-830-1645
                                     http://ldaco.org
                                     info@ldaco.com
Bobbi Neiss, Executive Director
Jill Marrs, President
The Learning Disabilities Association of Colorado is committed to supporting the potential of individuals with learning and attention disabilities through accurate identification, advocacy, and education.

155   PEAK Parent Center
611 N Weber St
Ste 200
Colorado Springs, CO 80903-1072   719-531-9400
                                         800-284-0251
                                     Fax: 719-531-9452
                                     www.peakparent.org
                                     info@peakparent.org
Barbara Buswell, Executive Director
Kent Willis, President
Sarah Billerbeck, Vice President
A federally-designated Parent Traning and Information Center (PTI). As a PTI, PEAK supports and empowers parents, providing them with information and strategies to use when advocating for their children with disabilities by expanding knowledge of special education and offering new strategies for success.

156 Rocky Mountain Disability and Business Technical Assistance Center
3630 Sinton Road
Suite 103
Colorado Springs, CO 80907-5072   719-444-0268
                                          800-949-4232
                                     Fax: 719-444-0269
                                     TTY: 719-444-0268
                                     www.adainformation.org
                                     rmdbtac@mtc-inc.com
Bob Gattis, Director of Evaluation
Randy Dipner, Senior Advisor
Chantal Woodyard, Outreach Coordinator
Provides information on the Americans with Disabilities Act to Colorado, Utah, Montana, Wyoming, North Dakota and South Dakota.

157 Rocky Mountain International Dyslexia Association
PO Box 745100
Arvada, CO 80006-5100   303-721-9425
                                     855-5-IDA-RM
                                Fax: 720-282-5748
                                www.dyslexia-rmbida.org
                                ida_rmb@yahoo.com
Karen Leopold, President
Ellen Hunter, Vice President
Lucinda Greene, Treasurer
The mission of the International Dyslexia Association of Colorado is to pursue and provide the most comprehensive range of evidence-based information, education, and services that address the full scope of dyslexia and other associated learning disabilities and to have a meaningful impact on the lives of individuals and families affected by dyslexia so they may advocate for themselves and achieve their highest potential.
300+ members 1949

Connecticut

158 Capitol Region Education Council
111 Charter Oak Ave
Hartford, CT 06106-1912   860-247-2732
                                     860-247-CREC
                                Fax: 860-246-3304
                                www.crec.org
                                tjohnsonsmith@crec.org
Bruce E. Douglas, Ph.D., Executive Director
Sandy Cruz-Serrano, COO & Interim CFO
Regina Terrell, Director of Human Resources
Will promote cooperation and collaboration with local school districts and other organizations committed to the improved quality of public education; provide cost-effective services to member districts and other clients; listen and respond to client needs for the improved quality of public education; and provide leadership in the region through the quality of its services and its ability to identify and share quality services of its member districts and other organizations to public education.
1966

159 Connecticut Association for Children and Adults with Learning Disabilities
25 Van Zant Street
Suite 15-5
Norwalk, CT 06855-1713   203-838-5010
                                Fax: 203-866-6108
                                www.cacld.org
                                cacld@optonline.net
Beryl Kaufman, Executive Director
A regional, non-profit organization that supports individuals, families and professionals by providing information, education, and consultation while promoting public awareness and understanding. CACLD's goal is to ensure access to the resources needed to help children and adults with learning disabilities and attention deficit disorders achieve their full potential.
1963

160 Connecticut Association of Private Special Education Facilities (CAPSEF)
330 Main Street
3rd Floor
Hartford, CT 06106 1851   860-525-1318
                                Fax: 860-541-6484
                                www.capsef.org
                                info@capsef.org
Pat Gerrity, President/Comm Co-Chair
Bernie Lindauer, Treasurer /Finace Co-Chair
Catherine Murphy - Brooks, Secretary
A voluntary association of provate schools which provides quality, cost effective, special education and related services to the special needs of children and adolescents (birth to 21 years) of Connecticut. The focus of these education services is social and vocation programs designed to enable students to succeed in the least restrictive environment
2,500 members 1974

161 Easter Seals - Capital Region & Eastern Connecticut
100 Deerfield Rd
Windsor, CT 06248-0100   800-270-0600
                                www.easterseals.com/hartford/
Richard W. Davidson, Chairman
Sandra L. Bouwman, 1st Vice Chairman
Joseph G. Kern, 2nd Vice Chairman
Easter Seals Connecticut creates solutions that change the lives of children and adults with disabilities or special needs, their families and communities.
1966

162 Nonverbal Learning Disorders Association
507 Hopmeadow St
Simsbury, CT 06070-2456   860-658-5522
                                Fax: 860-658-6688
                                www.nlda.org
                                info@nlda.org
Patricia Carrin, President
A non-profit corporation dedicated to research, education and advocacy for nonverbal learning disorders.

163 SpEd Connecticut
#105, 75 Charter Oak Ave
Hartford, CT 06106-2416   860-560-1711
                                Fax: 860-560-1750
                                www.spedconnecticut.com/spedindex.html
                                info@spedconnecticut.org
SpEd Connecticut is a non-profit organization of parents, professionals, and persons with learning disabilities. We are dedicated to promoting a better understanding of learning disabilities, securing appropriate educational and employment opportunities for children and adults with learning disabilities and improving the quality of life for this population. Formerly known as the Learning Disabilities Association of Connecticut.

164 State Education Resources Center of Connecticut
25 Industrial Park Rd
Middletown, CT 06457-1516   860-632-1485
                                Fax: 860-632-8870
                                www.ctserc.org
                                info@ctserc.org
Ingrid Canady, Interim Executive Director
Matthew Dugan, Program Services Director
Alice Henley, Director, Program Development
Non-profit educational organization. Provides high-quality Profession Development to teachers, educators, parents and families throughout the state of CT.
1969

Delaware

165 Easter Seals - Delaware & Maryland's Easten Shore, New Castle

61 Corporate Cir
Kearns Center
New Castle, DE 19720-2439   302-324-4444
                                   800-677-3800
                              Fax: 302-324-4441
                              TDD: 302-324-4442
                              www.easterseals.com/de

Kenan J. Sklenar, President/CEO
Cynthia Morgan, Chair
Martha Rees, Vice Chair
Provides exceptional services to ensure that all people with disabilities or special needs and their families have equal opportunities to live, learn, work and play in their communities.

166 Easter Seals - Georgetown

22317 DuPont Blvd
Georgetown, DE 19947-2153   302-253-1100
                              Fax: 302-856-7296
                              www.easterseals.com/de/

Pam Reuther, Contact
Provides exceptional services to ensure that all people with disabilities or special needs and their families have equal opportunities to live, learn, work and play in their communities.

167 Parent Information Center of Delaware

404 Larch Circle
Wilmington, DE 19804   302-999-7394
                                   888-547-4412
                              Fax: 302-999-7637
                              www.picofdel.org
                              picofdel@picofdel.org

Verna Wilkins Henley, President
Joan Y. French, Secretary
Keith Morton, Executive Director
A statewide non-profit organization dedicated to providing information, education and support, to families and caregivers of children with disabilites or special needs from birth to age 26. We strive to promote partnerships among families, educators, policy makers and the greater Delaware Community.

District of Columbia

168 Association for Childhood Education International (ACEI)

1200 18th St NW
Ste 700
Washington, DC 20036   202-372-9986
                                   800-423-3563
                              Fax: 202-372-9989
                              www.acei.org
                              headquarters@acei.org

Christine Chen, President
Diane Whitehead, Executive Director
Judy Singer, Director of Development
Mission is to promote and support in global community the optimal education and development of children, from birth through early adolescence, and to influence the professional growth of educators and the efforts of others who are committed to the needs of children in a changing society.

169 Center for Child and Human Development

Georgetown University
P.O.Box 571485
Washington, DC 20057-1485   202-687-5000
                              Fax: 202-687-8899
                              http://gucchd.georgetown.edu
                              gucdc@georgetown.edu

Phyllis Magrab, PhD, Executive Director

Established over four decades ago to improve the quality of life for all children and youth, especially those with, or at risk for, special needs and their families. Brings together policy, research and clincal practice for the betterment of individuals and families, especially childre, youth and those with special needs including: developmental disabilities and special health care needs, mental health needs, young children and those in the child welfare system.

170 Learning Ally: Washington Recording Studio

5225 Wisconsin Ave NW
Ste 312
Washington, DC 20015   202-244-8990
                              www.learningally.org
                              rdewey@learningally.org

Reed Dewey, Studio Leader
To create opportunities for individuals, from Kindergarten through Graduate Level, who cannot read standard print because of a visual impairment, learning disability or other physical disability, to succeed in school by providing accessible educational materials.

Florida

171 Florida Advocacy Center for Persons with Disabilities

2728 Centerview Dr
Ste 102
Tallahassee, FL 32301-6298   850-488-9071
                                   800-342-0823
                              Fax: 850-488-8640
                              TDD: 800-346-4127
                              www.advocacycenter.org
                              webmaster@advocacycenter.org

Gary Weston, Executive Director
The Advocacy Center for Persons with Disabilities is a nonprofit organization providing protection and advocacy services in the State of Florida. Our mission is to advance the dignity, equality, self-determination and expressed choices of individuals with disabilities.

172 International Dyslexia Association of Florida

2740 SW Martin Downs Blvd
Ste 189
Palm City, FL 34990   904-803-9591
                              www.idafla.org
                              info@idafla.org

Susan Sentell, President
David Howie, Treasurer
Frank McKeown, Secretary
A non-profit, scientific and educational organization, which was formed to increase public awareness of dyslexia in Florida.
1949

173 Learning Disabilities Association of Florida

7100 W Camino Real
Ste 215
Boca Raton, FL 33433   941-637-8957
                              Fax: 941-637-0617
                              www.lda-fl.org
                              cathyeldafl@gmail.com

Mark Halpert, Co-President
Cathy Einhorn, Co-President
A nonprofit volunteer organization of parents, professionals, and LD adults. It is devoted to defining and finding solutions to the broad spectrum of learning issues.

174 Miami Lighthouse for the Blind and Visually Impaired

601 SW 8th Ave
Miami, FL 33130-3209   305-856-2288
                              Fax: 305-285-6967
                              www.miamilighthouse.com
                              info@miamilighthouse.com

Virginia A. Jacko, President/CEO
Richard Fernandez, Chief Financial Officer
Carol Brady-Simmons, Chief Program Officer

The oldest and largest private agency in Florida to serve people of all ages who are blind or the visually impaired.

Georgia

175   Easter Seals - North Georgia
53 Perimeter Center E
Ste #550
Atlanta, GA 30319-1454
404-943-1070
Fax: 404-943-0890
http://northgeorgia.easterseals.com
Donna Davidson, President/CEO
Robert Gwaltney, VP of Early Education and Care
Bipin Nagar, Chief Financial Officer
Provides information and referral, physical, occupational, and speech therapy, child care, Head Start and teacher training.

176   Easter Seals - Southern Georgia
1906 Palmyra Rd
Albany, GA 31701-1598
229-439-7061
800-365-4583
Fax: 229-435-6278
http://southerngeorgia.easterseals.com
Kari Middleton, President
Matt Hatcher, Chief Operating Officer
Beth English, Executive Director
Creates solutions that change the lives of children, adults and families with disabilities or special needs by offering a variety of programs and services that enable individuals to lead lives of equality, dignity and independence.

177   International Dyslexia Association of Georgia
1951 Greystone Rd
Atlanta, GA 30318-2622
404-256-1232
www.idaga.org
info@idaga.org
Karen Huppertz, President
Renee Bernhardt, Vice-President
Meredith Chase, Treasurer
Formed to increase public awareness about dyslexia in the State of Georgia. The Branch encourages teachers to train in multisensory language instruction. Provides a network for individuals with dyslexia, their families and professionals in the educational and medical fields.
300 members

178   Learning Ally: Athens Recording Studio
320 S Hull St
Athens, GA 30605
706-549-1313
www.learningally.org
scourt@learningally.org
Michael Kaminer, Production Director
Wendy White, Production Assistant
To create opportunities for individuals, from Kindergarten through Graduate Level, who cannot read standard print because of a visual impairment, learning disability or other physical disability, to succeed in school by providing accessible educational materials.

179   Learning Disabilities Association of Georgia
4105 Briarcliff Rd NE
Ste 3
Atlanta, GA 30345
404-303-7774
Fax: 404-467-0190
www.ldag.org
ldaga@bellsouth.net
Tia Powell, President
One of 50 volunteer state organizations which comprise the Learning Disabilities Association of America. For over 30 years, LDAG has been enhancing the quality of life for individuals of all ages with Learning Disabilities and/or Attention Deficit and Hyperactivity Disorders.

Hawaii

180   Aloha Special Technology Access Center
710 Green St
Honolulu, HI 96813-2119
808-523-5547
Fax: 808-536-3765
www.alohastac.org
astachi@yahoo.com
Eric Anderson, Executive Director
Provide individuals with disabilities and their families access to computers, peripheral tools, and appropriate software. Aloha Stac aims to increase awareness, understanding, and implementation of microcomputer technology by establishing a program of activities and events to educate the community about what computers make possible for persons with disabilities.
1988

181   Assistive Technology Resource Centers of Hawaii (ATRC)
200 North Vineyard Boulevard
Ste 430
Honolulu, HI 96817-5362
808-532-7110
800-645-3007
Fax: 808-532-7120
TTY: 808-532-7110
www.atrc.org
atrc-info@atrc.org
Barbara Fischlowitz-Leong, MEd, Executive Director/CEO
Jodi Asato, MEd, Deputy Director/Program Manager
Edna Kaahaaina, Office Manager
A statewide, non-profit organization committed to ensuring access to assistive technology for persons with disabilities. ATRC links individuals with technology so all people can participate in every aspect of community life. Also empowers individuals to maintain dignity and control their lives by promoting technology thorough, advocacy, training, information, and education.

182   Easter Seals - Hawaii
710 Green St
Honolulu, HI 96813-2119
808-536-1015
888-241-7450
Fax: 808-536-3765
http://hawaii.easterseals.com
info@easterssealshawaii.org
Ron Brandvold, President & CEO
Esther Underwood, VP of Human Resources
Kelly Ikeda Ellis, Director of Development
Provide exceptional services to ensure that all people with disabilities of special needs and their families have equal opportunities to live, learn, work and play in their communities.

183   International Dyslexia Association of Hawaii
705 S King Street
Ste 206
Honolulu, HI 96813
808-538-7007
866-773-4432
Fax: 808-538-7009
www.dyslexia-hawaii.org
hida@dyslexia-hawaii.org
Ryan Masa, President
Laurie Moore, Secretary
Margaret J. Higa, MSCP, Executive Director
HIDA's mission is to increase awareness of dyslexia in the community, provide support for parents and teachers, and promote teacher training. We also provide tutoring and testing referrals and information about other resources in Hawaii.
1986

184 **Learning Disabilities Association of Hawaii (LDAH)**
245 N Kukui Street
Ste 205
Honolulu, HI 96817-3921   808-536-9684
                                 Fax: 808-537-6780
                                 www.ldahawaii.org
                                 MMoore@LDAHawaii.org
Neil Aoki, Esq., President
Tayne Sekimura, Vice President
Paul Singer, MEd, Secretary/Treasurer
A non-profit organization founded in 1968 by parents of
children with learning disabilities.
1968

Idaho

185 **Disability Rights - Idaho**
4477 Emerald St
Ste B-100
Boise, ID 83706-2066   208-336-5353
                              800-632-5125
                              Fax: 208-336-5396
                              TDD: 208-336-5353
                              www.disabilityrightsidaho.org
                              info@disabilityrightsidaho.org
Rick Huber, President
Sheree Cooper, Vice-President
Mary Robertson, Secretary
The designated Protection and Advocacy System for Idaho
provides advocacy for people with disabilities who have
been abused/neglected; denied services or benefits; have experienced rights violations or discrimination because of
their disability; or have voting accessibility problems. Also
provides information & referral; negotiation & mediation;
short term & technical assistance; legal
advice/representation.
1977

Illinois

186 **Child Care Association of Illinois**
413 West Monroe
1st Fl
Springfield, IL 62704-1885   217-528-4409
                                    Fax: 217-528-6498
                                    www.cca-il.org
                                    ilccamb@aol.com
Margaret M. Berglind, ACSW-LCSW, President & CEO
Pat Griffith, Chair
Zack Schrantz, 1st Vice Chair
A voluntary, not-for-profit organization dedicated to im-
proving the delivery of social services to the abused, ne-
glected, and troubled children, youth and families of
Illinois.
1964

187 **Easter Seals - Metropolitan Chicago**
1939 W 13th St
Ste 300
Chicago, IL 60608-1226   312-491-4110
                                866-GIV-2ESC
                                Fax: 312-733-0247
                                http://chicago.easterseals.com
                                mmorgan@eastersealschicago.org
F. Timothy Muri, President & CEO
Andrew Sprogis, Chair of the Board
Mark O'Toole, Vice Chair
Provides comprehensive services for individuals with dis-
abilities or other special needs and their families to improve
quality of life and maximize independence.

188 **Illinois Protection & Advocacy Agency: Equip for
Equality**
20 N Michigan Ave
Ste 300
Chicago, IL 60602-4861   312-341-0022
                                800-537-2632
                                Fax: 312-341-0295
                                TTY: 800-610-2779
                                www.equipforequality.org
                                contactus@equipforequality.org
Zena Naiditch, President & CEO
Deborah M. Kennedy, Vice President AIU
Barry C. Taylor, Vice President CRT
Advances the human and civil rights of children and adults
with physical and mental disabilities in Illinois. The only
statewide, cross-disability, comprehensive advocacy organization providing self-advocacy assistance, legal services,
and disability rights education while also engaging in public
policy and legislative advocacy and conducting abuse investigations and other oversight activities.
1985

189 **International Dyslexia Association of Illinois**
751 Roosevelt Rd
Ste 116
Glen Ellyn, IL 60137-5905   630-469-6900
                                   Fax: 630-469-6810
                                   www.readibida.org
                                   info@readibida.org
Dr. Suzanne O'Brien, President
Julia Nelson, Vice-President
John Bloomfield, Treasurer
Dedicated to the study and remediation of dyslexia and to the
support and encouragement of individuals with dyslexia and
their families.

190 **Jewish Child & Family Services Downtown Chicago -
Central Office**
216 W Jackson Blvd
Ste 800
Chicago, IL 60606-6920   312-357-4800
                                855-275-5237
                                Fax: 312-855-3754
                                www.jcfs.org
                                ask@jcfs.org
Howard Sitron, President & CEO
Margaret Vimont, EVP & COO
Vincent Everson, VP & CFO
Provides a range of comprehensive programs designed to en-
able individuals and families to grow and develop positively
throughout their lives.

191 **Learning Ally: Orland Pk Recording Studio**
14600 S Ravinia Ave
Orland Park, IL 60462   708-349-9356
                               www.learningally.org
                               selhenicky@learningally.org
Sandy Elhenicky, Studio Leader
To create opportunities for individuals, from Kindergarten
through Graduate Level, who cannot read standard print because of a visual impairment, learning disability or other
physical disability, to succeed in school by providing accessible educational materials.

192 **Learning Disabilities Association of Illinois**
10101 S Roberts Rd
Ste 205
Palos Hills, IL 60465-1556   708-430-7532
                                    Fax: 708-430-7592
                                    www.ldail.org
                                    ldaofil@ameritech.net
Sharon Schussler, Administrative Assistant
A resource office with information for parents, profession-
als and adults with learning disabilities.

193   National Council of Teachers of English
1111 W Kenyon Rd
Urbana, IL 61801-1096   217-328-3870
                                          877-369-6283
                                          Fax: 217-328-9645
                                          www.ncte.org
                                          executivecommittee@ncte.org
Doug Hesse, President
Susan Houser, President-Elect
Jocelyn Chadwick, Vice President
The National Council of Teachers of English, with over
30,000 members and subscribers worldwide, is dedicated to
improving the teaching and learning of English and the lan-
guage arts at all levels of education.

194   Second Sense
65 E Wacker Place
Ste 1010
Chicago, IL 60601-7463   312-236-8569
                                          Fax: 312-236-8128
                                          www.second-sense.org
                                          info@second-sense.org
Brett Christenson, President
Laura Rounce, Vice President
Michael P. Wagner, Treasurer
Support and information for families and individuals with
visual disabilities. Formerly Guild for the Blind.

Indiana

195   Easter Seals - Arc of Northeast Indiana
4919 Coldwater Rd
Fort Wayne, IN 46825-5532   260-456-4534
                                          800-234-7811
                                          Fax: 260-745-5200
                                          http://neindiana.easterseals.com
                                          delbrecht@esarc.org
Donna K. Elbrecht, President/CEO
Danielle K. Tips, Vice President Of Programs
Misty Woltman, CFO/Controller
Provides services to children and adults with disabilities and
other special needs, and support to their families.

196   Easter Seals - Southwestern Idiana
Rehabilitation Center
3701 Bellemeade Ave
The Rehabilitation Center
Evansville, IN 47714-0137   812-479-1411
                                          Fax: 812-437-2634
                                          www.in-sw.easterseals.com
Kelly Schneider, President
Guy Davis, Vice-President Of Administration
Laura Terhune, Vice-President Of Development
The Easter Seals Rehabilitation Center in Evansville, IN
provides services to children and adults with disabilities and
other special needs and support to their families.

197   International Dyslexia Association of Indiana
2511 E 46th St
Ste 2
Indianapolis, IN 46205-2460   317-926-1450
                                          Fax: 317-705-2067
                                          www.ida-indiana.org
                                          inbofida@hotmail.com
Mary Binnion, President
Tracy Brazda, Vice-President
Therese Rooney, Treasurer
A non-profit organization dedicatedt to helping individuals
with dyslexia, their families and the communities that support them. Promotes and disseminates researched-based
knowledge for early identification, effective teaching approaches and intervention strategies for dyslexics.
1971

198   Learning Disabilities Association of Indiana
1427 W 86th Street
Ste 110
Indianapolis, IN 46260   317-872-4331
                                          800-284-2519
                                          Fax: 574-272-3058
                                          www.ldaofindiana.net
Sharon Harris, President
A non-profit, volunteer organization of parents, educators,
and other individuals who are committed to promoting
awareness, knowledge and acceptance of individuals with
learning disabilities and associated disorders such as attention deficit/hyperactivity disorders.
1972

Iowa

199   Center for Disabilities and Development
University of Iowa Children's Hospital
100 Hawkins Dr
213 CDD
Iowa City, IA 52242-1011   319-353-6900
                                          877-686-0031
                                          Fax: 319-356-7700
                                          TTY: 877-686-0032
                                          www.uichildrens.org/cdd/
                                          cdd-scheduling@uiowa.edu
Dianne McBrien, MD, Medical Director
Jane Davis, RN, BSN, Manager
Lenore Holte, PhD, CCC-A, Manager
Improve the health and independence of people with disabil-
ities and advance the community systems on which they
rely.
1947

200   International Dyslexia Association of Iowa
P.O.Box 11188
Cedar Rapids, IA 52410-1188   765-507-9432
                                          866-782-2930
                                          www.ida-ia.org
                                          info@ida-ia.org
Denise Little, President
Tricia Krsek, Vice President
Genevieve Monthie, Secretary
Provides workshops, hands-on simulations, and resources to
incease public awareness of dyslexia.

201   Iowa Program for Assistive Technology
Center for Disabilities and Development (CDD)
CDD
100 Hawkins Drive
Iowa City, IA 52242-1011   319-353-8777
                                          800-779-2001
                                          Fax: 319-356-8284
                                          TDD: 877-686-0032
                                          TTY: 877-686-0032
                                          www.iowaat.org
                                          IPAT@uiowa.edu
Jane Gay, Director
Gary Johnson, Coordinator
Marlene Phipps, Office Clerk
IPAT's goals are to promote and create systems change in
the state with regards to assistive technology (AT) and it's
use. IPAT works with consumers and family members, service providers, and state and local agencies/organizations to
promote assistive technology through awareness, training,
and policy work. IPAT accomplishes this through five
specifi goal areas: education, employment, health, community living and recreation, telecommunication and
information technology.

202 Learning Disabilities Association of Iowa
5665 Greendale Rd
Ste D
Johnston, IA 50131-1903   515-280-8558
                                  888-690-5324
                              Fax: 515-243-1902
                                  www.lda-ia.org
                          kathylda@askresource.org

Paula Hamp, President
Patty Beyer, 1st Vice President
Gayle Slattery, 2nd Vice President
Dedicated to identifying causes and promoting prevention of learning disabilities and to enhancing the quality of life for all individuals with learning disabilities and their families by: encouraging effective identification and intervention, fostering research, and protecting the rights of individuals with learning disabilities under the law.

Kansas

203 Disability Rights Center of Kansas (DRC)
214 SW 6th Ave
Ste 100
Topeka, KS 66603-3726   785-273-9661
                                 877-776-1541
                             Fax: 785-273-9414
                             TDD: 877-335-3725
                             TTY: 877-335-3725
                                 www.drckansas.org
                                   info@ksadv.org

Rocky Nichols, MPA, Executive Director
Debbie White, CPA, Deputy Director
Lane Williams, JD, Deputy Director
Formerly Kansas Advocacy & Protection Services, a public interest legal advocacy agency empowered by federal law to advocate for the civil and legal rights of Kansans with disabilities.

204 Easter Seals - Capper Foundation
3500 SW 10th Ave
Topeka, KS 66604-1904   785-272-4060
                             Fax: 785-272-7912
                      http://capper.easterseals.com

Bruce Meyers, Chair
Jim Leiker, President & CEO
Sandy Warren, Executive Vice-President & CFO
A community resource providing services to enhance the independence of people with disabilities, primarily children.

205 Goodwill Industries of Kansas
3351 N Webb Rd
Wichita, KS 67226-3403   316-744-9291
                             Fax: 316-744-1428
                           http://goodwillks.org/

Emily Compton, President/CEO
Dave Chadick, VP, Industrial Services
Molly Fox, VP, Marketing & Development
Education, training and employment for people with disabilities and other barriers to employment.

206 Learning Disabilities Association of Kansas
2618 SW Arvonia Pl
Topeka, KS 66614-4603   785-273-4505
                             Fax: 785-228-9527
                                 www.ldakansas.org
                          acronin@olatheschools.com

Charity Ziegler, President
Kent Wiliams, Treasurer
LDAK is a nonprofit, volunteer organization whose purpose is to advance the education and general well-being of children and adults with learning disabilities.

Kentucky

207 Learning Disabilities Association of Kentucky
2210 Goldsmith Lane
Suite 118
Louisville, KY 40218-1038   502-473-1256
                                 877-587-1256
                             Fax: 502-473-4695
                                 www.ldaofky.org
                          LDAofKY@yahoo.com

Tim Woods, Executive Director
A non-profit organization of individuals with learning differences and attention difficulties, their parents, educators, and other service providers.

Louisiana

208 Advocacy Center of Louisiana: Lafayette
600 Jefferson Street
Suite 812
Lafayette, LA 70501-6982   337-237-7380
                                 800-960-7705
                             Fax: 337-237-0486
                             TTY: 855-861-3577
                                 www.advocacyla.org

Dale Higgins, President
James Thompson, Treasurer
Paget Bazile, Secretary
Protects and advocates for the human and legal rights of persons living in Louisiana who are elderly or disabled.

209 Advocacy Center of Louisiana: New Orleans
8325 Oak Street
New Orleans, LA 70118   504-237-2337
                                 800-960-7705
                             Fax: 504-522-5507
                             TTY: 855-861-3577
                                 www.advocacyla.org
                     advocacycenter@advocacyla.org
Reagan Toledano, President
James Thompson, Treasurer
Paget Bazile, Secretary
Protects and advocates for the human and legal rights of persons living in Louisiana who are elderly or disabled.

210 Advocacy Center of Louisiana: Shreveport
2620 Centenary Blvd
Bldg 2, Ste 248
Shreveport, LA 71104-3356   318-227-6186
                                 800-960-7705
                             Fax: 318-227-1841
                                 www.advocacyla.org

Dale Higgins, President
James Thompson, Treasurer
Paget Bazile, Secretary
Protects and advocates for the human and legal rights of persons living in Louisiana who are elderly or disabled.

Maine

211 Easter Seals - Maine
125 Presumpscot St
Portland, ME 04103-5225   207-828-0754
                             Fax: 207-828-5355
                      http://maine.easterseals.com
Kelly Couture, Director of Development
Jeremy Kendall, Director Of Military & Vetrans
Creates solutions that change lives of children and adults with disabilities or other special needs and their families.

212 Learning Disabilities Association of Maine (LDA)
PO Box 1013
Windham, ME 04062   207-861-7823
                                       877-208-4029
                                  Fax: 207-861-7823
                                   www.ldame.org
                                   info@ldame.org
Gene Maxim Randolph, President
Bruce Cort, Treasurer
Tracy Gregoire, Program Director
Dedicated to assisting individuals with learning and atten-
tion disabilities through support, education and advocacy.

213 Maine Parent Federation
PO Box 2067
Augusta, ME 04338   207-588-1933
                                       800-870-7746
                                  Fax: 207-588-1938
                                  TTY: 207-588-1933
                              www.startingpointsforme.org
                              parentconnnect@mpf.org
Janice LaChance, Executive Director
The Maine Parent Federation is a statewide organiztion that
provides information, advocacy, education, and training to
benefit all children. We promote individual aspirations and
community inclusion for people with disabilities.
1984

Maryland

214 Disability Support Services
University of Maryland, Shoemaker Bldg
#0106, 4281 Chapel Ln
College Park, MD 20740   301-314-7651
                                  Fax: 301-405-0813
                              www.counseling.umd.edu/dss
Jo Ann Hutchinson, RhD, Director
Coordinates services that ensure individuals with disabili-
ties equal access to University of Maryland College Park
programs.
800 members

215 Division of Rehabilitation Services
Maryland State Department of Education
2301 Argonne Dr
Baltimore, MD 21218-1628   410-554-9442
                                       888-554-0334
                                  Fax: 410-554-9412
                                  TTY: 410-554-9411
                              www.dors.state.md.us
                              dors@maryland.gov
Robert Burns, Director
Enables persons with disabilities to achieve employment,
economic self-sufficiency and independence.

216 Easter Seals - DC, MD, VA
1420 Spring St
Silver Spring, MD 20910-2701   301-588-8700
                                       800-886-3771
                                  Fax: 301-920-9770
                              http://gwbr.easterseals.com
Lisa Reeves, President and CEO
Jonathan Horowitch, Chief Operating Officer
Michael Piemonte, Chief Financial Officer
Provides exceptional services to ensure that all people with
disabilities or special needs and their families have equal opportunities to live, learn, work and play in their communities. Proudly servinf Washington-Balitmore Region and the
surrounding communities in Maryland, Northern Virginia
and West Virginia.

217 International Dyslexia Association of Maryland
40 York Rd
4th Fl
Baltimore, MD 21204   410-296-0232
                                  Fax: 410-321-5069
                                   www.interdys.org
                                   info@idamd.org
Rick Smith, Chief Executive Officer
Newton Guerin, Chief Operating Officer
David Holste, Chief Financial Officer
Believes that all individuals have the right to achieve their
full potential and that individual learning abilities can be
strengthen. MBIDA will promote and organize classes and
workshops to provide informtion and training for dyslexic
individuals, educators, parents and others.

218 International Dyslexia Association of DC Capital Area
501 McArthur Dr
Rockville, MD 20850   301-315-0563
                                   www.dcida.org
                                   info@dcida.org
Laurie Moloney, President
Sue Christakos, Secretary
Laurie Hauple, Treasurer
The DC Capital Area Branch of the International Dyslexia
Association is a 501 (c) (3) non-profit, scientific and educa-
tional organization dedicated to the study and treatment of
dyslexia. Our all volunteer board of directors seeks to in-
crease public awareness of dyslexia in the DC Metropolitan
Area.

219 Learning Disabilities Association of Maryland
PO Box 744
Dunkirk, MD 20754   888-265-6459
                                   www.ldamd.org
                                   ldamd@ldamd.org
Judy Lantz, President
Chris Casey, Vice President
Donna Bowling, Treasurer
Dedicated to enhancing the quality of life for all individuals
with learning disabilities and their families through aware-
ness, advocacy, education, service and collaborative efforts.

**220 Maryland Association of University Centers on Disabili-
ties**
1100 Wayne Ave
Ste 1000
Silver Spring, MD 20910-5646   301-588-8252
                                  Fax: 301-588-2842
                                   www.aucd.org
                              ljcohen@email.arizona.edu
Karen Edwards, MD, MPH, President
Brent Askvig, PhD, Secretary
Andrew J. Imparato, JD, Executive Director
The mission of AUCD is to advance policy and practice for
and with people living with developmental and other disabilities, their families, and communities by supporting our
members to engage in research, education, and service activities that achieve our vision

221 National Data Bank for Disabled Service
University of Maryland
Susquehanna Hall
4th Floor
College Park, MD 20742-0001   301-314-7651
                                  Fax: 301-314-9478
                              www.counseling.umd.edu/dss
                              jahutch@umd.edu
Jo Ann Hutchinson RhD, Director
Evalyn Hamilton, Customer Service Coordinator
Coordinates services that ensure individuals with disabili-
ties equal access to University of Maryland College Park
programs.
800 members 1976

222 National Federation of Families for Children's Mental Health
12320 Parklawn Dr
Rockville, MD 20852-6390
240-403-1901
Fax: 240-403-1909
www.ffcmh.org
ffcmh@ffcmh.org
Lynda Gargan, Interim Executive Director
Barbara Huff, Social Marketing TA Provider
Dedicated exclusively to helping children with mental health needs and their families achieve a better quality of life.

Massachusetts

223 Adaptive Environments
Institute for Human Centered Design
200 Portland St
Ste 1
Boston, MA 02114
617-695-1225
Fax: 617-482-8099
TTY: 617-695-1225
www.adaptiveenvironments.org
info@humancentereddesign.org
Ralph Jackson, FAIA, President
Chris Pilkington, Vice President
Gabriela Bonome-Sims, Director of Administration
Committed to advancing the role of design in expanding opportunity and enhancing experience for people of all ages and abiliites.
1978

224 Easter Seals - Massachusetts
484 Main St
Denholm Building
Worcester, MA 01608-1817
800-244-2756
Fax: 508-831-9768
www.ma.easterseals.com
info@eastersealsma.com
Peter Mahoney, Chairman
Louie Psallidas, Vice-Chair
Michael McManama, Vice-Chair
Statewide, community based organization that has been helping people with disabilities to live full and independent lives for over 60 years.

225 International Dyslexia Association of Massachusetts
PO Box 662
Lincoln, MA 01773
617-650-0011
http://ma.dyslexiaida.org
mabida@comcast.net
Janet Thibeau, President
Alexis Treat, Vice President
Caroline Legor, Secretary
The Massachusetts Branch of The International Dyslexia Association (MABIDA) is a 501 (c) (3) non-profit, scientific and educational organization dedicated to the study and treatment of dyslexia. This Branch was formed to increase public awareness of dyslexia in Massachusetts.

226 Learning Disabilities Worldwide (LDW)
14 Nason St
Maynard, MA 01754
978-897-5399
Fax: 978-897-5355
www.ldworldwide.org
info@ldworldwide.org
Emmanuel Chinweoke Aja, MD, Chairman
Nicholas D. Young, PhD, EdD, Vice-Chairman
Teresa Allissa Citro, Chief Executive Officer

Formerly the Learning Disabilities Association of Massachusetts, works to enhance the lives of individuals with learning disabilities, with a specail emphasis on the underserved. The purpose is to identify and support the unrecognized strengths and capabilities of a person with learning disabilities. We strive to increase awareness and understanding of learning disabilities through our multilingual media productions and publications that serve populations across cultures and nations.
15,000 members 1965

227 Massachusetts Association of Approved Private Schools (MAAPS)
607 North Avenue
15 Lakeside Office Park
Wakefield, MA 01880-1647
781-245-1220
Fax: 781-245-5294
TTY: 781-245-5145
www.maaps.org
info@maaps.org
Mark P. de Chabert, Chief Operating Officer
James V. Major IOM, CAE, Executive Director
Kristen Brown, Business Manager
Nonprofit association of Chapter 766 approved private schools dedicated to providing educational programs and services to students with special needs throughout Massachusetts. Concerned that children with special needs have appropriate, quality education and that they and their families know the rights, policies, procedures and options that make the education process a productive reality for special needs children.

Michigan

228 Easter Seals - Michigan
2399 E Walton Blvd
Auburn Hills, MI 48326-2759
248-475-6400
800-649-3777
www.mi.easterseals.com
Brent Wirth, President and CEO
Juliana Harper, Chief Program Officer/SVP
Robert Carlesimo, Chief Financial Officer/SVP
Offers programs and services for children and adults with disabilities and special needs.

229 International Dyslexia Association of Michigan
5735 Big Pine Dr
Ypsilanti, MI 48197-7184
888-432-6424
http://mi.dyslexiaida.org
info@idamichigan.org
Joanne Marttila Pierson, President
The purpose of the Michigan Branch of the International Dyslexia Association is to develop awareness and provide information about Dyslexia.

230 Learning Disabilities Association of Michigan (LDA)
PO Box 150015
Grand Rapids, MI 49515-1914
517-319-0370
888-597-7809
Fax: 517-485-8462
www.ldaofmichigan.org
ldaofmichigan@gmail.com
Regina Carey, President
Roseanne Renauer, President-Elect
Erin Rooney, Treasurer
A nonprofit, volunteer association that is dedicated to enhancing the quality of life for all individuals with learning disabilities and their families through advocacy, education, training, services and support of research. Our goal is to see LD understood and addressed and the individuals with learning disabilities will thrive and participate fully in society.
1,200 Members

Minnesota

231 International Dyslexia Association Upper Midwest Branch
5021 Vernon Ave
Ste 159
Minneapolis, MN 55436-2102   612-486-4242
http://umw.dyslexiaida.org
info@ida-umb.org

Tom Strewler, President
Brian Pittenger, Treasurer
Jennifer Bennett, Secretary
Informs and educates people about dyslexia and related difficulties in learning to read and write, in a way that supports and encourages, promotes effective change, and gives individuals the opportunity to lead productive and fulfilling lives, which benefits society with the resource that is liberated. this branch serves Minnesota, North Dakota, and South Dakota.

232 Learning Disabilities Association of Minnesota
6100 Golden Valley Rd
Golden Valley, MN 55422   952-582-6000
Fax: 952-582-6031
www.ldaminnesota.org
info@ldaminnesota.org

W. Brooks Donald, MD, President
Jeff Fox, Vice President
Luke Seifert, Treasurer
Nonprofit educational agency helping children, youth, and adults at risk for learning disabilities and other learning difficulties.

233 Technical Assistance Alliance for Parent Centers: PACER Center
8161 Normandale Blvd
Bloomington, MN 55437-1044   952-838-9000
888-248-0822
Fax: 952-838-0199
TTY: 952-838-0190
www.pacer.org
alliance@taalliance.org

Dan Levinson, Board President
Tammy Pust, Board Vice-President
Paula Goldberg, Executive Director
An innovative project that supports a unified technical assistance system for the purpose of developing, assisting and coordinating Parent Training Information Projects and Community Parent Resource Centers.

Mississippi

234 Learning Disabilities Association of Mississippi
4080 Old Canton Rd
PO Box 4477
Jackson, MS 39216   601-362-1667
Fax: 301-362-9180
www.ldams.org
ldams@bellsouth.net

Martha Kabbes Burns, Contact
A non-profit, volunteer organization that is an informational Support Center for parents of children with learning disabilities, adults with learning disabilities, and professionals providing services related to learning disabilities.

Missouri

235 Easter Seals - Heartland
13975 Manchester Rd
Ste 2
Manchester, MO 63011-4500   636-227-6030
800-664-5025
Fax: 636-779-2270
www.ucpheartland.org
forkoshr@ucpheartland.org

Richard Forkosh, President & CEO
Kathleen Fagin, Vice President Programs
Steve Staicoff, CFO
Provides exceptional services to ensure all people with disabilities have equal opportunities to live, learn, work and play in their communities.

236 Learning Disabilities Association of Missouri
1942 E Meadowmere
Ste 104, PO Box 3303
Springfield, MO 65808-3303   417-864-5110
Fax: 417-864-7290

Cathy Einhorn, President
Provides information and support to parents, individuals with learning disabilities and professionals.

237 Missouri Protection & Advocacy Services
925 S Country Club Dr
Ste 3
Jefferson City, MO 65109-4510   573-893-3333
866-777-7199
Fax: 573-893-4231
TDD: 800-735-2966
www.moadvocacy.org
mopasjc@earthlink.net

Joe Wrinkle, Chair
Barbara H. French, Vice-Chair
Susan Pritchard-Green, Secretary/Treasurer
A federally mandated system in the state which provides protection of the rights of persons with disabilities through leagally-based advocacy. The mission is to protect the rights of individuals with disabilities by providing advocacy and legal services.
1977

238 St. Louis Learning Disabilities Association
13537 Barrett Parkway Dr
Ste 110
Ballwin, MO 63021-5896   314-966-3088
Fax: 314-966-1806
www.ldastl.org
info@ldastl.org

Sheryl Silvey, President
Tina Roche, Treasurer
James Hartman, Vice-President
A non-profit organization dedicated to enhancing the understanding and acceptance of learning disabilities. Education, support, and consultation are provided to children, parents, and professionals to help reach their full potential.
1993

Montana

239 Learning Disabilities Association of Montana
3544 Toboggan Rd
Billings, MT 59101-9121   406-259-3110
info@ldaofmt.org

Mark Taylor, President
The Learning Disabilities Association of Montana assists individuals with learning disabilities through information, advocacy and support.

240 Montana Parents, Let's Unite for Kids (PLUK)
516 N 32nd St
Billings, MT 59101-6003   406-255-0540
800-222-7585
Fax: 406-255-0523
www.pluk.org
info@pluk@pluk.org

Roger Holt, Executive Director

PLUK is a private, nonprofit organization formed by parents of children with disabilities and chronic illnesses. Its purpose is to provide information, support, training and assistance to aid parents with their children at home, in school and as adults. We keep current on best practices in education, medicine, law, human services, rehabilitation, and technology to insure families with disabilites have access to high quality services.
1984

Nebraska

241   Easter Seals - Nebraska
A Subsidiary of Visiting Nurse Association
12565 W Center Rd
Ste 100
Omaha, NE 68144-8144   402-345-2200
                                     800-650-9880
                                Fax: 402-345-2500
                              www.ne.easterseals.com
James C. Summerfelt, President/CEO
Angela Howell, Vice-President
Lily Sughroue, Director of Camp, Respite, Rec.
Provides exceptional services to help ensure all people with disabilities have an equal opportunity to live, learn, work and play.

242   International Dyslexia Association of Nebraska
5921 Sunrise Rd
PO Box 6302
Lincoln, NE 68506-0302   402-434-6434
                                Fax: 410-321-5069
                                     www.ne-ida.com
                                     info@ne-ida.com
Joan Stoner, President
Nebraska Branch works to enhance the public's perception and understanding of dyslexia and related language/learning disabilities.
1984

243   Learning Disabilities Association of Nebraska
11118 N 62nd St
Omaha, NE 68152-4717   402-348-1567
                                Fax: 402-934-1479
             http://ldaamerica.org/lda-chapters/nebraska/
                              admin@ldanebraska.org
Deb Carlson, President
Support groups for parents and teachers, information for school and the community about ADHD and LD children/adults. Offers book and video library, educational seminars and conferences, parent panels. Quarterly newsletter.
1984

Nevada

244   Children's Cabinet
1090 S Rock Blvd
Reno, NV 89502-7116   775-856-6200
                                Fax: 775-856-6208
                              www.childrenscabinet.org
                              mail@childrenscabinet.org
Don Butterfield, Chair
Michael Russellield, Co-Chair
Grant D. Anderson, Treasurer
The Children's Cabinet strives to ensure every child and family in our community has the services and resources to meet fundamental development, care, and learning needs.

245   Easter Seals - Nevada
6200 W Oakey Blvd
Las Vegas, NV 89146-1103   702-870-7050
                                Fax: 702-870-7649
                              http://sn.easterseals.com
Kenny Allwein, Chairman
Neyda Becker, Vice-Chair
Karl Armstrong, Esq., Secretary

Provides services to children and adults with disabilities and other special needs, and support to their families.

246   Learning Disabilities Association of Nevada
2970 Idlewild Drive
Reno, NV 89509   888-300-6710
                                     www.ldaamerica.org
                                     info@ldaamerica.org
Nancie Payne, President
Ed Schlitt, First Vice President
Beth McGaw, Secretary
To create opportunities for success for all individuals affected by learning disabilities and to reduce the incidence of learning disabilities in future generations.

New Hampshire

247   Crotched Mountain
1 Verney Dr
Greenfield, NH 03047-5000   603-547-3311
                                Fax: 603-547-6212
                              www.crotchedmountain.org
                              info@crotchedmountain.org
Michael Coughlin, President/CEO
Andra Hall, EdD, Director Of Education
Frederick R. Bruch, Jr., MD, FACP, Chief Medical Officer
Serves individuals with disabilities and their families, embracing personal choice and development, and building communities of mutual support.

248   Easter Seals - New Hampshire
555 Auburn St
Manchester, NH 03103-4803   603-623-8863
                                     800-870-8728
                                Fax: 603-625-1148
                              www.nheasterseals.com
Larry J. Gammon, President & CEO
Elin A. Treanor, Chief Financial Officer
Karen Van Der Beken, Chief Development Officer
Easter Seals New Hampshire is one of the most comprehensive affiliates in the nation, assisting more than 18,000 children and adults with disabilities through a network of more than a dozen service sites around the state and in Vermont. Each center provides top-quality, family-focused and innovative services tailored to meet the specific needs of the particular community it serves.
1936

249   International Dyslexia Association of New Hampshire
PO Box 3724
Concord, NH 03302-3724   603-229-7355
                                     www.nhida.org
                                     info@nhida.org
Anne Eaton, President
Audrey Burke, Vice-President
Melissa Farrall, PhD, First Treasurer
The New Hampshire Branch of The International Dyslexia Association (NH/IDA) is a 501 (c) (3) non-profit, scientific and educational organization dedicated to the study and treatment of the learning disability, dyslexia. The New Hampshire Branch was formed in 2002 to increase public awareness of dyslexia. The New Hampshire Branch serves New Hampshire, Maine and Vermont

250   NH Family Ties
70 Pembroke Rd
Concord, NH 03301   800-499-4153
                                     www.nhfamilyties.org
                                     p2p@nhsupport.net
Phillip Eller, Executive Director

If you are a parent of a child with special challenges and you would like to speak to a parent whose child has similar needs - someone who will understand, Parent to Parent is a network of families willing to share experiences. Should you call a Supporting Parent will contact you by phone or visit within 24 hours. All information will be kept confidential and there is no cost for the service. Formerly known as Parent to Parent of New Hampshire.
1987

251   New Hampshire Disabilities Rights Center (DRC)
64 N Main St
Ste 2, 3 Fl
Concord, NH 03301-4913   603-228-0432
                                        800-834-1721
                                   Fax: 603-225-2077
                                   TDD: 800-834-1721
                                        www.drcnh.org
                                   advocacy@drcnh.org

Paul Levy, President
Joanne Malloy, Vice President
Cynthia Trottier, Treasurer
A statewide organization that is independent from state government or service providers and is dedicated to the full and equal enjoyment of civil and other legal rights by people with disabilities. The DRC is New Hampshire's designated Protection and Advocacy agency and authorized by federal statute to pursue legal, administrative and other appropriate remedies on behalf of individuals with disabilities.
1978

New Jersey

252   ASPEN Asperger Syndrome Education Network
9 Aspen Cir
Edison, NJ 08820-2832   732-321-0880
                                        www.aspennj.org
                                        info@aspennj.org

Lori Shery, President
Rich Meleo, Vice President
Elizabeth Yamashita, Vice President
Provides families and individuals whose lives are affected by Autism Spectrum Disorders (Asperger Syndrome, Pervasive Developmental Disorder-NOS, High Functioning Autism), and Nonverbal Learning Disabilities with education, support and advocacy.

253   Disability Rights New Jersey
210 S Broad S
3rd Fl
Trenton, NJ 08608   609-292-9742
                                        800-922-7233
                                   Fax: 609-777-0187
                                   TTY: 609-633-7106
                                        www.drnj.org
                                   advocate@drnj.org

Walter Anthony Woodberry, Chair
Andrew McGeady, Vice Chair
Joseph B. Young, Executive Director
A consumer-directed, non-profit organization that serves as New Jersey's designated protection and advocacy system for people with disabilities in the state.

254   Easter Seals - New Jersey
25 Kennedy Blvd
Ste 600
East Brunswick, NJ 08816   732-257-0882
                                   Fax: 732-257-7373
                                   TDD: 732-535-3217
                                        http://eastersealsnj.org

Brian J Fitzgerald, President/CEO
Cheryl Young, CFO, Assistant Treasurer
Shelley Samuels, Chief Program Officer
To enable individuals with disabilities or special needs and their families to live, learn, work and play in their communities with equality, dignity and independence.

255   Family Resource Associates, Inc.
35 Haddon Ave
Shrewsbury, NJ 07702-4007   732-747-5310
                                   Fax: 732-747-1896
                                        www.frainc.org
                                        info@frainc.org

Alan Proske, President
Bill Sheeser, Vice President
Nancy Phalanukorn, Executive Director
A non-profit agency with the mission of helping children, adolescents and people of all ages with disabilities to reach their fullest potenttial. Provides home-based early intervention for infants, therapeutic recreation programs and assistive technology services, along with family and sibling support groups.
1979

256   Family Support Center of New Jersey
1 AAA Dr
Ste 203
Trenton, NJ 08691   732-528-8080
                                        800-336-5843
                                   Fax: 609-392-5621
                                        www.fscnj.org
                                   jacqui.moskowitz@fscnj.org

Eric M. Joice, Executive Director
Liza Gundell, Deputy Director
Jessica Goldsmith Barzilay, Assistant Director
The Family Support Center of New Jersey (FSCNJ) is a clearing house of up-to-date information on national, state and local family support programs, services and disabilities. FSCNJ offers a one stop shopping approach to individuals seeking information on disabilities and services by providing them with easy acces to a comprehensive array of services.

257   International Dyslexia Association of New Jersey
PO Box 32
Long Valley, NJ 07853-0032   908-876-1179
                                   Fax: 908-876-3621
                                        www.njida.org
                                        njida@msn.com

Hal Malchow, President
Elsa Cardenas-Hagan, Vice President
Ben Shifrin, M.Ed., Vice President
An international nonprofit, scientific and educational organization dedicated to the study of dyslexia. We offer tutoring and testing referrals, as well as support teacher education and hold outreach programs. Teacher Scholarships are offered to our Annual Fall Conferences, Wilson Reading Overviews and Project Read programs. Newsletter published bi-annually.
700 members

258   Learning Disabilities Association of New Jersey
PO Box 6268
East Brunswick, NJ 08816   732-645-2738
                                   Fax: 973-265-4303
                                        www.ldanj.org
                                        info@ldanj.org

To create opportunities for success in all individuals affected by learning disabilities and to reduce the incidence of learning disabilities in future generations.

259   New Jersey Self-Help Group Clearinghouse
375 E McFarlan St
Dover, NJ 07801-3628   973-989-1122
                                        800-367-6274
                                   Fax: 973-989-1159
                                        www.njgroups.org
                                   wrodenbaugh@saintclares.org

Aimee Braca-Deo, Program Administrator
Barbara White, State Program Coordinator
Wendy Rodenbaugh, Information & Referral Assistant
Puts callers in touch with any of several hundred national and international self-help groups covering a wide range of illnesses, disabilities, addictions, bereavement and stressful life situations.

260 **Special Child Health and Early Intervention Services**
NJ Department of Health
50 E State St
6th Fl, PO Box 360
Trenton, NJ 08625-0360   609-984-0755
Fax: 609-292-9288
www.nj.gov/health/fhs/sch
Marilyn Gorney-Daley, DO, MPH, Director
Assists families caring for children with long-term medical and developmental disabilities. Programs include Early Intervention Services, Case Management, Special Child Health Services, Registry, Autism Registry, Early Hearing Detection & Intervention, and Newborn Screening and Genetics Services and Hemophilia Program.

New Mexico

261 **Easter Seals - Santa Maria El Mirador**
10 A-Van-Nu-Po
Santa Fe, NM 87508-1461   505-424-7700
Fax: 505-424-7707
http://smem.easterseals.com
Mark Johnson, CEO
Provides an array of quality supports for individuals with developmental disabilities in community integrated environments centered on personl choice, self value, and dignity.

262 **International Dyslexia Association Southwest Branch**
3915 Carlisle Blvd NE
Albuquerque, NM 87107-4503   505-255-8234
www.southwestida.org
swida@southwestida.org
Carolee Dean, President
Claudia Gutierrez, Vice-President
Cammie Archuleta, Treasurer
Deeply committed to the training of teachers, speech pathologists, parents, literacy volunteers, and other professionals in appropriate instructional methods for individuals with dyslexia. IDA's Southwest Branch encourages the use of Orton-Gilligham multisensory structured language based (MSL-based) methodology, which has proven to be the most effective way to teach individuals with dyslexia and related learning disabilities.
1985

263 **Learning Disabilities Association of New Mexico: Albuquerque**
6301 Menaul Blvd NE
Ste 556
Albuquerque, NM 87110-3323   505-821-2545
www.vivanewmexico.com/nm/nmlda
bp@peavler.org
Penny White, President
A nonprofit volunteer organization affiliated with the Learning Disabilities Association of America (LDAA). LDAA gives support and information to persons with learning disabilities, parents, teachers, and other professionals through 50 state affiliates and 800 local units.

264 **Learning Disabilities Association of New Mexico: Las Cruces**
6301 Menaul Blvd. NE
#556
Albuquerque, NM 87110-3323   505-821-2545
Fax: 505-867-3398
www.vivanewmexico.com/nmlda/about.html
epoel@nmsu.edu
Selma Nevarez, President
LDA is a non-profit organization of volunteers including individuals with learning disabilities, their families and professionals. LDA is dedicated to identifying causes and promoting prevention of learning disabilities and to enhancing the quality of life for all individuals with learning disabilities and their families by encouraging effective identification and intervention, fostering research, and protecting their rights under the law.

New York

265 **Advocates for Children of New York**
151 W 30th St
5th Fl
New York, NY 10001-4197   212-947-9779
Fax: 212-947-9790
www.advocatesforchildren.org
info@advocatesforchildren.org
Kim Sweet, Executive Director
Matthew Lenaghan, Deputy Director
Rebecca Shore, Director of Litigation
Works on behalf of children from infancy to age 21 who are at greatest risk for school-based discrimination and/or academic failure. AFC provides a full range of services: free individual case advocacy, technical assistance, and training for parents, students, and professionals about children's educational entitlements and due process rights in New York City.

266 **American Autism Association**
115 E - 34th St
Ste 1703
New York, NY 10156   877-654-4483
http://myautism.org
info@myautism.org
Eduard Rozenfeld, President
The American Autism Association offers educational services, financial aid, and informational resources to assist families of children with autism.

267 **Easter Seals - New York**
40 W 37th St
Ste 503
New York, NY 10018   212-220-2290
Fax: 212-695-4807
www.ny.easterseals.com
Craig Stenning, Executive Director
Aris Pavlides, Svp Development
Kevin Carey, Director of Finance
Provides programs and services to children and adults with disabilities and other special needs, and their families. The goal is to help individuals with special needs gain dignity, equality and independence. Also provide the highest quality services in the most caring and cost-effective manner.
1922

268 **International Dyslexia Association Long Island**
1488 Deer Park Ave
Ste 190
North Babylon, NY 11703   631-261-7441
Fax: 631-261-7834
www.lidyslexia.org
info@lidyslexia.org
Concetta Russo, EdD, President
Glenna Rubin, PhD, Vice-President
Randi Burns, 2nd Vice-President
Our objectives are to increase awareness of dyslexia in the community; provide support for parents and teachers; promote teacher training. We offer a telephone message system for information requests; sponsor an annual conference and four topic workshops as well as a summer Orton-Gillingham course. We have a network of local school officials, parents, attorneys and other professionals to help parents navigate the channels of the school system.

269 **International Dyslexia Association New York**
71 W 23rd St
Ste 1527
New York, NY 10010-4197   212-691-1930
Fax: 212-633-1620
http://everyonereading.org
info@everyonereading.org
Candace Carponter, Esq, President
Lavinia Mancuso, Executive Director
Rachel Levine, Esq, Program Director

This is a nonprofit organization whose mission is to provide continuing education in appropriate diagnostic remedial approaches and to support the rights of people with dyslexia in order that they may lead fulfilling lives. To this end, the NYB-IDA disseminates information, publishes a quarterly newsletter, and provides information and referral services, teacher training, conferences, adult support groups, and workshops for parents. Annual teen conference.

270 International Dyslexia Association of Western New York

2555 Elmwood Ave
Kenmore, NY 14217
716-874-7200
Fax: 716-874-7205
www.ldaofwny.org
info@ldaofwny.org

Michael Helman, President
Marc Hennig, Deputy Exec Director of Programs
Jamie Feliciano, Interim Director of Finance
Strives to be a resource for information and services that address the full scope of dyslexia in a way that builds cooperation, partnership and understanding among professional communities and dyslexic individuals so that everyone is valued and has the opportunity to be productive and fulfilled in life. Newsletter and teacher training scholarships.

271 LDA Life and Learning Services

Starbridge
1650 South Ave
Ste 200
Rochester, NY 14620
585-546-1700
Fax: 585-224-7100
www.starbridgeinc.org
info@starbridgeinc.org

Colin Garwood, President/CEO
Jason Blackwell, VP Programs & Services
Ida Jones, VP Org & Workplace Development
A non-profit agency that partners with individuals who seek hlep in learning, so that they can succeed in school, work, and community life. The primaty constituents include people who are working to overcome cognitive or developmental barriers to learning. Also serve as a resource to people who are involved in the lives of these individuals, such as family members, employers, teachers and health care professionals.

272 Learning Ally: New York Recording Studio

545 Fifth Ave
Ste 1005
New York, NY 10017
212-557-5720
www.learningally.org
dcasper@learningally.org

Daniel Casper, Studio Leader
To create opportunities for individuals, from Kindergarten through Graduate Level, who cannot read standard print because of a visual impairment, learning disability or other physical disability, to succeed in school by providing accessible educational materials.

273 Learning Disabilities Association of New York State (LDANYS)

1190 Troy-Schenectady Rd
Latham, NY 12110
518-608-8992
Fax: 518-608-8993
http://ldanys.org
info@ldaamerica.org

Michael Helman, President
Charles Giglio, Vice-President
LDANYS works with the Governor's office, members of the state legislature, Board of Regents, and key state agencies that oversee programs and services that touch the lives of individuals who have learning disabilities and their families to ensure policies are fair and provide equal access to programs and services for individuals who have learning disabilities.

274 Learning Disabilities Association of Central New York

722 West Manlius Street
East Syracuse, NY 13057-2178
315-432-0665
Fax: 315-431-0606
www.ldacny.org
ldacny@ldacny.org

Brannan Karg, President
Bill Patrick, Vice President
Paulette Purdy, Executive Director
Enhances the quality of life for children and adults with learning disabilities by providing advocacy, programs and educational resources. Serving the counties of Cayuga, Cortland, Madison, Onondaga and Owsego.

275 Learning Disabilities Association of New York City

722 West Manlius Street
East Syracuse, NY 13057
315-432-0665
Fax: 315-431-0606
www.ldanyc.org
ldacny@ldacny.org

Brannan Karg, President
Bill Patrick, Vice President
Paulette Purdy, Executive Director
Serves the counties of Brooklyn, Bronx, Manhattan, Queens and Staten Island. Facilitates access to needed services for all New Yorkers with Learning Disabilities, especially those in the more disadvantaged communities, and provides support to those individuals and their families.
1989

276 Learning Disabilities Association of Western New York

2555 Elmwood Ave
Kenmore, NY 14217-1939
716-874-7200
888-250-5031
Fax: 716-874-7205
www.ldaofwny.org
information@ldaofwny.org

Jane Bedore, President
Valerie Franczyk, Executive Vice-President
Pauli Chameli, Vice-President
To create conditions under which persons with learning disabilities, neurological impairments, and developmental disabilities are given opportunities to make choices and develop and achieve independence. The association also addresses each individual's health, future, participation in community, and personal relationships. LDA Southern Fredonia Tier branch can be reached at 716-679-1601.

277 Northeast ADA Center

201 Dolgen Hall
Ithaca, NY 14853
800-949-4232
Fax: 607-255-2763
http://northeastada.org
northeastada@cornell.edu

LaWanda H. Cook, Training Specialist
Carolina Harris, Program Evaluation Specialist
The Northeast ADA Center provides information and training on the Americans with Disabilities Act (ADA) in New York, New Jersey, Puerto Rico and the U.S. Virgin Islands.

278 Resources for Children with Special Needs

116 E 16th St
5th Fl
New York, NY 10003-2164
212-677-4650
Fax: 212-254-4070
www.resourcesnyc.org
info@resourcesnyc.org

Ellen Miller-Wachtel, Chair
Barbara A. Glassman, Executive Director
Emily Mann, Senior Director of Program
An information, referral, advocacy, tranining and support center for NYC parents/professionals looking for services for children-birth to 26 with learning, developmental, emotional of physical disabilities. Publications available on website.

279 Strong Center for Developmental Disabilities
Golisano Children's Hospital at Strong
601 Elmwood Ave
PO Box 671
Rochester, NY 14642-0001   585-275-0355
                              Fax: 585-275-3366
www.urmc.rochester.edu/childrens-hospita
steve_sulkes@urmc.rochester.edu
Stephen B. Sulkes, MD, Co-Director
Susan A. Hetherington, PhD, Co-Director
A University Center of Excellence for Developmental Disabilities, Education, Research and Service. Provides services, advocacy, education, technical assistance, and research to ensure full inclusion of persons with developmental disabilities in their communities and to maximize their potentional for leading independent and productive lives.

280 Westchester Institute for Human Development
Westchester Medical Center
Cedarwood Hall
20 Plaza W
Valhalla, NY 10595   914-493-8150
                        Fax: 914-493-1973
www.wihd.org
info@WIHD.org
Ansley Bacon, PhD, President/CEO
David O'Hara, PhD, Chief Operating Officer
Marianne Ventrice, CPA, Chief Financial Officer
WIHD advances policies and practices that foster the healthy development and ensure the safety of all children, strenghten families and communities, and promote health and well-being among people of all ages with disabilities and special health care needs.
1950

281 Yellin Center for Mind, Brain, and Education
104 W 29th St
12th Fl
New York, NY 10001   646-775-6646
                        Fax: 646-775-6602
www.yellincenter.com
info@yellincenter.com
Dr. Paul B. Yellin, MD, FAAP, Director
Comprehensive Neurodevelopmental and Psychoeducational Evaluation for students in Pre-K, K-12, College, Graduate and Professional Schools, and for adults. Ongoing support including Academic Coaching, Medication Management, Progress Monitoring and College Transition Support. Outreach to School, Teachers, and other providers where indicated. Professional development presentations for schools and parent organizations. Sliding scale available.

North Carolina

282 Mind Matters
Southeast Psych
6060 Piedmont Row Drive South
Ste 120
Charlotte, NC 28287   704-552-0116
                        Fax: 704-552-7550
www.southeastpsych.com
cpohlman@southeastpsych.com
Karen Amrhein, CFO
Allison Barnett, Assistant to the CFO
Britny Kirsner, Group Coordinator
Mind Matters at Southeast Psych believes in describing learners (not just labeling them), identifying strengths (not just weaknesses), explaining findings clearly (not just reporting scores), collaborating to support struggling learners, and improving the self-insight of all learners.

283 Success in Mind
324 Blackwell St
Ste 1240
Durham, NC 27701   919-680-8921
                          877-680-8921
                      Fax: 919-680-8949
www.success-in-mind.org
info@success-in-mind.org
Beth Briere, MD, Executive Director
Craig Pohlman, PhD, Learning Specialist
Marianne Zura, MD, Neurodevelopmentalist
Provides students, families, teachers and others involved in a student's educatoin with a deep understanding and a common language that demystifies learning, values individual learning differences, and promotes success for each learner.

North Dakota

284 Easter Seals - Bismarck-Mandan
1031 Interstate Ave
Frontier Bldg
Bismarck, ND 58503   701-751-0863
                          800-247-0698
www.esgwnd.org
info@al.easterseals.com
Easter Seals provides services to children and adults with disabilities and other special needs, and support to their families.

285 Easter Seals - Dickson
2125 Sims St
PO Box 361
Dickson, ND 58602-0361   701-264-1060
                              866-895-1587
                          Fax: 701-264-1099
www.esgwnd.org
info@al.easterseals.com
Easter Seals provides services to children and adults with disabilities and other special needs, and support to their families.

286 Easter Seals - Fargo
3333 7th Ave S
Ste 1
Fargo, ND 58102   701-373-8393
www.esgwnd.org
info@al.easterseals.com
Easter Seals provides services to children and adults with disabilities and other special needs, and support to their families.

287 Easter Seals - Jamestown
402 14th Ave NE
Ste 1
Jamestown, ND 58402-0756   701-251-1446
                              866-897-6004
                          Fax: 701-252-9527
www.esgwnd.org
info@al.easterseals.com
Easter Seals provides services to children and adults with disabilities and other special needs, and support to their families.

288 Easter Seals - Minot/Williston
800 12th Ave SW
Minot, ND 58701-9114   701-839-4121
                            866-895-1589
                        Fax: 701-838-5998
www.esgwnd.org
info@al.easterseals.com
Easter Seals provides services to children and adults with disabilities and other special needs, and support to their families.

289 Easter Seals Goodwill - Headquarters
211 Collins Ave
Mandan, ND 58554-7206   701-663-6828
                                     800-247-0698
                                Fax: 701 663 6859
                                     www.esgwnd.org
                                     info@al.easterseals.com
John Ives, Chairman
Randy Thomas, Chairman Elect
Lynne Stokley, Chief Executive Officer
Easter Seals provides services to children and adults with
disabilities and other special needs, and support to their fam-
ilies.

290 North Dakota Association For The Disabled (NDAD)
309 Washington Ave
Ste 303
Williston, ND 58801   701-355-4458
                                Fax: 701-227-8847
                                     www.ndcpd.org
                                     ndcpd@minotstateu.edu
Brent Askvig, Executive Director
Lori Garnes, Associate Director, Development
Susie Mack, Coordinator for Operations
The NDCPD provides services, education, and research de-
signed to encourage communities to welcome, value, and en-
sure the well-being of the differently abled. It is part of the
University Center of Excellence on Developmental Disabil-
ities, Education, Research and Services.

**291 North Dakota Association for Lifelong Learning
(NDALL)**
1605 E Capitol Ave
Bismarck, ND 58501   701-355-4458
                                Fax: 701-227-8847
                http://sites.google.com/site/northdakotaall/
                                     clearfour@btinet.net
Jennifer Kraft, President
Jennifer Frueh, Vice-President
Irene Mohn, Secretary/Treasurer
The North Dakota Association for Lifelong Learning
(NDALL) supports educators, adult students, and partners in
alternative education. Formerly it was known as the North
Dakota Association of Adult Basic & Secondary Education
(NDABSE).

292 North Dakota Autism Center
647 13th Ave E
West Fargo, ND 58078   701-277-8844
                                Fax: 701-227-8847
                                     www.ndautismcenter.org
                                     dkasprowicz@ndautismcenter.org
Darcy Kasprowicz, Contact
The Autism Center supports families and individuals affected by autism spectrum disorders through care, therapy,
advocacy, and more. Is also the home of the AuSome Kids
Day Program which focuses on the needs of preschool and
school age children with Autism Spectrum Disorders or related disabilities and behaviours.

**293 North Dakota Center for Persons with Disabilities
(NDCPD)**
Minot State University
500 University Ave W
Ste 203, Memorial Hall
Minot, ND 58707   701-355-4458
                                Fax: 701-227-8847
                                     www.ndcpd.org
                                     ndcpd@minotstateu.edu
Brent Askvig, Executive Director
Lori Garnes, Associate Director, Development
Susie Mack, Coordinator for Operations
The NDCPD provides services, education, and research de-
signed to encourage communities to welcome, value, and en-
sure the well-being of the differently abled. It is part of the
University Center of Excellence on Developmental Disabil-
ities, Education, Research and Services.

294 North Dakota Protection & Advocacy Project
400 E Broadway
Ste 409, Wells Fargo Bank Bldg
Bismarck, ND 58501-4071   701-328-2950
                                     800-472-2670
                                Fax: 701-328-3934
                                     www.ndpanda.org
                                     panda@nd.gov
Teresa Larsen, Executive Director
David Boeck, Director of Legal Services
Dotty Simes, Fiscal Manager
The Protection & Advocacy Project advocates for the rights
of North Dakotans with disabilities.

295 Pathfinder Services
7 3rd St SE
Ste 101
Minot, ND 58701   701-837-7500
                                     800-245-5840
                                Fax: 701-837-7548
                                TDD: 701-837-7548
                                     www.psnd.co/index.php
                                     info@pathfinder-nd.org
David King, Board President
Jacki Harasym, Interim Director
Daniel Griffith, Program Support
Pathfinder seeks to support North Dakota families of chil-
dren and youth with learning difficulties. Programs include
webinars, workshops, and parent advising.

Ohio

296 Easter Seals - Youngstown
299 Edwards St
Youngstown, OH 44502-1599   330-743-1168
                                Fax: 330-743-1616
                                TTY: 320-743-1616
                                     www.mtc.easterseals.com
Ken Sklenar, Executive Director
Easter Seals of Mahoning, Trumbull and Columbiana Counties pledges to help persons with disabilities or special needs
live with equality, dignity and independence.

297 International Dyslexia Association of Central Ohio
PO Box 1601
Westerville, OH 43086   614-899-5711
                                     http://cobida.org
                                     info@cobida.org
Martha G. Michael, PhD, President
Mike McGovern, Vice President
Diana McGovern, Treasurer
Increases awareness of dyslexia and related learning disabil-
ities; assist professionals, dyslexics and their families; pro-
mote use of effective teaching methods; and disseminate
research-based knowledge. Serves Central Ohio and parts of
West Virginia.

298 International Dyslexia Association of Northern Ohio
PO Box 549
Aurora, OH 44202-0141   216-556-0883
                                     http://noh.dyslexiaida.org
                                     info@dyslexia-nohio.org
May Jo O'Neil, MeD, President
A non-profit, scientific and educational organization dedi-
cated to the study and treatment of the language-based read-
ing disability, dyslexia.

299 International Dyslexia Association: Ohio Valley Branch
317 E 5th St
Cincinnati, OH 45202   513-651-4747
                                     www.cincinnatidyslexia.org
                                     info@interdys.org
Martha Chiodi, President

A non-profit, scientific and educational organization dedicated to the study and treatment of the learning disability, dyslexia. This Branch was formed to increase public awareness of dyslexia on the Southern Ohio, Southeast Indiana, Kentucky and Huntington, West Virginia areas.

300   Learning Disabilities Association of Cuyahoga County

4800 E 131st St
Ste B
Garfield Heights, OH 44105   216-581-4549
                                     Fax: 216-581-7076
                                     www.ldacc.org
                                     info@ldacc.org

Ellen Fishman, Executive Director
Empowers those with Specific Learning Disabilities to realize their potential and achieve their goals.

Oklahoma

301   Easter Seals - Oklahoma

701 NE 13th St
Oklahoma City, OK 73104-5003   405-239-2525
                                     Fax: 405-239-2278
                                     http://ok.easterseals.com

Matt Vance, Chairman
Lauri Monetti, Development Director
Paula K. Porter, President & CEO
Provides services to children and adults with disabilities and other special needs, and support to their families.

302   Learning Disabilities Association of Oklahoma

5150 E 101st St
PO Box 1134
Jenks, OK 74037-1134   918-298-1600
                                     www.ldao.org
                                     ldao@ldao.org

Evie Lindberg, President
Elana Grissom, Treasurer
Holly Rice, Second Vice-President
A nonprofit organization committed to enhancing the lives of individuals with learning disabilities and their families through education, advocacy, research, and service

Oregon

303   Easter Seals - Oregon

7300 SW Huntziker St
Ste 103
Portland, OR 97223-3797   503-228-5108
                                     800-556-6020
                                     Fax: 503-228-1352
                                     www.easterseals.com/oregon/

David Cheveallier, CEO
Provides services to children and adults with disabilities and other special needs, helping them to live with equality, dignity and independence.

304   International Dyslexia Association of Oregon

PO Box 2609
Portland, OR 97208-2609   503-228-4455
                                     800-530-2234
                                     Fax: 503-228-3152
                                     www.orbida.org
                                     info@orbida.org

Jane Cooper, President
Judy Wright, Vice-President
Gary Wright, Treasurer
The Oregon Branch of the International Dyslexia Association (ORBIDA) focuses on increasing public awareness of how dyslexia affects both children and adults.

305   Learning Disabilities Association of Oregon

10175 SW Barbur Blvd
Ste 214B
Portland, OR 97219   503-997-3181
                                     www.ldaor.org
                                     wisechoice@comcast.net

Myrna Soule, President
Works to promote the welfare of children and adults with learning disabilities. A non-profit organization that serves as a resource, referral, and information center for adults with learning disabilities, parents of children with learning disabilities, and profesionals working in the field of learning disabilities.

306   Oregon's Deaf and Hard of Hearing Services

500 Summer St NE
Ste E-16
Salem, OR 97301   503-947-5183
                                     800-521-9615
                                     Fax: 503-947-5184
                                     TTY: 800-521-9615
                                     www.odc.state.or.us
                                     odhhs.info@state.or.us

Patricia O'Sullivan, Manager
Provides information and referral source on deafness and hearing loss issues; training on deaf awareness and sensitivity, and how to communicate with those with hearing loss.

307   University of Oregon Center for Excellence in Developmental Disabilities

Center on Human Development College of Education
5252 University of Oregon
Eugene, OR 97403-5252   541-346-3591
                                     Fax: 541-346-2594
                                     http://ucedd.uoregon.edu
                                     uocedd@uoregon.edu

Jane Squires, PhD, Director
Debra Eisert, PhD, Associate Director
Leslie Martinez, Business Manager
The mission of our UCEDD in Developmental Disabilities is to be of assistance in improving the quality of life for Oregonians and all persons with developmental disabilities and their families. To accomplish this mission, we provide training, technical assistance, interdisciplinary training, dissemination, networking and model development that responds effectively, and in a culturally competent fashion, to the multiple needs of individuals and their families.

Pennsylvania

308   AAC Institute

1401 Forbes Ave
Ste 303
Pittsburgh, PA 15219-2627   412-402-0900
                                     www.aacinstitute.org
                                     khill@aacinstitute.org

Katya Hill, PhD, Clinic Director
Shannon Carney, Office Manager
Established in 2000, a resource for all who are interested in enhancing the communication of people who rely on AAC. A not-for-profit charitable organization, offers information and provides services worldwide.

309   Easter Seals - Eastern Pennsylvania

1501 Lehigh St
Ste 201
Allentown, PA 18103   610-289-0114
                                     Fax: 610-289-4282
                                     www.easterseals.com/esep/
                                     cgillen@esep.org

Elaine Stanko, Chairperson of the Board
Nancy Knowbel, President & CEO
Lisa Musselman, Vice-President, Programs

Speech, language, learning disabilities and hearing evaluations and therapy for all ages. PA licensed preschool on the premises. Open five days per week; 12 months. Call for an appointment or information on the programs provided.
1936

310   Easter Seals - Southeastern Pennsylvania

3975 Conshohocken Ave
Philadelphia, PA 19131-5484   215-879-1000
                                     800-587-3257
                                 Fax: 215-879-8424
                    www.easterseals.com/sepa/
                    development@easterseals-sepa.org
Roy Yaffe, Esq., President
Linda A. McDevitt, CPA/PFS, MT, Vice-President
Cummins Catherwood, Jr., Secretary
Speech, language, learning disabilities and hearing evaluations and therapy for all ages. PA licensed preschool on the premises. Open five days per week; 12 months. Call for an appointment or information on the programs provided.
1936

311   Easter Seals - Western & Central Pennsylvania

875 Greentree Rd, 6 Pkwy Center
Ste 150
Pittsburgh, PA 15220   412-281-7244
                                      800-587-3257
                                 Fax: 412-281-9333
                    www.easterseals.com/wcpenna/
                    development@eastersealswcpenna.org
C. James Zeszutek, Chairman
Ronald Palmer, 1st Vice Chairman
Peter J. Licastro, Treasurer
Speech, language, learning disabilities and hearing evaluations and therapy for all ages. PA licensed preschool on the premises. Open five days per week; 12 months. Call for an appointment or information on the programs provided.
1934

312   Huntingdon County PRIDE

1301 Mount Vernon Ave
Huntingdon, PA 16652-1149   814-643-5724
                                 Fax: 814-643-6085
                    www.huntingdonpride.org
                    apfingstl@huntingdonpride.org
Adam Pfingstl, Executive Director
Kathleen Renninger, Service Coordinator
Linda Weir, PRIDE Cares Coordinator
Provide programs which enable people who are developmentally and/or physically disabled to function at their optimal level of performance.

313   International Dyslexia Association of Pennsylvania

1062 E Lancaster Ave
Ste 15A
Rosemont, PA 19010-0251   610-527-1548
                                      855-220-8885
                                 Fax: 610-527-5011
                                 www.pbida.org
                                 dyslexia@pbida.org
Lisa Goldstein, MD, President
Tracy Ray Bowes, Manager
Betsy Boston, Simulation Coordinator
The Pennsylvania Branch of the International Dyslexia Association (PBIDA), serving Pennsylvania and Delaware provides support and information for individuals, families and educational professionals concerned with the issues of dyslexia and learning differences.

314   Learning Disabilities Association of Pennsylvania

4156 Library Rd
Ste 1
Pittsburg, PA 15234   412-341-1515
                                      888-775-3272
                                 www.ldapa.org
Debbie Rodes, President

A nonprofit organization dedicated to serving Pennsylvania residents by providing accurate, up-to-date information regarding learning disabilities as well as support.

315   Pennsylvania Center for Disability Law and Policy

1515 Market St
Ste 1300
Philadelphia, PA 19102-1819   215-557-7112
                                     888-745-2357
                                 Fax: 215-557-7602
                                 TDD: 215-557-7112
                    www.equalemployment.org
                    admin@equalemployment.org
Stephen S. Pennington, Executive Director
Jamie C. Ray-Leonetti, Co-Director
Margaret Passio-McKenna, Senior Advocate
An advocacy program for people with disabilities administered by the Center for Disability Law & Policy. CAP helps people who are seeking services from the Office of Vocational Rehabilitation, Blindness and Visual Services, Centers for Independent Living and other progrmas funded under federal law. Hep is provided to you at no charge, regardless of income. Dedicated to ensuring that the rehabilitation system in Pennsylvania is open and responsive to your needs.

Rhode Island

316   International Dyslexia Association of Rhode Island

PO Box 603144
Providence, RI 02906   401-521-0020
                                 Fax: 401-847-6720
                                 www.interdys.org
                                 ida.Rhodeisland@gmail.com
Hal Malchow, President
Elsa Cardenas-Hagan, Vice President
Ben Shifrin, MEd, Vice President
A non-profit, scientific and educational organization dedicated to the study and treatment of dyslexia.

South Carolina

317   Easter Seals - South Carolina

PO Box 5715
Columbia, SC 29250-5715   803-256-0735
                                      800-951-4090
                                 Fax: 803-356-6902
                                 http://sc.easterseals.com
Drew Royall, Chair
Deanna Lewis, President & CEO
Ellen Staubach, Director, Finance & HR
Provides services to children and adults with disabilities and other special needs, and support to their families.

318   International Dyslexia Association of South Carolina

30 Southhampton Dr
Charleston, SC 29407   864-256-1075
                                 http://scbida.org
                    southcarolinabranchida@gmail.com
Heidi Bishop, President
Marlene Reed, Treasurer
Becky Strange, Secretary
The South Carolina Branch provides general information about dyslexia and makes referrals to various professionals and schools serving individuals with learning disabilities.
130 members

South Dakota

319   Learning Disabilities Association of South Dakota
1021 S Courtland St
Chamberlin, SD 57325   605-234-0115
                                                888-388-5553
                                            Fax: 305-787-7848
                                              www.lda-sd.org
                                  maneugebauer@midstatesd.net
Mary Alice Larson, President
Margie Neugebauer, Executive Director
The Association conducts workshops and conferences, assists local communities, collaborates with other organizations with similar missions and concerns, and provides 1-on-1 assistance to individuals and families. Most visible among its efforts is the Association's statewide annual conference.
1996

320   South Dakota Center for Disabilities
Health Science Center
1400 W 22nd St
Sioux Falls, SD 57105-1505   605-357-1439
                                                800-658-3080
                                            Fax: 605-357-1438
                                            TDD: 800-658-3080
                                            TTY: 800-658-3080
                                              www.usd.edu/cd
                                                 cd@usd.edu
Wendy Parent-Johnson, PhD, Executive Director
John R. Johnson, PhD, Research & Development Director
Jana Richardson, Financie & Admin Director
A division of the Department of Pediatrics at the Sanford School pf Medicine at the University of South Dakota. The Center for Disabilities is South Dakota's University Center for Excellence in Developmental Disabilities Education, Research and Service sometimes referred to as University Centers for Excellence in Developmental Disabilities.

Tennessee

321   Easter Seals - Tennessee
750 Old Hickory Blvd
Ste 2-260
Brentwood, TN 37027-3721   615-292-6640
                                            Fax: 615-251-0994
                                            TDD: 615-385-3485
                                   www.easterseals.com/tennessee/
Tim Ryerson, President & CEO
Phillip Many, Chief Financial Officer
Christy Cochran, Vice-President Of Operations
Creates solutions that change the lives of children and adults with disabilities or other special needs and their families.

322   International Dyslexia Association: Tennessee Branch
6731 Ridgerock Lane
Knoxville, TN 37909   877-836-6432
                                            Fax: 931-528-3916
                                               www.tnida.org
                                   ivonne.tennent@gmail.com
Emily Dempster, President
Erin Alexander, Senior Vice President
Shannon Polk, Secretary
The Tennessee Branch of the International Dyslexia Association (TN-IDA) was formed to increase awareness about Dyslexia in the state of Tennessee. TN-IDA supports efforts to provide information regarding appropriate language arts instruction to those involved with language-based learning differences and to encourage the identity of these individuals at-risk for such disorders as soon as possible. This branch also serves individuals in the state of Kentucky.

323   Learning Disabilities Association of Tennessee
PO Box 40237
Memphis, TN 38174-0237   901-788-5328
                                www.learningdisabilitiesoftennessee.org
                                info@learningdisabilitiesoftennessee.org
Sue Marsh, President
Robin Stevens, Vice President
Whitney Wheeler, Secretary
The Learning Disabilities Association of Tennessee has a mission to provide information concerning awareness, advocacy, parent information, and community education to maximize the quality of life for individuals and families affected by Learning Disabilities and related disorders in the state of Tennessee.

Texas

324   Easter Seals - Central Texas
8505 Cross Park Dr
Ste 120
Austin, TX 78754-5165   512-615-6800
                                            Fax: 512-476-1638
                                   www.centraltx.easterseals.com
Tod Marvin, President & CEO
Mia Martin, Chief Financial Officer
Lucas Wells, Chief Program Officer
Easter Seals Central Texas provides exceptional services so people with disabilities and their families can fully participate in their communities.

325   Easter Seals - North Texas
1424 Hemphill St
Fort Worth, TX 76104-4703   817-332-7171
                                                888-617-7171
                                            Fax: 817-332-7601
                                   www.easterseals.com/northtexas/
                                        info@easterseals.com
Donna Dempsey, President & CEO
Nancy Quimby, Executive Vice-President & Cfo
Lenee Bassham, VP, Community Living Services
Created by the merger of Easter Seals of Greater Dallas and Easter Seals Greater Northwest Texas. Creates opportunities that advance the independence of individuals with disabilities and other special needs.

326   International Dyslexia Association of Austin
PO Box 92604
Austin, TX 78709-2604   512-452-7658
                                              www.austinida.org
Sharon McMichael, President
Whitney Bonner, Vice-President
Monica Wommack, Treasurer
The Austin Area Branch of the International Dyslexia Association is a 501 (c) (3) non profit organization dedicated to promoting reading excellence for all children through early identification of dyslexia, effective literacy education for adults and children with dyslexia, and teacher training.

327   International Dyslexia Association of Dallas
14070 Proton Rd
Ste 100
Dallas, TX 75244-3601   972-233-9107
                                            Fax: 972-490-4219
                                               www.dbida.org
                                   adminassistant@dbida.org
LaNaye Reid, President
The Dallas Branch of The International Dyslexia Association is committed to leadership and advocacy for people with dyslexia by providing: support for individuals and group interactions; programs to inform and educate; information for professionals and the general public.

328 International Dyslexia Association of Houston
PO Box 540504
Houston, TX 77254-0504   832-282-7154
                                Fax: 972-490-4219
                                www.houstonida.org
                          HoustonBIDA@gmail.com
Jessica Harris, LDT, CALT, President
Mary H. Yarus, MeD, LDT, CALT, Vice-President
Brock Griffiths, CPA, Treasurer
A non-profit organization dedicated to helping individuals
with dyslexia and related learning disorders, their families
and the communities that support them.

329 Learning Ally: Austin Recording Studio
1314 W 45th St
Austin, TX 78756   512-323-9390
                                www.learningally.org
                          tericson@learningally.org
Toni Ericson, Studio Leader
To create opportunities for individuals, from Kindergarten
through Graduate Level, who cannot read standard print because of a visual impairment, learning disability or other
physical disability, to succeed in school by providing accessible educational materials.

330 Learning Disabilities Association of Texas
PO Box 831392
Richardson, TX 75083-1392   800-604-7500
                                www.ldatx.org
                           contact@ldatx.org
Nancie Payne, President
Ed Schlitt, First Vice President
Beth McGaw, Secretary
Promotes the educational and general welfare of individuals
with learning disabilities.
1963

331 North Texas Rehabilitation Center
1005 Midwestern Pkwy
Wichita Falls, TX 76302-2211   940-322-0771
                                800-861-1322
                                Fax: 940-766-4943
                                www.ntrehab.org
                         sthompson@ntrehab.org
Mike Castles, President & CEO
Lesa Enlow, Program Director
Sheila Moeller, Financial Officer
A not-for-profit organization providing nationally accredited outpatient medical, academic, and developmental rehabilitation to North Texas and Southern Oklahoma. From the
Early Childhood Intervention program to the Aquatics programs, these services are designed to help our patients
acheive their highest level of independence.
1948

Utah

332 International Dyslexia Association of Utah
4649 W 10600 N
Highland, VT 84003   801-756-1933
                                Fax: 801-718-2222
                                www.ubida.org
                 dyslexiacenterofutah@comcast.net
Shelley Hatch, Director
Dedicated to ensuring that every student with the learning
difference of Dyslexia will receive scientifically based instruction and services consistent with his/her needs.

333 Learning Disabilities Association of Utah
PO Box 900726
Sandy, UT 84090-0726   801-553-9156
                                www.ldau.org
                           contact@ldau.org
Jennifer Cardinal, Executive

A non-profit volunteer organization supporting people with
learning disabilities and their families. Our mission is to create opportunities for individuals with learning abilities to
succeed and for their families to participate in their success.

Vermont

334 Vermont Protection & Advocacy
141 Main St
Ste 7
Montpelier, VT 05602-2916   802-229-1355
                                800-834-7890
                                Fax: 802-229-1359
                                TTY: 802-229-2603
                www.disabilityrightsvt.org/programs.html
                                info@vtpa.org
Ed Paquin, Executive Director
Dedicated to addressing problems, questions and complaints
brought to it by Vermonters with disabilities. VP&A's mission is to promote the equality, dignity, and self-determination of people with disabilities. VP&A provides
infomration, referral and advocacy services, including leagl
representation when appropriate, to individuals with
disabilities throughout Vermont.

Virginia

335 Easter Seals - UCP North Carolina & Virginia
5171 Glenwood Ave
Ste 400
Raleigh, NC 27612   804-287-1007
                                800-662-7119
                                Fax: 804-287-1008
                          http://eastersealsucp.com
                   info@nc.eastersealsucp.com
Luanne Welch, President & CEO
Sam Eberts, Chair
Michael O'Donnell, Treasurer
A lifelong partner fo people managing disabilities and men-
tal health challenges. Services are centered around each per-
son's individual needs to live, learn and participate fully in
his or her community.

336 International Dyslexia Association of Virginia
3126 W Cary St
Ste 102
Richmond, VA 23221   804-272-2881
                                866-893-0583
                                Fax: 804-272-0277
                                http://vbida.org
                                info@vbida.org
Cathy Gregory, President
Elsa Cardenas-Hagan, Vice President
Ben Shifrin, M.Ed., Vice President
Formed to increase public awareness of dyslexia in the State
of Virginia. We serve the entire state, with the exception of
Northern Virginia, which is part of the DC-Capital Branch in
Washington, DC. We serve individuals with dyslexia, their
families, and professionals in the field.

Washington

337 Disability Rights Washington
315 5th Ave S
Ste 850
Seattle, WA 98104-2691   206-324-1521
                                800-562-2702
                                Fax: 206-957-0729
                                TTY: 206-957-0728
                          www.disabilityrightswa.org
                                info@dr-wa.org
David Carlson, Director of Legal Advocacy
Andrea Kadlec, Director of Community Relations
Tom Hazeltine, Controller

Is a private, non-profit organization that has been protecting the rights of people with disabilities.
1974

338 Easter Seals - Washington
220 W Mercer St
Ste 210E
Seattle, WA 98119-3954   206-281-5700
                                800-678-5708
                           Fax: 206-284-0938
                    http://wa.easterseals.com
Kristopher Kohl, Board Chair
Cathy Bisaillon, President & CEO
Stephanie Nelson, Vice Chair
Provides exceptional services to ensure that people living with autism and other disabilities have equal opportunities to live, learn, work and play.

339 International Dyslexia Association Of Washington State
PO Box 27435
Seattle, WA 98165   206-382-1020
                              www.wabida.org
                              info@wabida.org
Kristie English, President
Kathleen Conklin, Vice-President
Dana Mott, Managing Director
The Washington State Branch of the International Dyslexia Association is a 501 (c) (3) non-profit, scientific and educational organization dedicated to the study and treatment of dyslexia. Our all volunteer board of directors seeks to increase public awareness of dyslexia in our branch's area which includes Washington, Idaho, and western Montana.

340 Learning Disabilities Association of Washington
Family Resource Center Campus
16315 NE 87th Street
Suite B11
Redmond, WA 98052-3537   425-882-0820
                                800-536-2343
                           Fax: 425-558-4773
                              www.ldawa.org
                             nsobich@ldawa.org
Nancy Sobich, Director
Elizabeth Smith, President
Promotes and provides services and support to improve the quality of life for individuals and families affected by learning and attentional disabilities
1965

341 Washington Parent Training Project: PAVE
6316 S 12th Street
Ste B
Tacoma, WA 98465-1900   253-565-2266
                                800-572-7368
                           Fax: 253-566-8052
                           TDD: 800-572-7368
                           TTY: 800-572-7368
                              www.wapave.org
                             pave@wapave.org
Tracy Kahlo, Executive Director
Heather Hebdon, Associate Director
Elma Rounds, CFO & Office Manager
PAVE, a parent directed organization, exists to increase independence, empowerment, future opportunities and choices for consumers with special needs, their families and communities, through training, information, referral and support.
1979

West Virginia

342 Easter Seals - West Virginia
Rehabilitation Center
1305 National Rd
Wheeling, WV 26003-5705   304-242-1390
                                800-677-1390
                           Fax: 304-243-5880
                         www.easterseals.com/wv/
Victor Greco, Chair of the Board
The Rehabilitaiton Center primary service area includes Ohio, Marshal, Wetzel, Tyler, Brooke and Hancock counties in West Virginia and Belmont, Monroe, Jefferson and Harrison Counties in Ohio.

Wisconsin

343 Easter Seals - Southeast Wisconsin
2222 S 114th St
Easter Seals Generations Center
West Allis, WI 53227   414-449-4444
                                800-470-5463
                           Fax: 414-571-5568
                           TTY: 414-571-9212
                         www.easterseals.com/wi-se/
Dale Van Dam, Chair
Robert Glowacki, Chief Executive Officer
Michelle Schaefer, Chief Operating Officer
Provides services across the lifespan to individuals with autism and other disabilities. Services include: autism therapies, early intervention, day services and work service training.

344 International Dyslexia Association of Wisconsin
1616 Graham Ave
Masonic Temple
Eau Claire, WI 54701   608-355-0911
                              www.wibida.org
                             wibida@gmail.com
Tammy Tillotson, President
Kimberly Chan, Treasurer
Pattie Huse, Secretary
We believe all individuals have the right to achieve their potential, that individual learning abilities can be strengthened and that social, educaitonal, and cultural barriers to language acquisition and use must be removed.

Wyoming

345 Cheyenne Habilitation & Theraputic Center (CHAT)
2000 Westland Road
Cheyenne, WY 82001   307-433-1110
                           Fax: 307-733-0478
                          www.chatcenterinc.com
Kim Elfering, Director
CHAT Center finds opportunities (employment and volunteer) for disabled participants in their programs to be involved in the community.
1972

346 Children's Learning Center
185 W Snow King Ave
PO Box 4100
Jackson, WY 83001   307-733-1616
                           Fax: 307-733-0478
                          www.childrenlearn.org
                       info@learningcenterwy.org
Audrey Cohen-Davis, Chair
Karen Horstmann, Vice-Chair
Lance Windey, Treasurer
Provide quality child development services to the Counties of Teton Sublette, for children age six weeks to three years. CLC has more than 80 staff, 14 classrooms, 3 therapy facilities and 6 campuses.
1972

347   Easter Seals - Wyoming
991 Joe St
Sheridan, WY 82801-1363   307-672-2816
                                          Fax: 307-672-3896
                        www.easterseals.com/wyoming/
Scott L Wilson, Board Chair
Michelle Belknap, President & CEO
Dawn Mellinger, Secretary
Provides life improving programs and services to benefit
children and adults with disabilities.

**348   Northwest Community Action Programs - Casper
        (NOWCAP)**
PO Box 51248
345 North Walsh Dr
Casper, WY 82609   307-237-9146
                                          Fax: 307-234-1029
                             www.nowcapservices.org
                        cboston@nowcapservices.org
Chris Boston, Executive Director
Kari Cornella, Opportunity Source Director
NOWCAP Services is a provider of services for people with
disabilities in Natrona County.
1972

**349   Northwest Community Action Programs - Cody
        (NOWCAP)**
PO Box 2527
337 Robert St
Cody, WY 82414   307-587-4046
                                          Fax: 307-587-8187
                             www.nowcapservices.org
                        jbarnes@nowcapservices.org
Jerry Barnes, Community Services Director
NOWCAP Services is a provider of services for people with
disabilities in Natrona County.
1972

**350   Northwest Community Action Programs - Rock Springs
        (NOWCAP)**
PO Box 1666
416 West Blair Ave
Rock Springs, WY 82901   307-382-2683
                                          Fax: 307-362-3035
                             www.nowcapservices.org
                        rlloyd@nowcapservices.org
Roy Lloyd, Southwest Community Services
NOWCAP Services is a provider of services for people with
disabilities in Natrona County.
1972

351   The Arc Of Natrona County
4070 Plaza Dr
Ste 106
Casper, WY 82604   307-577-4913
                                          Fax: 307-577-4014
                        http://arcofnatronacounty.org
Nathan Edwards, President
Beau Covert, Vice-President
Terri Weiner, Secretary & Arc President
The Arc provides education, research, advocacy, and sup-
port to individuals with cognitive, intellectual and develop-
mental disabilities, as well as for their families and friends in
the Natrona County.
1972

National Programs

352   Attention Deficit Disorder Association
PO Box 7557
Wilmington, DE 19803-9997   856-439-9099
                                              800-939-1019
                                         Fax: 800-939-1019
                                              www.add.org
                                              info@add.org

Evelyn Polk Green, MS.Ed, President
Linda Roggli, PCC, Vice President
Duane Gordon, Communications Committee Chair
The National Attention Deficit Disorder Association is an
organization focused on the needs of adults and young adults
with ADD/ADHD, and their children and families. We seek
to serve individuals with ADD, as well as those who love,
live with, teach, counsel and treat them.

353   Children and Adults with Attention Deficit Hyperactivity Disorder (CHADD)
4601 Presidents Drive
Suite 300
Lanham, MD 20706   301-306-7070
                                              800-233-4050
                                         Fax: 301-306-7090
                                              www.chadd.org
                                              help@chadd.org

Michael MacKay, President
M. Jeffry Spahr, MBA, JD, Secretary
Patricia Michel, CPA, MBA, Treasurer
Children and Adults with Attention-Deficit/Hyperactivity
Disorder (CHADD), is a national non-profit, tax-exempt
(Section 501) organization providing education, advocacy
and support for individuals with AD/HD. In addition to an
informative Web site, CHADD also publishes a variety of
printed materials to keep members and professionals current
on research advances, medications and treatments affecting
individuals with AD/HD.
16,000 members

354   Council for Exceptional Children (CEC)
2900 Crystal Drive
Suite 1000
Arlington, VA 22202-3557   888-232-7733
                                         Fax: 703-264-9494
                                         TTY: 866-915-5000
                                              www.cec.sped.org
                                              service@cec.sped.org

Robin D. Brewer, President
Alexander T. Graham, Executive Director
Deborah Ziegler, Associate Executive Director
The Council for Exceptional Children (CEC) is an international organization dedicated to improving educational outcomes for individuals with exceptionalities, students with
disabilities, and/or the gifted. CEC advocates for appropriate governmental policies, sets professional standards, provides continual professional development, advocates for
newly and historically underserved individuals with
exceptionalities, and helps professionals obtain resources
necessary for professional practice.

355   Council for Learning Disabilities CLD
11184 Antioch Rd
Box 405
Overland Park, KS 66210-2420   913-491-1011
                                         Fax: 913-491-1012
                                              www.cldinternational.org
                                              steve.chamberlain@utb.edu

Steve Chamberlain, President
Mary Beth Calhoon, Vice President
Linda Nease, Executive Director

The mission of the Council for Learning Disabilities/CLD is
to enhance the education and life span development of individuals with learning disabilities. CLD establishes standards of excellence and promotes innovative strategies on
research and practice through interdisciplinary education,
collaboration, and advocacy. CLD's publication, Learning
Disability Quarterly, focuses on the latest research in the
field of learning disabilities with an applied focus.

356   Dyslexia Research Institute
5746 Centerville Rd
Tallahassee, FL 32309-2893   850-893-2216
                                         Fax: 850-893-2440
                                              www.dyslexia-add.org
                                              dri@dyslexia-add.org

Patricia K. Hardman, Ph.D., Director
Robyn A Rennick MS, Director
Addresses academic, social and self-concept issues for dyslexic and ADD children and adults. College prep courses,
study skills, advocacy, diagnostic testing, seminars, teacher
training, day school, tutoring and an adult literacy and life
skills program is available using an accredited MSLE
approach.

357   Learning Disabilities Association of America
Learning Disabilities Association of America
4156 Library Rd
Pittsburgh, PA 15234-1349   412-341-1515
                                              888-300-6710
                                         Fax: 412-344-0224
                                              www.ldanatl.org
                                              info@ldaamerica.org

Nancie Payne, President
Ed Schlitt, First Vice President
Beth McGaw, Secretary
An information and referral center for parents and professionals dealing with Attention Deficit Disorders, and other
learning disabilities. Free materials and referral service to
nearest chapter.

358   National Alliance on Mental Illness (NAMI)
3803 N. Fairfax Drive
Suite 100
Arlington, VA 22203   703-524-7600
                                              888-999-6264
                                         Fax: 703-524-9094
                                              www.nami.org
                                              info@nami.org

David Levy, Chief Financial Officer
Lynn Borton, Chief Operating Officer
Jean-Michel Texier, Chief Information Officer
NAMI/National Alliance on Mental Illness is a mental
health organization dedicated to improving the lives of persons living with serious mental illness and their families.
NAMI members, leaders, and friends work across all levels
to meet a shared NAMI mission of support, education, advocacy, and research for people living with mental illness.

359   National Center for Learning Disabilities (NCLD)
381 Park Avenue South
Suite 1401
New York, NY 10016-8829   212-545-7510
                                              888-575-7373
                                         Fax: 212-545-9665
                                              www.ncld.com
                                              ncld@ncld.org?subject=Comments
James H. Wendorf, Executive Director
Kevin Hager, Chief Comm & Engagement Officer
Stevan J. Kukic, PhD, Director School Transformation
NCLD develops and delivers programs and promotes research to improve instruction, assessment and support services for individuals with learning disabilities. They create
and disseminate essential information for parents and educators, providing help and hope.

360 **National Clearinghouse of Rehabilitation Training Materials (NCRTM)**
Utah State University
6524 Old Main Hill
Logan, UT 84322-6524
866-821-5355
Fax: 435-797-7537
www.nchrtm.okstate.edu
ncrtm@cc.us.edu
Chenyong Zhu, M.S., Instructional Designer
Jared Schultz, Principal Investigator
Sylvia Sims, Office Assistant
The mission of the NCRTM is to advocate for the advancement of best practice in rehabilitation counseling through the development, collection, dissemination, and utilization of professional information, knowledge and skill.

361 **National Dissemination Center for Children with Disabilities**
1825 Connecticut Ave NW
Suite 700
Washington, DC 20009
202-884-8200
800-695-0285
Fax: 202-884-8441
www.nichcy.org
emulligan@fhi360.org
Suzanne Ripley, Director
National Dissemination Center for Children with Disabilities is a central source of information on: disabilities in infants, toddlers, children, and youth; IDEA, which is the law authorizing special education; No Child Left Behind (as it relates to children with disabilities); and research-based information on effective educational practices.

362 **National Institute of Mental Health (NIMH) Nat'l Institute of Neurological Disorders and Stroke**
NIMH Neurological Institute
P.O. Box 5801
Bethesda, MD 20824-0001
800-352-9424
Fax: 301-496-5751
TTY: 301-408-5981
www.ninds.nih.gov
nimhinfo@nih.gov
Story C Landis Ph.D, Director NINDS
Thomas Inseo, Director NIMH
NINDS is part of the National Institutes of Health which support research on developmental disorders such as ADHD. Research programs of the NINDS, the National Institute of Mental Health (NIMH), and the National Institute of Child Health and Human Development (NICHD) seek to address unanswered questions about the causes of ADHD, as well as to improve diagnosis and treatment.

363 **National Resource Center on AD/HD**
4601 Presidents Drive
Suite 300
Lanham, MD 20706
301-306-7070
800-233-4050
Fax: 301-306-7090
www.help4adhd.org/
Timothy J MacGeorge MSW, Director
The National Resource Center on AD/HD (NRC): A Program of CHADD (Children and Adults with Attention-Deficit/Hyperactivity Disorder), was established in 2002 to be the national clearinghouse for the latest evidence-based information on AD/HD. The NRC provides comprehensive information and support to individuals with AD/HD, their families and friends, and the professionals involved in their lives.

364 **U.S. Department of Health & Human Services Administration on Developmental Disabilities**
370 L'Enfant Promenade SW
Mailstop HHH 405-D
Washington, DC 20447-0001
202-690-6590
Fax: 202-690-6904
www.acf.hhs.gov/programs/add
fmccormick@acf.hhs.gov
Faith McCormick, Director

The Administration on Developmental Disabilities ensures that individuals with developmental disabilities and their families participate in the design of and have access to culturally competent services, supports, and other assistance and opportunities that promotes independence, productivity, and integration and inclusion into the community.

Publications/Videos

365 **A New Look at ADHD: Inhibition, Time, and Self-Control**
Guilford Publications
72 Spring St
New York, NY 10012-4019
212-431-9800
800-365-7006
Fax: 212-966-6708
www.guilford.com
info@guilford.com
Russell A. Barkley PhD, Author
This video provides an accessible introduction to Russell A. Barkley's influential theory of the nature and origins of ADHD. The companion manual reviews and amplifies key ideas and contains helpful suggestions for further reading. The package also includes a leader's guide, providing tips on the optimal use of the video with a variety of audiences. *$99.00*
Video & Manual
ISBN 1-593854-21-8

366 **AD/HD For Dummies**
American Psychiatric Publishing, Inc (APPI)
1000 Wilson Boulevard
Suite 1825
Arlington, VA 22209-3924
703-907-7322
800-368-5777
Fax: 703-907-1091
www.appi.org
appi@psych.org
John McDuffie, Associate Publisher
Jeff Strong, Author
Michael O Flanagan, Author
This book provides answers for parents of children who may have either condition, as well as for adult sufferers. Written in a friendly, easy-to-understand style, it helps people recognize and understand ADD and ADHD symptoms and offers an authoritative, balanced overview of both drug and non-drug therapies. *$29.95*
Paperback
ISBN 0-764537-12-7

367 **ADD and Creativity: Tapping Your Inner Muse**
Taylor Publishing
7211 Circle S Road
Austin, TX 78745
512-444-0571
800-225-3687
Fax: 512-440-2160
www.taylorpublishing.com
Yearbooks@balfour.com
Lynn Weiss PhD, Author
Raises and answers questions about the dynamic between the two components and shows how they can be a wonderful gift but also a painful liability if not properly handled. Real-life stories and inspirational affirmations throughout. *216 pages Paperback*
ISBN 0-878339-60-4

368 **ADD and Romance: Finding Fulfillment in Love, Sex and Relationships**
Taylor Publishing
7212 Circle S Road
Austin, TX 78745
512-444-0571
800-225-3687
Fax: 512-440-2160
www.taylorpublishing.com
Yearbooks@balfour.com
Jonathan Halverstadt, Author

A look at how attention deficit disorder can damage romantic relationships when partners do not take time, or do not know how to address this problem. This book provides the tools needed to build and sustain a more satisfying relationship.
240 pages Paperback
ISBN 0-878332-09-X

369   ADD and Success
Taylor Publishing
7213 Circle S Road
Austin, TX 78745   512-444-0571
                                            800-225-3687
                                      Fax: 512-440-2160
                                      www.taylorpublishing.com
                                      Yearbooks@balfour.com
Lynn Weiss PhD, Author
Presents the stories of 13 individuals and their experiences and challenges of living with adult attention disorder and achieving success.
224 pages Paperback
ISBN 0-878339-94-9

370   ADD in Adults
Taylor Publishing
7214 Circle S Road
Austin, TX 78745   512-444-0571
                                            800-225-3687
                                      Fax: 512-440-2160
                                      www.taylorpublishing.com
                                      Yearbooks@balfour.com
Lynn Weiss PhD, Author
Updated version of this best-selling book on the topic of ADD helps others to understand and live with the issues related to ADD. *$17.95*
192 pages Paperback
ISBN 0-878338-50-0

371   ADD/ADHD Behavior-Change Resource Kit:
Ready-to-Use Strategies & Activities for Helping Children
With Attention Deficit Disorder
1000 Wilson Boulevard
Suite 1825
Arlington, VA 22209-3924   703-907-7322
                                            800-368-5777
                                      Fax: 703-907-1091
                                      www.appi.org
                                      appi@psych.org
John McDuffie, Associate Publisher
Grad L Flick Ph.D, Author
Rebecca D. Rinehart, Publisher
For teachers, counselors and parents, this comprehensive new resource is filled with up-to-date information and practical strategies to help kids with attention deficits learn to control and change their own behaviors and build the academic, social, and personal skills necessary for success in school and in life. The Kit first explains ADD/ADHD behavior, its biological bases and basic characteristics and describes procedures used for diagnosis and various treatment options. *$29.95*
Paperback
ISBN 0-876281-44-4

372   ADHD - What Can We Do?
Guilford Publications
72 Spring St
New York, NY 10012-4019   212-431-9800
                                            800-365-7006
                                      Fax: 212-966-6708
                                      www.guilford.com
                                      info@guilford.com
Seymour Weingarten, Editor-in-Chief
Russell A. Barkley PhD, Author
Bob Matloff, President

This program introduces viewers to a variety of the most effective techniques for managing ADHD in the classroom, at home, and on family outings. Illustrated are ways that parents, teachers, and other professionals can work together to implement specific strategies that help children with the disorder improve their school performance and behavior. Informative interviews, demonstrations of techniques, and commentary from Dr. Barkley illuminate the significant difference that treatment can make. *$99.00*
Manual-DVD/VHS
ISBN 1-593854-25-0

373   ADHD - What Do We Know?
Guilford Publications
72 Spring St
New York, NY 10012-4019   212-431-9800
                                            800-365-7006
                                      Fax: 212-966-6708
                                      www.guilford.com
                                      info@guilford.com
Seymour Weingarten, Editor-in-Chief
Bob Matloff, President
Russell A. Barkley PhD, Author
Covering all the basic issues surrounding ADHD, this program is highly instructive. Through commentary from Dr. Barkley and interviews with parents, teachers, and children, viewers gain an understanding of: the causes and prevalence of ADHD; effects on children's learning and behavior; other conditions that may accompany ADHD; and, long-term prospects for children with the disorder. *$99.00*
Manual-DVD/VHS
ISBN 1-593854-17-X

374   ADHD Challenge Newsletter
PO Box 2277
Peabody, MA 01960-7277   800-233-2322
                                      Fax: 978-535-3276
                                      www.dyslexiacenter.org/ar/000039.shtml
                                      info@dyslexiacenter.org
Joan T Esposito, Founder and Program Director
Leslie V. Esposito, C.F.R.E, Development Director
Valerie Allen, Center Coordinator
National newsletter on ADD/ADHD that presents interviews with nationally-known scientists, as well as physicians, psychologists, social workers, educators, and other practitioners in the field of ADHD. *$35.00*
Bimonthly

375   ADHD Report
Guilford Publications
72 Spring St
New York, NY 10012-4019   212-431-9800
                                            800-365-7006
                                      Fax: 212-966-6708
                                      www.guilford.com
                                      info@guilford.com
Seymour Weingarten, Editor-in-Chief
Russell A. Barkley PhD, Author
Bob Matloff, President
Presents the most up-to-date information on the evaluation, diagnosis and management of ADHD in children, adolescents and adults. This important newsletter is an invaluable resource for all professionals interested in ADHD. *$79.00*
16 pages Bimonthly
ISSN 1065-8025

376   ADHD and the Nature of Self-Control
Guilford Publications
72 Spring St
New York, NY 10012-4019   212-431-9800
                                            800-365-7006
                                      Fax: 212-966-6708
                                      www.guilford.com
                                      info@guilford.com
Seymour Weingarten, Editor-in-Chief
Russell A. Barkley PhD, Author
Bob Matloff, President

This instructive program integrates information about ADHD with the experiences of adults from different walks of life who suffer from the disorder. Including interviews with these individuals, their family members, and the clinicians who treat them, the program addresses such important topics as the symptoms and behaviors that are characteristic of the disorder, how adult ADHD differs from the childhood form, the effects of ADHD on the family, and successful coping strategies. *$55.00*
Hardcover
ISBN 1-593853-89-0

377   ADHD in Adolescents: Diagnosis and Treatment
Guilford Publications
72 Spring St
New York, NY 10012-4019   212-431-9800
                                            800-365-7006
                                        Fax: 212-966-6708
                                          www.guilford.com
                                          info@guilford.com

Seymour Weingarten, Editor-in-Chief
Arthur L Robin, Author
Russell A Barkley PhD, Co-Author
This highly practical guide presents an empirically based approach to understanding, diagnosing, and treating ADHD in adolescents. Practitioners learn to conduct effective assessments and formulate goals that teenagers can comprehend, accept, and achieve. Educational, medical, and family components of treatment are described in depth, illustrated with detailed case material. Included are numerous reproducible handouts and forms. *$32.00*
Paperback
ISBN 1-572305-45-2

378   ADHD in Adults: What the Science Says
Guilford Publications
72 Spring St
New York, NY 10012-4019   212-431-9800
                                            800-365-7006
                                        Fax: 212-966-6708
                                          www.guilford.com
                                          info@guilford.com

Seymour Weigarten, Editor-in-Chief
Russell Barkley PhD, Author
Kevin R. Murphy, Author
Providing a new perspective on ADHD in adults, this book analyzes findings from two major studies directed by leading authority Russell A. Barkley. Information is presented on the significant impairments produced by the disorder across major functional domains and life activities, including educational outcomes, work, relationships, health behaviors, and mental health. Accessible tables, figures, and sidebars encapsulate the study results and offer detailed descriptions of the methods. *$50.00*
Hardcover
ISBN 1-593855-86-9

379   ADHD in the Schools: Assessment and Intervention Strategies
Guilford Publications
72 Spring St
New York, NY 10012-4019   212-431-9800
                                            800-365-7006
                                        Fax: 212-966-6708
                                          www.guilford.com
                                          info@guilford.com

Seymour Weigarten, Editor-in-Chief
George J DupPaul, Author
Gary Stoner, Author
This popular reference and text provides essential guidance for school-based professionals meeting the challenges of ADHD at any grade level. Comprehensive and practical, the book includes several reproducible assessment tools and handouts. A team-based approach to intervention is emphasized in chapters offering research-based guidelines for identifying and assessing children with ADHD and those at risk. *$29.00*
Paperback
ISBN 1-593850-89-1

380   ADHD/Hyperactivity: A Consumer's Guide For Parents and Teachers
P.O.Box 746
DeWitt, NY 13214-0746   315-446-4849
                                            800-550-2343
                                        Fax: 315-446-2012
                                           www.gsi-add.com
                                           info@gsi-add.com
The publication is designed to assist parents and teachers in understanding ADHD/Hyperactivity, providing guidance in the selection of educational programs, effective evaluations, and offers suggestions for choosing medications. Dr. Gordon discusses 30 easy-to-understand principles that will help parents, teachers, and clinicians avoid the many pitfalls along the path to effective diagnosis and treatment. *$14.95*

381   ADHD: Attention Deficit Hyperactivity Disorder in Children, Adolescents, and Adults
Oxford University Press
198 Madison Ave
New York, NY 10016-4308   212-726-6000
                                            800-445-9714
                                        Fax: 919-677-1303
                                          www.oup.com/us
                                       custserv.us@oup.com

Paul H. Wender, Author
ADHD provides parents and adults whose lives have been touched by this disorder an indispensable source of help, hope, and understanding. Explains the vital importance of drug therapy in treating ADHD; provides practical and extensive instructions for parents of ADHD sufferers; includes personal accounts of ADHD children, adolescents, and adults; and, offers valuable advice on where to find help. *$13.95*
ISBN 0-195113-49-7

382   Assessing ADHD in the Schools
Guilford Publications
72 Spring St
New York, NY 10012-4019   212-431-9800
                                            800-365-7006
                                        Fax: 212-966-6708
                                          www.guilford.com
                                          info@guilford.com

Seymour Weingarten, Editor-in-Chief
George J DuPaul, Author
Gary Stoner, Author
This dynamic program demonstrates an innovative model for assessing ADHD in the schools. In a departure from other approaches, DuPaul and Stoner depict assessment as a collaborative, problem-solving process that is inextricably linked to the planning of individualized interventions. A range of crucial assessment techniques are considered, including parent interviews, behavior and academic performance rating scales, and direct observation. *$99.00*
Manual-DVD/VHS
ISBN 1-572304-14-6

383   Attention Deficit Disorder Warehouse
300 Northwest 70th Avenue
Suite 102
Plantation, FL 33317-2360   954-792-8100
                                            800-233-9273
                                        Fax: 954-792-8545
                                        www.addwarehouse.com
                                    websales@addwarehouse.com
Roberta Parker, Co-Founder/Owner/Manager
Harvey Parker, PhD, Co-Founder/Owner/Manager
A comprehensive resource for the understanding and treatment of all developmental disorders, including ADHD and related problems, the ADD Warehouse provides a vast collection of ADHD-related books, videos, training programs, games, professional texts and assessment products.

384 Attention Deficit Disorder in Adults Workbook
Taylor Publishing
7214 Circle S Road
Austin, TX 78745   512-444-0571
                                     800-225-3687
                             Fax: 512-440-2160
                             www.taylorpublishing.com
                             Yearbooks@balfour.com
Lynn Weiss, Author
Dr. Lynn Weiss's best-selling Attention Deficit Disorder In Adults has sold over 125,000 copies since its publication in 1991. This updated volume still contains all the original information — how to tell if you have ADD, ways to master distraction, ADD's impact on the family, and more—plus the newest treatments available. *$17.99*
192 pages Paperback
ISBN 0-878338-50-0

385 Attention Deficit Disorder: A Concise Source of Information for Parents
Temeron Books
6531-111 Street
Edmonton, AB T6H 4R5   780-989-0910
                                      855-283-0900
                             Fax: 780-989-0930
                             www.brusheducation.ca
                             contact@brusheducation.ca
Hossein Moghadam MD, Author
Lauri Seidlitz, Managing Editor
Fraser Seely, Partner
The authors travel from a brief historical review of ADD, through a description of symptoms and consequences, to a discussion of treatment. *$12.95*
128 pages Paperback
ISBN 1-550590-82-0

386 Attention Deficit Hyperactivity Disorder: Handbook for Diagnosis & Treatment
Guilford Publications
72 Spring St
New York, NY 10012-4019   212-431-9800
                                     800-365-7006
                             Fax: 212-966-6708
                             www.guilford.com
                             info@guilford.com
Bob Matloff, President
Russell Barkley PhD, Author
Seymour Weingarten, Editor-in-Chief
This second edition helps clinicians diagnose and treat Attention Deficit Hyperactivity Disorder. Written by an internationally recognized authority in the field, it covers the history of ADHD, its primary symptoms, associated conditions, developmental course and outcome, and family context. A workbook companion manual is also available.
700 pages Hardcover

387 Attention Deficit/Hyperactivity Disorder Fact Sheet
National Dissemination Center for Children
1825 Connecticut Ave NW
Suite 700
Washington, DC 20009   202-884-8200
                                     800-695-0285
                             Fax: 202-884-8441
                             www.nichcy.org
                             emulligan@fhi360.org
Stephen F Moseley, President
An 8 page informational fact sheet, a publication of the National Dissemination Center for Children with Disabilities, that provides information on attention deficit/hyperactivity disorder in infants, toddlers, children, and youth. The brochure provides suggestions and tips for parents and teachers in addition to providing links to organizations where individuals can obtain further details on ADHD.

388 Attention-Deficit Disorders and Comorbidities in Children, Adolescents, and Adults
American Psychiatric Publishing, Inc (APPI)
1000 Wilson Boulevard
Suite 1825
Arlington, VA 22209-3924   703-907-7322
                                     800-368-5777
                             Fax: 703-907-1091
                             www.appi.org
                             appi@psych.org
John McDuffie, Associate Publisher
Thomas E. Brown, Editor
Rebecca D. Rinehart, Publisher
Book provides in-depth discussion of both ADD/Attention Deficit Disorders and that of ADHD/Attention Deficit-Hyperactivity Disorders, providing readers with information that focuses on several perspectives including learning disorders in children and adolescents; cognitive therapy for adults with ADHD; educational interventions for students with ADDs; tailoring treatments for individuals with ADHD; clinical and research perspectives, etc. *$82.00*
Hardcover
ISBN 0-880487-11-9

389 Attention-Deficit Hyperactivity Disorder: A Clinical Workbook
Guilford Publications
72 Spring St
New York, NY 10012-4019   212-431-9800
                                     800-365-7006
                             Fax: 212-966-6708
                             www.guilford.com
                             info@guilford.com
Seymour Weingarten, Editor-in-Chief
Russell A Barkley PhD, Author
Kevin R. Murphy, Co-Author
The revised and expanded third edition of this user-friendly workbook provides a master set of the assessment and treatment forms, questionnaires, and handouts recommended by Barkley in the third edition of the Handbook. Formatted for easy photocopying, many of these materials are available from no other source. Includes interview forms and rating scales for use with parents, teachers, and adult clients; checklists and fact sheets; daily school report cards for monitoring academic progress. *$34.00*
Paperback
ISBN 1-593852-27-4

390 Attention-Deficit/Hyperactivity Disorder: A Clinical Guide To Diagnosis and Treatment
American Psychiatric Publishing, Inc (APPI)
1000 Wilson Boulevard
Suite 1825
Arlington, VA 22209   703-907-7322
                                     800-368-5777
                             Fax: 703-907-1091
                             www.appi.org
                             appi@psych.org
Robert E Hales, M.D., M.B.A., Editor-in-Chief
Larry B Silver, Author
Rebecca D. Rinehart, Publisher
This new edition of Dr. Larry Silver's groundbreaking clinical book incorporates recent research findings on attention-deficit/hyperactivity disorder (ADHD), covering the latest information on diagnosis, associated disorders, and treatment, as well as ADHD in adults. The publication thoroughly reviews disorders often found to be comorbid with ADHD, including specific learning disorders, anxiety disorders, depression, anger regulation problems, obsessive-compulsive disorder, and tic disorders. *$52.00*
Paperback
ISBN 1-585621-31-6

391 CHADD Educators Manual
CHADD
4601 Presidents Drive
Suite 300
Lanham, MD 20706
301-306-7070
800-233-4050
Fax: 301-306-7090
www.chadd.org
help@chadd.org
Michael F. MacKay, JD, CPA, MSIA, President
Christine Hoch, Director of Development
Susan Buningh, MRE, Executive Editor
An in-depth look at Attention Deficit Disorders from an educational perspective. *$10.00*

392 Children with ADD: A Shared Responsibility
Council for Exceptional Children
2900 Crystal Drive
Suite 1000
Arlington, VA 22202-3557
703-620-3660
888-232-7733
Fax: 703-264-9494
TDD: 866-915-5000
TTY: 703-264-9446
www.cec.sped.org
service@cec.sped.org
George J DuPaul, Author
Gary Stoner, Co-Author
Robin D. Brewer, President
This book represents a consensus of what professionals and parents believe ADD is all about and how children with ADD may best be served. Reviews the evaluation process under IDEA and 504 and presents effective classroom strategies.
35 pages
ISBN 0-865862-33-8

393 Classroom Interventions for ADHD
Guilford Publications
72 Spring St
New York, NY 10012-4019
212-431-9800
800-365-7006
Fax: 212-966-6708
www.guilford.com
info@guilford.com
Seymour Weingarten, Editor-in-Chief
George J DupPaul, Author
Gary Stoner, Co-Author
This informative video provides an overview of intervention approaches that can be used to help students with ADHD enhance their school performance while keeping the classroom functioning smoothly. The video features an illuminating discussion among DuPaul, Stoner, and Russell A. Barkley, addressing provocative questions on the benefits of proactive, preventive measures, on the one hand, and reactive techniques, on the other. *$99.00*
Manual-DVD/VHS
ISBN 1-572304-15-4

394 Coping: Attention Deficit Disorder: A Guide for Parents and Teachers
Temeron Books
6531-111 Street
Edmonton, AB T6H 4R5
780-989-0910
855-283-0900
Fax: 780-989-0930
www.brusheducation.ca
contact@brusheducation.ca
Mary Ellen Beugin, Author
Lauri Seidlitz, Managing Editor
Fraser Seely, Partner
The author investigates medical and behavioral interventions that can be tried with ADD children and gives suggestions on coping with these children at home and at school.
$15.95
173 pages Paperback
ISBN 1-550590-13-8

395 Driven to Distraction: Attention Deficit Disorder from Childhood Through Adulthood
Hallowell Center
144 North Rd
Suite 2450
Sudbury, MA 01776-1142
978-287-0810
Fax: 978-287-5566
www.drhallowell.com
HallowellReferralsNYC@gmail.com
Edward M Hallowell, Author
John J. Ratey MD, Co-Author
Through vivid stories of the experience of their patients, Drs. Hallowell and Ratey show the varied forms ADD takes — from the hyperactive search for high stimulation to the floating inattention of daydreaming — and the transforming impact of precise diagnosis and treatment. *$10.40*
336 pages
ISBN 0-684801-28-0

396 E-ssential Guide: A Parent's Guide to AD/HD Basics
Schwab Learning
160 Spear Street
Suite 1020
San Francisco, CA 94105
650-655-2410
Fax: 650-655-2411
www.schwablearning.org
Bill Jackson, Founder, President, and CEO
Matthew Nelson, Chief Operating Officer
Gretchen Anderson, Vice President, Product
This guide covers the fundamental facts about Attention-Deficit/Hyperactivity Disorder (AD/HD) that will provide a better understanding of AD/HD. Included is: A general overview of AD/HD and helpful strategies for managing your child's AD/HD at home and at school.

397 Fact Sheet-Attention Deficit Hyperactivity Disorder
Attention Deficit Disorder Association
PO Box 7557
Wilmington, DE 19803-9997
856-439-9099
800-939-1019
Fax: 800-939-1019
www.add.org
info@add.org
Evelyn Polk Green, MS.Ed, President
Linda Roggli, PCC, Vice President
Duane Gordon, Communications Committee Chair
A pamphlet offering factual information on ADHD. *$10.00*

398 Family Therapy for ADHD - Treating Children, Adolescents, and Adults
Guilford Publications
72 Spring St
New York, NY 10012-4019
212-431-9800
800-365-7006
Fax: 212-966-6708
www.guilford.com
info@guilford.com
Seymour Weingarten, Editor-in-Chief
Craig A. Everett, Author
Sandra Volgy Everett, Co-Author
Presents an innovative approach to assessing and treating ADHD in the family context. Readers learn strategies for diagnosing the disorder and evaluating its impact not only on affected young persons but also on their parents and siblings. From expert family therapists, the volume outlines how professionals can help families mobilize their resources to manage ADHD symptoms; improve functioning in school and work settings; and develop more effective coping strategies.
$29.00
Paperback
ISBN 1-572307-08-0

399   Focus Magazine
Attention Deficit Disorder Association
PO Box 7557
Wilmington, DE 19803-9997   856-439-9099
                                             800-939-1019
                                        Fax: 800-939-1019
                                             www.add.org
                                             info@add.org

Evelyn Polk Green, MS.Ed, President
Linda Roggli, PCC, Vice President
Duane Gordon, Communications Committee Chair
Comprehensive magazine of the National Attention Deficit
Disorder Association. It focuses on the needs of adults and
young adults with ADD/ADHD, their children and families,
teachers and friends. Free with membership.
Quarterly

**400   Getting a Grip on ADD: A Kid's Guide to Understand-
ing & Coping with ADD**
Educational Media Corporation
1443 Old York Road
Warminster, PA 18974   763-781-0088
                                             800-448-2197
                                        Fax: 215-956-9041
                                             www.educationalmedia.com
                                             help@marcoproducts.com
Kim T. Frank, Author
Susan Smith, Co-Author
Help your elementary and middle school students cope more
effectively with Attention Deficit Disorders. *$9.95*
64 pages Paperback
ISBN 0-932796-60-5

401   How to Reach & Teach Teenagers With ADHD
John Wiley & Sons Inc
111 River Street
Hoboken, NJ 07030-5774   201-748-6000
                                             800-225-5945
                                        Fax: 201-748-6088
                                             http://as.wiley.com
                                             info@wiley.com
Grad L Flick PhD, Author
Stephen M. Smith, President/CEO
Ellis E. Cousens, EVP, COO
This comprehensive resource is pack with tested, up-to-date
information and techniques to help teachers, counselors and
parents understand and manage adolescents with attention
deficit disorder, including step-by-step procedures for behavioral intervention at school and home and reproducible
handouts, checklists and record-keeping forms. *$29.00*
ISBN 0-130320-21-6

402   Hyperactive Child Book
St. Martin's Press
175 5th Ave
New York, NY 10010-7703   646-307-5151
                                             888-330-8477
                                        Fax: 212-677-7456
                                             http://us.macmillan.com
                                             permissions@stmartins.com
Patricia Kennedy, Author
Lief G Terdal, Co-Author
The Hyperactive Child Book contains a comprehensive review of information about raising, treating, and educating a
child with Attention Deficit-Hyperactivity disorder. The
book will be useful to parents, teachers, and health care professionals in their efforts to provide for the ADHD child.
$12.95
288 pages
ISBN 0-312112-86-6

403   Hyperactive Child, Adolescent and Adult
Oxford University Press
198 Madison Ave
New York, NY 10016-4308   212-726-6000
                                             800-445-9714
                                        Fax: 919-677-1303
                                             www.oup.com/us
                                             custserv.us@oup.com

Paul H Wender, Author
How does one know if a youngster is hyperactive? How do
you know if you are hyperactive yourself? The answers may
lie in this easy-to-read and comprehensive volume written
by one of the leading researchers in the field. *$27.00*
172 pages Hardcover
ISBN 0-195042-91-3

**404   Hyperactive Children Grown Up: ADHD in Children,
Adolescents, and Adults**
Guilford Publications
72 Spring St
New York, NY 10012-4019   212-431-9800
                                             800-365-7006
                                        Fax: 212-966-6708
                                             www.guilford.com
                                             info@guilford.com
Seymour Weingarten, Editor-in-Chief
Gabrielle Weiss, Author
Lily Trokenberg Hechtman, Co-Author
Based on the McGill prospective studies, research that now
spans more than 30 years, the volume reports findings on the
etiology, treatment, and outcome of attention deficits and
hyperactivity at all stages of development. This second edi-
tion includes entirely new chapters that describes new devel-
opments in Attention Deficit Hyperactivity Disorder
(ADHD) in addition to the assessment, diagnosis, and treatment of ADHD adults. *$35.00*
Paperback
ISBN 0-898625-96-3

**405   I Would if I Could: A Teenager's Guide To ADHD/Hy-
peractivity**
PO Box 746
DeWitt, NY 13214   315-446-4849
                                             800-550-2343
                                        Fax: 315-446-2012
                                             www.gsi-add.com
                                             info@gsi-add.com
Michael Gordon Ph.D, Author
Janet H. Junco, Illustration
Arthur L. Robin, PhD., Co-Author
Provides youngsters with straightforward information about
the disorder in addition to exploring its impact on family relationships, self-esteem, and friendships. Dr. Gordon uses
humor and candor to educate and encourage teenagers who
too often find themselves confused and frustrated, providing
youngsters with straightforward information about the disorder and exploring its impact on family relationships,
self-esteem, and friendships. *$12.50*

**406   I'd Rather Be With a Real Mom Who Loves Me: A
Story for Foster Children**
PO Box 746
DeWitt, NY 13214   315-446-4849
                                             800-550-2343
                                        Fax: 315-446-2012
                                             www.gsi-add.com
                                             info@gsi-add.com
Michael Gordon Ph.D, Author
Janet H. Junco, Illustration
This book tells the story of a young boy who's lived most of
his life away from his birth parents. It's an honest, realistic
account of the frustrations and heartache he endures. This
fully illustrated book sensitively but forthrightly deals with
the entire range of concerns that confront foster children
with ADHD/Hyperactivity disorder. *$12.00*

**407   Identifying and Treating Attention Deficit Hyperactivity
Disorder: A Resource for School and Home**
U S Department of Education/Special Ed-Rehab Srvcs
PO Box 1398
Jessup, MD 20794-1398   877-433-7827
                                        Fax: 301-470-1244
                                        TDD: 877-576-7734
                                             www.ed.gov/rschstat/research/pubs/adhd
                                             edpubs@inet.ed.gov

Alexa Posny, Editor
Danny Harris, Chief Information Officer
Arne Duncan, Secretary of Education
Publication from the U S Department of Education that provides comprehensive information on attention deficit hyperactivity disorders, including causes, medical evaluation and treatment options in addition to helpful hints and tips for both the home and school environments. *$6.00*

408   International Reading Association Newspaper: Reading Today
International Reading Association
PO Box 8139
800 Barksdale Rd.
Newark, DE 19714-8139   302-731-1600
                                            800-336-7323
                                       Fax: 302-731-1057
                                          www.reading.org
                              customerservice@reading.org
Alan Farstrup, Editor
Jill Lewis-Spector, President
Diane Barone, Vice-President
Reading Today, the Association's bimonthly newspaper, is the first choice of IRA members for news and information on all these topics and more. It is available in print exclusively as an IRA membership benefit.
Bimonthly

409   Jumpin' Johnny
Gordon Systems, Inc.
PO Box 746
DeWitt, NY 13214   315-446-4849
                                            800-550-2343
                                       Fax: 315-446-2012
                                          www.gsi-add.com
                                         info@gsi-add.com
Michael Gordon Ph.D, Author
Janet H. Junco, Illustration and Design
Harvey C. Parker, PhD., Co-Author
This entertaining and informative book will help children understand the basic ideas about the evaluation of ADHD/Hyperactivity. Jumpin' Johnny tells what it is like to be inattentive and impulsive, and how his family and school work with him to make life easier. Children find this book amusing, educational, and accurate in its depiction of the challenges that confront them daily. *$11.00*

410   LD Child and the ADHD Child
1406 Plaza Dr
Winston Salem, NC 27103-1470   336-768-1374
                                            800-222-9796
                                       Fax: 336-768-9194
                                          www.blairpub.com
                                     sakowski@blairpub.com
Steve Kirk, Editor
Suzanne H Stevens, Author
Carolyn Sakowski, President
It is a brief, upbeat, always realistic look at what learning disabilities are and what problems LD children and parents face at home and at school. It contains a wealth of valuable suggestions, and its tempered optimism may dimish one's sense of futility and helplessness. *$12.95*
261 pages Paperback
ISBN 0-895871-42-4

411   Learning Times
Learning Disabilities Association of Georgia
2566 Shallowford Road
Suite 104 PMB 353
Atlanta, GA 30345-1200   404-303-7774
                                       Fax: 404-467-0190
                                            www.ldag.org
                                  ldaga@bellsouth.net
Tia Powell, Editor
Information and helpful articles on learning disabilities.
$40.00
Bimonthly

412   Making the System Work for Your Child with ADHD
Guilford Publications
72 Spring St
New York, NY 10012-4019   212-431-9800
                                            800-365-7006
                                       Fax: 212-966-6708
                                           www.guilford.com
                                         info@guilford.com
Seymour Weingarten, Editor-in-Chief
Perter S Jensen, Co-Author
Bob Matloff, President
Child psychiatrist Dr. Peter Jensen guides parents over the rough patches and around the hairpin curves in this empowering, highly informative book. Readers learn the whats, whys, and how-tos of making the system work and in getting their money's worth from the healthcare system, cutting through red tape at school, and making the most of fleeting time with doctors and therapists. *$17.95*
Paperback
ISBN 1-572308-70-2

413   Managing Attention Deficit Hyperactivity Disorder: A Guide for Practitioners
John Wiley & Sons Inc
111 River Street
Hoboken, NJ 07030-5774   201-748-6000
                                            800-225-5945
                                       Fax: 201-748-6088
                                          http://as.wiley.com
                                          info@wiley.com
Sam Goldstein, Author
Michael Goldstein, Co-Author
Stephen M. Smith, President/CEO
A valuable working resource for practitioners who manage children with ADHD, Managing Attention Deficit Hyperactivity in Children, Second Edition features: in-depth reviews of the latest research into the etiology and development of ADHD; Step-by-step guidelines on evaluating ADHD-medically, at home, and in school; a multidisciplinary approach to treating ADHD that combines medical, family, cognitive, behavioral, and school interventions; and critical discussions of controversial new treatments. *$130.00*
Hardcover
ISBN 0-471121-58-9

414   Mastering Your Adult ADHD A Cognitive-Behavioral Treatment Program
Oxford University Press
198 Madison Ave
New York, NY 10016-4308   212-726-6000
                                            800-445-9714
                                       Fax: 919-677-1303
                                          www.oup.com/us
                                    custserv.us@oup.com
Steven A Safren, Author
Used in conjunction with the corresponding client workbook, this therapist guide offers effective treatment strategies that follow an empirically-supported treatment approach. It provides clinicians with effective means of teaching clients skills that have been scientifically tested and shown to help adults cope with ADHD. *$35.00*
ISBN 0-195188-18-7

415   Maybe You Know My Kid: A Parent's Guide to Identifying ADHD
119 West 40th Street
New York, NY 10018   212-407-1500
                                            800-221-2647
                                       Fax: 212-935-0699
                                     www.kensingtonbooks.com/
                            SZacharius@kensingtonbooks.com
Mary Cahill Fowler, Author
Steven Zacharius, Chairman, President & CEO
A guide for parents of children diagnosed with ADD discusses the recent changes in the education of these children and offers practical guidelines for improving educational performance.

416 Meeting the ADD Challenge: A Practical Guide for Teachers
Research Press
P.O. Box 7886
Champaign, IL 61826-9177   217-352-3273
                                                        800-519-2707
                                                   Fax: 217-352-1221
                                               www.researchpress.com
                                            orders@researchpress.com
Steve B Gordon, Author
Michael J Asher, Co-Author
Provides educators with practical information about the needs and treatment of children and adolescents with ADD. The book addresses the defining characteristics of ADD, common treatment approaches, myths about ADD, matching intervention to student, use of behavior-rating scales and checklists evaluating interventions, regular verses, special class placement, helps students regulate their own behavior and more. Case examples are used throughout. *$17.95*
196 pages
ISBN 0-878223-45-2

417 My Brother is a World Class Pain A Sibling's Guide To ADHD/Hyperactivity
Gordon Systems, Inc.
P.O.Box 746
DeWitt, NY 13214-0746   315-446-4849
                                                        800-550-ADHD
                                                   Fax: 315-446-2012
                                                     www.gsi-add.com
                                                     info@gsi-add.com
Michael Gordon Ph.D, Author
A book for the often forgotten group of those affected by ADHD, the brothers and sisters of ADHD children, this story about an older sister's efforts to deal with her active and impulsive brother sends the clear message to siblings of the ADHD child that they can play an important role in a family's quest for change. *$11.00*

418 NIMH-Attention Deficit-Hyperactivity Disorder Information Fact Sheet
National Institute of Mental Health
6001 Executive Blvd.
Room 6200, MSC 9663
Bethesda, MD 20892-9663   301-443-4536
                                                        866-615-6464
                                                   Fax: 301-443-4279
                                                   TTY: 301-443-8431
                                                    www.nimh.nih.gov
                                                 nimhinfo@nih.gov
Thomas Insel MD, Director
Marlene Guzman, Senior Advisor to the Director
William Potter, Senior Advisor to the Director
NINDS (National Institute of Neurological Disorders and Stroke) is part of the National Institutes of Health several components of which support research on developmental disorders such as ADHD. Informational fact sheet provides data relative to research, symptons and diagnosis, in addition to links for organizational resources relative to the disorder.

419 National Alliance on Mental Illness (NAMI) Attention-Deficit/Hyperactivity Disorder Fact Sheet
3803 N. Fairfax Drive
Suite 100
Arlington, VA 22203   703-524-7600
                                                        888-999-6264
                                                   Fax: 703-524-9094
                                                   TDD: 703-516-7227
                                                        www.nami.org
                                                     info@nami.org
Jim Payne, J.D., Interim President, First VP
Linda E. Jensen, Second Vice President
Mary Giliberti, J.D., Executive Director

NAMI/National Alliance on Mental Illness is a mental health organization dedicated to improving the lives of persons living with serious mental illness and their families. ADHD fact sheet provides information on attention-deficit/hyperactivity disorder through NAMI's mission of support, education, advocacy, and research for people living with mental illness.

420 Natural Therapies for Attention Deficit Hyperactivity Disorder
Comprehensive Psychiatric Resources, Inc.
203 Crescent Street
Suite 110
Waltham, MA 02453-2741   781-647-0066
                                                   Fax: 781-899-4905
                                              www.integrativepsychmd.com
                                           office@integrativepsychmd.com
James M Greenblatt MD, Director
A full day workshop professionally recorded on six audio-tapes featuring Dr. James M. Greenblatt, M.D., neuropsychiatrist. Dr. Greenblatt explores updated research on nutrition and ADD, food additives, food allergies, fatty acids and more, provides practical treatment strategies and helps you make informed choices between effective and worthless therapies. *$59.95*

421 Nutritional Treatment for Attention Deficit Hyperactivity Disorder
Comprehensive Psychiatric Resources, Inc.
203 Crescent Street
Suite 110
Waltham, MA 02453   781-647-0066
                                                   Fax: 781-899-4905
                                              www.integrativepsychmd.com
                                           office@integrativepsychmd.com
James M Greenblatt MD, Director
A full day workshop professionally recorded on six audio-tapes featuring Dr. James M. Greenblatt, M.D., neuropsychiatrist. Dr. Greenblatt explores updated research on nutrition and ADD, food additives, food allergies, fatty acids and more, provides practical treatment strategies and helps you make informed choices between effective and worthless therapies.

422 Power Parenting for Children with ADD/ADHD A Parent's Guide for Managing Difficult Behaviors
111 River Street
Hoboken, NJ 07030-5774   201-748-6000
                                                   Fax: 201-748-6088
                                                        www.wiley.com
                                                     info@wiley.com
Grad L Flick, Author
A Practical Parent's Guide for Managing Difficult Behaviors. Written in clear, non-technical language, this much-needed guide provides practical, real-life techniques and activities to help parents. *$19.95*
ISBN 0-876288-77-1

423 Putting on the Brakes: Young People's Guide to Understanding ADHD
American Psychological Association
750 First Street Northeast
Washington, DC 20002-4242   202-336-5500
                                                        800-374-2721
                                                   TDD: 202-336-6123
                                                   TTY: 202-336-6123
                                       www.maginationpress.com/4414576.html
                                               executiveoffice@apa.org
Patricia O Quinn, Author
Judith Stern, Co-Author
This book allows children to put their understanding of ADHD into action. Using pictures, puzzles, and other techniques to assist in the learning of a range of skills, this book helps teach problem solving, organizing, setting priorities, planning, maintaining control — all of those hard-to-learn skills that make everyday life just a little more manageable. *$14.95*
ISBN 0-945354-57-6

424   Rethinking Attention Deficit Disorders
Brookline Books
8 Trumbull Rd
Suite B-001
Northampton, MA 01060   413-584-0184
                                          800-666-2665
                                       Fax: 413-584-6184
                                     www.brooklinebooks.com
                                      brbooks@yahoo.com
Susan Sharp, Author
Jonathan Stolzenberg, Author
This ground-breaking work argues that the two behavioral
manifestations of attention deficit disorder—hyperactivity
and impulsivity—represent a person's attempts at self-regulation. The authors view Attention Deficit Disorder as a
problem with control and fluency of attention; people with
ADD have sustaining focus when faced with novel and/or intense stimulae. *$27.95*
272 pages
ISBN 1-571290-37-0

**425   Ritalin Is Not The Answer: A Drug-Free Practical Pro-
gram for Children Diagnosed With ADD or ADHD**
John Wiley & Sons Inc
111 River Street
Hoboken, NJ 07030-5774   201-748-6000
                                       Fax: 201-748-6088
                                          www.wiley.com
                                        info@wiley.com
David P Stein, Author
Ritalin Is Not the Answer confronts and challenges what has
become common practice and teaches parents and educators
a healthy, comprehensive behavioral program that really
works as an alternative to the epidemic use of medication-without teaching children to use drugs in order to handle their behavioral and emotional problems. *$15.00*
Paperback
ISBN 0-787945-14-5

426   Shelley, the Hyperactive Turtle
Woodbine House
6510 Bells Mill Rd
Bethesda, MD 20817-1636   301-897-3570
                                          800-843-7323
                                       Fax: 301-897-5838
                                    www.woodbinehouse.com
                                   info@woodbinehouse.com
Deborah M Moss, Author
Shelley the turtle has a very hard time sitting still, even for
short periods of time. During a visit to the doctor, Shelley
learns that he is hyperactive, and that he can take medicine
every day to control his wiggly feeling. *$14.95*
20 pages Hardcover
ISBN 1-890627-75-5

**427   Stimulant Drugs and ADHD Basic and Clinical Neuro-
science**
Oxford University Press
198 Madison Ave
New York, NY 10016-4308   212-726-6000
                                          800-445-9714
                                       Fax: 919-677-1303
                                        www.oup.com/us
                                     custserv.us@oup.com
Mary Solanto, Editor
This volume is the first to integrate advances in the basic and
clinical neurosciences in order to shed new light on this important question. The chapter topics span basic research into
the neuroanatomy, neurophysiology and neuropsychology
of catecholamines, animal models of ADHD, and clinical
studies of neuroimaging, genetics, pharmacokinetics and
pharmacodynamics, and the cognitive pharmacology of
stimulants. *$81.50*
ISBN 0-195133-71-4

428   The ADD/ADHD Checklist
American Psychiatric Publishing, Inc (APPI)
1000 Wilson Boulevard
Suite 1825
Arlington, VA 22209   703-907-7322
                                          800-368-5777
                                       Fax: 703-907-1091
                                           www.appi.org
                                        appi@psych.org
Robert E Hales, M.D., M.B.A., Editor-in-Chief
Sandra F Rief MA, Author
Rebecca D. Rinehart, Publisher
Written by a nationally known educator with two decades of
experience in working with ADD/ADHD students. This
unique resource is packed with up-to-date facts, findings,
and proven strategies and techniques for understanding and
helping children and adolescents with attention deficit prob-
lems and hyperactivity- all in a handy list format. *$12.95*
Paperback
ISBN 0-137623-95-2

**429   The ADHD Book of Lists: A Practical Guide for Helping
Children and Teens With ADD**
American Psychiatric Publishing, Inc (APPI)
1000 Wilson Boulevard
Suite 1825
Arlington, VA 22209   703-907-7322
                                          800-368-5777
                                       Fax: 703-907-1091
                                           www.appi.org
                                        appi@psych.org
Robert E Hales, M.D., M.B.A., Editor-in-Chief
Sandra F Rief MA, Author
Rebecca D. Rinehart, Publisher
The ADHD Book of Lists is a comprehensive, reliable
source of answers, practical strategies, and tools written in a
convenient list format. Created for teachers (K-12), parents,
school psychologists, medical and mental health professionals, counselors, and other school personnel, this important
resource contains the most current information about Attention Deficit/Hyperactivity Disorder (ADHD). *$29.95*
Paperback
ISBN 0-787965-91-4

430   The Down & Dirty Guide to Adult ADD
Gordon Systems, Inc.
P.O.Box 746
DeWitt, NY 13214-0746   315-446-4849
                                          800-550-ADHD
                                       Fax: 315-446-2012
                                        www.gsi-add.com
                                      info@gsi-add.com
Michael Gordon Ph.D, Author
A book about Adult ADD that is informative, and uncomplicated. Drs. Gordon and McClure spare no effort or humor in
clearly describing concepts essential to understanding how
this disorder is best identified and treated. You'll find a re-
freshing absence of jargon and an abundance of common
sense, practical advice, and healthy skepticism. This fine
brew of scientific evidence and clinical wisdom is so clev-
erly presented that even the most inattentive reader will
breeze through its pages. *$16.95*

**431   The Hidden Disorder: A Clinician's Guide to Attention
Deficit Hyperactivity Disorder in Adults**
American Psychological Association
750 First Street Northeast
Washington, DC 20002-4242   202-336-5500
                                          800-374-2721
                                       Fax: 202-336-5500
                                       TTY: 202-336-6123
                                     www.apa.org/publications
                                     nkaslow@emory.edu
Robert J Resnick PhD, Author

Through accessible writing and engaging case studies, Robert J. Resnick, PhD, provides expert clinical guidance on etiology, differential diagnosis, assessment, and treatment. Adults with ADHD often require intermittent treatment at different points in their lives. This book provides various treatment interventions over the livespan. Also covered are the various co-morbid and look alike disorders that can confound diagnosis and lead to unsuccessful treatment. *$34.95*
Hardcover
ISBN 1-557987-24-2

432   Treating Huckleberry Finn: A New Narrative Approach to Working With Kids Diagnosed ADD/ADHD
John Wiley & Sons Inc
111 River Street
Hoboken, NJ 07030-5774   201-748-6000
                                  Fax: 201-748-6088
                                  www.wiley.com
                                  info@wiley.com
David Nylund, Author
Ritalin Is Not the Answer confronts and challenges what has become common practice and teaches parents and educators a healthy, comprehensive behavioral program that really works as an alternative to the epidemic use of medication-without teaching children to use drugs in order to handle their behavioral and emotional problems. *$32.00*
Paperback
ISBN 0-787961-20-6

433   Understanding and Teaching Children With Autism
John Wiley & Sons Inc
111 River Street
Hoboken, NJ 07030-5774   201-748-6000
                                  Fax: 201-748-6088
                                  www.wiley.com
                                  info@wiley.com
Rita Jordan, Author
Stuart Powell, Co-Author
The triad of impairment: social, language and communication and thought behavior aspects of development discussed. Difficulties in interacting, transfer of learning and bizarre behaviors are part of syndrome. Many LD are associated with autism. *$65.00*
188 pages Paperback
ISBN 0-471957-14-3

434   Understanding and Treating Adults With Attention Deficit Hyperactivity Disorder
American Psychiatric Publishing, Inc (APPI)
1000 Wilson Boulevard
Suite 1825
Arlington, VA 22209   703-907-7322
                               800-368-5777
                               Fax: 703-907-1091
                               www.appi.org
                               appi@psych.org
Robert E Hales, M.D., M.B.A., Editor-in-Chief
Brian B Doyle MD, Author
Rebecca D. Rinehart, Publisher
Understanding the evolution of the concept and treatment of ADHD in children illuminates current thinking about the disorder in adults. Dr. Doyle presents guidelines for establishing a valid diagnosis, including clinical interviews and standardized rating scales. He covers genetic and biochemical bases of the disorder. He also addresses the special challenges of forming a therapeutic alliance-working with coach caregivers; cultural, ethnic, and racial issues; and legal considerations. *$52.00*
Paperback
ISBN 1-585622-21-4

435   What Causes ADHD?: Understanding What Goes Wrong and Why
Guilford Press
72 Spring St
New York, NY 10012-4019   800-365-7006
                                   Fax: 212-966-6708
                                   www.guilford.com
                                   info@guilford.com

Seymour Weingarten, Editor
Joel T Nigg, Author
This book focuses on the multiple pathways by which attention-deficit/ hyperactivity disorder (ADHD) develops. Joel T. Nigg discusses the processes taking place within the symptomatic child's brain and the reasoning for such activity, tracing intersecting causal influences of genetic, neural, and environmental factors. Specific suggestions are provided for studies that might further refine the conceptualization of the disorder, with significant potential benefits for treatment and prevention. *$44.00*
Hardcover
ISBN 1-593852-67-3

436   Why Can't My Child Behave?
Feingold Association of the United States
11849 Suncatcher Drive
Fishers, IN 46037   631-369-9340
                             800-321-3287
                             Fax: 631-369-2988
                             www.feingold.org/book.html
                             janeFAUS@aol.com
Jane Hersey, Author & Director
This book shows how foods and food additives can trigger learning and behavior problems in sensitive people. It provides practical guidance on using a simple diet to uncover the causes of ADD and ADHD. *$22.00*
473 pages Paperback
ISBN 0-965110-50-8

437   You Mean I'm Not Lazy, Stupid or Crazy?
Simon & Schuster, Inc.
1230 Avenue of the Americas
New York, NY 10020-1513   212-698-7000
                                   800-622-6611
                                   Fax: 212-698-7007
                                   www.simonsays.com
Peggy Ramundo, Author
Kate Kelly, Co-Author
This book is written by ADD adults for other ADD adults. A comprehensive guide, it provides accurate information, practical how-to's, and moral support. Among other issues, readers will get information on: unique differences in ADD adults; the impact on their lives; up-to-date research findings; treatment options available for adults; and much more. *$16.00*
464 pages
ISBN 0-743264-48-7

Web Sites

438   www.add.org
Attention Deficit Disorder Association
The National Attention Deficit Disorder Association is an organization focused on the needs of adults and young adults with ADD/ADHD, and their children and families. We seek to serve individuals with ADD, as well as those who love, live with, teach, counsel and treat them.

439   www.addhelpline.org
ADD Helpline for Help with ADD
A site dedicated to providing information and support to all parents, regardless of their choice of treatment, belief or approach toward ADD/ADHD.

440   www.addritudemag.com
Attitude Magazine
Information and inspiration for adults and children with attention deficit disorder.

441   www.addvance.com
ADDvance Online Newsletter
A resource for individuals with ADD and ADHD.

442   **www.addwarehouse.com**
ADD Warehouse
The world's largest collection of ADHD-related books, videos, training programs, games, professional texts and assessment products.

443   **www.adhdnews.com/ssi.htm**
Guidance in applying for Social Security disability benefits on behalf of a child who has ADHD.

444   **www.cec.sped.org**
Council for Exceptional Children
Dedicated to improving educational outcomes for individuals with exceptionalities, students with disabilities, and/or the gifted.

445   **www.chadd.org**
National Resource Center on AD/HD
CHADD works to improve the lives of people affected by AD/HD.

446   **www.childdevelopmentinfo.com**
Child Development Institute
Online information on child development, child psychology, parenting, learning, health and safety as well as childhood disorders such as attention deficit disorder, dyslexia and autism. Provides comprehensive resources and practical suggestions for parents.

447   **www.dyslexia.com**
Davis Dyslexia Association International
Links to internet resources for learning. Includes dyslexia, Autism and Asperger's Syndrome, ADD/ADHD and other learning disabilities.

448   **www.ldonline.org**
LD Online
LD OnLine seeks to help children and adults reach their full potential by providing accurate and up-to-date information and advice about learning disabilities and ADHD. The site features hundreds of helpful articles, monthly columns by noted experts, first person essays, children's writing and artwork, a comprehensive resource guide, very active forums, and a Yellow Pages referral directory of professionals, schools, and products.

449   **www.ncgiadd.org**
National Center for Gender Issues and AD/HD
Offers knowledge and understanding of girls and women with ADHD to improve their lives.

450   **www.nichcy.org**
Nat'l Dissemination Center for Children Disabiliti
Provides information on disabilties in children and youth and programs and services.

451   **www.oneaddplace.com**
One A D D Place
A virtual neighborhood of information and resources relating to ADD, ADHD and learning disorders.

452   **www.therapistfinder.net**
Locate psychologists, psychiatrists, social workers, family counselors, and more specializing in all disorders.

453   **www.webmd.com**
Web MD Health
Medical website with information which includes learning disabilities, ADD/ADHD, etc.

Publications

454 Guide to ACA Accredited Camps
American Camping Association
5000 State Road 67 N
Martinsville, IN 46151-7902

765-342-8456
800-428-2267
Fax: 765-342-2065
TDD: 765-342-8456
www.acacamps.org
badkins@ACAcamps.org

Peg Smith, Chief Executive Officer
Brigitta Adkins, Executive Director
Rhonda Begley, Chief Financial Officer
A national listing of accredited camping programs. Listed by activity, special clientele, camp name, and specific disabilities. *$14.95*
285 pages Annually
ISBN 0-876031-66-1

455 Guide to Summer Programs
Porter Sargent Handbooks
2 LAN Drive
Suite 100
Westford, MA 01886

978-692-5092
800-342-7470
Fax: 978-692-4174
www.carnegiecomm.com
info@carnegiecomm.com

Joe Moore, President/CEO
Meghan Dalesandro, EVP, Operations
Mark Cunningham, SVP, Enrollment Marketing
Covers a broad spectrum of recreational and educational summer opportunities in the US and abroad. Current facts from 1650 camps and schools, as well as programs for those with special needs and disabilities. *$27.00*
960 pages Biannual/Paper
ISBN 9-780875-58-7

456 Resources for Children with Special Needs: Camp Guide
116 E 16th St
Fl 5
New York, NY 10003-2164

212-677-4650
Fax: 212-254-4070
www.resourcesnyc.org
info@resourcesnyc.org

Rachel Howard, Executive Director
Hilda Melendez, Program Manager
Eric Sweeting, Director of Family Support
Resources for Children with Special Needs' Camp Guide, includes new camps, expanding both the range of special needs camps beyond the New York area and the northeast, and the types of disabilities served. It provides up-to-date information on more than 300 camps and programs that provide a wide range of summer activities for children with emotional, developmental, learning and physical disabilities and special needs.

457 Summer Camps for Children with Disabilities
National Dissemination Center for Children
1825 Connecticut Ave NW
Suite 700
Washington, DC 20009

202-884-8200
800-695-0285
Fax: 202-884-8441
TTY: 800-695-0285
www.nichcy.org/pubs/genresc/camps.htm
nichcy@fhi360.org

Suzanne Ripley, Executive Director
Extensive listing of resources available providing information on a variety of summer camps for children with disabilities. Address and contact info in addition to Website links are included.

Alabama

458 Camp ASCCA
Easter Seals of Alabama
P.O.Box 21
5278 Camp ASCCA Dr.
Jacksons Gap, AL 36861-0021

256-825-9226
800-843-2267
Fax: 256-825-8332
www.campascca.org
info@campascca.org

Matt Rickman, Camp Director
Joe Spavone, R.N., Director of Health Services
Allison Wetherbee, Director of Community Relations
Helps children and adults with disabilities achieve equality, dignity and maximum independence. This is to be accomplished through a safe and quality program of camping, recreation and education in a year-round barrier-free environment. Founded 1976.

459 Camp Merrimack
Merrimack Hall Performing Arts Center
3320 Triana Blvd.
Huntsville, AL 35805

256-534-6455
www.merrimackhall.com
adinges@merrimackhall.com

Debra Jenkins, Founder
Ashley Dinges, Consultant
Melissa Reynolds, Program & Operations Director
Performing arts education camp for children ages 3-12 with Autism, Down Syndrome, Cerebral Palsy and cancer.

460 Good Will Easter Seals
2448 Gordon Smith Dr
Mobile, AL 36617-2319

251-471-1581
800-411-0068
Fax: 251-476-4303
TTY: 800-411-0068
www.gesgc.org
bill@gesgc.org

Frank Harkins, President/CEO
John McCain, Chief Operating Officer
Terri Bolin, VP Program Services
Easter Seals camping and recreation programs serve children, adults and families of all abilities. Various programs are available with the united purpose of giving disabled individuals a fun and safe camping or recreational experience. Camperships are available.

Arizona

461 Camp Civitan
Civitan Foundation
5008 N. Civitan Road
Williams, AZ 86046

602-953-2944
Fax: 602-953-2946
www.civitanfoundationaz.com
info@campcivitan.org

Shannon Valenzuela, Chair/Director of Shelter Oper
Randy Ewers, Vice Chairman
Rob Adams, Camp Director
Week-long camp sessions for developmentally disabled children and adults. The camp offers a variety of recreational programs that promote self-esteem, teamwork and socialization.

Arkansas

462   Easter Seals - Adult Services Center

Easter Seals - Arkansas
3920 Woodland Heights Rd
Little Rock, AR 72212-2406
                                        501-227-3600
                                        877-533-3600
                                   Fax: 501-227-7180
                                   TTY: 501-227-3686
                                   www.ar.easter-seals.com
                                   mail@easter-seals.org

Rick Fleetwood, Chairman
Angela Harrison-King, Vice Chairman
Elaine Eubank, President/CEO
Easter Seals camping and recreation programs serve children, adults and families of all abilities. Various programs are available with the united purpose of giving disabled individuals a fun and safe camping or recreational experience.

California

463   Camp Krem: Camping Unlimited

4610 Whitesands Ct
El Sobrante, CA 94803-1820
                                        510-222-6662
                                   Fax: 510-223-3046
                                   www.campingunlimited.com
                                   campkrem@gmail.com

Judy Simmons, President
Alex J. Krem, Treasurer
Mary Farfaglia, Executive Director
Provides year-round, recreation programs for children and adults with disabilities, Down Syndrome, Cerebral Palsy, Autism, wide range of physical/emotional disabilities.

464   Camp ReCreation

2110 Broadway
Sacramento, CA 95818-2518
                                        916-733-0136
                                   Fax: 916-733-0195
                                   http://camprecreation.org
                                   camprec@scd.org

Kathi Barber, Camp Administration
Camp ReCreation is a residential summer camp program for persons with developmental disabilities, offering participants opportunities for fun, social interaction, and spiritual growth while providing valuable respite for parents and care givers. Camp ReCreation is held at Camp Ronald McDonald at Eagle Lake, owned and operated by Ronald McDonald House Charities Northern California and is sponsored by the Catholic Diocese of Sacramento.

465   Camp Ronald McDonald at Eagle Lake

2555 49th St
Sacramento, CA 95817-2306
                                        916-734-4230
                                   Fax: 916-734-4238
                                   www.campronald.org
                                   vflaig@rmhcnc.org

Vicky Flaig MEd RD, Camp Director
Camp Ronald McDonald at Eagle Lake is a fully accessible residential summer camp for children who are at-risk with a variety of special medical needs, economic hardship and/or emotional, developmental or physical disabilities. Traditional camping activities include arts & crafts, hikes, fishing, canoeing, sports, swimming, talent show and campfires.

466   Easter Seals - Bay Area, San Jose

Easter Seals - Bay Area
180 Grand Ave
Ste 300
Oakland, CA 94612-3705
                                        510-835-2131
                                   Fax: 510-444-2340
                                   www.easterseals.com/bayarea
                                   info@easterseals.com.

Susan Armiger, President and CEO
Eric Broque, Chief Financial Officer
Robert Van Tuyl, Chief Operating Officer

Easter Seals camping and recreation programs serve children, adults and families of all abilities. Various programs are available with the united purpose of giving disabled individuals a fun and safe camping or recreational experience.

467   Easter Seals - Northern California

20 Pimentel Ct
Ste A-1
Novato, CA 94949-5656
                                        415-382-7450
                                        800-234-7325
                                   Fax: 415-382-6052
                                   TTY: 415-382-7454
                                   www.easterseals.com
                                   cking@noca.easterseals.com

Richard W. Davidson, Chairman
Sandra L. Bouwman, 1st Vice Chairman
Joseph G. Kern, 2nd Vice Chairman
Easter Seals camping and recreation programs serve children, adults and families of all abilities. arious programs are available with the united purpose of giving disabled individuals a fun and safe camping or recreational experience. The following are camping and recreational services offered: camp respite for adults, camperships, recreational services for adults and recreational services for children. Speech and language therapy and occupational therapy for children ages 0-3.

468   Easter Seals - Northern California, Rohnert Park

5440 State Farm Dr
Rohnert Park, CA 94928
                                        707-584-1443
                                        800-234-7325
                                   Fax: 707-584-3438
                                   TDD: 707-584-1889
                                   TTY: 707-584-1889
                                   www.easterseals.com
                                   skreuzer@ca-no.easter-seals.org

Richard W. Davidson, Chairman
Sandra L. Bouwman, 1st Vice Chairman
Joseph G. Kern, 2nd Vice Chairman
Easter Seals camping and recreation programs serve children, adults and families of all abilities. Various programs are available with the united purpose of giving disabled individuals a fun and safe camping or recreational experience. The folllowing are camping and recreational services offered: Camp respite for adults, camperships, day camping for children, recreational services for children and residential camping programs.

469   Easter Seals - Superior California, Stockton

7273 Murray Dr
Ste 1
Stockton, CA 95210
                                        916-485-6711
                                        888-887-3257
                                   Fax: 916-485-2653
                                   www.superiorca.easterseals.com
                                   info@easterseals.com

Richard W. Davidson, Chairman
Sandra L. Bouwman, 1st Vice Chairman
Joseph G. Kern, 2nd Vice Chairman
Easter Seals camping and recreation programs serve children, adults and families of all abilities. Various programs are available with the united purpose of giving disabled individuals a fun and safe camping or recreational experience. Camping and recreational services offered are: Swim programs.

470   Easter Seals - Tri-Counties California

National Organization of Easter Seals
10730 Henderson Rd
Ventura, CA 93004-1898
                                        805-647-1141
                                   Fax: 805-647-1148
                                   www.easterseals.com
                                   ca-tr.easterseals.com

Richard W. Davidson, Chairman
Sandra L. Bouwman, 1st Vice Chairman
Joseph G. Kern, 2nd Vice Chairman

Easter Seals camping and recreation programs serve children, adults and families of all abilities. Various programs are available with the united purpose of giving disabled individuals a fun and safe camping or recreational experience. Camping and recreational services offered are: Camperships and swim programs.

471   Easterseals Camp Harmon Easter Seals Of Central California
16403 Highway 9
Boulder Creek, CA 95006-9696   831-338-3383
                                       Fax: 831-338-0200
                                       www.campharmon.org
                                       campharmon@es-cc.org
Scott Webb, Director
The following are camping and recreational services offered: Easter Seals own and operated camps and residential camping programs.

472   Grizzly Creek Camp
Easter Seals Northern California
20 Pimentel Court
Suite A-1
Novato, CA 94949   415-382-7450
                                             800-234-7325
                                       www.noca.easterseals.com
                                       kjohnson@noca.easterseals.com
Helen Gale, Manager
Easter Seals camping and recreation programs serve children, adults and families of all abilities. Various programs are available with the united purpose of giving disabled individuals a fun and safe camping or recreational experience. Camperships are available.

473   Kaleidoscope After School Program
Easter Seals - Bay Area
7425 Larkdale Ave
Dublin, CA 94568-1500   925-828-8857
                                       Fax: 925-828-5245
                                       www.easterseals.com
                                       info@easterseals.com
Richard W. Davidson, Chairman
Sandra L. Bouwman, 1st Vice Chairman
Joseph G. Kern, 2nd Vice Chairman
Easter Seals camping and recreation programs serve children, adults and families of all abilities. Various programs are available with the united purpose of giving disabled individuals a fun and safe camping or recreational experience.

474   Via West
2851 Park Ave
Santa Clara, CA 95050-6006   408-243-7861
                                       Fax: 408-243-0452
                                       www.viaservices.org
                                       camp@viaservices.org
Leslie Davis, MA, Chief Executive Officer
Leslie Leger, Vice President of Administration
Jacqueline Forsythe, MBA, Vice President of Advancement
Camp Costanoan is a residential, respite and recreational camp for children and adults, ages 5 and older, with physical and/or developmental disabilities. Camp Costanoan enhances camper self-esteem, improves socialization skills and provide hands-on learning and therapeutic recreation opportunities. Additionally, Camp provides respite for families of individuals with disabilities.

Colorado

475   Rocky Mountain Village Camp
Easter Seals of Colorado
P.O.Box 115
Empire, CO 80438-0115   303-569-2333
                                       Fax: 303-569-3857
                                       www.easterseals.com
                                       kkoev@eastersealscolorado.org

Krasimir Koev, Camp Director
Richard W. Davidson, Chairman
Sandra L. Bouwman, 1st Vice Chairman
Camping and recreational services are: Adventure, camp respite for adults, camp respite for children, camperships, conference rental, family retreats, recreational services for adults, recreational services for children, residential camping programs, swim programs and therapeutic horseback riding.

476   The Learning Camp
P.O.Box 1146
Vail, CO 81658-1146   970-524-2706
                                       Fax: 970-524-4178
                                       www.learningcamp.com
                                       information@learningcamp.com
Ann Cathcart, Director
Summer camp that focuses on helping children with learning disabilities, such as dyslexia, ADD, ADHD and other learning challenges. The Learning Camp provides adventurous summer camp fun for boys and girls ages 7 - 14 combined with carefully designed academic programs. Camp activities include swimming, horseback riding, backpacking, archery, arts and crafts, fishing, canoeing, board games, and Colorado River rafting.

Connecticut

477   Camp Shriver
The ARC Of Greater Enfield
75 Hazard Avenue
Enfield, CT 06082-4001   860-763-5411
                                       www.arcct.com
                                       enfieldarc@sbcglobalnet.com
John Gallacher, Superintendent
Year round recreational programs for children and young adults with cognitive, intellectual and developmental delays.

478   Cyber Launch Pad Camp
Learning Incentive/American School for the Deaf
141 North Main Street
West Hartford, CT 06107-1264   860-236-5807
                                       Fax: 860-233-9945
                                       www.benbronzacademy.org
                                       Inquire@learningincentive.com
Aileen Stan-Spence, Director
Susan Sharp, Ph.D., Education Director
Ian Spence, Ph.D., M.S.W., Executive Director
Half days camp where children and their parents learn to use CyberSlate which is learning keyboarding, word processing, programming and remedial sessions in reading, writing and arithmetic for learning disabled children.

479   Eagle Hill Summer Program
Eagle Hill School
45 Glenville Rd
Greenwich, CT 06831-5331   203-622-9240
                                       Fax: 203-622-0914
                                       www.eaglehillschool.org
                                       info411@eaglehill.org
Nelson Dorta, Director
Brian Dayton, Summer Activities Director
Designed for children experiencing academic difficulty. Open to boys and girls ages 5-11. Some of the programs offered are mathematics, spelling, reading tutorials, writing workshops, oral language, handwriting, and study skills. Students attending the morning classes may also sign up for the Summer Activities Extended Program which is held in the afternoon.

480   Easter Seals - Camp Hemlocks
Easter Seals - Connecticut
85 Jones St
PO Box 198
Hebron, CT 06248-0198   860-228-9496
                                          800-832-4409
                                     Fax: 860-228-2091
                                     TTY: 860-228-2091
                                     www.ct.easterseals.com
                                     campinfo@eastersealsct.org
Sunny Ku, Director
Offers an environment that allows campers with disabilities
optimal independence. Camping and recreational services
are: Aquatics, Family Camp, Recreational Services for
Adults and Children, Residential Camping Programs, Ad-
venture/Traveling Program.

481   Horizons, Inc.
127 Babcock Hill Road
P.O. Box 323
South Windham, CT 06266-0323   860-456-1032
                                     Fax: 860-456-4721
                                     www.horizonsct.org
                                     staffpage@camphorizons.org
Adam Milne, Board Chairman
Chris Mcnaboe, Board President
Kathleen Mcnaboe, Board Vice President
The mission of Horizons is to provide high quality residen-
tial, recreational support and work programs for people who
have developmental disabilties or who have other challeng-
ing social and emotional needs.

482   Our Victory Day Camp
46 Vineyard Ln
Stamford, CT 06902-1112   203-329-3394
                                          800-329-3394
                                     Fax: 203-569-6171
                                     www.ourvictory.com/
                                     ourvictory@aol.com
Fred Tunick, Executive Director
Our Victory Day Camp is a 7-week day camping program for
children from 5 to 12 years of age. It is oriented toward children with learning disabilities and/or attention deficit disorder. The program is designed to expose each camper to a
wide variety of activities. The goal is to create an opportunity for each camper to achieve success, whatever the
camper's ability. Activities include arts and crafts, drama,
music, nature, dancing, hiking, jewelry making, swimming,
and sports.

483   Summer Day Programs
Middletown Parks and Recreation Department
100 Riverview Ctr
Suite 140
Middletown, CT 06457-3401   860-343-6620
                                     Fax: 860-344-3319
                                     www.cityofmiddletown.com
                                     john.milardo@cityofmiddletown.com
Raymond Santostefano, Director
These camps offer a variety of recreational and social activi-
ties. Each camp will be integrated with at least 12% popula-
tion of children with disabilities. Campers must be
Middletown residents.

484   Timber Trails Camps
Connecticut Valley Girl Scout Council
340 Washington St
Hartford, CT 06106-3317   860-522-0163
                                          800-922-2770
                                     Fax: 860-548-0325
                                     www.gsofct.org
                                     camp@gsofct.org
Theresa Miller, Camp Director
All girls age 6 to 17 who can function in a group in a mainstream environment are welcome, including those with
chronic illnesses, learning disabilities, and physical or emotional needs.

485   Valley-Shore YMCA
201 Spencer Plains Road
P.O. Box 694
Westbrook, CT 06498-0694   860-399-9622
                                     Fax: 860-399-8349
                                     www.vsymca.org
                                     vsymca@vsymca.org
Lenny Goldberg, 1st Vice President/Treasurer
John Duhig, Secretary
Chris Pallatto, CEO/Executive Director
Family Play Dates, an adaptive recreation program designed
for special language need children ages 3-7 years. (Perva-
sive Developmental Disorder and high functioning Autism,
Asperger's, Down Syndrome). Daycamp with swimming,
hiking, sports, games, nature study, archery and low ropes
course.

486   Wheeler Regional Family YMCA
149 Farmington Avenue
149 Farmington Ave.
Plainville, CT 06062   860-793-9631
                                     www.ghymca.org
                                     wheeler.membership@ghymca.org
Michelle Hill, Director
The Wheeler Regional Family YMCA is a non-profit chari-
table community organization. The YMCA provides a wide
variety of programs for all ages. The YMCA's main pro-
grams include Child Care, Aquatic Programs, Day Camp,
Teen programs, Wellness and Fitness Programs. The
Wheeler Regional Family YMCA serves Plainville, Bristol,
Farmington, Burlington and Plymouth.

487   Winston Prep School Summer Program
57 West Rocks Road
Norwalk, CT 06851-2213   203-229-0465
                                     www.winstonprep.edu
                                     ctopenhouse@winstonprep.edu
Scott Bezsylko, Executive Director
Stephanie Mori, Director
For 6th through 12th grade students with learning differences such as dyslexia, nonverbal learning disabilities, expressive or receptive language disorders and attention
deficit problems. The Summer Enrichment Program at their
New York City branch school is designed to enhance academic skills. Students from area parochial, public and private schools attend the program every year. They receive
daily one-on-one instruction in addition to attending class in
the courses they have selected.

Florida

488   3D Learner Program
3D Learner, Inc.
7100 W. Camino Real
Suite 215
Boca Raton, FL 33433-7049   561-361-7495
                                          561-361-7497
                                     Fax: 954-796-3883
                                     www.3dlearner.com
                                     parents@3dlearner.com
Mira Stulberg-Halpert M.Ed, Educational Director
Julie Halpert, Lead Trainer
Mark Halpert, Director
3D Learner Program, a one-week program for struggling students who learn best when they see and experience information. We have had students from all over the US. We address
attention, self esteem and reading with a natural and effective method. Our students make immediate gains and often
see significant gains with 3 months. Free learning survey
and 10 minute consult. Also speak toparents and
professionals.

489 Camp Challenge
Easter Seals Florida
31600 Camp Challenge Rd
Sorrento, FL 32776-9729
352-383-4711
800-377-3257
Fax: 321-383-0744
www.fl.easterseals.com/campchallenge
camp@fl.easter-seals.com
Susan Ventura, CEO
Suzanne Caporina, Primary Contact
At Easter Seals Camp Challenge, campers participate in arts & crafts, nature activities, a universal high and low ropes course, music and dancing, outside entertainers, farm animals and other camp activities.

490 Camp Kavod
Adolph & Rose Levis Jewish Community Center
9801 Donna Klein Blvd
Boca Raton, FL 33428-1755
561-852-3200
www.levisjcc.org/special-needs/camp-kavo
mariannej@levisjcc.org
Andrea Platt, Director
Marianne Jacobs, Director
Programs at the Center preserve and strengthen Jewish continuity by enriching personal, cultural, social and physical development. The Center shall foster leadership, enhance education, create a neighborhood of commonality for Jews of all beliefs, promote the welfare of the Jewish community and the community as a whole, and affirm the significance of the State of Israel.

491 Camp Thunderbird
909 E Welch Road
Apopka, FL 32712
407-889-8088
888-807-8378
Fax: 407-889-8072
www.questinc.org
rcage@questinc.org
Dustin Schwab, Interim Director
Rosa Figueroa, LPN, Site Coordinator
Since 1969, Quest's Camp Thunderbird has been dedicated to providing a real summer camp experience for people with special needs. Because of the physical and behavioral challenges associated with Down syndrome, autism, Cerebral Palsy and other developmental disabilities, these children and adults aren't typically eligible to attend traditional camps. Quest's Camp Thunderbird is their chance to learn new skills and focus on the remarkable things they can do, while making new friends and unforgett

492 Easter Seals - Florida
2010 Mizell Ave
Winter Park, FL 32792-2405
407-629-4565
Fax: 407-644-7373
www.fl.easterseals.com
Susan Ventura, President and CEO
Gladys Epps, CFO/COO
Rob Porcaro, Senior VP of Operations
Easter Seals camping and recreation programs serve children, adults and families of all abilities. Various programs are available with the united purpose of giving disabled individuals a fun and safe camping or recreational experience. Camping and recreational services are: Day camping for children.

Georgia

493 Camp Hollywood
FOCUS
3825 Presidential Parkway
Suite 103
Atlanta, GA 30340
770-234-9111
Fax: 770-234-9131
www.focus-ga.org
inquiry@focus-ga.org
Saxon Dasher, President
Lucy Cusick, Executive Director
Joy Trotti, Associate Director

Unique camp for children with developmental delays, neurological involvement, cerebral palsy, heart problems and immune deficiencies. Campers enjoy art projects and games. FOCUS also hosts Camp TEAM and Camp Infinity.

494 Easter Seals - Southern Georgia
1906 Palmyra Rd
Albany, GA 31701-1598
229-439-7061
800-365-4583
Fax: 229-435-6278
www.southerngeorgia.easterseals.com
benglish@swga-easterseals.org
Beth English, CEO & Executive Director
Matt Hatcher, Chief Operating Officer
Amanda Hobbs, Director of Human Resources
Easter Seals camping and recreation programs serve children, adults and families of all abilities. Various programs are available with the united purpose of giving disabled individuals a fun and safe camping or recreational experience. Camping and recreational services offered are: Camp respite for adults, camp respite for children, day camping for children and therapeutic horseback riding.

495 United Cerebral Palsy Of Georgia
3300 Northeast Expy NE
Building 9
Atlanta, GA 30341
770-676-2000
888-827-9455
Fax: 770-455-8040
www.ucp.org
info@ucpga.org
Stephen Bennett, President and CEO
Diane Wilush, Executive Director
Laura Heise, CPA, Director of Finance
UCP offers afterschool programs that help to develop cognitive, motors, language and communication skills, while fostering self-image and independence.

Hawaii

496 Easter Seals Hawaii - Oahu Service Center
710 Green St
Honolulu, HI 96813-2119
808-536-1015
888-241-7450
Fax: 808-536-3765
www.eastersealshawaii.org
info@eastersealshawaii.org
Christopher Blanchard, President and CEO
Esther Underwood, VP of Human Resources
Iwalani Dayton, VP, Development
Easter Seals camping and recreation programs serve children, adults and families of all abilities. Various programs are available with the united purpose of giving disabled individuals a fun and safe camping or recreational experience. Camping and recreational services offered are: Residential camping programs.

Idaho

497 SUWS Wilderness Program
Aspen Education Group
911 Preacher Creek Rd
Shoshone, ID 83352-5061
208-886-2565
888-879-7897
Fax: 208-886-2153
www.suws.com
Kathy Rex, CTRS, Executive Director
Programs specialize in helping troubled teens and defiant teens with behavioral and emotional problems. Operating in southern Idaho since 1981, SUWS wilderness programs have assisted young people to identify and work through internal conflicts and emotional obstacles that have kept them from responding to parental efforts, schools, and treatment.

Illinois

498   Camp Free To Be
UCP Easter Seals In Southwestern Illinois
2730 North Center
Maryville, IL 62067   618-288-2218
                                          Fax: 618-288-2249
www.ucpheartland.org/services/illinois-s
plunkf@ucpheartland.org
Stephen Bennett, President and CEO
Connie Garner, Executive Vice President
Michael E. Hill, Senior Vice President
Day camp for ages 5-12 with disabilities and their siblings.
Activities include picnicking, swimming, fishing, outdoor
games, and arts & crafts.

**499   Camp Little Giant: Touch of Nature Environmental
Center**
Southern Illinois University
1208 Touch of Nature Rd
Carbondale, IL 62901   618-453-5348
                                          Fax: 618-453-1188
                                          http://ton.siu.edu
                                          tonec@siu.edu
Randy Osborn, Program Coordinator
A residential camp program designed to meet the recreational needs of adults and children with disabilities. The
programs are designed for individuals with physical/devel-
opmental disabilities, visual & hearing impairments, mus-
cular dystrophy, cerebral palsy, autism, ADD/ADHD,
traumatic brain injury and special needs.

500   Camp Timber Pointe
Easter Seals Central Illinois
20 Timber Pointe Lane
Hudson, IL 61748   309-365-8021
                                          Fax: 309-365-8934
                                          http://ci.easterseals.com
Steven Thompson, President & CEO
Seshadri Guha, Chair
Brad Halverson, Vice Chairman
Camping and respite program for children and adults ages 7
& up with disabilities or special needs and their families.
Campers can participate in recreational activities susch as
fishing, boating, swimming, music, sports, horseback riding
and arts and crafts.

501   Easter Seals - Camping & Recreation List
National Easter Seals Society
233 S Wacker Dr
Ste 400
Chicago, IL 60606-4851   800-221-6827
                                          TTY: 312-726-4258
                                          info@easter-seals.com
James E Williams Jr, CEO
Various programs with the united purpose of giving disabled
children a fun and safe camping or recreational experience.
Call for information on activities in your state.

502   Easter Seals - Central Illinois
Easter Seals Peoria & Bloomington-Normal & Decatur
2715 N 27th St
Decatur, IL 62526-2171   217-429-1052
                                          Fax: 217-423-7605
                                          www.easterseals-ci.org
Steven Thompson, CEO
Seshadri Guha, Chair
Brad Halverson, Vice Chairman
Easter Seals camping and recreation programs serve chil-
dren, adults and families of all abilities. Various programs
are available with the united purpose of giving disabled individuals a fun and safe camping or recreational experience.
The following are Camping and Recreational services offered: Recreational services for adults and recreational
services for children.

503   Easter Seals - Joliet
Easter Seals Joliet Region, Inc.
212 Barney Dr
Regional Pediatric Center and Corporate
Joliet, IL 60435-2830   815 725 2194
                                          Fax: 815-725-5150
                                          www.joliet.easterseals.com
dcondotti@il-wg.easter-seals.org
Debbie Condotti, CEO
Deb Shimanis, Chairman
Wayne Chesson, Vice Chairman
Easter Seals camping and recreation programs serve chil-
dren, adults and families of all abilities. Various programs
are available with the united purpose of giving disabled indi-
viduals a fun and safe camping or recreational experience.
The following are camping and recreational services
offered: Camperships.

504   Easter Seals - UCP, Peoria
Easter Seals of Peoria Bloomington
507 E Armstrong Ave
Peoria, IL 61603-3197   309-686-1177
                                          Fax: 306-686-7722
                                          www.ci.easterseals.com
Steven Thompson, CEO
Seshadri Guha, Chair
Brad Halverson, Vice Chairman
Easter Seals camping and recreation programs serve chil-
dren, adults and families of all abilities. Various programs
are available with the united purpose of giving disabled indi-
viduals a fun and safe camping or recreational experience.
The following are Camping and Recreational services offered: Recreational services for adults and recreational
services for children.

505   Jayne Shover Center
Easter Seals DuPage and the Fox Valley Region
799 S McLean Blvd
Elgin, IL 60123-6704   847-742-3264
                                          Fax: 847-742-9436
                                          www.dfvr.easterseals.com
                                          admin@il-js.easterseals.com
Theresa Forthofer, President/CEO
Erik Johnson, Vice President of Development
Kathy Schrock, VP of Clinical Services
Easter Seals camping and recreation programs serve chil-
dren, adults and families of all abilities. Various programs
are available with the united purpose of giving disabled individuals a fun and safe camping or recreational experience.
The following are Camping and Recreational services offered: Recreational services for adult and recreational
services for children.

Indiana

506   Easter Seals - ARC of Northeast Indiana
4919 Coldwater Rd
Fort Wayne, IN 46825-5532   260-456-4534
                                          800-234-7811
                                          Fax: 260-745-5200
                                          http://neindiana.easterseals.com
                                          damstutz@esarc.org
Donna K. Elbrecht, President/CEO
Susan K. Klug, Chief Operating Officer
Misty Woltman, CFO/Controller
Easter Seals camping and recreation programs serve children, adults and families of all abilities. Various programs
are available with the united purpose of giving disabled individuals a fun and safe camping or recreational experience.
The following are recreational services of-
fered: Recreational services for adults and camp respite for
adults and children.

507 Easter Seals - Crossroads
4740 Kingsway Dr
Indianapolis, IN 46205-1521
317-466-1000
Fax: 317-466-2000
TTY: 317-479-3232
www.eastersealscrossroads.org
J. Patrick Sandy, President/CEO
Susan Saunders, CFO/Security Officer
Angela Danner, Director, Human Resources
Easter Seals camping and recreation programs serve children, adults and families of all abilities. Various programs are available with the united purpose of giving disabled individuals a fun and safe camping or recreational experience. The following are camping and recreational services offered: Camperships and recreational services for children.

Iowa

508 Camp Albrecht Acres
14837 Sherrill Road
P.O. Box 50
Sherrill, IA 52073
563-552-1771
Fax: 563-552-2732
www.albrechtacres.org
info@albrechtacres.org
Deb Rahe, Executive Director
Heidi Zwack Goin, President
Terry Mozena, Vice President
For children with special needs. Activities include cookouts, swimming, fishing, hay wagon rides, volleyball, dances and arts and crafts.

509 Camp Sunnyside
Easter Seals Of Iowa
401 NE 66th Ave
Des Moines, IA 50313-1243
515-289-1933
Fax: 515-289-1281
TTY: 515-289-4069
www.ia.easterseals.com
clecroy@eastersealsia.org
Sherri Nielsen, President/CEO
Krable Mentzer, Chief Development Officer
Kevin Small, Chief Financial Officer
Easter Seals camping and recreation programs serve children, adults and families of all abilities. Various programs are available with the united purpose of giving disabled individuals a fun and safe camping or recreational experience. The following are Camping and Recreational services offered: Adventure, camp respite for children, day camping for children, easter seals own and operated camps and residential camping programs.

Louisiana

510 Camp Without Barriers
Easter Seals Of Louisiana
1010 Common Street
Suite 2000
New Orleans, LA 70112-2411
504-523-3465
800-695-7325
Fax: 504-523-3465
www.louisiana.easterseals.com
Tracy Garner, President/CEO
Donald Cowdin, Sr. Vice President
Ddawn Huber, Vice President
A non-profit, community-based health agency whose mission is to help children and adults with disabilities achieve independence through a variety of programs and services. Campers enjoy boating, nature walks, swimming, arts & crafts and campfire sing-a-longs.
1951

511 Easter Seals - Louisiana
New Orleans Corporate Office
1010 Common St
Ste 2000
New Orleans, LA 70112-2411
504-523-7325
800-695-7325
Fax: 504-523-3465
www.louisiana.easterseals.com
info@easterseals.org
Tracy Garner, President/CEO
Donald Cowdin, Sr. Vice President
Ddawn Huber, Vice President
Easter Seals camping and recreation programs serve children, adults and families of all abilities. Various programs are available with the united purpose of giving disabled individuals a fun and safe camping or recreational experience. The following are camping and recreational services offered: Camperships.

Maryland

512 Camp Fairlee Manor
Easter Seals of Delaware-Maryland
Fairlee Manor Recreation/Education
22242 Bay Shore Road
Chestertown, MD 21620
410-778-0566
Fax: 410-778-0567
www.easterseals.com
contact@esdel.org
Richard W. Davidson, Chairman
Sandra L. Bouwman, 1st Vice Chairman
Joseph G. Kern, 2nd Vice Chairman
For children with physical disabilities and/or cognitive impairments. Activities include arts & crafts, sports, games, nature walks, fishing, swimming and much more.

513 Kamp A-Kom-plish
9035 Ironsides Rd
Nanjemoy, MD 20662-3432
301-870-3226
Fax: 301-870-2620
www.melwoodrecreation.org
recreation@melwood.org
Michael Glanz, VP, Community Services
Doria Fleisher, Associate Director, Recreation
Hannah Rutt, Travel Coordinator
A sleep-away camp for for children and teens aged 8 to 16 years old. Located on 108 acres there are air-conditioned cabins, fishing, boating and trails for hiking. We welcome children with a variety of disabilities, such as developmental, physical and emotional however we are not able to support children with extreme behavioral issues or intense medical needs.

Massachusetts

514 Bridges To Independence Programs
The Bridge Center
470 Pine Street
Bridgewater, MA 02324-2112
508-697-7557
Fax: 508-697-1529
www.thebridgectr.org
info@TheBridgeCtr.og
Tom Walsh, President
Neal Andelman, First Vice President
Andrew Musto, Second Vice President
Program offers teens and young adults the skills necessary for independent living and vocational success, as well as structured social and recreational opportunities

515 Camp Connect
The Bridge Center
470 Pine Street
Bridgewater, MA 02324-2112
508-697-7557
Fax: 508-697-1529
www.thebridgectr.org
info@TheBridgeCtr.org

Tom Walsh, President
Neal Andelman, First Vice President
Andrew Musto, Second Vice President
Camp for children and teens with high functioning Autism and Asperger's Syndrome. The programs offers to help support social skills and thinking development and practice.

516 **Camp Discovery**
The Bridge Center
470 Pine Street
Bridgewater, MA 02324   508-697-7557
                               Fax: 508-697-1529
                               www.thebridgectr.org
                               info@TheBridgeCtr.org
Tom Walsh, President
Neal Andelman, First Vice President
Andrew Musto, Second Vice President
For campers with intellectual and developmental disabilities who benefit from extensive or pervasive support. Campers have access to all activities and also have staff support with daily living activities.

517 **Camp Endeavor**
The Bridge Center
470 Pine Street
Bridgewater, MA 02324   508-697-7557
                               Fax: 508-697-1529
                               www.thebridgectr.org
                               info@TheBridgeCtr.org
Tom Walsh, President
Neal Andelman, First Vice President
Andrew Musto, Second Vice President
For children and adolescents with learning, intellectual and developmental disabilities. The program offers campers the chance to meet new people, try new activities and feel successfull.

518 **Camp Joy**
Boston Centers for Youth & Families
1483 Tremont St
Boston, MA 02120-2908   617-635-4920
                               Fax: 617-635-4524
                               TTY: 617-635-5041
                               www.cityofboston.gov/bcyf
                               BCYF@cityofboston.gov
Daphne Griffin, Executive Director
A therapeutic recreational program for special needs children and adults. Currently serving over 700 participants with a professionally qualified staff of 290 at 15 sites throughout the city. Serves the physically and cognitively challenged, multi-handicapped, behaviorally involved, legally blind/visually impaired, deaf/hearing impaired, learning disabled, and pre-school special needs children.

519 **Camp Lapham**
119 Myrtle Street
Duxbury, MA 02332   781-834-2700
                               Fax: 781-834-2701
                               www.crossroads4kids.org
                               samantha@crossroads4kids.org
Kevin Phelan, Chair of the Board
Deb Samuels, President
Malcolm Huckaby, Board Governance Co-Chair
Designed to meet the needs of children who thrive in a small, structured environment. The program emphasis includes anger and behavior management, along with strong self-image building all in a fun, noncompetitive camp atmosphere. With a maximum of 50 children enrolled per session and a low camper to counselor ratio of 1 to 4, the campers experience success in a more family-like atmosphere which enables each child to focus on personal goals and nonviolent methods of interaction.

520 **Camp Ramah**
2 Commerce Way
Norwood, MA 02062-3056   781-702-5290
                               Fax: 781-702-5239
                               www.campramahne.org
                               info@campramahne.org

Rabbi Ed Gelb, Director
Josh Edelglass, Assistant Director
Young people have fun while developing skills, strong friendships and a Jewish conciousness that lasts a lifetime through a variety of experiences such as sports, nature, music, arts and crafts, boating, study, Shabbat and Judaica. Campers have developmental disabilities. Some campers with LD are included in typical divisions.

521 **Camp Starfish**
1121 Main Street
Lancaster, MA 01523   978-368-6580
                               Fax: 978-368-6578
                               www.campstarfish.org
                               info@campstarfish.org
Dr. Alisha Pollastri, PhD, Co-President
Carrie Endries, Co-President
Bryn Dunn, Treasurer
Year round camp for children and young adults with ADHD, Aspergers, behavioral issues and learning disabilities. The focus is on teaching the children how to interact appropriately in a soocial group, and work on individual goals, while developing self-esteem and self-confidence.

522 **Camp Summit**
The Bridge Center
470 Pine Street
Bridgewater, MA 02324   508-697-7557
                               Fax: 508-697-1529
                               www.thebridgectr.org
                               info@TheBridgeCtr.org
Tom Walsh, President
Neal Andelman, First Vice President
Andrew Musto, Second Vice President
For children and adolescents ages 4-22 who struggle with behavior control.

523 **Creative Expressions Program**
The Bridge Center
470 Pine St
Bridgewater, MA 02324-2112   508-697-7557
                               Fax: 508-697-1529
                               www.bridgectr.org
                               info@TheBridgeCtr.org
Mary Gallant, Director
Visual and performing arts, music, drama and dance. Children learn how to express themselves with art specific skills.

524 **Crossroads for Kids**
119 Myrtle St
Duxbury, MA 02332-2903   781-834-2700
                               888-543-7284
                               Fax: 781-834-2701
                               www.crossroads4kids.org
                               samantha@crossroads4kids.org
Kevin Phelan, Chair of the Board
Deb Samuels, President
Malcolm Huckaby, Board Governance Co-Chair
The daily programs provide a good balance between active and quiet, sport, cultural, group and individual activities. We place campers into smaller, age appropriate groups so they receive the extra support, care and encouragement they need to feel at home here at camp.

525 **Explorer Camp**
Easter Seals Massachusetts
484 Main St
Worcester, MA 01608-1893   800-244-2756
                               Fax: 508-831-9768
                               TTY: 800-564-9700
                               www.eastersealsma.org
                               camp@eastersealsma.org
Colleen Flanagan, Camp & Youth Leadership Manager
Kirk Joslin, CEO
Thomas Sanglier II, Chairman

The following are camping and recreational services offered: Camp respite for adults, camp respite for children, canoeing, computer camp, computer program, day camping for children, residential camping programs, sailing, swim programs, therapeutic horseback riding and water skiing.

526 Handi Kids Camp
The Bridge Center
470 Pine Street
Bridgewater, MA 02324-2112   508-697-7557
                                     Fax: 508-697-1529
                                     www.thebridgectr.org
                                     info@TheBridgeCtr.org

Tom Walsh, President
Neal Andelman, First Vice President
Andrew Musto, Second Vice President
Handi Kids is a non-profit, recreational facility for children and young adults with physical and cognitive disabilities. Handi Kids provides therapeutic recreation to hundreds of individuals on a year-round basis, the goal of which is to benefit each child emotionally, physically and socially while helping those who require individualized attention and guidance enjoy and participate in recreational activities.

527 Hillside School Summer Program
404 Robin Hill Road
Marlborough, MA 01752-1099   508-485-2824
                                     Fax: 508-485-4420
                                     www.hillsideschool.net
                                     admissions@hillsideschool.net
David Beecher, Director
Hillside School is an independent boarding and day school for boys, grades 5-9. Hillside provides educational and residential services to boys needing to develop their academic and social skills while building self-confidence and maturity. The 200-acre school is located in a rural section of Marlborough and includes a working farm. Hillside accommodates both traditional learners who want a more personalized education, and those boys with learning difficulties and/or attention problems.

528 Hippotherapy Camp Program
The Bridge Center
470 Pine Street
Bridgewater, MA 02324-2112   508-697-7557
                                     Fax: 508-697-1529
                                     www.thebridgectr.org
                                     info@TheBridgeCtr.org

Tom Walsh, President
Neal Andelman, First Vice President
Andrew Musto, Second Vice President
Occupational & Physical Therapists use horseback activities to help clients meet individual clinical goals such as mobility, strength, improved gait & balance, endurance and independence. The center also offers Therapeutic Riding which helps to improve posture, balance, communication & sensory processing. The Therapeutic Carriage Driving program allows those who do not ride horses the opportunity to sit with their instructor and learn how to control a horse when it is pulling a carriage.

529 Horse Camp
The Bridge Center
470 Pine Street
Bridgewater, MA 02324   508-697-7557
                                     Fax: 508-687-1529
                                     www.thebridgectr.org
                                     info@TheBridgeCtr.org

Tom Walsh, President
Neal Andelman, First Vice President
Andrew Musto, Second Vice President
For ages 8 and up who love to ride horses. The camp offers riding center activities and mounted riding lessons.

530 Landmark School Summer Boarding Program
Landmark School
429 Hale Street
P.O. Box 227
Prides Crossing, MA 01965   978-236-3216
                                     Fax: 978-921-7268
                                     www.landmarkoutreach.org
                                     admission@landmarkschool.org
Robert Broudo, President and Headmaster
Mark R. Brislin, Vice President
Dan Ahearn, Director
Our Summer Program accepts boys and girls age 7-20, in grades 1-12, who possess average to superior intelligence, a history of healthy emotional development, and have been diagnosed with a language-based learning disability. Landmark's Summer Boarding Program excels at providing a safe, fun, and exciting summer experience.

531 Landmark Summer Program: Exploration and Recreation
429 Hale Street
P.O. Box 227
Prides Crossing, MA 01965   978-236-3010
                                     Fax: 978-927-7268
                                     www.landmarkschool.org
                                     admission@landmarkschool.org
Robert Broudo, President and Headmaster
Mark R. Brislin, Vice President
David Seiter, Director of Facilities
For students in grades 3-6, Landmark's Exploration Program provides the opportunity to combine a half-day of academic classes with a half-day Marine Science/Adventure Ropes experience. Students entering grades 1-5 may choose the Recreation Program which combines a half-day of academics with an afternoon of recreational activities. Both programs provide intensive academic study for students with language-based learning disabilities, and daily one-to-one tutorials.

532 Landmark Summer Program: Marine Science
429 Hale Street
P.O. Box 227
Prides Crossing, MA 01965   978-236-3010
                                     Fax: 978-927-7268
                                     www.landmarkschool.org
                                     admission@landmakrschool.org
Robert Broudo, President and Headmaster
Mark R. Brislin, Vice President
David Seiter, Director of Facilities
Landmark's Marine Science Summer Program enrolls students in grades 7-12, who have been diagnosed with a language-based learning disability, and are interested in marine studies. Students spend half the day exploring local coastal ecosystems, working on research teams and collecting data. The other half of the day is spent developing their language skills in an academic classroom setting and in one-to-one tutorial sessions.

533 Landmark Summer Program: Musical Theater
429 Hale Street
P.O. Box 227
Prides Crossing, MA 01965   978-236-3010
                                     Fax: 978-927-7268
                                     www.landmarkschool.org
                                     admission@landmarkschool.org
Robert Broudo, President and Headmaster
Mark R. Brislin, Vice President
David Seiter, Director of Facilities
Landmark's new Musical Theater program gives students the opportunity to perform on stage or develop technical theater skills behind-the-scenes. The class culminates in a full-scale theatrical production at the end of six weeks. On-stage performers learn to act, dance, and sing as part of a musical company. Technical theater students try their hand at set-design and building, sound and lighting, and produce the summer's musical production.

534 Linden Hill School & Summer Program
154 S Mountain Rd
Northfield, MA 01360-9701   413-498-2906
                                    Fax: 413-498-2908
                                    www.lindenhs.org/
                                    office@lindenhs.org
James Mc Daniel, Headmaster
The Linden Hill Summer Program provides a balance of academic work and traditional camp experiences. Support and remdiation is offered through a multi-sensory approach to language training based in the renowned and clinically-proven Orton-Gillingham method. Honesty, integrity and pride in their success are goals for each of our participants. Linden Hill has hundreds of acres of fields, woods, ponds and streams, as well as a comfortable dormitory lodging and healthy, delicious home-cooked meals.

535 Moose Hill Nature Day Camp
293 Moose Hill Street
Sharon, MA 02067   781-784-5691
                                    www.massaudubon.org
                                    moosehillcamp@massaudubon.org
Henry Tepper, President
Bancroft Poor, Vice President
Kay Andberg, Camp Director
Nature Day Camp is a welcoming environment with fewer than one hundred campers in each weekly session. The goal is to educate children and enrich their lives through outdoor exploration, focused activities, games, hikes, and crafts. Most weeks include special visitors and camp-wide theme days. The camp day runs from 9 a.m. to 3 p.m. with before and after camp programs available. The camp uses the Nature Center of Moose Hill Wildlife Sanctuary as its base.

536 Patriots' Trail Girl Scout Council Summer Camp
95 Berkeley St
Boston, MA 02116-6239   617-350-8335
                                    800-882-1662
                                    Fax: 617-482-9045
                                    TDD: 800-882-1662
                                    www.ptgirlscouts.org/properties_camps/
                                    info@ptgirlscouts.org
Elizabeth Stevenson,, President
Mary Shapiro, First Vice Chair
Dawn Morris, Second Vice Chair
Canoeing, swimming, windsurfing, life-saving, sailing, biking and trips.

537 Summer@Carroll
The Carroll School
25 Baker Bridge Rd
Lincoln, MA 01773-3199   781-259-8342
                                    Fax: 781-259-8842
                                    www.carrollschool.org
                                    summer@carrollschool.org
Stephen Wilkins, Headmaster
Sam Foster, Chair
Josh Levy, Co-Vice Chair
Summer at Carroll is designed to offer academic intervention and remediation to children diagnosed with primary language learning difficulties, such as dyslexia. Small group teaching, individualized instruction and attention to the needs of goals of the students are what Carroll prides themselves on.

538 The Drama Play Connection, Inc.
298 Crescent St
Waltham, MA 02453-3803   781-899-1160
                                    Fax: 781-899-1180
                                    www.dramaplayconnection.com
                                    info@dramaplayconnection.com
Liana P Morgens, Ph.D., President
Sean Hyde O'Brien, Psy.D., Board Member
Carol Singer, Ed.D., Board Member

The Summer Pragmatic Language Drama Program serves primarily children and adolescents with Asperger's Disorder, Nonverbal Learning Disabilities, and those with related social pragmatic difficulties. The pragmatic program is designed to help children acquire the skills necessary to function more competently with their peers. The program includes drama curriculum that focuses on teaching nonverbal language skills through the use of improvisation and other drama techniques.

539 The Kolburne School Summer Program
Kolburne School
343 NM Southfield Rd
New Marlborough, MA 01230-2035   413-229-8787
                                    Fax: 413-229-4165
                                    www.kolburne.net
                                    info@kolburne.net
Jeane K Weinstein, Executive Director
A family operated residential treatment center located in the Berkshire Hills of Massachusetts. Through integrated treatment services, effective behavioral management, recreational programming, and positive staff relationships, our students develop the emotional stability, interpersonal skills and academic/vocational background necessary to return home with success.

Michigan

540 Adventure Learning Center at Eagle Village
4507 170th Ave
Hersey, MI 49639-8785   231-832-2234
                                    800-748-0061
                                    Fax: 231-832-1729
                                    www.eaglevillage.org
                                    info@eaglevillage.org
Pauk Liabenow, Chair & Ambassador
James Giroux, Secretary and Ambassador
Merle Ross, Treasurer & Ambassador
Adventure Learning Center at Eagle Village offers a variety of fun camp experiences for any child, including those with emotional and/or behavioral impairments. Challenging activities make the camps rewarding experiences.

541 Camp Barefoot
The Fowler Center For Outdoor Learning
2315 Harmon Lake Road
Mayville, MI 48744   989-673-2050
                                    Fax: 989-673-6355
                                    www.thefowlercenter.org
                                    director@thefowlercenter.org
Jack Fowler, Chairman/Founder
Kyle L. Middleton, CTRS, Executive Director
Lynn M. Seeloff, CTRS, Assistant Director
Specifically designed for teens and young adults age 18 and older with traumatic brain injuries or closed head injuries. Campers can request their daily activities.

542 Children's Therapy Programs
Easter Seals - Michgan, Inc.
2399 E. Walton Avenue
Auburn Hills, MI 48326-4761   248-475-6400
                                    800-757-3257
                                    www.easterseals.com/michigan/
Brent Wirth, President and CEO
Juliana Harper, Chief Program Officer/SVP
Rich Hollis, CFO/Senior Vice President
Various programs designed for children with autism, speech and language delays, amotional, motor and social skill issues.

543 Easter Seals - Genesee County Greater Flint Therapy Center
1420 University Ave
Flint, MI 48504-6208   810-238-0475
                                    Fax: 810-238-9270
                                    http://mi.easterseals.com
Diane Austin, Program Manager

Children and adults with mental and physical disabilities and other special needs have access to services designed to meet their individual needs. Health professionals from a variety of disciplines work with each person to overcome obstacles to independence, and to reach his/her personal goals through person centered planning. The following are camping and recreational services offered: Recreational services for adults and children, residential camping programs, therapeutic horseback riding.

544   Easter Seals - Michigan
2399 E Walton Blvd
Auburn Hills, MI 48326-6249   248-475-6400
www.easterseals.com/michigan/
Brent Wirth, President and CEO
Juliana Harper, Chief Program Officer/SVP
Rich Hollis, CFO/Senior Vice President
Offers a variety of programs to individuals with disabilities and special needs.

545   The Fowler Center For Outdoor Learning
2315 Harmon Lake Rd
Mayville, MI 48744-9737   989-673-2050
                                   Fax: 989-673-6355
                              www.thefowlercenter.org
                              info@thefowlercenter.org
Lynn Sealoff, Director
The Fowler Center is an outdoor recreation and education facility that provides programs for children, teens and adults with disabilities. Along with day camp programs, the camp also offers autism weekend camps and respite camps.

546   The JCC Center
Jewish Community Center of Metropolitan Detroit
D. Dan & Betty Kahn Building
6600 West Maple
West Bloomfield, MI 48322-3022   248-661-1000
                                   Fax: 248-661-3680
                                      www.jccdet.org
                                     dstone@jccdet.org
Brian D. Siegel, Chair
Florine Mark, President
Ilana Glazier, Vice President
Programs that support Jewish unity, ensure Jewish continuity and enrich Jewish life while conveying the importance of well-being within the Jewish and general community and the people of Israel.

Minnesota

547   Camp Buckskin
4124 Quebec Avenue North
Suite 300
Minneapolis, MN 55427   763-208-4805
                                   Fax: 763-208-8668
                               www.campbuckskin.com
                               info@campbuckskin.com
Tom Bauer, Director
Mary Bauer, Director
Jared Griffin, Program Director
Overnight summer camp program that specializes in serving boys and girls ages 6 - 18 who are experiencing social skill and academic difficulties. While not an entrance requirement, the majority of our campers have a primary diagnosis of AD/HD, Learning Disabilities, or Aspergers while others may have a secondary or related diagnosis.

548   Camp Confidence
1620 Mary Fawcett Memorial Dr
East Gull Lake, MN 56401-7538   218-828-2344
                                   Fax: 218-828-2618
                               www.campconfidence.com
                               info@campconfidence.com
Jeff Olson, Executive Director
Bob Slaybaugh, Program Director
Kelly Brooking, Director of Finance

A year-round center for persons with developmental disabilities specializing in recreation and outdoor education. Aimed at promoting self confidence and self esteem and the necessary skills to become full, contributing members of society.

549   Camp Friendship
Friendship Ventures
10509 108th St NW
Annandale, MN 55302-2912   952-852-0101
                                       800-450-8376
                                   Fax: 952-852-0123
                                   http://truefriends.org
                                   fv@friendshipventures.org
Floyd Adelman, Chairman
Jeff Bangsberg, Board Member
Jerry Caruso, Board Member
A summer resident camp that is open to anyone five or older who has developmental and/or physical disabilities.

550   Camp New Hope
Friendship Ventures
10509 108th Street NW
Annandale, MN 55302-4598   952-852-0101
                                       800-450-8376
                                   Fax: 952-852-0123
                                   http://truefriends.org
                                   fv@friendshipventures.org
Floyd Adelman, Chairman
Jeff Bangsberg, Board Member
Jerry Caruso, Board Member
A summer resident camp that is open to anyone five or older who has developmental and/or physical disabilities.

551   Camp Winnebago
19708 Camp Winnebago Rd
Caledonia, MN 55921-5738   507-724-2351
                                   Fax: 507-724-3786
                                www.campwinnebago.org
                                director@campwinnebago.org
Terry Chiglo, President
Eileen Loken, Vice President
Jane Palen, Secretary
Individuals with developmental disabilities, six years of age and older, are eligible to attend Camp Winnebago. A variety of traditional summer camp activities abound: swimming, cooking over a fire, games, arts and crafts, hay-wagon rides, dancing and more. Activities are adapted to the age and ability of each camper to ensure maximum participation.

Missouri

552   Camp Encourage
208 West Linwood Boulevard
Kansas City, MO 64111   816-830-7171
                                www.campencourage.org
                                info@campencourage.org
Jenny Hines, Board President/Parent Liason
Kelly Lee, M.S.Ed., Executive Director
Marita Burrow, Ph.D., Secretary
For children and young adults with Autism Spectrum disorders. The camp offers activities such as horseback riding, archery, fishing, swimming, hayrides, horseback riding, and art activities.

553   H.O.R.S.E.
C/O BJ Wright
19021 Long Grove Road
Higginsville, MO 64037   660-909-5381
                                www.horsehelpspeople.org
                                Brenda@HORSEhelpspeople.org
Brenda Wright, Executive Director
Athena Sharp, Director
Colleen White, Director

Combines the healing power of horses to deliver alternative therapeutic services to children with autism spectrum disorders and emotionally troubled individuals. The programs help to develop emotional awareness & expression, social skills and relationship building, as well as to help them build more self-esteem and self confidence.

Nebraska

554 Camp Kitaki
YMCA Of Lincoln Nebraska
570 Fallbrook Blvd.
Suite 210
Lincoln, NE 68521-3110   402-434-9200
                                  Fax: 402-434-9226
                                www.ymcalincoln.org
                          CampKitaki@ymcalincoln.org
Barb Bettin, President/CEO
J.P. Lauterbach, Chief Operations Officer
Misty Muff, Chief Administrative Officer
A Christian camp for children with ADD and other disabilities. Archery, climbing, horseback riding, fishing and aquatic activities are some of the activities.

555 Easter Seals - Nebraska
12565 W Center Rd
Ste 100
Omaha, NE 68144-8144   402-345-2200
                                       800-650-9880
                                  Fax: 402-345-2500
                          http://ne.easterseals.com
                              mtufte@ne.easterseals.com
James C. Summerfelt, President & CEO
Lily Howell, Director
Angela Howell, Vice President of Employment
The following are camping and recreational services offered: Camp respite for adults, camp respite for children, camperships, recreational services for children and residential camping programs.

New Hampshire

556 Calumet Camp
Calumet Lutheran Ministries
1090 Ossipee Lake Road
P.O. Box 236
West Ossipee, NH 03890-0236   603-539-4773
                                  Fax: 603-539-5343
                                      www.calumet.org
                                karl@Calumet.org
Brian Eckblom, Chair
Jim Nye, Treasurer
Karl Ogren, Executive Director of Calumet Lu
Camp Calumet is for kids, adults, seniors, singles, church groups, families and the developmentally disabled.

557 Easter Seals - New Hempshire
555 Auburn St
Manchester, NH 03103-4803   603-623-8863
                                       800-870-8728
                                  Fax: 603-625-1148
                              www.eastersealsnh.org
                          vbottino@eastersealsnh.org
Larry J. Gammon, President & CEO
Elin A. Treanor, COO/CFO
Karen Van Der Beken, Chief Development Officer
Easter Seals camping and recreation programs serve children, adults and families of all abilities. Various programs are available with the united purpose of giving disabled individuals a fun and safe camping or recreational experience. The following are camping and recreational services offered: Camp respite for adults, camperships, day camping for children, recreational services for children and residential camping programs.

New Jersey

558 Camp Merry Heart
Easter Seals Of New Jersey
21 O Brien Rd
Hackettstown, NJ 07840-4839   908-852-3896
                                  Fax: 908-852-9263
                                www.easterseals.com/nj
                          msimpson@nj.easterseals.org
Richard W. Davidson, Chairman
Sandra L. Bouwman, 1st Vice Chairman
Joseph G. Kern, 2nd Vice Chairman
Camp Merry Heart provides a safe, supervised and beautiful setting for iindividuals with disabilities and special needs. Activities include swimming, boating, fishing, arts and crafts, singing, dance and nature studies.

559 Camp Moore
New Jersey State Elks Association
P.O. Box 1596
Woodbridge, NJ 07095   732-326-1300
                                  Fax: 732-326-1319
                                   TDD: 609-271-0138
                                      www.njelks.org
                          elkscampmoore@njelks.org
Todd Garmer, Camp Director
Elks Camp Moore offers a fun filled vacation away from home for children with special needs. A week at Elks Camp Moore is a remarkable experience not soon to be fogotten. The primary goal of the camp is to further develop the recreational and social skills of each child. In a relaxed and accepting atmosphere, each camper experiences new adventures, lasting friendships, and opportunities that promote independence and greater self-confidence.

560 Round Lake Camp
21 Plymouth St
Fairfield, NJ 07004-1615   973-575-3333
                                  Fax: 973-575-4188
                              www.roundlakecamp.org
                                  rlc@njycamps.org
David Friedman, Camp Director
A camp for children with learning differences and social communication disorders. The camp is designed so that all the educational, recreational and social activities are planned to meet the capabilities of each child.

561 Summit Camp
Summit Camp & Travel Programs
322 Route 46 West
Suite 210
Parsippany, NJ 07054-6266   973-732-3230
                                  Fax: 973-732-3226
                                  www.summitcamp.com
                              info@summitcamp.com
Mayer Stiskin, Executive Director
Eugene Bell, Senior Director
Leah Love, Assistant Director
Summit offers co-ed 4 week and 8 week programs, along with a 10 day Mini-Camp, providing many camp activities that feature a heated swimming pool, complete lake activities, climbing wall, go-karts, computer labs, adventure programs, field trips, etc. The programs and staffing are tailored to the needs of the children dealing with social/emotional challenges, Aspergers, Tourette's, Non-verbal LD, Bipolar Disorder. The camp serves 300 children and provides a staff of 270.

New Mexico

562 Camp Without Barriers
Easter Seals Of New Mexico - Santa Fe
2041 S. Pacheco Street
Suite 100
Santa Fe, NM 87505   505-424-7700
                                  Fax: 505-424-7707
                              www.smem.easterseals.com

Jane Carr, Camp Director
Camp Easter Seals New Mexico provides fun for children and adults with disabilities. Its unique combination of comfortable accessible facilities and energetic, outgoing staff offers a fun, exciting, summer experience with memories to last a lifetime. Camp Easter Seals is held at Kamp Kiwanis' site, located in Vanderwagen, New Mexico.

New York

563 Adirondack Leadership Expeditions
82 Church St
Saranac Lake, NY 12983-1858   518-897-5011
Fax: 518-897-5017
www.adirondackleadership.com
rtheisen@adkle.com
Robert Theisen, Ph.D, Executive Director
Specializes in helping young adults age 13 to 17 who are experiencing / exhibiting any of the following: entitlement, manipulation, family conflict, isolation, low self-esteem, substance use, defiant behavior, attention deficit, learning differences, school failure, and negative peer relationships.

564 Camp Akeela
3 New King Street
White Plains, NY 10604   866-680-4744
Fax: 866-462-2828
www.campakeela.com
info@campakeela.com
Eric Sasson, Director
Debbie Sasson, Director
Kevin Trimble, Assistant Director
Akeela campers thrive in a world in which they are surrounded by peers with similar experiences and a staff who understands and embraces them. Not only do they have the time of their lives at camp, but they return home with skills and a newfound self-confidence that they carry with them throughout the year.

565 Camp Bari Tov
92ny Street Y
1395 Lexington Ave
New York, NY 10128-1612   212-415-5500
Fax: 212-415-5788
www.92y.org
Stuart J. Ellman, President
Laurence D. Belfer, Vice President
Marc S. Lipschultz, Vice President
Summer recreational program for children and young adults ages 5-13 with severe developmental disabilities. Campers participate in a variety of camp activities which include adaptive sports, music, art, nature and more.

566 Camp Colonie
Easter Seals New York
292 Washington Avenue Ext.
Suite 112
Albany, NY 12203-6385   212-220-2290
800-727-8785
Fax: 518-456-5094
www.ny.easterseals.com
info@ny.easter-seals.org
John McGrath, MPA, Chief Executive Director
Aris Pavlides, SVP, Development
Thomas Renart, M.A., M.S., SVP Program Services
Week long sessions for children and young adults age 5-21 years of age with developmental, emotional or physical disabilities.

567 Camp Dunnabeck at Kildonan School
425 Morse Hill Rd
Amenia, NY 12501-5240   845-373-8111
Fax: 845-373-9793
www.kildonan.org
admissions@kildonan.org
Kevin Pendergast, Head Master

Specializes in helping intelligent children with specific reading, writing and spelling disabilities. Provides Orton-Gillingham tutoring with camp activities, including swimming, sailing, waterskiing, horseback riding, ceramics, tennis and woodworking.

568 Camp Huntington
Registration & Billing Office
P.O. Box 37
High Falls, NY 12440-0037   866-514-5281
Fax: 845-853-1172
www.camphuntington.com
dfalk@camphuntington.com
Michael Bednarz, Executive Director
Alex Mellor, Program Director
Cathy Crowley, Program Supervisor
Coed camp for children and young adults ages 6-21 who have learning and developmental disabililties, Autism Spectrum Disorders, Apsperger's, and ADD/ADHD. Programs emphasize development of social skills and independent living, vocational orientation, speech and language.

569 Camp Kehilla
Sid Jacobson JCC
300 Forest Dr
East Hills, NY 11548-1231   516-484-1545
Fax: 516-484-7354
www.campkehilla.org
pzimmer@sjjcc.org
Pam Zimmer, MS Ed., Camp Director
Karen Kiernan, LMSW., Director
Marissa Gonta, Assistant Director
A summer day camp for children and teens with special needs.

570 Camp Northwood
132 State Route 365
Remsen, NY 13438-5700   315-831-3621
Fax: 315-831-5867
www.nwood.com
northwoodprograms@hotmail.com
Gordon Felt, Camp Director
Coed camp providing structured programs and activities to children and young adults ages 8-18 with Asperger's Syndrome, HFA, and Attention Deficit Disorders.

571 Camp Sunshine-Camp Elan
Mosholu Montefiore Community Center
3450 Dekalb Ave
Bronx, NY 10467-2302   718-882-4000
Fax: 718-882-6369
www.mmcc.org
info@mmcc.org
Natly Esnard, Co-Chair
Jon Lefkowitz, Co-Chair
Helen Kornblau, Vice-President
Provides programs, services and seasonal camping for children and adults. The camp serves children who are intellectually limited, emotionally impaired, and/or those who demonstrate special learniing disabilities.

572 Camp Tova
1395 Lexington Avenue
New York, NY 10128   212-415-5500
Fax: 212-415-5788
www.92y.org
Stuart J. Ellman, President
Laurence D. Belfer, Vice President
Marc S. Lipschultz, Vice President
Camp Tova is for children and young adults ages 6-13 with learning and other developmental disabilities. Campers develop a wide variety of social and creative skills while enjoying a variety of camp activites.

573 **Clover Patch Camp**
55 Helping Hand Ln
Glenville, NY 12302-5801 518-384-3081
Fax: 518-384-3001
www.cloverpatchcamp.org
cloverpatchcamp@cfdsny.org
Laura Taylor, Camp Director
Clover Patch is a summer camp for individuals with disabilities where each camper is encouraged to reach his or her fullest potential. Campers enjoy a wide variety of programs and are able to make new friends and create everlasting memories.

574 **EBL Coaching Summer Programs**
17 E 89th St
Ste 1D
New York, NY 10128-0615 212-249-0147
Fax: 212-937-2305
www.eblcoaching.com
info@eblcoaching.com
Emily Levy, Director
Lauren Hosking, Education Coordinator
Provides one-on-one tutoring and small group summer programs for students with learning disabilities and ADHD. They use all research-based, multi-sensory strategies, including the Orton Gillingham technique.

575 **Easter Seals - Albany**
292 Washington Avenue Ext
Ste 112
Albany, NY 12203-6385 518-456-0828
800-727-8785
Fax: 518-456-5094
http://ny.easterseals.com
info@ny.easter-seals.org
John McGrath, MPA, Chief Executive Director
Aris Pavlides, SVP Development
Thomas Renart, M.A., M.S., SVP Program Services
Easter Seals camping and recreation programs serve children, adults and families of all abilities. Various programs are available with the united purpose of giving disabled individuals a fun and safe camping or recreational experience. The following are camping and recreational services offered: Camp respite for children, camperships, day camping for children and recreational services for children.

576 **Gow School Summer Programs**
PO Box 85
South Wales, NY 14139-0085 716-652-3450
Fax: 716-652-3457
www.gow.org
summer@gow.org
David Mendlewski, Director
Doug Cotter, Admissions Director
M. Bradley Rogers, Jr., Headmaster
For boys and girls who have experienced past academic difficulties and have learning differences but possess the potential for success. The five week co-educational Gow School Summer Program (GSSP) serves students ages 8-16. Academic classes are combined with traditional camp activities and weekend trips.

577 **Kamp Kiwanis**
NY District Kiwanis Foundation
9020 Kiwanis Rd
Taberg, NY 13471-2727 315-336-4568
Fax: 315-336-3845
www.kiwanis.org
kamp@kiwanis-ny.org
Rebecca Lopez, Executive Director
Jessica Dymond, Chief Development Officer
Jerry Huncosky, CEO
Coed camp for children aged 8-14 who have special needs, are austistic, or physically/mentally challenged.

578 **Mainstreaming at Camp**
Frost Valley YMCA
2000 Frost Valley Rd
Claryville, NY 12725-5221 845-985-2291
Fax: 845-985-0056
www.frostvalley.org
nfo@frostvalley.org
Joe Medler, Camp Director
Serves children with developmental disabilities. The YMCA's 'Mainstreaming at Camp' allows campers to integrate with other campers throughout the day and reside in their own village with specially trained staff in the evenings.

579 **Rockland County Association for the Learning Disabled (YAI/RCALD)**
2 Crosfield Avenue
Suite 411
West Nyack, NY 10994-2212 845-358-2032
Fax: 845-358-6119
www.yai.org
link@yai.org
Melissa Yu, MD, CEO
YAI/RCALD conducts a wide variety of programs, supervised by experienced and professional staff, designed to build life skills, promote self-esteem, provide information exchange and offer other support services for individuals with learning and other developmental disabilities. The programs include, vocational evaluation and placements, recreational, residential, camping, service coordination and support groups.

580 **Samuel Field Y**
58-20 Little Neck Pkwy
Little Neck, NY 11362-2595 718-225-6750
Fax: 718-255-3910
http://sfysummercamps.org
sfy@sfy.org
Danielle Hersch, Program Director
Andy Gavora, Assistant Director
Robin Topol, Director of Special Services
Day camps specialize in serving children who have developmental disabilities 5-21 years old. Younger campers enjoy the center-based Childhood Program where they swim, play in the gym, cook, dance, as well as share arts and crafts activities and music. Activities for older campers include swimming, nature fun, an overnight at the Little Neck Site, community field trips, as well as a wide variety of specialty activities, such as drama, music, sports and arts and crafts.

581 **School Vacation Camps: Youth with Developmental Disabilities**
YWCA of White Plains-Central Westchester
515 North St
White Plains, NY 10605-3002 914-949-6227
Fax: 914-949-8903
http://ywcawpcw.org
frontdesk@ywcawpcw.org
Maria L. Imperial, CEO
L. Danielle Cylich, Chief Operating Officer
Mary Lee, Director Information Technology
Camp for people with developmental disabilities.

582 **Shield Summer Play Program**
144-61 Roosevelt Avenue
Flushing, NY 11354-6252 718-939-8700
Fax: 718-961-7669
www.shield.org
sprovenzano@shield.org
Dr. Susan Provenzano, Ed.D, Executive Director
Beth Anisman, B&Co., LLC, President
Michael E. Katz, Treasurer
The School Program provides a school for children, adolescents, and young adults, ages 6 to 21, who have been diagnosed with either mental retardation or other developmental disabilities. The program provides special education and related services based on each student's skills and potential for independence. Instruction focuses on developing and enhancing skills in community, recreational, and vocational settings. Year-round services are available.

North Carolina

583 Camp Sky Ranch
634 Sky Ranch Rd
Blowing Rock, NC 28605-8231
828-264-8600
Fax: 828-265-2339
www.campskyranchevents.com
jsharp1@triad.rr.com
Jack Sharp, Director
Serves developmentally and mentally disabled individuals of all ages, from all over the world. Children and adults with Down Syndrome, Prader-Willie Syndrome, ADD/HD, Fragile X Syndrome, and Autism attend our camp each year.

584 Discovery Camp
Talisman Camps & Programs
64 Gap Creek Rd
Zirconia, NC 28790-8791
828-697-6313
855-588-8254
Fax: 828-697-6249
www.talismancamps.com
info@talismancamps.com
Linda Tatsapaugh, Operations Director & Owner
Doug Smathers, Camp Director & Owner
Robiyn Mims, Admissions Director
Discovery Camp is a 2-week program designed for children ages 8-11, who may have ADD, learning disabilities, or experiencing some social anxiety. The activity packed schedule and 1:2.5 staff-camper ratio allows campers to have a positive experience at camp. In a nurturing yet structured environment, campers are challenged to become more independent and outgoing within the emotionally and physically safe setting that small group living provides. A good introduction to camp for younger kids.

585 SOAR Adventure Camps - Balsam
SOAR, Inc.
226 SOAR Lane
PO Box 388
Balsam, NC 28707-0388
828-456-3435
Fax: 828-456-3449
www.soarnc.org
admissions@soarnc.org
John Willson, MS, Executive Director
Laura Pate, Director of Operations
Joseph Geier, Balsam Base Associate Director
Emphasis is placed on developing self-confidence, social skills, problem-solving techniques, a willingness to attempt new challenges and the motivation which comes through successful goal orientation. Full semester and summer programs are available.

586 Talisman Camps & Programs
64 Gap Creek Rd
Zirconia, NC 28790-8791
828-697-6313
855-588-8254
Fax: 828-697-6249
www.talismancamps.com
info@talismancamps.com
Linda Tatsapaugh, Operations Director & Owner
Doug Smathers, Camp Director & Owner
Robiyn Mims, Admissions Director
Programs are co-educational, for children ages 9-13 who have been diagnosed with LD, ADD, ADHD, and mild behavior issues. Participants live on campus in rustic cabins participating in a variety of activities designed to promote better communication and cooperation skills. Limited enrollment helps to facilitate an extended-family environment. The 2.5 to 1 camper-to-staff ratio ensures that no child is lost in the crowd.

587 Talisman Summer Camp
64 Gap Creek Rd
Zirconia, NC 28790-8791
828-697-6313
855-588-8254
Fax: 828-697-6249
www.talismancamps.com
info@talismancamps.com
Linda Tatsapaugh, Operations Director & Owner
Doug Smathers, Camp Director & Owner
Robiyn Mims, Admissions Director
Includes three programs for children with learning disabilities, high functioning Autism and Asperger's Snydrome.

588 Victory Junction Gang Camp
4500 Adams Way
Randleman, NC 27317-8242
336-498-9055
Fax: 336-498-9090
www.victoryjunction.org
info@victoryjunction.org
Mark Schumacher, Chief Development Officer
Lisa Weber, Chief Financial Officer
Austin Petty, Chief Operating Officer
Enriches the lives of children with chronic medical conditions or serious illnesses by providing life-changing camping experiences that are exciting, fun, and empowering, in a safe and medically sound environment.

589 Wilderness Experience
Ashe County 4-H
512 Brickhaven Rd.
Raleigh, NC 27606
336-219-2650
Fax: 919-515-7812
www.nc4h.org
larry_hancock@ncsu.edu
Ken Burgess, Extension Associate
Larry Hancock, Extension Associate
Keith Russell, Director
The type of 4-H Camp program operating in North Carolina offers campers a greater chance to learn, develop life skills and form attitudes that will help them to become self-directing and productive members of society. At camp, youth focus on subjects that might be difficult to handle at home due to need for special equipment. Camp then becomes a learning laboratory that allows youth to apply their new knowledge to real-life situations.

Ohio

590 Academic Fun & Fitness Camp
Creative Education Institute
120 North Main Street
Chagrin Falls, OH 44022
440-914-0200
Fax: 440-542-1504
www.cei4learning.org
caroler@cei4learning.org
Sharon Miles, BS, MA, Camp Director
For children ages 6-18 with special needs and learning differences such as ADD/ADHD, Asperger's Syndrome, and Dyslexia. 6 weeks in June & July; 5 to 1 camper/counselor ratio.

591 Akron Rotary Camp
4460 Rex Lake Dr
Akron, OH 44319-3430
330-644-4512
Fax: 330-644-1013
www.akronymca.org
rotarycamp@akronymca.org
Dan Reynolds, Camp Director
Laura Bennett, Trustee
Nicholas P. Capotosto, Trustee
Rotary Camp was founded in 1924 with the purpose of providing children with special needs a place to spend their summers - a place where disabilities and limits do not hold kids back. Children ages 6-17 and who have physical or developmental disabilities are eligible to participate in this fun-filled camping experience.

592 Camp Courageous
12701 Waterville-Swanton Road
Whitehouse, OH 43571
419-875-6828
Fax: 419-875-5598
www.campcourageous.com
camping@campcourageous.com
Charlie Becker, Executive Director
Jeanne Muellerleile, Camp Director

Camp Courageous is a year-round recreational and respite facility for individuals with disabilities. The camp provides the opportunity to campers for social and personal growth within a supportive environment while helping them to develop enhanced self-esteem. Some of the recreational activities include bocce ball, canoeing, games, hikes, scavenger hunts and arts & crafts.

593   Camp Echoing Hills

36272 County Road 79
Warsaw, OH 43844-9770   740-327-2311
                                                800-419-6513
                                         Fax: 740-327-6371
                              www.echoinghillsvillage.org
                          ckuhns@echoinghillsvillage.org
Buddy Busch, Camp Director
Buddy Busch, President/CEO
Camp Echoing Hills is a ministry of Echoing Hills Village, which specializes in providing various programs for individuals with developmental disabilities in six locations across Ohio and Ghana West Africa. Camp Echoing Hills provides a safe and encouraging residential camping experience where campers develop friendships, skills and life-long memories.

594   Camp Happiness

Catholic Charities Disability Services
7911 Detroit Ave
Cleveland, OH 44102-2815   216-334-2963
                                          Fax: 216-334-2905
                         www.clevelandcatholiccharities.org
                       mjscott@clevelandcatholiccharities.org
Patrick Gareau, President/CEO
Glenda Buzzelli, Chief Administrative Officer
Wayne Peel, Chief Financial Officer
A summer camp program for persons with developmental disabilities, Camp Happiness is a six-week day camp offered at several sites throughout the Diocese of Cleveland that provides educational, social and recreational services to children and adults with developmental disabilities during the summer months.

595   Camp Nuhop

404 Hillcrest Dr
Ashland, OH 44805-4152   419-289-2227
                                          Fax: 419-289-2227
                                         www.campnuhop.org
                          campnuhop@zoominternet.net
Trevor Dunlap, Executive Director
A residential camp for all children with learning disabilities, attention deficit disorders and behavior disorders.

596   Easter Seals - Broadview Heights

Easter Seals North East Ohio
1929 A East Royalton Rd
Broadview Heights, OH 44147-2809   440-838-0990
                                                888-325-8532
                                         Fax: 440-838-8440
                                         TTY: 440-838-0990
                              www.easterseals.com/noh
                          spowers@noh.easterseals.com
Sheila Dunn, CEO
Chris Clyde, Associate Director
Kristin Feldman, Director of Outdoor Education
The following are camping and recreational services offered: Camperships and day camping for children. Through our summer campership program, funding is available to children and adults with disabilities so they can select a summer day or residential camp of their choice. The program provides individuals with the opportunity to attend a camp specifically designed for their special needs and optimal enjoyments.

597   Easter Seals - Central & Southeast Ohio

3830 Trueman Ct
Hilliard, OH 43026   614-228-5523
                                                800-860-5523
                                         Fax: 614-228-8249
                           www.easterseals.com/centralohio
                          info@easterseals-cseohio.org
Pandora Shaw-Dupras, CEO
Rob DuVall, Director
Kristy Emch-Roby, Director of Giving and Events
The following are camping and recreational services offered: Aquatics. Summer Day Camp is open to toddlers, ages 18 months to 2 years, and preschoolers and young school-aged children from 3-8 years of age with and without disabilities.

598   Easter Seals - Cincinnati

2901 Gilbert Ave
Cincinnati, OH 45206-1211   513-281-2316
                                                800-288-1123
                                         Fax: 513-475-6787
                              www.easterseals.com/swohio
                          buildingability@easterdealswrc.org
Pam Green, President and CEO
David Dreith, Executive Vice President
Easter Seals camping and recreation programs serve children, adults and families of all abilities. Various programs are available with the united purpose of giving disabled individuals a fun and safe camping or recreational experience. The following are camping and recreational services offered: Adventure.

599   Easter Seals - Marietta

Easter Seals
PO Box 31
Marietta, OH 45750   740-374-8876
                                                800-860-5523
                                         Fax: 740-374-4501
                           www.eastersealscentralohio.org
                          matt@campascca.org
Karin A Zuckerman, CEO
Colleen Flanagan, Camp Manager
Alex Barge, Camp Director
Easter Seals camping and recreation programs serve children, adults and families of all abilities. Various programs are available with the united purpose of giving disabled individuals a fun and safe camping or recreational experience. The following are camping and recreational services offered: Camp respite for children and therapeutic horseback riding.

600   Easter Seals - Northeast Ohio

3085 W Market St
Ste 124
Akron, OH 44333-3651   330-836-9741
                                                800-589-6834
                                         Fax: 330-836-4967
                           http://neohio.easterseals.com
                          spowers@noh.easterseals.com
Patrick Dunphy, Chairman
Sheila Dunn, CEO
Rhonda Sims, Primary Contact
Easter Seals camping and recreation programs serve children, adults and families of all abilities. Various programs are available with the united purpose of giving disabled individuals a fun and safe camping or recreational experience. The following are camping and recreational services offered: Swim programs.

601   Easter Seals - Youngstown

299 Edwards St
Youngstown, OH 44502-1599   330-743-1168
                                         Fax: 330-743-1616
                                         TTY: 330-743-1616
                              www.easterseals.com/mtc
                          matt@campascca.org
Vickie Villano, Director
Colleen Flanagan, Camp Manager
Alex Barge, Camp Director

Easter Seals camping and recreation programs serve children, adults and families of all abilities. Various programs are available with the united purpose of giving disabled individuals a fun and safe camping or recreational experience. The following are camping and recreational services offered: Recreationsl/Day care for Ages 6-12.

602 Marburn Academy Summer Programs

1860 Walden Dr
Columbus, OH 43229-3627
614-433-0822
Fax: 614-433-0812
www.marburnacademy.org
marburnadmission@marburnacademy.org

Earl B Oremus, Headmaster
Scott Burton, Associate Head of School
Beth Weakley, Director of Finance & Facilities
A four program academic day camp for children with LD and dyslexia, offering remediation in reading, math, phonemic awareness, or writing.

603 Pilgrim Hills Camp

Ohio Conference United Church of Christ
33833 Township Road 20
Brinkhaven, OH 43006
740-599-6314
800-282-0740
Fax: 740-599-9790
www.ocucc.org
campregistrar@ocucc.org

Jeff Thompson, Camp Director
Pamela Brown, Communications Director
Daniel Busch, Association Ministe
Many camp programs for all children including learning disabled. Pilgrim Hills Camp is located on 375 acres of woodlands, meadows, ponds and trails. The facilities includes a large dining hall and full kitchen to feed up to 300 with full food service and menu options available.

604 Recreation Unlimited Farm and Fun

Recreation Unlimited Foundation
7700 Piper Rd
Ashley, OH 43003-9741
740-548-7006
Fax: 740-747-2640
www.recreationunlimited.org
info@recreationunlimited.org

Jeremy James, Director
Provides year round programs in recreation, sports and education for individuals with developmental or physical disabilities. Campers build self-confidence and self-esteem while gaining positive relationships, attitudes and behaviors.

Oklahoma

605 Easter Seals - Oklahoma

701 NE 13th St
Oklahoma City, OK 73104-5003
405-239-2525
Fax: 405-239-2278
http://ok.easterseals.com
esok1@coxinet.net

Matt Vance, Chairman
Lauri Monetti, Development Director
Paula K. Porter, President & CEO
Easter Seals camping and recreation programs serve children, adults and families of all abilities. Various programs are available with the united purpose of giving disabled individuals a fun and safe camping or recreational experience. The following are camping and recreational services offered: Camperships.

Oregon

606 Easter Seals - Medford

406 S Riverside Ave
Ste 101
Medford, OR 97501
541-842-2199
800-244-5289
Fax: 541-842-4048
www.or.easterseals.com
matt@campascca.org

Richard W. Davidson, Chairman
J. David Cheveallier, CEO
Katie Shepard, Primary Contact
Programs offered in Medford include summer day camp, Recreation & Respite, and the popular First Saturday dance and social event. Programs are held at various community centers in Medford.

607 Easter Seals - Oregon

Easter Seals National
5757 SW Macadam Ave
Portland, OR 97239-3797
503-228-5108
800-556-6020
Fax: 503-228-1352
www.or.easterseals.com
matt@campascca.org

J. David Cheveallier, President
Colleen Flanagan, Camp Manager
Alex Barge, Camp Director
Easter Seals camping and recreation programs serve children, adults and families of all abilities. Various programs are available with the united purpose of giving disabled individuals a fun and safe camping or recreational experience. The following are camping and recreational services offered: Residential camping programs. In addition, the Portland program center hosts a warm water aquatic facility.

Pennsylvania

608 Camp Lee Mar

805 Redgate Road
Dresher, PA 19025-9612
215-658-1708
Fax: 215-658-1710
www.leemar.com
gtour400@aol.com

Ariel Segal, MSW, Director
Lynsey Trohoske, BA, Assistant Director
Laura Leibowitz, BA, M.Ed, Assistant Director
Private residential special needs camp for children and young adults with mild to moderate learning and developmental challenges, including but not limited to the following: mental retardation, developmental disabilities, down syndrome, autism, learning disabilities, Williams Syndrome, Asperger Syndrome, ADD, Prader Willi, and ADHD. A structured environment, individual attention and guidance are emphasized at all times.

Texas

609 Charis Hills

498 Faulkner Rd
Sunset, TX 76270-6683
940-964-2145
888-681-2173
Fax: 940-964-2147
www.charishills.org
info@charishills.org

Rand Southard, Director
Colleen Southard, Director
Chelsea Skinner, Program Director
Those with special learning needs have an opportunity to come to a place of acceptance. Here they meet others, both children and their counselors, who share similar experiences who are on the road to success. They have the opportunity to learn new activities in an environment that is safe, physically and socially.

Utah

610   **Summer Reading Camp at Reid Ranch**
2965 East 3435 South
Salt Lake City, UT 84109   801-466-4214
Fax: 801-466-4214
www.reidschool.com
ereid@xmission.com

Dr. Mervin R Reid, President
Dr. Ethna R. Reid, Director
The camp offers daily reading and language arts programs for children and young adults. Recreational activities include horseback riding, swimming, paddle boats and canoes, mountain climbing, volleyball and other other sports.

Virginia

611   **Summer PLUS Program**
Blue Ridge Autism and Achievement Center
312 Whitwell Drive
Roanoke, VA 24019   540-366-7399
Fax: 540-366-5523
www.achievementcenter.org
braac.roanoke@gmail.com

Angela Leonard, BA Education, Executive Director
Lisa Hensley, BS Accounting, Business Manager
Patti Cook, BS Business, Administrative Director
Summer camp program for children with learning disabilities and Autism. Programs put emphasis on social play and social skill development, communication and social skills all while targeting learning goals.

Wisconsin

612   **YMCA Camp Glacier Hollow**
Stevens Point Area YMCA
1000 Division St
Stevens Point, WI 54481-2700   715-342-2999
Fax: 715-342-2987
www.glacierhollow.com
pmatthai@spymca.org

Pete Matthai, Camp Director
Tiffany Praeger, Summer Camp Program Director
Offers a one week camp for children with learning disabilities.

Wyoming

613   **SOAR Adventure Camps - Dubois**
SOAR, Inc.
Eagle View Ranch
184 Uphill Rd
Dubois, WY 82513   307-455-3084
Fax: 801-820-3050
www.soarnc.org
evr@soarnc.org

Jeremy Neidens, Director
Emphasis is placed on developing self-confidence, social skills, problem-solving techniques, a willingness to attempt new challenges and the motivation which comes through successful goal orientation. Full semester and summer programs are available.

Language Arts

614 Analogies 1, 2 & 3
Educators Publishing Service
PO Box 9031
Cambridge, MA 02139-9031   617-547-6706
   800-225-5750
Fax: 617-547-3805
www.epsbooks.com
CustomerService.EPS@schoolspecialty.com
Arthur Liebman, Author
Rick Holden, President
Jeff Belanger, Regional Sales Manager
Studying analogies helps students to sharpen reasoning ability, develop critical thinking, understand relationships between words and ideas, learn new vocabulary, and prepare for the SAT's and for standardized tests.

615 AtoZap!
Sunburst Technology
1550 Executive Dr
Elgin, IL 60123-9311   800-321-7511
Fax: 888-608-0344
http://store.sunburst.com
service@sunburst.com
Michael Guillory, Channel Sales/Marketing Manager
A whimsical world of magical talking alphabet blocks and energetic playful characters this program provides young children with exciting opportunities to explore new concepts through open-ended activities and games. Mac/Win CD-ROM

616 Basic Signing Vocabulary Cards
Harris Communications
15155 Technology Dr
Eden Prairie, MN 55344-2273   952-906-1180
   800-825-6758
Fax: 952-906-1099
TTY: 800-825-9187
www.harriscomm.com
info@harriscomm.com
Dr. Robert Harris, President
Darla Hudson, Customer Service
Lori Foss, Marketing Director
Harris Communications is the sign language superstore and sells a full line of sign language materials for children, students, teachers and interpreters. Please visit us on-line to view all of our sign language products. Catalog is also available to view on-line or sent via USPS. *$7.95*
100 cards/set

617 Bubbleland Word Discovery
Sunburst Technology
1550 Executive Dr
Elgin, IL 60123-9311   800-321-7511
Fax: 888-608-0344
http://store.sunburst.com
service@sunburst.com
Michael Guillory, Channel Sales/Marketing Manager
Build and sharpen language arts skills with this multimedia dictionary. Students explore ten familiar locations that include a pet shop, zoo, toy store, hospital, playground, beach and airport where they engage in 40 activities that build word recognition, pronunciation and spelling skills.

618 Carolina Picture Vocabulary Test (CPVT): For Deaf and Hearing Impaired Children
Pro-Ed
8700 Shoal Creek Blvd
Austin, TX 78757-6897   512-451-3246
   800-897-3202
Fax: 800-397-7633
www.proedinc.com
info@proedinc.com
Cheri Richardson, Permissions Editor
Thomas Layton, Author
David Holmes, Co-Author

A norm-referenced, validated, receptive sign vocabulary test for deaf and hearing-impaired children. *$147.00*

619 Curious George Pre-K ABCs
Sunburst Technology
1550 Executive Dr
Elgin, IL 60123-9311   800-321-7511
Fax: 888-608-0344
http://store.sunburst.com
service@sunburst.com
Michael Guillory, Channel Sales/Marketing Manager
Children go on a lively adventure with Curious George visiting six multi level activities that provide an animated introduction to letters and their sounds. Students discover letter names and shapes, initial letter sounds, letter pronunciations, the order of the alphabet and new vocabulary words during the fun exursions with Curious George. Mac/Win CD-ROM

620 Early Communication Skills for Children with Down Syndrome
Therapro
225 Arlington St
Framingham, MA 01702-8773   508-872-9494
   800-257-5376
Fax: 508-875-2062
www.therapro.com
info@therapro.com
Libby Kumin PhD, Author
Karen Conrad, President
Provides professional expertise in understandable terms. Parents and professionals learn how their skills are evaulated by professionals, and what activities they can practice with a child immediately to encourage a childs's communication skill development. *$19.95*
368 pages

621 Early Listening Skills
Therapro
225 Arlington St
Framingham, MA 01702-8773   508-872-9494
   800-257-5376
Fax: 508-875-2062
www.therapro.com
info@therapro.com
Diana Williams, Author
Karen Conrad, President
Two hundred activities designed to be photocopied for classroom or home. Includes materials on auditory detection, discrimination, recognition, sequencing and memory. Describes listening projects and topics for the curriculum. Activity sheets for parents are included. A practical, comprehensive and effective manual for professionals working with preschool children or the older child with special needs. *$63.50*

622 Earobics Step 2: Home Version
Abilitations Speech Bin
PO Box 1579
Appleton, WI 54912-1579   419-589-1600
   888-388-3224
Fax: 888-388-6344
www.schoolspecialty.com
orders@schoolspecialty.com
Joseph M. Yorio, President, CEO
Rick Holden, Executive Vice President
Kevin Baehler, Vice President, Acting CFO
Step 2 teaches critical language comprehension skills and trains the critical auditory skills children need for success in learning. It offers hundreds of levels of play, appealing graphics, and entertaining music to train the critical auditory skills young children need for success in learning. Item number C483. *$58.99*

623   Earobics Step 2: Specialist/Clinician Version
Abilitations Speech Bin
PO Box 1579
Appleton, WI 54912-1579   419-589-1600
                                 888-388-3224
                                 Fax: 888-388-6344
                                 www.schoolspecialty.com
                                 orders@schoolspecialty.com
Joseph M. Yorio, President, CEO
Rick Holden, Executive Vice President
Kevin Baehler, Vice President, Acting CFO
Earobics features: tasks and level counter with real time display; adaptive training technology for individualized programs; and reporting to track and evaluate each individual's progress. Step 2 teaches critical language comprehension skills and trains the critical auditory skills children need for success in learning. Item number C484. *$298.99*

624   Every Child a Reader
Sunburst Technology
1550 Executive Dr
Elgin, IL 60123-9311   800-321-7511
                               Fax: 888-608-0344
                               http://store.sunburst.com
                               service@sunburst.com
Michael Guillory, Channel Sales/Marketing Manager
Traditional reading strategies in a rich literary context. Designed to promote independent reading and develop oral and written language expression.

625   Explode the Code: Wall Chart
Educators Publishing Service
PO Box 9031
Cambridge, MA 02139-9031   617-547-6706
                                   800-225-5750
                                   Fax: 617-547-3805
                                   www.epsbooks.com
                        CustomerService.EPS@schoolspecialty.com
Nancy M Hall, Author
Rick Holden, President
Jeff Belanger, Regional Sales Manager
Learning sounds is exciting with the new Explode The Code alphabet chart! Each letter is represented by a colorful character from the series and is stored inside a felt pocket embroidered with the letter's name.

626   First Phonics
Sunburst Technology
1550 Executive Dr
Elgin, IL 60123-9311   800-321-7511
                               Fax: 888-608-0344
                               http://store.sunburst.com
                               service@sunburst.com
Michael Guillory, Channel Sales/Marketing Manager
Targets the phonics skills that all children need to develop, sounding out the first letter of a word. This program offers four different engaging activities that you can customize to match each child's specific need.

627   Fun with Language: Book 1
Therapro
225 Arlington St
Framingham, MA 01702-8773   508-872-9494
                                    800-257-5376
                                    Fax: 508-875-2062
                                    www.therapro.com
                                    info@therapro.com
Kathleen Yardley, Author
Karen Conrad, President
A wonderful reproducible workbook of thinking and language skill exercises for children ages 4-8. Perfect when you need something on a moment's notice. Over 100 beautifully illustrated exercises in the following categories: Spatial Relationships; Opposites; Categorizing; Following Directions; Temporal Concepts; Syntax & Morphology; Same and Different; Plurals; Memory; Reasoning; Storytelling; and Describing. Targets both receptive and expressive language as well as problem-solving skills. *$59.50*

628   Goldman-Fristoe Test of Articulation: 2nd Edition
Abilitations Speech Bin
PO Box 1579
Appleton, WI 54912-1579   419-589-1600
                                  888-388-3224
                                  Fax: 888-388-6344
                                  www.schoolspecialty.com
                                  orders@schoolspecialty.com
Joseph M. Yorio, President, CEO
Ronald Goldman, Author
Macalyne Fristoe, Co-Author
It systematically measures a child's production of 39 consonant sounds and blends. Its age range is 2-21 years, and age based standard scores have separate gender norms. In this revised edition, inappropriate stimulus words have been replaced based on multicultural review, and all new artwork is featured. Item number 190915116. *$229.99*

629   HearFones
Abilitations Speech Bin
PO Box 1579
Appleton, WI 54912-1579   419-589-1600
                                  888-388-3224
                                  Fax: 888-388-6344
                                  www.schoolspecialty.com
                                  orders@schoolspecialty.com
Joseph M. Yorio, President, CEO
Rick Holden, Executive Vice President
Kevin Baehler, Vice President, Acting CFO
This unique nonelectronic self-contained headset is made of composite and plastic materials, and it's easy to clean. It lets users hear themselves more directly and clearly so they can analyze their own speech sound production and voice quality. Item number N261. *$28.99*

630   I Can Say R
Abilitations Speech Bin
PO Box 1579
Appleton, WI 54912-1579   419-589-1600
                                  888-388-3224
                                  Fax: 888-388-6344
                                  www.schoolspecialty.com
                                  orders@schoolspecialty.com
Joseph M. Yorio, President, CEO
Rick Holden, Executive Vice President
Kevin Baehler, Vice President, Acting CFO
Helping children overcome problems saying R sounds is one of the most perplexing dilemmas speech and language pathologists face in their caseloads. Here's a terrific book packed with innovative practice materials to make that task easier. Item number 190728116. *$26.99*

631   Idiom's Delight
Academic Therapy Publications
20 Leveroni Court
Novato, CA 94949-5746   415-883-3314
                                800-422-7249
                                Fax: 888-287-9975
                                www.academictherapy.com
                                sales@academictherapy.com
Jim Arena, President
Joanne Urban, Manager
Cynthia Coverston
Offers 75 idioms and accompanying reproducible activities. Delightful illustrations portraying humorous literal interpretations of idioms are sprinkled throughout the book to enhance enjoyment. *$14.00*
64 pages
ISBN 0-878798-89-7

632   Island Reading Journey
Sunburst Technology
1550 Executive Dr
Elgin, IL 60123-9311   800-321-7511
                               Fax: 888-608-0344
                               http://store.sunburst.com
                               service@sunburst.com
Michael Guillory, Channel Sales/Marketing Manager

Enhance your reading program with meaningful summary and extension activities for 100 intermediate level books. Students read for meaning while they engage in activities that test for comprehension, build writing skills with reader response and essay questions, develop usage skills with cloze activities and improve vocabulary/word attack skills.

633   Kaufman Speech Praxis Test
Abilitations Speech Bin
PO Box 1579
Appleton, WI 54912-1579   419-589-1600
                                 888-388-3224
                            Fax: 888-388-6344
                         www.schoolspecialty.com
                         orders@schoolspecialty.com
Nancy R. Kaufman, Author
Joseph M. Yorio, President, CEO
Rick Holden, Executive Vice President
This standardized test utlilizes a hierarchy of simple to complex motor-speech movements, from oral movement and simple phonemic/syllable to complex phonemic/syllable level. The complete kit contains manual, guide, and 25 test booklets. Item number 192126116. *$185.00*

634   LILAC
Abilitations Speech Bin
PO Box 1579
Appleton, WI 54912-1579   419-589-1600
                                 888-388-3224
                            Fax: 888-388-6344
                         www.schoolspecialty.com
                         orders@schoolspecialty.com
Joseph M. Yorio, President, CEO
Rick Holden, Executive Vice President
Kevin Baehler, Vice President, Acting CFO
LILAC uses direct and naturalistic teaching in a creative approach that links spoken language learning to reading and writing. Activities to develop semantic, syntactic, expressive, and receptive language skills are presented sequentially from three-to five-year-old developmental levels. Item number 190825116. *$27.99*

635   Language Activity Resource Kit: LARK
Abilitations Speech Bin
PO Box 1579
Appleton, WI 54912-1579   419-589-1600
                                 888-388-3224
                            Fax: 888-388-6344
                         www.schoolspecialty.com
                         orders@schoolspecialty.com
Joseph M. Yorio, President, CEO
Richard A Dressler, Author
Kevin Baehler, Vice President, Acting CFO
The LARK: Language Activity Resource Kit has been revised! This perennially popular language kit is now more portable and versatile for use with persons who have moderate to severe language disorders. Item number 190613116. *$217.99*

636   Max's Attic: Long & Short Vowels
Sunburst Technology
1550 Executive Dr
Elgin, IL 60123-9311   800-321-7511
                            Fax: 888-608-0344
                         http://store.sunburst.com
                            service@sunburst.com
Michael Guillory, Channel Sales/Marketing Manager
Filled to the rafters with phonics fun, this animated program builds your students' vowel recognition skills.

637   Pair-It Books: Early Emergent Stage 2
Houghton Mifflin Harcourt
222 Berkeley Street
Boston, MA 02116   617-351-5000
                                 855-969-4642
                            Fax: 800-269-5232
                            www.hmhco.com
                         school.permissions@hmhco.com

Michael Opitz, Author
Linda K. Zecher, President, CEO & Director
Eric Shuman, Chief Financial Officer
John K. Dragoon, EVP and Chief Marketing Officer
A series of 20 books, each containing 16 pages, that gradually become more difficult and reflect more complex text structures such as dialogue, content vocabulary and question and answer formats. All stories are available on audio cassette, and four are available in big book format.

638   PhonicsMart CD-ROM
HMH Supplemental Publishers
222 Berkeley Street
Boston, MA 02116   617-351-5000
                                 855-969-4642
                            Fax: 800-269-5232
                            www.hmhco.com
                         school.permissions@hmhco.com
Linda K. Zecher, President, CEO & Director
Eric Shuman, Chief Financial Officer
John K. Dragoon, EVP and Chief Marketing Officer
Five interactive games offer practice and reinforcement in 19 phonics skills at a variety of learning levels! Over 700 key words are vocalized, and each is accompanied by sound effects, colorful illustrations, animation, or video clips!

639   Polar Express
Sunburst Technology
1550 Executive Dr
Elgin, IL 60123-9311   800-321-7511
                            Fax: 888-608-0344
                         http://store.sunburst.com
                            service@sunburst.com
Michael Guillory, Channel Sales/Marketing Manager
Share the magic and enchantment of the holiday season with this CD-ROM version of Chris Van Allsburg's Caldecott-winning picture book.

640   Python Path Phonics Word Families
Sunburst Technology
1550 Executive Dr
Elgin, IL 60123-9311   800-321-7511
                            Fax: 888-608-0344
                         http://store.sunburst.com
                            service@sunburst.com
Michael Guillory, Channel Sales/Marketing Manager
Your students improve their word-building skills by playing three fun strategy games that involve linking one-or two-letter consonant beginnings to basic word endings.

641   Ridgewood Grammar
Educators Publishing Service
PO Box 9031
Cambridge, MA 02139-9031   617-547-6706
                                 800-225-5750
                            Fax: 617-547-3805
                            www.epsbooks.com
                      CustomerService.EPS@schoolspecialty.com
Terri Wiss, Author
Nancy Bison, Co-Author
Rick Holden, President
Grammar is an important part of any student's education. This new series, from the school district that developed the popular Ridgewood Analogies books, teaches 3rd, 4th, and 5th graders about the parts of speech and their use in sentences.

642   Sequential Spelling 1-7 with Student Respose Book
AVKO Educational Research Foundation
3084 Willard Rd
Birch Run, MI 48415-9404   810-686-9283
                                 866-285-6612
                            Fax: 810-686-1101
                            www.avko.org
                         webmaster@avko.org
Don McCabe, President/Research Director
Linda Heck, Vice-President
Michael Lane, Treasurer

Sequential Spelling uses immediate student self-correction. It builds from easier words of a word family such as all and then builds on them to teach; all, tall, stall, install, call, fall, ball, and their inflected forms such as: stalls, stalled, stalling, installing, installment. *$89.95*
72 pages
ISBN 1-664003-00-0

643 Soaring Scores CTB: TerraNova Reading and Language Arts
HMH Supplemental Publishers
222 Berkeley Street
Boston, MA 02116   617-351-5000
                                                   855-969-4642
                                            Fax: 800-269-5232
                                               www.hmhco.com
                              school.permissions@hmhco.com
Linda K. Zecher, President, CEO & Director
Eric Shuman, Chief Financial Officer
John K. Dragoon, EVP and Chief Marketing Officer
Through a combination of targeted instructional practice and test-taking tips, these workbooks help students build better skills and improve CTB-TerraNova test scores. Initial lessons address reading comprehension and language arts. The authentic practice test mirrors the CTB's format and content.

644 Soaring Scores in Integrated Language Arts
HMH Supplemental Publishers
222 Berkeley Street
Boston, MA 02116   617-351-5000
                                                   855-969-4642
                                            Fax: 800-269-5232
                                               www.hmhco.com
                              school.permissions@hmhco.com
Linda K. Zecher, President, CEO & Director
Eric Shuman, Chief Financial Officer
John K. Dragoon, EVP and Chief Marketing Officer
Help your students develop the right skills and strategies for success on integrated arts assessments. Soaring Scores presents three sets of two lengthy, thematically linked literature selections. Students develop higher-order thinking skills as they respond to open-ended questions about the selections.

645 Soaring Scores on the CMT in Language Arts& on the CAPT in Reading and Writing Across Disciplines
HMH Supplemental Publishers
222 Berkeley Street
Boston, MA 02116   617-351-5000
                                                   855-969-4642
                                            Fax: 800-269-5232
                                               www.hmhco.com
                              school.permissions@hmhco.com
Linda K. Zecher, President, CEO & Director
Eric Shuman, Chief Financial Officer
John K. Dragoon, EVP and Chief Marketing Officer
Make every minute count when you are preparing for the CMT or CAPT. Fine tune your language arts test preparation with the program developed specifically for the Connecticut's assessments. Questions are correlated to Connecticut's content standards for reading and responding, producing text, applying English language conventions, and exploring and responding to texts.

646 Soaring Scores on the NYS English Language Arts Assessment
HMH Supplemental Publishers
222 Berkeley Street
Boston, MA 02116   617-351-5000
                                                   855-969-4642
                                            Fax: 800-269-5232
                                               www.hmhco.com
                              school.permissions@hmhco.com
Linda K. Zecher, President, CEO & Director
Eric Shuman, Chief Financial Officer
John K. Dragoon, EVP and Chief Marketing Officer
With these workbooks, students receive instructional practice for approaching the assessment's reading, listening and writing questions.

647 Soaring on the MCAS in English Language Arts
HMH Supplemental Publishers
222 Berkeley Street
Boston, MA 02116   617-351-5000
                                                   855-969-4642
                                            Fax: 800-269-5232
                                               www.hmhco.com
                              school.permissions@hmhco.com
Linda K. Zecher, President, CEO & Director
Eric Shuman, Chief Financial Officer
John K. Dragoon, EVP and Chief Marketing Officer
Instructional practice in the first section builds skills for the MCAS language, literacy, and composition questions. A practice test models the MCAS precisely in design and length.

648 Spelling: A Thematic Content-Area Approach
HMH Supplemental Publishers
222 Berkeley Street
Boston, MA 02116   617-351-5000
                                                   855-969-4642
                                            Fax: 800-269-5232
                                               www.hmhco.com
                              school.permissions@hmhco.com
Linda K. Zecher, President, CEO & Director
Eric Shuman, Chief Financial Officer
John K. Dragoon, EVP and Chief Marketing Officer
Help students master the words they will use most frequently in the classroom. Organized lessons incorporate word analysis of letter patterns, correlations to appropriate literature, writing exercises, and application and extension activities.

649 Stories and More: Time and Place
Riverdeep, Inc.
100 Pine Street
Suite 1900
San Francisco, CA 94111-5205   415-659-2000
                                            Fax: 415-659-2020
                                     http://web.riverdeep.net
                                           info@riverdeep.net
Barry O'Callaghan, Executive Chairman/CEO
Jim Rudy, Chief Revenue Officer
Tom Mulderry, Executive Vice President
Combines three well-loved stories - The House on Maple Street, Roxaboxen, and Galimoto with engaging activities that strengthen students' reading comprehension.

650 Sunken Treasure Adventure: Beginning Blends
Sunburst Technology
1550 Executive Dr
Elgin, IL 60123-9311   800-321-7511
                                            Fax: 888-608-0344
                                    http://store.sunburst.com
                                         service@sunburst.com
Michael Guillory, Channel Sales/Marketing Manager
Focus on beginning blends sounds and concepts with three high-spirited games that invite students to use two letter consonant blends as they build words.

651 Teaching Phonics: Staff Development Book
HMH Supplemental Publishers
222 Berkeley Street
Boston, MA 02116   617-351-5000
                                                   855-969-4642
                                            Fax: 800-269-5232
                                               www.hmhco.com
                              school.permissions@hmhco.com
Linda K. Zecher, President, CEO & Director
Eric Shuman, Chief Financial Officer
John K. Dragoon, EVP and Chief Marketing Officer
Fine-tune your instructional approach with fresh insights from phonics experts. This resource offers informative articles and timely tips for teaching phonics in the integrated language arts classroom.

652 Test of Early Language Development
Pro-Ed, Inc.
8700 Shoal Creek Blvd
Austin, TX 78757-6897
512-451-3246
800-897-3202
Fax: 800-397-7633
www.proedinc.com
info@proedinc.com

Wayne Hresko, Author
D Kim Reid, Co-Author
Don Hammill, Co-Author
A normed test appropriate for children 0-2 through 7-11. It quickly and easily measures Receptive and Expressive language and yields an overall Spoken Language Score. *$295.00*

653 Vocabulary Connections
HMH Supplemental Publishers
222 Berkeley Street
Boston, MA 02116
617-351-5000
855-969-4642
Fax: 800-269-5232
www.hmhco.com
school.permissions@hmhco.com

Linda K. Zecher, President, CEO & Director
Eric Shuman, Chief Financial Officer
John K. Dragoon, EVP and Chief Marketing Officer
Keep students engaged in building vocabulary through crossword puzzles and cloze passages, and by using words in context and making analogies. Lessons build around thematically organized literature and nonfiction selections provide meaningful context for essential vocabulary words.

654 Workbook for Aphasia
Wayne State University Press
4809 Woodward Ave
Detroit, MI 48201-1309
313-577-6120
800-978-7323
Fax: 313-577-6131
www.wsupress.wayne.edu
bookorders@wayne.edu

Susan Howell Brubaker, Author
Jane Hoehner, Director
Gabe Gloden, Community Engagement Officer
This book gives you materials for adults who have recovered a significant degree of speaking, reading, writing, and comprehension skills. It includes 106 excercises divided into eight target areas. *$65.00*
500 pages

655 Workbook for Language Skills
Wayne State University Press
4809 Woodward Ave
Detroit, MI 48201-1309
313-577-6120
800-978-7323
Fax: 313-577-6131
http://wsupress.wayne.edu
bookorders@wayne.edu

Susan Howell Brubaker, Author
Jane Hoehner, Director
Gabe Gloden, Community Engagement Officer
This workbook features 68 real-world exercises designed for use with mildly to severely cognitive and language-impaired individuals. The workbook is divided in seven target areas: Sentence Completion; General Knowledge; Word Recall; Figurative Language; Sentence Comprehension; Sentence Construction and Spelling. *$50.00*
288 pages

Life Skills

656 Activities for the Elementary Classroom
Curriculum Associates
153 Rangeway Rd
North Billerica, MA 01862-2013
978-667-8000
800-225-0248
Fax: 800-366-1158
www.curriculumassociates.com
cainfo@curriculumassociates.com

Ernest L Kern, Editor
Robert Waldron, President and CEO
Dave Caron, Chief Financial Officer
Challenge your students to make a hole in a 3x5 index card large enough to poke their heads through. Or offer to pour them a glass of air. You'll have their attenion — the first step toward learning — when you use the high-interest, hands-on activities in these exciting teacher resource books.

657 Activities of Daily Living: A Manual of Group Activities and Written Exercises
Therapro
225 Arlington St
Framingham, MA 01702-8773
508-872-9494
800-257-5376
Fax: 508-875-2062
www.therapro.com
info@therapro.com

Karen McCarthy COTA, Author
Karen Conrad, President
Designed to provide group leaders easy access to structured plans for Activities of Daily Living (ADL) Groups. Organized into five modules: Personal Hygiene; Laundry Skills; Money Management; Leisure Skills and Nutrition. Each includes introduction, assessment guidelines, worksheets to copy, suggested board work, and wrap-up discussions. Appropriate for adult or adolescent programs, school systems and programs for the learning disabled. *$25.00*
136 pages

658 Aids and Appliances for Independent Living
Maxi-Aids
42 Executive Blvd
Farmingdale, NY 11735-4710
631-752-0521
800-522-6294
Fax: 631-752-0689
TTY: 631-752-0738
www.maxiaids.com

Elliot Zaretsky, President
Thousands of products to make life easier. Eating, dressing, communications, bed, bath, kitchen, writing aids and more.

659 Changes Around Us CD-ROM
222 Berkeley Street
Boston, MA 02116
617-351-5000
855-969-4642
Fax: 800-269-5232
www.hmhco.com
school.permissions@hmhco.com

Linda K. Zecher, President, CEO & Director
Eric Shuman, Chief Financial Officer
John K. Dragoon, EVP and Chief Marketing Officer
Nature is the natural choice for observing change. By observing and researching dramatic visual sequences such as the stages of development of a butterfly, children develop a broad understanding of the concept of change. As they search this multimedia database for images and information about plant and animal life cycles and seasonal change, students strengthen their abilities in research, analysis, problem-solving, critical thinking and communication.

660 Classroom Visual Activities
Therapro
225 Arlington St
Framingham, MA 01702-8773
508-872-9494
800-257-5376
Fax: 508-875-2062
www.therapro.com
info@therapro.com

Regina G Richards MA, Author
Karen Conrad, President
This work presents a wealth of activities for the development of visual skills in the areas of pursuit, scanning, aligning, and locating movements; eye hand coordination, and fixation activity. Each activity lists objectives and criteria for success and gives detailed instuctions. *$15.00*
80 pages

661   Cognitive Strategy Instruction for Middleand High Schools
Brookline Books
PO Box 1209
Brookline, MA 02446
617-734-6772
800-666-2665
Fax: 617-734-3952
www.brooklinebooks.com
brbooks@yahoo.com

Eileen Wood, Editor
Vera E Woloshyn, Editor
Teena Willoughby, Editor
Presents cognitive strategies empirically validated for middle and high school students, with an emphasis for teachers on how to teach and support the strategies. *$26.95*
286 pages
ISBN 1-571290-07-9

662   Fine Motor Activities Guide and Easel Activities Guide
Therapro
225 Arlington St
Framingham, MA 01702-8773
508-872-9494
800-257-5376
Fax: 508-875-2062
www.therapro.com
info@therapro.com

Jayne Berry OTR, Author
Carol Ann Meyers OTR, Co-Author
Karen Conrad, President
Useful for activity plans or teacher-educator-parent consultations. Perfect hand-outs as part of your inservice packet (no need to write out ideas, photocopy materials, etc). Package of 10 booklets. *$19.00*

663   Finger Frolics: Fingerplays
Therapro
225 Arlington St
Framingham, MA 01702-8773
508-872-9494
800-257-5376
Fax: 508-875-2062
www.therapro.com
info@therapro.com

Liz Cromwell, Author
Dixie Hibner, Co-Author
John Faitel, Editor
Invaluable for occupational therapists, speech/language pathologists and teachers. Over 350 light and humorous fingerplays help children with rhyming and performing actions which develop fine motor and language skills. *$13.25*

664   Hands-On Activities for Exceptional Students
Sage/Corwin Press
2455 Teller Rd
Thousand Oaks, CA 91320-2218
805-499-9734
800-233-9936
Fax: 805-499-5323
www.corwinpress.com
order@corwin.com

Mike Soules, President
Beverly Thorne, Author
Lisa Shaw, Executive Director Editorial
This execptional new release is developed for educators of students who have cognitive delays who will eventually work in a sheltered employment environment. If you need new ideas at your fingertips, this practical book is for you. *$25.95*
112 pages Special Ed
ISBN 1-890455-31-8

665   Health
HMH Supplemental Publishers
222 Berkeley Street
Boston, MA 02116
617-351-5000
855-969-4642
Fax: 800-269-5232
www.hmhco.com
school.permissions@hmhco.com

Linda K. Zecher, President, CEO & Director
Eric Shuman, Chief Financial Officer
John K. Dragoon, EVP and Chief Marketing Officer
Lessons and projects focus on nutrition, outdoor safety, smart choices, and exercise. Designed to make children more health conscious. Activity formats include fill in the blank, word puzzles, multiple choice, crosswords, and more.

666   Life-Centered Career Education Training
Council for Exceptional Children
2900 Crystal Drive
Ste 1000
Arlington, VA 22202-3557
703-620-3660
888-232-7733
Fax: 703-264-9494
TDD: 866-915-5000
TTY: 866-915-5000
www.cec.sped.org
service@cec.sped.org

Robin D. Brewer, President
James P. Heiden, President Elect
Christy A. Chambers, Immediate Past President
LCCE teaches you to prepare students to function independently and productively as family members, citizens, and workers, and to enjoy fulfilling personal lives. LCCE is a motivating and effective classroom, home, and community-based curriculum.

667   MORE: Integrating the Mouth with Sensory & Postural Functions
Therapro
225 Arlington St
Framingham, MA 01702-8773
508-872-9494
800-257-5376
Fax: 508-875-2062
www.therapro.com
info@therapro.com

Patricia Oetter OTR, Author
Eileen Richter OTR, Co-Author
Karen Conrad, President
MORE is an acronym for Motor components, Oral organization, Respiratory demands and Eye contact and control; elements of toys and items that can be used to facilitate integration of the mouth with sensory and postural development, as well as self-regulation and attention. A theoretical framework for the treatment of both sensorimotor and speech/language problems is presented, methods for evaluating therapeutic potential of motor toys, and activities designed to improve functions. *$49.95*

668   Memory Workbook
Therapro
225 Arlington St
Framingham, MA 01702-8773
508-872-9494
800-257-5376
Fax: 508-875-2062
www.therapro.com
info@therapro.com

Karen Conrad, President
Kathleen Anderson, Author
Pamela Crow Miller, Co Author
Recalling daily activities, seasons, months of the year, shapes, words and pictures. *$12.50*

669   One-Handed in a Two-Handed World
Therapro
225 Arlington St
Framingham, MA 01702-8773
508-872-9494
800-257-5376
Fax: 508-875-2062
www.therapro.com
info@therapro.com

Tommye K Mayer, Author
Karen Conrad, President
A personal guide to managing single handed. Written by a woman who has lived one-handed for many years, this book shares a methodology and mindset necessary for managing. It details a wide array of topics including personal care, daily chores, office work, traveling, sports, relationships and many more. A must for patients and therapists. *$19.95* *250 pages*

670   **People at Work**
Pearson AGS Globe
PO Box 2500
Lebanon, IN 46052-3009   800-992-0244
                                       Fax: 877-260-2530
                                       www.pearsonschool.com

Marjorie Scardino, CEO
Victor Coira, Sales Representative
Victoria Ramos, Digital Sales Rep
With an interest level of High School through Adult, ABE and ESL and a reading level of Grades 3-4, this program is a simple, thorough teaching plan for every day of the school year. The program's 180 sessions are divided into eighteen study units that each survey an entire occupational cluster of eight jobs while focusing on one or two writing skills. *$26.95*

671   **Responding to Oral Directions**
Pro-Ed
8700 Shoal Creek Blvd
Austin, TX 78757-6897   512-451-3246
                                       800-897-3202
                                       Fax: 800-397-7633
                                       www.proedinc.com
                                       info@proedinc.com

Robert A Mancuso, Author
Help children of all ages who function at first through sixth-grade levels learn to identify unclear directions and ask for clarification. Nine units teach them how to handle: recognizing directions, carryover and generalization; unreasonable, distorted, vague, unfamiliar, lengthy, unknown, and mixed directions. Item number 190575116. *$59.00*

672   **So What Can I Do?**
Therapro
225 Arlington St
Framingham, MA 01702-8773   508-872-9494
                                       800-257-5376
                                       Fax: 508-875-2062
                                       www.therapro.com
                                       info@therapro.com

Gail Kushnir, Author
Karen Conrad, President
A book to help children develop their own solutions to everyday problems. Cartoon illustrations feature common situations for children to analyze. The adult asks the child, so what can you do? The child is then encouraged to think of creative solutions, developing their emotional intelligence and improving coping skills. 58 problems to solve. *$10.95*

673   **Special Needs Program**
Dallas Metro Care
1380 River Bend Drive
Dallas, TX 75247   214-743-1200
                                       877-283-2121
                                       Fax: 214-630-3469
                                       www.metrocareservices.org
                                       metrocare@metrocareservices.org
Jill Martinez, Chairman
Judy N. Myers, Vice Chairman
Corey Golomb, Secretary
The special needs curriculum teaches students with disabilities the life skills they need to achieve self-sufficiency. The program focuses on and enhances coping skills.

674   **Stepwise Cookbooks**
Therapro
225 Arlington St
Framingham, MA 01702-8773   508-872-9494
                                       800-257-5376
                                       Fax: 508-875-2062
                                       www.therapro.com
                                       info@therapro.com

Beth Jackson, Author
Karen Conrad, President
A chance for children and adults at all developmental levels to participate in fun-filled hands-on cooking activities while developing independence. These cookbooks were developed by an OT working with children and teenagers with cognitive and physical challenges. Only one direction is presented on a page to reduce confusion. Recipes are represented by large Boardmaker symbols from Mayer Johnson. Large, easy-to-read text with dividing lines for visual clarity. *$52.50*

675   **Strategies for Problem-Solving**
Houghton Mifflin Harcourt
222 Berkeley Street
Boston, MA 02116   617-351-5000
                                       855-969-4642
                                       Fax: 800-269-5232
                                       www.hmhco.com
                                       school.permissions@hmhco.com

Arnold Yellin, Author
Linda K. Zecher, President, CEO & Director
Eric Shuman, Chief Financial Officer
Show students more than one way to approach a problem, and you hand them the key to effective problem solving. These reproducible activities build math reasoning and critical thinking skills, reinforce core concepts, and reduce math anxiety too. *$11.99*

676   **Survey of Teenage Readiness and Neurodevelopmental Status**
Educators Publishing Service
PO Box 9031
Cambridge, MA 02139-9031   617-547-6706
                                       800-225-5750
                                       Fax: 617-547-3805
                                       www.epsbooks.com
                                       CustomerService.EPS@schoolspecialty.com
Melvin D Levine MD FAAP, Author
Stephen R. Hooper, Ph.D., Co-Author
Rick Holden, President
Developed by Dr. Mel Livine and Dr.Stephen Hooper, The Survey of Teenage Readiness and Neurodevelopmental Status capitalizes on adolescents' evolving metacognitive abilities by directly asking them for their perceptions of how they are functioning in school and how they process information across a variety of neurocognitive and psychosocial domains.

677   **Swallow Right 2nd Edition**
Therapro
225 Arlington St
Framingham, MA 01702-8773   508-872-9494
                                       800-257-5376
                                       Fax: 508-875-2062
                                       www.therapro.com
                                       info@therapro.com

Roberta B Pierce, Author
Karen Conrad, President
This 12-session program evaluates and treats oral myofunctional disorders. 40 reproducible sequential exercises train individuals from five years to adult how to swallow correctly. Easy-to-use evaluation and tracking forms, checklist, and carryover strategies make this book a real time-saver! Item number Q858. *$55.00*

678 Target Spelling
Houghton Mifflin Harcourt
222 Berkeley Street
Boston, MA 02116

617-351-5000
855-969-4642
Fax: 800-269-5232
www.hmhco.com
school.permissions@hmhco.com
Linda K. Zecher, President, CEO & Director
Eric Shuman, Chief Financial Officer
John K. Dragoon, EVP and Chief Marketing Officer
You can differentiate instructions to address a variety of
learning styles and profiles and meet the needs of special education students.

679 Teaching Dressing Skills: Buttons, Bowsand More
Therapro
225 Arlington St
Framingham, MA 01702-8773

508-872-9494
800-257-5376
Fax: 508-875-2062
www.therapro.com
info@therapro.com
Marcy Coppelman Goldsmith, Author
Karen Conrad, President
Consists of 5 fold-out pamphlets for teaching children and
adults of varying abilities the basic dressing skills: shoe tying, buttoning, zippering, dressing and undressing. Each
task is broken down with every step clearly illustrated and
specific verbal directions given to avoid confusion and to
eliminate excess verbiage that can distract the learner. The
author, an experienced OT, has included the needed prerequisites for each task, many great teaching tips and more.
$10.50
5 Pamphlets

680 ThemeWeavers: Animals Activity Kit
Riverdeep
14046 Collections Center Drive
Chicago, IL 60693

855-969-4642
Fax: 800-269-5232
www.hmhinnovation.com
school.permissions@hmhco.com
Linda K. Zecher, President and CEO
Eric Shuman, Chief Financial Officer
John K. Dragoon, EVP
ThemeWeavers: Animals is the essential companion for
theme-based teaching. Dozens of animal-themed, interactive activities immediately engage your students to practice
fundamental skills in math, language arts, science, social
studies and more. Easy-to-use tools allow you to modify
these activities or create your own to meet specific
classroom needs.

681 ThemeWeavers: Nature Activity Kit
Riverdeep
14046 Collections Center Drive
Chicago, IL 60693

855-969-4642
Fax: 800-269-5232
www.hmhinnovation.com
school.permissions@hmhco.com
Linda K. Zecher, President and CEO
Eric Shuman, Chief Financial Officer
John K. Dragoon, EVP
ThemeWeavers: Nature Activity Kit is an all-in-one solution for theme-based teaching. In just a few minutes, you can
select from dozens of ready-to-use activities centering on
the seasons and weather and be ready for the next day's lesson! Interactive and engaging activities cover multiple subject areas such as language arts, math, science, social studies
and art.

682 Thinkin' Science ZAP
Riverdeep
14046 Collections Center Drive
Chicago, IL 60693

855-969-4642
Fax: 800-269-5232
www.hmhinnovation.com
school.permissions@hmhco.com

Linda K. Zecher, President and CEO
Eric Shuman, Chief Financial Officer
John K. Dragoon, EVP
It is a dark and stormy night as you step backstage to be guest
director at the Wonder Dome, the world-famous auditorium
of light, sound, and electricity. But great zotz! The Theater
has been zapped by lightning, and the Laser Control System
is on the fritz! Can you learn all about light, sound and electricity to rescue the show? *$69.95*

683 Time: Concepts & Problem-Solving
Houghton Mifflin Harcourt
222 Berkeley Street
Boston, MA 02116

617-351-5000
855-969-4642
Fax: 800-269-5232
www.hmhco.com
school.permissions@hmhco.com
Linda K. Zecher, President, CEO & Director
Eric Shuman, Chief Financial Officer
John K. Dragoon, EVP and Chief Marketing Officer
Develop concepts of telling time, identifying intervals, calculating elapsed time, and solving problems that deal with
time changes, lapses, and changes over the AM/PM cusp.

684 Travel the World with Timmy Deluxe
Riverdeep
14046 Collections Center Drive
Chicago, IL 60693

855-969-4642
Fax: 800-269-5232
www.hmhinnovation.com
school.permissions@hmhco.com
Linda K. Zecher, President and CEO
Eric Shuman, Chief Financial Officer
John K. Dragoon, EVP
France and Russia are the newest destinations for Edmark's
favorite world traveler, Timmy! In this delightful and improved program, students will enjoy expanding their understanding of the world around them. With wonderful stories,
songs, games, and printable crafts, early learners discover
how their international neighbors live, dress, sing, eat and
play.

685 Workbook for Reasoning Skills
Wayne State University Press
4809 Woodward Ave
Detroit, MI 48201-1309

313-577-6120
800-978-7323
Fax: 313-577-6131
http://wsupress.wayne.edu
bookorders@wayne.edu
Susan Howell Brubaker, Author
Jane Hoehner, Director
Gabe Gloden, Community Engagement Officer
This workbook is designed for adults and children who need
practice in reasoning, thinking, and organizing. Includes 67
exercises created for individuals with closed head injuries
and mild to moderate cognitive deficits. Item number W332.
$60.00
328 pages

Math

686 Algebra Stars
Sunburst Technology
1550 Executive Dr
Elgin, IL 60123-9311

800-321-7511
Fax: 888-608-0344
http://store.sunburst.com
service@sunburst.com
Michael Guillory, Channel Sales/Marketing Manager
Students build their understanding of algebra by constructing, categorizing, and solving equations and classifying
polynomial expressions using algebra tiles.

687 Attack Math
Educators Publishing Service
PO Box 9031
Cambridge, MA 02139-9031   617-547-6706
                                          800-225-5750
                                          Fax: 617-547-3805
                                          www.epsbooks.com
          CustomerService.EPS@schoolspecialty.com
Carole Greenes, Author
George Immerzeel, Co-Author
Linda Schulman, Co-Author
This series, for grades 1-6, teaches the four arithmetic operations: addition, subtraction, multiplication and division. Each operation is covered in three books, with book one teaching the basic facts and books two and three teaching multi-digit computation with whole numbers. A checkpoint and testpoint monitor progress at the middle and end of each book.

688 Awesome Animated Monster Maker Math
Sunburst Technology
1550 Executive Dr
Elgin, IL 60123-9311   800-321-7511
                                          Fax: 888-608-0344
                                          http://store.sunburst.com
                                          service@sunburst.com
Michael Guillory, Channel Sales/Marketing Manager
With an emphasis on building core math skills, this humorous program incorporates the monstrous and the ridiculous into a structured learning environment. Students choose from six skill levels tailored to the 3rd to 8th grade.

689 Basic Essentials of Math: Whole Numbers, Fractions, & Decimals Workbook
Houghton Mifflin Harcourt
222 Berkeley Street
Boston, MA 02116   617-351-5000
                                          855-969-4642
                                          Fax: 800-269-5232
                                          www.hmhco.com
                                          school.permissions@hmhco.com
James T Shea, Author
Linda K. Zecher, President, CEO & Director
Eric Shuman, Chief Financial Officer
Ideal for basic math skill instruction, test practice, or any situation requiring a thorough, confidence-building review. It provides a complete lesson - instruction, examples, and computation exercises. *$19.00*

690 Building Mathematical Thinking
Educators Publishing Service
PO Box 9031
Cambridge, MA 02139-9031   617-547-6706
                                          800-225-5750
                                          Fax: 617-547-3805
                                          www.epsbooks.com
          CustomerService.EPS@schoolspecialty.com
Marsha Stanton, Author
Rick Holden, President
Jeff Belanger, Regional Sales Manager
In this new math program, the units covered are presented as a series of Skinny Concepts that serve as manageable building blocks that eventually become entire topics. The Students Journal provides exercises for each Skinny Concept, encourages students to seek their own conclusions for problem solving, and provides space for the students ideas.

691 Building Perspective
Sunburst Technology
1550 Executive Dr
Elgin, IL 60123-9311   800-321-7511
                                          Fax: 888-608-0344
                                          http://store.sunburst.com
                                          service@sunburst.com
Michael Guillory, Channel Sales/Marketing Manager
Develop spatial perception and reasoning skills with this award-winning program that will sharpen your students' problem-solving abilities.

692 Building Perspective Deluxe
Sunburst Technology
1550 Executive Dr
Elgin, IL 60123-9311   800-321-7511
                                          Fax: 888-608-0344
                                          http://store.sunburst.com
                                          service@sunburst.com
Michael Guillory, Channel Sales/Marketing Manager
New visual thinking challenges await your students as they engage in three spacial reasoning activities that develop their 3D thinking, deductive reasoning and problem solving skills

693 Combining Shapes
Sunburst Technology
1550 Executive Dr
Elgin, IL 60123-9311   800-321-7511
                                          Fax: 888-608-0344
                                          http://store.sunburst.com
                                          service@sunburst.com
Michael Guillory, Channel Sales/Marketing Manager
Students discover the properties of simple geometric figures through concrete experience combining shapes. Measurements, estimating and operation skills are part of this fun program.

694 Concert Tour Entrepreneur
Sunburst Technology
1550 Executive Dr
Elgin, IL 60123-9311   800-321-7511
                                          Fax: 888-608-0344
                                          http://store.sunburst.com
                                          service@sunburst.com
Michael Guillory, Channel Sales/Marketing Manager
Your students improve math, planning and problem solving skills as they manage a band in this music management business simulation.

695 Creating Patterns from Shapes
Sunburst Technology
1550 Executive Dr
Elgin, IL 60123-9311   800-321-7511
                                          Fax: 888-608-0344
                                          http://store.sunburst.com
                                          service@sunburst.com
Michael Guillory, Channel Sales/Marketing Manager
Students discover patterns by exploring the properties of radiating and tiling patterns through Native American basket weaving and Japanese fish print themes.

696 Data Explorer
Sunburst Technology
1550 Executive Dr
Elgin, IL 60123-9311   800-321-7511
                                          Fax: 888-608-0344
                                          http://store.sunburst.com
                                          service@sunburst.com
Michael Guillory, Channel Sales/Marketing Manager
This easy-to-use CD-ROM provides the flexibility needed for eleven different graph types including tools for long-term data analysis projects.

697 Decimals: Concepts & Problem-Solving
Houghton Mifflin Harcourt
222 Berkeley Street
Boston, MA 02116   617-351-5000
                                          855-969-4642
                                          Fax: 800-269-5232
                                          www.hmhco.com
                                          school.permissions@hmhco.com
Linda K. Zecher, President, CEO & Director
Eric Shuman, Chief Financial Officer
John K. Dragoon, EVP and Chief Marketing Officer
This easy to implement, flexible companion to the classroom mathematics curriculum emcompasses decimal concepts such as values and names, equivalent decimals, mixed decimals, patterns, comparing, ordering, estimating and more.

698   Equation Tile Teaser
Sunburst Technology
1550 Executive Dr
Elgin, IL 60123-9311   800-321-7511
                                               Fax: 888-608-0344
                                        http://store.sunburst.com
                                          service@sunburst.com
Michael Guillory, Channel Sales/Marketing Manager
Students develop logic thinking and pre-algebra skills solving sets of numbers equations in three challenging problem-solving activities.

699   Factory Deluxe
Sunburst Technology
1550 Executive Dr
Elgin, IL 60123-9311   800-321-7511
                                               Fax: 888-608-0344
                                        http://store.sunburst.com
                                          service@sunburst.com
Michael Guillory, Channel Sales/Marketing Manager
Five activities explore shapes, rotation, angles, geometric attributes, area formulas, and computation. Includes journal, record keeping, and on-screen help. This program helps sharpen geometry, visual thinking and problem solving skills.

700   Focus on Math
Houghton Mifflin Harcourt
222 Berkeley Street
Boston, MA 02116   617-351-5000
                                               855-969-4642
                                               Fax: 800-269-5232
                                               www.hmhco.com
                                    school.permissions@hmhco.com
Linda K. Zecher, President, CEO & Director
Eric Shuman, Chief Financial Officer
John K. Dragoon, EVP and Chief Marketing Officer
omnsists of four sections and in each you will learn more about addition and subtraction, multiplication and division, fractions, decimals, measurements, geometry and problem solving.

701   Fraction Attraction
Sunburst Technology
1550 Executive Dr
Elgin, IL 60123-9311   800-321-7511
                                               Fax: 888-608-0344
                                        http://store.sunburst.com
                                          service@sunburst.com
Michael Guillory, Channel Sales/Marketing Manager
Build the fraction skills of ordering, equivalence, relative sizes and multiple representations with four, multi-level, carnival style games.

702   Fractions: Concepts & Problem-Solving
Houghton Mifflin Harcourt
222 Berkeley Street
Boston, MA 02116   617-351-5000
                                               855-969-4642
                                               Fax: 800-269-5232
                                               www.hmhco.com
                                    school.permissions@hmhco.com
Linda K. Zecher, President, CEO & Director
Eric Shuman, Chief Financial Officer
John K. Dragoon, EVP and Chief Marketing Officer
This companion to the classroom mathematics curriculum emcompasses many of the standards established at each grade level. Each activity page targets a specific skill to help bolster students who need additional work in a particular area of fractions.

703   GEPA Success in Language Arts Literacy and Mathematics
Houghton Mifflin Harcourt
222 Berkeley Street
Boston, MA 02116   617-351-5000
                                               855-969-4642
                                               Fax: 800-269-5232
                                               www.hmhco.com
                                    school.permissions@hmhco.com
Estell Kleinman, Author
Linda K. Zecher, President, CEO & Director
Eric Shuman, Chief Financial Officer
Build skills as you improve scores on the GEPA. Better test scores don't always mean better skills. With these workbooks, you can ensure that your students are becoming more proficient users of language and math as well as more skilled test-takers. Your students will gain valuable practice answering the types of questions found on the GEPA, such as open-ended and enhanced multiple-choice items. *$17.60*

704   Geometry for Primary Grades
Houghton Mifflin Harcourt
222 Berkeley Street
Boston, MA 02116   617-351-5000
                                               855-969-4642
                                               Fax: 800-269-5232
                                               www.hmhco.com
                                    school.permissions@hmhco.com
Linda K. Zecher, President, CEO & Director
Eric Shuman, Chief Financial Officer
John K. Dragoon, EVP and Chief Marketing Officer
Self-explanatory lessons ideal for independent work or as homework. Transitions from concrete to pictorial to abstract.

705   Get Up and Go!
Sunburst Technology
1550 Executive Dr
Elgin, IL 60123-9311   800-321-7511
                                               Fax: 888-608-0344
                                        http://store.sunburst.com
                                          service@sunburst.com
Michael Guillory, Channel Sales/Marketing Manager
Students interpret and construct timelines through three descriptive activities in the animated program. Students are introduced to timelines as they participate in an interactive story.

706   Grade Level Math
Houghton Mifflin Harcourt
222 Berkeley Street
Boston, MA 02116   617-351-5000
                                               855-969-4642
                                               Fax: 800-269-5232
                                               www.hmhco.com
                                    school.permissions@hmhco.com
Linda K. Zecher, President, CEO & Director
Eric Shuman, Chief Financial Officer
John K. Dragoon, EVP and Chief Marketing Officer
Easy to understand practice exercises help students build conceptual knowledge and computation skills together. Each book addresses essential grade appropriate math areas.

707   Graphers
Sunburst Technology
1550 Executive Dr
Elgin, IL 60123-9311   800-321-7511
                                               Fax: 888-608-0344
                                        http://store.sunburst.com
                                          service@sunburst.com
Michael Guillory, Channel Sales/Marketing Manager
Students develop data analysis skills with this easy to use graphing tool. With over 30 pictorial data sets and 16 lessons, students learn to construct and interpret six different graph types.

708 **Green Globs & Graphing Equations**
Sunburst Technology
1550 Executive Dr
Elgin, IL 60123-9311

800-321-7511
Fax: 888-608-0344
http://store.sunburst.com
service@sunburst.com

Michael Guillory, Channel Sales/Marketing Manager
As students explore parabolas, hyperbolas, and other graphs, they discover how altering an equation changes a graph's shape or position.

709 **Hidden Treasures of Al-Jabr**
Sunburst Technology
1550 Executive Dr
Elgin, IL 60123-9311

800-321-7511
Fax: 888-608-0344
http://store.sunburst.com
service@sunburst.com

Michael Guillory, Channel Sales/Marketing Manager
Beginning algebra students undertake three challenges that develop skills in the areas of solving linear equations, substituting variables, grouping like variables, using systems of equations and translating algebra word problems into equations.

710 **High School Math Bundle**
Sunburst Technology
1550 Executive Dr
Elgin, IL 60123-9311

800-321-7511
Fax: 888-608-0344
http://store.sunburst.com
service@sunburst.com

Michael Guillory, Channel Sales/Marketing Manager
Each program in this bundle focuses on a specific area to ensure that your students master the math skills they need. This bundle allows students to master basics of Algebra, explore equations and graphs, practice learning with algebra graphs, use trigonometric functions, apply math concepts to practical situations and improve problem solving and data analysis skills.

711 **Higher Scores on Math Standardized Tests**
Harcourt Achieve
222 Berkeley Street
Boston, MA 02116

617-351-5000
855-969-4642
Fax: 800-269-5232
www.hmhco.com
school.permissions@hmhco.com

Linda K. Zecher, President, CEO & Director
Eric Shuman, Chief Financial Officer
John K. Dragoon, EVP and Chief Marketing Officer
These grade level math test preparation series provide focused practice in areas where students have shown a weakness in previous standardized tests. Improves test scores by zeroing in on the skills requiring remediation.

712 **Hot Dog Stand: The Works**
Sunburst Technology
1550 Executive Dr
Elgin, IL 60123-9311

800-321-7511
Fax: 888-608-0344
http://store.sunburst.com
service@sunburst.com

Michael Guillory, Channel Sales/Marketing Manager
Students practice math, problem-solving, and communication skills in a multimedia business simulation that challenges students with unexpected events.

713 **How the West Was 1+3x4**
Sunburst Technology
1550 Executive Dr
Elgin, IL 60123-9311

800-321-7511
Fax: 888-608-0344
http://store.sunburst.com
service@sunburst.com

Michael Guillory, Channel Sales/Marketing Manager
Students use order of operations to construct equations and race along number line trails.

714 **Ice Cream Truck**
Sunburst Technology
1550 Executive Dr
Elgin, IL 60123-9311

800-321-7511
Fax: 888-608-0344
http://store.sunburst.com
service@sunburst.com

Michael Guillory, Channel Sales/Marketing Manager
Elementary students learn important problem solving, strategic planning and math operation skills, as they become owners of a busy ice cream truck.

715 **Intermediate Geometry**
Houghton Mifflin Harcourt
222 Berkeley Street
Boston, MA 02116

617-351-5000
855-969-4642
Fax: 800-269-5232
www.hmhco.com
school.permissions@hmhco.com

Linda K. Zecher, President, CEO & Director
Eric Shuman, Chief Financial Officer
John K. Dragoon, EVP and Chief Marketing Officer
Prepares intermediate and middle school students for a successful experience in high school geometry. Intermediate geometry provides a study of the concepts, computation, problem-solving, and enrichment of topics identified by NCTM standards. This three-book series links the informal explorations of geometry in primary grades to more formalized processes taught in high school.

716 **Introduction to Patterns**
Sunburst Technology
1550 Executive Dr
Elgin, IL 60123-9311

800-321-7511
Fax: 888-608-0344
http://store.sunburst.com
service@sunburst.com

Michael Guillory, Channel Sales/Marketing Manager
Students discover patterns found in art and nature, exploring linear and geometric designs, predicting outcomes and creating patterns of their own.

717 **Mastering Math**
Houghton Mifflin Harcourt
222 Berkeley Street
Boston, MA 02116

617-351-5000
855-969-4642
Fax: 800-269-5232
www.hmhco.com
school.permissions@hmhco.com

Linda K. Zecher, President, CEO & Director
Eric Shuman, Chief Financial Officer
John K. Dragoon, EVP and Chief Marketing Officer
Now low level readers can succeed at math with this easy to read presentation. Makes basic math concepts accessible to all students.

718 **Measurement: Practical Applications**
Houghton Mifflin Harcourt
222 Berkeley Street
Boston, MA 02116

617-351-5000
855-969-4642
Fax: 800-269-5232
www.hmhco.com
school.permissions@hmhco.com

Linda K. Zecher, President, CEO & Director
Eric Shuman, Chief Financial Officer
John K. Dragoon, EVP and Chief Marketing Officer
Concentrated practice on the measurement skills we use on a daily basis. This practical presentation of both customary and metric units helps the student to understand the importance of measurement skills in everyday life. Hands on activities and real life situations create logical applications so measurements make sense.

719 Memory Fun!
Sunburst Technology
1550 Executive Dr
Elgin, IL 60123-9311
800-321-7511
Fax: 888-608-0344
http://store.sunburst.com
service@sunburst.com
Michael Guillory, Channel Sales/Marketing Manager
Welcome to Tiny's attic where students build memory, matching, counting and money sense through a variety of fun matching activities.

720 Middle School Math Bundle
Sunburst Technology
1550 Executive Dr
Elgin, IL 60123-9311
800-321-7511
Fax: 888-608-0344
http://store.sunburst.com
service@sunburst.com
Michael Guillory, Channel Sales/Marketing Manager
This bundle helps improve student's logical thinking, number sense and operation skills. This product comes with Math Arena, Building Perspective Deluxe, Equation Tile Teasers and Easy Sheet.

721 Middle School Math Collection Geometry Basic Concepts
Houghton Mifflin Harcourt
222 Berkeley Street
Boston, MA 02116
617-351-5000
855-969-4642
Fax: 800-269-5232
www.hmhco.com
school.permissions@hmhco.com
Linda K. Zecher, President, CEO & Director
Eric Shuman, Chief Financial Officer
John K. Dragoon, EVP and Chief Marketing Officer
Provides students with enough comprehensive, skill specific practice in the key areas of geometry to ensure mastery. Ideal for junior high or high school students in need of remediation.

722 MindTwister Math
Riverdeep
14046 Collections Center Drive
Chicago, IL 60693
855-969-4642
Fax: 800-269-5232
www.hmhinnovation.com
school.permissions@hmhco.com
Linda K. Zecher, President and CEO
Eric Shuman, Chief Financial Officer
John K. Dragoon, EVP
MindTwister Math provides a challenging review of third grade math and problem-solving skills in a fast-paced, multi-player game show format. Thousands of action-packed challenges encourage students to practice essential math facts including addition, subtraction, mutiplication and division and develop more advanced mathematical problem-solving skills such as visualization, deduction, sequencing, estimating and pattern recognition.

723 Mirror Symmetry
Sunburst Technology
1550 Executive Dr
Elgin, IL 60123-9311
800-321-7511
Fax: 888-608-0344
http://store.sunburst.com
service@sunburst.com
Michael Guillory, Channel Sales/Marketing Manager
Students advance their understanding of geometric properties and spatial relationships by exploring lines of symmetry within a single geometric shape.

724 Multiplication & Division
Houghton Mifflin Harcourt
222 Berkeley Street
Boston, MA 02116
617-351-5000
855-969-4642
Fax: 800-269-5232
www.hmhco.com
school.permissions@hmhco.com
Linda K. Zecher, President, CEO & Director
Eric Shuman, Chief Financial Officer
John K. Dragoon, EVP and Chief Marketing Officer
Skill specific activities focus on the concepts and inverse relationships of multiplication and division. Explains in simplified terms how the process of multiplication undoes the process of division, and vice versa.

725 My Mathematical Life
Sunburst Technology
1550 Executive Dr
Elgin, IL 60123-9311
800-321-7511
Fax: 888-608-0344
http://store.sunburst.com
service@sunburst.com
Michael Guillory, Channel Sales/Marketing Manager
Students discover the math involved in everyday living as they take a character from high school graduation to retirement, advising on important health, education, career, and financial decisions.

726 Nimble Numeracy: Fluency in Counting and Basic Arithmetic
Oxton House Publishers
PO Box 209
Farmington, ME 04938
207-779-1923
800-539-7323
Fax: 207-779-0623
www.oxtonhouse.com
info@oxtonhouse.com
Dr. Phyllis E. Fischer, Author
William Berlinghoff PhD, Managing Editor
Bobby Brown, Marketing Director
Dr. Phyllis Fischer, Author
This is a richly detailed handbook for teachers, tutors, and parents who want to help children develop fluent arithmetic skills. It provides explicit techniques for teaching counting and basic arithmetic, with special emphasis on the language of our base-ten, place-value system for speaking about and writing numbers. *$19.95*
136 pages
ISBN 1-881929-19-1

727 Number Meanings and Counting
Sunburst Technology
1550 Executive Dr
Elgin, IL 60123-9311
800-321-7511
Fax: 888-608-0344
http://store.sunburst.com
service@sunburst.com
Michael Guillory, Channel Sales/Marketing Manager
Students develop their understanding of number meaning and uses with experiences practicing estimating, using number meanings, and making more-and-less comparisons.

728 Number Sense & Problem Solving CD-ROM
Sunburst Technology
1550 Executive Dr
Elgin, IL 60123-9311
800-321-7511
Fax: 888-608-0344
http://store.sunburst.com
service@sunburst.com
Michael Guillory, Channel Sales/Marketing Manager
Build number and operation skills with these three programs: How the West Was One + Three x Four, Divide and Conquer and Puzzle Tanks.

729 Numbers Undercover
Sunburst Technology
1550 Executive Dr
Elgin, IL 60123-9311

800-321-7511
Fax: 888-608-0344
http://store.sunburst.com
service@sunburst.com
Michael Guillory, Channel Sales/Marketing Manager
As children try to solve the case of missing numbers, they practice telling time, measuring and estimating, counting, and working with money.

730 Penny Pot
Sunburst Technology
1550 Executive Dr
Elgin, IL 60123-9311

800-321-7511
Fax: 888-608-0344
http://store.sunburst.com
service@sunburst.com
Michael Guillory, Channel Sales/Marketing Manager
Students learn about money as they count combinations of coins in this engaging program.

731 Problemas y mas
Houghton Mifflin Harcourt
222 Berkeley Street
Boston, MA 02116

617-351-5000
855-969-4642
Fax: 800-269-5232
www.hmhco.com
school.permissions@hmhco.com
Alan Handel, Author
Linda K. Zecher, President, CEO & Director
Eric Shuman, Chief Financial Officer
This ESL math practice and strategy tool is in three levels the same as Problems Plus, but expressly for your Spanish fluent ESL learners. *$13.40*
ISBN 0-811495-93-0

732 Problems Plus Level H
Houghton Mifflin Achieve
222 Berkeley Street
Boston, MA 02116

617-351-5000
855-969-4642
Fax: 800-269-5232
www.hmhco.com
school.permissions@hmhco.com
Francis J Gardella, Author
Linda K. Zecher, President, CEO & Director
Eric Shuman, Chief Financial Officer
A one-of-a-kind guide to solving open-ended math problems. Doesn't just give answers to test questions. With its innovative problem-solving plan, this series teaches math thinking and problem attack strategies, plus offers practice in higher order thinking skills students need to solve open-ended math problems successfully. *$15.10*

733 Puzzle Tanks
Sunburst Technology
1550 Executive Dr
Elgin, IL 60123-9311

800-321-7511
Fax: 888-608-0344
http://store.sunburst.com
service@sunburst.com
Michael Guillory, Channel Sales/Marketing Manager
A problem-solving program that uses logic puzzles involving liquid measurements.

734 Representing Fractions
Sunburst Technology
1550 Executive Dr
Elgin, IL 60123-9311

800-321-7511
Fax: 888-608-0344
http://store.sunburst.com
service@sunburst.com
Michael Guillory, Channel Sales/Marketing Manager
In this investigation students work with one interpretation of a fraction and the relationship between parts and wholes by working with symbolic and visual representations.

735 Sequencing Fun!
Sunburst Technology
1550 Executive Dr
Elgin, IL 60123-9311

800-321-7511
Fax: 888-608-0344
http://store.sunburst.com
service@sunburst.com
Michael Guillory, Channel Sales/Marketing Manager
Text, pictures, animation, and video clips provide a fun-filled program that encourages critical thinking skills.

736 Shape Up!
Sunburst Technology
1550 Executive Dr
Elgin, IL 60123-9311

800-321-7511
Fax: 888-608-0344
http://store.sunburst.com
service@sunburst.com
Michael Guillory, Channel Sales/Marketing Manager
Students actively create and manipulate shapes to discover important ideas about mathematics in an electronic playground of two and three dimensional shapes.

737 Shapes Within Shapes
Sunburst Technology
1550 Executive Dr
Elgin, IL 60123-9311

800-321-7511
Fax: 888-608-0344
http://store.sunburst.com
service@sunburst.com
Michael Guillory, Channel Sales/Marketing Manager
Students identify shapes within shapes, then rearrange them to develop spatial sense and deepen their understanding of the properties of shapes.

738 Spatial Relationships
Sunburst Technology
1550 Executive Dr
Elgin, IL 60123-9311

888-492-8817
Fax: 888-608-0344
http://store.sunburst.com
service@sunburst.com
Michael Guillory, Channel Sales/Marketing Manager
Students explore location by identifying the positions of objects and creating paths between places. Children develop spatial abilities and language needed to communicate about our world.

739 Speed Drills for Arithmetic Facts
Oxton House Publishers
PO Box 209
Farmington, ME 04938

207-779-1923
800-539-7323
Fax: 207-779-0623
www.oxtonhouse.com
info@oxtonhouse.com
William Berlinghoff PhD, Managing Editor
Bobby Brown, Marketing Director
Dr. Phyllis Fischer, Author
This looseleaf packet is a set of 48 pages of carefully constructed exercises to promote automaticity with basic arithmetic facts. The worksheets reinforce the interrelationship of three numbers in addition/subtraction and multiplication/division statements. Also included are six pages of detailed teaching advice and a chart template for tracking student progress. *$24.95*
54 pages
ISBN 1-881929-16-7

740 Splish Splash Math
Sunburst Technology
1550 Executive Dr
Elgin, IL 60123-9311

800-321-7511
Fax: 888-608-0344
http://store.sunburst.com
service@sunburst.com
Michael Guillory, Channel Sales/Marketing Manager

Students learn and practice basic operation skills as they engage in this high interest program that keeps them motivated. Great visual rewards and three levels of difficulty keep students challenged.

741 Strategies for Problem-Solving
Houghton Mifflin Harcourt
222 Berkeley Street
Boston, MA 02116
617-351-5000
855-969-4642
Fax: 800-269-5232
www.hmhco.com
school.permissions@hmhco.com
Arnold Yellin, Author
Linda K. Zecher, President, CEO & Director
Eric Shuman, Chief Financial Officer
Show students more than one way to approach a problem, and you hand them the key to effective problem solving. These reproducible activities build math reasoning and critical thinking skills, reinforce core concepts, and reduce math anxiety, too. *$11.99*
ISBN 0-817267-61-1

742 Strategies for Success in Mathematics
Houghton Mifflin Harcourt
222 Berkeley Street
Boston, MA 02116
617-351-5000
855-969-4642
Fax: 800-269-5232
www.hmhco.com
school.permissions@hmhco.com
June Coultas, Author
Linda K. Zecher, President, CEO & Director
Eric Shuman, Chief Financial Officer
Teach your students specific problem-solving skills and test taking strategies for success with math and math assessments. Practice thoroughly covers five math clusters: numerical operations, patterns and functions, algebraic concepts, measurement and geometry, and data analysis. *$16.60*

743 Sunbuddy Math Playhouse
Sunburst Technology
1550 Executive Dr
Elgin, IL 60123-9311
800-321-7511
Fax: 888-608-0344
http://store.sunburst.com
service@sunburst.com
Michael Guillory, Channel Sales/Marketing Manager
An entertaining play, hidden math-related animations, and four multi-level interactive activities encourage children to explore math and reading.

744 Ten Tricky Tiles
Sunburst Technology
1550 Executive Dr
Elgin, IL 60123-9311
800-321-7511
Fax: 888-608-0344
http://store.sunburst.com
service@sunburst.com
Michael Guillory, Channel Sales/Marketing Manager
Students develop their arithmetic and logic skills with three levels of activities that involve solving sets of numbers sentences.

745 Tenth Planet: Combining and Breaking Apart Numbers
Sunburst Technology
1550 Executive Dr
Elgin, IL 60123-9311
800-321-7511
Fax: 888-608-0344
http://store.sunburst.com
service@sunburst.com
Michael Guillory, Channel Sales/Marketing Manager
Students develop their number sense as they engage in real life dilemmas, which demonstrates the basic concepts of operations.

746 Tenth Planet: Comparing with Ratios
Sunburst Technology
1550 Executive Dr
Elgin, IL 60123-9311
800-321-7511
Fax: 888-608-0344
http://store.sunburst.com
service@sunburst.com
Michael Guillory, Channel Sales/Marketing Manager
Students learn that ratio is a way to compare amounts by using multiplication and division. Through five engaging activities, students recognize and describe ratios, develop proportional thinking skills, estimate ratios, determine equivalent ratios, and use ratios to analyze data.

747 Tenth Planet: Equivalent Fractions
Sunburst Technology
1550 Executive Dr
Elgin, IL 60123-9311
800-321-7511
Fax: 888-608-0344
http://store.sunburst.com
service@sunburst.com
Michael Guillory, Channel Sales/Marketing Manager
This exciting investigation develops students' conceptual understanding that every fraction can be named in many different but equivalent ways.

748 Tenth Planet: Fraction Operations
Sunburst Technology
1550 Executive Dr
Elgin, IL 60123-9311
800-321-7511
Fax: 888-608-0344
http://store.sunburst.com
service@sunburst.com
Michael Guillory, Channel Sales/Marketing Manager
Students build on their concepts of fraction meaning and equivalence as they learn how to perform operations with fractions.

749 Tenth Planet: Grouping and Place Value
Sunburst Technology
1550 Executive Dr
Elgin, IL 60123-9311
800-321-7511
Fax: 888-608-0344
http://store.sunburst.com
service@sunburst.com
Michael Guillory, Channel Sales/Marketing Manager
Students develop their understanding of our number system, learning to think about numbers in groups of ones, tens, and hundreds, and discovering the meaning of place value.

750 Zap! Around Town
Sunburst Technology
1550 Executive Dr
Elgin, IL 60123-9311
800-321-7511
Fax: 888-608-0344
http://store.sunburst.com
service@sunburst.com
Michael Guillory, Channel Sales/Marketing Manager
Students develop mapping and direction skills in this easy-to-use, animated program featuring Shelby, your friendly Sunbuddy guide.

Preschool

751 2's Experience Fingerplays
Building Blocks
38w567 Brindlewood Ln
Elgin, IL 60124-7976
800-233-2448
Fax: 847-742-1054
www.bblocksonline.com
sales@bblocksonline.com

Liz Wilmes, Author
Dick Wilmes, Co-Author

A wonderful collection of fingerplays, songs and rhymes for the very young child. Fingerplays are short, easy to learn, and full of simple movement. Chant or sing the fingerplays and then enjoy the accompanying games and activities. *$12.95*
144 pages

752   Curious George Preschool Learning Games
Sunburst Technology
1550 Executive Dr
Elgin, IL 60123-9311   800-321-7511
                                        Fax: 888-608-0344
                                    http://store.sunburst.com
                                    service@sunburst.com
Michael Guillory, Channel Sales/Marketing Manager
Join Curious George in Fun Town and play five arcade-style games that promote the visual and auditory discrimination skills all students need before they begin to read. Mac/Win CD-ROM

753   Devereux Early Childhood Assessment (DECA)
Kaplan Early Learning Company
1310 Lewisville Clemmons Rd
Lewisville, NC 27023-9635   336-766-7374
                                             800-334-2014
                                        Fax: 800-452-7526
                                        www.kaplanco.com
                                        info@kaplanco.com
Paul A. LeBuffe, Author
Jack A Naglieri, Co-Author
Hal Kaplan, President & CEO
Strength-based standardized, norm-referenced behavior rating scale designed to promote resilience and measure protective factors in children ages 2-5. Through the program, early childhood professionals and families learn specific strategies to support young children's social and emotional development and to enhance the ovall quality of early childhood programs. *$125.95*

754   Devereux Early Childhood Assessment: Clinical Version (DECA-C)
Kaplan Early Learning Company
1310 Lewisville Clemmons Rd
Lewisville, NC 27023-9635   336-766-7374
                                             800-334-2014
                                        Fax: 800-452-7526
                                        www.kaplanco.com
                                        info@kaplanco.com
Paul A. LeBuffe, Author
Jack A Naglieri, Co-Author
Hal Kaplan, President & CEO
DECA-C is designed to support early intervention efforts to reduce or eliminate significant emotional and behavioral concerns in preschool children. This can be used for guide interventions, identify children needing special services, assess outcomes and help programs meet Head Start, IDEA, and similar requirements. Kit includes: 1 Manual, 30 Record Forms, and 1 Norms Reference Card. *$125.95*

755   Early Movement Skills
Therapro
225 Arlington St
Framingham, MA 01702-8773   508-872-9494
                                             800-257-5376
                                        Fax: 508-875-2062
                                        www.therapro.com
                                        info@therapro.com
Naomi Benari, Author
Karen Conrad, President
Easy to follow, reproducible gross motor activities are graded from very simple (even for the passive child) to more demanding (folk dancing). Each of the 150 pages offers an activity with its objective, a clear instruction of the activity, rationale, and alternative movements and games. Many activities involve music and rythm. A great source for early intervention and early childhood programs. *$58.00*

756   Early Screening Inventory: Revised
Pearson Assessments
5601 Green Valley Dr
Bloomington, MN 55437-1099   800-627-7271
                                        Fax: 800-232-1223
                                    www.pearsonassessments.com
                            clinicalcustomersupport@pearson.com
Samuel J Meisels, Author
Martha S Wiske, Co-Author
Laura W Henderson, Co-Author
A developmental screening instrument for 3-to-6-year olds. Provides a norm-referenced overview of visual-motor/adaptive, language and cognition, and gross motor development. Meets IDEA and Head Start requirements for early identification and parental involvement. Test in English or Spanish in 15-20 minutes. Training video and materials available.

757   Early Sensory Skills
Therapro
225 Arlington St
Framingham, MA 01702-8773   508-872-9494
                                             800-257-5376
                                        Fax: 508-875-2062
                                        www.therapro.com
                                        info@therapro.com
Jackie Cooke, Author
Karen Conrad, President
A wonderful book filled with practical and fun activities for stimulating vision, touch, taste and smell. Invaluable for anyone working with children 6 months to 5 years, this manual outlines basic principals followed by six sections containing activities, games and topics to excite the senses. Introductions are easy to follow, and materials for the sensory work are readily accessible in the everyday environment. *$57.75*

758   Early Visual Skills
Therapro
225 Arlington St
Framingham, MA 01702-8773   508-872-9494
                                             800-257-5376
                                        Fax: 508-875-2062
                                        www.therapro.com
                                        info@therapro.com
Diana Williams, Author
Karen Conrad, President
A beautifully designed, easy to follow reproducible book for working with young children on visual perceptual skills. Most of the activities are nonverbal and can be used with children who have limited language. Each section has both easy and challenging activities for school and for parents working with children at home. Activities include sorting, color and shape matching, a looking walk, games to develop visual memory and concentration and many more. *$62.50*
208 pages

759   HELP for Preschoolers at Home
Therapro
225 Arlington St
Framingham, MA 01702-8773   508-872-9494
                                             800-257-5376
                                        Fax: 508-875-2062
                                        www.therapro.com
                                        info@therapro.com
Karen Conrad, President
Three hundred pages of practical, home-based activities that can be easily administered by the parents or the child's home-care provider. Upon completion of their assessments, teachers and therapists provide parents with these handouts to help them work on skills at home in conjunction with the program. *$72.50*

760   LAP-D Kindergarten Screen Kit
Kaplan Early Learning Company
1310 Lewisville Clemmons Rd
Lewisville, NC 27023-9635   336-766-7374
                                             800-334-2014
                                        Fax: 800-452-7526
                                        www.kaplanco.com
                                        info@kaplanco.com

Hal Kaplan, President & CEO
Concise, standardized screening deice normed on 5 year old children. Tasks are in four domains: fine, motor, gross motor, cognitive, and language. The Kindergarten Kit includes the technical manual, examiners, manual, and materials to assist in determining pure outcomes. *$124.95*

761 Learning Accomplishment Profile Diagnostic Normed Screens for Age 3-5
Kaplan Early Learning Company
1310 Lewisville Clemmons Rd
Lewisville, NC 27023-9635

336-766-7374
800-334-2014
Fax: 800-452-7526
www.kaplanco.com
info@kaplanco.com

Hal Kaplan, President & CEO
For 3-5 years. Create reliable developmental snapshots in fine motor, gross motor, cognitive, language, personal/social, and self-help skill domains. *$349.95*

762 Learning Accomplishment Profile (LAP-R) KIT
Kaplan Early Learning Company
1310 Lewisville Clemmons Rd
Lewisville, NC 27023-9635

336-766-7374
800-334-2014
Fax: 800-452-7526
www.kaplanco.com
info@kaplanco.com

Hal Kaplan, President & CEO
Mike Mathers, Author
A criterion-referenced assessment instrument measuring development in six domains: gross motor, fine motor, cognitive, language, self-help and social/emotional. Kit includes all materials necessary for assessing 20 children. *$299.95*

763 Learning Accomplishment Profile Diagnostic Normed Assessment (LAP-D)
Kaplan Early Learning Company
1310 Lewisville Clemmons Rd
Lewisville, NC 27023-9635

336-766-7374
800-334-2014
Fax: 800-452-7526
www.kaplanco.com
info@kaplanco.com

Belinda J. Hardin, Ph.D., Author
Ellen S. Peisner-Feinberg, Ph.D, Co-Author
Stephanie W. Weeks, Ph.D., Co-Author
A comprehensive developemtal assessment tool for children between the ages of 30 and 72 months. LAP-D consists of a hierarchy of developmental skills arranged in four developmental domains: fine motor, gross motor, cognitive and language. *$624.95*

764 Partners for Learning (PFL)
Kaplan Early Learning Company
1310 Lewisville Clemmons Rd
Lewisville, NC 27023-9635

336-766-7374
800-334-2014
Fax: 800-452-7526
www.kaplanco.com
info@kaplanco.com

Hal Kaplan, President & CEO
This resource uses cards, books, posters, and support materials to supply teaching ideas and to support child development. PARTNERS for Learning encourages cognitive, social, motor, and language development. The kit provides materials for curriculum planning and self-assessment. *$199.95*

765 Right from the Start: Behavioral Intervention for Young Children with Autism
Therapro
225 Arlington St
Framingham, MA 01702-8773

508-872-9494
800-257-5376
Fax: 508-875-2062
www.therapro.com
info@therapro.com

Sandra Harris PhD, Author
Mary Jane Weiss PhD, Co-Author
Karen Conrad, President
This informative and user-friendly guide helps parents and service providers explore programs that use early intensive behavioral intervention for young children with autism and related disorders. Within these programs, many children improve in intellectual, social and adaptive functioning, enabling them to move on to regular elementary and preschools. Benefits all children, but primarily useful for children age five and younger. *$16.95*
138 pages

766 Sensory Motor Activities for Early Development
Therapro
225 Arlington St
Framingham, MA 01702-8773

508-872-9494
800-257-5376
Fax: 508-875-2062
www.therapro.com
info@therapro.com

Chia Swee Hong, Author
Helen Gabriel, Co-Author
Cathy St John, Co-Author
A complete package of tried and tested gross and fine motor activities. Many activities to stimulate sensory and body awareness, encourage basic movement, promote hand skills, and enhance spatial/early perceptual skills. Master handouts throughout to give to parents for home practice activities for working in small groups. *$51.50*
93 pages

Reading

767 Animals of the Rainforest Classroom Library
HMH Supplemental Publishers
222 Berkeley Street
Boston, MA 02116

617-351-5000
855-969-4642
Fax: 800-269-5232
www.hmhco.com
school.permissions@hmhco.com

Linda K. Zecher, President and CEO
Eric Shuman, Chief Financial Officer
John K. Dragoon, EVP and Chief Marketing Officer
When reading is a struggle, academic success is even harder to achieve. Now you can put social studies and science curriculum content within reach of every student with this series. Designed specifically for limited readers. *$46.50*
ISBN 0-739849-32-8

768 Ants in His Pants: Absurdities and Realities of Special Education
Sage Publications
2455 Teller Rd
Thousand Oaks, CA 91320-2218

805-499-9774
800-818-7243
Fax: 800-583-2665
www.sagepub.com
orders@sagepub.com

Michael Giangreco, Author
Kevin Ruelle, Co-Author
Blaise R. Simqu, President
With wit, humor and profound one liners, Michael Giangreco will transform your thinking as you take a lighter look at the sometimes comical and occasionally harsh truths in the ever changing field of special education. *$20.95*
128 pages
ISBN 1-890455-42-3

769 **AppleSeeds**
Cobblestone Publishing
Ste C
30 Grove St
Peterborough, NH 03458-1453   603-924-7209
                                      800-821-0115
                                 Fax: 603-924-7380
                              www.cobblestonepub.com
                        customerservice@caruspub.com
Susan Buckley, Editor
An award winning magazine of adventure and exploration
for children ages 7 to 9. Provides kids with themed issues
that explore a different topic with insightful articles, cool
photographs, and a unique you-are-there perspective on culture and history. *$29.95*
36 pages 9 times a year

770 **Basic Level Workbook for Aphasia**
Wayne State University Press
4809 Woodward Ave
Detroit, MI 48201-1309   313-577-6120
                                      800-978-7323
                                 Fax: 313-577-6131
                             http://wsupress.wayne.edu
                              bookorders@wayne.edu
Susan Howell Brubaker MS, Author
Jane Hoehner, Director
Gabe Gloden, Community Engagement Officer
If you work with adolescents and adults with mild to moder-
ate language deficits or limited, impaired, or emerging read-
ing skills, this workbook is what you've been waiting for!
The mMaterial is relevant to their lives, interests, experi-
ences, and vocabulary. Item number W324. *$50.00*
360 pages
ISBN 0-814326-20-X

771 **Beyond the Code**
Educators Publishing Service
PO Box 9031
Cambridge, MA 02139-9031   617-547-6706
                                      800-225-5750
                                 Fax: 617-547-3805
                                   www.epsbooks.com
                  CustomerService.EPS@schoolspecialty.com
Nancy M Hall, Author
Rick Holden, President
Jeff Belanger, Regional Sales Manager
Beyond the Code gives beginning readers experience read-
ing original stories as well as thinking about what they have
read. This companion series follows the same phonetic pro-
gression as the frist 4 books of the popular Explode the Code
program.

772 **Chess with Butterflies**
Oxton House Publishers
PO Box 209
Farmington, ME 04938   207-779-1923
                                      800-539-7323
                                 Fax: 207-779-0623
                                  www.oxtonhouse.com
                                 info@oxtonhouse.com
William Berlinghoff PhD, Managing Editor
Bobby Brown, Marketing Director
Sandi Hawkins, Representative
This is a phoneticaly controlled sequel to 'Fishing with Bal-
loons.' It continues the adventures of the main character as it
develops more sophisticated word families. Lists for those
word families and notes on using them for reading instruction are included in the back of the book. *$5.95*
66 pages
ISBN 1-881929-43-4

773 **Claims to Fame**
Educators Publishing Service
PO Box 9031
Cambridge, MA 02139-9031   617-547-6706
                                      800-225-5750
                                 Fax: 617-547-3805
                                   www.epsbooks.com
                  CustomerService.EPS@schoolspecialty.com
Carol Einstein, Author
Rick Holden, President
Jeff Belanger, Regional Sales Manager
The three exercises after each reading are tailored to the con-
tent of each story. In Thinking About What You Have Read,
students check and extend their understanding of the story.
Working with Words asks students to think about and experi-
ment with vaious word meanings.

774 **Clues to Meaning**
Educators Publishing Service
PO Box 9031
Cambridge, MA 02139-9031   617-547-6706
                                      800-225-5750
                                 Fax: 617-547-3805
                                   www.epsbooks.com
                  CustomerService.EPS@schoolspecialty.com
Ann L Staman, Author
Rick Holden, President
Jeff Belanger, Regional Sales Manager
A versatile series which teaches beginning readers to use the
sounds of letters as one strategy among many in learning to
read.

775 **Concept Phonics**
Oxton House Publishers
PO Box 209
Farmington, ME 04938   207-779-1923
                                      800-539-7323
                                 Fax: 207-779-0623
                                  www.oxtonhouse.com
                                 info@oxtonhouse.com
William Berlinghoff PhD, Managing Editor
Bobby Brown, Marketing Director
Dr. Phyllis Fischer, Author
This is a remarkably effective, research-based, multisensory
program for teaching reading-decoding and speech to stu-
dents with learning disabilities at any age or grade level. Its
13 component pieces include a book on understanding phonics, detailed teacher's guides, and sets of contrast cards,
speed drills, worksheets, visual teaching aids, and comprehensive word lists. *$315.00*
ISBN 1-881929-36-1

776 **Cosmic Reading Journey**
Sunburst Technology
1550 Executive Dr
Elgin, IL 60123-9311   800-321-7511
                                 Fax: 888-608-0344
                               http://store.sunburst.com
                                 service@sunburst.com
Michael Guillory, Channel Sales/Marketing Manager
This reading comprehension program provides meaningful
summary and writing activities for the 100 books that early
readers and their teachers love most.

777 **Creepy Cave Initial Consonants**
Sunburst Technology
1550 Executive Dr
Elgin, IL 60123-9311   800-321-7511
                                 Fax: 888-608-0344
                               http://store.sunburst.com
                                 service@sunburst.com
Michael Guillory, Channel Sales/Marketing Manager
Help your students develop letter recognition and phonemic
awareness skills matching words with the same initial conso-
nant letter in a Creepy Cave.

778 Decoding Automaticity Materials for Reading Fluency
Oxton House Publishers
PO Box 209
Farmington, ME 04938
207-779-1923
800-539-7323
Fax: 207-779-0623
www.oxtonhouse.com
info@oxtonhouse.com
William Berlinghoff PhD, Managing Editor
Bobby Brown, Marketing Director
Dr. Phyllis Fischer, Author
This six-part set is designed to bring students from decoding to automaticity in reading words. The two sets of worksheets train the brain's visual processor to recognize letter units in words; the contrast cards train the brain's speech processor to say the sounds for the letter units; and the speed drills put these two tasks together for reading whole words automatically. Also included are comprehensive sets of lists of one-and two syllable words for designing customized materials. *$150.00*
ISBN 1-881929-37-X

779 Dyslexia Training Program
Educators Publishing Service
PO Box 9031
Cambridge, MA 02139-9031
617-547-6706
800-225-5750
Fax: 617-547-3805
www.epsbooks.com
CustomerService.EPS@schoolspecialty.com
Kathryn Hansen, Key Accounts Coordinator
Ryan Todd, Sales Consultant
Jeff Belanger, Regional Sales Manager
Introduces reading and writing skills to dyslexic children through a two-year, cumulative series of daily one-hour videotaped lessons and accompanying student's books and teacher's guides.

780 Earobics® Clinic Version Step 1
Abilitations Speech Bin
PO Box 1579
Appleton, WI 54912-1579
419-589-1600
888-388-3224
Fax: 888-388-6344
www.schoolspecialty.com
orders@schoolspecialty.com
Joseph M. Yorio, President, CEO
Rick Holden, Executive Vice President
Kevin Baehler, Vice President, Acting CFO
Earobics is a dazzling software that teaches phonological awareness and auditory processing. It systematically — anf enjoyably — trains these critical skills for development ages four to seven years. Item number C482. *$298.99*

781 EarobicsM® Step 1 Home Version
Abilitations Speech Bin
PO Box 1579
Appleton, WI 54912-1579
419-589-1600
888-388-3224
Fax: 888-388-6344
www.schoolspecialty.com
orders@schoolspecialty.com
Joseph M. Yorio, President, CEO
Rick Holden, Executive Vice President
Kevin Baehler, Vice President, Acting CFO
Step 1 offers hundreds of levels of play, appealing graphics, and entertaining music to train the critical auditory skills young children need for success in learning. Item number C481. *$58.99*

782 Emergent Reader
Sunburst Technology
1550 Executive Dr
Elgin, IL 60123-9311
800-321-7511
Fax: 888-608-0344
http://store.sunburst.com
service@sunburst.com
Michael Guillory, Channel Sales/Marketing Manager
This story-reading program supports the efforts of beginning readers by developing their sight word vocabularies.

783 Every Child a Reader
Sunburst Technology
1550 Executive Dr
Elgin, IL 60123-9311
800-321-7511
Fax: 888-608-0344
http://store.sunburst.com
service@sunburst.com
Michael Guillory, Channel Sales/Marketing Manager
Traditional reading strategies in a rich literary context. Designed to promote independent reading and develop oral and written language expression.

784 Explode the Code
Educators Publishing Service
PO Box 9031
Cambridge, MA 02139-9031
617-547-6706
800-225-5750
Fax: 617-547-3805
www.epsbooks.com
CustomerService.EPS@schoolspecialty.com
Nancy M Hall, Author
Rick Holden, President
Jeff Belanger, Regional Sales Manager
Explode the Code provides a sequential, systematic approach to phonics in which students blend sounds to build vocabulary and read words, phrases, sentences, and stories.

785 Fishing with Balloons
Oxton House Publishers
PO Box 209
Farmington, ME 04938
207-779-1923
800-539-7323
Fax: 207-779-0623
www.oxtonhouse.com
info@oxtonhouse.com
William Burlinghoff PhD, Owner
Bobby Brown, Marketing Director
Dion , Author
This is a phonetically controlled chapter book about a 10 year old who learns how his physical disability need not be a barrier to his aspirations. As the story holds the reader's interest, it also emphasizes certain families of words. Lists for those word families and notes on using them for reading instruction are included in the back of the book. *$5.95*
68 pages
ISBN 1-881929-34-5

786 Great Series Great Rescues
HMH Supplemental Publishers
222 Berkeley Street
Boston, MA 02116
617-351-5000
855-969-4642
Fax: 800-269-5232
www.hmhco.com
school.permissions@hmhco.com
Henry Billings, Author
Linda K. Zecher, President, CEO & Director
Eric Shuman, Chief Financial Officer
Human drama makes beginning reading worth the effort. Eight exciting titles build confidence as they build skills. Short, easy-to-read selections enable limited readers to succeed with material that matters. *$15.00*
ISBN 0-811441-76-8

787 Handprints
Educators Publishing Service
PO Box 9031
Cambridge, MA 02139-9031
617-547-6706
800-225-5750
Fax: 617-547-3805
www.epsbooks.com
CustomerService.EPS@schoolspecialty.com
Ann L Staman, Author
Rick Holden, President
Jeff Belanger, Regional Sales Manager

Handprints is a set of 50 storybooks and 4 workbooks for beginning readers in kindergarten and first grade. The storybooks increase in difficulty very gradually and encourage the new readers to use meaning, language, and print cues as they read.

788   High Noon Books
Academic Therapy Publications
20 Leveroni Court
Novato, CA 94949-5746

415-883-3314
800-422-7249
Fax: 888-287-9975
www.academictherapy.com
sales@academictherapy.com

Jim Arena, President
Joanne Urban, Manager
Cynthia Coverston
Serving the field of learning disabilities for the past 25 years. High-interest books for reluctant readers. Reading solution programs, phonics, spelling, writing, visual tracking materials.

789   I Can Read
Teddy Bear Press
3703 S Edmunds St
Ste 67
Seattle, WA 98118

206-402-6947
Fax: 866-870-7323
www.teddybearpress.com
fparker@teddybearpress.net

Fran Parker, Author
A series of 7 reading books and 7 workbooks, a set of 52 flashcards and teacher manual which uses a sight word approach to teach beginning readers. These teacher created books and workbooks present an easy to use beginning reading program which provides repetition, visual motor, visual discrimination and word comprehension activities. It was created to teach young, learning disabled children and has been successfully employed to teach beginning readers of varying ages and abilities. *$90.00*

790   I Can See the ABC's
Teddy Bear Press
3703 S Edmunds St
Ste 67
Seattle, WA 98118

206-402-6947
Fax: 866-870-7323
www.teddybearpress.com
fparker@teddybearpress.net

Fran Parker, Author
A big 11x17 which contains the pre-primer words found in the I Can Read program while introducing the alphabet. *$25.00*

791   Inclusion: Strategies for Working with Young Children
Corwin Press
2455 Teller Road
Thousand Oaks, CA 91320-2218

805-499-9734
800-233-9936
Fax: 805-499-5323
www.corwinpress.com
webmaster@corwin.com

Lorraine O Moore PhD, Author
Mike Soules, President
Lisa Shaw, Executive Director
This exceptional resource is a gold mine of developmentally based ideas to help children between the ages of 3-7 or older students who may be developmentally delayed. This is a very practical and easy-to-use publication which is appropriate for early childhood teachers, K-2 general and special education teachers. *$28.95*
144 pages Educators
ISBN 1-890455-33-4

792   Island Reading Journey
Sunburst Technology
1550 Executive Dr
Elgin, IL 60123-9311

800-321-7511
Fax: 888-608-0344
http://store.sunburst.com
service@sunburst.com

Michael Guillory, Channel Sales/Marketing Manager
Enhance your reading program with meaningful summary and extension activities for 100 intermediate level books. Students read for meaning while they engage in activities that test for comprehension, build writing skills with reader response and essay questions, develop usage skills with cloze activities and improve vocabulary/word attack skills.

793   Kids Media Magic 2.0
Sunburst Technology
1550 Executive Dr
Elgin, IL 60123-9311

800-321-7511
Fax: 888-608-0344
http://store.sunburst.com
service@sunburst.com

Michael Guillory, Channel Sales/Marketing Manager
The first multimedia word processor designed for young children. Help your child become a fluent reader and writer. The Rebus Bar automatically scrolls over 45 vocabulary words as students type.

794   Let's Go Read 1: An Island Adventure
Riverdeep
14046 Collections Center Drive
Chicago, IL 60693

855-969-4642
Fax: 800-269-5232
www.hmhinnovation.com
school.permissions@hmhco.com

Linda K. Zecher, President, CEO & Director
Eric Shuman, Chief Financial Officer
John K. Dragoon, EVP and Chief Marketing Officer
Take off with Robby the Raccoon, Emily the Squirrel and the Reading Rover on an exciting adventure to an island inhabited by the alphabet. Motivated by the delight of mastering new challenges, your child will play through more than 35 fun activties that install and reinforce the essential skills for successful reading.

795   Let's Go Read 2: An Ocean Adventure
Riverdeep
14046 Collections Center Drive
Chicago, IL 60693

855-969-4642
Fax: 800-269-5232
www.hmhinnovation.com
school.permissions@hmhco.com

Linda K. Zecher, President, CEO & Director
Eric Shuman, Chief Financial Officer
John K. Dragoon, EVP and Chief Marketing Officer
Building upon your child's mastery of letters, Let's Go Read: 2 explores how letters combine to form words, and how words combine to express meaning. Dozens of captivating, skill-building activities teach your child the skills to sound out, recognize, build and comprehend hundreds of new words. It's an endlessly fun voyage toward reading fluency!

796   Let's Read
Educators Publishing Service
PO Box 9031
Cambridge, MA 02139-9031

617-547-6706
800-225-5750
Fax: 617-547-3805
www.epsbooks.com
CustomerService.EPS@schoolspecialty.com

Leonard Bloomfield, Author
Clarence L Barnhart, Co-Author
Robert K Barnhart, Co-Author
Using a linguistic approach to teaching reading skills, this series emphasizes relationship of spelling to sound, presenting the concepts together, and providing nine reading books and accompanying workbooks for practice. Provides classroom directions and suggestions for supplementary exercises.

797 Lighthouse Low Vision Products
Lighthouse International
111 E 59th St
New York, NY 10022-1202   212-821-9200
                               800-829-0500
                          Fax: 212-821-9707
                          TTY: 212-821-9713
                               www.lighthouse.org
                               info@lighthouse.com
Mark G. Ackermann, President, CEO
Maura J. Sweeney, SVP/COO
John Vlachos, SVP, Chief Financial Officer
Empowers people of all ages who are visually impaired to
lead safe, active and independent lives

798 Megawords
Educators Publishing Service
PO Box 9031
Cambridge, MA 02139-9031   617-547-6706
                               800-225-5750
                          Fax: 617-547-3805
                               www.epsbooks.com
         CustomerService.EPS@schoolspecialty.com
Kristin Johnson, Author
Polly Baird, Co-Author
Rick Holden, President
A series with a systematic, multisensory approach to learn-
ing the longer words encountered from fourth grade on. Stu-
dents first work with syllables, then combine the syllables
into words, use them in context, and work to increase their
reading and spelling proficiency. Teacher's Guide and Answer Key available.

799 Mike Mulligan & His Steam Shovel
Houghton Mifflin
222 Berkeley Street
Boston, MA 02116   617-351-5000
                               855-969-4642
                          Fax: 800-269-5232
                               www.hmhco.com
                               school.permissions@hmhco.com
Virginia Lee Burton, Author
Linda K. Zecher, President, CEO & Director
Eric Shuman, Chief Financial Officer
This CD-ROM version of the Caldecott classic lets students
experience interactive book reading and participate in four
skills-based extension activities that promote memory,
matching, sequencing, listening, pattern recognition and
map reading skills.
ISBN 0-395664-99-3

800 More Primary Phonics
Educators Publishing Service
PO Box 9031
Cambridge, MA 02139-9031   617-547-6706
                               800-225-5750
                          Fax: 617-547-3805
                               www.epsbooks.com
         CustomerService.EPS@schoolspecialty.com
Barbara W Makar, Author
Rick Holden, President
Jeff Belanger, Regional Sales Manager
Reinforces and expands skills developed in Primary Pho-
nics. Workbooks and storybooks contain the same phonetic
elements, sight words and phonetic sequences as workbooks
1 and 2.

**801 Multi-Sequenced Speed Drills for Fluency Multi-Se-
quenced Speed Drills for Fluency in Decoding**
Oxton House Publishers
PO Box 209
Farmington, ME 04938   207-779-1923
                               800-539-7323
                          Fax: 207-779-0623
                               www.oxtonhouse.com
                               info@oxtonhouse.com
William Burlinghoff PhD, Owner
Bobby Brown, Marketing Director
Dr. Phyllis Fischer, Author

This 179-page set of reading speed drills are carefully constructed to promote decoding automaticity and the fluent
recognition of words. They follow the traditional
Orton-Gillingham spelling and sound sequences. The set
also includes eight pages of teaching advice and a master
chart fro tracking student programs. *$29.95*
195 pages
ISBN 1-881929-14-0

802 Next Stop
Educators Publishing Service
PO Box 9031
Cambridge, MA 02139-9031   617-547-6706
                               800-225-5750
                          Fax: 617-547-3805
                               www.epsbooks.com
         CustomerService.EPS@schoolspecialty.com
Tanya Auger, Author
Rick Holden, President
Jeff Belanger, Regional Sales Manager
Increase reading and language skills while exploring differ-
ent literacy genres. This series is intended for students who
are ready to move beyond phonetically controlled readers to
the nest stop-real chapter books that will help prepare them
for the more challenging literature they will encounter in
later grades.

803 Patterns of English Spelling
AVKO Educational Research Foundation
3084 Willard Rd
Birch Run, MI 48415-9404   810-686-9283
                               866-285-6612
                          Fax: 810-686-1101
                               www.avko.org
                               webmaster@avko.org
Don Mc Cabe, President/Research Director
Linda Heck, Vice-President
Michael Lane, Treasurer
Use the index to locate the page upon which you can find all
the words that share the same patterns. If you look up the
word cat, you will find all the pages where all the at words
are located. If you look up the word precious you will find all
the words ending in cious. There are ten volumes which can
be purchased all together or separately. *$119.95*
Whole set

804 Phonemic Awareness: The Sounds of Reading
Corwin Press
2455 Teller Rd
Thousand Oaks, CA 91320-2218   805-499-9734
                               800-233-9936
                          Fax: 805-499-5323
                               www.corwinpress.com
                               order@corwin.com
Victoria Groves Scott, Author
Mike Soules, President
Lisa Shaw, Executive Director Editorial
In this dynamic new video, Dr. Scott demonstrates the principal components of phonemic awareness: identification;
comparison; segmentation; blending and rhyming. This
video will help you to better understand phonemic awareness training and will show you how to apply these components not only to the reading curriculum but to all subjects
through the school day. Filmed in actual classroom settings.
$69.95
25 minute video
ISBN 1-890455-29-6

805 Polar Express
Houghton Mifflin
222 Berkeley Street
Boston, MA 02116   617-351-5000
                               855-969-4642
                          Fax: 800-269-5232
                               www.hmhco.com
                               school.permissions@hmhco.com
Chris Van Allsburg, Author
Linda K. Zecher, President, CEO & Director
Eric Shuman, Chief Financial Officer

Share the magic and enchantment of the holiday season with this CD-ROM version of the Caldecott-winning picture book.

806 Prehistoric Creaures Then & Now
HMH Supplemental Publishers
222 Berkeley Street
Boston, MA 02116　　　617-351-5000
　　　855-969-4642
Fax: 800-269-5232
www.hmhco.com
school.permissions@hmhco.com
K S Rodriguez, Author
Linda K. Zecher, President, CEO & Director
Eric Shuman, Chief Financial Officer
When reading is a struggle, academic success is even harder to achieve. Now you can put social studies and science curriculum content within reach of every students with Steadwell Books — the series designed specifically for limited readers. Attention-getting photos and informative illustrations, maps, and time lines communicate the social studies and science concepts found in the text.
ISBN 0-739821-47-4

807 Primary Phonics
Educators Publishing Service
PO Box 9031
Cambridge, MA 02139-9031　　　617-547-6706
　　　800-225-5750
Fax: 617-547-3805
www.epsbooks.com
CustomerService.EPS@schoolspecialty.com
Barbara W Makar, Author
Rick Holden, President
Jeff Belanger, Regional Sales Manager
This revised program of storybooks and coordinated workbooks teaches reading for grades K-2. There is a set of ten storybooks to go with each of the first five workbooks. A Primary Phonics Picture Dictionary contains 2,500 commonly used words, including most of the words in the series. This series' individualized nature permits students to progress at their own speed. Teacher's manual available.

808 Read On! Plus
Sunburst Technology
1550 Executive Dr
Elgin, IL 60123-9311　　　800-321-7511
Fax: 888-608-0344
http://store.sunburst.com
service@sunburst.com
Michael Guillory, Channel Sales/Marketing Manager
Promote skills and strategies that improve reading comprehension, and build appreciation for literature and the written word.

809 Reader's Quest I
Sunburst Technology
1550 Executive Dr
Elgin, IL 60123-9311　　　800-321-7511
Fax: 888-608-0344
http://store.sunburst.com
service@sunburst.com
Michael Guillory, Channel Sales/Marketing Manager
These reading workshops provide students with direct reading instruction, interactive practice activities, and practical strategies to ensure reading success.

810 Reader's Quest II
Sunburst Technology
1550 Executive Dr
Elgin, IL 60123-9311　　　800-321-7511
Fax: 888-608-0344
http://store.sunburst.com
service@sunburst.com
Michael Guillory, Channel Sales/Marketing Manager
These reading workshops provide students with direct reading instruction, interactive practice activities, and practical strategies to ensure reading success.

811 Reading Comprehension Bundle
Sunburst Technology
1550 Executive Dr
Elgin, IL 60123-9311　　　800-321-7511
Fax: 888-608-0344
http://store.sunburst.com
service@sunburst.com
Michael Guillory, Channel Sales/Marketing Manager
This collection for the intermediate-level classroom develops the skills students need to read for meaning and understanding.

812 Reading Comprehension in Varied Subject Matter
Educators Publishing Service
PO Box 9031
Cambridge, MA 02139-9031　　　617-547-6706
　　　800-225-5750
Fax: 617-547-3805
www.epsbooks.com
CustomerService.EPS@schoolspecialty.com
Jane Ervin, Author
Rick Holden, President
Jeff Belanger, Regional Sales Manager
Ten workbooks that present a wide range of people and situations with new reading selections, new vocabulary, and a new writing exercise. Each book contains 31 selections in the subject areas of social studies, science, literature, mathematics, philosophy, logic, language, and the arts.

813 Reading Pen
Wizcom Technologies
20 Haganan St.
Einav Industrial Park　　　073-290-6133
www.wizcomtech.com
customer_service@wizcomtech.com
Isaac Soibelman, President
Tiran Fartouk, CEO
Portable assitive reading device that reads words aloud and can be used anywhere. Scans a word from printed text, displays the word in large characters, reads the word aloud from built-in speaker or ear phones and defines the word with the press of a button. Displays syllables, keeps a history of scanned words, adjustable for left or right-handed use. Includes a tutorial video and audio cassette. Not recommended for persons with low vision or impaired fine motor control.
$279.00

814 Reading Who? Reading You!
Sunburst Technology
1550 Executive Dr
Elgin, IL 60123-9311　　　800-321-7511
Fax: 888-608-0344
http://store.sunburst.com
service@sunburst.com
Michael Guillory, Channel Sales/Marketing Manager
Teach beginning reading skills effectively with phonics instruction built into engaging games and puzzles that have children asking for more.

815 Reading for Content
Educators Publishing Service
PO Box 9031
Cambridge, MA 02139-9031　　　617-547-6706
　　　800-225-5750
Fax: 617-547-3805
www.epsbooks.com
CustomerService.EPS@schoolspecialty.com
Carol Einstein, Author
Rick Holden, President
Jeff Belanger, Regional Sales Manager
Reading for Content is a series of 4 books designed to help students improve their reading comprehension skills. Each book contains 43 pasages followed by 4 questions. Two questions ask for a recall of main ideas, and two ask the student to draw conclusions from what they have just read.

816 Reading for Job and Personal Use
PO Box 2500
Lebanon, IN 46052-3009
800-848-9500
Fax: 877-260-2530
www.pearsonschool.com
k12cs@custhelp.com
Marjorie Scardino, CEO
Victor Coira, Sales Representative
Victoria Ramos, Digital Sales Rep
The practical, real-life exercises in these texts teach students how to read and comprehend catalogs, training manuals, letters and memos, signs, reports, charts, and more.

817 Reasoning & Reading Series
Educators Publishing Service
PO Box 9031
Cambridge, MA 02139-9031
617-547-6706
800-225-5750
Fax: 617-547-3805
www.epsbooks.com
CustomerService.EPS@schoolspecialty.com
Joanne Carlisle, Author
Rick Holden, President
Jeff Belanger, Regional Sales Manager
These workbooks develop basic language and thinking skills that build the foundation for reading comprehension. Exercises reinforce reading as a critical reasoning activity. Many exercises encourage students to come up with their own response in instances where there is no single correct answer. In other cases, exercises lend themselves to students working collaboratively to see how many different answers satisfy a question.

818 Right into Reading: A Phonics-Based Reading and Comprehension Program
Educators Publishing Service
PO Box 9031
Cambridge, MA 02139-9031
617-547-6706
800-225-5750
Fax: 617-547-3805
www.epsbooks.com
CustomerService.EPS@schoolspecialty.com
Jane Ervin, Author
Rick Holden, President
Jeff Belanger, Regional Sales Manager
Right into Reading introduces phonics skills in a carefully ordered sequence of bite-size lessons so that students can progress easily and successfully from one reading level to the next. The stories and selections are unusually diverse and interactive.

819 See Me Add
Teddy Bear Press
3703 S Edmunds St
Ste 67
Seattle, WA 98118
206-402-6947
Fax: 866-870-7323
www.teddybearpress.com
fparker@teddybearpress.net
Fran Parker, Author
Introduces the concept of addition using simple story problems and the basic sight word vocabulary found in the I Can Read and Reading Is Fun programs. *$25.00*

820 See Me Subtract
Teddy Bear Press
3703 S Edmunds St
Ste 67
Seattle, WA 98118
206-402-6947
Fax: 866-870-7323
www.teddybearpress.com
fparker@teddybearpress.net
Fran Parker, Author
Introduces the concept of subtraction using simple story problems. *$25.00*

821 Sounds and Spelling Patterns for English
Oxton House Publishers
PO Box 209
Farmington, ME 04938
207-779-1923
800-539-7323
Fax: 207-779-0623
www.oxtonhouse.com
info@oxtonhouse.com
William Burlinghoff PhD, Owner
Bobby Brown, Marketing Director
Dr. Phyllis Fischer, Author
This book is a clear, concise, practical, jargon-free overview of the sounds that make up the English languate and the symbols that we use to represent them in writing. It includes an explanatory chapter on phonological and phonemic awareness and a broad range of strategies for helping beginning readers develop fluent decoding skills. *$24.95*
140 pages
ISBN 1-881929-01-9

822 Specialized Program Individualizing Reading Excellence (SPIRE)
Educators Publishing Service
PO Box 9031
Cambridge, MA 02139-9031
617-547-6706
800-225-5750
Fax: 617-547-3805
www.epsbooks.com
CustomerService.EPS@schoolspecialty.com
Sheila Clark Edmands, Author
Rick Holden, President
Jeff Belanger, Regional Sales Manager
SPIRE is a comprehensive multisensory reading and language arts program for students with learning differences.

823 Starting Comprehension
Educators Publishing Service
PO Box 9031
Cambridge, MA 02139-9031
617-547-6706
800-225-5750
Fax: 617-547-3805
www.epsbooks.com
CustomerService.EPS@schoolspecialty.com
Ann L Staman, Author
Rick Holden, President
Jeff Belanger, Regional Sales Manager
A reading series of 12 workbooks that develops essential comprehension skills at the earliest reading level. It is divided into two different strands, one for students who have a strong visual sense, the other for those who learn sounds easily. Vocabulary introduced within context of exercises, using most of the words in the books. Student relates the details of the passage to the main idea.

824 Stories and More: Animal Friends
Riverdeep, Inc.
14046 Collections Center Drive
Chicago, IL 60693
855-969-4642
Fax: 800-269-5232
www.hmhinnovation.com
school.permissions@hmhco.com
Linda K. Zecher, President, CEO & Director
Eric Shuman, Chief Financial Officer
John K. Dragoon, EVP and Chief Marketing Officer
Stories and More: Animal Friends features three well-known stories — The Gunnywolf, The Trek, and Owl and the Moon — with engaging activities that strengthen students reading comprehension. A scaffolding of pre-reading, reading, and post-reading activities for each story helps kindergarten and 1st grade students practice prediction and sequencing skills; appreciate the importance of character and setting; and respond to literature through writing, drawing, and speaking. *$69.95*

825 Stories and More: Time and Place
Riverdeep, Inc.
14046 Collections Center Drive
Chicago, IL 60693
855-969-4642
Fax: 800-269-5232
www.hmhinnovation.com
school.permissions@hmhco.com
Linda K. Zecher, President, CEO & Director
Eric Shuman, Chief Financial Officer
John K. Dragoon, EVP and Chief Marketing Officer
Stories and More: Time and Place combines three well-loved stories — The House on Maple Street, Roxaboxen, and Galimoto — with — angaging activities that strengthen students' reading comprehension. In these books, the setting plays a primary role. Second and third grade students learn the importance of time, culture, and place in our lives.

826 Stories from Somerville
Oxton House Publishers
PO Box 209
Farmington, ME 04938
207-779-1923
800-539-7323
Fax: 207-779-0623
www.oxtonhouse.com
info@oxtonhouse.com
William Berlinghoff PhD, Managing Editor
Bobby Brown, Marketing Director
Kim Ramsey, Author
This set of two readers and three workbooks contains a total of 75 separate but interconnected, phonetically-controlled stories that follow a careful pattern of skill development. They are compatible with most phonics-based reading programs. The realistic personal interactions of the characters also provide opportunities for rich class discussion about various social skills that may be troublesome for many students, including those with learning disabilities. *$69.95*
ISBN 1-881929-40-4

827 Take Me Home Pair-It Books
Harcourt Achieve
222 Berkeley Street
Boston, MA 02116
617-351-5000
855-969-4642
Fax: 800-269-5232
www.hmhco.com
school.permissions@hmhco.com
Linda K. Zecher, President and CEO
Eric Shuman, Chief Financial Officer
John K. Dragoon, EVP and Chief Marketing Officer
Make reading time a family favorite. Our most popular Pair-It Book titles in convenient take-home packages make it easy to get parents involved in reinforcing reading. *$346.10*

828 Taking Your Camera To...Steadwell
Harcourt Achieve
222 Berkeley Street
Boston, MA 02116
617-351-5000
855-969-4642
Fax: 800-269-5232
www.hmhco.com
school.permissions@hmhco.com
Linda K. Zecher, President, CEO
Eric Shuman, Chief Financial Officer
John K. Dragoon, EVP and Chief Marketing Officer
Give limited readers unlimited access to major countries! Each title devotes a spread to the land, the people, major cities, lifestyles, places to visit, government and religion, earning a living, sports and school, food and holidays, quick facts, statistics and maps, and the future. *$7.80*

829 Teaching Comprehension: Strategies for Stories
Oxton House Publishers
PO Box 209
Farmington, ME 04938
207-779-1923
800-539-7323
Fax: 207-779-0623
www.oxtonhouse.com
info@oxtonhouse.com
William Burlinghoff PhD, Managing Editor
Bobby Brown, Marketing Director
Dr. Phyllis Fischer, Author
This handbook gives teachers a richly detailed roadmap for providing students with effective strategies for comprehending and remembering stories. It inlcudes story-line masters for helping students to organize their thinking about a story and to accurately depict characters and sequence events. *$24.95*
62 pages
ISBN 1-881929-27-2

830 Tenth Planet: Roots, Suffixes, Prefixes
Sunburst Technology
1550 Executive Dr
Elgin, IL 60123-9311
800-321-7511
Fax: 888-608-0344
http://store.sunburst.com
service@sunburst.com
Michael Guillory, Channel Sales/Marketing Manager
Students learn to decode difficult and more complex words as they engage in six activities where they construct and dissect words with roots, prefixes and suffixes.

831 Transition Stage 2-3
Harcourt Achieve
222 Berkeley Street
Boston, MA 02116
617-351-5000
855-969-4642
Fax: 800-269-5232
www.hmhco.com
school.permissions@hmhco.com
Linda K. Zecher, President and CEO
Eric Shuman, Chief Financial Officer
John K. Dragoon, EVP and Chief Marketing Officer
A series of 20 books, each containing 16 pages, that provide readers with a gradual transition into early fluency. All stories are available on audio cassette, and four are available in big book format. *$951.80*

832 Vowels: Short & Long
Sunburst Technology
1550 Executive Dr
Elgin, IL 60123-9311
800-321-7511
Fax: 888-608-0344
http://store.sunburst.com
service@sunburst.com
Michael Guillory, Channel Sales/Marketing Manager
Introduce students to vowels and the role they play in the structure of words. By engaging in word building activities, students learn to identify short and long vowels and regular spelling patterns.

833 Wilson Language Training
47 Old Webster Rd
Oxford, MA 01540-2705
508-368-2399
800-899-8454
Fax: 508-368-2300
www.wilsonlanguage.com
info@wilsonlanguage.com
Barbara A Wilson, Co-Founder/President
Ed Wilson, Co-Founder/Publisher
Dedicated to providing educators with the resources they need to help their students become fluent, independent readers. Provides professional development and research-based reading and spelling curricula for all ages.

834 Wordly Wise 3000 ABC 1-9
Educators Publishing Service
PO Box 9031
Cambridge, MA 02139-9031
617-547-6706
800-225-5750
Fax: 617-547-3805
www.epsbooks.com
CustomerService.EPS@schoolspecialty.com
Kenneth Hodkinson, Author
Sandra Adams, Co-Author
Rick Holden, President

Three thousand new and carefully selected words taken from literature, textbooks and SAT-prep books, are the basis of this new series that teaches vocabulary through reading, writing, and a variety of exercises for grades 4-12.

835   Wordly Wise ABC 1-9
Educators Publishing Service
PO Box 9031
Cambridge, MA   02139-9031   617-547-6706
                                            800-225-5750
                                         Fax: 617-547-3805
                                          www.epsbooks.com
         CustomerService.EPS@schoolspecialty.com
Kenneth Hodkinson, Author
Sandra Adams, Co-Author
Rick Holden, President
Vocabulary workbook series employs crossword puzzles, riddles, word games and a sense of humor to make the learning of new words an interesting experience.

Science

836   Learn About Life Science: Animals
Sunburst Technology
1550 Executive Dr
Elgin, IL   60123-9311   800-321-7511
                                         Fax: 888-608-0344
                                       http://store.sunburst.com
                                        service@sunburst.com
Michael Guillory, Channel Sales/Marketing Manager
Learn about animal classification, adaptation to climate, domestication and special relationships between humans and animals.

837   Learn About Life Science: Plants
Sunburst Technology
1550 Executive Dr
Elgin, IL   60123-9311   800-321-7511
                                         Fax: 888-608-0344
                                       http://store.sunburst.com
                                        service@sunburst.com
Michael Guillory, Channel Sales/Marketing Manager
Students explore the world of plants. From small seeds to tall trees students learn what plants are and what they need to grow.

838   Learn About Physical Science: Simple Machines
Sunburst Technology
1550 Executive Dr
Elgin, IL   60123-9311   800-321-7511
                                         Fax: 888-608-0344
                                       http://store.sunburst.com
                                        service@sunburst.com
Michael Guillory, Channel Sales/Marketing Manager
Students delve into the mechanical world learning about the ways simple machines make our work easier.

839   Life Cycles Beaver
HMH Supplemental Publishers
222 Berkeley Street
Boston, MA   02116   617-351-5000
                                            855-969-4642
                                         Fax: 800-269-5232
                                           www.hmhco.com
                                   school.permissions@hmhco.com
Sabrina Crewe, Author
Linda K. Zecher, President, CEO & Director
Eric Shuman, Chief Financial Officer
Dramatic photos tell the story of animal growth and development. This softcover series enriches any classroom science curriculum. Animal development is a complex subject but this series makes it understandable for young readers with simple text and informative images that follow each animal from birth to maturity. *$8.80*

840   Maps & Navigation
Sunburst Technology
1550 Executive Dr
Elgin, IL   60123-9311   800-321-7511
                                         Fax: 888-608-0344
                                       http://store.sunburst.com
                                        service@sunburst.com
Michael Guillory, Channel Sales/Marketing Manager
This exciting nautical simulation provides students with opportunities to use their math and science skills.

841   Our Universe
HMH Supplemental Publishers
222 Berkeley Street
Boston, MA   02116   617-351-5000
                                            855-969-4642
                                         Fax: 800-269-5232
                                           www.hmhco.com
                                   school.permissions@hmhco.com
Gregory Vogt, Author
Linda K. Zecher, President, CEO & Director
Eric Shuman, Chief Financial Officer
Unravel the mysteries of space! A complex universe becomes amazingly clear in these easy-to-read titles. *$96.00*
ISBN 0-739833-55-3

842   Prehistoric Creaures Then & Now
HMH Supplemental Publishers
222 Berkeley Street
Boston, MA   02116   617-351-5000
                                            855-969-4642
                                         Fax: 800-269-5232
                                           www.hmhco.com
                                   school.permissions@hmhco.com
K S Rodriguez, Author
Linda K. Zecher, President, CEO & Director
Eric Shuman, Chief Financial Officer
Now limited readers can dig into the details of dinosaurs! Each information-packed title includes a special spread with a project, a profile of a dinosaur expert, or a description of a recent dinosaur discovery.
ISBN 0-739821-47-4

843   Space Academy GX-1
Riverdeep
14046 Collections Center Drive
Chicago, IL   60693   855-969-4642
                                         Fax: 800-269-5232
                                        www.hmhinnovation.com
                                   school.permissions@hmhco.com
Linda K. Zecher, President, CEO & Director
Eric Shuman, Chief Financial Officer
John K. Dragoon, EVP and Chief Marketing Officer
Explore the solar system with Space Academy GX-1! Fully aligned with national science standards and state curricula, Space Academy GX-1, students investigate the astronomical basis for seasons, phases of the moon, gravity, orbits, and more. As students succeed, Grow Slides adjust to offer more advanced topics and problems.

844   Talking Walls
Riverdeep
14046 Collections Center Drive
Chicago, IL   60693   855-969-4642
                                         Fax: 800-269-5232
                                        www.hmhinnovation.com
                                   school.permissions@hmhco.com
Linda K. Zecher, President, CEO & Director
Eric Shuman, Chief Financial Officer
John K. Dragoon, EVP and Chief Marketing Officer
The Talking Walls Software Series is a wonderful springboard for a student's journey of exploration and discovery. This comprehensive collection of researched resources and materials enables students to focus on learning while conducting a guided search for information.

845 Talking Walls: The Stories Continue
Riverdeep
14046 Collections Center Drive
Chicago, IL 60693   855-969-4642
                          Fax: 800-269-5232
                        www.hmhinnovation.com
                  school.permissions@hmhco.com
Linda K. Zecher, President, CEO & Director
Eric Shuman, Chief Financial Officer
John K. Dragoon, EVP and Chief Marketing Officer
Using the Talking Walls Software Series, students discover the stories behind some of the world's most fascinating walls. The award-winning books, interactive software, carefully chosen Web sites, and suggested classroom activities build upon each other, providing a rich learning experience that includes text, video, and hands-on projects.

846 ThemeWeavers: Nature Activity Kit
Riverdeep
14046 Collections Center Drive
Chicago, IL 60693   855-969-4642
                          Fax: 800-269-5232
                        www.hmhinnovation.com
                  school.permissions@hmhco.com
Linda K. Zecher, President, CEO & Director
Eric Shuman, Chief Financial Officer
John K. Dragoon, EVP and Chief Marketing Officer
ThemeWeavers: Nature Activity Kit is an all-in-one solution for theme-based teaching. In just a few minutes, you can select from dozens of ready-to-use activities centering on the seasons and weather and be ready for the next day's lesson! Interactive and engaging activities cover multiple subject areas such as language arts, math, science, social studies and art.

847 Thinkin' Science
Sunburst Technology
1550 Executive Dr
Elgin, IL 60123-9311   800-321-7511
                            Fax: 888-608-0344
                        http://store.sunburst.com
                          service@sunburst.com
Michael Guillory, Channel Sales/Marketing Manager
Five environments introduce students to the scientific methods and concepts needed to understand basic earth, life and physical sciences. Students learn to think like scientists as they solve problems using hypothesis, experimentation, observation and deduction.

848 Thinkin' Science ZAP!
Sunburst Technology
1550 Executive Dr
Elgin, IL 60123-9311   800-321-7511
                            Fax: 888-608-0344
                        http://store.sunburst.com
                          service@sunburst.com
Michael Guillory, Channel Sales/Marketing Manager
Working with laser beams, electrical circuits, and visible sound waves, students practice valuable thinking skills, observation, prediction, dedutive reasoning, conceptual modeling, theory building and hypothesis testing while experimenting within scientifically accurate learning environment.

849 True Tales
HMH Supplemental Publishers
222 Berkeley Street
Boston, MA 02116   617-351-5000
                          855-969-4642
                          Fax: 800-269-5232
                        www.hmhco.com
                  school.permissions@hmhco.com
Henry Billings, Author
Linda K. Zecher, President, CEO & Director
Eric Shuman, Chief Financial Officer

If you have been looking for reading comprehension materials for limited readers, your search is over. True Tales presents powerful real-lfe events with direct connections to geography and science at reading level 3. Gripping accounts of personal triumph and tragedy put geography and science in a very real context. Accompanying activities develop reading and language arts, science, and geography skills students need to boost test scores. *$205.00*
ISBN 0-739834-49-5

850 Virtual Labs: Electricity
Riverdeep
14046 Collections Center Drive
Chicago, IL 60693   855-969-4642
                          Fax: 800-269-5232
                        www.hmhinnovation.com
                  school.permissions@hmhco.com
Linda K. Zecher, President, CEO & Director
Eric Shuman, Chief Financial Officer
John K. Dragoon, EVP and Chief Marketing Officer
Five environments introduce students to the scientific methods and conepts needed to understand basic Earth, life, and physical sciences. Students will learn to think like scientists as they solve problems using hypothesis, experimentation, observation, and deduction. *$69.95*

Social Skills

851 Activities Unlimited
Therapro
225 Arlington St
Framingham, MA 01702-8773   508-872-9494
                                  800-257-5376
                                Fax: 508-875-2062
                                www.therapro.com
                                info@therapro.com
A Cleveland, Author
B Caton, Co-Author
L Adler, Co-Author
Helps young children develop fine and gross motor skills, increase their language, become self-reliant and play cooperatively. An innovative resource that immediately attracts and engages children. Short of time? Need a good idea? Count on Activites Unlimited. *$17.95*

852 Activity Schedules for Children with Autism: Teaching Independent Behavior
Therapro
225 Arlington St
Framingham, MA 01702-8773   508-872-9494
                                  800-257-5376
                                Fax: 508-875-2062
                                www.therapro.com
                                info@therapro.com
Lynn McClannahan PhD, Author
Patricia Krantz PhD, Co-Author
Karen Conrad, President
An activity schedule is a set of pictures or words that cue a child to follow a sequence of activities. When mastered, the children are more self-directed and purposeful at home, school and leisure activites. In this book, parents and professionals can find detailed instructions and examples, assess a child's readiness to use activity schedules, and understand graduated guidance and progress monitoring. Great for promoting independence in children with autism. *$16.95*
117 pages

853 Alert Program with Songs for Self-Regulation
Therapro
225 Arlington St
Framingham, MA 01702-8773   508-872-9494
                                  800-257-5376
                                Fax: 508-875-2062
                                www.therapro.com
                                info@therapro.com
Mary Sue Williams OTR, Author
Sherry Shellenberger OTR, Co-Author
Karen Conrad, President

This program compares the body to an engine, running either high, low, or just right. Side A is an overview, Side B has 15 songs for self-regulation. Extremely successful in helping kids recognize and change their own engine speeds. *$23.95*
Audio Tape

854   An Introduction to How Does Your Engine Run?
Therapro
225 Arlington St
Framingham, MA 01702-8773   508-872-9494
                                           800-257-5376
                                    Fax: 508-875-2062
                                    www.therapro.com
                                    info@therapro.com

Mary Sue Williams OTR, Author
Sherry Shellenberger OTR, Co-Author
Karen Conrad, President
Introduces the entire Alert Program, which explains how we regulate our arousal states. Describes the use of sensorimotor strategies to manage levels of alertness. This program is fun for students and the adults working with them, and translates easily into real life. *$7.95*

855   Andy and His Yellow Frisbee
Woodbine House
6510 Bells Mill Rd
Bethesda, MD 20817-1636   301-897-3570
                                           800-843-7323
                                    Fax: 301-897-5838
                                    www.woodbinehouse.com
                                    info@woodbinehouse.com

Mary Thompson, Author
A heartwarming story about Andy, a boy with autism. Like many children with autism, Andy has a fascination with objects in motion. His talent for spinning his Frisbee and a new classmate's curiosity set this story in motion. Rosie, the watchful and protective sister, supplies backround on Andy and autism, as well as a sibling's perspective. *$14.95*
24 pages

856   Breakthroughs Manual: How to Reach Students with Autism
Therapro
225 Arlington St
Framingham, MA 01702-8773   508-872-9494
                                           800-257-5376
                                    Fax: 508-875-2062
                                    www.therapro.com
                                    info@therapro.com

Karen Sewell, Author
Karen Conrad, President
This manual features practical suggestions for everyday use with preschool through high school students. Covers communication, behavior, academics, self-help, life and social skills. Includes reproducible lesson plans and up to date listing of classroom materials and catalog supply companies. *$49.50*
243 pages

857   Busy Kids Movement
Therapro
225 Arlington St
Framingham, MA 01702-8773   508-872-9494
                                           800-257-5376
                                    Fax: 508-875-2062
                                    www.therapro.com
                                    info@therapro.com

Karen Conrad, President
Full of ideas for developing youngsters' gross motor skills. Games, dramatics, action songs, music and rythm activities. *$9.95*
64 pages

858   Calm Down and Play
Childswork
PO Box 1246
Wilkes-Barre, PA 18703-1246   800-962-1141
                                    Fax: 800-262-1886
                                    www.childswork.com

Sally Germain, Editor
Loretta Oleck Berger, Author
Filled with fun and effective activities to help children: calm down and control their impulses; focus, concentrate, and organize their thoughts; identify and verbalize feelings; channel and release excess energy appropriately; and build self-esteem and confidence. *$17.95*

859   Courageous Pacers Classroom Chart
Therapro
225 Arlington St
Framingham, MA 01702-8773   508-872-9494
                                           800-257-5376
                                    Fax: 508-875-2062
                                    www.therapro.com
                                    info@therapro.com

Karen Conrad, President
Tim Erson, Author
Highly recommended to accompany the Courageous Pacers Program. Assists in keeping record of 12 students' progress in walking and lifting. A great visual tool to view progress.

860   Courageous Pacers Program
Therapro
225 Arlington St
Framingham, MA 01702-8773   508-872-9494
                                           800-257-5376
                                    Fax: 508-875-2062
                                    www.therapro.com
                                    info@therapro.com

Karen Conrad, President
Tim Erson, Author
This fun and easy program was developed to help students become more active. Research shows that students who are more active, do better in school. The goal of the program is simple: get students to walk 100 miles and lift 10,000 pounds in a year.
92 pages

861   Face to Face: Resolving Conflict Without Giving in or Giving Up
820 S. Monaco Parkway
#255
Denver, CO 80224   602-633-4213
                                    Fax: 202-667-8629
                                    www.nafcm.org
                                    mphillips@nafcm.org

Matt Phillips, Executive Director
Jan Bellard, Author
Jilda Gutierrez, Co-Author
Modular curriculum for training program for AmeriCorps members. Addresses conflict at the personal level, interpersonal level, and group collaboration. Includes workbook.

862   Forms for Helping the ADHD Child
Childswork
PO Box 1246
Wilkes-Barre, PA 18703-1246   800-962-1141
                                    Fax: 800-262-1886
                                    www.childswork.com

Sally Germain, Editor
Lawrence E. Shapiro, Author
Forms, charts, and checklists for treating children with Attention Deficit Hyperactivity Disorder cover a wide range of approaches. Includes effective aids in assessing, treating, and monitoring the progress of the ADHD child. *$31.95*
100 pages

863   Funsical Fitness With Silly-cise CD: Motor Development Activities
Therapro
225 Arlington St
Framingham, MA 01702-8773   508-872-9494
                                           800-257-5376
                                    Fax: 508-875-2062
                                    www.therapro.com
                                    info@therapro.com

Karen Conrad, President

This unique blending of developmentally appropriate gross motor, sensory integration, and aerobic activities is guaranteed to build children's strength, balance endurance, coordination, and self confidence. Leads children through four 15-minute classes of Wacky Walking, Grinnastics, Brain Gym, Warm Ups, Adventurobics, and Chill Out activities. *$15.00*

864 Games we Should Play in School
Therapro
225 Arlington St
Framingham, MA 01702-8773   508-872-9494
                                    800-257-5376
                                    Fax: 508-875-2062
                                    www.therapro.com
                                    info@therapro.com
Frank Aycox, Author
Karen Conrad, President
Includes over 75 interactive, fun, social games; describes how to effectively lead Social Play sessions in the classroom. Students become more cooperative, less antagonistic and more capable of increased attentiveness. Contains the secrets to enriching the entire school environment. *$16.50*
154 pages

865 Jarvis Clutch: Social Spy
Educators Publishing Service
PO Box 9031
Cambridge, MA 02139-9031   617-547-6706
                                    800-225-5750
                                    Fax: 617-547-3805
                                    www.epsbooks.com
                   CustomerService.EPS@schoolspecialty.com
Melvin D Levine MD FAAP, Author
Rick Holden, President
Jeff Belanger, Regional Sales Manager
In Jarvis Clutch social spy, Dr. Mel Levine teams up with eight grader Jarvis Clutch for an insider's look at life on the middle school social scene. Jarvis's wry and insightful observations of student interactions at Eastern Middle School bring to light the myriad social challenges that adolescents face every day, including peer pressure, the need to seem cool, the perils of dating., Include the commentary in Jarivs' Spy Notes!

866 Learning in Motion
Therapro
225 Arlington St
Framingham, MA 01702-8773   508-872-9494
                                    800-257-5376
                                    Fax: 508-875-2062
                                    www.therapro.com
                                    info@therapro.com
Patricia Angermeir OTR BCP, Author
Joan Krzyzanowski OTR MS, Co-Author
Kristina Keller Moir OTR BCP, Co-Author
Written by 3 OTs, this book is for the busy therapist or teacher of preschoolers to second graders. Provides group activities using gross, fine andsensory motor skills in theme based curricula. Every lesson plan contains goals, objectives, materials and adaptations to facilitate inclusion and multilevel instructions. Includes 130 lesson plans with corresponding parent letters that explain the lesson and provide home follow-up activities. *$39.95*
379 pages

867 New Language of Toys: Teaching Communication Skills to Children with Special Needs
Therapro
225 Arlington St
Framingham, MA 01702-8773   508-872-9494
                                    800-257-5376
                                    Fax: 508-875-2062
                                    www.therapro.com
                                    info@therapro.com
Karen Conrad, President
Sue Schwarz PhD, Author
Joan Heller Miller EdM, Co-Author

Play time becomes a fun and educational experience with this revised hands-on approach for developing communication skills using everyday toys. Includes a fresh assortment of toys, books and new chapters on computer technology, language learning, videotapes and television. *$18.95*
289 pages

868 Reaching Out, Joining In: Teaching Social Skills to Young Children with Autism
Therapro
225 Arlington St
Framingham, MA 01702-8773   508-872-9494
                                    800-257-5376
                                    Fax: 508-875-2062
                                    www.therapro.com
                                    info@therapro.com
Mary Jane Weiss PhD BCBA, Author
Sandra Harris PhD, Co-Author
Karen Conrad, President
Describes how to help young children diagnosed within the autism spectrum with one of their most challenging areas of development, social behavior. Focuses on four broad topics: play skills; the language of social skills; undestanding another person's perspective; and using these skills in an inclusive classroom. The authors present concrete strategies to teach basic play skills, how to play with others, to recognize social cues and engage in social conversation. Practical and accessible. *$16.95*
215 pages

869 Right from the Start: Behavioral Intervention for Young Children with Autism
Therapro
225 Arlington St
Framingham, MA 01702-8773   508-872-9494
                                    800-257-5376
                                    Fax: 508-875-2062
                                    www.therapro.com
                                    info@therapro.com
Mary Jane Weiss PhD BCBA, Author
Sandra L Harris PhD, Co-Author
Karen Conrad, President
This informative and user-friendly guide helps parents and service providers explore programs that use early intensive behavioral intervention for young children with autism and related disorders. Within these programs, many children improve in intellectual, social and adaptive functioning, enabling them to move on to regular elementary and preschools. Benefits all children, but primarily useful for children age five and younger. *$16.95*
215 pages

870 S'Cool Moves for Learning: A Program Designed to Enhance Learning Through Body-Mind
Therapro
225 Arlington St
Framingham, MA 01702-8773   508-872-9494
                                    800-257-5376
                                    Fax: 508-875-2062
                                    www.therapro.com
                                    info@therapro.com
Debra M Heiberger MA, Author
Margot C Heiniger White MA OTR, Co-Author
Karen Conrad, President
The movement activities described in this book are organized in a way that is easy to integrate into the class routine throughout the day. The Minute Moves for the Classroom included in several chapters is a handy reference of movement activities which help make the transition from one activity to another fun and smooth. *$35.00*

871 Simple Steps: Developmental Activities for Infants, Toddlers & Two Year Olds
Therapro
225 Arlington St
Framingham, MA 01702-8773   508-872-9494
                                 800-257-5376
                                 Fax: 508-875-2062
                                 www.therapro.com
                                 info@therapro.com

Karen Miller, Author
Karen Conrad, President
Three hundred activities linked to the latest research in brain development. Outlines a typical developmental sequence in 10 domains: social/emotional, fine motor; gross motor; language; cognition; sensory; nature; music and movement; creativity and dramatic play. Chapters on curriculum development and learning environment also included. *$24.95*
293 pages

872 Solutions Kit for ADHD
Childswork
PO Box 1246
Wilkes-Barre, PA 18703-1246   800-962-1141
                                   Fax: 800-262-1886
                                   www.childswork.com

Sally Germain, Editor
Dana Regan, Author
Lawrence E Shapiro, Co-Author
This comprehensive kit is packed with hands-on materials for a multi-modal approach to working with ADHD kids aged 5 through 12. *$105.00*

873 Song Games for Sensory Integration
Therapro
225 Arlington St
Framingham, MA 01702-8773   508-872-9494
                                 800-257-5376
                                 Fax: 508-875-2062
                                 www.therapro.com
                                 info@therapro.com

Karen Conrad, President
Aubrey Carton, Author
Lois Hickman, Co-Author
For young children with sensory processing challenges, 15 play-along routines help remediate everything from bilateral skills to vestibular dysfunction. Narrative is helpful for parents. Includes an 81 page book filled with ideas for extending therapeutic value of these activites. 87 minute CD. *$21.00*
Audio Tape

874 Start to Finish: Developmentally Sequenced Fine Motor Activities for Preschool Children
Therapro
225 Arlington St
Framingham, MA 01702-8773   508-872-9494
                                 800-257-5376
                                 Fax: 508-875-2062
                                 www.therapro.com
                                 info@therapro.com

Nory Marsh, Author
Karen Conrad, President
Seventy stimulating activities target 4 areas of fine motor development normally acquired between 3 and 5: hand manipulation, pencil grasp, scissors skill and grasp, and visual motor skills. Each 30 minute activity has skills, projected goal, supplies needed, instructions and modifications provided and needs limited preparation time. *$59.50*

875 Stop, Relax and Think
Childswork
PO Box 1246
Wilkes Barre, PA 18703-1246   800-962-1141
                                   Fax: 800-262-1886
                                   www.childswork.com

Sally Germain, Editor

In this board game, active impulsive children learn motor control, relaxation skills, how to express their feelings, and how to problem-solve. Can be used both as a diagnostic and a treatment tool, and behaviors learned in the game can be generalized into the home or classroom. *$52.00*

876 Stop, Relax and Think Ball
Childswork
PO Box 1246
Wilkes-Barre, PA 18703-1246   800-962-1141
                                   Fax: 800-262-1886
                                   www.childswork.com

Sally Germain, Editor
This ball teaches children to control their impulsivity by helping them understand and control their actions. *$22.00*

877 Stop, Relax and Think Card Game
Childswork
PO Box 1246
Wilkes-Barre, PA 18703-1246   800-962-1141
                                   Fax: 800-262-1886
                                   www.childswork.com

Sally Germain, Editor
Becky Bridges, Author
Players are dealt Stop, Relax and Think cards and also Stressed Out, Confused, and Discouraged cards. As they acquire more cards, they must choose different self-control skills, and they learn the value of patience and cooperating with others to achieve a goal. *$21.95*

878 Stop, Relax and Think Scriptbook
Childswork
PO Box 1246
Wilkes-Barre, PA 18703-1246   800-962-1141
                                   Fax: 800-262-1886
                                   www.childswork.com

Sally Germain, Editor
Hennie Shore, Author
In this uniquely designed book, children can practice what to say and how to act in eight different scenarios common to children with behavioral problems. The counselor and the child sit across from each other and read the scripts. *$24.95*

879 Stop, Relax and Think Workbook
Childswork
PO Box 1246
Wilkes-Barre, PA 18703-1246   800-962-1141
                                   Fax: 800-262-1886
                                   www.childswork.com

Sally Germain, Editor
Lisa M. Schab, LCSW, Author
This new workbook contains more than 60 paper and pencil activities that teach children such important skills as: thinking about consequences, staying focused and completing a task, engaging in quiet activities without disturbing others, and more. *$19.95*

880 Successful Movement Challenges
Therapro
225 Arlington St
Framingham, MA 01702-8773   508-872-9494
                                 800-257-5376
                                 Fax: 508-875-2062
                                 www.therapro.com
                                 info@therapro.com

Jack Capon, Author
Karen Conrad, President
Extensive and exciting movement activities for children in preschool, elementary and special education. Includes movement exploration challenges using parachutes, balls, hoops, ropes, bean bags, rythm sticks, scarves and much more. This popular publication also includes body conditioning, mat activities and playground apparatus activities. Everyone enjoys the creative and carefully designed movement experiences. *$14.25*
127 pages

881 Teaching Kids with Mental Health and Learning Disorders in the Regular Classroom
Free Spirit Publishing
217 5th Ave N
Suite 200
Minneapolis, MN 55401-1299

800-735-7323
866-703-7322
Fax: 866-419-5199
www.freespirit.com
help4kids@freespirit.com

Judy Galbraith, Founder/President
Myles L. Cooley, Author
Generalized Anxiety Disorder (GAD), depression, Asperger's Syndrome, and ADHD. Many students have these and other mental health issues and learning problems. Written by a clinical psychologist, this guide describes mental health and learning disorders often observed in school children, explains how each might be exhibited in the classroom, and offers expert suggestions on what to do (and sometimes what not to do). *$34.95*
256 pages
ISBN 1-575420-89-9

882 Understanding Argumentative Communication: How Many Ways Can You Ask for a Cookie?
Therapro
225 Arlington St
Framingham, MA 01702-8773

508-872-9494
800-257-5376
Fax: 508-875-2062
www.therapro.com
info@therapro.com

Christine Derse MEd, Author
Janice Lopes MSEd, Co-Author
Karen Conrad, President
Ten uncomplicated lesson plans for classroom use. Teach a complete overview of all that Argumentative Communication encompasses or give students a brief awareness lesson about just one type of communication. Lessons can be used either consecutively or singly. Includes defining communication, gestures, sign language, object boards, picture boards, headsticks, eye pointing, scanning with picture boards, picture boards in sentence format and computers for argumentative communication. *$18.95*
142 pages

883 Updown Chair
R.E.A.L. Design
187 S Main St
Dolgeville, NY 13329-1455

315-429-3071
800-696-7041
Fax: 315-429-3071
www.realdesigninc.com
rdesign@twcny.rr.com

Kris Wohnsen, Co-Owner
Sam Camarello, Co-Owner
The updown chair is designed for children from 43-63 in height. It combines optimal positioning and sitting comfort with ease of adjustment. Changing the seat height can be done quickly and safely with our exclusive foot lever activation which uses a pneumatic cylinder assist. Children can be elevated to just the right position for floor or table top activities.

884 Wikki Stix Hands On-Learning Activity Book
Therapro
225 Arlington St
Framingham, MA 01702-8773

508-872-9494
800-257-5376
Fax: 508-875-2062
www.therapro.com
info@therapro.com

Karen Conrad, President
Loaded with great ideas for using Wikki Stix. For all ages and curriculums. *$3.50*

885 Workbook for Verbal Expression
PO Box 1579
Appleton, WI 54912-1579

419-589-1600
888-388-3224
Fax: 888-388-6344
www.schoolspecialty.com
orders@schoolspecialty.com

Joseph M. Yorio, President, CEO
Beth M Kennedy, Author
Kevin Baehler, Vice President, Acting CFO
A book of 100s of excercises from simple naming, automatic speech sequences, and repetition exercises to complex tasks in sentence formulation and abstract verbal reasoning. Item number 1435.

Social Studies

886 American Government Today
HMH Supplemental Publishers
222 Berkeley Street
Boston, MA 02116

617-351-5000
855-969-4642
Fax: 800-269-5232
www.hmhco.com
school.permissions@hmhco.com

Mark Sanders, Author
Linda K. Zecher, President, CEO & Director
Eric Shuman, Chief Financial Officer
Give limited readers unlimited access to social studies and citizenship topics! Whether applying for citizenship or studying for GED Test, learners need to know about our nation's capital and the democracy it hosts. In this series, even limited readers can get a clear picture of a complex system. *$52.00*
ISBN 0-139822-03-9

887 Calliope
Cobblestone Publishing
30 Grove St
Suite C
Peterborough, NH 03458-1453

603-924-7209
800-821-0115
Fax: 603-924-7380
www.cobblestonepub.com
customerservice@caruspub.com

Rosalie Baker, Editor
Kid's world history magazine written for kids ages 9 to 14, goes beyond the facts to explore provocative issues. *$33.95 9x/year*

888 Discoveries: Explore the Desert Ecosystem
Sunburst Technology
1550 Executive Dr
Elgin, IL 60123-9311

800-321-7511
Fax: 888-608-0344
http://store.sunburst.com
service@sunburst.com

Michael Guillory, Channel Sales/Marketing Manager
This program invites students to explore the plants, animals, culture and georgraphy of the Sonoran Desert by day and by night.

889 Discoveries: Explore the Everglades Ecosystem
Sunburst Technology
1550 Executive Dr
Elgin, IL 60123-9311

800-321-7511
Fax: 888-608-0344
http://store.sunburst.com
service@sunburst.com

Michael Guillory, Channel Sales/Marketing Manager
This multi curricular research program takes students to the Everglades where they anchor their exploration photo realistic panaramas of the habitiat.

890 **Discoveries: Explore the Forest Ecosystem**
Sunburst Technology
1550 Executive Dr
Elgin, IL 60123-9311   800-321-7511
                                   Fax: 888-608-0344
                                http://store.sunburst.com
                                   service@sunburst.com
Michael Guillory, Channel Sales/Marketing Manager
This theme based CD-ROM enables students of all abilities to actively research a multitude of different forest ecosystems in the Appalachian National Park.

891 **Easybook Deluxe Writing Workshop: Colonial Times**
Sunburst Technology
1550 Executive Dr
Elgin, IL 60123-9311   800-321-7511
                                   Fax: 888-608-0344
                                http://store.sunburst.com
                                   service@sunburst.com
Michael Guillory, Channel Sales/Marketing Manager
Writing workshops combine theme-based activities with the award-winning EasyBook Deluxe.

892 **Easybook Deluxe Writing Workshop: Immigration**
Sunburst Technology
1550 Executive Dr
Elgin, IL 60123-9311   800-321-7511
                                   Fax: 888-608-0344
                                http://store.sunburst.com
                                   service@sunburst.com
Michael Guillory, Channel Sales/Marketing Manager
Writing workshops combine theme-based activities with the award-winning EasyBook Deluxe.

893 **Easybook Deluxe Writing Workshop: Rainforest & Astronomy**
Sunburst Technology
1550 Executive Dr
Elgin, IL 60123-9311   800-321-7511
                                   Fax: 888-608-0344
                                http://store.sunburst.com
                                   service@sunburst.com
Michael Guillory, Channel Sales/Marketing Manager
Writing workshops combine theme-based activities with the award-winning EasyBook Deluxe.

894 **Explorers & Exploration: Steadwell**
HMH Supplemental Publishers
222 Berkeley Street
Boston, MA 02116   617-351-5000
                                     855-969-4642
                                   Fax: 800-269-5232
                                      www.hmhco.com
                             school.permissions@hmhco.com
Linda K. Zecher, President and CEO
Eric Shuman, Chief Financial Officer
John K. Dragoon, EVP and Chief Marketing Officer
Long ago adventures are still a thrill in these vividly illustrated titles. Maps, diagrams, and contemporary prints lend an authenic air. A time line and list of events in the appropriate century put history in perspective. *$44.40*
ISBN 0-739822-05-5

895 **First Biographies**
HMH Supplemental Publishers
222 Berkeley Street
Boston, MA 02116   617-351-5000
                                     855-969-4642
                                   Fax. 800-269-3232
                                      www.hmhco.com
                             school.permissions@hmhco.com
Linda K. Zecher, President, CEO
Eric Shuman, CFO
John K. Dragoon, EVP and Chief Marketing Officer
True stories of true legends! Legendary figures triumph over tough challenges in these brief biographies. Beginning readers learn about favorite heroes and heroines in books they can read for themselves. *$98.80*
ISBN 0-817268-91-X

896 **Imagination Express Destination Time Trip USA**
Sunburst Technology
1550 Executive Dr
Elgin, IL 60123-9311   800-321-7511
                                   Fax: 888-608-0344
                                http://store.sunburst.com
                                   service@sunburst.com
Michael Guillory, Channel Sales/Marketing Manager
Student's travel through time to explore the history and development of a fictional New England town. An online scrapbook lets them learn about architecture, fashion, entertainment and events of the six major periods in U.S. history.

897 **Make-a-Map 3D**
Sunburst Technology
1550 Executive Dr
Elgin, IL 60123-9311   800-321-7511
                                   Fax: 888-608-0344
                                http://store.sunburst.com
                                   service@sunburst.com
Michael Guillory, Channel Sales/Marketing Manager
Students learn basic mapping, geography and navigation skills. Students design maps of their immediate surroundings by dragging and dropping roads and buildings and adding landmarks, land forms and traffic signs.

898 **Maps & Navigation**
Sunburst Technology
1550 Executive Dr
Elgin, IL 60123-9311   800-321-7511
                                   Fax: 888-608-0344
                                http://store.sunburst.com
                                   service@sunburst.com
Michael Guillory, Channel Sales/Marketing Manager
This exciting nautical simulation provides students with opportunities to use their math and science skills.

899 **Prehistoric Creaures Then & Now**
HMH Supplemental Publishers
222 Berkeley Street
Boston, MA 02116   617-351-5000
                                     855-969-4642
                                   Fax: 800-269-5232
                                      www.hmhco.com
                             school.permissions@hmhco.com
K S Rodiguez, Author
Linda K. Zecher, President, CEO & Director
Eric Shuman, Chief Financial Officer
Now limited readers can dig into the details of dinosaurs! Each information-packed title includes a special spread with a project, a profile of a dinosaur expert, or a description of a recent dinosaur discovery.
ISBN 0-739821-47-4

900 **Story of the USA**
Educators Publishing Service
PO Box 9031
Cambridge, MA 02139-9031   617-547-6706
                                     800-225-5750
                                   Fax: 617-547-3805
                                      www.epsbooks.com
                        CustomerService.EPS@schoolspecialty.com
Franklin Escher Jr, Author
Rick Holden, President
Jeff Belanger, Regional Sales Manager
A series of four workbooks for grades 4-8 which presents basic topics in American History: Book 1, Explorers and Settlers - Book 2, A Young Nation Solves Its Problems - Book 3, America Becomes A Giant and Book 4, Modern America. A list of vocabulary words introduces each chapter and study questions test students' knowledge.

901 **Talking Walls Bundle**
Sunburst Technology
1550 Executive Dr
Elgin, IL 60123-9311   800-321-7511
                                   Fax: 888-608-0344
                                http://store.sunburst.com
                                   service@sunburst.com

Michael Guillory, Channel Sales/Marketing Manager
Broaden students' perspective of cultures around the world with this two program CD-ROM bundle. From the Great Wall of China to the Berlin Wall to the Vietnam Memorial, students explore 28 walls that represent examples of the greatest human achievements to the most intimate expressions of individuality.

902 Test Practice Success: American History
HMH Supplemental Publishers
222 Berkeley Street
Boston, MA 02116   617-351-5000
                                   855-969-4642
                              Fax: 800-269-5232
                                   www.hmhco.com
                     school.permissions@hmhco.com
Linda K. Zecher, President and CEO
Eric Shuman, Chief Financial Officer
John K. Dragoon, EVP and Chief Marketing Officer
When you are trying to meet history standards, standardized test preparation is hard to schedule. Now you can do both at the same time. Steck-Vaughn/Berrent Test Practice Success: American History refreshes basic skills, familiarizes students with test formats and directions, and teaches test-taking strategies, while drawing on the material students are studying in class. *$16.30*
ISBN 0-739831-31-3

903 True Tales
HMH Supplemental Publishers
222 Berkeley Street
Boston, MA 02116   617-351-5000
                                   855-969-4642
                              Fax: 800-269-5232
                                   www.hmhco.com
                     school.permissions@hmhco.com
Henry Billings, Author
Linda K. Zecher, President, CEO & Director
Eric Shuman, Chief Financial Officer
If you have been looking for reading comprehension materials for limiteed readers, your search is over. True Tales presents powerful real-lfe events with direct connections to geography and science at reading level 3. Gripping accounts of personal triumph and tragedy put geography and science in a very real context. Accompanying activities develop reading and language arts, science, and geography skills students need to boost test scores. *$205.00*
ISBN 0-739834-49-5

Study Skills

904 Experiences with Writing Styles
Harcourt Achieve
222 Berkeley Street
Boston, MA 02116   617-351-5000
                                   855-969-4642
                              Fax: 800-269-5232
                                   www.hmhco.com
                     school.permissions@hmhco.com
Linda K. Zecher, President and CEO
Eric Shuman, Chief Financial Officer
John K. Dragoon, EVP and Chief Marketing Officer
Give your students experience applying the writing process in nine relevant situations, from personal narratives to persuasive paragraphs to research reports. Units provide a clear definition of each genre and plenty of practice with prewriting, writing, revising, proofreading, and publishing. *$11.99*

905 Keyboarding Skills
Educators Publishing Service
PO Box 9031
Cambridge, MA 02139-9031   617-547-6706
                                   800-225-5750
                              Fax: 617-547-3805
                                   www.epsbooks.com
             CustomerService.EPS@schoolspecialty.com

Diana Hanbury King, Author
Rick Holden, President
Jeff Belanger, Regional Sales Manager
This innovative touch typing method enables students of all ages to learn to type quickly and easily. After learning the alphabet, students can practice words, phrases, numbers, symbols and punctuation.

906 Learning Strategies Curriculum
Edge Enterprises
708 W 9th St
Suite 107
Lawrence, KS 66044-2846   785-749-1473
                                   877-767-1487
                              Fax: 785-749-0207
                     www.edgeenterprisesinc.com
                    eeinfo@edgeenterprisesinc.com
Jean B. Schumaker Ph.D., President
Jacqueline Schafer, Editor
A learning strategy is an individual's approach to a learning task. It includes how a person thinks and acts when planning, executing and evaluating performance on the task and its outcomes. In short, learning strategy instruction focuses on how to learn and how to effectively use what has been learned. Manuals range from sentence writing to test taking. All require training. For information, contact the Kansas Center for Research on Learning, 3061 Dole Center, Lawrence 66045 (785-864-4780)

907 Super Study Wheel: Homework Helper
Therapro
225 Arlington St
Framingham, MA 01702-8773   508-872-9494
                                   800-257-5376
                              Fax: 508-875-2062
                                   www.therapro.com
                              info@therapro.com
Karen Conrad, President
The fun and simple way to find study tips. Developed by learning specialists and an occupational therapist, the Super Study Wheel is an idea-packed resource (with 101 tips) to improve study skills in 13 areas. As a visual, motor and kinesthetic tool, it is very helpful to students with unique learning styles. *$6.95*

Toys & Games, Catalogs

908 Maxi Aids
42 Executive Blvd
Farmingdale, NY 11735-4710   631-752-0521
                                   800-522-6294
                              Fax: 631-752-0689
                              TTY: 631-752-0738
                                   www.maxiaids.com
Elliot Zaretsky, President
Aids and appliances for independent living with products designed especially for the visually impaired, blind, hard of hearing, deaf, deaf-blind, arthritic and the physically challenged. New educational games and toys section.

909 PCI Educational Publishing
8700 Shoal Creek Boulevard
San Antonio, TX 78757-6897   512-451-3246
                                   800-897-3202
                              Fax: 512-451-8542
                                   www.pcieducation.com
                         jberger@pcieducation.com
Lee Wilson, President and CEO
Janie Haugen-McLane, Founder
Randy Pennington, Executive Vice President
Offers 14 programs in a gameboard format to improve life and social skills including Cooking Class, Community Skills, Looking Good, Eating Skills, Workplace Skills, Behavior Skills, Time Skills, Money Skills, Safety Skills, Household Skills, Social Skills, Health Skills, Survival Skills and Recreation Skills. Also offers a Life Skills catalog with over 140 additional products.

Toys & Games, Products

910 Beads and Baubles
Therapro
225 Arlington St
Framingham, MA 01702-8773

508-872-9494
800-257-5376
Fax: 508-875-2062
www.therapro.com
info@therapro.com

Karen Conrad, President
A basic stringing activity great for developing fine motor skills. Over 100 pieces in various shapes, colors, and sizes to string on a lace. Three laces included. *$7.99*

911 Beads and Pattern Cards
Therapro
225 Arlington St
Framingham, MA 01702-8773

508-872-9494
800-257-5376
Fax: 508-875-2062
www.therapro.com
info@therapro.com

Karen Conrad, President
Colorful wooden sphers, cubes, cylinders and laces provide pre-reading/early math practice and help develop shape/color sorting and recognition skills. *$27.95*

912 Big Little Pegboard Set
Therapro
225 Arlington St
Framingham, MA 01702-8773

508-872-9494
800-257-5376
Fax: 508-875-2062
www.therapro.com
info@therapro.com

Karen Conrad, President
Kids love to play with this set of 25 safe, brightly colored hardwood pegs and a durable foam rubber board. *$18.95*

913 Busy Box Activity Centers
Enabling Devices
50 Broadway
Hawthorne, NY 10532

914-747-3070
800-832-8697
Fax: 914-747-3480
www.enablingdevices.com
customer_support@enablingdevices.com
Steven E. Kanor PhD, President/Founder
With their bright colors and exciting variety of textures and shapes that are designed to invite exploration that results in rewards including buzzers, music box melodies, radio, vibrations, puffs of air, flashing lights, and even a model that talks. Encourages hand-eye coordination, fine motor skills, gross arm movement. A full line of activity centers are available to meet the needs of the learning disabled, hearing impaired, visually impaired and multisensory impaired. *$163.95*

914 Colored Wooden Counting Cubes
Therapro
225 Arlington St
Framingham, MA 01702-8723

508-872-9494
800-257-5376
Fax: 508-875-2062
www.therapro.com
info@therapro.com

Karen Conrad President
100 cubes in 6 colors are perfect for counting, patterning, and building activities. Activity Guide included. *$19.95*

915 Disc-O-Bocce
Therapro
225 Arlington St
Framingham, MA 01702-8723

508-872-9494
800-257-5376
Fax: 508-875-2062
www.therapro.com
info@therapro.com

Karen Conrad, President
Requested by therapists working with adults, this item is also great for children. Hundreds of uses include tossing the discs onto the ground and stepping on them to follow their path, tossing and trying to hit the same color disc on the floor, or using the discs to toss in a game of tic-tac-toe on the floor. Includes 12 colorful bocce discs in a storage box with handle. *$29.95*

916 Earobics® Clinic Version
Abilitations Speech Bin
PO Box 1579
Appleton, W 54912-1579

419-589-1600
888-388-3224
Fax: 888-388-6344
www.schoolspecialty.com
orders@schoolspecialty.com
Joseph M. Yorio, President, CEO
Rick Holden, Executive Vice President
Kevin Baehler, Vice President, Acting CFO
Earobics features: Tasks and Level Counter with real time display, adaptive training technology for individualized programs and reporting to track and evaluate each individual's progress. Step 2 teaches critical language comprehension skills and trains the critical auditory skills children need for success in learning. Item number C484. *$298.99*

917 Earobics® Home Version
Abilitations Speech Bin
PO Box 1579
Appleton, W 54912-1579

419-589-1600
888-388-3224
Fax: 888-388-6344
www.schoolspecialty.com
orders@schoolspecialty.com
Joseph M. Yorio, President, CEO
Rick Holden, Executive Vice President
Kevin Baehler, Vice President, Acting CFO
Step 2 teaches critical language comprehension skills and trains the critical auditory skills children need for success in learning. It offers hundreds of levels of play, appealing graphics, and entertaining music to train the critical auditory skills young children need for success in learning. Item number C483. *$58.99*

918 Earobics® Step 1 Home Version
School Specialty
PO Box 1579
Appleton, WI 54912-1579

419-589-1600
888-388-3224
Fax: 888-388-6344
www.schoolspecialty.com
orders@schoolspecialty.com
Joseph M. Yorio, President, CEO
Rick Holden, Executive Vice President
Kevin Baehler, Vice President, Acting CFO
Step 1 offers hundreds of levels of play, appealing graphics, and entertaining music to train the critical auditory skills young children need for success in learning. Item number C481. *$58.99*

919 Eye-Hand Coordination Boosters
Therapro
225 Arlington St
Framingham, MA 01702-8723

508-872-9494
800-257-5376
Fax: 508-875-2062
www.therapro.com
info@therapro.com

Karen Conrad, President
L. Jay Lev, Author
A book of 92 masters that can be used over and over again with work sheets that are appropriate for all ages. These are perceptual motor activities that involve copying and tracing in the areas of visual tracking, discrimination and spatial relationships. *$21.50*

920 Familiar Things
Therapro
225 Arlington St
Framingham, MA 01702-8723

508-872-9494
800-257-5376
Fax: 508-875-2062
www.therapro.com
info@therapro.com

Karen Conrad, President
Identify and match shapes of common objects with these large square, rubber pieces. *$19.99*

921 Flagship Carpets
PO Box 1779
Calhoun, GA 30701

800-848-4055
www.flagshipcarpets.com
info@flagshipcarpets.com

Offers a variety of carpet games like hopscotch, the alphabet, geography maps, custom logo mats and more.

922 GeoSafari Wonder World USA
Educational Insights
152 W. Walnut St
Suite 201
Gardena, CA 90248

800-955-4436
Fax: 888-892-8731
www.educationalinsights.com
CS@educationalinsights.com

Navigate the United States in a thrilling, interactive tour across this giant, beautifully detailed 4' x 6' cloth map embroidered with state boundaries. As children learn about American geography, they will love attaching the 78 self-stick felt pieces that identify the states and their unique features. *$199.99*

923 Geoboard Colored Plastic
Therapro
225 Arlington St
Framingham, MA 01702-8723

508-872-9494
800-257-5376
Fax: 508-875-2062
www.therapro.com
info@therapro.com

Karen Conrad, President
Teach eye/hand coordination skills while strengthening pincher grasp with rubber bands. *$3.25*

924 Geometrical Design Coloring Book
Therapro
225 Arlington St
Framingham, MA 01702-8723

508-872-9494
800-257-5376
Fax: 508-875-2062
www.therapro.com
info@therapro.com

Karen Conrad, President
Spyros Horemis, Author
Color these 46 original designs of pure patterns and abstract shapes for a striking and beautiful result, regardless of skill level. Most designs are made of a combination of small and large areas. *$3.95*

925 Get in Shape to Write
Therapro
225 Arlington St
Framingham, MA 01702-8723

508-872-9494
800-257-5376
Fax: 508-875-2062
www.therapro.com
info@therapro.com

Karen Conrad, President
Phillip Bongiorno MA OTR, Author
Lorette Konezny, Editor
Practice the visual perceptual motor skills needed for writing with these colorful, fun, and engaging activities. The 23 reusable activities will keep a student's interest while they learn to process auditory, visual, and motor movement patterns. In addition, learn concepts of matching and sorting colors, shapes and familiar objects. *$12.95*

926 Half 'n' Half Design and Color Book
Therapro
225 Arlington St
Framingham, MA 01702-8723

508-872-9494
800-257-5376
Fax: 508-875-2062
www.therapro.com
info@therapro.com

Karen Conrad, President
Elaine Heller, Author
Geometric designs appropriate for all ages. The client draws over dotted lines to finish the other half of the printed design. *$15.00*

927 Link N' Learn Activity Book
Therapro
225 Arlington St
Framingham, MA 01702-8723

508-872-9494
800-257-5376
Fax: 508-875-2062
www.therapro.com
info@therapro.com

Karen Conrad, President
Carol A. Thornton, Author
A nice accompaniment to the color rings. There are great cognitive activities included. *$9.99*

928 Link N' Learn Activity Cards
Therapro
225 Arlington St
Framingham, MA 01702-8723

508-872-9494
800-257-5376
Fax: 508-875-2062
www.therapro.com
info@therapro.com

Karen Conrad, President
Learn patterning, sequencing and color discrimination and logic skills with this set of 20 cards that show life-sized links. An instructor's guide is included. *$7.99*

929 Link N' Learn Color Rings
Therapro
225 Arlington St
Framingham, MA 01702-8723

508-872-9494
800-257-5376
Fax: 508-875-2062
www.therapro.com
info@therapro.com

Karen Conrad, President
These easy to hook and separate colorful 1-1/2 inch plastic rings can be used in color sorting, counting, sequencing, and other perceptual/cognitive activities. *$5.99*

930 Magicatch Set
Therapro
225 Arlington St
Framingham, MA 01702-8723

508-872-9494
800-257-5376
Fax: 508-875-2062
www.therapro.com
info@therapro.com

Karen Conrad, President
This Velcro catch game offers a much higher degree of success and feeling of security than traditional ball tossing games. 7 1/2 inch neon catching paddles and 2 1/2 inch ball, in a mesh bag. No latex. *$7.50*

931 Magnetic Fun
Therapro
225 Arlington St
Framingham, MA 01702-8723

508-872-9494
800-257-5376
Fax: 508-875-2062
www.therapro.com
info@therapro.com

Karen Conrad, President
One swipe of the magic wand can pick up small objects without the need for a refined pincher grasp. *$13.95*

932   Maze Book
Therapro
225 Arlington St
Framingham, MA 01702-8723

508-872-9494
800-257-5376
Fax: 508-875-2062
www.therapro.com
info@therapro.com

Karen Conrad, President
Paul McCreary, Author
Significantly more challenging than the ABC Mazes; rich in perceptual activities. *$10.95*
32 pages

933   Opposites Game
Therapro
225 Arlington St
Framingham, MA 01702-8723

508-872-9494
800-257-5376
Fax: 508-875-2062
www.therapro.com
info@therapro.com

Karen Conrad, President
Children can explore the concept of opposites by matching and then joining these tiles. Self correcting feature allows for both independent and supervised play. Helps build observation and recognition skills. *$8.50*

934   Parquetry Blocks & Pattern Cards
Therapro
225 Arlington St
Framingham, MA 01702-8723

508-872-9494
800-257-5376
Fax: 508-875-2062
www.therapro.com
info@therapro.com

Karen Conrad, President
Encourages visual perceptual skills and challenges a person's sense of design and color with squares, triangles, and rhombuses in six colors. *$28.90*

935   Pegboard Set
Therapro
225 Arlington St
Framingham, MA 01702-8723

508-872-9494
800-257-5376
Fax: 508-875-2062
www.therapro.com
info@therapro.com

Karen Conrad, President
Encourage development of fine motor skills while teaching color, sorting, patterning and counting! Pegboard is 10.75 inches square and made of durable plastic featuring 100 holes in a 10 x 10 array. *$10.50*

936   Plastic Cones
Therapro
225 Arlington St
Framingham, MA 01702-8723

508-872-9494
800-257-5376
Fax: 508-875-2062
www.therapro.com
info@therapro.com

Karen Conrad, President
The 12-inch versions of the construction project cones are bright orange and made of lightweigth vinyl. Hole in top. *$8.25*

937   Primer Pak
Therapro
225 Arlington St
Framingham, MA 01702-8723

508-872-9494
800-257-5376
Fax: 508-875-2062
www.therapro.com
info@therapro.com

Karen Conrad, President

A challenging sampler of manipulatives. Four Fit-A-Space disk puzzles with basic shapes, an 8x8 Alphabet Puzzle, three Lacing Shapes for primary lacing, and 24 Locktagons to form structures. *$14.99*

938   Rhyming Sounds Game
Therapro
225 Arlington St
Framingham, MA 01702-8723

508-872-9494
800-257-5376
Fax: 508-875-2062
www.therapro.com
info@therapro.com

Karen Conrad, President
Introduces 32 different rhyming sounds as players match the ending sound of the picture tile to the corresponding object on the category boards. Includes sorting/storage tray, 56 picture tiles, and 4 category cards with self-checking feature. No reading required. *$9.99*

939   Shape and Color Sorter
Therapro
225 Arlington St
Framingham, MA 01702-8723

508-872-9494
800-257-5376
Fax: 508-875-2062
www.therapro.com
info@therapro.com

Karen Conrad, President
This simple and safe task of perception includes 25 crepe foam rubber pieces to sort by shape or color. Comes in five bright colors, each color representing a shape. Shapes fit nicely onto five large pegs. *$14.99*

940   Shapes
Therapro
225 Arlington St
Framingham, MA 01702-8723

508-872-9494
800-257-5376
Fax: 508-875-2062
www.therapro.com
info@therapro.com

Karen Conrad, President
Muncie Hendler, Author
This 8 1/2 x 11 inch high quality coloring book will help children learn to recognize shapes while improving their fine motor and perceptual skills. *$1.50*
30 pages

941   Snail's Pace Race Game
Therapro
225 Arlington St
Framingham, MA 01702-8723

508-872-9494
800-257-5376
Fax: 508-875-2062
www.therapro.com
info@therapro.com

Karen Conrad, President
This classic, easy color game is back and is fun for all to play. Roll the colored dice to see which wooden snail will move closer to the finish line. Promotes color recognition, understanding of taking turns, and sharing. *$19.95*

942   Speak & Learn Communicator
Enabling Devices
50 Broadway
Hawthorne, NY 10532

914-747-3070
800-832-8697
Fax: 914-747-3480
www.enablingdevices.com
customer_support@enablingdevices.com

Steven E. Kanor PhD, President/Founder
Memory game! Have fun individualizing this matching memory game. Pre-record your questions and answers and you're ready to play. This is an exciting way to reinforce identification and matching numbers, letters, shapes, and words. *$390.95*

943 Spider Ball
Therapro
225 Arlington St
Framingham, MA 01702-8723

508-872-9494
800-257-5376
Fax: 508-875-2062
www.therapro.com
info@therapro.com

Karen Conrad, President
Easy to catch, won't roll away! This foam rubber ball has rubber legs that make it incredibly easy to catch. Invented by a PE teacher to help children improve their ball playing skills. The Spiderball's legs act as brakes bringing it to a stop when rolled and minimizing the time needed to chase a missed ball. 2 1/4 inch diameter. *$4.50*

944 Squidgie Flying Disc
Therapro
225 Arlington St
Framingham, MA 01702-8723

508-872-9494
800-257-5376
Fax: 508-875-2062
www.therapro.com
info@therapro.com

Karen Conrad, President
This is a great flexible flying disc that is amazingly easy to throw and travels over long distances. It is soft and easy to catch. It will even float in the pool! *$5.50*

945 String A Long Lacing Kit
Therapro
225 Arlington St
Framingham, MA 01702-8723

508-872-9494
800-257-5376
Fax: 508-875-2062
www.therapro.com
info@therapro.com

Karen Conrad, President
A lacing activity that develops hand eye coordination and concentration as children create 2 colorful bead buddies. Each buddy has 4 laces attached to its painted heal now build the body with 23 beads! *$15.00*

946 Things in My House: Picture Matching Game
Therapro
225 Arlington St
Framingham, MA 01702-8723

508-872-9494
800-257-5376
Fax: 508-875-2062
www.therapro.com
info@therapro.com

Karen Conrad, President
Strengthen visual discrimination, sorting, and organizing skills. Young children enjoy finding correct matches in this fun first game. The colorful graphics depicting familiar household objects and activities encourage verbalization and imaginative play. *$9.99*

947 Toddler Tote
Therapro
225 Arlington St
Framingham, MA 01702-8723

508-872-9494
800-257-5376
Fax: 508-875-2062
www.therapro.com
info@therapro.com

Karen Conrad, President
Offers one Junior Fit-A-Space panel that has large geometric shapes; 4 Shape Squares providing basic shapes in a more challenging size; 2 Peg Play Vehicles and Pegs introducing early peg board skills; 3 Familiar Things and 2 piece puzzles and a handy take-along bag. *$14.99*

948 Whistle Kit
Therapro
225 Arlington St
Framingham, MA 01702-8723

508-872-9494
800-257-5376
Fax: 508-875-2062
www.therapro.com
info@therapro.com

Karen Conrad, President
The whistles in this collection are colorful and sturdy. Most feature moving parts as well as noise-makers to stimulate both ocular and oral motor skills. Includes nine whistles. Respiratory demand ranges from easy to difficult. *$18.95*

949 Wikki Stix
Therapro
225 Arlington St
Framingham, MA 01702-8723

508-872-9494
800-257-5376
Fax: 508-875-2062
www.therapro.com
info@therapro.com

Karen Conrad, President
Colorful, nontoxic waxed strings which are easily molded to create various forms, shapes and letters. Combine motor planning skill with fine motor skill by following simple shapes with Wikki Stix and then coloring in the shape. *$5.99*

950 Windup Fishing Game
Therapro
225 Arlington St
Framingham, MA 01702-8723

508-872-9494
800-257-5376
Fax: 508-875-2062
www.therapro.com
info@therapro.com

Karen Conrad, President
Encourages eye-hand coordination. Rubber hook safely catches velcro on chipboard fish. *$3.99*

951 Wonder Ball
Therapro
225 Arlington St
Framingham, MA 01702-8723

508-872-9494
800-257-5376
Fax: 508-875-2062
www.therapro.com
info@therapro.com

Karen Conrad, President
This 3 inch ball made of many small suction cups feels good in the palm of the hand and, when thrown against a smooth surface, will firmly stick. Pulling it from the surface requires strength, resulting in proprioceptive stimulation. *$5.99*

Writing

952 ABC's, Numbers & Shapes
Therapro
225 Arlington St
Framingham, MA 01702-8723

508-872-9494
800-257-5376
Fax: 508-875-2062
www.therapro.com
info@therapro.com

Karen Conrad, President
Do-A-Dot Activity Books are great for pre-writing skill books, printed on heavy paper stock, with each page perforated for easy removal. They promote eye-hand coordination and visual recognition. *$4.95*

953 Author's Toolkit
Sunburst Technology
1550 Executive Dr
Elgin, IL 60123-9311

800-321-7511
Fax: 888-608-0344
http://store.sunburst.com
service@sunburst.com

Students can use this comprehensive tool to organize ideas, make outlines, rough drafts, edit and print all their written work.

954 Callirobics: Advanced Exercises
Therapro
225 Arlington St
Framingham, MA 01702-8723

508-872-9494
800-257-5376
Fax: 508-875-2062
www.therapro.com
info@therapro.com

Karen Conrad, President
Liora Laufer, Author
Allows those who have finished earlier Callirobics programs to continue improving their handwriting in a fun and creative way. Callirobics Advanced lets one create shapes to popular music from around the world. *$29.95*
Book and CD

955 Callirobics: Exercises for Adults
Therapro
225 Arlington St
Framingham, MA 01702-8723

508-872-9494
800-257-5376
Fax: 508-875-2062
www.therapro.com
info@therapro.com

Karen Conrad, President
Liora Laufer, Author
Callirobics-for-Adults is a program designed to help adults regain handwriting skills to music. The music assists as an auditory cue in initiating writing movements, and will help develop a sense of rhythm in writing. The program consists of two sections: exercises of simple graphical shapes that help adults gain fluency in the writing movement, and exercises of various combinations of cursive letters. *$35.95*

956 Callirobics: Handwriting Exercises to Music
Therapro
225 Arlington St
Framingham, MA 01702-8723

508-872-9494
800-257-5376
Fax: 508-875-2062
www.therapro.com
info@therapro.com

Karen Conrad, President
Liora Laufer, Author
Ten structured sessions, each with 2 exercises and 2 pieces of music. Includes stickers and a certificate book. *$29.95*
Book and CD

957 Callirobics: Prewriting Skills with Music
Therapro
225 Arlington St
Framingham, MA 01702-8723

508-872-9494
800-257-5376
Fax: 508-875-2062
www.therapro.com
info@therapro.com

Karen Conrad, President
Liora Laufer, Author
These 11 handwriting exercises are a series of simple and enjoyable graphical patterns to be traced by the child while listening to popular melodies. *$29.95*
Book and CD

958 Caps, Commas and Other Things
Academic Therapy Publications
20 Leveroni Court
Novato, CA 94949-5746

415-883-3314
800-422-7249
Fax: 888-287-9975
www.academictherapy.com
sales@academictherapy.com

Jim Arena, President
Joanne Urban, Manager
Sheryl Pastorek, Author

A writing program for regular, remedial and ESL students in grades 3 through 12 and adults in basic education classes remedial ESL. Six levels on capitalization and punctuation, four levels on written expression. Specific lesson plans with reproducible worksheets. *$20.00*
264 pages
ISBN 0-878793-25-9

959 Dysgraphia: Why Johnny Can't Write
Therapro
225 Arlington St
Framingham, MA 01702-8723

508-872-9494
800-257-5376
Fax: 508-875-2062
www.therapro.com
info@therapro.com

Karen Conrad, President
Diane Walton Cavey, Author
Dysgraphia is a serious writing difficulty. This book provides guidelines for recognizing dysgraphic children and explains their special writing needs. Offers valuable tips, ideas and methods to promote success and self regard. *$13.95*

960 Easybook Deluxe
Sunburst Technology
1550 Executive Dr
Elgin, IL 60123-9311

800-321-7511
Fax: 888-608-0344
http://store.sunburst.com
service@sunburst.com

Designed to support the needs of a wide range of writers, this book publishing tool provides students with a creative environment to write, design and illustrate stories and reports, and to print their work in book formats.

961 Easybook Deluxe Writing Workshop: Colonial Times
Sunburst Technology
1550 Executive Dr
Elgin, IL 60123-9311

800-321-7511
Fax: 888-608-0344
http://store.sunburst.com
service@sunburst.com

Writing workshops combine theme-based activities with the award-winning EasyBook Deluxe.

962 Easybook Deluxe Writing Workshop: Immigration
Sunburst Technology
1550 Executive Dr
Elgin, IL 60123-9311

800-321-7511
Fax: 888-608-0344
http://store.sunburst.com
service@sunburst.com

Writing workshops combine theme-based activities with the award-winning EasyBook Deluxe.

963 Easybook Deluxe Writing Workshop: Rainforest & Astronomy
Sunburst Technology
1550 Executive Dr
Elgin, IL 60123-9311

800-321-7511
Fax: 888-608-0344
http://store.sunburst.com
service@sunburst.com

Writing workshops combine theme-based activities with the award-winning EasyBook Deluxe.

964 Easybook Deluxe Writing Workshop: Whales & Oceans
Sunburst Technology
1550 Executive Dr
Elgin, IL 60123-9311

800-321-7511
Fax: 888-608-0344
http://store.sunburst.com
service@sunburst.com

Writing workshops combine theme-based activities with the award-winning EasyBook Deluxe.

965 Fonts 4 Teachers
Therapro
225 Arlington St
Framingham, MA 01702-8723   508-872-9494
                                    800-257-5376
                                    Fax: 508-875-2062
                                    www.therapro.com
                                    info@therapro.com

Karen Conrad, President
A software collection of 31 True Type fonts for teachers, parents and students. Fonts include Tracing, lined and unlined Traditional Manuscript and Cursive (similar to Zaner Blouser and D'Nealian), math, clip art, decorative, time, American Sign Language symbols and more. The included manual is very informative, with great examples of lesson plans and educational goals. *$39.95*
Windows/Mac

966 From Scribbling to Writing
Therapro
225 Arlington St
Framingham, MA 01702-8723   508-872-9494
                                    800-257-5376
                                    Fax: 508-875-2062
                                    www.therapro.com
                                    info@therapro.com

Karen Conrad, President
Ideas, exercises and practice pages for all children preparing to write. Contains line drawing exercises, forms to complete, and forms for encouraging good flow of movement during writing. *$32.50*
99 pages

967 Fun with Handwriting
Therapro
225 Arlington St
Framingham, MA 01702-8723   508-872-9494
                                    800-257-5376
                                    Fax: 508-875-2062
                                    www.therapro.com
                                    info@therapro.com

Karen Conrad, President
One hundred and one ways to improve handwriting. Includes key to writing legibly, chalkboard activities, evaluation tips, and real world handwriting projects. *$16.00*
160 pages Spiral-bound

968 Getting Ready to Write: Preschool-K
Therapro
225 Arlington St
Framingham, MA 01702-8723   508-872-9494
                                    800-257-5376
                                    Fax: 508-875-2062
                                    www.therapro.com
                                    info@therapro.com

Karen Conrad, President
A wonderful little book for any handwriting program. Includes many basic skills needed for beginning writing such as matching like objects, finding differences, writing basic strokes, left to right sequence, etc. *$6.50*
97 pages

969 Getting it Write
Therapro
225 Arlington St
Framingham, MA 01702-8723   508-872-9494
                                    800-257-5376
                                    Fax: 508-875-2062
                                    www.therapro.com
                                    info@therapro.com

Karen Conrad, President
A 6-week course for individuals or groups of 4-10 children, 6-12 years. Weekly, 1/2 hour classes begin with a short orientation followed by 25 minutes of games and sensory motor activities, from prewriting to writing practice, from basic strokes to letter formation. Reproducible manuscript and cursive worksheets are included along with homework assignments. *$58.95*
215 pages

970 Handwriting Without Tears
806 W. Diamond Avenue
Suite 230
Gaithersburg, MD 20878   301-263-2700
                                    Fax: 301-263-2707
                                    www.hwtears.com
                                    info@hwtears.com

Jan Z Olsen, OTR, Founder and Developer
An easy and fun method for children of all abilities to learn printing and cursive.

971 Handwriting: Manuscript ABC Book
Therapro
225 Arlington St
Framingham, MA 01702-8723   508-872-9494
                                    800-257-5376
                                    Fax: 508-875-2062
                                    www.therapro.com
                                    info@therapro.com

Karen Conrad, President
Illustrated rhymes, practice letters and words, coloring and tear out alphabet cards teach letter formation. *$11.95*
56 pages

972 Home/School Activities Manuscript Practice
Therapro
225 Arlington St
Framingham, MA 01702-8723   508-872-9494
                                    800-257-5376
                                    Fax: 508-875-2062
                                    www.therapro.com
                                    info@therapro.com

Karen Conrad, President
Directions for forming lower and upper case letters, and numbers, with space for practice. Activities use letters in words and sentences. *$11.95*
64 pages

973 Let's Write Right: Teacher's Edition
AVKO Educational Research Foundation
3084 Willard Rd
Birch Run, MI 48415-9404   810-686-9283
                                    866-285-6612
                                    Fax: 810-686-1101
                                    www.avko.org
                                    webmaster@avko.org

Don Mc Cabe, President/Research Director
Linda Heck, Vice-President
Michael Lane, Treasurer
This is a teacher's lesson plan book which uses an approach designed specifically for dyslexics to teach reading and spelling skills through the side door of penmanship exercises with an empasis on legibility. Student books are handy but are not required. *$19.95*

974 Let's-Do-It-Write: Writing Readiness Workbook
Therapro
225 Arlington St
Framingham, MA 01702-8723   508-872-9494
                                    800-257-5376
                                    Fax: 508-875-2062
                                    www.therapro.com
                                    info@therapro.com

Karen Conrad, President
A great variety of prewriting activities and exercises focusing on development of eye-hand coordination and motor, sensory and cognitive skills. Also, helps improve sitting posture, cutting skills, pencil grasp, spatial orientation and problem-solving. Written by an occupational therapist who is a special educator. *$19.95*
112 pages

975 Making Handwriting Flow
Oxton House Publishers
PO Box 209
Farmington, ME 04938

207-779-1923
800-539-7323
Fax: 207-779-0623
www.oxtonhouse.com
info@oxtonhouse.com

William Burlinghoff PhD, Owner
This packet inlcudes a 16-page booklet, 'Using Models and Drills for Fluency,' and 28 pages of tracing models of numerals, whole words, phrases, and sentences for both manuscript and cursive handwriting, along with a chart for tracking student progress. *$24.95*
ISBN 1-881929-15-9

976 Media Weaver 3.5
Sunburst Technology
1550 Executive Dr
Elgin, IL 60123-9311

800-321-7511
Fax: 888-608-0344
http://store.sunburst.com
service@sunburst.com

Publishing becomes a multimedia event with this dynamic word processor that contains hundreds of media elements and effective process writing resources.

977 Middle School Writing: Expository Writing
HMH Supplemental Publishers
222 Berkeley Street
Boston, MA 02116

617-351-5000
855-969-4642
Fax: 800-269-5232
www.hmhco.com
school.permissions@hmhco.com

Linda K. Zecher, President and CEO
Eric Shuman, Chief Financial Officer
John K. Dragoon, EVP and Chief Marketing Officer
An effective comprehensive review and reinforcement of the writing and research skills students will need. Effectively used in both school and home setting. Ideal for junior high or high school students in need of remediation. *$7.99*
ISBN 0-739829-28-9

978 PAF Handwriting Programs for Print, Cursive (Right or Left-Handed)
Educators Publishing Service
PO Box 9031
Cambridge, MA 02139-9031

617-547-6706
800-435-7728
Fax: 888-440-2665
www.epsbooks.com
CustomerService.EPS@schoolspecialty.com

Rick Holden, President
Eileen Perlman, Co-Author
These workbooks can be used in conjunction with the PAF curriculum or independently as a classroom penmanship program. They were specifically designed to accommodate all students including those with fine-motor, visual-motor and graphomotor weaknesses. The workbooks contain both large models for introducing motor patterns and smaller models to facilitate the transition to primary and loose-leaf papers. A detailed instruction booklet accompanies each workbook. *$25.00*

979 StartWrite
Therapro
225 Arlington St
Framingham, MA 01702-8723

508-872-9494
800-257-5376
Fax: 508-875-2062
www.therapro.com
info@therapro.com

Karen Conrad, President

With this easy-to-use software package, you can make papers and handwriting worksheets to meet individual student's needs. Type letters, words, or numbers and they appear in a dot format on the triple line guide. Change letter size, add shading, turn on or off guide lines and arrow strokes and place provided clipart. Fonts include Manuscript and Cursive, Modern Manuscript and Cursive and Italic Manuscript and Cursive. Useful manual included. *$42.50*
Windows/Mac

980 Strategies for Success in Writing
HMH Supplemental Publishers
222 Berkeley Street
Boston, MA 02116

617-351-5000
855-969-4642
Fax: 800-269-5232
www.hmhco.com
school.permissions@hmhco.com

Linda K. Zecher, President and CEO
Eric Shuman, Chief Financial Officer
John K. Dragoon, EVP and Chief Marketing Officer
Help your students gain success and master all the steps in writing through essay-writing strategies and exercises in proofreading, editing, and revising written work. This program also helps students approach tests strategically. *$16.60*
ISBN 0-739810-47-2

981 Sunbuddy Writer
Sunburst Technology
1550 Executive Dr
Elgin, IL 60123-9311

800-321-7511
Fax: 888-608-0344
http://store.sunburst.com
service@sunburst.com

An easy-to-use picture and word processor designed especially for young writers.

982 Tool Chest: For Teachers, Parents and Students
Therapro
225 Arlington St
Framingham, MA 01702-8723

508-872-9494
800-257-5376
Fax: 508-875-2062
www.therapro.com
info@therapro.com

Karen Conrad, President
Diana A. Henry, Author
Ideas for self-regulation and handwriting skills. 26+ activities, each on its own page, with rationale, supplies needed, instructions and related projects. Provides a fast way to prepare for OT activities. Supports the videotapes Tools for Teachers and Tools for Students. *$19.95*

983 Type-It
Educators Publishing Service
PO Box 9031
Cambridge, MA 02139-9031

617-547-6706
800-435-7728
Fax: 888-440-2666
www.epsbooks.com
CustomerService.EPS@schoolspecialty.com

Rick Holden, President
A linguistically oriented beginning 'touch-system' typing manual. A progress chart allows students to pace their progress in short, easily attainable units, often enabling them to proceed with little or no supervision.

984 Write On! Plus: Beginning Writing Skills
Sunburst Technology
1550 Executive Dr
Elgin, IL 60123-9311

800-321-7511
Fax: 888-608-0344
http://store.sunburst.com
service@sunburst.com

This classic process writing series teaches a wide range of core writing and literature skills through hundreds of motivating and challenging activities.

985 Write On! Plus: Elementary Writing Skills
Sunburst Technology
1550 Executive Dr
Elgin, IL 60123-9311   800-321-7511
                                    Fax: 888-608-0344
                              http://store.sunburst.com
                                  service@sunburst.com
This classic process writing series teaches a wide range of core writing and literature skills through hundreds of motivating and challenging activities.

986 Write On! Plus: Essential Writing
Sunburst Technology
1550 Executive Dr
Elgin, IL 60123-9311   800-321-7511
                                    Fax: 888-608-0344
                              http://store.sunburst.com
                                  service@sunburst.com
This classic process writing series teaches a wide range of core writing and literature skills through hundreds of motivating and challenging activities.

987 Write On! Plus: Growing as a Writer
Sunburst Technology
1550 Executive Dr
Elgin, IL 60123-9311   800-321-7511
                                    Fax: 888-608-0344
                              http://store.sunburst.com
                                  service@sunburst.com
This classic process writing series teaches a wide range of core writing and literature skills through hundreds of motivating and challenging activities.

988 Write On! Plus: High School Writing Skills
Sunburst Technology
1550 Executive Dr
Elgin, IL 60123-9311   800-321-7511
                                    Fax: 888-608-0344
                              http://store.sunburst.com
                                  service@sunburst.com
This classic process writing series teaches a wide range of core writing and literature skills through hundreds of motivating and challenging activities.

989 Write On! Plus: Literature Studies
Sunburst Technology
1550 Executive Dr
Elgin, IL 60123-9311   800-321-7511
                                    Fax: 888-608-0344
                              http://store.sunburst.com
                                  service@sunburst.com
This classic process writing series teaches a wide range of core writing and literature skills through hundreds of motivating and challenging activities.

990 Write On! Plus: Middle School Writing Skills
Sunburst Technology
1550 Executive Dr
Elgin, IL 60123-9311   800-321-7511
                                    Fax: 888-608-0344
                              http://store.sunburst.com
                                  service@sunburst.com
This classic process writing series teaches a wide range of core writing and literature skills through hundreds of motivating and challenging activities.

991 Write On! Plus: Responding to Great Literature
Sunburst Technology
1550 Executive Dr
Elgin, IL 60123-9311   800-321-7511
                                    Fax: 888-608-0344
                              http://store.sunburst.com
                                  service@sunburst.com
This classic process writing series teaches a wide range of core writing and literature skills through hundreds of motivating and challenging activities.

992 Write On! Plus: Spanish/ English Literacy Series
Sunburst Technology
1550 Executive Dr
Elgin, IL 60123-9311   800-321-7511
                                    Fax: 888-608-0344
                              http://store.sunburst.com
                                  service@sunburst.com
This classic process writing series teaches a wide range of core writing and literature skills through hundreds of motivating and challenging activities.

993 Write On! Plus: Steps to Better Writing
Sunburst Technology
1550 Executive Dr
Elgin, IL 60123-9311   800-321-7511
                                    Fax: 888-608-0344
                              http://store.sunburst.com
                                  service@sunburst.com
This classic process writing series teaches a wide range of core writing and literature skills through hundreds of motivating and challenging activities.

994 Write On! Plus: Writing with Picture Books
Sunburst Technology
1550 Executive Dr
Elgin, IL 60123-9311   800-321-7511
                                    Fax: 888-608-0344
                              http://store.sunburst.com
                                  service@sunburst.com
This classic process writing series teaches a wide range of core writing and literature skills through hundreds of motivating and challenging activities.

995 Writer's Resources Library 2.0
Sunburst Technology
1550 Executive Dr
Elgin, IL 60123-9311   800-321-7511
                                    Fax: 888-608-0344
                              http://store.sunburst.com
                                  service@sunburst.com
Students quickly access seven reference resources with this indispensable writing tool.

996 Writing Trek Grades 4-6
Sunburst Technology
1550 Executive Dr
Elgin, IL 60123-9311   800-321-7511
                                    Fax: 888-608-0344
                              http://store.sunburst.com
                                  service@sunburst.com
Enhance your students' experience in your English language arts classroom with twelve authentic writing projects that build students' competence while encouraging creativity.

997 Writing Trek Grades 6-8
Sunburst Technology
1550 Executive Dr
Elgin, IL 60123-9311   800-321-7511
                                    Fax: 888-608-0344
                              http://store.sunburst.com
                                  service@sunburst.com
Twelve authentic language arts projects, activities, and assignments develop your students' writing confidence and ability.

998 Writing Trek Grades 8-10
Sunburst Technology
1550 Executive Dr
Elgin, IL 60123-9311   800-321-7511
                                    Fax: 888-800-3028
                              http://store.sunburst.com
                                  service@sunburst.com
Michael Guillory, Channel Sales/Marketing Manager
Help your students develop a concept of genre as they become familiar with the writing elements and characteristics of a variety of writing forms.

Learning Disabilities

999   ACA Charlotte
ACA Membership Division
5999 Stevenson Ave
Alexandria, VA 22304-3304   800-347-6647
                                              Fax: 800-473-2329
                                              www.counseling.org
                                              membership@counseling.org
Robert L. Smith, President
Thelma Duffey, President-Elect
Brian Canfield, Treasurer
Keynote speakers and workshops as well as exhibits are offered.
March

1000   ACRES -American Council on Rural Special Education Conference
Montana Center On Disabilities/MSU-Billings
1500 University Drive
Billings, MT 59101   406-657-2312
                                              888-866-3822
                                              Fax: 406-657-2313
                                              www.acressped.org
                                              inquiries@acres-sped.org
Ben Lignugaris-Kra, Manager
Conference of special educators, teachers and professors working with exceptional needs students. Keynote speakers, silent auction.
March

1001   AR-CEC Annual Conference
Arkansas Council for Exceptional Children
1201 West Center
Beebe, AR 72012   479-967-6025
                                              Fax: 479-967-6056
                                              http://cec.k12.ar.us
                                              sheidelberg@raider.k12.ar.us
Stephanie Lawrence, President & Conference Planner
Stephanie Heidelberg, Vice President
Mary Pearson, President-Elect
The council is dedicated to meeting the needs of it's members through serving as an effective advocate, fostering involvement of the membership and advancing the professional and ethical growth of it's members. The conference is held annually at the Hot Springs Convention Center in Hot Springs, AR.
November

1002   ASHA Convention
American Speech-Language-Hearing Association
2200 Research Blvd
Rockville, MD 20850-3289   301-296-5700
                                              800-498-2071
                                              Fax: 301-296-8580
                                              TTY: 301-296-5650
                                              www.asha.org
                                              partners@asha.org
Elizabeth S. McCrea, PhD, CCC-SLP, President
Judith L. Page, PhD, CCC-SLP, President-Elect
Barbara K. Cone, PhD, CCC-A, Vice President
ASHA is the nation's leading organization for speech-language pathologists, speech/language/hearing scientists and audiologists. Topics addressed include hearing impairments, special education and speech communication. 10,000 attendees.
November

1003   Active Parenting Publishers
1220 Kennestone Circle
Suite 130
Marietta, GA 30066-6022   770-429-0565
                                              800-825-0060
                                              Fax: 770-429-0334
                                              www.activeparenting.com
                                              cservice@activeparenting.com
Michael Popkin PhD, President/Founder

Provides parenting education curricula, including one for parents of ADD/ADHD children.

1004   Annual Postsecondary Disability Training Institute
University of Connecticut
249 Glenbrook Rd
Unit 2064
Storrs Mansfield, CT 06269-2064   860-486-3321
                                              Fax: 860-486-5799
                                              www.cped.uconn.edu
                                              joseph.madaus@uconn.edu
Dr. Joseph Madaus, Director
Carroll Waite, Program Assistant
Joseph Madaus, Institute Coordinator
Assists concerned professionals to meet the unique needs of college students with disabilities.
June

1005   Assessing Learning Problems Workshop
Learning Disabilities Resources
2775 S. Quincy St.
Arlington, VA 22206   FAX 703-998-2060
                                              www.ldonline.org
Noel Gunther, Executive Director
Christian Lindstrom, Director, Learning Media
Shalini Anand, Senior Manager, Web Development
This workshop includes behavioral manifestations of information processing problems and how to relate these to learning processes.

1006   Assistive Technology Training Program
Calfornia State University, Northridge
Cntr On Disabilities Training Prog.
18111 Nordhoff St., Bayramian Hall 110
Northridge, CA 91330-8340   818-677-2578
                                              Fax: 818-677-4929
                                              TTY: 818-677-2684
                                              www.csun.edu
                                              conference@csun.edu
Dan Duran, Counselor
Sean Goggin, Equipment Systems Specialist
Paras Davoodi, Counselor/Learning Specialist
Sponsor of national and international assistive technology training programs. The programs help to expand the knowledge of professionals and also introduces newcomers to the field. Participants learn about all forms of assistive technology and their potential areas of application.

1007   Association Book Exhibit: Brain Research
Association Book Exhibit
9423 Old Mount Vernon Rd
Alexandria, VA 22309-2716   703-619-5030
                                              Fax: 703-619-5035
                                              www.bookexhibit.com
                                              info@bookexhibit.com
Mark Terotchi, President
Attendence is 800-1,000. Every serious publisher of Neuroscience material represented.

1008   Behavioral Institute for Children and Adolescents
1711 County Rd B W
Ste 110S
Roseville, MN 55113   651-484-5510
                                              Fax: 651-483-3879
                                              www.behavioralinstitute.org
                                              mknoll@behavioralinstitute.org
Sheldon Braaten, Executive Director
Mitchell Yell, Director & President
Jackie Baroch, Director/Treasurer
Promoting improved services for troubled children and youths. Provides a wide variety of supporting services to professionals and parents who work with children with emotional and behavioral challenges. Services include professional development, discounted publications and materials, conferences, workshops, consultation, program design and evaluation, a professional library and scholarship program.

1009 CACLD Spring & Fall Conferences
Connecticut Assoc for Children and Adults with LD
25 Van Zant Street
Suite 15-5
East Norwalk, CT 06855-1719
203-838-5010
Fax: 203-866-6108
www.CACLD.org
cacld@optonline.net
Beryl Kaufman, Executive Director
Elaine Eckenrode, Conference Coordinator
Offers speakers, workshops, presentations and more for professionals and parents of individuals with a learning disability or attention deficit disorder. CACLD has also donated hundreds of books and tapes to libraries, schools, and parent centers which help in training teachers and paraprofessionals.

1010 CASE Conference
Council Of Administrators Of Special Education
Osigian Office Centre
101 Katelyn Circle, Suite E
Warner Robbins, GA 31088
478-333-6892
Fax: 478-333-2453
www.casecec.org
lpurcell@casecec.org
Laurie VanderPloeg, President
Luann Purcell, Executive Director
Tom Adams, Finance Committee Chariman
International educational organization dedicated to the enhancement of worth, dignity, and the potential of each individual in society.
January

1011 CEC Federation Conference: Virginia
Council for Exceptional Children
1110 N. Glebe Road
Suite 300
Arlington, VA 22201
888-232-7733
Fax: 703-264-9494
TDD: 866-915-5000
www.cec.sped.org
victore@cec.sped.org
Robin D. Brewer, President
James P. Heiden, President Elect
Christy A. Chambers, Immediate Past President
Find a wealth of information targeted just for educators. Choose from more than 600 workshops, lectures, demonstrations, mini workshops, panels and poster sessions.
April

1012 CEC/KASP Federation Conference: Kansas
Council for Exceptional Children

www.kansascec.org
dmplunkett@fhsu.edu
Dr. Diane Plunkett, Ph.D., President
Angela Harris, Vice President
Frances Strieby, Treasurer/Finance
Exhibits and workshop sessions for educators building a brighter tomorrow.
October

1013 CSUN Conference
California State University, Northridge
18111 Nordhoff St
Bayramian Hall 110
Northridge, CA 91330-8200
818-677-2578
Fax: 818-677-4929
TTY: 818-677-2684
www.csun.edu
conference@csun.edu
Dan Duran, Counselor
Sean Goggin, Equipment Systems Specialist
Paras Davoodi, Counselor/Learning Specialist
Comprehensive, international conference, where all technologies across all ages, disabilities, levels of education and training, employment and independent living are addressed. It is the largest conference of its kind with exhibit halls open free to public.

1014 Center on Disabilities Conference
California State University, Northridge
18111 Nordhoff St
Bayramian Hall 110
Northridge, CA 91330-8340
818-677-2578
Fax: 818-677-4929
TTY: 818-677-2684
www.csun.edu
conference@csun.edu
Dan Duran, Counselor
Sean Goggin, Equipment Systems Specialist
Paras Davoodi, Counselor/Learning Specialist
Focuses on issues pertaining to the disabled learner and gifted education. 2,000 attendees.

1015 Closing the Gap Conference
526 Main Street
P.O. Box 68
Henderson, MN 56044-0068
507-248-3294
Fax: 507-248-3810
www.closingthegap.com
info@closingthegap.com
Budd Hagen, Co-Founder
Dolores Hagen, Co-Founder
Connie Kneip, Vice President/General Manager
Annual international conference with over 100 exhibitors concerned with the use of assistive technology in special education and rehabilitation.
October

1016 College Students with Learning Disabilities Workshop
Learning Disabilities Resources
2775 S. Quincy St.
Arlington, VA 22206
FAX 703-998-2060
www.ldonline.org
Noel Gunther, Executive Director
Christian Lindstrom, Director, Learning Media
Shalini Anand, Senior Manager, Web Development
This workshop is designed to provide both information and motivation to both students and college personnel.

1017 ConnSENSE Conference
University of Connecticut
233 Glenbrook Rd
Unit 4174
Storrs Mansfield, CT 06269-4174
860-486-2020
Fax: 860-486-4412
TDD: 860-486-2077
www.csd.uconn.edu
csd@uconn.edu
Donna Korbel, Director
Jennifer H. Lucia, Associate Director
Christine M. Wenzel, Associate Director
Annual conference on technology for people with special needs.

1018 Creative Mind: Building Foundations that will Last Forever
P Buckley Moss Foundation for Children's Education
108 S. Wayne Avenue
Waynesboro, VA 22980-7485
540-932-1728
Fax: 540-941-8865
www.mossfoundation.org
foundation@mossfoundation.org
Patricia Moss, President/Artist Representative
Marion G. Roark, Treasurer
Douglas Ball, Director
The mission of the foundation is to integrate art into all educational programs, with a special focus on children who learn in different ways.

1019 EDU Therapeutics Annual Conference
14401 Roland Canyon Rd
Salinas, CA 93908
831-484-0994
Fax: 831-484-0998
www.edu-therapeutics.com
joan@EDU-Therapeutics.com

Terry McHenry, President
Martin Donald, Specialist
Dr. Joan Smith, Program Director
Provides diagnositc assessment for LD, ADD, head-trauma (Cognitive), and dyslexia. Provides teacher/clinical training in LD, ADD, dyslexia with EDU-therapeutics.

1020 Eden Family of Services
Eden Services
2 Merwick Road
Princeton, NJ 08540-5711

609-987-0099
Fax: 609-987-0243
http://edenautism.org
info@edenservices.org

Peter H. Bell, President & CEO
Jennifer Bizub, Chief Operating Officer
John Inzilla, Chief Financial Officer
Provides year-round educational services, early intervention, parent training and workshops, respite care, outreach services, community based residential services and employment opportunities for individuals with autism.

1021 Educating Children Summer Training Institute (ECSTI)
Muskingum College-Graduate & Continuing Studies
117 Montgomery Hall
163 Stormont Street
New Concord, OH 43762-1118

740-826-8211
Fax: 740-826-6038
www.muskingum.edu
ecsti@muskingum.edu

Bonnie Callahan, Director of Marketing
ECSIT offers graduate teacher education and continuing professional development through a series of week long courses. An innovative immersion program, ECSTI offers over 40 course options.

1022 Educational Options for Students with Learning Disabilities and LD/HD
Connecticut Assoc for Children and Adults with LD
25 Van Zant St
Norwalk, CT 06855-0719

203-838-5010
Fax: 203-866-6108
www.cacld.org
cacld@optonline.net

Beryl Kaufman, Executive Director
Elaine Eckenrode, Conference Coordinator
Annual conference held for parents, students and professionals. Features workshops, panels, exhibitors and a bookstore.
Spring

1023 IDA Conference
International Dyslexia Association
40 York Road
4th Floor
Baltimore, MD 21204-5243

410-296-0232
Fax: 410-321-5069
www.interdys.org
info@interdys.org

Hal Malchow, President
Elsa Cardenas-Hagan, Vice President
Ben Shifrin, M.Ed., Vice President
The conference promotes effective teaching approaches and strives to pursue and provide the most comprehensive range of information and services that address dyslexia and related difficulties with learning to read and write.
November

1024 Inclusion of Learning Disabled Students in Regular Classrooms Workshop
Learning Disabilities Resources
2775 S. Quincy St.
Arlington, VA 22206

FAX 703-998-2060
www.ldonline.org

Noel Gunther, Executive Director
Christian Lindstrom, Director, Learning Media
Shalini Anand, Senior Manager, Web Development

This workshop provides teachers with practical suggestions and techniques for including students with learning problems.

1025 Interest Driven Learning Master Class Workshop
199 NE Burr Oak Ct
Lees Summit, MO 64064-1962

816-478-4824
800-245-5733
Fax: 816-478-4824
www.drpeet.com
drpeet@drpeet.com

Bill Peet MD, President
Provides master classes or workshops on how to use talking word processors and interactive fiction to create highly effective supplemental reading and writing activities for learners of varying abilities aged three to eight. Assistive technology access channels provided for all disabilities. All strategies taught reference the results of 25 years or research.

1026 International Conference on Learning Disabilities
Council for Learning Disabilities
11184 Antioch Road
P.O. Box 405
Overland Park, KS 66210-0405

913-491-1011
Fax: 913-491-1012
www.cldinternational.org
lneaseCLD@aol.com

Steve Chamberlain, President
Mary Beth Calhoon, Vice President
Rebbeca Shankland, Secretary
Focuses on all aspects pertaining to learning disabled individuals from a teaching and research perspective.
October

1027 LDA Annual International Conference
Learning Disabilities Association of America
4156 Library Rd
Pittsburgh, PA 15234-1349

412-341-1515
Fax: 412-344-0224
www.LDAAmerica.org
info@ldaamerica.org

Nancie Payne, President
Ed Schlitt, Vice President
Beth McGaw, Secretary
Topics addressed at the conference include advocacy, adult literacy and classroom for individuals with learning disabilities..
March

1028 LDAT Annual State Conference
1011 West 31st Street
Austin, TX 78705-2099

512-458-8234
800-604-7500
Fax: 512-458-3826
www.ldat.org
contact@ldat.org

Jean Kueker, President
Promotes the education and general welfare of individuals with learning disabilities.

1029 LDR Workshop: What Are Learning Disabilities, Problems and Differences?
Learning Disabilities Resources
2775 S. Quincy St.
Arlington, VA 22206

FAX 703-998-2060
www.ldonline.org

Noel Gunther, Executive Director
Christian Lindstrom, Director, Learning Media
Shalini Anand, Senior Manager, Web Development
In this workshop, Dr. Cooper draws on personal experiences with a learning disability and on his clinical work with thousands of individuals with a wide variety of learning problems to provide the participants with an understanding of the positive and negative aspects of being, living and learning differently.

1030 Landmark School Outreach Program
Landmark School
429 Hale Street
P.O. Box 227
Prides Crossing, MA 01965-0227   978-236-3216
                                    Fax: 978-927-7268
                                  www.landmarkoutreach.org
                                  outreach@landmarkschool.org
Dan Ahearn, Director
Kaia Cunningham, Assistant Director/teacher
Lisa Besen, Teacher
Provides consultation and professional development to schools, professional organizations, parent groups, and businesses on topics related to individuals with learning disabilities. Services are individually designed to meet the client's specific needs and can range from a two-hour workshop to a year-long collaboration. Options include: annual Professional Development Institute at Landmark School; on-site professional development programs at schools; online professional development program.

1031 Learning Disabilities and the World of Work Workshop
Learning Disabilities Resources
2775 S. Quincy St.
Arlington, VA 22206   FAX 703-998-2060
                              www.ldonline.org
Noel Gunther, Executive Director
Christian Lindstrom, Director, Learning Media
Shalini Anand, Senior Manager, Web Development
This workshop is designed for employers, parents or professionals working with individuals with learning disabilities.

1032 Learning Problems and Adult Basic Education Workshop
Learning Disabilities Resources
2775 S. Quincy St.
Arlington, VA 22206   FAX 703-998-2060
                              www.ldonline.org
Noel Gunther, Executive Director
Christian Lindstrom, Director, Learning Media
Shalini Anand, Senior Manager, Web Development
This workshop for adult educators discusses the manifestations of learning problems in adults.

1033 Lindamood-Bell Learning Processes Professional Development
416 Higuera St
San Luis Obispo, CA 93401-3833   805-541-3836
                                            800-233-1819
                                       Fax: 805-541-8756
                                     www.lindamoodbell.com
Nanci Bell, Co-founder and the Director
Offers workshops nationwide for educators in the internationally acclaimed Lindamood-Bell teaching methods. Approximately 40 workshops hosted annually across the United State and Internationally. Inservices also available.

1034 NCFL Conference
National Center For Family Literacy
325 W. Main Street
Suite 300
Louisville, KY 40202-4237   502-584-1133
                                Fax: 502-584-0172
                                  www.famlit.org
                              notify@familieslearning.org
Sharon Darling, President & Founder
George R. Siemens, Vice President, External Affairs
Mary Anne O. Cronan, Vice President & Director
Comprehensive conference serving family literacy professionals and practitioners who are in the field of improving literacy skills and the lives of the parents and children. Attendees will learn about the latest research in the education industry, and hear from celebrity advocates and authors.
March

1035 National Head Start Association
1651 Prince St
Alexandria, VA 22314-2818   703-739-0875
                                      866-677-8724
                                 Fax: 703-739-0878
                                    www.nhsa.org
                                  yvinci@nhsa.org
Vanessa Rich, Chairman
Alvin Jones, Vice-Chairperson
Mary Rose Cox, Secretary
Both Adminstrator and Mid-Manager credentials are offered in a six day, institute style setting, workshop. Family Services and Health credentials are offered through a self study format.
September

1036 National Head Start Association Parent Conference
1651 Prince St
Alexandria, VA 22314-2818   703-739-0875
                                      866-677-8724
                                 Fax: 703-739-0878
                                    www.nhsa.org
                                 asmith@nhsa.orgrg
Vanessa Rich, Chairman
Alvin Jones, Vice-Chairperson
Mary Rose Cox, Secretary
Newest information on enhancing parent involvement, child development, and sharpening parenting skills. More than 100 workshops.

1037 North American Montessori Teachers' Association Conference
13693 Butternut Rd
Burton, OH 44021-9571   440-834-4011
                             Fax: 440-834-4016
                          www.montessori-namta.org
                          staff@montessori-namta.org
David Kahn, Director
Montessori method of teaching is discussed as well as topics pertaining to all levels of special education. This and other conferences are held in different locations and months throughout the year. Please contact us for more information.
Quarterly

1038 Pacific Rim Conference on Disabilities
University of Hawaii Center on Disability Studies
1410 Lower Campus Rd.
#171F
Honolulu, HI 96822-2447   808-956-7539
                               Fax: 808-956-7878
                             www.pacrim.hawaii.edu
                               prinfo@hawaii.edu
Valerie Shearer, Director
Charmaine Crockett, Conference Organizer
Participants from the US and other Pacific Rim nations study such topics in disabilities as lifelong inclusion in education and community, new technology, family support, employment and adult services.
March

1039 Pennsylvania Training and Technical Assistance Network Workshops
PaTTAN
6340 Flank Drive
Suite 600
Harrisburg, PA 17112-2764   717-541-4960
                                      800-360-7282
                                 Fax: 717-541-4968
                                   www.pattan.net
                               askpattan@pattan.net
Angela Kirby-Wehr, Director
Victor Rodriguez-Diaz, Ph.D., Assistant Director
Chris Cherny, Assistant Director

Supports the Department of Education's efforts to lead and serve the educational community by offering professional development that builds the capacity of loacl educational agencies to meet students' needs. PaTTAN's primary focus is special education. However, services are also provided to support Early Intervention, student assessment, tutoring and other partnership efforts, all designed to help students succeed.

1040 Social Skills Workshop
Learning Disabilities Resources
2775 S. Quincy St.
Arlington, VA 22206   FAX 703-998-2060
                                        www.ldonline.org

Noel Gunther, Executive Director
Christian Lindstrom, Director, Learning Media
Shalini Anand, Senior Manager, Web Development
This workshop is relevant for individuals with learning disabilities, parents or professionals.

1041 Son-Rise Program®
Autism Treatment Center of America
2080 Undermountain Rd
Sheffield, MA 01257-9643   413-229-2100
                                        877-766-7473
                                    Fax: 413-229-3202
                                www.autismtreatment.com
                                     autism@option.org
Barry Kaufman, Founder
Raun Kaufman, Director of Global Education
Since 1983, the Autism Treatment Center of America has provided innovative training programs and workshops for parents and professionals caring for children challenged by Autism, Autism Spectrum Disorders, Pervasive Developmental Disorder (PDD) and other developmental difficulties.
1983

1042 TASH Annual Conference Social Justice inthe 21st Century
2013 H Street
NW
Washington, DC 20006   202-540-9020
                                        888-221-9425
                                    Fax: 202-540-9019
                                        www.tash.org
                                        info@tash.org
Barb Trader, Executive Director
Bethany Alvare, Advocacy Communications Manager
Edwin Canizalez, Training and Events Manager
Progressive international conference that focuses on strategies for achieving full inclusion for people with disabilities. This invigorating conference, which brings together the best hearts and minds in the disability movement, features over 450 breakout sessions, exhibits, roundtable discussions, poster sessions and much more.
December

1043 Teaching Math Workshop
Learning Disabilities Resources
2775 S. Quincy St.
Arlington, VA 22206   FAX 703-998-2060
                                        www.ldonline.org
Noel Gunther, Executive Director
Christian Lindstrom, Director, Learning Media
Shalini Anand, Senior Manager, Web Development
A workshop for teachers on how to teach math to individuals with learning problems.

1044 Teaching Reading Workshop
LD OnLine/Learning Disabilities Resource
WETA Public Television
2775 S. Quincy Street
Arlington, VA 22206   FAX 703-998-2060
                                        www.ldonline.org
Noel Gunther, Executive Director
Christian Lindstrom, Director, Learning Media
Shalini Anand, Senior Manager, Web Development

This workshop explains how to teach individuals with reading problems, dyslexia, ADD, and specific learning disabilities.

1045 Teaching Spelling Workshop
LD OnLine/Learing Disabilities Resource
WETA Public Television
2775 S. Quincy Street
Arlington, VA 22206   FAX 703-998-2060
                                        www.ldonline.org
Noel Gunther, Executive Director
Christian Lindstrom, Director, Learning Media
Shalini Anand, Senior Manager, Web Development
A workshop that focuses on how to spell, which directly affects an individual's ability to write.

1046 Technology & Persons with Disabilities Conference
California State University Northridge
18111 Nordhoff St
Bayramian Hall 110
Northridge, CA 91330-8340   818-677-2578
                                  Fax: 818-677-4929
                                  TTY: 818-677-2684
                                        www.csun.edu
                                 conference@csun.edu
Dan Duran, Counselor
Sean Goggin, Equipment Systems Specialist
Paras Davoodi, Counselor/Learning Specialist
A major training venue held yearly for professionals from around the world who are involved in the field of disabilities and assistive technology that helps disabled individuals in the fields of education, employment and independent living.
March

1047 Wilson Language Training
47 Old Webster Rd
Oxford, MA 01540-2705   508-368-2399
                                        800-899-8454
                                  Fax: 508-368-2300
                                 www.wilsonlanguage.com
                                 info@wilsonlanguage.com
Barbara Wilson, Director
Jay LaRoche, Vice President of Outreach
Dr. Tim Odegard, Director
Our workshops instruct teachers, or other professionals in a related field, how to succeed with students who have not learned to read, write and spell despite great effort. Established in order to provide training in the Wilson Reading System, the Wilson staff provides Two-Day Overview Workshops as well as certified Level I and II training.

1048 Young Adult Institute Conference on Developmental Disabilities
460 W 34th St
New York, NY 10001-2382   212-273-6100
                                        866-292-4546
                                  Fax: 212-268-1083
                                        www.yai.org
Matthew Sturiale, L.C.S.W., Chief Executive Officer
Roberta G. Koenigsberg, Chief Compliance Officer
Sanjay Dutt, Chief Financial Officer
Annual conference of developmental disabilities. In-depth sessions on the keys to success in developmental and learning disabilities.
May

Assistive Devices

1049 AbleData National Institute on Disability & Rehab. Research
U.S. Department of Education
103 West Broad St.
Suite 400
Falls Church, MD 22046
703-356-8035
800-227-0216
Fax: 703-356-8314
TTY: 703-992-8313
www.abledata.com
abledata@neweditions.net
Katherine Belknap, Project Director
Juanita Hardy, Information Specialist
David Johnson, Publications Director
AbleData is a free resource offering information on more than 40,000 assistive technology products for people with disabilities. Our listings include commercially available products and do-it-yourself solutions.

1050 Ablenet
2625 Patton Road
Roseville, MN 55113-1308
651-294-2200
800-322-0956
Fax: 651-294-2259
www.ablenetinc.com
customerservice@ablenetinc.com
Jennifer Thalhuber, President/CEO
Bill Sproull, Chairman
William Mills, Director
Dedicated to making a difference in the lives of people with disabilities.

1051 Adaptive Device Locator System (ADLS)
Academic Software
3504 Tates Creek Rd
Lexington, KY 40517-2601
859-552-1020
Fax: 253-799-4012
www.acsw.com
asistaff@acsw.com
Warren E Lacefield, President
Penelope D Ellis, COO/Dir Sales/Marketing
Sylvia B. Lacefield, Graphic Artist
System describes thousands of devices, cross references over 1000 vendors and illustrates devices graphically. The ADLS databases include a full spectrum of living aids, products ranging from specialized eating utensils to dressing aids, electronic switches, computer hardware and software, adapted physical education devices and much more. Now accessible on the internet through Adaptworld.com and Acsw.com *$195.00*

1052 Alliance for Technology Access
1119 Old Humboldt Road
Jackson, TN 38305
731-554-5282
800-914-3017
Fax: 731-554-5283
TTY: 731-554-5284
www.ataccess.org
atainfo@ataccess.org
James Allison, President
Mike Hewitt, Secretary/Treasurer
Bob Van der Linde, Vice President
The mission of the Alliance for Technology Access (ATA) is to increase the use of technology by children and adults with disabilities and functional limitations.

1053 Braille Keyboard Sticker Overlay Label Kit
Hooleon Corporation
PO Box 589
304 West Denby Ave
Melrose, NM 88124
575-253-4503
800-937-1337
Fax: 505-253-4299
www.hooleon.com
sales@hooleon.com

Joan Crozier, Founder
Bob Crozier, Founder
Transparent with raised braille allows both sighted and nonsighted users to use same keyboard.

1054 Connect Outloud
Freedom Scientific
11800 31st Ct N
St Petersburg, FL 33716-1805
727-803-8000
800-444-4443
Fax: 727-803-8001
www.freedomscientific.com
info@freedomscientific.com
John Blake, President, CEO
Designed to allow beginners through experienced blind or low vision computer users to access the Internet through speech and Braille output. Based on our JAWS for Windows technology, and offers additional access to Windows XP. *$249.00*

1055 Controlpad 24
Genovation
17741 Mitchell N
Irvine, CA 92614-6028
949-833-3355
800-822-4333
Fax: 949-833-0322
www.genovation.com
max@genovation.com
Fully programmable 24 key pad. Its principal purpose is to provide single keystroke macros.

1056 Dyna Vox Technologies
2100 Wharton St
Suite 400
Pittsburgh, PA 15203-1942
412-381-4883
866-396-2869
Fax: 412-381-5241
www.dynavoxtech.com
Ray.Merk@dynavoxtech.com
Sherry Bertner, Managing Director
DynaVox Technologies develops, manufactures, distributes and supports a variety of speech-output devices that allow individuals challenged by speech, lanuage and learning disabilities to make meaningful connections with their world. The company's products allow individuals of all ages and abilities to initiate and participate in conversations at home, work, in school and throughout the community. *$4500.00*

1057 EZ Keys XP
Words+
42505 10th St W
Lancaster, CA 93534-7059
661-723-7723
800-869-8521
Fax: 661-723-2114
www.words-plus.com
info@word-plus.com
Assistance program that provides keyboard control, dual word prediction, abbreviation-expansion and speech output while running standard software. *$695.00*

1058 Enabling Devices
50 Broadway
Hawthorne, NY 10532
914-747-3070
800-832-8697
Fax: 914-747-3480
www.enablingdevices.com
customer_support@enablingdevices.com
Steven E. Kanor PhD, President/Founder
A designer, manufacturer and distributor of unique and affordable assitive and adaptive technologies for the physically and mentally challenged, ED/TFSC's products are sought by parents, teachers, and professionals alike.

1059 Genie Color TV
TeleSensory
417 Cypress Street
Bakersfield, CA 93304
650-743-9515
800-804-8004
Fax: 661-327-2478
www.telesensory.com
info@telesensory.com
Brings clarity and comfort to reading and writing. Since many people with low vision find that specific color combinations enhance legibility, VersiColor offers 24 customized foreground and background color combinations to choose from in addition to a full color mode. Genie can also connect to a computer for use with Telesensory's Vista screen magnification system. *$2995.00*

1060 Genovation
17741 Mitchell N
Irvine, CA 92614-6028
949-833-3355
800-822-4333
Fax: 949-833-0322
www.genovation.com
max@genovation.com
Produces a wide variety of computer input devices for data-entry, and custom applications. Produces the Function Keypad 682 for people with limited dexterity. It is programmable, allowing the user to store macros (selected patterns of key strokes) into memory, and relegendable keys allow easy labeling of user-programmed functions. Additional options such as larger keys (1x2), allow reconfiguration to meet the user's needs. Call toll-free for pricing and availability.

1061 Handbook of Adaptive Switches and Augmentative Communication Devices, 3rd Ed
3504 Tates Creek Road
Lexington, KY 40517-2601
895-552-1020
Fax: 253-799-4012
www.acsw.com
asistaff@acsw.com

Warren E Lacefield, President
Penelope D Ellis, COO/Dir Sales/Marketing
Sylvia B. Lacefield, Graphic Artist
An essential sourcebook for assistive technology specialists, teacheers, therapists, and others who select adaptive swicthes and augmentative communication devices for persons with disabilities.

1062 Home Row Indicators
Hooleon Corporation
PO Box 589
304 West Denby Ave
Melrose, NM 88124
575-253-4503
800-937-1337
Fax: 505-253-4299
www.hooleon.com
sales@hooleon.com

Joan Crozier, Founder
Bob Crozier, Founder
Plastic adhesive labels with a raised bump in the center allowing the user to designate home row keys, or any other key, for quick recognition.

1063 IntelliKeys
IntelliTools
2625 Patton Road
Roseville, MN 55113-1308
651-294-2200
800-322-0956
Fax: 651-294-2259
www.ablenetinc.com
customerservice@ablenetinc.com

Jennifer Thalhuber, President/CEO
Bill Sproull, Chairman
William Mills, Director
Alternative, touch-sensitive keyboard. Plugs into any MAC, APPLE, or IBM compatible computer, no interface needed. *$395.00*

1064 JAWS Screen Reading Software
Freedom Scientific
11800 31st Ct N
St Petersburg, FL 33716-1805
727-803-8000
800-444-4443
Fax: 727-803-8001
www.freedomscientific.com
info@freedomscientific.com

John Blake, President, CEO
JAWS is a powerful accessibility solution for the blind & people with low vision that reads information from computer screens using synthesised speech. This advanced & versitile software was specifically designed to meet the needs of blind and visually impaired computer users. WIth JAWS, users can access their computer applications and the Internet via text-to-speech technology. Through the use of a refreshable braille display, JAWS can provide braille output in addition to or instead of speech

1065 JAWS for Windows
Freedom Scientific
11800 31st Ct N
St Petersburg, FL 33716-1805
727-803-8000
800-444-4443
Fax: 727-803-8001
www.freedomscientific.com
info@freedomscientific.com

John Blake, President, CEO
Works with your PC to provide access to today's software applications and the internet. With its internal software speech synthesizer and the computer's sound card, information from the screen is read aloud, providing technology to access a wide variety of information, education and job related applications.

1066 Large Print Keyboard
Hooleon Corporation
PO Box 589
304 West Denby Ave
Melrose, NM 88124
575-253-4503
800-937-1337
Fax: 505-253-4299
www.hooleon.com
sales@hooleon.com

Joan Crozier, Founder
Bob Crozier, Founder
Keyboard with 104 keys features large print on all the keys. *$49.95*

1067 Large Print Lower Case Key Label Stickers
Hooleon Corporation
PO Box 589
304 West Denby Ave
Melrose, NM 88124
575-253-4503
800-937-1337
Fax: 505-253-4299
www.hooleon.com
sales@hooleon.com

Joan Crozier, Founder
Bob Crozier, Founder
For children learning the keyboard. Made of durable rigid plastic and are die cut to fit exactly.

1068 Lekotek of Georgia Shareware
Lekotek of Georgia
1955 Cliff Valley Way NE
Suite 102
Atlanta, GA 30329-2437
404-633-3430
Fax: 404-633-1242
www.lekotekga.org
info@lekotekga.org

Helene Prokesch, Executive Director and Founder
Peggy McWilliams, Director of Technology Services
Ellen Lindemann, Assistant Director

Software created by our staff using Intellipics, Intellipics Studio or Hyperstudio. Players are included to run this shareware. Color overlays for intellemusic are included. Input methods are mouse, switch, touch window, head mouse and intellikeys if applicable. Subjects are colors and emotions, early childhood music in English and Spanish, shapes and sounds, pictures and letters.

1069 **Open Book**
Freedom Scientific
11800 31st Ct N
St Petersburg, FL 33716-1805
727-803-8000
800-444-4443
Fax: 727-803-8001
www.freedomscientific.com
info@freedomscientific.com
John Blake, President, CEO
Allows you to convert printed documents or graphic based text into an electronic text format using accurate optical character recognition and quality speech. The many powerful low vision tools allow you to customize how the document appears on your screen, while other features provide portability. *$995.00*

1070 **Phonic Ear Auditory Trainers**
Phonic Ear
2080 Lakeville Hwy
Petaluma, CA 94954-6713
707-769-1110
800-227-0735
Fax: 707-769-9624
www.phonicear.com
mail@phonicear.com
Paul Hickey, Director
A line of learning disabled communication equipment.

1071 **QuicKeys**
Startly Technologies
PO Box 65580
West Des Moines, IA 50265
515-221-1801
800-523-7638
Fax: 515-221-1806
www.startly.com
Assigns Macintosh & Windows functions to one keystroke.

1072 **Reading Pen**
Wizcom Technologies
Boston Post Rd W 33
Ste 320
Marlborough, MA 01752-1829
508-251-5388
888-777-0552
Fax: 508-251-5394
www.wizcomtech.com
usa.info@wizcomtech.com
Michael Kenan, President
Portable assistive reading device that reads words aloud and can be used anywhere. Scans a word from printed text, displays the word in large characters, reads the word aloud from built-in speaker or ear phones and defines the word with the press of a button. Displays syllables, keeps a history of scanned words, adjustable for left or right-handed use. Includes a tutorial video and audio cassette. Not recommended for persons with low vision or impaired fine motor control.

1073 **Switch Accessible Trackball**
Lekotek of Georgia
1955 Cliff Valley Way NE
Suite 102
Atlanta, GA 30329-2437
404-633-3430
Fax: 404-633-1242
www.lekotekga.org
info@lekotekga.org
Helene Prokesch, Executive Director and Founder
Peggy McWilliams, Director of Technology Services
Ellen Lindemann, Assistant Director
Universal to Mac or Windows, this device aids computer navigation where traditional devices are not used. Trackball guards available. *$125.00*

1074 **Unicorn Expanded Keyboard**
2625 Patton Road
Roseville, MN 55113-1308
651-294-2200
800-322-0956
Fax: 651-294-2259
www.ablenetinc.com
customerservice@ablenetinc.com
Jennifer Thalhuber, President/CEO
Bill Sproull, Chairman
William Mills, Director
Alternative keyboard with large, user-defined keys, requires interface. Smaller version is also available.

1075 **Unicorn Smart Keyboard**
2625 Patton Road
Roseville, MN 55113-1308
651-294-2200
800-322-0956
Fax: 651-294-2259
www.ablenetinc.com
customerservice@ablenetinc.com
Jennifer Thalhuber, President/CEO
Bill Sproull, Chairman
William Mills, Director
Works with any standard keyboard and offers seven overlays and a cable for one type of computer.

1076 **Universal Numeric Keypad**
Genovation
17741 Mitchell N
Irvine, CA 92614-6028
949-833-3355
800-822-4333
Fax: 949-833-0322
www.genovation.com
max@genovation.com
A 21 key numeric keypad that works with any laptop or portable computer.

1077 **Up and Running**
IntelliTools
2625 Patton Road
Roseville, MN 55113-1308
651-294-2200
800-322-0956
Fax: 651-294-2259
www.ablenetinc.com
customerservice@ablenetinc.com
Jennifer Thalhuber, President/CEO
Bill Sproull, Chairman
William Mills, Director
A custom overlay kit for the IntelliKeys Keyboard that provides instant access to a wide range of software including over 60 popular educational programs. *$69.95*

1078 **VISTA**
TeleSensory
417 Cypress Street
Bakersfield, CA 93304
650-743-9515
800-8048004
Fax: 661-327-2478
www.telesensory.com
info@telesensory.com
Image enlarging system that magnifies the print and graphics on the screen from three to 16 times. *$2495.00*

1079 **VisagraphIII Eye-Movement Recording System& Reading Plus**
Taylor Associated Communications
110 West Canal Street
Suite 301
Winooski, VT 05404
802-735-1942
800-732-3758
Fax: 802-419-4786
www.readingplus.com
info@readingplus.com
Mark Taylor, Chief Executive Officer
Kelly Scannell, Chief Operating Officer
Stan Taylor, Founder/Chairman
Measures reading performance efficiency, visual and functional proficiency, perceptual development, and information processing competence.

1080   Window-Eyes
GW Micro
725 Airport North Office Park
Fort Wayne, IN 46825-6707

260-489-3671
Fax: 260-489-2608
www.gwmicro.com
support@gwmicro.com

Erik Deckers, Director of Sales and Marketing
Screen reader that is adaptable to your specific needs and preferances. Works automatically so you can focus on your application program, not so much on operating the screen reader.

Books & Periodicals

1081   AppleWorks Education
AACE
P.O. Box 719
Waynesville, NC 28786

757-366-5606
Fax: 828-246-9557
www.aace.org
info@aace.org

Gary H. Marks, Executive Director
Tracy Jacobs, Office Manager
Covers educational uses of AppleWorks software. *$25.00*

1082   Bibliography of Journal Articles on Microcomputers & Special Education
Special Education Resource Center
25 Industrial Park Rd
Middletown, CT 06457-1516

860-632-1485
800-842-8678
Fax: 860-632-8870
www.ctserc.org
info@ctserc.org

Marianne Kirner, Executive Director
Ingrid Canady, Assistant Director for Program
Mathew Dugan, Assistant Director
This pamphlet offers information on a wide variety of professional journals in the fields of microcomputers and special education.

1083   Closing the Gap Newsletter
Closing the Gap Solutions
526 Main Street
P.O. Box 68
Henderson, MN 56044-0068

507-248-3294
Fax: 507-248-3810
www.closingthegap.com
info@closingthegap.com

Budd Hagen, Co-Founder
Dolores Hagen, Co-Founder
Connie Kneip, Vice President/General Manager
Bimonthly newsletter on the use of computer technology in special education and rehabilitation. CTG also sponsors an annual international conference. *$34.00*
40 pages
ISSN 0886-1935

1084   Computer Access-Computer Learning
Special Needs Project

818-718-9900
Fax: 818-349-2027
www.specialneeds.com

Hod Gray, Editor
Ginny LaVine, Author
A resource manual in adaptive technology. *$22.50*
226 pages

1085   MACcessories: Guide to Peripherals
Western Illinois University: Macomb Projects
1 University Cir
Macomb, IL 61455-1367

309-298-1414
800-322-3905
Fax: 309-298-2305
www.wiu.edu
info@wiu.edu

Amanda B. Silberer, Audiology Clinic Coordinator
Joyce Johanson, Associate Director
Beverly Stuckwisch, Chief Clerk
Designed to help the Macintosh user understand peripheral devices. Includes descriptions of each device, advantages and disadvantages of each, procedures for installation, troubleshooting tips, suggested software and company resources. *$15.00*
41 pages

1086   Switch to Turn Kids On
Western Illinois University: Macomb Projects
Horrabin Hall 71b 1 University Cir
Macomb, IL 61455-1390

309-298-1414
800-322-3905
Fax: 309-298-2305
www.wiu.edu/users/micpc
info@wiu.edu

Amanda B. Silberer, Audiology Clinic Coordinator
Carrie Lowderman, Clerk
Beverly Stuckwisch, Chief Clerk
Guide to homemade switches gives information on conducting a switch workshop and constructing a battery interrupter as well as various kinds of switches (tread switches, ribbon switches, mercury switches, pillow switches). Contains illustrations and step-by-step instructions. *$12.00*
47 pages

Centers & Organizations

1087   American Foundation for the Blind
2 Penn Plaza
Suite 1102
New York, NY 10121

212-502-7600
800-232-5463
Fax: 888-545-8331
www.afb.org
afbinfo@afb.net

Carl R. Augusto, President/CEO
Kelly Bleach, Chief Administrative Officer
Rick Bozeman, Chief Financial Officer
Is a national nonprofit that expands possibilities for people with vision loss. AFB's priorities include broadening access to technology; elevating the quality of information and tools for the professionals who serve people with vision loss; and promoting independent and healthy living for people with vision loss by providing them and their families with relevant and timely resources.

1088   Artificial Language Laboratory
Michigan State University
405 Computer Ctr
East Lansing, MI 48824-1042

517-353-0870
Fax: 517-353-4766
www.msu.edu

John Eulenberg PhD, Director
Multidisciplinary teaching and research center involved in basic and applied research concerning the computer processing of formal linguistic structures.

1089   Association for Educational Communications and Technology
320 W. 8th St.
Ste 101
Bloomington, IN 47404-3745

812-335-7675
877-677-2328
Fax: 812-335-7678
www.aect.org
aect@aect.org

Stephen Harmon, President
Ellen Hoffman, Executive Secretary
Robert Maribe Branch, President-Elect
Provides leadership in educational communications and technology by linking professionals holding a common interest in the use of educational technology and its application to the learning process.

1090 Birmingham Alliance for Technology Access Center
Birmingham Independent Living Center
206 13th St S
Birmingham, AL 35233-1317 205-251-2223
Fax: 205-251-0605
TTY: 205-251-2223
www.ilrgb.org
bilc@bellsouth.net
Daniel G Kessler, Executive Director
Information dissemination, network, referral service, support services, and training. Disabilities served are cognitive, hearing, learning, physical, speech and vision.

1091 Bluegrass Technology Center
409 Southland Drive
Lexington, KY 40503 859-294-4343
800-209-7767
Fax: 866-576-9625
www.bluegrass-tech.org
office@bluegrass-tech.org
Bruce W. Turley, President
Robin Rice, Vice President
Odetta Carlisle, Secertary
Provides support to all persons with disabilities in their efforts to access technology and to increase awareness and understanding of how that technology can enhance their abilities to participate more fully in their community, assisting individuals directly or indirectly by working with their caregivers, therapists, vocational counselors, case managers, educators, employers, and community members.

1092 CAST
Center for Applied Special Technology
40 Harvard Mill Sq
Suite 3
Wakefield, MA 01880-3233 781-245-2212
Fax: 781-245-5212
TDD: 781-245-9320
www.cast.org
cast@cast.org
Stephen P. Crosby, Chairman
Sheldon H. Berman, Director
David Flink, Director
A nonprofit organization that works to expand learning opportunities for all individuals, especially those with disabilities, through the research and development of innovative, technology-based educational resources and strategies.

1093 Center for Accessible Technology
3075 Adeline
Suite 220
Berkeley, CA 97403 510-841-3224
Fax: 510-841-7956
www.cforat.org
info@cforat.org
Guy Thomas, President
Sara Armstrong Ph.D, Treasurer
Carol Cody, Executive Director
Resource center for parents, professionals, developers and individuals with disabilities, filled with computers, software, adapted toys and adaptive technology.

1094 Center for Enabling Technology
College of New Jersey
PO Box 7718
2000 Pennington Road
Ewing, NJ 08628-718 609-771-3016
Fax: 609-637-5172
TTY: 609-771-2309
www.tcnj.edu
R. Barbara Gitenstein, President
Lisa Angeloni, Vice President
Thomas Mahoney, General Counsel/VP
Ongoing projects that match assistive devices to the children who need them. Training and educational workshops.

1095 Comprehensive Services for the Disabled
PO Box 1605
Wall, NJ 07719-1605 732-681-5632
800-784-2919
Fax: 732-681-5632
Donald DeSanto, Executive Director
Helps special students realize their potential and bring college admission a step closer. Program designed to meet the needs and maximize the unique talents of each individual. The staff consists of highly qualified teachers who see beyond labels and reach the person inside. By pacing scholastics to each student's ability, the college increases understanding and makes learning a positive experience. Instruction is tailored to each individual.

1096 Computer Access Center
Empowertech
P.O. Box 12464
Albuquerque, NM 87195 505-242-9588
www.cac.org
info@cacradicalgrace.org
Richard Barlow, Director
Mark Cavanaugh, Director
Phil Robers, Director
Computer resource center serving primarily as a place where people with all types of disabilities can preview equipment. Workshops, seminars, after school clubs for children and individual consultations are provided.

1097 Council for Exceptional Children Annual Convention & Expo
Council for Exceptional Children
2900 Crystal Drive
Suite 1000
Arlington, VA 22202-3557 703-264-9454
800-224-6830
Fax: 703-620-2521
TDD: 866-915-5000
TTY: 866-915-5000
www.cec.sped.org
victore@cec.sped.org
Robin D. Brewer, President
James P. Heiden, President Elect
Christy A. Chambers, Immediate Past President
This database contains citations and abstracts of print and nonprint materials dealing with exceptional children, those who have disabilities and those who are gifted. Resources in all areas of special education and related services (including services provided by audiologists, speech therapists, occupational therapists, physical therapists, and educational psychologists) are covered in ECER.

1098 Dialog Information Services
2250 Perimeter Park Drive
Suite 300
Morrisville, NC 27560 919-804-6493
888-809-6193
Fax: 919-804-6410
www.proquest.com
Andy Snyder, Chairman
Kurt Sanford, CEO
Jonathan Collins, CFO
Offers access to over 390 data bases containing information on various aspects of disabling conditions and services to disabled individuals.

1099 HEATH Resource Center
2134 G St NW
Washington, DC 20052
www.heath.gwu.edu
AskHEATH@gwu.edu
Jessica Queener, Project Director
Reina Guartico, Research Assistant
Dr. Juliana Taymans, Professor

The HEATH Resource Center is an online clearinghouse on postsecondary education for individuals with disabilities. The HEATH Resource Center Clearinghouse has information for students with disabilities on educational disability support services, policies, procedures, adaptations, accessing college or university campuses, career-technical schools, and other postsecondary training entities.

1100   High Tech Center Training Unit
21050 McClellan Rd
Cupertino, CA 95014-4276   408-996-4636
                                          800-411-8954
                                     Fax: 408-996-6042
                                     TTY: 408-252-4938
                                     www.htctu.fhda.edu
                                       info@htctu.net

Gaeir Dietrich, Director
Michael Fosnaugh, Administrative Assistant
Dale Kan, Network Specialist
Provides training for faculty and staff of the California community colleges in access technologies.

1101   Iowa Program for Assistive Technology
IA University Assistive Technology
100 Hawkins Dr
Iowa City, IA 52242-1011   800-779-2001
                                        http://iowaat.org
                                        IPAT@uiowa.edu

Jane Gay, Director
Gary Johnson, Coordinator, Community Program
Marlene Phipps, Office Clerk
Computer accesssed solutions for physically challenged students.

1102   Learning Independence through Computers
LINC
2301 Argonne Drive
Baltimore, MD 21218-4325   410-554-9134
                                     Fax: 410-261-2907
                                          www.linc.org

Theo Pinette, Executive Director
Jessica Robles, Volunteer Services Manager
Justin Creamer, Sr. Assistive Technology
Resource center that offers specially adapted computer technology to children and adults with a variety of disabilities. State-of-the-art systems allow consumers to achieve their potential for productivity and independence at home, school, work and in the community. Also offers a quarterly newsletter called Connections.

1103   Lighthouse Central Florida
215 E New Hampshire St
Orlando, FL 32804-6403   407-898-2483
                                     Fax: 407-895-5255
                          www.lighthousecentralflorida.org
                                     lighthouse@lcf-fl.org

Lee Nasehi, President/CEO
Donna Esbensen, VP/CFO
Provides life-changing services for children and adults who are blind and sight-impaired. Offers a comprehensive array of professional vision rehabilitation services in the Central Florida area.
1976

1104   Project TECH
Massachusetts Easter Seal Society
6th Fl
484 Main St
Worcester, MA 01608-1893   800-244-2756
                                     Fax: 508-831-9768
                                     TTY: 800-564-9700
                                     www.eastersealsma.org
                                     info@eastersealsma.org

David S. Hoffman, Vice Chair
Harry E. Salerno, Chairman
Anthony A. Tambone, Treasurer
Assistive technology services, suited to an individual's needs. Transition from school to work, employment planning, occupational skills and more are coached here.

1105   RESNA Technical Assistance Project
Ste 1540
1700 N Moore St
Arlington, VA 22209-1917   703-524-6686
                                     Fax: 703-524-6639
                                          www.resna.org
                                     membership@resna.org

Nell Bailey, Executive Director
Alex Mihailidis, PhD, P.Eng, President
Paul J. Schwartz, MSIE, ATP, R, Treasurer
Provides technical assistance to states in the development and implementation of consumer responsive statewide programs of technology-related assistance under the Technology Related Assistance for Individuals with Disabilities Act of 1988.

1106   Ruth Eason School
648 Old Mill Rd
Millersville, MD 21108-1373   410-222-3815
                                     Fax: 410-222-3817
                                          www.aacps.org
                                     schoolsite@aacps.org

Cathy Larner, Principal
Linda Abey, Principal
Tracy D Angelo, Secretary

1107   Star Center
1119 Old Humboldt Rd
Jackson, TN 38305-1752   731-668-3888
                                          800-464-5619
                                     Fax: 731-668-1666
                                     TTY: 731-668-9664
                                     www.starcenter.tn.org
                                 information@starcenter.tn.org

Jane Gay, Executive Director
Johnson Gay, Coordinator
Marlene Phipps, Office Clerk
Technology center for people with disabilities. Some of the services are: music therapy, art therapy, augmentative communication evaluation and training, vocational evaluation, job placement, vision department, environmental controls.

1108   Tech-Able
1451 Klondike Road
Suite D
Conyers, GA 30094-5982   770-922-6768
                                     Fax: 770-992-6769
                                          www.techable.org
                                     c.b.wright@techable.org

Cassandra Baker-Wright, Executive Director
Patricia Hanus, Program Assistant
Erika Ruffin-Mosley, Assistive Technology Trainer
Assistive technology demonstration and information center. Provides demonstrations of computer hardware and software specially designed to assist people with disabilities. Serves a wide range of disabilities and virtually all age groups. Also custom fabrication of key guards and switches.

1109   Technology Access Center
475 Metroplex Dr
Ste 301
Nashville, TN 37211-3142   615-248-6733
                                          800-368-4651
                                     Fax: 615-259-2536
                                     TDD: 615-248-6733
                                     www.tacnashville.org
                                     techaccess@tacnashville.org

Bob Kibler, Director
Lynn Magner, Service Coordinator
Linda Judeich, Director of Services
Serves the community as a resource center and carries out specific projects related to assistive technology.

1110 Technology Access Foundation
605 SW 108th St
Seattle, WA 98146   206-725-9095
                                   Fax: 206-725-9097
                                   www.techaccess.org
                                   taf@techaccess.org
Jill Scheuerman, President
Kelly Evans, Vice President
Harish Nanda, Treasurer
Provides information, consultation and technical assistance
on assistive technology for people with disabilities, includ-
ing computer hardware and software technology, and adap-
tive and assistive equipment.

1111 Technology Assistance for Special Consumers
1856 Keats Dr NW
Huntsville, AL 35810-4465   256-859-8300
                                   Fax: 256-859-4332
                                   www.ucptasc.org
                                   tracyc@ucphuntsville.org
Cathy Scholl, President
Nicole Schroer, President Elect
Dr. Adam Hott, Secretary
Offers a computer resource center which has both computers
and software for use at the center or for short-term.

1112 Technology Utilization Program
National Aeronautics and Space Administration
Suite 5K39
Washington, DC 20546   202-358-0000
                                   Fax: 202-358-4338
                                   www.nasa.gov
                                   public-inquiries@hq.nasa.gov.
Charles F. Bolden, Jr., Administrator
David Radzanowski, Chief of Staff
Michael French, Deputy Administrator
Adapts aerospace technology to the development of equip-
ment for the disabled, sick and elderly persons.

1113 Technology for Language and Learning
PO Box 327
East Rockaway, NY 11518   516-625-4550
                                   Fax: 516-621-3321
                                   ForTLL@aol.com
Joan Tanenhaus, Executive Director
An organization dedicated to advancing the use of comput-
ers and technology for children and adults with special lan-
guage and learning needs. Public domain computer software
for special education.

Games

1114 A Day at Play
Don Johnston
26799 W Commerce Dr
Volo, IL 60073-9675   847-740-0749
                                   800-999-4660
                                   Fax: 847-740-7326
                                   www.donjohnston.com
                                   info@donjohnston.com
Ruth Ziolkowski, President
A Day at Play and Out and About, programs in the UKanDu
Little Books Series, are early literacy programs that consist
of several create-your-own four-page animated stories that
help build language experience for early readers. Students
fill in the blanks to complete a sentence on each page and
then watch the page come alive with animation and sound.
After completing the story, students can print it out to make a
book which can be read over and over again.

1115 Academic Drill Builders: Wiz Works
SRA Order Services
PO Box 182605
Columbus, OH 43218   800-334-7344
                                   Fax: 614-860-1877
                                   www.sraonline.com
                                   SEG_CustomerService@mcgraw-hill.com

The McGraw-Hill Education Urban Advisory Resource
works with large urban districts across the country to help
them provide better quality instruction, curriculum, and assessment to their students. *$49.00*

1116 Adaptive Physical Education Program
2 Merwick Road
Princeton, NJ 08540-5711   609-987-0099
                                   www.edenservices.org
Tom Mc Cool, Executive Director
Anne Holmes, Outreach/Support Director
This volume contains teaching programs in the area of sen-
sory integration and adaptive physical education for stu-
dents with autism. *$50.00*

1117 Alpine Tram Ride
Merit Software
121 W 27th St
Suite 603
New York, NY 10011-6262   212-675-8567
                                   800-753-6488
                                   Fax: 212-675-8607
                                   www.meritsoftware.com
                                   sales@meritsoftware.com
Ben Weintraub, CEO
Teaches cognitive redevelopment skills. *$12.95*

1118 Blocks in Motion
Don Johnston
26799 W Commerce Dr
Volo, IL 60073-9675   847-740-0749
                                   800-999-4660
                                   Fax: 847-740-7326
                                   www.donjohnston.com
                                   info@donjohnston.com
Ruth Ziolkowski, President
An art and motion program that makes drawing, creating and
animating fun and educational for all users. Based on the
Piagetian theory for motor-sensory development, this program promotes the concept that the process is as educational
and as much fun as the end result. Good fine motor skills are
not required for students to be successful and practice critical thinking. *$99.00*

1119 CONCENTRATE! On Words and Concepts
Laureate Learning Systems
110 E Spring St
Winooski, VT 05404-1898   802-655-4755
                                   800-562-6801
                                   Fax: 802-655-4757
                                   www.laureatelearning.com
                                   laureate-webmaster@laureatelearning.com
Mary Sweig Wilson Ph.D., President/CEO/Author
Bernard J. Fox, Vice President/Author
Marion Blank, Ph.D, Developmental Psychologist
A series of educational games that reinforces the lessons of
the Words and Concepts Series while developing short term
memory skills. *$105.00*

1120 Camp Frog Hollow
Don Johnston
26799 W Commerce Dr
Volo, IL 60073-9675   847-740-0749
                                   800-999-4660
                                   Fax: 847-740-7326
                                   www.donjohnston.com
                                   info@donjohnston.com
Ruth Ziolkowski, President
Camp Frog Hollow chronicles the further adventures of K.C.
and Clyde as they head off to summer camp. This entertaining approach to reading, literacy and learning can be beneficial for individual reading lessons or large group activities.
The journaling feature provides students the opportunity to
record their thoughts and feelings while the tracking feature
provides a record of progress for the teacher/parent.

1121 Create with Garfield
SRA Order Services
PO Box 182605
Columbus, OH 43218   800-843-8855
                                    Fax: 972-228-1982
                                    www.sraonline.com
            SEG_CustomerService@mcgraw-hill.com
The McGraw-Hill Education Urban Advisory Resource
works with large urban districts across the country to help
them provide better quality instruction, curriculum, and as-
sessment to their students.

1122 Create with Garfield: Deluxe Edition
SRA Order Services
PO Box 182605
Columbus, OH 43218   800-843-8855
                                    Fax: 972-228-1982
                                    www.sraonline.com
            SEG_CustomerService@mcgraw-hill.com
The McGraw-Hill Education Urban Advisory Resource
works with large urban districts across the country to help
them provide better quality instruction, curriculum, and as-
sessment to their students.

1123 Dino-Games
Academic Software
3504 Tates Creek Rd
Lexington, KY 40517-2601   859-552-1020
                                    Fax: 253-799-4012
                                    www.acsw.com
                                    asistaff@acsw.com

Dr Warren E Lacefield, President
Penelope D Ellis, COO/Dir Sales/Marketing
Sylvia B. Lacefield, Graphic Artist
Single switch software programs designed for early switch
practice. CD-ROM for Mac or PC. Visit web site for demon-
strations. *$39.00*

1124 Early Games for Young Children
Software to Go-Gallaudet University
800 Florida Ave NE
Washington, DC 20002-3600   202-651-5220
                                    Fax: 202-651-5109
                                    www.gallaudet.edu
                                    clerc.center@gallaudet.edu

Ken Kurlychek, Information Specialist
Ed Bosso, Vice President

1125 Garfield Trivia Game
SRA Order Services
PO Box 182605
Columbus, OH 43218   800-843-8855
                                    Fax: 972-228-1982
                                    www.sraonline.com
            SEG_CustomerService@mcgraw-hill.com
The McGraw-Hill Education Urban Advisory Resource
works with large urban districts across the country to help
them provide better quality instruction, curriculum, and as-
sessment to their students.

1126 KC & Clyde in Fly Ball
Don Johnston
26799 W Commerce Dr
Volo, IL 60073-9675   847-740-0749
                                        800-999-4660
                                    Fax: 847-740-7326
                                    www.donjohnston.com
                                    info@donjohnston.com

Ruth Ziolkowski, President
In the UKanDu Series of interactive software which is designed to promote learning, independence, and accommodate special needs. Word interaction and context are stressed
as students progress through the story and make decisions on
how the storyline will advance. Active interaction at the
word level is encouraged by UKanDu the wordbird, the tour
guide to language in this story. *$95.00*

1127 Mind Over Matter
World Class Learning
PO Box 639
Candler, NC 28715   800-638-6470
                                    Fax: 800-638-6499
                                    www.wclm.com
                                    dealers@wclm.com
A game program that challenges students to solve 185 visual
word puzzles or create their own puzzles, using symbols and
graphics.

1128 Monkey Business
Merit Software
121 W 27th St
Suite 603
New York, NY 10001-6262   212-675-8567
                                        800-753-6488
                                    Fax: 212-675-8607
                                    www.meritsoftware.com
                                    sales@meritsoftware.com

Ben Weintraub, CEO
Choose one of the three levels of difficulty and play until a
minimum score is reached. *$10.95*

1129 Multi-Scan
Academic Software
3504 Tates Creek Rd
Lexington, KY 40517-2601   859-552-1020
                                    Fax: 253-799-4012
                                    www.acsw.com
                                    asistaff@acsw.com

Warren E Lacefield, President
Penelope D Ellis, COO/Dir Sales/Marketing
Sylvia B. Lacefield, Graphic Artist
Single switch activity center containing educational games
such as numerical dot to dot, concentration, mazes, and
matching, for PCs and Macintosh CD-ROM. Handbook for
adaptive switches available. *$149.00*

1130 On a Green Bus
Don Johnston
26799 W Commerce Dr
Volo, IL 60073-9675   847-740-0749
                                        800-999-4660
                                    Fax: 847-740-7326
                                    www.donjohnston.com
                                    info@donjohnston.com

Ruth Ziolkowski, President
An early literacy program in the UKandDu Little Books Series consisting of several create-your-own four-page animated stories that help build language experience for early
readers. Students fill in the blanks, completing sentences on
each page. After completing the story, students can print it
out to make a book which can be read over and over again.

1131 Teddy Barrels of Fun
SRA Order Services
PO Box 182605
Columbus, OH 43218   1-888-772-45
                                    Fax: 972-228-1982
                                    www.sraonline.com
            SEG_CustomerService@mcgraw-hill.com
The McGraw-Hill Education Urban Advisory Resource
works with large urban districts across the country to help
them provide better quality instruction, curriculum, and as-
sessment to their students. *$42.00*

Language Arts

1132 Alphabet Circus
SRA Order Services
PO Box 182605
Columbus, OH 43218   1-888-772-45
                                    Fax: 972-228-1982
                                    www.sraonline.com
            SEG_CustomerService@mcgraw-hill.com

The McGraw-Hill Education Urban Advisory Resource works with large urban districts across the country to help them provide better quality instruction, curriculum, and assessment to their students. *$35.00*

1133 American Sign Language Dictionary: Software
Speech Bin
PO Box 1579
Appleton, WI 54912-1579
419-589-1600
888-388-3224
Fax: 888-388-6344
www.schoolspecialty.com
orders@schoolspecialty.com
Joseph M. Yorio, President, CEO
Rick Holden, Executive Vice President
Kevin Baehler, Vice President, Acting CFO
The CD includes captivating video clips that show 2,500+ words, phrases, and idioms in sign language. The videos may be played at normal speed, slow motion, and stop action. Animations explain origins of selected signs; drills and games are provided to reinforce learning. Item number M545 for Windows $24.95 Item number M540 for MAC. *$29.95*

1134 American Sign Language Video Dictionary & Inflection Guide
Harris Communications
15155 Technology Dr
Eden Prairie, MN 55344-2273
952-906-1180
800-825-6758
Fax: 952-906-1099
TTY: 800-825-9187
www.harriscomm.com
info@harriscomm.com
Dr. Robert Harris, President
Darla Hudson, Customer Service
Lori Foss, Marketing Director
Combines text, video, and animation to create a leading interactive reference tool that makes learning ASL easy and fun. Contains 2700 signs, searching capabilities in 5 languages, new learning games, and expanded sections in fingerspelling. Part #CD 144. *$49.95*
448 pages Video

1135 AtoZap!
Sunburst Technology
3150 W Higgins Rd
Suite 140
Hoffman Estates, IL 60619
800-321-7511
www.sunburst.com
Service@sunburst.com
When users select an A, little airplanes that fly madly about appear. Users select T and students have their own telephone to talk to any one of nine animated friends. This program for prereaders has an activity for every letter.

1136 Auditory Skills
Psychological Software Services
3304 W 75th St
Indianapolis, IN 46268
317-257-9672
Fax: 317-257-9674
www.neuroscience.cnter.com
nsc@neuroscience.cnter.com
Odie L Bracy, Clinical Neuropsychologist
Nancy Bracy, Office Manager
Andrea Oakes, Clinical Assistant
Four computer programs designed to aid in the remediation of auditory discrimination problems. *$50.00*

1137 Basic Skills Products
EDCON Publishing Group
P.O. Box 383759
Waikoloa, HI 96738
415-580-0953
888-553-3266
Fax: 877-597-6376
www.edconpublishing.com
Deals with basic math and language arts. Free catalog available.

1138 Challenging Our Minds
Psychological Software Services
3304 W 75th St
Indianapolis, IN 46268
317-257-9672
Fax: 317-257-9674
www.challenging-our-minds.com
info@challenging-our-minds.com
Odie L Bracy, President
Nancy Bracy, Office Manager
Challenging our Minds (COM) is a cognitive enhancement system designed by a neuropsychologist to develop and enhance cognitive functions across the domains of attention, executive skills, memory, visuospatial skills, problem solving skills, communication and psychosocial skills. COM is a subscription website providign online cognitive enhancement applications for all children.

1139 Character Education:Life Skills Online Education
Phillip Roy Inc.
PO Box 130
Indian Rocks Beach, FL 33785
727-593-2700
800-255-9085
Fax: 727-595-2685
www.philliproy.com
info@philliproy.com
Ruth Bragman, President
Includes 77 CDs, 77 books and unlimited interactive online access, per purchasing site. All print materials are also available to be Brailled and all CDs come with complete audio components along with interactive graphics. Pre/post tests included along with teacher's guide and lesson plans. All materials can be duplicated at purchasing site. No yearly fees. *$3950.00*

1140 Cognitive Rehabilitation
Technology for Language and Learning
PO Box 327
East Rockaway, NY 11518
516-625-4550
Fax: 516-621-3321
A series of public domain programs that strengthen cognitive skills, memory, language and visual motor skills. *$20.00*

1141 Construct-A-Word I & II
SRA Order Services
PO Box 182605
Columbus, OH 43218
800-334-7344
Fax: 800-953-8691
www.mheducation.com
SEG_CustomerService@mheducation.com
David Levin, President/CEO
David Stafford, SVP/General Counsel
Maryellen Valaitis, SVP, Human Resources
The McGraw-Hill Education Urban Advisory Resource works with large urban districts across the country to help them provide better quality instruction, curriculum, and assessment to their students. *$99.00*

1142 Crypto Cube
Software to Go-Gallaudet University
800 Florida Ave NE
Washington, DC 20002-3695
202-651-5031
Fax: 202-651-5109
TTY: 202-651-5855
http://clerccenter.gallaudet.edu
clerc.center@gallaudet.edu
Ed Bosso, Vice President
Ken Kurlychek, Electronic Information

1143 Curious George Pre-K ABCs
Sunburst Technology
3150 W Higgins Rd
Suite 140
Hoffman Estates, IL 60619
800-321-7511
www.sunburst.com
service@sunburst.com

Children go on a lively adventure with Curious George visiting six multi level activities that provide an animated introduction to letters and their sounds. Students discover letter names and shapes, initial letter sounds, letter pronunciations, the order of the alphabet and new vocabulary words during the fun exursions with Curious George. Mac/Win CD-ROM

1144 Eden Institute Curriculum: Classroom
2 Merwick Road
Princeton, NJ 08540   609-987-0099
                                         Fax: 609-987-0243
                                         http://edenautism.org
Peter H. Bell, President/CEO
John Inzilla, Chief Financial Officer
Jennifer Bizub, Chief Operating Officer
This volume is geared toward students with autism who have mastered some basic academic skills and are able to learn in a small group setting. Teaching programs include academics, domestic and social skills. *$100.00*

1145 Elephant Ears: English with Speech
Ballard & Tighe
471 Atlas Street
PO Box 219
Brea, CA 92822-0219   714-990-4332
                                             800-321-4332
                                         Fax: 714-255-9828
                                         www.ballard-tighe.com
                                         info@ballard-tighe.com
Dorothy Roberts, Chairperson
Dr. Sari Luoma, Vice President, Assessment
Fred Tan, VP, Information Technology
Features instruction and assessment of prepositions in a 3-part diskette. *$49.00*

1146 Emerging Literacy
Technology for Language and Learning
PO Box 327
East Rockaway, NY 11518   516-625-4550
                                         Fax: 516-621-3321
A five-volume set of stories. *$25.00*

1147 Essential Learning Systems
Creative Education Institute
4567 Lake Shore Drive
P.O. Box 7306
Waco, TX 76710   254-751-1188
                                             800-234-7319
                                         Fax: 888-475-2402
                                         www.ceilearning.com
                                         info@ceilearning.com
Enables special education, learning disabled and dyslexic students to develop the skills they need to learn. Using computer exercises to appropriately stimulate the brain's language areas, the lagging learning skills can be developed and patterns of correct language taught.

1148 First Phonics
Sunburst Technology
3150 W Higgins Rd
Suite 140
Hoffman Estates, IL 60619   800-321-7511
                                         www.sunburst.com
                                         service@sunburst.com
Targets the phonics skills that all children need to develop, sounding out the first letter of a word. This program offers four different engaging activities that you can customize to match each child's specific need.

1149 Gremlin Hunt
Merit Software
121 West 27th Street
Suite 1200
New York, NY 10001   212-675-8567
                                             800-753-6488
                                         Fax: 800-918-9336
                                         www.meritsoftware.com
                                         sales@meritsoftware.com

Ben Weintraub, CEO
Gremlins test visual discrimination and memory skills at three levels. *$9.95*

1150 High Frequency Vocabulary
Technology for Language and Learning
PO Box 327
East Rockaway, NY 11518   516-625-4550
                                         Fax: 516-621-3321
Each volume of the series has 10 stories that teach specific vocabulary. *$35.00*

1151 Hint and Hunt I & II
SRA Order Services
PO Box 182605
Columbus, OH 43218   800-334-7344
                                         Fax: 800-953-8691
                                         www.mheducation.com
                          SEG_CustomerService@mheducation.com
David Levin, President/CEO
David Stafford, SVP/General Counsel
Maryellen Valaitis, SVP, Human Resources
The McGraw-Hill Education Urban Advisory Resource works with large urban districts across the country to help them provide better quality instruction, curriculum, and assessment to their students. *$99.00*

1152 HyperStudio Stacks
Technology for Language and Learning
PO Box 327
East Rockaway, NY 11518   516-625-4550
                                         Fax: 516-621-3321
Offers various volumes in language arts, social studies and reading. *$10.00*

1153 IDEA Cat I, II and III
Ballard & Tighe
471 Atlas Street
PO Box 219
Brea, CA 92822-0219   714-990-4332
                                             800-321-4332
                                         Fax: 714-255-9828
                                         www.ballard-tighe.com
                                         info@ballard-tighe.com
Dorothy Roberts, Chairperson
Dr. Sari Luoma, Vice President, Assessment
Fred Tan, VP, Information Technology
Computer-assisted teaching of English language lessons reinforces skills of Level I, II, and III of the IDEA Oral Program. *$142.00*

1154 Improving Reading/Spelling Skills via Keyboarding
AVKO Educational Research Foundation
3084 Willard Road
Birch Run, MI 48415-9404   810-686-9283
                                             866-285-6612
                                         Fax: 810-686-1101
                                         www.avko.org
                                         webmaster@avko.org
Don McCabe, President, Research Director
Linda Heck, Vice President, Clio, Michigan
Michael Lane, Treasurer, Clio, Michigan
Students learn spelling patterns and acquire important word recognition skills as they slowly and methodically learn proper fingering and keystrokes on a typewriter or computer keyboard. *$12.95*
ISBN 1-564004-01-5

1155 Katie's Farm
Lawrence Productions
6146 West Main St.
Suite A
Kalamazoo, MI 49009   269-903-2395
                                         www.lpi.com
                                         sales@lpi.com
Karen Morehouse, Operations Manager
Designed to encourage exploration and language development. *$29.95*

1156 Kid Pix
Riverdeep
222 Berkeley Street
Boston, MA 02116

617-351-5000
888-242-6747
Fax: 877-892-9820
www.hmhco.com
IIEcustomerservice@hmhpub.com

Linda K. Zecher, President, CEO, Director
James G. Nicholson, President, Riverside Publishing
William Bayers, EVP, General Counsel
Houghton Mifflin Harcourt offers a wide array of technology-driven pre-k-12 solutions that inspire excellence and innovation in education, and raise student achievement. *$59.95*

1157 Kids Media Magic 2.0
Sunburst Technology
3150 W Higgins Rd
Suite 140
Hoffman Estates, IL 60619

800-321-7511
www.sunburst.com
service@sunburst.com

The first multimedia word processor designed for young children. Help your child become a fluent reader and writer. The Rebus Bar automatically scrolls over 45 vocabulary words as students type.

1158 Language Carnival I
SRA Order Services
PO Box 182605
Columbus, OH 43218

800-334-7344
Fax: 800-953-8691
www.mheducation.com
SEG_CustomerService@mheducation.com

David Levin, President/CEO
David Stafford, SVP and General Counsel
Maryellen Valaitis, SVP Human Resources
The McGraw-Hill Education Urban Advisory Resource works with large urban districts across the country to help them provide better quality instruction, curriculum, and assessment to their students.

1159 Language Carnival II
SRA Order Services
PO Box 182605
Columbus, OH 43218

800-334-7344
Fax: 800-953-8691
www.mheducation.com
SEG_CustomerService@mheducation.com

David Levin, President/CEO
David Stafford, SVP and General Counsel
Maryellen Valaitis, SVP Human Resources
The McGraw-Hill Education Urban Advisory Resource works with large urban districts across the country to help them provide better quality instruction, curriculum, and assessment to their students.

1160 Language Master
Franklin Learning Resources
2 Manhattan Drive
Burlington, NJ 08016

609-386-2500
800-266-5626
Fax: 609-239-5950
www.franklin.com
service@franklin.com

A language master without speech defining over 83,000 words, spelling correction capability, pick/edit feature, vocabulary enrichment activities and advanced word list. *$79.95*

1161 Learn to Match
Technology for Language and Learning
PO Box 327
East Rockaway, NY 11518

516-625-4550
Fax: 516-621-3321

Joan Tanenhaus, Founder
Ten volume set of picture-matching disks. *$50.00*

1162 Letter Sounds
Sunburst Technology
3150 W Higgins Rd
Suite 140
Hoffman Estates, IL 60619

800-321-7511
www.sunburst.com
service@sunburst.com

Students develop phonemic awareness skills as they make the connection between consonant letters and their sounds.

1163 Letters and First Words
C&C Software
5713 Kentford Cir
Wichita, KS 67220-3131

316-683-6056
800-752-2086

Carol Clark, President
Helps children learn to identify letters and recognize their associated sounds. *$30.00*

1164 Lexia Phonics Based Reading
Lexia Learning Systems
200 Baker Avenue Ext
Concord, MA 01742

978-405-6200
800-435-3942
Fax: 978-287-0062
www.lexialearning.com
info@lexialearning.com

Nicholas C Gaehde, President
Collin Earnst, Vice President of Marketing
Peter Koso, Vice President of Operations
Five activity areas with 64 branching units and practice with 535 one-syllable words and 90 two-syllable words, sentences and stories. *$250.00*

1165 Look! Listen! & Learn Language!
Abilitations Speech Bin
PO Box 1579
Appleton, WI 54912-1579

419-589-1425
888-388-3224
Fax: 888-388-6344
www.schoolspecialty.com
orders@schoolspecialty.com

Joseph M. Yorio, President, CEO
Patrick T. Collins, EVP, Distribution
Rick Holden, EVP
Interactive activities for children with autism, PDD, Down syndrome, language delay, or apraxia include: hello; Match Same to Same; Quack; Let's talk About It; visual scanning/attention and match ups! Item number L177. *$98.99*

1166 M-ss-ng L-nks Single Educational Software
Sunburst Technology
3150 W Higgins Rd
Suite 140
Hoffman Estates, IL 60619

800-321-7511
www.sunburst.com
service@sunburst.com

This award-winning program is an engrossing language puzzle. A passage appears with letters or words missing. Students complete it based on their knowledge of word structure, spelling, grammar, meaning in context, and literary style.

1167 Max's Attic: Long & Short Vowels
Sunburst Technology
3150 W Higgins Rd
Suite 140
Hoffman Estates, IL 60619

800-321-7511
www.sunburst.com
service@sunburst.com

Filled to the rafters with phonics fun, this animated program builds your students' vowel recognition skills.

1168 **Memory I**
Psychological Software Services
3304 W 75th St
Indianapolis, IN 46268
317-257-9672
Fax: 317-257-9674
www.neuroscience.cnter.com
nsc@neuroscience.cnter.com
Odie L Bracy, PhD, HSPP, Clinical Neuropsychologist
Nancy Bracy, Office Manager
Andrea Oakes, Clinical Assistant
Consists of four computer programs designed to provide verbal and nonverbal memory exercises. *$110.00*

1169 **Memory II**
Psychological Software Services
3304 W 75th St
Indianapolis, IN 46268
317-257-9672
Fax: 317-257-9674
www.neuroscience.cnter.com
nsc@neuroscience.cnter.com
Odie L Bracy, PhD, HSPP, Clinical Neuropsychologist
Nancy Bracy, Office Manager
Andrea Oakes, Clinical Assistant
These programs allow for work with encoding, categorizing and organizing skills. *$150.00*

1170 **Microcomputer Language Assessment and Development System**
Laureate Learning Systems
110 East Spring Street
Winooski, VT 05404-1898
802-655-4755
800-562-6801
Fax: 802-655-4757
www.laureatelearning.com
laureate-webmaster@laureatelearning.com
Dr. Mary Sweig Wilson Ph.D., President/CEO, Founder
Bernard J. Fox, Co-Founder, Vice President
Marion Blank, Ph.D, Developmental Psychologist
A series of seven diskettes designed to teach over 45 fundamental syntactic rules. Students are presented two or three pictures, depending on the grammatical construction being trained with optional speech and/or text and asked to select the picture which represents the correct construction. *$775.00*

1171 **Mike Mulligan & His Steam Shovel**
Sunburst Technology
3150 W Higgins Rd
Suite 140
Hoffman Estates, IL 60619
800-321-7511
www.sunburst.com
service@sunburst.com
This CD-ROM version of the Caldecott classic lets students experience interactive book reading and participate in four skills-based extension activities that promote memory, matching, sequencing, listening, pattern recognition and map reading skills.

1172 **My Own Bookshelf**
Soft Touch
12301 Central Ave NE Ste 205
P.O. Box 490215
Blaine, MN 55449
763-502-0440
888-755-1402
Fax: 763-862-2920
www.marblesoft.com
support@marblesoft.com
Joyce Meyer, President
Mark Larson, CEO, Product Development
Research indicates that when students select their own books to read, their literacy levels improve. My Own Bookshelf gives students the ability to select their own books and to read them as often as they wish. *$30.00*

1173 **Optimum Resource**
1 Mathews Drive
Suite 107
Hilton Head Island, SC 29926
843-689-8000
888-784-2592
Fax: 843-689-8008
www.stickybear.com
info@stickybear.com
Richard Hefter, President
An educational software publishing company for grades K-12. Our software titles are available in Consumer, School, Labpack or Site License versions. Please call for further details. Prices range from $59.95 for Consumer to $699.95 for Site Licenses.

1174 **Phonology: Software**
Abilitations Speech Bin
PO Box 1579
Appleton, WI 54912-1579
419-589-1425
888-388-3224
Fax: 888-388-6344
www.schoolspecialty.com
orders@schoolspecialty.com
Joseph M. Yorio, President, CEO
Patrick T. Collins, EVP, Distribution
Rick Holden, EVP
This unique software gives you six entertaining games to treat children's phonological disorders. The program uses target patterns in a pattern cycling approach to phonological processess. Item number L183. *$98.99*

1175 **Python Path Phonics Word Families**
Sunburst Technology
3150 W Higgins Rd
Suite 140
Hoffman Estates, IL 60619
800-321-7511
www.sunburst.com
service@sunburst.com
Your child improves their word-building skills by playing three fun strategy games that involve linking one- or two-letter consonant beginnings to basic word endings.

1176 **Read, Write and Type! Learning System**
Talking Fingers
830 Rincon Way
San Rafael, CA 94903
415-472-3103
800-674-9126
www.readwritetype.com
contact@talkingfingers.com
Jeannine Herron, Developer
Leslie Grimm, Developer
This 40-lesson adventure is a powerful tool for 6-8 year-olds just learning to read, for children of other cultures learning to read and write in English, and for students of any age who are struggling to become successful readers and writers.

1177 **Same or Different**
Merit Software
121 West 27th Street
Suite 1200
New York, NY 10001
212-675-8567
800-753-6488
Fax: 800-918-9336
www.meritsoftware.com
sales@meritsoftware.com
Ben Weintraub, CEO
Requires students to make important visual discriminations which involve shape, color and whole/part relationships. *$9.95*

1178 **Sequencing Fun!**
Sunburst Technology
3150 W Higgins Rd
Suite 140
Hoffman Estates, IL 60619
800-321-7511
www.sunburst.com
service@sunburst.com
Text, pictures, animation and video clips provide a fun filled program that encourages critical thinking skills.

1179 Show Time
Software to Go-Gallaudet University
800 Florida Ave NE
Washington, DC 20002-3695 202-651-5031
Fax: 202-651-5109
http://clerccenter.gallaudet.edu
clerc.center@gallaudet.edu
Ed Bosso, Vice President
Ken Kurlychek, EI Specialist

1180 Soft Tools
Psychological Software Services
3304 W 75th St
Indianapolis, IN 46268-1664 317-257-9672
Fax: 317-257-9674
www.neuroscience.cnter.com
nsc@neuroscience.cnter.com
Odie L Bracy, PhD, HSPP, Clinical Neuropsychologist
Nancy Bracy, Office Manager
Andrea Oakes, Clinical Assistant
Menu-driven disk versions of the computer programs published in the Cognitive Rehabilitation Journal. *$50.00*

1181 Sound Match
Enable/Schneier Communication Unit
1603 Court Street
Syracuse, NY 13208 315-455-7591
Fax: 315-455-5989
TTY: 315-455-1794
www.enablecny.org
info@enablecny.org
Michael Wolfson, Chief Financial Officer
Prudence York, Executive Director
Mary DiBiase, Program Director
Presents a variety of sounds/noises requiring gross levels of auditory discrimination and matching. *$25.00*

1182 Speaking Language Master Special Edition
Franklin Learning Resources
2 Manhattan Drive
Burlington, NJ 08016 609-386-2500
800-266-5626
Fax: 609-239-5950
www.franklin.com
service@franklin.com
A language master with speech defining over 110,000 words, spelling correction capability, pick/edit feature, vocabulary enrichment activities and advanced word list. *$79.95*

1183 Spell-a-Word
RJ Cooper & Associates
22600-A Lambert St.
Suite 708
Lake Forest, CA 92630 949-582-2571
800-752-6673
Fax: 949-582-3169
www.rjcooper.com
info@rjcooper.com
R J Cooper, Owner
A large print, talking, spelling program. It uses an errorless learning method. It has both a drill and test mode, which a supervisor can set. Letters, words or phrases are entered by a supervisor and recorded by supervisor, peer, or sibling. Available for Mac, Windows. *$99.00*

1184 Spellagraph
Software to Go-Gallaudet University
800 Florida Ave NE
Washington, DC 20002-3695 202-651-5031
Fax: 202-651-5109
http://clerccenter.gallaudet.edu
clerc.center@gallaudet.edu
Ed Bosso, Vice President
Ken Kurlychek, EI Specialist

1185 Spelling Ace
Franklin Learning Resources
2 Manhattan Drive
Burlington, NJ 08016 609-386-2500
800-266-5626
Fax: 609-239-5950
www.franklin.com
service@franklin.com
The basic spelling corrector with 80,000 words. Sound-Alikes feature identifies commonly confused words. *$25.00*

1186 Spelling Mastery
SRA/McGraw-Hill
PO Box 182605
Columbus, OH 43218 800-334-7344
Fax: 800-953-8691
www.mheducation.com
SEG_CustomerService@mheducation.com
David Levin, President/CEO
David Stafford, SVP and General Counsel
Maryellen Valaitis, SVP, Human Resources
The McGraw-Hill Education Urban Advisory Resource works with large urban districts across the country to help them provide better quality instruction, curriculum, and assessment to their students.

1187 Stanley Sticker Stories
Riverdeep
222 Berkeley Street
Boston, MA 02116 617-351-5000
855-969-4642
Fax: 877-892-9820
www.hmhco.com
IIEcustomerservice@hmhpub.com
Linda K. Zecher, President, CEO, Director
James G. Nicholson, President, Riverside Publishing
John K. Dragoon, EVP, Chief Marketing Officer
Houghton Mifflin Harcourt offers a wide array of technology-driven pre-k-12 solutions that inspire excellence and innovation in education, and raise student achievement. *$59.95*

1188 Sunken Treasure Adventure: Beginning Blends
Sunburst Technology
3150 W Higgins Rd
Suite 140
Hoffman Estates, IL 60619 800-321-7511
www.sunburst.com
service@sunburst.com
Focus on beginning blends sounds and concepts with three high-spirited games that invite students to use two letter consonant blends as they build words.

1189 Syllasearch I, II, III, IV
SRA Order Services
PO Box 182605
Columbus, OH 43218 800-334-7344
Fax: 800-953-8691
www.mheducation.com
SEG_CustomerService@mheducation.com
David Levin, President/CEO
David Stafford, SVP and General Counsel
Maryellen Valaitis, SVP, Human Resources
The McGraw-Hill Education Urban Advisory Resource works with large urban districts across the country to help them provide better quality instruction, curriculum, and assessment to their students. *$99.00*

1190 Talking Nouns II: Sterling Edition
Laureate Learning Systems
110 East Spring Street
Winooski, VT 05404-1898 802-655-4755
800-562-6801
Fax: 802-655-4757
www.laureatelearning.com
laureate-webmaster@laureatelearning.com

Dr. Mary Sweig Wilson Ph.D., President/CEO, Founder
Bernard J. Fox, Co-Founder, Vice President
Marion Blank, Ph.D, Developmental Psychologist
Designed to build expressive language and augmentative communication skills. *$130.00*

1191 Talking Nouns: Sterling Edition
Laureate Learning Systems
110 East Spring Street
Winooski, VT 05404-1898   802-655-4755
800-562-6801
Fax: 802-655-4757
www.laureatelearning.com
laureate-webmaster@laureatelearning.com
Dr. Mary Sweig Wilson Ph.D., President/CEO, Founder
Bernard J. Fox, Co-Founder, Vice President
Marion Blank, Ph.D, Developmental Psychologist
An interactive communication product that helps build expressive language and augmentative communication skills. *$130.00*

1192 Talking Verbs Sterling Edition
Laureate Learning Systems
110 East Spring Street
Winooski, VT 05404-1898   802-655-4755
800-562-6801
Fax: 802-655-4757
www.laureatelearning.com
laureate-webmaster@laureatelearning.com
Dr. Mary Sweig Wilson Ph.D., President/CEO, Founder
Bernard J. Fox, Co-Founder, Vice President
Marion Blank, Ph.D, Developmental Psychologist
Builds expressive language and augmentative communication skills. *$130.00*

1193 Twenty Categories
Laureate Learning Systems
110 East Spring Street
Winooski, VT 05404-1898   802-655-4755
800-562-6801
Fax: 802-655-4757
www.laureatelearning.com
laureate-webmaster@laureatelearning.com
Dr. Mary Sweig Wilson Ph.D., President/CEO, Founder
Bernard J. Fox, Co-Founder, Vice President
Marion Blank, Ph.D, Developmental Psychologist
Designed to use with children and adults, these two diskettes provide instruction in both abstracting the correct category for a noun and placing a noun in the appropriate category. *$100.00*

1194 Type to Learn 3
Sunburst Technology
3150 W Higgins Rd
Suite 140
Hoffman Estates, IL 60619   800-321-7511
www.sunburst.com
service@sunburst.com
With the 25 lessons in this animated update of Type to Learn, students embark on time travel missions to learn keyboarding skills.

1195 Type to Learn Jr
Sunburst Technology
3150 W Higgins Rd
Suite 140
Hoffman Estates, IL 60619   800-321-7511
www.sunburst.com
service@sunburst.com
One of the first steps to literacy is learning how to use the keyboard. Age appropriate instruction and three practice activities help students use the computer with greater ease.

1196 Type to Learn Jr New Keys for Kids
Sunburst Technology
3150 W Higgins Rd
Suite 140
Hoffman Estates, IL 60619   800-321-7511
www.sunburst.com
service@sunburst.com

With new keys to learn, your early keyboarders focus on using the letter and number keys, the shift key, home row and are introduced to selected internet symbols.

1197 Vowel Patterns
Sunburst Technology
3150 W Higgins Rd
Suite 140
Hoffman Estates, IL 60619   800-321-7511
www.sunburst.com
service@sunburst.com
Some vowels are neither long nor short. In this investigation, students explore and learn to use abstract vowels.

1198 Word Invasion: Academic Skill Builders in Language Arts
SRA Order Services
PO Box 182605
Columbus, OH 43218   800-334-7344
Fax: 800-953-8691
www.mheducation.com
SEG_CustomerService@mheducation.com
David Levin, President/CEO
David Stafford, SVP and General Counsel
Maryellen Valaitis, SVP, Human Resources
The McGraw-Hill Education Urban Advisory Resource works with large urban districts across the country to help them provide better quality instruction, curriculum, and assessment to their students. *$49.00*

1199 Word Master: Academic Skill Builders in Language Arts
SRA Order Services
PO Box 182605
Columbus, OH 43218   800-334-7344
Fax: 800-953-8691
www.mheducation.com
SEG_CustomerService@mheducation.com
David Levin, President/CEO
David Stafford, SVP and General Counsel
Maryellen Valaitis, SVP, Human Resources
The McGraw-Hill Education Urban Advisory Resource works with large urban districts across the country to help them provide better quality instruction, curriculum, and assessment to their students. *$49.00*

1200 Word Wise I and II: Better Comprehension Through Vocabulary
SRA Order Services
PO Box 182605
Columbus, OH 43218   800-334-7344
Fax: 800-953-8691
www.mheducation.com
SEG_CustomerService@mheducation.com
David Levin, President/CEO
David Stafford, SVP and General Counsel
Maryellen Valaitis, SVP, Human Resources
The McGraw-Hill Education Urban Advisory Resource works with large urban districts across the country to help them provide better quality instruction, curriculum, and assessment to their students.

Life Skills

1201 Bozons' Quest
110 East Spring Street
Winooski, VT 05404-1898   802-655-4755
800-562-6801
Fax: 802-655-4757
www.laureatelearning.com
laureate-webmaster@laureatelearning.com
Dr. Mary Sweig Wilson Ph.D., President/CEO, Founder
Bernard J. Fox, Co-Founder, Vice President
Marion Blank, Ph.D, Developmental Psychologist
A computer game designed to teach cognitive skills and strategies and left/right discrimination skills.

1202 Calendar Fun with Lollipop Dragon
SVE & Churchill Media
700 Indian Springs Drive
Lancaster, PA 17601   888-892-3484
                            Fax: 877-324-6830
http://store.discoveryeducation.com
education_info@discovery.com
Young students learn the calendar basics. *$84.00*

1203 Comparison Kitchen
SRA Order Services
PO Box 182605
Columbus, OH 43218   800-334-7344
                            Fax: 800-953-8691
                            www.mheducation.com
SEG_CustomerService@mheducation.com
David Levin, President/CEO
David Stafford, SVP and General Counsel
Maryellen Valaitis, SVP, Human Resources
The McGraw-Hill Education Urban Advisory Resource
works with large urban districts across the country to help
them provide better quality instruction, curriculum, and as-
sessment to their students. *$35.00*

1204 Early Learning: Preparing Children for School, Phillip Roy, Inc.
PO Box 130
Indian Rocks Beach, FL 33785   727-593-2700
                            800-255-9085
                            Fax: 727-595-2685
                            www.philliproy.com
                            info@philliproy.com
Ruth Bragman, President
This program includes unlimited online access to 42 interactive lessons per individual. This pre-kindergarten curriculum has over 250 activities which include: Math,
Problem-Solving, Reading, Language Development, Physical Skills, Self-Esteem, Your Community, and Healthy Habits. Includes audio and interactive graphics. Allows parents
to work with their children at home or any place. Can be duplicated at the purcashing school. No yearly fees.

1205 Electric Crayon
Merit Software
121 West 27th Street
Suite 1200
New York, NY 10001   212-675-8567
                            800-753-6488
                            Fax: 800-918-9336
                            www.meritsoftware.com
                            sales@meritsoftware.com
Ben Weintraub, CEO
A tool to help preschool and primary aged children learn
about and enjoy the computer. *$14.95*

1206 First Categories Sterling Edition
Laureate Learning Systems
110 East Spring Street
Winooski, VT 05404-1898   802-655-4755
                            800-562-6801
                            Fax: 802-655-4757
                            www.laureatelearning.com
laureate-webmaster@laureatelearning.com
Dr. Mary Sweig Wilson Ph.D., President/CEO, Founder
Bernard J. Fox, Co-Founder, Vice President
Marion Blank, Ph.D, Developmental Psychologist
A computer program that trains 6 early categories using 60
nouns. Eleven innovative, activities, hundreds of drawings,
and photographs and exciting 3-D animation make this program fun and effective. *$230.00*

1207 First R
Milliken Publishing
501 East Third Street
Box 802
Dayton, OH 45401-0802   937-228-6118
                            800-444-1144
                            Fax: 937-223-2042
                            www.lorenzeducationalpress.com
                            lep@lorenz.com
Thomas Moore, President
Evan Gould, Author
Barbara Meeks, Author
A phonetically-based word recognition program with em-
phasis on comprehension. *$325.00*

1208 First Verbs Sterling Edition
Laureate Learning Systems
110 East Spring Street
Winooski, VT 05404-1898   802-655-4755
                            800-562-6801
                            Fax: 802-655-4757
                            www.laureatelearning.com
laureate-webmaster@laureatelearning.com
Dr. Mary Sweig Wilson Ph.D., President/CEO, Founder
Bernard J. Fox, Co-Founder, Vice President
Marion Blank, Ph.D, Developmental Psychologist
A computer program that trains and tests 40 early develop-
ing verbs using animated pictures and a natural sounding fe-
male voice. *$225.00*

1209 First Words II Sterling Edition
Laureate Learning Systems
110 East Spring Street
Winooski, VT 05404-1898   802-655-4755
                            800-562-6801
                            Fax: 802-655-4757
                            www.laureatelearning.com
laureate-webmaster@laureatelearning.com
Dr. Mary Sweig Wilson Ph.D., President/CEO, Founder
Bernard J. Fox, Co-Founder, Vice President
Marion Blank, Ph.D, Developmental Psychologist
Continues the training of First Words with training and test-
ing of an additional 50 early developing nouns presented
within the same 10 categories as used in First Words.
$235.00

1210 First Words Sterling Edition
Laureate Learning Systems
110 East Spring Street
Winooski, VT 05404-1898   802-655-4755
                            800-562-6801
                            Fax: 802-655-4757
                            www.laureatelearning.com
laureate-webmaster@laureatelearning.com
Dr. Mary Sweig Wilson Ph.D., President/CEO, Founder
Bernard J. Fox, Co-Founder, Vice President
Marion Blank, Ph.D, Developmental Psychologist
A talking program that trains and tests 50 early developing
nouns presented within 10 categories. *$235.00*

1211 Fish Scales
SRA Order Services
PO Box 182605
Columbus, OH 43218   800-334-7344
                            Fax: 800-953-8691
                            www.mheducation.com
SEG_CustomerService@mheducation.com
David Levin, President/CEO
David Stafford, SVP and General Counsel
Maryellen Valaitis, SVP, Human Resources
The McGraw-Hill Education Urban Advisory Resource
works with large urban districts across the country to help
them provide better quality instruction, curriculum, and as-
sessment to their students. *$35.00*

1212 Following Directions: Left and Right
Laureate Learning Systems
110 East Spring Street
Winooski, VT 05404-1898

802-655-4755
800-562-6801
Fax: 802-655-4757
www.laureatelearning.com
laureate-webmaster@laureatelearning.com
Dr. Mary Sweig Wilson Ph.D., President/CEO, Founder
Bernard J. Fox, Co-Founder, Vice President
Marion Blank, Ph.D, Developmental Psychologist
This computer program uses ten activities to improve your ability to follow directions and develop left/right discrimination skills. *$125.00*

1213 Following Directions: One and Two-Level Commands
Laureate Learning Systems
110 East Spring Street
Winooski, VT 05404-1898

802-655-4755
800-562-6801
Fax: 802-655-4757
www.laureatelearning.com
laureate-webmaster@laureatelearning.com
Dr. Mary Sweig Wilson Ph.D., President/CEO, Founder
Bernard J. Fox, Co-Founder, Vice President
Marion Blank, Ph.D, Developmental Psychologist
Designed for a broad range of students experiencing difficulty in processing, remembering and following oral commands, a program of exercises on short and long-term memory highlighting specific spatial, directional and ordinary terms. *$175.00*

1214 Functional Skills System and MECA
Conover Company
4 Brookwood Court
Appleton, WI 54914

800-933-1933
Fax: 800-933-1943
www.conovercompany.com
sales@conovercompany.com
Functional Skills System software assists in the transition from school to the community and workplace. Functional literary, functional life skills, functional social skills, functional work skills. MECA - The system for creating post-secondary transition outcomes and the instructional services to support them. *$2535.00*

1215 Information Station
SVE & Churchill Media
700 Indian Springs Drive
Lancaster, PA 17601

888-892-3484
Fax: 877-324-6830
http://store.discoveryeducation.com
education_info@discovery.com
Students who boot up this software will find themselves floating miles above the earth orbiting the planet in an information station satellite. *$144.00*

1216 Lion's Workshop
Merit Software
121 West 27th Street
Suite 1200
New York, NY 10001

212-675-8567
800-753-6488
Fax: 800-918-9336
www.meritsoftware.com
sales@meritsoftware.com
Ben Weintraub, CEO
Presents various objects with parts missing or with like objects to be matched. *$9.95*

1217 Marsh Media
Marshware
PO Box 8082
Shawnee Mission, KS 66208-0082

800-821-3303
Fax: 866-333-7421
www.marshmedia.com
info@marshmedia.com
Joan K Marsh, President

Marsh Media publishes closed captioned health and guidance videos for the classroom and school library. Catalog available.

1218 Math Spending and Saving
World Class Learning
PO Box 639
Candler, NC 28715

800-638-6470
Fax: 800-638-6499
www.wclm.com
jdash@wclm.com
Designed for secondary students and adults, this program focuses on personal financial management, comparison shopping and calculation of essential banking transactions.

1219 Money Skills
MarbleSoft
12301 Central Ave NE Ste 205
P.O. Box 490215
Blaine, MN 55449

763-502-0440
888-755-1402
Fax: 763-862-2920
www.marblesoft.com
support@marblesoft.com
Joyce Meyer, President
Mark Larson, CEO, Product Development
Vicki Larson, Sales
Money Skills 2.0 includes five activities that teach counting money and making change: Coins and Bills; Counting Money; Making Change; how much change? and the Marblesoft Store. Teaches American, Canadian and European money using clear, realistic pictures of the money. Single and dual-switch scanning options on all difficulty levels. Runs on Macintosh and Windows computers. *$60.00*

1220 My House: Language Activities of Daily Living
Laureate Learning Systems
110 East Spring Street
Winooski, VT 05404-1898

802-655-4755
800-562-6801
Fax: 802-655-4757
www.laureatelearning.com
laureate-webmaster@laureatelearning.com
Dr. Mary Sweig Wilson Ph.D., President/CEO, Founder
Bernard J. Fox, Co-Founder, Vice President
Marion Blank, Ph.D, Developmental Psychologist
Train over 300 functional vocabulary items, increase understanding of objects and their functions while building independence in the home, community, and school. *$150.00*

1221 Optimum Resource
1 Mathews Drive
Suite 107
Hilton Head Island, SC 29926

843-689-8000
888-784-2592
Fax: 843-689-8008
www.stickybear.com
info@stickybear.com
Richard Hefter, President
An educational software publishing company for grades K-12. Our software titles are available in Consumer, School, Labpack or Site License versions. Please call for further details. Prices range from $59.95 for Consumer to $699.95 for Site Licenses.

1222 PAVE: Perceptual Accuracy/Visual Efficiency
Software to Go-Gallaudet University
800 Florida Ave NE
Washington, DC 20002-3695

202-651-5031
Fax: 202-651-5109
http://clerccenter.gallaudet.edu
clerc.center@gallaudet.edu
Ed Bosso, Vice President
Ken Kurlychek, EI Specialist

1223 Print Shop Deluxe
Riverdeep
222 Berkeley Street
Boston, MA 02116
617-351-5000
855-969-4642
Fax: 877-892-9820
www.hmhco.com
IIEcustomerservice@hmhpub.com
Linda K. Zecher, President, CEO, Director
James G. Nicholson, President, Riverside Publishing
John K. Dragoon, EVP, Chief Marketing Officer
Houghton Mifflin Harcourt offers a wide array of technology-driven pre-k-12 solutions that inspire excellence and innovation in education, and raise student achievement.

1224 Quiz Castle
Software to Go-Gallaudet University
800 Florida Ave NE
Washington, DC 20002-3695
202-651-5031
Fax: 202-651-5109
http://clerccenter.gallaudet.edu
clerc.center@gallaudet.edu
Ed Bosso, Vice President
Ken Kurlychek, EI Specialist

1225 Secondary Print Pack
Failure Free
140 Cabarrus Ave W
Concord, NC 28025-5150
704-786-7838
800-542-2170
Fax: 704-785-8940
www.failurefree.com
info@failurefree.com
Joseph Lockavitch, President
Thousands of independent activities teaching over 750 words. *$1929.00*

1226 Stickybear Software
Optimum Resource
1 Mathews Drive
Suite 107
Hilton Head Island, SC 29926
843-689-8000
888-784-2592
Fax: 843-689-8008
www.stickybear.com
info@stickybear.com
Richard Hefter, President
An educational software publishing company for grades K-12. Our software titles are available in Consumer, School, Labpack or Site License versions. Please call for further details. Prices range from $59.95 for Consumer to $699.95 for Site Licenses.

1227 Teenage Switch Progressions
RJ Cooper & Associates
22600-A Lambert St.
Suite 708
Lake Forest, CA 92630
949-582-2571
800-752-6673
Fax: 949-582-3169
www.rjcooper.com
info@rjcooper.com
R J Cooper, Owner
Five activities for teenage persons working on switch training, attention training, life skills simulation and following directions. *$75.00*

1228 TeleSensory
417 Cypress Street
Bakersfield, CA 93304
650-743-9515
800-804-8004
Fax: 661-327-2478
www.telesensory.com
info@telesensory.com
Helps visually impaired people become more independent with the most comprehensive products available anywhere for reading, writing, taking notes and using computers.

Math

1229 2+2
RJ Cooper & Associates
22600-A Lambert St.
Suite 708
Lake Forest, CA 92630
949-582-2571
800-752-6673
Fax: 949-582-3169
www.rjcooper.com
info@rjcooper.com
R J Cooper, Owner
This large print, talking, early academic program is for drilling math facts, including addition, subtraction, multiplication and division. It uses an errorless learning method. Available for Mac, Windows. *$89.00*

1230 Access to Math
Don Johnston
26799 West Commerce Drive
Volo, IL 60073
847-740-0749
800-999-4660
Fax: 847-740-7326
www.donjohnston.com
info@donjohnston.com
Don Johnston, Founder
Ruth Ziolkowski, President
The Macintosh talking math worksheet program that's two products in one. For teachers, it makes customized worksheets in a snap. For students who struggle, it provides individualized on-screen lessons.

1231 Algebra Stars
Sunburst Technology
3150 W Higgins Rd
Suite 140
Hoffman Estates, IL 60619
800-321-7511
www.sunburst.com
service@sunburst.com
Students build their understanding of algebra by constructing, categorizing, and solving equations and classifying polynomial expressions using algebra tiles.

1232 Alien Addition: Academic Skill Builders in Math
SRA Order Services
PO Box 182605
Columbus, OH 43218
800-334-7344
Fax: 800-953-8691
www.mheducation.com
SEG_CustomerService@mheducation.com
David Levin, President/CEO
David Stafford, SVP and General Counsel
Maryellen Valaitis, SVP, Human Resources
The McGraw-Hill Education Urban Advisory Resource works with large urban districts across the country to help them provide better quality instruction, curriculum, and assessment to their students. *$49.00*

1233 Awesome Animated Monster Maker Math
Sunburst Technology
3150 W Higgins Rd
Suite 140
Hoffman Estates, IL 60619
800-321-7511
www.sunburst.com
service@sunburst.com
With an emphasis on building core math skills, this humorous program incorporates the monstrous and the ridiculous into a structured learning environment. Students choose from six skill levels tailored to the 3rd to 8th grade.

1234 Awesome Animated Monster Maker Math and Monster Workshop
Sunburst Technology
3150 W Higgins Rd
Suite 140
Hoffman Estates, IL 60619
800-321-7511
www.sunburst.com
service@sunburst.com

Students develop money and strategic thinking skills with this irresistable game that has them tinker about making monsters.

1235 Awesome Animated Monster Maker Number Drop
Sunburst Technology
3150 W Higgins Rd
Suite 140
Hoffman Estates, IL 60619   800-321-7511
www.sunburst.com
service@sunburst.com
Your students will think on their mathematical feet estimating and solving thousands of number problems in an arcade-style game designed to improve their performance in numeration, money, fractions, and decimals.

1236 Basic Math Competency Skill Building
Educational Activities Software
PO Box 220790
Saint Louis, MO 63122   866-243-8464
Fax: 239-225-9299
www.ea-software.com
jwest@siboneylg.com
Jan West, Sales Director
Michael Conlon, Author
An interactive, tutorial and practice program to teach competency with arithmetic operations, decimals, fractions, graphs, measurement and geometric concepts. (stand alone version) MA02 *$369.00*

1237 Basic Skills Products
EDCON Publishing Group
30 Montauk Blvd
Oakdale, NY 11769   631-567-7227
888-553-3266
Fax: 631-567-8745
www.edconpublishing.com
Deals with basic math and language arts. Free catalog available.

1238 Building Perspective
Sunburst Technology
3150 W Higgins Rd
Suite 140
Hoffman Estates, IL 60619   800-321-7511
www.sunburst.com
service@sunburst.com
Develop spatial perception and reasoning skills with this award-winning program that will sharpen your students' problem-solving abilities.

1239 Building Perspective Deluxe
Sunburst Technology
3150 W Higgins Rd
Suite 140
Hoffman Estates, IL 60619   800-321-7511
www.sunburst.com
service@sunburst.com
New visual thinking challenges await your students as they engage in three spacial reasoning activities that develop their 3D thinking, deductive reasoning and problem solving skills

1240 Combining Shapes
Sunburst Technology
3150 W Higgins Rd
Suite 140
Hoffman Estates, IL 60619   800-321-7511
www.sunburst.com
service@sunburst.com
Students discover the properties of simple geometric figures through concrete experience combining shapes. Measurements, estimating and operation skills are part of this fun program.

1241 Conceptual Skills
Psychological Software Services
3304 W 75th St
Indianapolis, IN 46268-1664   317-257-9672
Fax: 317-257-9674
www.neuroscience.cnter.com
nsc@neuroscience.cnter.com
Odie L Bracy, PhD, HSPP, Clinical Neuropsychologist
Nancy Bracy, Office Manager
Andrea Oakes, Clinical Assistant
Twelve programs designed to enhance skills involved in relationships, comparisons and number concepts. *$50.00*

1242 Concert Tour Entrepreneur
Sunburst Technology
3150 W Higgins Rd
Suite 140
Hoffman Estates, IL 60619   800-321-7511
www.sunburst.com
service@sunburst.com
Your students improve math, planning and problem solving skills as they manage a band in this music management business simulation.

1243 Counters
Software to Go-Gallaudet University
800 Florida Ave NE
Washington, DC 20002-3695   202-651-5031
Fax: 202-651-5109
http://clerccenter.gallaudet.edu
clerc.center@gallaudet.edu
Ed Bosso, Vice President
Ken Kurlychek, EI Specialist

1244 Counting Critters
Software to Go-Gallaudet University
800 Florida Ave NE
Washington, DC 20002-3695   202-651-5031
Fax: 202-651-5109
http://clerccenter.gallaudet.edu
clerc.center@gallaudet.edu
Ed Bosso, Vice President
Ken Kurlychek, EI Specialist

1245 DLM Math Fluency Program: Addition Facts
SRA Order Services
PO Box 182605
Columbus, OH 43218   800-334-7344
Fax: 800-953-8691
www.mheducation.com
SEG_CustomerService@mheducation.com
David Levin, President/CEO
David Stafford, SVP and General Counsel
Maryellen Valaitis, SVP, Human Resources
The McGraw-Hill Education Urban Advisory Resource works with large urban districts across the country to help them provide better quality instruction, curriculum, and assessment to their students. *$32.00*

1246 DLM Math Fluency Program: Division Facts
SRA Order Services
PO Box 182605
Columbus, OH 43218   800-334-7344
Fax: 800-953-8691
www.mheducation.com
SEG_CustomerService@mheducation.com
David Levin, President/CEO
David Stafford, SVP and General Counsel
Maryellen Valaitis, SVP, Human Resources
The McGraw-Hill Education Urban Advisory Resource works with large urban districts across the country to help them provide better quality instruction, curriculum, and assessment to their students.

1247 DLM Math Fluency Program: Multiplication Facts
SRA Order Services
PO Box 182605
Columbus, OH 43218   800-334-7344
Fax: 800-953-8691
www.mheducation.com
SEG_CustomerService@mheducation.com
David Levin, President/CEO
David Stafford, SVP and General Counsel
Maryellen Valaitis, SVP, Human Resources
The McGraw-Hill Education Urban Advisory Resource
works with large urban districts across the country to help
them provide better quality instruction, curriculum, and as-
sessment to their students. *$32.00*

1248 DLM Math Fluency Program: Subtraction Facts
SRA Order Services
PO Box 182605
Columbus, OH 43218   800-334-7344
Fax: 800-953-8691
www.mheducation.com
SEG_CustomerService@mheducation.com
David Levin, President/CEO
David Stafford, SVP and General Counsel
Maryellen Valaitis, SVP, Human Resources
The McGraw-Hill Education Urban Advisory Resource
works with large urban districts across the country to help
them provide better quality instruction, curriculum, and as-
sessment to their students. *$32.00*

1249 Data Explorer
Sunburst Technology
3150 W Higgins Rd
Suite 140
Hoffman Estates, IL 60619   800-321-7511
www.sunburst.com
service@sunburst.com
This easy-to-use CD-ROM provides the flexibility needed
for eleven different graph types including tools for
long-term data analysis projects.

1250 Dragon Mix: Academic Skill Builders in Math
SRA Order Services
PO Box 182605
Columbus, OH 43218   800-334-7344
Fax: 800-953-8691
www.mheducation.com
SEG_CustomerService@mheducation.com
David Levin, President/CEO
David Stafford, SVP and General Counsel
Maryellen Valaitis, SVP, Human Resources
The McGraw-Hill Education Urban Advisory Resource
works with large urban districts across the country to help
them provide better quality instruction, curriculum, and as-
sessment to their students. *$49.00*

1251 Elementary Math Bundle
Sunburst Technology
3150 W Higgins Rd
Suite 140
Hoffman Estates, IL 60619   800-321-7511
www.sunburst.com
service@sunburst.com
Number sense and operations are the focus of the Elementary Math Bundle. Students engage in activities that reinforce basic addition and subtraction skills. This product
comes with Splish Splash Math, Ten Tricky Tiles and
Numbers Undercover.

1252 Equation Tile Teasers
Sunburst Technology
3150 W Higgins Rd
Suite 140
Hoffman Estates, IL 60619   800-321-7511
www.sunburst.com
service@sunburst.com
Students develop logic thinking and pre-algebra skills solving sets of numbers equations in three challenging problem-solving activities.

1253 Equations
Software to Go-Gallaudet University
800 Florida Ave NE
Washington, DC 20002-3695   202-651-5031
Fax: 202-651-5109
http://clerccenter.gallaudet.edu
clerc.center@gallaudet.edu
Ed Bosso, Vice President
Ken Kurlychek, EI Specialist

1254 Factory Deluxe
Sunburst Technology
3150 W Higgins Rd
Suite 140
Hoffman Estates, IL 60619   800-321-7511
www.sunburst.com
service@sunburst.com
Five activities explore shapes, rotation, angles, geometric
attributes, area formulas, and computation. Includes journal, record keeping, and on-screen help. This program helps
sharpen geometry, visual thinking and problem solving
skills.

1255 Fast-Track Fractions
SRA Order Services
PO Box 182605
Columbus, OH 43218   800-334-7344
Fax: 800-953-8691
www.mheducation.com
SEG_CustomerService@mheducation.com
David Levin, President/CEO
David Stafford, SVP and General Counsel
Maryellen Valaitis, SVP, Human Resources
The McGraw-Hill Education Urban Advisory Resource
works with large urban districts across the country to help
them provide better quality instruction, curriculum, and as-
sessment to their students. *$46.00*

1256 Fraction Attraction
Sunburst Technology
3150 W Higgins Rd
Suite 140
Hoffman Estates, IL 60619   800-321-7511
www.sunburst.com
service@sunburst.com
Build the fraction skills of ordering, equivalence, relative
sizes and multiple representations with four, multi-level,
carnival style games.

1257 Fraction Fuel-Up
SRA Order Services
PO Box 182605
Columbus, OH 43218   800-334-7344
Fax: 800-953-8691
www.mheducation.com
SEG_CustomerService@mheducation.com
David Levin, President/CEO
David Stafford, SVP/General Counsel
Maryellen Valaitis, SVP Human Resources
The McGraw-Hill Education Urban Advisory Resource
works with large urban districts across the country to help
them provide better quality instruction, curriculum, and as-
sessment to their students. *$46.00*

1258 Get Up and Go!
Sunburst Technology
3150 W Higgins Rd
Suite 140
Hoffman Estates, IL 60619   800-321-7511
www.sunburst.com
service@sunburst.com
Students interpret and construct timelines through three descriptive activities in the animated program. Students are introduced to timelines as they participate in an interactive
story.

1259 Learning About Numbers
C&C Software
5713 Kentford Cir
Wichita, KS 67220-3131   316-683-6056
                                800-752-2086
Carol Clark, President
Three segments use computer graphics to provide students
with an experience in working with numbers. *$25.00*

1260 Math Machine
Software to Go-Gallaudet University
800 Florida Ave NE
Washington, DC 20002-3695   202-651-5031
                           Fax: 202-651-5109
                  http://clerccenter.gallaudet.edu
                       clerc.center@gallaudet.edu
Ed Bosso, Vice President
Ken Kurlychek, EI Specialist

1261 Math Masters: Addition and Subtraction
SRA Order Services
PO Box 182605
Columbus, OH 43218   800-334-7344
                           Fax: 800-953-8691
                       www.mheducation.com
              SEG_CustomerService@mheducation.com
David Levin, President/CEO
David Stafford, SVP/General Counsel
Maryellen Valaitis, SVP Human Resources
The McGraw-Hill Education Urban Advisory Resource
works with large urban districts across the country to help
them provide better quality instruction, curriculum, and as-
sessment to their students.

1262 Math Masters: Multiplication and Division
SRA Order Services
PO Box 182605
Columbus, OH 43218   800-334-7344
                           Fax: 800-953-8691
                       www.mheducation.com
              SEG_CustomerService@mheducation.com
David Levin, President/CEO
David Stafford, SVP/General Counsel
Maryellen Valaitis, SVP Human Resources
The McGraw-Hill Education Urban Advisory Resource
works with large urban districts across the country to help
them provide better quality instruction, curriculum, and as-
sessment to their students.

1263 Math Shop
Software to Go-Gallaudet University
800 Florida Ave NE
Washington, DC 20002-3695   202-651-5031
                           Fax: 202-651-5109
                  http://clerccenter.gallaudet.edu
                       clerc.center@gallaudet.edu
Ed Bosso, Vice President
Ken Kurlychek, EI Specialist

1264 Math Skill Games
Software to Go-Gallaudet University
800 Florida Ave NE
Washington, DC 20002-3695   202-651-5031
                           Fax: 202-651-5109
                  http://clerccenter.gallaudet.edu
                       clerc.center@gallaudet.edu
Ed Bosso, Vice President
Ken Kurlychek, EI Specialist

1265 Math for Everyday Living
Educational Activities Software
PO Box 87
Baldwin, NY 11510   800-797-3223
                           Fax: 516-623-9282
                                www.edact.com
                               learn@edact.com
Rose Falco, Educational Activities

Designed for secondary students, a tutorial and practice program with simulated activities for applying math skills in
making change, working with sales slips, unit pricing, computing gas mileage and sales tax. *$89.00*

1266 Mighty Math Astro Algebra
Riverdeep
222 Berkeley Street
Boston, MA 02116   617-351-5000
                                855-969-4642
                           Fax: 877-892-9820
                                www.hmhco.com
                   IIEcustomerservice@hmhpub.com
Linda K. Zecher, President, CEO, Director
James G. Nicholson, President, Riverside Publishing
John K. Dragoon, EVP, Chief Marketing Officer
Houghton Mifflin Harcourt offers a wide array of technol-
ogy-driven pre-k-12 solutions that inspire excellence and in-
novation in education, and raise student achievement.
$59.95

1267 Mighty Math Calculating Crew
Riverdeep
222 Berkeley Street
Boston, MA 02116   617-351-5000
                                855-969-4642
                           Fax: 877-892-9820
                                www.hmhco.com
                   IIEcustomerservice@hmhpub.com
Linda K. Zecher, President, CEO, Director
James G. Nicholson, President, Riverside Publishing
John K. Dragoon, EVP, Chief Marketing Officer
Houghton Mifflin Harcourt offers a wide array of technol-
ogy-driven pre-k-12 solutions that inspire excellence and in-
novation in education, and raise student achievement.
$59.95

1268 Mighty Math Carnival Countdown
Riverdeep
222 Berkeley Street
Boston, MA 02116   617-351-5000
                                855-969-4642
                           Fax: 877-892-9820
                                www.hmhco.com
                   IIEcustomerservice@hmhpub.com
Linda K. Zecher, President, CEO, Director
James G. Nicholson, President, Riverside Publishing
John K. Dragoon, EVP, Chief Marketing Officer
Houghton Mifflin Harcourt offers a wide array of technol-
ogy-driven pre-k-12 solutions that inspire excellence and in-
novation in education, and raise student achievement.
$59.95

1269 Mighty Math Cosmic Geometry
Riverdeep
222 Berkeley Street
Boston, MA 02116   617-351-5000
                                855-969-4642
                           Fax: 877-892-9820
                                www.hmhco.com
                   IIEcustomerservice@hmhpub.com
Linda K. Zecher, President, CEO, Director
James G. Nicholson, President, Riverside Publishing
John K. Dragoon, EVP, Chief Marketing Officer
Houghton Mifflin Harcourt offers a wide array of technol-
ogy-driven pre-k-12 solutions that inspire excellence and in-
novation in education, and raise student achievement.
$59.95

1270 Mighty Math Number Heroes
Riverdeep
222 Berkeley Street
Boston, MA 02116   617-351-5000
                                855-969-4642
                           Fax: 877-892-9820
                                www.hmhco.com
                   IIEcustomerservice@hmhpub.com
Linda K. Zecher, President, CEO, Director
James G. Nicholson, President, Riverside Publishing
John K. Dragoon, EVP, Chief Marketing Officer

Houghton Mifflin Harcourt offers a wide array of technology-driven pre-k-12 solutions that inspire excellence and innovation in education, and raise student achievement. *$59.95*

1271 Mighty Math Zoo Zillions
Riverdeep
222 Berkeley Street
Boston, MA 02116

617-351-5000
855-969-4642
Fax: 877-892-9820
www.hmhco.com
IIEcustomerservice@hmhpub.com
Linda K. Zecher, President, CEO, Director
James G. Nicholson, President, Riverside Publishing
John K. Dragoon, EVP, Chief Marketing Officer
Houghton Mifflin Harcourt offers a wide array of technology-driven pre-k-12 solutions that inspire excellence and innovation in education, and raise student achievement. *$59.95*

1272 Millie's Math House
Riverdeep
222 Berkeley Street
Boston, MA 02116

617-351-5000
855-969-4642
Fax: 877-892-9820
www.hmhco.com
IIEcustomerservice@hmhpub.com
Linda K. Zecher, President, CEO, Director
James G. Nicholson, President, Riverside Publishing
John K. Dragoon, EVP, Chief Marketing Officer
Houghton Mifflin Harcourt offers a wide array of technology-driven pre-k-12 solutions that inspire excellence and innovation in education, and raise student achievement. *$59.95*

1273 Number Farm
Software to Go-Gallaudet University
800 Florida Ave NE
Washington, DC 20002-3695

202-651-5031
Fax: 202-651-5109
http://clerccenter.gallaudet.edu
clerc.center@gallaudet.edu
Ed Bosso, Vice President
Ken Kurlychek, EI Specialist

1274 Number Please
Merit Software
121 West 27th Street
Suite 1200
New York, NY 10001

212-675-8567
800-753-6488
Fax: 800-918-9336
www.meritsoftware.com
sales@meritsoftware.com
Ben Weintraub, CEO
Students are challenged to remember combinations of 4, 7 and 10 digit numbers. *$9.95*

1275 Number Sense and Problem Solving
Sunburst Technology
3150 W Higgins Rd
Suite 140
Hoffman Estates, IL 60619

800-321-7511
www.sunburst.com
service@sunburst.com
Build number and operation skills with these three programs: How the West Was One + Three x Four, Divide and Conquer and Puzzle Tank.

1276 Number Stumper
Software to Go-Gallaudet University
800 Florida Ave NE
Washington, DC 20002-3695

202-651-5031
Fax: 202-651-5109
http://clerccenter.gallaudet.edu
clerc.center@gallaudet.edu
Ed Bosso, Vice President
Ken Kurlychek, EI Specialist

1277 Race Car 'rithmetic
Software to Go-Gallaudet University
800 Florida Ave NE
Washington, DC 20002-3695

202-651-5031
Fax: 202-651-5109
http://clerccenter.gallaudet.edu
clerc.center@gallaudet.edu
Ed Bosso, Vice President
Ken Kurlychek, EI Specialist

1278 Read and Solve Math Problems #1
Educational Activities
PO Box 87
Baldwin, NY 11510

800-797-3223
Fax: 516-623-9282
www.edact.com
learn@edact.com
Rose Falco, Educational Activities
A tutorial and practice program for students which focuses on recognition of key words in solving arithmetic word problems, writing equations and solving word problems. *$109.00*

1279 Read and Solve Math Problems #2
Educational Activities
PO Box 87
Baldwin, NY 11510

800-797-3223
Fax: 516-623-9282
www.edact.com
learn@edact.com
Rose Falco, Educational Activities
A tutorial and practice program for students which focuses on recognition of key words in solving two-step arithmetic problems, writing equations and solving two-step word problems. *$109.00*

1280 Read and Solve Math Problems #3
Educational Activities
PO Box 87
Baldwin, NY 11510

800-797-3223
Fax: 516-623-9282
www.edact.com
learn@edact.com
Rose Falco, Educational Activities
Designed for students, this tutorial and practice program provides initial instruction and experience in critical thinking and problem-solving using fractions and mixed numbers. *$109.00*

1281 Shape Up!
Sunburst Technology
3150 W Higgins Rd
Suite 140
Hoffman Estates, IL 60619

800-321-7511
www.sunburst.com
service@sunburst.com
Students actively create and manipulate shapes to discover important ideas about mathematics in an electronic playground of two and three dimensional shapes.

1282 Spatial Relationships
Sunburst Technology
3150 W Higgins Rd
Suite 140
Hoffman Estates, IL 60619

800-321-7511
www.sunburst.com
service@sunburst.com
Your students will strenghten their spatial perception, spatial reasoning and problem-solving skills with three great programs now on one CD-ROM.

1283 Splish Splash Math
Sunburst Technology
3150 W Higgins Rd
Suite 140
Hoffman Estates, IL 60619

800-321-7511
www.sunburst.com
service@sunburst.com

Students learn and practice basic operation skills as they engage in this high interest program that keeps them motivated. Great visual rewards and three levels of difficulty keep students challanged.

1284   Tenth Planet: Combining & Breaking Apart Numbers
Sunburst Technology
3150 W Higgins Rd
Suite 140
Hoffman Estates, IL 60619   800-321-7511
www.sunburst.com
service@sunburst.com
Students explore part-whole relationships and develop number sense by combining and breaking apart numbers in a variety of problem-solving situations.

1285   Tenth Planet: Comparing with Ratios
Sunburst Technology
3150 W Higgins Rd
Suite 140
Hoffman Estates, IL 60619   800-321-7511
www.sunburst.com
service@sunburst.com
Students learn that ratio is a way to compare amounts by using multiplication and division. Through five engaging activities, students recognize and describe ratios, develop proportional thinking skills, estimate ratios, determine equivalent ratios, and use ratios to analyze data.

1286   Tenth Planet: Equivalent Fractions
Sunburst Technology
3150 W Higgins Rd
Suite 140
Hoffman Estates, IL 60619   800-321-7511
www.sunburst.com
service@sunburst.com
This exciting investigation develops students' conceptual understanding that every fraction can be named in many different but equivalent ways.

1287   Tenth Planet: Fraction Operations
Sunburst Technology
3150 W Higgins Rd
Suite 140
Hoffman Estates, IL 60619   800-321-7511
www.sunburst.com
service@sunburst.com
Students build on their concepts of fraction meaning and equivalence as they learn how to perform operations with fractions.

1288   World Class Learning Materials
World Class Learning
PO Box 639
Candler, NC 28715   800-638-6470
Fax: 800-638-6499
www.wclm.com
jdash@wclm.com
Designed for secondary students and adults, this program focuses on personal financial management, comparison shopping and calculation of essential banking transactions.

1289   Zap! Around Town
Sunburst Technology
3150 W Higgins Rd
Suite 140
Hoffman Estates, IL 60619   800-321-7511
www.sunburst.com
service@sunburst.com
Students develop mapping and direction skills in this easy-to-use, animated program featuring Shelby, your friendly Sunbuddy guide.

Preschool

1290   Creature Series
Laureate Learning Systems
110 East Spring Street
Winooski, VT 05404-1898   802-655-4755
800-562-6801
Fax: 802-655-4757
www.laureatelearning.com
laureate-webmaster@laureatelearning.com
Dr. Mary Sweig Wilson Ph.D., President/CEO, Founder
Bernard J. Fox, Co-Founder, Vice President
Marion Blank, Ph.D, Developmental Psychologist
Six different computer programs designed to improve visual and auditory attention and teach cause and effect, turn taking, and switch use. *$95.00*

1291   Curious George Visits the Library
Software to Go-Gallaudet University
800 Florida Ave NE
Washington, DC 20002-3695   202-651-5031
Fax: 202-651-5109
http://clerccenter.gallaudet.edu
clerc.center@gallaudet.edu
Ed Bosso, Vice President
Ken Kurlychek, EI Specialist

1292   Early Discoveries: Size and Logic
Software to Go-Gallaudet University
800 Florida Ave NE
Washington, DC 20002-3695   202-651-5031
Fax: 202-651-5109
http://clerccenter.gallaudet.edu
clerc.center@gallaudet.edu
Ed Bosso, Vice President
Ken Kurlychek, EI Specialist

1293   Early Emerging Rules Series
Laureate Learning Systems
110 East Spring Street
Winooski, VT 05404-1898   802-655-4755
800-562-6801
Fax: 802-655-4757
www.laureatelearning.com
laureate-webmaster@laureatelearning.com
Dr. Mary Sweig Wilson Ph.D., President/CEO, Founder
Bernard J. Fox, Co-Founder, Vice President
Marion Blank, Ph.D, Developmental Psychologist
Three programs that introduce early developing grammatical constructions and facilitate the transition from single words to word combinations. *$175.00*

1294   Early Learning I
MarbleSoft
12301 Central Ave NE Ste 205
P.O. Box 490215
Blaine, MN 55449   763-502-0440
888-755-1402
Fax: 763-862-2920
www.marblesoft.com
support@marblesoft.com
Joyce Meyer, President
Mark Larson, CEO, Product Development
Vicki Larson, Sales
Early Learning 2.0 includes four activities that teach prereading skills. Single and dual-switch scanning are built in and special prompts allow blind students to use all levels of difficulty. Includes Matching Colors, Learning Shapes, Counting Numbers and Letter Match. Runs on Macintosh and Windows computers. *$70.00*

1295 Early and Advanced Switch Games
RJ Cooper & Associates
22600-A Lambert St.
Suite 708
Lake Forest, CA 92630
949-582-2571
800-752-6673
Fax: 949-582-3169
www.rjcooper.com
info@rjcooper.com

R J Cooper, Owner
Thirteen single switch games that start at cause/effect, work through timing and selection and graduate with matching and manipulation tasks. *$75.00*

1296 Edustar's Early Childhood Special Education Programs
Edustar America
Ste 186
6220 S Orange Blossom Trl
Orlando, FL 32809-4627
561-638-8733
800-952-3041
Fax: 561-330-0849
www.orlandomedicalinstitute.com
info@omi.edu

David Zeldin, Marketing Manager
Stewart Holtz, Curriculum Director
Integrated software program that incorporates manipulatives and special tables for learning early childhood subjects. Features include an illuminated six key keyboard. A special U-shaped touch table for the physically challenged and changeable mats and keys for different subject areas.

1297 Joystick Games
Technology for Language and Learning
PO Box 327
East Rockaway, NY 11518
516-625-4550
Fax: 516-621-3321

Joan Tanenhaus, Founder
Five volumes of public domain joystick programs. *$28.50*

1298 Kindercomp Gold
Software to Go-Gallaudet University
800 Florida Ave NE
Washington, DC 20002-3695
202-651-5031
Fax: 202-651-5109
http://clerccenter.gallaudet.edu
clerc.center@gallaudet.edu

Ed Bosso, Vice President
Ken Kurlychek, EI Specialist

1299 Old MacDonald's Farm Deluxe
KidTECH
12301 Central Ave NE Ste 205
P.O. Box 490215
Blaine, MN 55449
763-502-0440
888-755-1402
Fax: 763-862-2920
www.marblesoft.com
support@marblesoft.com

Joyce Meyer, President
Mark Larson, CEO, Product Development
Vicki Larson, Sales
Utilizes the all-time favorite children's song to teach vocabulary and animal sounds to young children. *$30.00*

1300 Shape and Color Rodeo
SRA Order Services
PO Box 182605
Columbus, OH 43218
800-334-7344
Fax: 800-953-8691
www.mheducation.com
SEG_CustomerService@mheducation.com

David Levin, President/CEO
David Stafford, SVP/General Counsel
Maryellen Valaitis, SVP Human Resources
The McGraw-Hill Education Urban Advisory Resource works with large urban districts across the country to help them provide better quality instruction, curriculum, and assessment to their students. *$35.00*

1301 Trudy's Time and Place House
Riverdeep
222 Berkeley Street
Boston, MA 02116
617-351-5000
855-969-4642
Fax: 877-892-9820
www.hmhco.com
IIEcustomerservice@hmhpub.com

Linda K. Zecher, President, CEO, Director
James G. Nicholson, President, Riverside Publishing
John K. Dragoon, EVP, Chief Marketing Officer
Houghton Mifflin Harcourt offers a wide array of technology-driven pre-k-12 solutions that inspire excellence and innovation in education, and raise student achievement. *$59.95*

1302 Word Pieces
Software to Go-Gallaudet University
800 Florida Ave NE
Washington, DC 20002-3695
202-651-5031
Fax: 202-651-5109
http://clerccenter.gallaudet.edu
clerc.center@gallaudet.edu

Ed Bosso, Vice President
Ken Kurlychek, EI Specialist

Problem Solving

1303 Captain's Log
BrainTrain
727 Twinridge Lane
North Chesterfield, VA 23235
804-320-0105
800-822-0538
Fax: 804-320-2491
www.braintrain.com
info@braintrain.com

Joseph A Sandford, Ph.D., Founder
Virginia Sandford, VP, Sales & Marketing
A comprehensive, multilevel computerized mental gym to help people with brain injuries, learning disabilities, developmental disabilities, ADD, ADHD and psychiatric disorders improve their cognitive skills. *$2695.00*
ISBN 3-490019-95-0

1304 Changes Around Us CD-ROM
222 Berkeley Street
Boston, MA 02116
617-351-5000
855-969-4642
Fax: 877-892-9820
www.hmhco.com
IIEcustomerservice@hmhpub.com

Linda K. Zecher, President, CEO, Director
James G. Nicholson, President, Riverside Publishing
John K. Dragoon, EVP, Chief Marketing Officer
Nature is the natural choice for observing change. By observing and researching dramatic visual sequences such as the stages of development of a butterfly, children develop a broad understanding of the concept of change. As they search this multimedia database for images and information about plant and animal life cycles and seasonal change, students strengthen their abilities in research, analysis, problem-solving, critical thinking and communication.

1305 Factory Deluxe: Grades 4 to 8
Sunburst Technology
3150 W Higgins Rd
Suite 140
Hoffman Estates, IL 60619
800-321-7511
www.sunburst.com
service@sunburst.com

Five activities explore shapes, rotation, angles, geometric attributes, area formulas, and computation. Includes journal, record keeping, and on-screen help. This program helps sharpen geometry, visual thinking and problem solving skills.

1306   Freddy's Puzzling Adventures
SRA Order Services
PO Box 182605
Columbus, OH 43218   800-334-7344
                                  Fax: 800-953-8691
                              www.mheducation.com
          SEG_CustomerService@mheducation.com
David Levin, President/CEO
David Stafford, SVP/General Counsel
Maryellen Valaitis, SVP Human Resources
The McGraw-Hill Education Urban Advisory Resource
works with large urban districts across the country to help
them provide better quality instruction, curriculum, and as-
sessment to their students. *$34.00*

1307   Guessing and Thinking
Software to Go-Gallaudet University
800 Florida Ave NE
Washington, DC 20002-3695   202-651-5031
                                  Fax: 202-651-5109
                    http://clerccenter.gallaudet.edu
                         clerc.center@gallaudet.edu
Ed Bosso, Vice President
Ken Kurlychek, EI Specialist

1308   High School Math Bundle
Sunburst Technology
3150 W Higgins Rd
Suite 140
Hoffman Estates, IL 60619   800-321-7511
                                  www.sunburst.com
                              service@sunburst.com
Each program in this bundle focuses on a specific area to ensure that your students master the math skills they need. This
bundle allows students to master basics of Algebra, explore
equations and graphs, practice learning with algebra graphs,
use trigonometric functions, apply math concepts to practical situations and improve problem solving and data analysis
skills.

1309   Ice Cream Truck
Sunburst Technology
3150 W Higgins Rd
Suite 140
Hoffman Estates, IL 60619   800-321-7511
                                  www.sunburst.com
                              service@sunburst.com
Elementary students learn important problem solving, stra-
tegic planning and math operation skills, as they become
owners of a busy ice cream truck.

1310   Memory Match
Software to Go-Gallaudet University
800 Florida Ave NE
Washington, DC 20002-3695   202-651-5031
                                  Fax: 202-651-5109
                    http://clerccenter.gallaudet.edu
                         clerc.center@gallaudet.edu
Ed Bosso, Vice President
Ken Kurlychek, EI Specialist

1311   Memory: A First Step in Problem Solving
Software to Go-Gallaudet University
800 Florida Ave NE
Washington, DC 20002-3695   202-651-5031
                                  Fax: 202-651-5109
                    http://clerccenter.gallaudet.edu
                         clerc.center@gallaudet.edu
Ed Bosso, Vice President
Ken Kurlychek, EI Specialist

1312   Merit Software
Merit Software
121 West 27th Street
Suite 1200
New York, NY 10001   212-675-8567
                                       800-753-6488
                                  Fax: 800-918-9336
                              www.meritsoftware.com
                           sales@meritsoftware.com
Ben Weintraub, CEO
Deductive logic and problem solving are the primary skills
developed in the variation of the game MASTERMIND.
$9.95

1313   Middle School Math Bundle
Sunburst Technology
3150 W Higgins Rd
Suite 140
Hoffman Estates, IL 60619   800-321-7511
                                  www.sunburst.com
                              service@sunburst.com
This bundle helps improve student's logical thinking, num-
ber sense and operation skills. This product comes with
Math Arena, Building Perspective Deluxe, Equation Tile
Teasers and Easy Sheet.

1314   Nordic Software
P.O. Box 5403
Lincoln, NE 68505   402-489-1557
                                       800-306-6502
                                  Fax: 402-489-1560
                              www.nordicsoftware.com
                    webmaster@nordicsoftware.com
Develops and publishes entertaining, educational software.
Children ages three and up can build math skills, expand
their vocabulary and increase proficiency in spelling, among
other subjects. *$59.95*

1315   Number Sense & Problem Solving CD-ROM
Sunburst Technology
3150 W Higgins Rd
Suite 140
Hoffman Estates, IL 60619   800-321-7511
                                  www.sunburst.com
                              service@sunburst.com
Build number and operation skills with these three pro-
grams: How the West Was One + Three x Four, Divide and
Conquer and Puzzle Tank.

1316   Problem Solving
Psychological Software Services
3304 W 75th St
Indianapolis, IN 46268-1664   317-257-9672
                                  Fax: 317-257-9674
                         www.neuroscience.cnter.com
                         nsc@neuroscience.cnter.com
Odie L Bracy, PhD, HSPP, Clinical Neuropsychologist
Nancy Bracy, Office Manager
Andrea Oakes, Clinical Assistant
Nine computer programs designed to challenge high func-
tioning patients/students with tasks requiring logic. *$150.00*

1317   Single Switch Games
MarbleSoft
12301 Central Ave NE Ste 205
P.O. Box 490215
Blaine, MN 55449   763-502-0440
                                       888-755-1402
                                  Fax: 763-862-2920
                              www.marblesoft.com
                           support@marblesoft.com
Joyce Meyer, President
Mark Larson, CEO, Product Development
Vicki Larson, Sales

There's a lot of educational software for single switch users, but how about something that's just for fun? We've taken some games similar to the ones you enjoyed as a kid and made them work just right for single switch users. Includes Single Switch Maze, A Frog's Life, Switching Lanes, Switch Invaders, Slingshot Gallery and Scurry. Runs on Macintosh and Windows computers. *$30.00*

1318 Sliding Block
Merit Software
121 West 27th Street
Suite 1200
New York, NY 10001   212-675-8567
                        800-753-6488
                        Fax: 800-918-9336
                        www.meritsoftware.com
                        sales@meritsoftware.com
Ben Weintraub, CEO
Learners rearrange one of the four pictures which can be scrambled at five separate levels to test visual discrimination and problem solving skills. *$9.95*

1319 SmartDriver
BrainTrain
727 Twinridge Lane
North Chesterfield, VA 23235   804-320-0105
                                 800-822-0538
                                 Fax: 804-320-2491
                                 www.braintrain.com
                                 info@braintrain.com
Joseph A Sandford, Ph.D., Founder
Virginia Sandford, VP, Sales & Marketing
Visual attention building software where you 'win' by driving defensively and following the rules of the road. Children love this driving game that teaches visual attention, visual tracking, patience, following the rules, planning, and hand-eye coordination.

1320 SoundSmart
BrainTrain
727 Twinridge Lane
North Chesterfield, VA 23235   804-320-0105
                                 800-822-0538
                                 Fax: 804-320-2491
                                 www.braintrain.com
                                 info@braintrain.com
Joseph A Sandford, Ph.D., Founder
Virginia Sandford, VP, Sales & Marketing
Auditory Attention Building software to help improve phonemic awareness, listening skills, working memory, mental processing speech and self-control. *$549.00*

1321 Strategy Challenges Collection: 1
Riverdeep
222 Berkeley Street
Boston, MA 02116   617-351-5000
                      855-969-4642
                      Fax: 877-892-9820
                      www.hmhco.com
                      IIEcustomerservice@hmhpub.com
Linda K. Zecher, President, CEO, Director
James G. Nicholson, President, Riverside Publishing
John K. Dragoon, EVP, Chief Marketing Officer
Houghton Mifflin Harcourt offers a wide array of technology-driven pre-k-12 solutions that inspire excellence and innovation in education, and raise student achievement. *$39.95*

1322 Strategy Challenges Collection: 2
Riverdeep
222 Berkeley Street
Boston, MA 02116   617-351-5000
                      855-969-4642
                      Fax: 877-892-9820
                      www.hmhco.com
                      IIEcustomerservice@hmhpub.com
Linda K. Zecher, President, CEO, Director
James G. Nicholson, President, Riverside Publishing
John K. Dragoon, EVP, Chief Marketing Officer

1323 Thinkin' Things Collection: 3
Riverdeep
222 Berkeley Street
Boston, MA 02116   617-351-5000
                      855-969-4642
                      Fax: 877-892-9820
                      www.hmhco.com
                      IIEcustomerservice@hmhpub.com
Linda K. Zecher, President, CEO, Director
James G. Nicholson, President, Riverside Publishing
John K. Dragoon, EVP, Chief Marketing Officer
Houghton Mifflin Harcourt offers a wide array of technology-driven pre-k-12 solutions that inspire excellence and innovation in education, and raise student achievement.

1324 Thinkin' Things: All Around Frippletown
Riverdeep
222 Berkeley Street
Boston, MA 02116   617-351-5000
                      855-969-4642
                      Fax: 877-892-9820
                      www.hmhco.com
                      IIEcustomerservice@hmhpub.com
Linda K. Zecher, President, CEO, Director
James G. Nicholson, President, Riverside Publishing
John K. Dragoon, EVP, Chief Marketing Officer
Houghton Mifflin Harcourt offers a wide array of technology-driven pre-k-12 solutions that inspire excellence and innovation in education, and raise student achievement.

1325 Thinkin' Things: Collection 1
Riverdeep
222 Berkeley Street
Boston, MA 02116   617-351-5000
                      855-969-4642
                      Fax: 877-892-9820
                      www.hmhco.com
                      IIEcustomerservice@hmhpub.com
Linda K. Zecher, President, CEO, Director
James G. Nicholson, President, Riverside Publishing
John K. Dragoon, EVP, Chief Marketing Officer
Houghton Mifflin Harcourt offers a wide array of technology-driven pre-k-12 solutions that inspire excellence and innovation in education, and raise student achievement.

1326 Thinkin' Things: Collection 2
Riverdeep
222 Berkeley Street
Boston, MA 02116   617-351-5000
                      855-969-4642
                      Fax: 877-892-9820
                      www.hmhco.com
                      IIEcustomerservice@hmhpub.com
Linda K. Zecher, President, CEO, Director
James G. Nicholson, President, Riverside Publishing
John K. Dragoon, EVP, Chief Marketing Officer
Houghton Mifflin Harcourt offers a wide array of technology-driven pre-k-12 solutions that inspire excellence and innovation in education, and raise student achievement.

1327 Thinkin' Things: Sky Island Mysteries
Riverdeep
222 Berkeley Street
Boston, MA 02116   617-351-5000
                      855-969-4642
                      Fax: 877-892-9820
                      www.hmhco.com
                      IIEcustomerservice@hmhpub.com
Linda K. Zecher, President, CEO, Director
James G. Nicholson, President, Riverside Publishing
John K. Dragoon, EVP, Chief Marketing Officer
Houghton Mifflin Harcourt offers a wide array of technology-driven pre-k-12 solutions that inspire excellence and innovation in education, and raise student achievement.

Professional Resources

1328 **Accurate Assessments**
18047 Oak Street
Omaha, NE 68130   402-341-8880
                                       800-324-7966
                                   Fax: 402-341-8911
                                 www.myaccucare.com
                             info@orionhealthcare.com
Accurate Assessments offers a full range of superior innovative technological services and expertise to the behavioral health industry. Our premier product, AccuCare Behavioral Healthcare System, was developed by teams of experts in their respective fields, insuring our products are truly useful to clinicians and are easy to use. This innovative software program is a comprehensive and adaptable approach to the behavioral health practice environment.

1329 **Beyond Drill and Practice: Expanding the Computer Mainstream**
Council for Exceptional Children
Suite 500
655 Tyee Road
Victoria, BC   250-412-3258
                                    www.abebooks.com
                              sellbooks@abebooks.com
Susan Jo Russell, Author
Rebecca Corwin, Author
Janice R. Mokros, Author
Provides informative guidelines and examples for teachers who want to expand the use of the computer as a learning tool. *$10.00*
120 pages

1330 **CE Software**
PO Box 65580
West Des Moines, IA 50265   515-221-1801
                                       800-523-7638
                                   Fax: 515-221-1806
                                   http://startly.com
International software developer. Many products for adaptive technology.

1331 **Compass Learning**
203 Colorado Street
Austin, TX 78701   512-478-9600
                                       800-678-1412
                                   Fax: 512-492-6193
                             www.compasslearning.com
                         support@compasslearning.com
Tammy Deal, Vice President, Human Resources
Arthur Vanderveen, VP, Development
Eileen Shihadeh, VP, Marketing
Educational software for teachers of K-12.

1332 **Computer Retrieval of Information on Scientific Project (CRISP)**
National Institute of Health
9000 Rockville Pike
Building 12A
Bethesda, MD 20892   301-496-5703
                                       866-319-4357
                                  TTY: 301-496-8294
                                   http://cit.nih.gov
                                 commons@od.nih.gov
Andrea T. Norris, Director
Alfred H. Whitley, Deputy Director of Admin
A major scientific information system containing data on the research programs supported by the US Public Health Service.

1333 **Conover Company**
4 Brookwood Court
Appleton, WI 54914   920-882-1272
                                       800-933-1933
                                   Fax: 800-933-1943
                               www.conovercompany.com
                            sales@conovercompany.com

Becky Schmitz, President
Mike Schmitz, Vice President of Operations
Provides off-the-shelf as well as custom sales and marketing, training, presentation, and application programs that connect learning to the workplace. Delivery platforms include workshops, print, custom software, CD-ROM, multimedia, internet, and intranet.

1334 **Developmental Profile**
Western Psychological Services
625 Alaska Avenue
Torrance, CA 90503-5124   424-201-8800
                                       800-648-8857
                                   Fax: 424-201-6950
                                  www.wpspublish.com
                         customerservice@wpspublish.com
Jeffrey Manson, President, CEO
Dave Herzberg, Ph.D., VP, Research & Development
Amanda Wynn, Marketing Director
This computer program substantially reduces the time educators spend on preparing Individualized Educational Plans (IEPs). The system allows the user to use any IEP format. Simply type the format into the computer, and the program will customize the system to your district's specifications. *$115.00*

1335 **FileMaker Inc.**
5201 Patrick Henry Drive
Santa Clara, CA 95054   408-987-7000
                                       800-325-2747
                                   Fax: 408-987-3002
                                    www.filemaker.com
                           filemaker_pr@filemaker.com
Dominique Goupil, President
Bill Epling, SVP/CAO
Frank Lu, Vice President of Engineering
Company that produces a variety of Macintosh Documentation.

1336 **International Society for Technology in Education (ISTE)**
University of Oregon
180 West 8th Ave
Suite 300
Eugene, OR 97401-2916   541-302-3777
                                       800-336-5191
                                   Fax: 541-302-3778
                                       www.iste.org
                                      iste@iste.org
Brian Lewis, M.A., C.A.E., CEO
Tracee Aliotti, Chief Marketing Officer
Anne Tully, Chief Operating Officer
A nonprofit professional organization dedicated to promoting appropriate uses of information technology to support and improve learning, teaching, and administration in K-12 education and teacher education.

1337 **KidDesk**
Riverdeep
222 3rd Ave SE
4th Floor
Cedar Rapids, IA 52401   319-395-9626
                                       800-825-4420
                                   Fax: 319-395-0217
              http://web.riverdeep.net/portal/page?_pageid=81
                                   info@riverdeep.net
Barry O'Callaghan, Executive Chairman & CEO
Tony Mulderry, EVP, Corporate Development
Jim Ruddy, Chief Revenue Officer
A hard disk security program, KidDesk makes it easy for kids to launch their programs, but impossible for them to access adult programs. Includes interactive desktop accessories including desktop-to-desktop electronic mail, and voice mail. *$24.95*

1338   KidDesk: Family Edition
Riverdeep
222 3rd Ave SE
4th Floor
Cedar Rapids, IA 52401   319-395-9626
                                       800-825-4420
                              Fax: 319-395-0217
http://web.riverdeep.net/portal/page?_pageid=81
                              info@riverdeep.net
Barry O'Callaghan, Executive Chairman & CEO
Tony Mulderry, EVP, Corporate Development
Jim Ruddy, Chief Revenue Officer
Now kids can launch their programs, but can't access yours!
With KidDesk Family Edition, you can give your children
the keys to the computer without putting your programs and
files at risk! The auto-start option provides constant hard
drive security — any time your computer is turned on,
KidDesk will appear. *$24.95*

1339   Laureate Learning Systems
110 East Spring Street
Winooski, VT 05404-1898   802-655-4755
                                       800-562-6801
                              Fax: 802-655-4757
                        www.laureatelearning.com
            laureate-webmaster@laureatelearning.com
Dr. Mary Sweig Wilson Ph.D., President/CEO, Founder
Bernard J. Fox, Co-Founder, Vice President
Marion Blank, Ph.D, Developmental Psychologist
Provides resources for people with learning disabilities.

1340   Learning Company
Riverdeep
100 Pine Street
Suite 1900
San Francisco, CA 94111   415-659-2000
                                       800-825-4420
                              Fax: 415-659-2020
http://web.riverdeep.net/portal/page?_pageid=81
                              info@riverdeep.net
Barry O'Callaghan, Executive Chairman & CEO
Tony Mulderry, EVP, Corporate Development
Jim Ruddy, Chief Revenue Officer

1341   Microsoft Corporation
1 Microsoft Way
Redmond, WA 98052-6399   425-882-8080
                                       800-642-7676
                              Fax: 425-936-7329
                              www.microsoft.com
Steve Ballmer, CEO
Lisa Brummel, Chief People Officer
Tony Bates, President
Our mission is to enable people and businesses throughout
the world to realize their full potential.

1342   Print Module
Failure Free
140 Cabarrus Ave West
Concord, NC 28025   704-786-7838
                                       888-233-READ
                              Fax: 704-785-8940
                              www.failurefree.com
                              info@failurefree.com
Dr. Joseph Lockavitch, Author and President
Joe Lockavitch, VP Sales and Marketing
Includes teacher's manual, instructional readers, flashcards,
independent activities and illustrated independent reading
booklets. *$499.00*

1343   PsycINFO Database
American Psychological Association
750 First St. NE
Washington, DC 20002-4242   202-336-5500
                                       800-374-2721
                              Fax: 202-336-5997
                              TDD: 202-336-6123
                              TTY: 202-336-6123
                                       www.apa.org
                                       mis@apa.org
Norman B. Anderson, PhD, EVP, Chief Executive Officer
Archie Turner, VP, Chief Financial Officer
Tony Habash, DSc, Chief Information Officer
An online abstract database that provides access to citations
to the international serial literature in psychology and re-
lated disciplines from 1887 to present. Available via
PsycINFO Direct at www.psycinfo.com.

1344   Public Domain Software
Kentucky Special Ed TechTraining Center
229 Taylor Education Building
UK College of Education
Lexington, KY 40506-0017   859-257-6076
                              Fax: 859-257-1325
                              TDD: 859-257-4714
                        http://2b.education.uky.edu
                              amanda.nelson@uky.edu
Mary John O'Hair, Dean and Professor
Parker Fawson, Associate Dean
Steve R. Parker, Associate Professor
Entire collections of Macintosh, MS-DOS or Apple II soft-
ware.

1345   Riverdeep
100 Pine Street
Suite 1900
San Francisco, CA 94111   415-659-2000
                                       800-825-4420
                              Fax: 415-659-2020
http://web.riverdeep.net/portal/page?_pageid=81
                              info@riverdeep.net
Barry O'Callaghan, Executive Chairman & CEO
Tony Mulderry, EVP, Corporate Development
Jim Ruddy, Chief Revenue Officer
Developer of educational software, including software for
mathematics instruction.

1346   Scholastic
2931 E McCarty St
Jefferson City, MO 65101-4468   573-636-5271
                                       800-724-6527
                              Fax: 573-636-0549
                              www.scholastic.com
                              custserv@scholastic.com
Faye Edwards, Executive VP/CAO/CEO
Larry Holland, Human Resources Director
Dick Robinson, President & CEO
For more than 90 years, Scholastic has been delivering outstanding books, magazines and educational programs directly to schools and families through channels that have
become childhood traditions - Scholastic Book Fairs,
monthly Book Clubs, and Scholastic News classroom
magazines.

1347   Speech Bin Abilitations
PO Box 1579
Appleton, WI 54912-1579   419-589-1425
                                       888-388-3224
                              Fax: 888-388-6344
                              www.schoolspecialty.com
                              orders@schoolspecialty.com
Joseph M. Yorio, President, CEO
Patrick T. Collins, EVP, Distribution
Rick Holden, Executive Vice President
The Speech Bin offers materials to help persons of all ages
who have special needs. We specialize in products for chil-
dren and adults who have communication disorders.

1348 Sunburst
3150 W Higgins Rd
Suite 140
Hoffman Estates, IL 60619   800-321-7511
                                              www.sunburst.com
                                              service@sunburst.com

Dan Figurski, President
Michael Guillroy, Channel Sales/Marketing Manager

Reading

1349 Adaptive Technology Tools
Freedom Scientific
11800 31st Court North
St Petersburg, FL 33716-1805   727-803-8000
                                              800-444-4443
                                              Fax: 727-803-8001
                                              www.freedomscientific.com
                                              info@FreedomScientific.com
John Blake, President, CEO
Peggy Dalton, Director, Professional Services
Bryan Carver, Inside Sales Director
A wide variety of adaptive technology tools for the visually
or reading impaired person.

1350 An Open Book
Freedom Scientific
11800 31st Court North
St Petersburg, FL 33716-1805   727-803-8000
                                              800-444-4443
                                              Fax: 727-803-8001
                                              www.freedomscientific.com
                                              info@FreedomScientific.com
John Blake, President, CEO
Peggy Dalton, Director, Professional Services
Bryan Carver, Inside Sales Director
The stand-alone reading machine, An Open Book, is an
easy-to-use appliance for noncomputer users that comes
equipped with a Hewlett Packard ScanJet IIP scanner,
DECtalk PC speech synthesizer and a 17 key keypad. An
Open Book uses Calera WordScan optical character recogni-
tion (OCR) to convert pages into text, then reads it aloud
with a speech synthesizer.

1351 An Open Book Unbound
Freedom Scientific
11800 31st Court North
St Petersburg, FL 33716-1805   727-803-8000
                                              800-444-4443
                                              Fax: 727-803-8001
                                              www.freedomscientific.com
                                              info@FreedomScientific.com
John Blake, President, CEO
Peggy Dalton, Director, Professional Services
Bryan Carver, Inside Sales Director
PC-based OCR and reading software. Together with a scanner and a speech synthesizer, this software provides everything needed to make an IBM-compatible PC into a talking
reading machine. The system includes automatic page orientation, automatic contrast control, decolumnization of
multicolumn documents and recognition of a wide variety of
type fonts and sizes. *$995.00*

1352 Bailey's Book House
Riverdeep
222 3rd Ave SE
4th Floor
Cedar Rapids, IA 52401   319-395-9626
                                              800-825-4420
                                              Fax: 319-395-0217
                        http://web.riverdeep.net/portal/page?_pageid=81
                                              info@riverdeep.net
Barry O'Callaghan, Executive Chairman & CEO
Tony Mulderry, EVP, Corporate Development
Jim Ruddy, Chief Revenue Officer

The award-winning Bailey's Book House now features 2
new activities! Bailey and his friends encourage young children to build important literacy skills while developing a
love for reading. In seven activities, kids explore the sounds
and meanings of letters, words, sentences, rhymes and stories. No reading skills are required: all directions and written
words are spoken. *$59.95*

1353 Comprehension Connection
Milliken Publishing
501 East Third Street
Box 802
Dayton, OH 45401-0802   937-228-6118
                                              800-444-1144
                                              Fax: 937-223-2042
                                              www.lorenzeducationalpress.com
                                              lep@lorenz.com
Thomas Moore, President
Comprehension Connection improves reading comprehen-
sion by stressing basic skills that combine the reading process with relevant activities and interesting,
thought-provoking stories. This award-winning software
package spans six reading levels that increase in difficulty.
Passages range from 150-300 words. *$150.00*

1354 Cosmic Reading Journey
Sunburst Technology
3150 W Higgins Rd
Suite 140
Hoffman Estates, IL 60619   800-321-7511
                                              www.sunburst.com
                                              service@sunburst.com
Michael Guillroy, Channel Sales/Marketing Manager
Dan Figurski, President
This reading comprehension program provides meaningful
summary and writing activities for the 100 books that early
readers and their teachers love most.

1355 Don Johnston Reading
Don Johnston
26799 West Commerce Drive
Volo, IL 60073   847-740-0749
                                              800-999-4660
                                              Fax: 847-740-7326
                                              www.donjohnston.com
                                              info@donjohnston.com
Don Johnston, Founder
Ruth Ziolkowski, President
Mindy Brown, Marketing Director
Don Johnston Inc. is a provider of quality products and services that enable people with special needs to discover their
potential and experience success. Products are developed
for the areas of computer access and for those who struggle
with reading and writing.

1356 Failure Free Reading
140 Cabarrus Ave West
Concord, NC 28025   704-786-7838
                                              888-233-READ
                                              Fax: 704-785-8940
                                              www.failurefree.com
                                              info@failurefree.com
Dr. Joseph Lockavitch, Author and President
Joe Lockavitch, VP Sales and Marketing
Curriculum areas covered: reading for those with learning
disabilities and moderate mentally disabled/emotionally
disabled.

1357 Judy Lynn Software
PO Box 373
East Brunswick, NJ 08816   732-390-8845
                                              Fax: 732-390-8845
                                              www.judylynn.com
                                              techsupt@judylynn.com
Elliot Pludwinski, Founder/President
Offers switch computer programs for windows. The pro-
grams are geared towards students with a cognitive age level
from 9 months and up. Programs are reasonably priced from
$39-$79. Recipient of a Parents' Choice Honor.

1358 Kurzweil 3000
Kurzweil Educational Systems
24 Prime Parkway
Suite 303
Natick, MA 01760

508-647-1340
800-894-5374
Fax: 781-276-0650
www.kurzweiledu.com
customerservice@cambiumtech.com

Mike Sokol, President/CEO
Kurzweil Educational's flagship product for struggling readers and writers. It is widely recognized as the most comprehensive and integrated solution for addressing language and literacy difficulties. The software uses a multisensory approach — presenting printed or electronic text on the computer screen with added visual and audible accessibility. The product incorporates a host of dynamic features including powerful decoding, study skills tools and test taking tools.

1359 Lexia Cross-Trainer
Lexia Learning Systems
200 Baker Avenue Ext
Concord, MA 01742

978-405-6200
800-435-3942
Fax: 978-287-0062
www.lexialearning.com
info@lexialearning.com

Nick Gaehde, President
Paul More, Vice President, Finance
Collin Earnst, Vice President of Marketing
Interactive software with an engaging video-gme interface that is designed to strengthen cognitive skills. Activities that advance visual-spatial and logical reasoning skills are designed to improve the memory, critical thinking, and problem solving abilities necessary for academic success in all subjects. *$250.00*

1360 Lexia Early Reading
Lexia Learning Systems
200 Baker Avenue Ext
Concord, MA 01742

978-405-6200
800-435-3942
Fax: 978-287-0062
www.lexialearning.com
info@lexialearning.com

Nick Gaehde, President
Paul More, Vice President, Finance
Collin Earnst, Vice President of Marketing
Engaging, interactive software fochildren aged four to six that introduces and develops proficiency with phonological principles and the alphabet - both proven indicators of later reading success.

1361 Lexia Primary Reading
Lexia Learning Systems
200 Baker Avenue Ext
Concord, MA 01742

978-405-6200
800-435-3942
Fax: 978-287-0062
www.lexialearning.com
info@lexialearning.com

Nick Gaehde, President
Paul More, Vice President, Finance
Collin Earnst, Vice President of Marketing
Interactive software designed to ensure mastery of basic phonological skills and introduce more advanced phonics principles. five levels of engaging activities deliver practice in phonemic awareness, sight-word recognition, word attack strategies, sound-symbol correspondence, listening and reading comprehension. *$50.00*

1362 Lexia Strategies for Older Students
Lexia Learning Systems
200 Baker Avenue Ext
Concord, MA 01742

978-405-6200
800-435-3942
Fax: 978-287-0062
www.lexialearning.com
info@lexialearning.com

Nick Gaehde, President
Paul More, Vice President, Finance
Collin Earnst, Vice President of Marketing
Reading skills software program specifically designed for ages 9-adult. Five levels of activities provide extensive practice in everything from basic phonological awareness to advanced word attack strategy and vocabulary development based on Greek and Laitn word roots. *$250.00*

1363 Mike Mulligan & His Steam Shovel
Sunburst Technology
3150 W Higgins Rd
Suite 140
Hoffman Estates, IL 60619

800-321-7511
www.sunburst.com
service@sunburst.com

Dan Figurski, President
Michael Guillory, Channel Sales/Marketing Manager
This CD-ROM version of the Caldecott classic lets students experience interactive book reading and participate in four skills-based extension activities that promote memory, matching, sequencing, listening, pattern recognition and map reading skills.

1364 Optimum Resource
1 Mathews Drive
Suite 107
Hilton Head Island, SC 29926

843-689-8000
888-784-2592
Fax: 843-689-8008
www.stickybear.com
info@stickybear.com

Richard Hefter, President
An educational software publishing company for grades K-12. Our software titles are available in Consumer, School, Labpack or Site License versions. Please call for further details. Prices range from $59.95 for Consumer to $699.95 for Site Licenses.

1365 Polar Express
Sunburst Technology
3150 W Higgins Rd
Suite 140
Hoffman Estates, IL 60619

800-321-7511
www.sunburst.com
service@sunburst.com

Dan Figurski, President
Michael Guillory, Channel Sales/Marketing Manager
Share the magic and enchantment of the holiday season with this CD-ROM version of Chris Van Allsburg's Caldecott-winning picture book.

1366 Prolexia
4726 13th Ave NW
Rochester, MN 55901-2631

507-780-1859
888-776-5394
Fax: 507-252-0131
www.prolexia.com
info@prolexia.com

John Rylander, President
UltraPhonics Tutor software teaches reading, spelling, handwriting, & pronunciation to beginners and those with dyslexia via multisensory structured phonics.

1367 Read On! Plus
Sunburst Technology
3150 W Higgins Rd
Suite 140
Hoffman Estates, IL 60619

800-321-7511
www.sunburst.com
service@sunburst.com

Dan Figurski, President
Michael Guillory, Channel Sales/Marketing Manager
Promote skills and strategies that improve reading comprehension, and build appreciation for literature and the written word.

1368 Read, Write and Type! Learning Systems
Talking Fingers
830 Rincon Way
San Rafael, CA 94903 415-472-3103
800-674-9126
Fax: 415-472-7812
TDD: 415-472-3106
www.readwritetype.com
contact@talkingfingers.com
Dr. Jeannine Herron, Co-Founder
Dr. Leslie Grimm, Co-Founder
A 40-level software adventure providing highly motivating instruction and practice in phonics, reading, writing, spelling and typing. This multisensory program includes 9 levels of assessment and reports. Classroom packs available.

1369 Reading Power Modules Books
Steck-Vaughn Company
9400 Southpark Center Loop
Orlando, FL 32819 407-345-2000
800-225-5425
Fax: 800-699-9459
www.hmhco.com
IIEcustomerservice@hmhpub.com
Linda K. Zecher, President, CEO, Director
James G. Nicholson, President, Riverside Publishing
John K. Dragoon, EVP, Chief Marketing Officer
Supplementary reading based on 4 decades of reading research. Companion books give students and teachers a choice of formats. High interest stories reinforce reading comprehension skills while building vocabulary, spelling skills, reading fluency, and speed.

1370 Reading Skills Bundle
Sunburst Technology
3150 W Higgins Rd
Suite 140
Hoffman Estates, IL 60619 800-321-7511
www.sunburst.com
service@sunburst.com
Dan Figurski, President
Michael Guillory, Channel Sales/Marketing Manager
Teach beginning reading with teacher-developed programs that sequentially present phonics, phonemic awareness, word recognition, and reading comprehension concepts.

1371 Reading Who? Reading You!
Sunburst Technology
3150 W Higgins Rd
Suite 140
Hoffman Estates, IL 60619 800-321-7511
www.sunburst.com
service@sunburst.com
Dan Figurski, President
Michael Guillory, Channel Sales/Marketing Manager
Teach beginning reading skills effectively with phonics instruction built into engaging games and puzzles that have children asking for more.

1372 Sentence Master: Level 1, 2, 3, 4
Laureate Learning Systems
110 East Spring Street
Winooski, VT 05404-1898 802-655-4755
800-562-6801
Fax: 802-655-4757
www.laureatelearning.com
laureate-webmaster@laureatelearning.com
Dr. Mary Sweig Wilson Ph.D., President/CEO, Founder
Bernard J. Fox, Co Founder, Vice President
Marion Blank, Ph.D, Developmental Psychologist
A revolutionary way to teach beginning reading. Avoiding the confusing rules of phonics and the complexity of whole language, The Sentence Master focuses on the most frequently-used words of our language; i.e. the, is, but, and, etc., by truly teaching these little words, The Sentence Master gives students control over the majority of text they will ever encounter. *$495.00*

1373 Simon Sounds It Out
Don Johnston
26799 West Commerce Drive
Volo, IL 60073 847-740-0749
800-999-4660
Fax: 847-740-7326
www.donjohnston.com
info@donjohnston.com
Don Johnston, Founder
Ruth Ziolkowski, President
Mindy Brown, Marketing Director
Struggling students who can recite the alphabet and recognize letters on a page may still have trouble making connections between letters and sounds. This creates a barrier to recognizing and learning words which prevents your students from reading and writing successfully. Simon Sounds It Out provides the vital practice and repetition they need to overcome the letter-to-sound barrier. *$59.00*

1374 Stickybear Software
Optimum Resource
1 Mathews Drive
Suite 107
Hilton Head Island, SC 29926 843-689-8000
888-784-2592
Fax: 843-689-8008
www.stickybear.com
info@stickybear.com
Richard Hefter, President
An educational software publishing company for grades K-12. Our software titles are available in Consumer, School, Labpack or Site License versions. Please call for further details. Prices range from $59.95 for Consumer to $699.95 for Site Licenses.

1375 Tenth Planet Roots, Prefixes & Suffixes
Sunburst Technology
3150 W Higgins Rd
Suite 140
Hoffman Estates, IL 60619 800-321-7511
www.sunburst.com
service@sunburst.com
Dan Figurski, President
Michael Guillory, Channel Sales/Marketing Manager
Students learn to decode difficult and more complex words as they engage in six activities where they construct and dissect words with roots, prefixes and suffixes.

1376 Time for Teachers Online
Stern Center for Language and Learning
183 Talcott Road
Suite 101
Williston, VT 05495 802-878-2332
800-544-4863
Fax: 802-878-0230
www.sterncenter.org
learning@sterncenter.org
Blanche Podhajski, Ph.D., President
Janna Osman, M.Ed., VP, Programs
Michael Shapiro, M.B.A., Chief Financial Officer
A 45 hour course completed entirely on the internet, designed to help teachers implement research-based best practices in reading instruction. *$525.00*

Science

1377 Changes Around Us CD-ROM
9400 Southpark Center Loop
Orlando, FL 32819 407-345-2000
800-225-5425
Fax: 800-699-9459
www.hmhco.com
IIEcustomerservice@hmhpub.com
Linda K. Zecher, President, CEO, Director
James G. Nicholson, President, Riverside Publishing
John K. Dragoon, EVP, Chief Marketing Officer

Nature is the natural choice for observing change. By observing and researching dramatic visual sequences such as the stages of development of a butterfly, children develop a broad understanding of the concept of change. As they search this multimedia database for images and information about plant and animal life cycles and seasonal change, students strengthen their abilities in research, analysis, problem-solving, critical thinking and communication.

1378 Exploring Heat
TERC
2067 Massachusetts Ave
Cambridge, MA 02140
617-873-9600
Fax: 617-873-9601
www.terc.edu
contactus@terc.edu

Arthur Nelson, Founder
George E. Hein, Chairman
Chris Dede, Board Member
A combination of lessons, software, temperature probes and activity sheets, specifically designed for the learning disabled child. *$160.00*

1379 Field Trip Into the Sea
Sunburst Technology
3150 W Higgins Rd
Suite 140
Hoffman Estates, IL 60619
800-321-7511
www.sunburst.com
service@sunburst.com

Dan Figurski, President
Michael Guillory, Channel Sales/Marketing Manager
Visit a kelp forest and the rocky shore with this information packed guide that lets your students learn about the plants, animals and habitats of coastal environments.

1380 Field Trip to the Rain Forest
Sunburst Technology
3150 W Higgins Rd
Suite 140
Hoffman Estates, IL 60619
800-321-7511
www.sunburst.com
service@sunburst.com

Dan Figurski, President
Michael Guillory, Channel Sales/Marketing Manager
Visit a Central American rainforest to learn more about its plants and animals with this dynamic research program that includes a useful information management tool.

1381 Learn About Life Science: Animals
Sunburst Technology
3150 W Higgins Rd
Suite 140
Hoffman Estates, IL 60619
800-321-7511
www.sunburst.com
service@sunburst.com

Dan Figurski, President
Michael Guillory, Channel Sales/Marketing Manager
Learn about animal classification, adaptation to climate, domestication and special relationships between humans and animals.

1382 Learn About Life Science: Plants
Sunburst Technology
3150 W Higgins Rd
Suite 140
Hoffman Estates, IL 60619
800-321-7511
www.sunburst.com
service@sunburst.com

Dan Figurski, President
Michael Guillory, Channel Sales/Marketing Manager
Students explore the world of plants. From small seeds to tall trees students learn what plants are and what they need to grow.

1383 Milliken Science Series: Circulation and Digestion
Milliken Publishing
501 East Third Street
Box 802
Dayton, OH 45401-0802
937-228-6118
800-444-1144
Fax: 937-223-2042
www.lorenzeducationalpress.com
lep@lorenz.com

Thomas Moore, President
Delores Boufard, Author
A program designed to introduce students to two subsystems of the human body. Provides practice using the correct terms for the various organs that make up each system, illustrating how the parts of each subsystem work together, and ensuring that students can explain the functions of the subsystems and their parts.

1384 Sammy's Science House
Riverdeep
222 3rd Ave SE
4th Floor
Cedar Rapids, IA 52401
319-395-9626
800-825-4420
Fax: 319-395-0217
http://web.riverdeep.net/portal/page?_pageid=81
info@riverdeep.net

Barry O'Callaghan, Executive Chairman & CEO
Tony Mulderry, EVP, Corporate Development
Jim Ruddy, Chief Revenue Officer
Developed by early learning experts, the award-winning Sammy's Science House builds important early science skills, encourages wonder and joy as children discover the world of science around them. Five engaging activities help children practice sorting, sequencing, observing, predicting and constructing. They'll learn about plants, animals, minerals, fun seasons and weather, too! *$59.95*

1385 Talking Walls
Riverdeep
222 3rd Ave SE
4th Floor
Cedar Rapids, IA 52401
319-395-9626
800-825-4420
Fax: 319-395-0217
http://web.riverdeep.net/portal/page?_pageid=81
info@riverdeep.net

Barry O'Callaghan, Executive Chairman & CEO
Tony Mulderry, EVP, Corporate Development
Jim Ruddy, Chief Revenue Officer
The Talking Walls Software Series is a wonderful springboard for a student's journey of exploration and discovery. This comprehensive collection of researched resources and materials enables students to focus on learning while conducting a guided search for information.

1386 Talking Walls: The Stories Continue
Riverdeep
222 3rd Ave SE
4th Floor
Cedar Rapids, IA 52401
319-395-9626
800-825-4420
Fax: 319-395-0217
http://web.riverdeep.net/portal/page?_pageid=81
info@riverdeep.net

Barry O'Callaghan, Executive Chairman & CEO
Tony Mulderry, EVP, Corporate Development
Jim Ruddy, Chief Revenue Officer
Using the Talking Walls Software Series, students discover the stories behind some of the world's most fascinating walls. The award-winning books, interactive software, carefully chosen Web sites, and suggested classroom activities build upon each other, providing a rich learning experience that includes text, video, and hands-on projects.

Social Studies

1387 Discoveries: Explore the Desert Ecosystem
Sunburst Technology
3150 W Higgins Rd
Suite 140
Hoffman Estates, IL 60619   800-321-7511
                                     Fax: 888-800-3028
                                     www.sunburst.com
                                     service@sunburst.com
Dan Figurski, President
Michael Guillory, Channel Sales/Marketing Manager
This program invites students to explore the plants, animals,
culture and georgraphy of the Sonoran Desert by day and by
night.

1388 Discoveries: Explore the Everglades Ecosystem
Sunburst Technology
3150 W Higgins Rd
Suite 140
Hoffman Estates, IL 60619   800-321-7511
                                     Fax: 888-800-3028
                                     www.sunburst.com
                                     service@sunburst.com
Dan Figurski, President
Michael Guillory, Channel Sales/Marketing Manager
This multi curricular research program takes students to the
Everglades where they anchor their exploration photo realis-
tic panaramas of the habitiat.

1389 Discoveries: Explore the Forest Ecosystem
Sunburst Technology
3150 W Higgins Rd
Suite 140
Hoffman Estates, IL 60619   800-321-7511
                                     Fax: 888-800-3028
                                     www.sunburst.com
                                     service@sunburst.com
Dan Figurski, President
Michael Guillory, Channel Sales/Marketing Manager
This theme based CD-ROM enables students of all abilities
to actively research a multitude of different forest ecosys-
tems in the Appalachian National Park.

1390 Imagination Express Destination: Castle
Riverdeep
222 3rd Ave SE
4th Floor
Cedar Rapids, IA 52401   319-395-9626
                                          800-825-4420
                                     Fax: 319-395-0217
          http://web.riverdeep.net/portal/page?_pageid=81
                                     info@riverdeep.net
Barry O'Callaghan, Executive Chairman & CEO
Tony Mulderry, EVP, Corporate Development
Jim Ruddy, Chief Revenue Officer
Kids enter a medieval kingdom where knights, jesters, wild
boars and falconers become actors in their own interactive
stories. As kids cast characters, develop plots, narrate and
write and record dialogue, they become enthusiastic writers,
editors, producers and publishers! *$59.95*

1391 Imagination Express Destination: Neighborhood
Riverdeep
222 3rd Ave SE
4th Floor
Cedar Rapids, IA 52401   319-395-9626
                                          800-825-4420
                                     Fax: 319-395-0217
          http://web.riverdeep.net/portal/page?_pageid=81
                                     info@riverdeep.net
Barry O'Callaghan, Executive Chairman & CEO
Tony Mulderry, EVP, Corporate Development
Jim Ruddy, Chief Revenue Officer

In Destination: Neighborhood, familiar settings and characters encourage kids to write about actual or imagined adventures. Kids enjoy developing creativity, writing and
communication skills as they explore the neighborhood and
all the people who live there. As kids select scenes, choose
and animate stickers, write, narrate, add music and record dialogue, their stories, journals, letters and poems come alive!
$59.95

1392 Imagination Express Destination: Ocean
Riverdeep
222 3rd Ave SE
4th Floor
Cedar Rapids, IA 52401   319-395-9626
                                          800-825-4420
                                     Fax: 319-395-0217
          http://web.riverdeep.net/portal/page?_pageid=81
                                     info@riverdeep.net
Barry O'Callaghan, Executive Chairman & CEO
Tony Mulderry, EVP, Corporate Development
Jim Ruddy, Chief Revenue Officer
The fascinating shores and depths of Destination: Ocean inspire kids to create interactive stories and movies. Using exciting new technology, kids make stickers move across each
scene: sharks swim through the sea kelp while dolphins leap
above waves! With Destination: Ocean, your child's writing
and creativity will soar! *$59.95*

1393 Imagination Express Destination: Pyramids
Riverdeep
222 3rd Ave SE
4th Floor
Cedar Rapids, IA 52401   319-395-9626
                                          800-825-4420
                                     Fax: 319-395-0217
          http://web.riverdeep.net/portal/page?_pageid=81
                                     info@riverdeep.net
Barry O'Callaghan, Executive Chairman & CEO
Tony Mulderry, EVP, Corporate Development
Jim Ruddy, Chief Revenue Officer
Kids can create interactive electronic books and movies featuring pharaohs, mummies and life on the Nile. Builds writing, creativity and communication skills as they learn about
and explore this captivating destination. Kids select scenes,
choose and animate characters, plan plots, write stories, narrate pages and add music, dialogue and sound effects to
make their own adventures. *$59.95*

1394 Imagination Express Destination: Rain Forest
Riverdeep
222 3rd Ave SE
4th Floor
Cedar Rapids, IA 52401   319-365-6108
                                          800-825-4420
                                     Fax: 319-395-0217
          http://web.riverdeep.net/portal/page?_pageid=81
                                     info@riverdeep.net
Barry O'Callaghan, Executive Chairman & CEO
Tony Mulderry, EVP, Corporate Development
Jim Ruddy, Chief Revenue Officer
Rain Forest invities kids to step into a Panamanian rain forest, where they craft exciting, interactive adventures filled
with exotic plants, insects, waterfalls and Kuna Indians.
Kids build essential communication skills as they select
scenes and characters, plan plots, write, narrate, animate and
record dialogue to create remarkable adventures! *$59.95*

1395 Imagination Express Destination: Time Trip USA
Riverdeen
222 3rd Ave SE
4th Floor
Cedar Rapids, IA 52401   319-395-9626
                                          800-825-4420
                                     Fax: 319-395-0217
          http://web.riverdeep.net/portal/page?_pageid=81
                                     info@riverdeep.net
Barry O'Callaghan, Executive Chairman & CEO
Tony Mulderry, EVP, Corporate Development
Jim Ruddy, Chief Revenue Officer

Children will love traveling through time to create interactive electronic books and movies set in a fictional New England town. As students select scenes, cast charcters, develop plots, narrate, write and record dialogue, they'll bring the town's history to life through their own exciting adventures. *$59.95*

Speech

1396 Eden Institute Curriculum: Speech and Language
2 Merwick Road
Princeton, NJ 08540-5711
609-987-0099
Fax: 609-987-0243
www.edenservices.org
info@edenservices.org

Dr. Tom Mc Cool, President/CEO
Melinda McAleer, Chief Development Officer
Anne Holmes, M.S., C.C.C.,, Chief Clinical Officer
Peceptive, expressive and pragmatic language skills programs for students with autism. *$170.00*

1397 Spectral Speech Analysis: Software
Speech Bin
PO Box 1579
Appleton, WI 54912-1579
419-589-1425
888-388-3224
Fax: 888-388-6344
www.schoolspecialty.com
orders@schoolspecialty.com

Joseph M. Yorio, President, CEO
Patrick T. Collins, EVP, Distribution
Rick Holden, Executive Vice President
This exciting new software uses visual feedback as an effective speech treatment tool. Speech-language pathologists can record speech and corresponding visual displays for clients who then try to match either auditory or visual targets. These built-in visual patterns can be displayed as either sophisticated spectrograms or real-time waveforms. Item number P227. *$159.95*

Word Processors

1398 Dr. Peet's TalkWriter
Interest Driven Learning
Apt 303
446 Bouchelle Dr
New Smyrna Beach, FL 32169-5429
816-478-4824
800-245-5733
Fax: 816-478-4824
www.drpeet.com
lpeet@drpeet.com

Bill William Peet, PhD, CEO
Libby Peet EdD, Adaptive Access Specialist
A talking, singing word processor designed to meet the needs of young learners from three to eight. Runs on Windows.

1399 Kids Media Magic 2.0
Sunburst Technology
3150 W Higgins Rd
Suite 140
Hoffman Estates, IL 60619
800-321-7511
Fax: 888-800-3028
www.sunburst.com
service@sunburst.com

Dan Figurski, President
Michael Guillory, Channel Sales/Marketing Manager
The first multimedia word processor designed for young children. Help your child become a fluent reader and writer. The Rebus Bar automatically scrolls over 45 vocabulary words as students type.

1400 Media Weaver 3.5
Sunburst Technology
3150 W Higgins Rd
Suite 140
Hoffman Estates, IL 60619
800-321-7511
Fax: 888-800-3028
www.sunburst.com
service@sunburst.com

Dan Figurski, President
Michael Guillory, Channel Sales/Marketing Manager
Publishing becomes a multimedia event with this dynamic word processor that contains hundreds of media elements and effective process writing resources.

1401 Sunbuddy Writer
Sunburst Technology
3150 W Higgins Rd
Suite 140
Hoffman Estates, IL 60619
800-321-7511
Fax: 888-800-3028
www.sunburst.com
service@sunburst.com

Dan Figurski, President
Michael Guillory, Channel Sales/Marketing Manager
An easy-to-use picture and word processor designed especially for young writers.

1402 Write: Outloud to Go
Don Johnston
26799 West Commerce Drive
Volo, IL 60073
847-740-0749
800-999-4660
Fax: 847-740-7326
www.donjohnston.com
info@donjohnston.com

Don Johnston, Founder
Ruth Ziolkowski, President
Mindy Brown, Marketing Director
A flexible and user-friendly talking word processor that offers multisensory learning and positive reinforcement for writers of all ages and ability levels. Powerful features include a talking spell checker, on-screen speech and file management and color capabilities that allow for customization to meet individual needs or preferences. Requires Macintosh computer. Voted Best Special Needs Product by the Software Publishers Association. *$99.00*

Writing

1403 Abbreviation/Expansion
Zygo Industries
48834 Kato Road
Suite 101-A
Fremont, CA 94538
510-249-9660
800-234-6006
Fax: 510-770-4930
www.zygo-usa.com
zygo@zygo-usa.com

Lawrence H. Weiss, President
Adam D. Weiss, VP, Sales & Marketing
Allows the individual to define and store word/phrase abbreviations to achieve efficiency and accelerated entry rate of text. *$95.00*

1404 Author's Toolkit
Sunburst Technology
3150 W Higgins Rd
Suite 140
Hoffman Estates, IL 60619
800-321-7511
Fax: 888-800-3028
www.sunburst.com
service@sunburst.com

Dan Figurski, President
Michael Guillory, Channel Sales/Marketing Manager
Students can use this comprehensive tool to organize ideas, make outlines, rough drafts, edit and print all their written work.

1405 Dr. Peet's Picture Writer
Interest Driven Learning
Apt 303
446 Bouchelle Dr
New Smyrna Beach, FL 32169-5429   386-427-4473
                                        800-245-5733
                                        Fax: 816-478-4824
                                        www.drpeet.com
                                        lpeet@drpeet.com

Bill William Peet, PhD, CEO
Libby Peet EdD, Adaptive Access Specialist
A talking picture-writer. It guides novice writers, regardless of age, motivation or ability, in creating simple talking picture sentences about things that are interesting and important to them. *$500.00*

1406 Easybook Deluxe
Sunburst Technology
3150 W Higgins Rd
Suite 140
Hoffman Estates, IL 60619   800-321-7511
                                  Fax: 888-800-3028
                                  www.sunburst.com
                                  service@sunburst.com

Dan Figurski, President
Michael Guillory, Channel Sales/Marketing Manager
Designed to support the needs of a wide range of writers, this book publishing tool provides students with a creative environment to write, design and illustrate stories and reports, and to print their work in book formats.

1407 Fonts4Teachers
Therapro
225 Arlington Street
Framingham, MA 01702-8723   508-872-9494
                                  800-257-5376
                                  Fax: 508-875-2062
                                  www.theraproducts.com
                                  info@therapro.com

Karen Conrad, President
A software collection of 31 True Type fonts for teachers, parents and students. Fonts include Tracing, lined and unlined Traditional Manuscript and Cursive (similar to Zaner Blouser and D'Nealian), math, clip art, decorative, time, American Sign Language symbols and more. The included manual is very informative, with great examples of lesson plans and educational goals. *$39.95*
Windows/Mac

1408 Great Beginnings
Teacher Support Software
5600 West 83rd Street
Suite 300, 8200 Tower
Bloomington, MN 55437   888-351-4199
                              800-447-5286
                              Fax: 800-896-1760
                              www.edmentum.com
                              info@edmentum.com

Vin Riera, President, CEO
Dan Juckniess, Senior Vice President
Stacey Herteux, Vice President, Human Resources
From a broad selection of topics and descriptive words, students may create their own stories and illustrate them with colorful graphics. *$69.95*

1409 Language Experience Recorder Plus
Teacher Support Software
5600 West 83rd Street
Suite 300, 8200 Tower
Bloomington, MN 55437   888-351-4199
                              800-447-5286
                              Fax: 800-896-1760
                              www.edmentum.com
                              info@edmentum.com

Vin Riera, President, CEO
Dan Juckniess, Senior Vice President
Stacey Herteux, Vice President, Human Resources

This program provides students with the opportunity to read, write and hear their own experience stories. Analyzes student writing. Cumulative word list, word and sentence counts and readability estimate. *$99.95*

1410 Mega Dots 2.3
Duxbury Systems
270 Littleton Rd
Unit 6
Westford, MA 01886-3523   978-692-3000
                                Fax: 978-692-7912
                                www.duxburysystems.com
                                info@duxsys.com

Joe Sullivan, President
Peter Sullivan, VP of Software Development
Neal Kuniansky, Marketing Director
MegaDots is a mature DOS braille translator with powerful features for the volume transcriber and producer. Its straightforward, style based system and automated features let you create great braille with only a few keystrokes, yet it is sophisticated enough to please the fussiest braille producers. You can control each step MegaDots follows to format, translate and produce braille documents. *$540.00*

1411 Once Upon a Time Volume I: Passport to Discovery
Compu-Teach
16541 Redmond Way
Suite C
Redmond, WA 98052   425-885-0517
                          800-448-3224
                          Fax: 425-883-9169
                          www.compu-teach.com
                          info@compu-teach.com

David Urban, President
Features familiar objects associated with three unique themes. These graphic images offer limitless possibilities for new stories and illustrations. As children author books from one to hundreds of pages, they can either display them on screen or print them out. Themes: Farm Life; Down Main Street; and On Safari. *$59.95*

1412 Once Upon a Time Volume II: Worlds of Enchantment
Compu-Teach
16541 Redmond Way
Suite C
Redmond, WA 98052   425-885-0517
                          800-448-3224
                          Fax: 425-883-9169
                          www.compu-teach.com
                          info@compu-teach.com

David Urban, President
Makes writing, reading and vocabulary skills easy to learn. While building their illustrations, children experiment with perspective and other spatial relationships. This volume features familiar objects associated with three unique themes: Underwater; Dinosaur Age; and Forest Friends. *$59.95*

1413 Once Upon a Time Volume III: Journey Through Time
Compu-Teach
16541 Redmond Way
Suite C
Redmond, WA 98052   425-885-0517
                          800-448-3224
                          Fax: 425-883-9169
                          www.compu-teach.com
                          info@compu-teach.com

David Urban, President
Makes writing, reading and vocabulary skills easy to learn. With imagination as a youngster's only guide, the important concepts of story creation and illustration are naturally discovered. Themes: Medieval Times, Wild West and Outer Space. *$59.95*

1414 Once Upon a Time Volume IV: Exploring Nature
Compu-Teach
16541 Redmond Way
Suite C
Redmond, WA 98052
425-885-0517
800-448-3224
Fax: 425-883-9169
www.compu-teach.com
info@compu-teach.com
David Urban, President
The latest in award-winning creative writing series. Kids just hear, click and draw as the state of the art graphics and digitized voice make writing, reading and vocabulary skills easy to learn. Themes: Rain Forest; African Grasslands; Ocean; Desert; and Forest. *$59.95*

1415 Read, Write and Type Learning System
Talking Fingers, California Neuropsych Services
830 Rincon Way
San Rafael, CA 94903
415-472-3103
800-674-9126
Fax: 415-472-7812
TDD: 415-472-3106
www.readwritetype.com
contact@talkingfingers.com
Dr. Jeannine Herron, Co-Founder
Dr. Leslie Grimm, Co-Founder
A 40-level software adventure providing highly motivating instruction and practice in phonics, reading, writing, spelling and typing. This multisensory program includes 9 levels of assessment and reports. Classroom packs available.

1416 StartWrite Handwriting Software
Therapro
225 Arlington Street
Framingham, MA 01702-8723
508-872-9494
800-257-5376
Fax: 508-875-2062
www.theraproducts.com
info@therapro.com
Karen Conrad, President
With this easy-to-use software package, you can make papers and handwriting worksheets to meet individual student's needs. Type letters, words, or numbers and they appear in a dot format on the triple line guide. Change letter size, add shading, turn on or off guide lines and arrow strokes and place provided clipart. Fonts include Manuscript and Cursive, Modern Manuscript and Cursive and Italic Manuscript and Cursive. Useful manual included. *$39.95*
Windows/Mac

1417 Writing Trek Grades 4-6
Sunburst Technology
3150 W Higgins Rd
Suite 140
Hoffman Estates, IL 60619
800-321-7511
Fax: 888-800-3028
www.sunburst.com
service@sunburst.com
Dan Figurski, President
Michael Guillory, Channel Sales/Marketing Manager
Enhance your students' experience in your English language arts classroom with twelve authentic writing projects that build students' competence while encouraging creativity.

1418 Writing Trek Grades 6-8
Sunburst Technology
3150 W Higgins Rd
Suite 140
Hoffman Estates, IL 60619
800-321-7511
Fax: 888-800-3028
www.sunburst.com
service@sunburst.com
Dan Figurski, President
Michael Guillory, Channel Sales/Marketing Manager
Twelve authentic language arts projects, activities, and assignments develop your students' writing confidence and ability.

1419 Writing Trek Grades 8-10
Sunburst Technology
3150 W Higgins Rd
Suite 140
Hoffman Estates, IL 60619
800-321-7511
Fax: 888-800-3028
www.sunburst.com
service@sunburst.com
Dan Figurski, President
Michael Guillory, Channel Sales/Marketing Manager
Help your students develop a concept of genre as they become familiar with the writing elements and characteristics of a variety of writing forms.

General

1420 American Institute for Foreign Study
1 High Ridge Park
Stamford, CT 06905
203-399-5000
866-906-2437
Fax: 203-399-5590
www.aifs.com
info@aifs.com

Sir Cyril Taylor, Founder and Chairman
William L. Gertz, President and CEO
Organizes cultural exchange programs throughout the world for more than 50,000 students each year, and arranges insurance coverage for our own participants as well as those of other organizations. Also provides summer travel programs overseas and in the U.S. ranging from 1 week to a full academic year.

1421 American-Scandinavian Foundation
58 Park Avenue
38th Street
New York, NY 10016
212-779-3587
Fax: 212-686-1157
www.scandinaviahouse.org
info@amscan.org

Edward P. Gallagher, President, CEO
Lynn Carter, EVP, Corporate Secretary
Lynda Selde, Director of Development
Promotes international understanding through educational and cultural exchange between the United States and Denmark, Finalnd, Iceland, Norway and Sweden.

1422 Andeo International Homestays
620 SW 5th Avenue
Suite 625
Portland, OR 97204
503-274-1776
800-274-6007
Fax: 503-274-9004
www.andeo.org
info@andeo.org

Melinda Samis, Director
Julie Padbury, Programs Coordinator
Kellie Irish, Programs Coordinator
Formerly International Summerstays, an international network of families, students, teachers, independent travelers and homestay specialists who are dedicated to exploring cross-cultural friendship and understanding.

1423 Arcadia University, College of Global Studies
450 South Easton Road
Glenside, PA 19038-3295
215-572-2901
866-927-2234
Fax: 215-572-2174
www.arcadia.edu/abroad
educationabroad@arcadia.edu

Lorna Stern, VP
Dennis Dutschke, Founding Academic Dean
Colleen Burke, Chief Operating Officer
The College offers study abroad programs for undergraduate and graduate students, internship and research opportunities, student and faculty exchanges and service learning programs, all ranging in length from semester, year, and short-term study/research abroad programs.

1424 Army & Air Force Exchange Services
3911 S. Walton Walker Blvd
PO Box 660202
Dallas, TX 75236-1598
214-465-6690
800-527-2345
Fax: 800-446-0163
TDD: 800-423-2011
www.aafes.com

Thomas C. Shull, Director/Chief Executive Officer
Michael P. Howard, Chief Operating Officer
Joseph S. Ward Jr., Deputy Director

Brings tradition of value, service and support to its 11.5 million authorized customers at military installations in the United States, Europe and in the Pacific.

1425 Association for International Practical Training
10400 Little Patuxent Parkway
Suite 250
Columbia, MD 21044
410-997-2200
800-994-2443
Fax: 410-992-3924
http://culturalvistas.org
aipt@aipt.org

Rob Fenstermacher, President and CEO
Linda Boughton, EVP, Chief Financial Officer
Dan Ewert, VP, Program Research
Nonprofit organization dedicated to encouraging and facilitating the exchange of qualified individuals between the US and other countries so they may gain practical work experience and improve international understanding.

1426 Basic Facts on Study Abroad
International Education
809 United Nations Plaza
New York, NY 10017
212-883-8200
Fax: 212-984-5452
www.iie.org
publications@un.org

Allen E Goodman, President and CEO
Peter Thompson, Executive Vice President
Jaye Chen, Executive Vice President
Information book including foreign study planning, educational choices, finances, and study abroad programs.

1427 Council on International Educational Exchange
300 Fore Street
Portland, ME 04101
207-553-4000
Fax: 207-553-4299
www.ciee.org
contact@ciee.org

James P. Pellow, ED.D., President, CEO
Brenda Majeski, SVP, Marketing & Communications
Nancy Kittredge, VP, Human Resources
CIEE creates and administers programs that allow high school and university students and educators to study and teach abroad. Programs and literature address participants with disabilities.

1428 Earthstewards Network
PO Box 10697
Bainbridge Island, WA 98110
206-842-7986
800-561-2909
Fax: 206-842-8918
www.earthstewards.org
outreach@earthstewards.org

Danaan Parry, Co-Founder
Bruce Haley, Director
Charlie Olson, Director
Hundreds of active, caring people in the US, Canada and other countries. Puts North American teenagers working alongside Northern Irish teenagers and more.

1429 Educational Foundation for Foreign Study
1 Education St
Cambridge, MA 02141-1805
800-447-4273
Fax: 617-619-1401
www.efexchangeyear.org
foundation@ef.com

Offers an opportunity to study and live for a year in a foreign country for students between the ages of 15 and 18.

1430 High School Student's Guide To Study, Travel and Adventure Abroad
Council on International Education Exchange
300 Fore Street
Portland, ME 04101
207-553-4000
800-407-8839
Fax: 207-553-4299
www.ciee.org
contact@ciee.org

James P. Pellow, ED.D., CEO and President
Brenda Majeski, SVP, Marketing & Communications
Nancy Kittredge, VP, Human Resources
This guide provides high school students with all the information they need for a successful trip abroad. Included are sections to help students find out if they're ready for a trip abroad, make the necessary preparations, and get the most rom their experience. Over 200 programs are described including language study, summer camps, homestays, study tours, and work camps. The program descriptions include information for people with disabilities.

1431 Higher Education Consortium for Urban Affairs

2233 University Avenue West
Suite 210
Saint Paul, MN 55114

651-287-3300
Fax: 651-659-9421
www.hecua.org
hecua@hecua.org

Jenny Keyser, Executive Director
Patrick Mulvihill, Director of Operations
Sarah Pradt, Director of Programs
Consortium of 15 Midwest colleges and universities offering undergraduate, academic programs, both international and domestic that incorporate field study and internships in the examination of urban and global issues.

1432 International Cultural Youth Exchange (ICYE)

134 W 26th Street
New York, NY 10001

212-206-7307
Fax: 212-633-9085
www.icye.org
icye@icye.org

A nonprofit youth exchange promoting youth mobility, intercultural learning and international voluntary service. ICYE organizes long- and short-term exchanges combining home stays with voluntary service in 34 countries around the world.

1433 International Partnership for Service-Learning and Leadership

1515 SW 5th Ave.
Suite 606
Portland, OR 97201

503-954-1812
Fax: 503-954-1881
www.ipsl.org
info@ipsl.org

Thomas Winston Morgan, President
Arianne Newton, Director of Programs
Dr. Erin Barnhart, Graduate Program Director
A not-for-profit educational organization incorporated in NYS serving students, collegs, universities, service agencies and related organizations around the world by fostering programs that link volunteer service to the community and academic study.

1434 Lions Club International

300 West 22nd Street
Oak Brook, IL 60523-8842

630-571-5466
Fax: 630-571-8890
www.lionsclub.org
districtadministration@lionsclub.org

Joseph Preston, International President
Jitsuhiro Yamada, First Vice President
Robert E. Corlew, Second Vice President
Over 46,000 individual clubs in over 190 countries and geographical areas, providing community service and promoting improved international relations. Clubs work with local communities to provide needed and useful programs for sight, diabetes and hearing, and aid in study abroad.

1435 Lisle

900 County Road 269
PO Box 1932
Leander, TX 78646

512-259-4404
800-477-1538
www.lisleinternational.org
office@lisleinternational.org

Dr. Dewitt Baldwin, Founder
Lori Bratton, VP
Barbara Bratton, Treasurer/Operations Mgr
Educational organization which works toward world peace and a better quality of human life through increased understanding between persons of similar and different cultures.

1436 Mobility International (MIUSA)

132 E Broadway
Suite 343
Eugene, OR 97401

541-343-1284
Fax: 541-343-6812
TTY: 541-343-1284
www.miusa.org

Susan Sygall, CEO, Co-Founder
Cerise Roth Vinson, Chief Operating Officer
Cindy Lewis, Director of Programs
MIUSA offers short-term international exchange programs in the US and abroad for people with and without disabilities, including non-apparent disabilities.

1437 National Society for Experimental Education

19 Mantua Road
Mount Royal, NJ 08061

856-423-3427
Fax: 856-423-3420
www.nsee.org
nsee@talley.com

Ron Kovach, President
James Walters, Past President
Jim Colbert, VP
A nonprofit membership association of educators, businesses, and community leaders. Also serves as a national resource center for the development and improvement of experimental education programs nationwide.

1438 No Barriers to Study

Lock Haven University
401 N Fairview Street
Lock Haven, PA 17745

570-484-2011
www.lhup.edu
admissions@lhup.edu

Dr. Donna Wilson, Provost/SVP for Academic Affairs
William Hanelly, Vice President
Rodney Jenkins, Vice President
A regional consortium committed to facilitating study abroad for college students with disabilities.

1439 People to People International

911 Main Street
Suite 2110
Kansas City, MO 64105

816-531-4701
800-676-7874
Fax: 816-561-7502
www.ptpi.org
ptpi@ptpi.org

Rosanne Rosen, SVP, Operations
Brian Hueben, Vice President, Finance
Clark Plexico, CEO
Nonpolitical, nonprofit organization working outside the government to advance the cause of international understanding through international contact.

1440 SUNY Buffalo Office of International Education

1300 Elmwood Avenue
South Wing 410
Buffalo, NY 14222

716-878-4620
Fax: 716-878-3054
www.buffalostate.edu/studyabroad
intleduc@buffalostate.edu

Hal D. Payne, Vice President, Student Affairs
Robert Summers, PhD, Assistant Dean
Josephine Zagarella Behrens, Director

1441 Sister Cities International
915 15th Street, NW
4th Floor
Washington, DC 20005   202-347-8630
                                    Fax: 202-393-6524
                                    www.sister-cities.org
                                    info@sister-cities.org
Patrick Madden, President
Launa Kowalski, Chair
Nancy Eidam, Operating Officer
A nonprofit citizen diplomacy network; creating and
strengthening partnerships between the US and international communities in an effort to increase global cooperation at the municipal level, to promote cultural
understanding, and to stimulate economic development. Encourages local community development and volunteer action by motivating and empowering private citizens,
municipal officials and business leaders to conduct
long-term programs of mutual benefit, including exchange
situations.

1442 Study Abroad
Davidson College
Box 7155
Davidson, NC 28035   704-894-2000
                                        800-768-0380
                                    Fax: 704-894-2120
                                    www.davidson.edu
                                    abroad@davidson.edu
Carol Quillen, President
Eileen Keeley, VP, College Relations
Deb Rutkowski, VP, College Relations

1443 World Experience
2440 S Hacienda Blvd
Suite 116
Hacienda Heights, CA 91745-4763   626-330-5719
                                        800-633-6653
                                    Fax: 626-333-4914
                                    www.worldexperience.org
                                    info@worldexperience.org
Kerry Gonzales, President
Marge Archambault, President
Offers a quality and affordable program for over three decades and continues to provide students and host families a
youth exchange program based on individual attention, with
the help of an international network of overseas directors
and USA coordinators

1444 Youth for Understanding USA
6400 Goldsboro Road
Suite 100
Bethesda, MD 20817   240-235-2100
                                        800-833-6243
                                    Fax: 240-235-2104
                                    www.yfu-usa.org
                                    admissions@yfu.org

Daryl Weinert, Chairman
William Dant, Vice Chairman
Michael E. Hill, President & CEO
Nonprofit international exchange program, prepares young
people for their responsibilities and opportunities in todays
changing, interdependent world through homestay exchange programs. Offers year, semester, and summer study
abroad and scholarship opportunities in 40 countries
worldwide.

Federal

1445 ABLE DATA
USDE National Institution on Disability/Rehab
103 West Broad St.
Suite 400
Falls Church, VA 22046
703-356-8035
800-227-0216
Fax: 703-356-8314
TDD: 301-608-8912
TTY: 703-992-8313
www.abledata.com
abledata@neweditions.net
Katherine Belknap, Project Director
Juanita Hardy, Information Specialist
David Johnson, Publications Director
Sponsored by the National Institute on Disability and Rehabilitation Research (NIDRR) of the US Department of Education; provides information on more than 34,000 assistive technology products, including detailed descriptions of each product, price and company information.

1446 ADA Information Line
US Department of Justice
950 Pennsylvania Avenue, NW
Washington, DC 20530
202-307-0663
800-514-0301
Fax: 202-307-1197
TTY: 800-514-0383
www.ada.gov
Rebecca B. Bond, Chief
James Bostrom, Deputy Chief
Jana Erickson, Deputy Chief
Answers questions about Title II (public services) and Title III (public accommodations) of the Americans with Disabilities Act (ADA). Provides materials and technical assistance on the provisions of the ADA.

1447 ADA Technical Assistance Programs
US Department of Justice
950 Pennsylvania Avenue, NW
Washington, DC 20530-0001
202-514-2000
800-514-0301
TTY: 800-514-0383
www.justice.gov
AskDOJ@usdoj.gov
Eric Holder, Attorney General
James Cole, Deputy Attorney General
Tony West, Associate Attorney General
Federally funded regional resource centers that provide information and referral, technical assistance, public awareness, and training on all aspects of the Americans with Disabilities Act (ADA).

1448 Americans with Disabilities Act (ADA) Resource Center
National Center for State Courts
300 Newport Avenue
Williamsburg, VA 23185
757-259-1525
800-616-6164
Fax: 757-220-0449
www.ncsc.org
webmaster@ncsc.dni.us
Mary McQueen, President
Robert Baldwin, EVP & General Counsel
Thomas Clarke, VP, Research & Technology
Disseminates information on ADA compliance to state and local court systems. Will develop a diagnostic checklist and strategies for compliance specifically relevant to the state and local courts.

1449 Civil Rights Division: US Department of Justice
Office of the Assistant Attorney General
950 Pennsylvania Avenue, NW
Washington, DC 20530-0001
202-514-2000
800-514-0301
Fax: 202-514-0293
TDD: 202-514-0716
www.justice.gov
AskDOJ@usdoj.gov
Eric Holder, Attorney General
James Cole, Deputy Attorney General
Tony West, Associate Attorney General
The program institution within the federal government responsible for enforcing federal statutes prohibiting discrimination on the basis of race, sex, disability, religion, and national origin.

1450 Clearinghouse on Adult Education and Literacy
US Department of Education
400 Maryland Avenue, SW
Washington, DC 20202
800-872-5327
Fax: 202-401-0689
TTY: 800-437-0833
www.ed.gov
Emma Vadehra, Chief of Staff
Eric Waldo, Senior Advisor
John Easton, Director
The Clearinghouse was established in 1981 to link the adult education community with existing resources in adult education, provide information which deals with state administered adult education programs funded under the Adult Education and Family Literacy Act, and provide resources that support adult education activities.

1451 Clearinghouse on Disability Information
Office of Special Education/Rehabilitative Service
400 Maryland Avenue, SW
Washington, DC 20202
202-245-7307
800-872-5327
Fax: 202-245-7636
TDD: 202-205-5637
www.ed.gov
Emma Vadehra, Chief of Staff
Eric Waldo, Senior Advisor
John Easton, Director
Provides information to people with disabilities, or anyone requesting information, by doing research and providing documents in response to inquiries. Information provided includes areas of federal funding for disability-related programs. Staff is trained to refer requests to other sources of disability-related information, if necessary.

1452 Employment and Training Administration: US Department of Labor
Frances Perkins Building
200 Constitution Ave NW
Washington, DC 20210
202-693-2700
866-487-2365
Fax: 202-693-2726
TTY: 866-487-2365
www.doleta.gov
webmaster@dol.gov
Thomas E. Perez, Secretary of Labour
Christopher Lu, Deputy Secretary of Labor
Matthew Colangelo, Chief of Staff
Administers federal government job training and worker dislocation programs, federal grants to states for public employment service programs, and unemployment insurance benefits. These services are primarily provided through state and local workforce development systems.

1453 Equal Employment Opportunity Commission
131 M Street, NE
Washington, DC 20507
202-663-4900
800-669-4000
TTY: 202-663-4494
www.eeoc.gov
info@eeoc.gov

Milton A. Mayo Jr., Inspector General
Stuart Ishimaru, Acting Chair
Enforces Section 501 which prohibits discrimination on the basis of disability in Federal employment, and requires that all Federal agencies establish and implement affirmative action programs for hiring, placing and advancing individuals with disabilities. Also oversees Federal sector equal employment opportunity complaint processing system.

1454 Eunice Kennedy Shriver National Institute of Child Health and Human Development (NICHD)
National Institutes of Health
31 Center Drive
Building 31, Room 2A32
Bethesda, MD 20892-2425

800-370-2943
Fax: 866-760-5947
TTY: 888-320-6942
www.nichd.nih.gov
NICHDInformationResourceCenter@mail.nih.gov

Alan Guttmacher, MD, Acting Director
The mission of the Eunice Kennedy Shriver National Institute of Child Health and Human Development (NICHD) is to ensure that every person is born healthy and wanted, that women suffer no harmful effects from the reproductive process, that all children have the chance to fulfill their potential to live healthy and productive lives free from disease or disability, and to ensure the health, productivity, independence and well-being of all people through optimal rehabilitation.

1455 National Council on Disability
1331 F Street, NW
Suite 850
Washington, DC 20004

202-272-2004
Fax: 202-272-2022
TTY: 202-272-2074
www.ncd.gov
executivedirector@ncd.gov

Rebecca Cokley, Executive Director
Joan M. Durocher, General Counsel
Anne Sommers, Director
An independent federal agency comprised of 15 members appointed by the President and confirmed by the Senate.

1456 National Institute of Mental Health
Science Writing, Press & Dissemination Branch
6001 Executive Boulevard
Room 6200, MSC 9663
Bethesda, MD 20892-9663

301-443-4536
866-615-6464
Fax: 301-443-4279
TTY: 301-443-8431
www.nimh.nih.gov
NIMHpress@mail.nih.gov

Ann D. Huston, Acting Associate Director
Dianne M. Rausch, Ph.D., Director, Office on AIDS
Kevin Quinn, Ph.D., Acting Director
Mission is to diminish the burden of mental illness through research. This public health mandate demands that we harness powerful scientific tools to achieve better understanding, treatment and eventually prevention of mental illness.

1457 National Institute on Disability and Rehabilitation Research
US Department of Education
400 Maryland Avenue, SW
Washington, DC 20202

202-245-7640
800-872-5327
Fax: 202-245-7323
www.ed.gov

Emma Vadehra, Chief of Staff
Eric Waldo, Senior Advisor
John Easton, Director
Provides leadership and support for a comprehensive program of research related to the rehabilitation of individuals with disabilities. All of the programmatic efforts are aimed to improving the lives of individuals with disabilities from birth through adulthood.

1458 National Library Services for the Blind and Physically Handicapped
1291 Taylor Street, NW
Washington, DC 20011

202-707-5100
888-657-7323
Fax: 202-707-0712
TDD: 202-707-0744
www.loc.gov/nls
nls@loc.gov

Karen Keninger, Director
Marsha Jackson, Administrative Section Head
Jane Caulton, Publications & Media Head
Administers a national library service that provdies braille and recorded books and magazines on free loan to anyone who cannot read standard print becuase of visual or physical disabilities.

1459 National Technical Information Service: US Department of Commerce
5301 Shawnee Rd
Alexandria, VA 22312

703-605-6050
888-584-8332
Fax: 703-605-6900
www.ntis.gov
info@ntis.gov

John J. Regazzi, Chairman of the Advisory Board
MacKenzie Smith, Advisory Board
Bruce Borzino, Director
Serves the nation as the largest central resource for government-funded scientific, technical, engineering, and business related information available today.

1460 Office for Civil Rights: US Department of Health and Human Services
200 Independence Avenue, SW
Room 509F, HHH Building
Washington, DC 20201

800-368-1019
TDD: 800-537-7697
www.hhs.gov/ocr
OCRMail@hhs.gov

Leon Rodriguez, Director
Juliet Choi, Chief of Staff
Promotes and ensures that people have equal access to an dopportunity to participate in and receive services from all HHS programs without facing unlawful discrimination, and that the privacy of their health information is protectec while ensuring access to care.

1461 Office for Civil Rights: US Department of Education
400 Maryland Avenue, SW
Washington, DC 20202

202-453-6100
800-421-3481
Fax: 202-453-6012
TTY: 800-877-8339
www.ed.gov/ocr
ocr@ed.gov

Catherine E. Lhamon, Assistant Secretary
James Ferg-Cadina, Dep. Assistant Secretary, Policy
To ensure equal access to education and to promote educational excellence throughout the nation through vigourous enforcement of civil rights.

1462 Office of Disability Employment Policy: US Department of Labor
200 Constitution Ave NW
Washington, DC 20210

202-693-2700
866-487-2365
Fax: 202-693-2726
TTY: 866-487-2365
www.dol.gov
webmaster@dol.gov

Thomas E. Perez, Secretary of Labour
Christopher Lu, Deputy Secretary of Labor
Matthew Colangelo, Chief of Staff
Provides national leadership by developing and influencing disability-related employment policy as well as practice affecting the employment of people with disabilities.

1463 **Office of Federal Contract Compliance Programs: US Department of Labor**
200 Constitution Ave NW
Washington, DC 20210

202-693-2700
866-487-2365
Fax: 202-693-2726
TTY: 866-487-2365
www.dol.gov
webmaster@dol.gov

Thomas E. Perez, Secretary of Labour
Christopher Lu, Deputy Secretary of Labor
Matthew Colangelo, Chief of Staff
Responsible for ensuring that employers doing business with the Federal government comply with the laws and regulations requiring nondiscrimination and affirmative action in employment.

1464 **Office of Personnel Management**
1900 E Street, NW
Washington, DC 20415-1000

202-606-1800
TTY: 202-606-2532
www.opm.gov
general@opm.gov

Angela Bailey, Chief Operating Officer
Amen Mashariki, Chief Technology Officer
Katherine Archuleta, Director
The central personnel agency of the federal government. Provides information on the selective placement program for persons with disabilities.

1465 **Rehabilitation Services Administration State Vocational Program**
US Department of Education
400 Maryland Avenue, SW
Washington, DC 20202

202-245-7488
800-872-5327
www.ed.gov

Emma Vadehra, Chief of Staff
Eric Waldo, Senior Advisor
John Easton, Director
State and local vocational rehabilitation agencies provide comprehensive services of rehabilitation, training and job-related assistance to people with disabilities and assist employers in recruiting, training, placing, accommodating and meeting other employment-related needs of people with disabilities.

1466 **Social Security Administration**
Office of Public Inquiries
6401 Security Blvd
Baltimore, MD 21235-6401

410-965-6114
800-772-1213
Fax: 410-966-2027
TTY: 800-325-0778
www.socialsecurity.gov

Bill Vitek, Commissioner
Provides financial assistance to those with disabilities who meet eligibility requirements.

1467 **US Bureau of the Census**
4600 Silver Hill Road
Washington, DC 20233

301-763-4636
800-923-8282
Fax: 301-457-3670
TTY: 800-877-8339
www.census.gov
pio@census.gov

Nancy Potok, Deputy Director and COO
John H. Thompson, Director
Thomas E Zebelsky, Director
The principal statistical agency of the federal government. It publishes data on persons with disabilities, as well as other demographic data derived from censuses and surveys.

1468 **US Department of Health & Human Services**
200 Independence Avenue, SW
Room 509F, HHH Building
Washington, DC 20201

202-690-7650
800-368-1019
TDD: 800-537-7697
www.hhs.gov
OCRMail@hhs.gov

Leon Rodriguez, Director
Juliet Choi, Chief of Staff/Senior Advisor
Councils in each state provide training and technical assistance to local and state agencies, employers and the public, improving services to people with developmental disabilities.

Alabama

1469 **Alabama Council for Developmental Disabilities**
100 North Union Street
P.O. Box 301410
Montgomery, AL 36130-1410

334-242-3973
800-232-2158
Fax: 334-242-0797
www.acdd.org
Myra.Jones@mh.alabama.gov

Elmyra Jones-Banks, Executive Director
Sophia Whitted, Fiscal Manager
Wendy Dean, Council Member, Self-Advocate
Serves as an advocate for Alabama's citizens with developmental disabilities and their families; to empower them with the knowledge and opportunity to make informed choices and exercise control over their own lives; and to create a climate for positive social change to enable them to be respected, independent and productive integrated members of society.

1470 **Alabama Department of Industrial Relations**
649 Monroe Street
Montgomery, AL 36131

334-242-8495
Fax: 334-242-2048
http://labor.alabama.gov
webmaster@labor.alabama.gov

Tom Surtees, Director
Bettye Folks Johnson, EEO Officer, Human Resources
To effectively use tax dollars to provide state and federal mandated workforce protection programs promoting a positive economic environment for Alabama employers and workers and to produce and disseminate information on the Alabama economy.

1471 **Alabama Disabilities Advocacy Program**
P.O.Box 870395
Tuscaloosa, AL 35487-0395

205-348-4928
800-826-1675
Fax: 205-348-3909
www.adap.net
adap@adap.ua.edu

Ellen Gillespie, Director
Angie Allen, Case Advocate
Christy Johnson, Sr., Case Advocate
To provide quality, legally-based advocacy services to Alabamians with disabilities in order to protect, promote and expand their rights.

1472 **Employment Service Division: Alabama**
Department of Industrial Relations
649 Monroe Street
Montgomery, AL 36131

334-242-8495
Fax: 334-242-2048
http://labor.alabama.gov
webmaster@labor.alabama.gov

Bob Brantley, Director
Bettye Folks Johnson, EEO Officer, Human Resources

Alaska

1473 Alaska State Commission for Human Rights
550 West 7th Avenue
Suite 1700
Anchorage, AK 99501
907-269-7450
800-478-4692
Fax: 907-269-7461
TDD: 907-276-3177
http://gov.alaska.gov
Sean Parnell, Governor
Anne Keene, Administrative Officer
The state agency which enforces the Alaska Human Rights Law. Consists of seven persons appointed by the governor and confirmed by the legislature.

1474 Assistive Technology of Alaska (ATLA)
Ste 4
2217 E Tudor Rd
Anchorage, AK 99507-1068
907-563-2599
800-723-2852
Fax: 907-563-0699
http://atlaak.com
atla@atlaak.org
Kathy Privratsky, Executive Director
To enhance the quality of life for Alaskans through education, demonstration, consultation, acquisition and implementation of assistive technologies. ATLA is Alaska's only assistive technology project for the Tech Act.

1475 Center for Community
600 Telephone Ave.
Anchorage, AK 99503
907-747-6960
855-907-7005
Fax: 907-747-4868
www.alaskacommunications.com
Connie Sipe, Executive Director
Margaret Andrews, Deputy Executive Director
Center for Community is a multiservice agency that provides early intervention, respite, futures planning, functional skills training, and vocational assistance and personal care for people with disabilities.

1476 Correctional Education Division: Alaska
Department of Corrections/Division of Institutions
550 West 7th Avenue
Suite 1700
Anchorage, AK 99501
907-269-7397
Fax: 907-269-7390
www.correct.state.ak.us/
anna.herzberger@alaska.gov
Anna Herberger, Criminal Justice Planner
Leslie Houston, Director
Charlie Huggins, Senate President

1477 Disability Law Center of Alaska
3330 Arctic Blvd.
Suite 103
Anchorage, AK 99503
907-565-1002
800-478-1234
Fax: 907-565-1000
www.dlcak.org
akpa@dlcak.org
Doug Harris, President, Board of Director
Julie Renwick, VP, Board of Director
Cristin Cowles-Brunton, Treasurer, Board of Director
An independent non-profit organization that provides legal advocacyservices for people with disabilities anywhere in Alaska. To promote and protect the legal and human rights of individuals with physical and/or mental disabilities.

1478 Employment Security Division
Alaska Department of Labor & Workforce Development
P.O.Box 115509
Juneau, AK 99811-5509
907-465-2712
Fax: 907-465-4537
http://labor.state.ak.us
esd.director@alaska.gov

Tom Nelson, Director
Promotes employment, economic stability, and growth by operating a no-fee labor exchange that meets the needs of employers, job seekers, and veterans.

1479 State Department of Education & Early Development
State of Alaska
801 West 10th Street, Suite 200
P.O. Box 110500
Juneau, AK 99811-0500
907-465-2800
Fax: 907-465-4156
TTY: 907-465-2815
www.eed.state.ak.us
eed.webmaster@alaska.gov
Sean Parnell, Governor
Esther J Cox, State Board of Education Chair
State education agency

1480 State GED Administration: GED Testing Program
Alaska Department of Education
801 West 10th Street, Suite 200
P.O. Box 110500
Juneau, AK 99811-0500
907-465-2800
Fax: 907-465-4156
TTY: 907-465-2815
www.eed.state.ak.us
eed.webmaster@alaska.gov
Sean Parnell, Governor
Karen Rehfeld, Executive Director
Barbara Thompson, TLS Director

Arizona

1481 Arizona Center for Disability Law
5025 E. Washington St.
Suite 202
Phoenix, AZ 85034
602-274-6287
800-927-2260
Fax: 602-274-6779
TTY: 602-274-6287
www.azdisabilitylaw.org
center@azdisabilitylaw.org
Art Gode, VP, Family Member
J.J. Rico, Interim Executive Director
Sharon Fabian, Attorney
Advocates for the leagl rights of persons with disabilities to be free from abuse, neglect and discrimination; and to have access to education, healthcare, housing and jobs, and other services in order to maximize independence and achieve equality.

1482 Arizona Center for Law in the Public Interest
2205 E Speedway
Tucson, AZ 85719
520-529-1798
Fax: 520-529-2927
www.aclpi.org
jherrcardillo@aclpi.org
Bruce Samuels, President
Timothy M Hogan, Executive Director
Anne C. Ronan, Staff
A non-profit law firm dedicated to ensuring government accountability and protecting the legal rights of Arizonans.

1483 Arizona Department of Economic Security
Rehabilitation Services Administration
Suite 200
3221 N 16th St
Phoenix, AZ 85016-7159
602-266-6752
800-563-1221
Fax: 602-241-7158
TTY: 855-475-8194
www.azdes.gov/rsa
cfitzgerald@azdes.gov
Tracy Wareing, Director
Sharon Sergent, Deputy Director
Chuck Fitzgerald, Community Team
Promotes the safety, well-being, and self sufficiency of children, asults and families.

1484 Arizona Department of Education
1535 West Jefferson Street
Phoenix, AZ 85007   602-542-5393
    800-352-4558
    www.ade.az.gov
    adeinbox@azed.gov

Peter Laing, Director
Lynn Tuttle, Director of Arts Education
Cynthia Bolewski, Director of Operations
To ensure academic excellence for all students.

1485 Arizona Governor's Committee on Employment of the Handicapped
ALS Association Arizona Chapter
360 E. Coronado Rd.
Suite 140
Phoenix, AZ 85004   602-297-3800
    866-350-2572
    Fax: 602-297-3804
    www.alsaz.org
    info@alsaz.org

Mark Kittredge, Chair
Dale Sparks, Vice Chair
Tom Avery, Treasurer
To lead the fight to cure and treat ALS through global, cutting-edge research, and to empower people with Lou Gehrig's disease and their families to live fuller lives by providing them with compassionate care and support.

1486 Correctional Education
Arizona Department of Corrections
1601 W Jefferson St
Phoenix, AZ 85007-3002   602-542-1160
    Fax: 602-364-0259
    bkilian@adc.state.az.us

Dora Schriro, Manager

1487 Division of Adult Education
Arizona Department of Education
1535 West Jefferson Street
Phoenix, AZ 85007   602-542-5393
    800-352-4558
    Fax: 602-258-4977
    www.ade.az.gov
    adeinbox@azed.gov

Peter Laing, Director
Lynn Tuttle, Director of Arts Education
Cynthia Bolewski, Director of Operations
To ensure that learners 16 years of age and older have access to quality educational opportunities.

1488 Fair Employment Practice Agency
Office of the Arizona Attorney General
1275 West Washington Street
Phoenix, AZ 85007-2926   602-542-5025
    800-352-8431
    Fax: 602-542-4085
    TDD: 602-542-5002
    TTY: 602-542-5002
    www.azag.gov
    consumerinfo@azag.gov

Tom Home, Attorney General

1489 GED Testing Services
Arizona Department of Education
1535 West Jefferson Street
Phoenix, AZ 85007   602-542-5393
    800-352-4558
    Fax: 602-258-4977
    www.ade.az.gov
    adeinbox@azed.gov

Peter Laing, Director
Lynn Tuttle, Director of Arts Education
Cynthia Bolewski, Director of Operations

1490 Governor's Council on Developmental Disabilities
Ste 201
1740 West Adams
Phoenix, AZ 85007   602-542-8970
    877-665-3176
    Fax: 602-542-8978
    TTY: 602-542-8979
    www.azgcdd.org
    djohnson@azdes.gov

Stephen W Tully, Chairman
Karla Phillips, Vice Chairman
To work in partnership with individuals with developmental disabilities and their families through systems change, advocacy and capacity building activities that promote indpendence, choice and the ability to pursue their own dreams.

Arkansas

1491 Arkansas Department of Corrections
425 W. Capitol
Suite 1620
Little Rock, AR 72201   501-324-8900
    877-727-3468
    Fax: 501-324-8904
    www.arkansas.gov

Ray Hobbs, Director
To provide public safety by carrying out the mandates of the courts; provide a safe humane environment for staff and inmates; provide programs to strengthen the work ethic; and provide opportunities for spiritual, mental, and physical growth.

1492 Arkansas Department of Education
Four Capitol Mall
Room 403-A
Little Rock, AR 72201   501-682-4475
    Fax: 501-682-1079
    http://arkansased.org

Tony Wood, Commissioner
Mike Hernandez, Deputy Commissioner
Deborah Coffman, Chief of Staff
Strives to ensure that all children in the state have acess to a quality education by providing educators, administrators anad staff with leadership, resources and training.

1493 Arkansas Department of Special Education
1401 West Capitol Ave
Victory Bldg., Suite 450
Little Rock, AR 72201   501-682-4221
    Fax: 501-682-5159
    TTY: 501-682-4222
    http://arksped.k12.ar.us
    spedsupport@arkansas.gov

Marcia Harding, Associate Director

1494 Arkansas Department of Workforce Education
Three Capitol Mall
Luther Hardin Bldg.
Little Rock, AR 72201   501-682-1500
    Fax: 501-682-1509
    http://dwe.arkansas.gov

Mike Beebe, Governor
William L. Walker, Jr., Director
James H. Smith, Jr., Deputy Director
To provide the leadership and contribute resources to serve the diverse and changing workforce training needs of the youth and adults in Arkansas.

1495 Arkansas Department of Workforce Services
#2 Capitol Mall
P.O. Box 2981
Little Rock, AR 72201
501-682-2121
855-225-4440
Fax: 501-682-8845
TDD: 501-296-1669
www.dws.arkansas.gov
ADWS.Info@arkansas.gov
Artee Williams, Director
Ron Snead, Deputy Director
Cindy Varner, Assistant Director

1496 Arkansas Governor's Developmental Disabilities Council
5800 West 10th Street
Suite 805
Little Rock, AR 72204
501-661-2589
855-627-7580
Fax: 501-661-2399
www.ddcouncil.org
brenda.mercer@arkansas.gov
Brenda Mercer, Executive Director
Teresa Sander, Family Services Coordinator
Michelle Boyd, Administrative Assistant
Supports people with developmental disabilities in the achievement of independence, productivity, integration and inclusion in the community.

1497 Assistive Technology Project
Increasing Capabilities Access Network (ICAN)
525 W. Capitol
Little Rock, AR 72201
501-666-8868
800-828-2799
Fax: 501-666-5319
TTY: 800-828-2799
www.arkansas-ican.org
rick.anderson@arkansas.gov
A consumer responsive statewide program promoting assistive technology devices and resources for persons of all ages and all disabilities.

1498 Client Assistance Program (CAP) Disability Rights Center of Arkansas
1100 N University
Suite 201
Little Rock, AR 72207
501-296-1775
800-482-1174
Fax: 501-296-1779
TTY: 800-482-1174
www.arkdisabilityrights.org
Info@arkdisabilityrights.org
Traci Perrin, President, Jonesboro
Kim Weser, Vice President, Redfield
Kimberly Marshall, Treasurer, Jonesboro
The purpose of CAP is to protect the rights of persons receiving or seeking services funded under the federal Rehabilitation Act. According to thise law, CAP services are available for all clients or applicants of the following services: Vocational Rehabilitation Services, Independent Living Services, Supported Employment, Independent Living Centers, and Projects with Industry.

1499 Increasing Capabilities Access Network
525 W. Capitol
Little Rock, AR 72201
501-666-8868
800-828-2799
Fax: 501-666-5319
TDD: 501-666-8868
TTY: 800-828-2799
www.arkansas-ican.org
rick.anderson@arkansas.gov
Linda Morgan, Project Administrator
A federally funded program of Arkansas Rehabilitation Services, is designed to make technology available and accessible for all who need it. ICAN is a funding information resource and provides information on new and existing technology free to any person regardless of age or disability.

1500 Office of the Governor
500 Woodlane Street
Suite 250
Little Rock, AR 72201
501-682-2345
Fax: 501-682-1382
www.governor.arkansas.gov
Mike Beebe, Governor
William L. Walker, Jr., Director
James H. Smith, Jr., Deputy Director

1501 Protection & Advocacy Agency
Disability Rights Center
1100 N University
Suite 201
Little Rock, AR 72207
501-296-1775
800-482-1174
Fax: 501-296-1779
TTY: 800-482-1174
www.arkdisabilityrights.org
Info@arkdisabilityrights.org
Traci Perrin, President, Jonesboro
Kim Weser, Vice President, Redfield
Kimberly Marshall, Treasurer, Jonesboro
Carry out activities under several Federal programs to provide a range of services to adocate for and protect the rights of persons with disabilities throughout the state

1502 State GED Administration
Arkansas Department of Workforce Education
Three Capitol Mall
Luther Hardin Bldg.
Little Rock, AR 72201
501-682-1500
Fax: 501-682-1509
http://dwe.arkansas.gov
tambra.nicholson@mail.state.ar.us
Mike Beebe, Governor
William L. Walker, Jr., Director
James H. Smith, Jr., Deputy Director
Serves all Arkansans who are 16 years or older, not enrolled in or graduated from high school, and who meet other state requirements regarding residency and testing eligibility.

California

1503 California Department of Fair Employment and Housing
2218 Kausen Drive
Suite 100
Elk Grove, CA 95758
916-478-7251
Fax: 916-478-7329
TDD: 800-700-2320
www.dfeh.ca.gov
contact.center@dfeh.ca.gov
Nelson Chan, Esq., Civil Rights Officer
Annmarie Billotti, Esq., Chief of Dispute Resolution
Phyllis W. Cheng, Director
To protect the people of California from unlawful discrimination in employment, housing and public accomodations, and from the perpetration of acts of hate violence.

1504 California Department of Rehabilitation
721 Capitol Mall
P.O. Box 944222
Sacramento, CA 95814
916-324-1313
800-952-5544
TTY: 916-558-5807
www.rehab.cahwnet.gov
externalaffairs@dor.ca.gov
Tony Sauer, Director
Works in partnership with consumers and other stakeholders to provide services and advocacy resulting in employment, independent living and equality for individuals with disabilities.

1505 California Department of Special Education

1430 N Street
Sacramento, CA 95814-5901   916-319-0800
                                   TTY: 916-445-4556
                                   www.cde.ca.gov
                                   scheduler@cde.ca.gov
Karen Stapf Walters, Executive Director
Patricia de Cos, Deputy Executive Director
Judy M. Cias, Chief Counsel
Information and reesources to serve the unique needs of persons with disabilities so that each person will meet or exceed high standards of achivment in academic and nonacademic skills.

1506 California Employment Development Department

P.O. BOX 826880, MIC 83
Sacramento, CA 94280-0001   916-654-7241
                                   Fax: 916-657-5294
                                   www.edd.ca.gov
Patrick W. Henning, Jr., Director
Sharon Hilliard, Chief Deputy Director
Greg Williams, Deputy Director, Administration
Promotes California's economic growth by providing services to keep employers, employees, and job seekers competitive.

1507 California State Board of Education

1430 N Street
Sacramento, CA 95814-5901   916-319-0800
                                   Fax: 916-319-0175
                                   TTY: 916-445-4556
                                   www.cde.ca.gov
                                   scheduler@cde.ca.gov
Karen Stapf Walters, Executive Director
Patricia de Cos, Deputy Executive Director
Judy M. Cias, Chief Counsel
The State Board of Education (SBE) is the governing and policy making body of the California Department of Education. The SBE sets K-12 education policy in the areas of standards, instructional materials, accessment, and accountability.

1508 California State Council on Developmental Disabilities

1507 21st Street
Suite 210
Sacramento, CA 95811   916-322-8481
                              866-802-0514
                              Fax: 916-443-4957
                              TTY: 916-324-8420
                              www.scdd.ca.gov
                              council@dss.ca.gov
Christofer Arroyo, Executive Director
Joseph Bowling, Executive Director
Susan Eastman, Executive Director
Advocates, promotes and implements policies and practices that achieve self-determination, independence, productivity and inclusion in all aspects of community life for Californians with developmental disabilities and their families.

1509 Career Assessment and Placement Center Whittier Union High School District

9401 Painter Ave
Whittier, CA 90605-2729   562-698-8121
                                 Fax: 562-693-5354
Daniel Hubert
Provides job placement programs, remunerative work services and work adjustment training programs.

1510 Clearinghouse for Specialized Media

California Department of Education
1430 N Street
Sacramento, CA 95814-5901   916-319-0800
                                   Fax: 916-319-0175
                                   TTY: 916-445-4556
                                   www.cde.ca.gov
                                   scheduler@cde.ca.gov

Karen Stapf Walters, Executive Director
Patricia de Cos, Deputy Executive Director
Judy M. Cias, Chief Counsel
Provides accessible formats of adopted curriculum to qualified students with disabilities in California.

1511 DBTAC: Pacific ADA Center

555 12th Street
Suite 1030
Oakland, CA 94607-4046   510-285-5600
                                800-949-4232
                                Fax: 510-285-5614
                                TTY: 800-949-4232
                                www.adapacific.org
Erica C. Jones, MPH, Director
To build a partnership between the disability and business communities and to promote full and unrestricted participation in society for persons with disabilities through education and technical assistance.

1512 Disability Rights California (California's Protection and Advocacy System)

1831 K Street
Sacramento, CA 95811-4114   916-504-5800
                                   800-776-5746
                                   Fax: 916-504-5801
                                   TTY: 800-719-5798
                                   www.disabilityrightsca.org
                                   legalmail@disabilityrightsca.org
Catherine Blakemore, Executive Director
Rick Guidara, IT Director
Milanka Radosavljevic, Administrative Services Director
A private, nonprofit organization that protects the legal, civil and service rights of Californians with disabilities.
1978

1513 Education & Inmate Programs Unit

P.O.Box 942883
Sacramento, CA 94283-0001   916-445-8035
                                   800-952-5544
                                   Fax: 916-324-1416
                                   www.corr.ca.gov
Jan Stuter, Manager
Gary Sutherland, Federal Grand Administrator
Adrianne Johnson, Secretary

1514 Employment Development Department: Employment Services Woodland

P.O. BOX 826880, MIC 83
Sacramento, CA 94280-0001   916-654-7241
                                   Fax: 916-657-5294
                                   www.edd.ca.gov
Patrick W. Henning, Jr., Director
Sharon Hilliard, Chief Deputy Director
Greg Williams, Deputy Director, Administration
The Employment Development Department promote's California's economic growth by providing services to keep employers, employees, and job seekers competitive.

1515 Employment Development Department: Employment Services W Sacramento

California Health & Human Services Agency
P.O. BOX 826880, MIC 83
Sacramento, CA 94280-0001   916-654-7241
                                   Fax: 916-657-5294
                                   www.edd.ca.gov
Patrick W. Henning, Jr., Director
Sharon Hilliard, Chief Deputy Director
Greg Williams, Deputy Director, Administration

1516 Office of Civil Rights: California

US Department of Education
400 Maryland Avenue, SW
Washington, DC 20202   202-245-7488
                              800-872-5327
                              www.ed.gov
                              ocr.sanfrancisco@ed.gov

Emma Vadehra, Chief of Staff
Eric Waldo, Senior Advisor
John Easton, Director

1517   Region IX: US Department of Education
US Department of Education
400 Maryland Avenue, SW
Washington, DC 20202   202-245-7488
                                         800-872-5327
                                    Fax: 415-437-7540
                                         www.ed.gov

Emma Vadehra, Chief of Staff
Eric Waldo, Senior Advisor
John Easton, Director
The Office of Federal Contract Compliance Programs is part
of the US Department of Labor's Employment Standards
Administration. It has a national network of six regional of-
fices, each with district and area offices in major
metropolitan centers.

**1518   Region IX: US Department of Health and Human Ser-
vices**
200 Independence Avenue, S.W.
Washington, DC 20201   415-437-8500
                                         877-696-6775
                                    Fax: 415-437-8505
                                         www.hhs.gov
                                    thomas.lorentzen@hhs.gov
Kathleen Falk, Regional Director
Kim Gillan, Regional Director
Stephene Moore, Regional Director

1519   Sacramento County Office of Education
P.O.Box 269003
Sacramento, CA 95826-9003   916-228-2500
                                    Fax: 916-228-2403
                                         www.scoe.net
David Gordon, Superintendent
A customer-driven educational leader and agent got change
in the country, region and state, is to support the preparation
of students for a changing and global 21st century society,
through a continuously improving system of aprtnerships
and coordinated services for our diverse community.

Colorado

1520   Assistive Technology Partners
601 East 18th Avenue
Pearl Plaza, Suite 130
Denver, CO 80203   303-315-1280
                                         800-255-3477
                                    Fax: 303-837-1208
                                    TTY: 303-837-8964
              www.ucdenver.edu/academics/colleges/medi
                             GeneralInfo@AT-Partners.org
Bill Caile, Chair
Cathy Bodine, Ph.D., CCC-SLP, Executive Director
Mike Dino, Advisory Council Member
Designed to support capacity building and advocacy activi-
ties, and to assist states in maintaining permanent, compre-
hensive statewide programs of technology related assistance
for all people with disabilities living in Colorado.

1521   Colorado Civil Rights Division
1560 Broadway
Suite 250
Denver, CO 80202   303-894-2000
                                         800-888-0170
                                    Fax: 303-894-2065
                             www.dora.state.co.us/puc.
                                    ccrd@dora.state.co.us
Steven Chavez, Executive Director

1522   Colorado Department of Labor and Employment
633 17th St
#201
Denver, CO 80202   303-318-8700
                                         888-390-7936
                                    Fax: 303-318-8710
              www.coworkforce.com/dwc/contactnumbers/d
                                    workers.comp@state.co.us
Brian Aggeler, Executive Director

1523   Colorado Developmental Disabilities
Colorado Department of Human Services
4055 S Lowell Blvd
Denver, CO 80236-3120   303-866-7450
                                    Fax: 303-866-7470
                             www.cdhs.state.co.us/ddd/
Sharon Jacksi, Director
Provides leadership for the direction, funding, and operation
of services to persons with developmental disabilities within
Colorado.

1524   Correctional Education Division
Colorado Department of Corrections
Ste 400
2862 S Circle Dr
Colorado Springs, CO 80906-4101   719-579-9580
                                    Fax: 719-226-4755
                                         www.doc.state.co.us
                             executive.director@doc.state.co.us
Rick Raemisch, Executive Director
Kellie Wasko, Deputy Executive Director
Steve Hager, Director of Prisons
To meet the diverse educational needs of inmates through
the provision of quality academic, vocational, life skills, and
transitional services whereby inmates can successfully integrate into society, gain and maintain employment and become responsible, productive individuals.

**1525   Legal Center for People with Disabilities and Older Peo-
ple**
455 Sherman Street
Suite 130
Denver, CO 80203   303-722-0300
                                         800-288-1376
                                    Fax: 303-722-0720
                                    TTY: 303-722-3619
                                         www.thelegalcenter.org
                                    tlcmail@thelegalcenter.org
Mary Anne Harvey, Executive Director
Randy Chapman, Esq., Director of Legal Services
Julie Z. Busby, Director of Development
The Legal Center protects and promotes the rights of people
with disabilities and older people in Colorado through direct
legal representation, advocacy, education and legislative
analysis.

1526   Region VIII: US Department of Education
Office of Civil Rights
400 Maryland Avenue, SW
Washington, DC 20202   202-245-7488
                                         800-872-5327
                                    Fax: 303-844-4303
                                         www.ed.gov
                                    ocr.denver@ed.gov
Emma Vadehra, Chief of Staff
Eric Waldo, Senior Advisor
John Easton, Director
This office covers the states of Arizona, Colorado, New
Mexico, Utah, and Wyoming.

**1527   Region VIII: US Department of Health and Human Ser-
vices**
200 Independence Avenue, S.W.
Washington, DC 20201   877-696-6775
                                         877-696-6775
                                    Fax: 877-696-6775
                                         www.hhs.gov
                                    joe.nunez@hhs.gov

Kathleen Falk, Regional Director
Kim Gillan, Regional Director
Stephene Moore, Regional Director

1528   Region VIII: US Department of Labor-Office of Federal Contract Compliance
US Department of Labor
Ste 950
1809 California St
Denver, CO 80202   303-844-1600
                                   Fax: 303-844-1616
These regional offices of agencies enforce laws prohibiting employment discrimination on the basis of disability.

1529   State Department of Education
201 E Colfax Ave
Denver, CO 80203-1704   303-866-6600
                                   Fax: 303-830-0793
                                   www.cde.state.co.us
                                   commissioner@cde.state.co.us
Dwight D Jones, Commissioner
The administrative arm of the Colorado Board of Education. CDE serves colorado's 178 local school districts, providing them with leadership, consultation and administrative services on a statewide and regional basis.

Connecticut

1530   Bureau of Special Education & Pupil Services
Department of Education
165 Capitol Avenue
Hartford, CT 06106   860-713-6543
                                   Fax: 860-713-7014
                                   www.state.ct.us/sde/
                                   annelouise.thompson@ct.gov
Stefan Pryor, Commissioner of Education
Charlene Russell Tucker, Chief Operating Officer
Adam Goldfarb, Chief of Staff
Offers information on educational programs and services. The Complaint Resolution Process Office answers and processes parent complaints regarding procedural violations by local educational agencies and facilities. The Due Process Office is responsible for the management of special education and due process proceedings which are available to parents and school districts.

1531   CHILD FIND of Connecticut
25 Industrial Park Road
Middletown, CT 06457-1520   860-632-1485
                                   800-445-2722
                                   Fax: 860-632-8870
                                   www.ctserc.org
                                   info@ctserc.org
Ingrid Canady, Associate Director for Program
Matthew Dugan, Assistant Director
Alice Henley, Assistant Director
A service under the direction of The Connecticut State Department of Education and operated by the Special Education Resource Center. The primary goal is the identification, diagnosis and programming of all unserved disabled children.

1532   Connecticut Bureau of Rehabilitation Services
Department of Social Services
55 Farmington Avenue
12th Floor
Hartford, CT 06105   860-424-4844
                                   800-537-2549
                                   Fax: 860-424-4850
                                   TDD: 860-424-4839
                                   www.ct.gov/brs
                                   brs.dss@ct.gov
Michael P Starkowski, Commissioner
Amy Porter, Bureau Director

Creates opportunities that enable individuals with significant disabilities to work competitively and live independently. Strive to provide appropriate, individualized services, develop effective partnerships, and share sufficient information so that consumers and their families may make informed choices about the rehabilitation process and employment options.

1533   Connecticut Department of Social Services
55 Farmington Avenue
12th Floor
Hartford, CT 06105   860-424-4844
                                   800-537-2549
                                   Fax: 860-424-4850
                                   TDD: 860-424-4839
                                   TTY: 800-842-4524
                                   www.ct.gov/brs
                                   brs.dss@ct.gov
Michael P Starkowski, Commissioner
Provides a broad range of services to the elderly, disabled, families and individuals who need assistance in maintaining or achieving their full potential for self-director, self-reliance and independent living.

1534   Connecticut Office of Protection and Advocacy for Persons with Disabilities
55 Farmington Avenue
12th Floor
Hartford, CT 06105   860-424-4844
                                   800-537-2549
                                   Fax: 860-424-4850
                                   TDD: 860-424-4839
                                   TTY: 860-297-4380
                                   www.ct.gov/brs
                                   brs.dss@ct.gov
James Mc Gaughey, Executive Director
Supports families and individuals who are affected by developmental disabilities.

1535   Connecticut State Department of Education
165 Capitol Avenue
Hartford, CT 06106   860-713-6543
                                   Fax: 860-713-7014
                                   www.sde.ct.gov
                                   annelouise.thompson@ct.gov
Stefan Pryor, Commissioner of Education
Charlene Russell Tucker, Chief Operating Officer
Adam Goldfarb, Chief of Staff
The adminstrative arm of the Connecticut State Board of Education. Through leadership, curriculum, research, planning, evaluation, assessment, data analyses and other assistance, the Department helps to ensure equal opportunity and excellence in education for all Connecticut students.

1536   Connecticut Tech Act Project
Dept of Social Services/Bureau of Rehab Services
25 Sigourney Street
11th Floor
Hartford, CT 06106   860-424-4881
                                   800-537-2549
                                   Fax: 860-424-4850
                                   TTY: 860-424-4839
                                   www.cttechact.com
Arlene Lugo, Program Coordinator
Terese Mayor, AT Council Chair
Fran Sinish, Advisory Council Member
Increasing independence and improve the lives of individuals with disabilities through increased access to Assistive Technology for work, school and community living.

1537   Correctional Education Division: Connecticut
Unified School District #1
24 Wolcott Hill Road
Wethersfield, CT 06109   860-692-7480
                                   Fax: 860-692-7783
                                   www.state.ct.us/doc/
                                   DOC.PIO@ct.gov

Angela J Jalbert, Superintendent
Leo Amone, Commissioner
Education continues to be one of the Department's more valuable assets in providing opportunities that will support an offender's successful community reintegration. Education programming is available to inmates through the Unified School District (USD)#1, a legally vested school district within the Department of Correction (DOC).

1538   Protection & Advocacy Agency
Office of P&A for Persons with Disabilities
60B Weston Street
Hartford, CT 06120-1551   860-297-4300
                                    800-842-7303
                               Fax: 860-566-8714
                               TTY: 860-297-4380
                                    www.ct.gov/opapd

Dannel P. Malloy, Governor
James Mc Gaughey, Executive Director
To advnace the cause of equal rights for persons with disabilities and their families.

1539   State GED Administration
Bureau of Adult Education and Training
25 Industrial Park Road
Middletown, CT 06457   860-807-2125
                               Fax: 860-807-2112
www.gedtestingservice.com/testers/ged-te
            ged@ct.govwloski@po.state.ct.us
Paul F Flinter, Bureau Chief
Sabrina Mancini, GED Administrator
The primary aid of the GED testing program in Connecticut is to provide a second opportunity for individuals to obtain their high school diplomas.

1540   State of Connecticut Board of Education & Services for the Blind
184 Windsor Avenue
Windsor, CT 06095   860-602-4000
                               Fax: 860-602-4020
                               TDD: 860-602-4002
                                    www.ct.go
                                    besb@po.state.ct.us

Dannel P. Malloy, Governor
Brian S Sigman, Executive Director
Provide quality educational and rehabilitative service to all people who are legally blind or deaf-blind and children who are visually impaired at no cost to our clients or their families.

Delaware

1541   Client Assistance Program (CAP)
254 E Camden Wyoming Ave
Camden, DE 19934-1303   302-698-9336
                                     800-640-9336
                               Fax: 302-698-9338
www.manta.com/c/mmpgrv5/client-assistanc
                charlesdmoore@comcast.net
Melissa Shahan, Executive Director
Provides free services to consumers and applicants for projects, programs and facilities funded under the Rehabilitation Act.

1542   Community Legal Aid Society
100 W 10th St
Suite 801
Wilmington, DE 19801   302-575-0660
                                     800-292-7980
                               Fax: 302-575-0840
                               TDD: 302-575-0696
                               TTY: 302-575-0696
                                    www.declasi.org
                                    clasincc@declasi.org

Keith Criddell, CAO & CFO
William J. Dunne, Esq., Executive Director
Jason D. Stoehr, Director of Development

Community Legal Aid Society is a private, non-profit law firm dedicated to equal justice for all. Prodive civil legal services to assist clients in becoming self sufficient and meeting basic needs with dignity. Clients include members of the community who have low incomes, who have disabilities, or who are age 60 and over.

1543   Correctional Education Division
Department of Corrections
245 McKee Road
Dover, DE 19904   302-857-5440
                               Fax: 302-739-8220
        http://doc.delaware.gov/victimServices.shtml
                          Gail.Stallings@state.de.us
Robert M. Coupe, Commissioner
Renee Buskirk, Victim Services Coordinator
Michael Records, PREA Coordinator

1544   Delaware Assistive Technology Initiative (DATI)
University of Delaware
461 Wyoming Road
Newark, DE 19716   302-831-0354
                                     800-870-3284
                               Fax: 302-831-4690
                               TDD: 302-651-6794
                                    www.dati.org
                                    dati-ud@udel.edu

Beth Mineo, Director
Joann McCafferty, Staff Assistant
DATI connects Delawareans who have disabilities with the tools they need in order to learn, work, play, and participate in community life safely and independently. DATI also operates Assistive Technology Resource Centers that offer training as well as no-cost equipment demonstrations and loans. DATI also provides funding information, develops partnerships with state agencies and organizations, and publishes resource materials and event calendars.

1545   Delaware Department of Education
401 Federal Street
John G. Townsend Building
Dover, DE 19901   302-735-4000
                               Fax: 302-739-4654
                                    www.doe.k12.de.us
                                    deeds@doe.k12.de.us

Jack Markell, Governor
Mary Kate McLaughlin, Chief of Staff
Valerie Woodruff, Secretary
Committed to promoting the highest quality education for every Delaware student by providing visionary leadership and superior service.

1546   Delaware Department of Labor
4425 N Market St
Wilmington, DE 19802-1307   302-761-8085
                               Fax: 302-761-6634
                                    www.delawareworks.com
                                    dlabor@state.de.us

Thomas Sharp, Secretary
Connects people to jobs, resources, monetary benefits, workplace protections and labor market information to promote financial independence, workplace justice and a strong economy.

1547   State GED Administration: Delaware
Department of Education
401 Federal Street
John G. Townsend Building
Dover, DE 19901   302-735-4000
                               Fax: 302-739-4654
                                    www.doe.k12.de.us
                                    deeds@doe.k12.de.us

Jack Markell, Governor
Mary Kate McLaughlin, Chief of Staff
Valerie Woodruff, Secretary
The primary aid of the GED testing program in Delaware is to provide a second opportunity for individuals to obtain their high school diplomas.

District of Columbia

1548 Client Assistance Program (CAP): District of Columbia
University Legal Services
220 I Street, N.E.
Suite 130
Washington, DC 20002 202-547-0198
Fax: 202-547-2662
www.uls-dc.org
jcooney@uls-dc.org
Jane M. Brown, Esq., Executive Director
Sandy Bernstein, Esq., Legal Director
Alicia C. Johns, AT Program Director
A federally funded program authorized under the amended Rehabilitation Act of 1973. University Legal Services administers the CAP program i the District of Columbig under contract with the District of Columbia Rehabilitation Services Administration. The goal of CAP is to identify, explain, and resolve the problems residents of the District of Columbia may be having with the rehabilitation program as quickly as possible.

1549 DC Department of Employment Services
Government of the District of Columbia
Ste 3000
64 New York Ave NE
Washington, DC 20002-3320 202-724-7000
Fax: 202-673-6993
TDD: 202-673-6994
TTY: 202-673-6994
www.does.dc.gov
does@dc.gov
Vincent C. Gray, Mayor
Summer Spencer, Director
The mission of the Department of Employment Services is to plan, develop and administer employment-related services to all segments of the Washington, DC metropolitan population. We achieve our mission through empowering and sstaining a diverse workforce, which enables all sectors of the community to achieve economic and social stability.

1550 District of Columbia Department of Corrections
Government of the District of Columbia
Room 203 N
1923 Vermont Ave NW
Washington, DC 20001-4125 202-673-7316
Fax: 202-671-2043
http://doc.dc.gov
doc@dc.gov
Vincent C. Gray, Mayor
Devon Brown, Director
Provides public safety by ensuring the safe, secure, and human confinement of pertrial detainees and sentenced misdemeanant prisoners.

1551 District of Columbia Fair Employment Practice Agencies
DC Office of Human Rights
Suite 570 N
414 4th St NW
Washington, DC 20001 202-727-4559
Fax: 202-727-9589
TTY: 202-727-8673
www.ohr.dc.gov
ohr@dc.gov
Vincent C. Gray, Mayor
Gustavo F Velasquez, Director
The DC Office of Human Rights is an agency of the District of Columbia government that seeks to eradicate discrimination, increase equal opportunity, and protect human rights in the city. The Office is also the advocate for the practice of good human relations and mutual understanding among the various racial ethnic and religious groups in the District of Columbia.

1552 Office of Civil Rights: District of Columbia
US Department of Education
400 Maryland Avenue, SW
Washington, DC 20202 202-245-7488
800-872-5327
Fax: 303-844-4303
TDD: 877-521-2172
www.ed.gov.ocr
ocr.dc@ed.gov
Emma Vadehra, Chief of Staff
Eric Waldo, Senior Advisor
John Easton, Director
This office covers the states of District of Columbia, North Carolina, South Carolina and Virginia.

1553 Office of Human Rights: District of Columbia
Government of the District of Columbia
Ste 570 N
441 4th St NW
Washington, DC 20001-2714 202-727-4559
Fax: 202-724-3786
http://ohr.dc.gov
ohr@dc.gov
Vincent C. Gray, Mayor
Gustavo F Velasquez, Director
The DC Office of Human Rights is an agency of the District of Columbia government that seeks to eradicate discrimination, increase equal opportunity, and protect human rights in the city.

1554 Protection and Advocacy Program: Districtof Columbia
University Legal Services
220 I Street, N.E.
Suite 130
Washington, DC 20002 202-547-0198
Fax: 202-547-2662
www.uls-dc.org
jbrown@uls-dc.org
Jane M. Brown, Esq., Executive Director
Sandy Bernstein, Esq., Legal Director
Alicia C. Johns, AT Program Director
A program authorized by federal law to help the District of Columbia residents with developemntal disabilities exercise their full rights as citizens.

Florida

1555 Client Assistance Program (CAP): Advocacy Center for Persons with Disabilities
2728 Centerview Drive
Suite 102
Tallahassee, FL 32301 850-488-9071
800-342-0823
Fax: 850-488-8640
TDD: 800-346-4127
www.disabilityrightsflorida.org
Catherine Beth Piecora, Chair
Minerva Vazquez, Vice Chair
Gary Weston, Executive Director
Assists anyone with a disability that is interested in applying for and receiving services from rehabilitation programs, projects or facilities funded under the Rehabilitation Act.

1556 Florida Department of Labor and Employment Security
2571 Executive Center Dr
Tallahassee, FL 32301 850-414-4615
Fax: 850-921-1459
Sandra Bell, Manager

1557   **Florida Fair Employment Practice Agency**
Florida Commission on Human Relations
2009 Apalachee Parkway
Suite 100
Tallahassee, FL 32301   850-488-7082
                                          800-342-8170
                                     Fax: 850-488-5291
                                  http://fchr.state.fl.us
                           fchrinfo@fchr.myflorida.com
Michelle Wilson, Executive Director
To prevent unlawful discrimination by ensuring people in
Florida are treated fairly and are given access to opportuni-
ties in employment, housing, and certain public accommo-
dations; and to promote mutual respect among groups
through education and partnerships.

Georgia

1558   **Client Assistance Program (CAP): Georgia Division of
Persons with Disabilities**
123 N. McDonough Street
Decatur, GA 30030   404-373-2040
                                          800-822-9727
                                     Fax: 404-373-4110
                                     TTY: 404-373-2040
                                  www.georgiacap.com
                           acarraway@georgiacap.com
Charles L Martin, Director
Ashley Carraway, Assistant Director
Jennifer Page, Counselor
Advocacy counseling and other services for persons with
disabilities.

1559   **Georgia Advocacy Office**
150 East Ponce de Leon Avenue
Suite 430
Decatur, GA 30030   404-885-1234
                                          800-537-2329
                                     Fax: 404-378-0031
                                     TDD: 800-537-2329
                                      www.thegao.org
                                      info@thegao.org
Ruby Moore, Executive Director
Mona Givens, Director of Investigations
Stacey Smith, Advocate
Our mission is to work with and for oppressed and vulnera-
ble individuals in Georgia who are labeled as disabled of
mentally ill of secure their protection and advocacy.

1560   **Georgia Department of Technical & Adult Education**
Technical College System of Georgia
Ste 400
1800 Century Pl NE
Atlanta, GA 30345-4304   404-679-1625
                                     Fax: 404-679-1630
                                      www.dtae.org
Ron Jackson, Commissioner
The Georgia Department of Technical and Adult Education
oversees the state's system of technical colleges, the adult
literacy program, and a host of economic and workforce de-
velopment programs

1561   **Governor's Council on Developmental Disabilities**
2 Peachtree St NW
Suite 26-246
Atlanta, GA 30303   404-657-2126
                                          888-273-4233
                                     Fax: 404-657-2132
                                     TDD: 404-657-2133
                                      www.gcdd.org
                           eric.jacobson@gcdd.ga.gov
Gary Childers, Chief Financial Officer
Eric Jacobson, Executive Director
D'Arcy Robb, Public Policy Director

To collaborate with Georgia citizens, public and private advocacy organizations, and policy makers to positively influence ppublic policies that enhance the quality of life for
people with developmental disabilities and their families.

1562   **Office of Civil Rights: Georgia**
US Department of Education
400 Maryland Avenue, SW
Washington, DC 20202   202-245-7488
                                          800-872-5327
                                     Fax: 303-844-4303
                                     TDD: 877-521-2172
                                      www.ed.gov
                                  ocr.atlanta@ed.gov
Emma Vadehra, Chief of Staff
Eric Waldo, Senior Advisor
John Easton, Director
This office covers the states of Florida, Georgia and Tennes-
see

1563   **Region IV: Office of Civil Rights**
Sam Nun Atlanta Federal Center
200 Independence Avenue, S.W.
Washington, DC 20201   877-696-6775
                                          877-696-6775
                                     Fax: 877-696-6775
                                      www.hhs.gov
                           chris.downing@hhs.gov
Kathleen Falk, Regional Director
Kim Gillan, Regional Director
Stephene Moore, Regional Director

1564   **State Department of Education**
Department of Technical and Adult Education
205 Jesse Hill Jr. Drive SE
Atlanta, GA 30334   404-656-2800
                                          800-311-3627
                                     Fax: 404-651-8737
                           www.gadoe.org/Pages/Home.aspx
                                  askdoe@gadoe.org
Jean DeVard-Kem MD, Assistant Commissioner
Debbie Caputo, Administrative Assistant

1565   **State GED Administration: Georgia**
GA Department of Technical and Adult Education
Ste 555
1800 Century Pl NE
Atlanta, GA 30345-4311   404-679-1621
                                     Fax: 404-679-4911
                                  www.dtae.tec.ga.us
                                      klee@dtae.org
Kimberly Lee, Director GED
The primary aid of the GED testign program in Georgia is to
provide a second opportunity for individuals to obtain their
high school diplomas.

1566   **Tools for Life, the Georgia Assistive Technology Act
Program**
Georgia Institute of Technology/AMAC
512 Means Street
Suite 250
Atlanta, GA 30318   404-894-0541
                                          800-497-8665
                                     TDD: 866-373-7778
                                      www.gatfl.org
                                      info@gatfl.org
Carolyn P Phillips M.Ed., ATP, Program Director
Ben Jacobs, Accommodations Specialist
Liz Persaud, Coordinator
The Tools for Life lists local and national training opportu-
nities coming to Georgia.

Hawaii

1567   Correctional Education
Department of Public Safety
919 Ala Moana Boulevard
Suite 405
Honolulu, HI 96814   808-587-1279
                                  Fax: 808-587-1280
                    http://hawaii.gov/psd/corrections
                              maureen@smsii.com
Martha Torney, Deputy Director of Admin
Ted Sakai, Director
Max Otani, Deputy Director of Corrections

1568   Hawaii Disability Rights Center
1132 Bishop Street
Suite 2102
Honolulu, HI 96813   808-949-2922
                                       800-882-1057
                                  Fax: 808-949-2928
                    www.hawaiidisabilityrights.org
                    info@hawaiidisabilityrights.org
Sharon Smockhoffmann, President
Kirby Shaw, VP
Pauline Arellano, Treasurer

1569   Hawaii State Council on Developmental Disabilities
919 Ala Moana Blvd.
Suite 113
Honolulu, HI 96814   808-586-8100
                                  Fax: 808-586-7543
                                       www.hiddc.org
                                  council@hiddc.org
Waynette Cabral, Executive Administrator
El Doi, Program Specialist - Kaua'i
Susan Kawano, Secretary
To support people with developmental disabilities to control
their own destiny and determine the quality of life they
desire.

1570   State GED Administration: Hawaii
Community Education Section
475 22nd Avenue
Room 202
Honolulu, HI 96816   808-203-5511
                                  Fax: 808-733-9154
                    www.gedtestingservice.com/testers/ged-te
Annette Young-Ogata, GED Administrator

Idaho

1571   Disability Rights Idaho
Comprehensive Advocacy (Co-Ad)
4477 Emerald Street
Suite B-100
Boise, ID 83706-2066   208-336-5353
                                       800-632-5125
                                  Fax: 208-336-5396
                                  TDD: 208-336-5353
                        www.disabilityrightsidaho.org
                        info@disabilityrightsidaho.org
James R Baugh, Executive Director
Mary Jo Butler, Legal Director
Dina Flores Brewer, Advocacy Director
Comprehensive Advocacy, Inc is the designated Protection
and Advocacy System for Idaho. Co-Ad provides advocacy
for people with disabilities who have been abused/ne-
glected; denied services or benefits; have experienced rights
violations or discrimination because of their disability; or
have voting accessibility problems. Co-Ad provides information & referral; negotitation & mediation; short term &
technical assistance; legal advice/representation.

1572   Idaho Assistive Technology Project
121 W. Sweet Avenue
Moscow, ID 83843   208-885-3557
                                       800-432-8324
                                  Fax: 208-885-6145
                                       www.idahoat.org
                                  idahoat@uidaho.edu
Ron Seiler, Project Director
Cathy Hart, Advisory Council Member
Larry Henrie, Advisory Council Member
The Idaho Assistive Technology Project)IATP) is a federally funded program managed by the Center on Disabilities
and Human Development at the University of Idaho. The
goal of IATP is to increase the availability of assistive technology devices and services for Idahoans with disabilities.
The IATP offers free trainings and technical assistance, a
low-interest loan program, assistive technology assessments for children and agriculture workers, and free
informational materials.

1573   Idaho Department of Education
650 West State Street
PO Box 83720
Boise, ID 83720-0027   208-332-6800
                                       800-432-4601
                                  Fax: 208-334-2228
                                       www.sde.idaho.gov
                                  cwells@sde.idaho.gov
Camille Wells, Communications Director
Tom Luna, Superintendent
Determined to create a customer-driven education system
that meets the needs of every student in Idaho and prepares
them to live, work and succeed in the 21st century.

1574   Idaho Division of Vocational Rehabilitation
650 W. State St.
Room 150
Boise, ID 83720   208-334-3390
                                  Fax: 208-334-5305
                                       www.vr.idaho.gov
                        department.info@vr.idaho.gov
Dr Michael Graham, Administrator
A state-federal program whose goal is to assist people with
disabilities to prepare for, secure, retain or regain employ-
ment.

1575   Idaho Fair Employment Practice Agency
Idaho Human Rights Commission
317 West Main Street
Second Floor
Boise, ID 83735-0660   208-334-2873
                                       888-249-7025
                                  Fax: 208-334-2664
                        www.humanrights.idaho.gov
                          inquiry@ihrc.idaho.gov
Pamela Parks, Administrator
Tracey Rolfsen, Deputy Attorney General
Sarah Mae Fisher, Senior Civil Rights Investigator

1576   Idaho Human Rights Commission
317 West Main St
Second Floor
Boise, ID 83735-0660   208-334-2873
                                       888-249-7025
                                  Fax: 208-334-2664
                                  TDD: 208-334-4751
                                  TTY: 208-334-4751
                                       www.state.id.us
                          inquiry@ihrc.idaho.gov
Leslie L Goddard, Director
To administer state and federal andti-discrimination laws in
Idaho in a manner that is fair, accurate, and timely; and to
work towards ensuring that all people within the state are
treated with dignity and respect in their places of employment, housing, education and public accommodations.

1577 Idaho Professional Technical Education
650 West State Street
Len B. Jordan Building, Room 324
Boise, ID 83720-0095   208-334-3216
                                  Fax: 208-334-2365
                                  www.pte.idaho.gov
                                  csengel@pte.idaho.gov
Dwight Johnson, Administrator
Vera McCrink, Associate Administrator
Susan Johnson, Director, Program Standards
The primary aid of the GED testing program in Idaho is to
provide a second opportunity for individuals to obtain their
high school equivalency certificate.

1578 State Department of Education: Special Education
650 West State Street
PO Box 83720
Boise, ID 83720-0027   208-332-6800
                                       800-432-4601
                                  Fax: 208-334-2228
                                  www.sde.idaho.gov
                                  cwells@sde.idaho.gov
Camille Wells, Communications Director
Tom Luna, Superintendent
Our mission is to enable all students to achieve high aca-
demic standards and quality of life. The Special Education
Team works collaboratively with districts, agencies, and
parents to ensure students receive quality, meaningful, and
needed services.

Illinois

1579 Chicago Board of Education
Office of the Board of Education
Fl 6
125 S Clark St
Chicago, IL 60603-4016   773-553-1000
                                  Fax: 773-553-1502
                                  www.cps.edu/Pages/home.aspx
                                  kmartin@cps.k12.il.us
Rufus Williams, President
Offers instruction and information services, curriculum in-
formation and government relations advocacy.

**1580 Client Assistance Program (CAP): Illinois Department
of Human Services**
100 South Grand Avenue East
Springfield, IL 62762   217-557-1601
                                       800-843-6154
                                  TTY: 217-557-2134
                                  www.dhs.state.il.us
                                  dhscap@dhs.state.il.us
Michelle R. Saddler, Secretary
Provides free services to consumers and applicants for projects, programs and facilities funded under the Rehabilitation Act.

1581 Correctional Education
Illinois Department of Corrections
1301 Concordia Court
PO Box 19277
Springfield, IL 62794-9277   217-558-2200
                                       800-546-0844
                                  Fax: 217-522-0355
                                  www.idoc.state.il.us
                                  info@doc.illinois.gov
Pat Quinn, Governor
Jared Brunk, Chief Financial Officer
S.A. Godinez, Director

1582 DBTAC: Great Lakes ADA Center
University of Illinois at Chicago
1640 West Roosevelt Road
Room 405
Chicago, IL 60608   312-413-1407
                                       800-949-4232
                                  Fax: 312-413-1856
                                  TTY: 312-413-1407
                                  www.adagreatlakes.org
                                  adata@adagreatlakes.org
Robin Jones, Project Director
Peter Berg, Technical Assistance Coordinator
Increases awareness and knowledge with the ultimate goal
of achieving voluntary compliance with the Americans with
Disabilities Act. This is accomplished within targeted audiences through provision of customized training, expert assistance, and dissemination of information developed by
various sources, including the federal agencies responsible
for enforcement of the ADA.

**1583 Illinois Affiliation of Private Schools for Exceptional
Children**
Lawrence Hall Youth Services
4833 N. Francisco Avenue
Lawrence Hall Youth Services
Chicago, IL 60625   773-769-3500
                                  Fax: 773-769-0106
                                  www.lawrencehall.org
                                  information@lawrencehall.org
Vicki Hicks, VP, Educational Services
Greg Meadors, VP, Information Technology
Mitchell Sandy, VP, Health Services

1584 Illinois Assistive Technology
1 West Old State CapitolPlaza
Suite 100
Springfield, IL 62701   217-522-7985
                                       800-852-5110
                                  Fax: 217-522-8067
                                  TTY: 212-522-9966
                                  www.iltech.org
                                  iatp@iltech.org
Horacio Esparza, President
Celestine Willis, VP
Wilhelmina Gunther, Executive Director
The primary focus is on education, employment, community
living, information technology and telecommunications.
The mission is to enable people iwth disabilities so they can
fully participate in all aspects of life.

1585 Illinois Council on Developmental Disabilities
207 State House
Springfield, IL 62706   217-782-0244
                                  Fax: 217-524-5339
                                  TTY: 888-261-3336
                                  www.state.il.us
                                  sheila.romano@illinois.gov
Pat Quinn, Governor
Sheila Romano, Director
Dedicated to improving the lives of people with developmental disabilities through advocacy, systemic change and
capacity building. Focuses its efforts across a person's life
span so that people with developmental disabilities can enjoy life as any other Illinoisan. The Council completes its
work through a variety of methods including grant awards,
technical assistance and collaboration.

**1586 Illinois Department of Commerce and Community Af-
fairs**
JTPA Programs Division
500 E Monroe
Springfield, IL 62701-1316   217-525-9308
                                       800-785-6055
                                  Fax: 800-785-6055
                                  TDD: 800-785-6055
                                  www.commerce.state.il.us
Adam Pollet, Director
Dan Seals, Assistant Director
Kent Bozarth, Deputy Director

1587 Illinois Department of Employment Security
33 S State St
Chicago, IL 60603-2808

312-793-5280
800-244-5631
Fax: 312-793-9834
TTY: 866-322-8357
www.ides.state.il.us

James P Sledge, Director
IDES helps job seekers find jobs and employers find workers. We also analyze and publish a gold mine of information on careers and the Illinois economy.

1588 Illinois Department of Human Rights
100 W. Randolph Street
10th Floor, Intake Unit
Chicago, IL 60601

312-814-6200
Fax: 312-814-1436
TDD: 312-263-1579
TTY: 866-740-3953
www.state.il.us/dhr
susan.allen@illinois.gov

Pat Quinn, Governor
Rocco Claps, Director
Civil rights enforcement agency covering employment, housing, financial credit, public accomodation, sexual harassment in education in the State of Illinois.

1589 Illinois Department of Rehabilitation Services
100 South Grand Avenue East
Springfield, IL 62762

217-557-1601
800-843-6154
TTY: 217-557-2134
www.dhs.state.il.us
dhscap@dhs.state.il.us

Michelle R. Saddler, Secretary
Karen Engstrom, Manager

1590 Illinois Office of Rehabilitation Services
Illinois Department of Human Services
100 S Grand Avenue East
Springfield, IL 62704

217-557-1601
800-843-6154
Fax: 217-557-1647
TTY: 217-557-2134
www.dhs.state.il.us
dhscap@dhs.state.il.us

Michelle R. Saddler, Secretary
DHS' Office of Rehabilitation Services is the state's lead agency serving individuals with disabilities.

1591 Illinois State Board of Education
100 N 1st St
Springfield, IL 62777-0001

217-782-4321
866-262-6663
Fax: 217-782-9224
www.isbe.net

Christopher Koch EdD, State Superintendent, Education
Elizabeth Hanselman, Super. Specialized Instruct.
Sets educational policies and guidelines for public and private schools, preschool through grade 12, as well as vocational education. Analyzes the aims, needs and requirements of edcuation and recommends legislation to the General Assembly and Governor for the benefit of the more than 2 million school children in Illinois.

1592 Office of Civil Rights: Illinois
US Department of Education
400 Maryland Avenue, SW
Washington, DC 20202

202-245-7488
800-872-5327
Fax: 303-844-4303
TDD: 877-521-2172
www.ed.gov
ocr.atlanta@ed.gov

Emma Vadehra, Chief of Staff
Eric Waldo, Senior Advisor
John Easton, Director
This office covers the states of Illinois, Indiana, Iowa, Minnesota, North Dakota, and Wisconsin.

1593 Protection & Advocacy Agency
Equip for Equality
20 North Michigan Avenue
Suite 300
Chicago, IL 60602

312-341-0022
800-537-2632
Fax: 312-341-0295
TTY: 800-610-2779
www.equipforequality.org
contactus@equipforequality.org

Zena Naiditch, President, CEO
Deborah M. Kennedy, VP, Abuse Investigation Unit
Barry C. Taylor, VP, Civil Rights Team
The mission of Equip for Equality is to advance the human and civil rights of children and adults with physical and mental disabilities. The only state-wide cross-disability, comprehensive advocacy organization providing self-advocacy assistance, legal services, and disability rights education while also engaging in publi policy and legislative advocacy and conducting abuse investigation and other oversight activities.

1594 Region V: Civil Rights Office
US Department of Health & Human Services
200 Independence Avenue, S.W.
Washington, DC 20201

877-696-6775
877-696-6775
Fax: 877-696-6775
www.hhs.gov
chris.downing@hhs.gov

Kathleen Falk, Regional Director
Kim Gillan, Regional Director
Stephene Moore, Regional Director

1595 Region V: US Department of Labor: Office of Federal Contract Compliance
US Department of Labor
200 Constitution Ave. NW
Washington, DC 20210

312-596-7010
866-4-USA-DO
Fax: 312-596-7044
www.dol.gov
ofccp-mw-preaward@dol.gov

Thomas E. Perez, Secretary of Labor
Christopher Lu, Deputy Secretary of Labor
Matthew Colangelo, Chief of Staff
These regional offices of agencies enforce laws prohibiting employment discrimination on the basis of disability.

1596 Region V: US Small Business Administration
500 W. Madison Street
Suite 1150
Chicago, IL 60661

312-353-4528
Fax: 312-886-5688
www.sba.gov
answerdesk@sba.gov

Robert S. Steiner, District Director
Mark Quinn, District Director, California
Ralph Ross, District Director, Kentucky
These regional offices of agencies enforce laws prohibiting employment discrimination on the basis of disability.

Indiana

1597 Assistive Technology
Ste G
5333 Commerce Square Dr
Indianapolis, IN 46237-8627

800-528-8246
www.attaininc.org
attaininfo@attaininc.org

Gary Hand, Executive Director
Mary Duffer, Executive Assistant
Provide direct service programs and creates structural change in the public and private sectors to promote the availability and use of Assistive Technology.

1598 Indiana ATTAIN Project
Indiana Family and Social Services Administration
P.O.Box 7083
Indianapolis, IN 46207-7083
317-233-0800
800-457-8283
www.in.gov/fssa

Mike Pence, Governor
Mitch Robb, Director
Rita Anderson, Executive Director

1599 Indiana Department of Correction
Rm E334
302 W Washington St
Indianapolis, IN 46204-2762
317-232-1746
800-457-8283
Fax: 317-233-4948
www.in.gov
rkoester@idoc.in.gov

Mike Pence, Governor
Mitch Robb, Director
Rita Anderson, Executive Director
To maintain public safety and provide offenders with self
improvement programs, job skills and family values in an efficient and cost effective manner for a successful return to
the community as law-abiding citizens.

**1600 Indiana Department of Workforce Development Dis-
ability Program Navigator**
10 N Senate Ave
Indianapolis, IN 46204-2277
317-232-6702
800-891-6499
Fax: 317-233-4793
www.in.gov/dwd
bcarvin@dwd.in.gov

Scott B. Sanders, Commissioner
Randy Gillespie, Chief Financial Officer
Jeff Gill, General Counsel
Provides guidance to employers on the hiring of individuals
with disabilities as well as additional tax credits and assistance for their employers. Also provide assistance to schools
on transition to work needs of students with disabilities.
Guides individuals with disabilities through the career services available in our WorkOne Centers as they obtain
employment.

1601 Indiana Protection & Advocacy Services
Ste 222
4701 N Keystone Ave
Indianapolis, IN 46205-1561
317-722-5555
800-457-8283
Fax: 317-722-5564
TTY: 800-838-1131
www.in.gov
kpedevilla@ipas.IN.gov

Mike Pence, Governor
Thomas Gallagher, Executive Director
Mitch Robb, Director
Created to protect and advocate the rights of people with disabilities and is Indiana's federally designated Protection and
Advocacy system and client assistance program. An independent state agency, which recieves no state funding and is
independent from all service providers, as required by
federal and state law.

1602 State Department of Education
115 W. Washington Street
South Tower, Suite 600
Indianapolis, IN 46204
317-232-6610
800-527-4931
Fax: 317-232-8004
www.doe.in.gov
webmaster@doe.in.gov

Glenda Ritz, Superintendent
John Barnes, Director of Legislative Affairs
Jeffrey Coyne, Director of Federal Relations
Mission is to fulfill its statutory responsibilty by establish-
ing policies that promote excellence in learning for all
students.

1603 State GED Administration
Office of Adult Education
115 W. Washington Street
South Tower, Suite 600
Indianapolis, IN 46204
317-232-6610
Fax: 317-232-8004
www.doe.in.gov
webmaster@doe.in.gov

Glenda Ritz, Superintendent
John Barnes, Director of Legislative Affairs
Jeffrey Coyne, Director of Federal Relations

Iowa

**1604 Client Assistance Program (CAP): Iowa Division of Per-
sons with Disabilities**
2nd Floor
Lucas State Office Building
Des Moines, IA 50319
888-219-0471
Fax: 515-242-6119
TTY: 888-219-0471
www.iowa.gov
dhr.disabilities@iowa.gov

Jill Fulitano-Avery, Administrator
Exists to promote the employment of Iowans with disabilities and reduce barriers to employment by providing information, referral, assessment and guidance, training and
negotiation services to employers and citizens with
disabilities.

1605 Governor's Council on Developmental Disabilities
617 E 2nd St
Des Moines, IA 50309-1831
515-281-9082
866-432-2846
Fax: 515-281-9087
http://idaction.com
fmorris@dhs.state.ia.us

Becky Harker, Executive Director
Identifies, develops and promotes public policy and support
practices through capacity building, advocacy, and systems
change activities. The purpose is to ensure that people with
developmental disabilities and their families are included in
planning, decision making, and development of policy related to services and supports that affect their quality of life
and full participation in communities of their choice.

1606 Iowa Department of Education
400 E 14th Street
Des Moines, IA 50319-0146
515-281-5294
Fax: 515-242-5988
www.iowa.gov/educate
judy.jeffrey@iowa.gov

Brad Buck, Director
Nicole Proesch, Legal Director
Ryan Wise, Deputy Director, Communications
Champion excellence in education through superior leadership and services. Committed to high levels of learning,
achievement and performance for all students, so they will
become successful members of their community and the
workforce.

1607 Iowa Employment Service
1000 East Grand Avenue
Des Moines, IA 50319-0209
515-281-5387
800-562-4692
TTY: 800-562-4692
www.iowajobs.gov
IWD.CustomerService@iwd.iowa.gov

1608 Iowa Welfare Programs
Iowa Department of Human Services
5th Floor
Hoover State Building
Des Moines, IA 50319
    515-281-5452
Fax: 515-281-4940
TDD: 800-735-2942
www.dhs.state.ia.us
kconcan@dhs.state.ia.us
Kevin Concannon, Executive Director
Sally Cunningham, Deputy Director
Dan Gilbert, Administrator
To provide assistance to families in need in the Des Moines area.

1609 Iowa Workforce Investment Act
Department of Economic Development
200 E Grand Ave
Des Moines, IA 50309-1856
    515-725-3000
Fax: 515-725-3010
TDD: 800-735-2934
www.iowalifechanging.com
info@iowa.gov
David Lyons, Executive Director
Mike Blouin, Director
Deb Townsend, Web Specialist
Job placement and training services. Especially for those workers who have been laid off, or have other barriers to steady employment.

1610 Learning Disabilities Association of Iowa
321 E 6th St
Des Moines, IA 50329-0001
    515-280-8558
888-690-5324
Fax: 515-243-1902
www.lda-ia.org
kathylda@askresource.org
Vicki Goshon, President
Dr Richard Owens, Past President
Joy Hauge, Treasurer
Dedicated to identifying causes and promoting prevention of learning disabilities and to enhancing the quality of life for all individuals with learning disabilities and their families.

1611 Protection & Advocacy Services
Ste 300
400 East Court Ave
Des Moines, IA 50309-2548
    515-278-2502
800-779-2502
Fax: 515-278-0539
TTY: 515-278-0571
www.ipna.org
info@ipna.org
Sylvia Piper, President
A federally funded program that will protect and advocate for the human and legal rights that ensure individuals with disabilities and/or mental illness a free, appropriate public education, employment opportunities and residence or treatment in the least restricitve environment or method and for freedom from stigma.

Kansas

1612 Disability Rights Center of Kansas
635 SW Harrison St.
Suite 100
Topeka, KS 66603-3726
    785-273-9661
877-776-1541
Fax: 785-273-9414
TDD: 877-335-3725
www.drckansas.org
Rocky Nichols, M.P.A., Executive Director
Debbie White, C.P.A., Deputy Director
Lane Williams, J.D., Deputy Director, Legal Division

Provides free services to consumers and applicants for projects, programs and facilities funded under the rehabilitation act.

1613 Kansas Adult Education Association
Barton County Community College
Barton Community College
245 NE 30 Rd
Great Bend, KS 67530
    620-792-2701
800-748-7594
www.bartonccc.edu
Dr. Carl Heilman, Ph.D., President
Todd Moore, Director for Admission
Cassandra Montoya, Student Work Services
The Kansas Adult Education Association has been the professional association for adult educators at community colleges, school districts, and non-profit organizations.

1614 Kansas Department of Labor
401 SW Topeka Blvd
Topeka, KS 66603-3182
    785-296-5000
Fax: 785-296-0179
www.dol.ks.gov
Jim Garner, Secretary
Formerly the Kansas Department of Human Resources, advances the economic well being of all Kansans through responsive workforce services.

1615 Kansas Department of Social and Rehabilitation Services
500 SW VanBuren
Topeka, KS 66603-1505
    785-296-2500
Fax: 785-296-5895
TDD: 785-296-4026
TTY: 785-296-4026
www.srskansas.org
Robbie Berry, Secretary
To protect children and promote adult self-sufficiency.

1616 Kansas Human Rights Commission
900 SW Jackson
Suite 568-S
Topeka, KS 66612-1258
    785-296-3206
888-793-6874
Fax: 785-296-0589
TTY: 785-296-0245
www.khrc.net
khrc@ink.org
Melvin Neufeld, Chair
Terry Crowder, Vice Chair
Ruth Glover, Executive Director
To prevent and eliminate discrimination and assure equal opportunities in all employment relations, to eliminate profiling in conjunction with traffic stops, to eliminate and prevent discrimination, segregation or separation, and assure equal opportunities in all places of public accommodations an in housing.

1617 Kansas State Department of Education
120 SE 10th Ave
Topeka, KS 66612-1182
    785-291-3097
Fax: 785-296-6715
www.ksde.org
contact@ksde.org
Alexa Posney, Commissioner
Promotes the mission of the Kansas State Board of Education through leadership and support for student learning in Kansas.

1618 Kansas State GED Administration
Kansas Board of Regents
1000 SW Jackson Street
Suite 520
Topeka, KS 66612-1368
    785-296-3421
Fax: 785-296-0983
www.kansasregents.org
cpuderbaugh@ksbor.org
Reginald L Robinson, President/CEO
Crystal Puderbaugh, State GED Administrator

Promotes adult education.

1619 Office of Disability Services
Wichita State University
1845 Fairmount
P.O. Box 0132
Wichita, KS 67260-0132

316-978-3309
Fax: 316-978-3114
TDD: 316-978-3391
www.wichita.edu
grady.landrum@wichita.edu

Grady Landrum, Director
Kathy Stewart, Assistant Director
Christina Gregory, Senior Administrative Assistant
To enable students, staff, faculty and guests of Wichita State University to achieve their educational goals, both personal and academic, to the fullest of their abilities by providing and coordinating accessibility services which afford individuals with learning, mental or physical disabilities the equal opportunity to attain these goals.

1620 State Literacy Resource Center
Kansas Board of Regents Adult Education
1000 SW Jackson Street
Suite 520
Topeka, KS 66612-1368

785-296-3421
Fax: 785-296-0983
www.kansasregents.org
dglass@ksbor.org

Reginald L Robinson, President/CEO
Michelle Carson, Associate Director
Dianne Glass, Director

Kentucky

1621 Assistive Technology Office
200 Juneau Drive
Suite 200
Louisville, KY 40243

502-429-4484
800-327-5287
Fax: 502-429-7114
www.katsnet.org
chase.forrester@ky.gov

Derrick Cox, Director
To make assistive technology information, devices and services easily obtainable for people of any age and/or disability.

1622 Kentucky Adult Education
Council on Postsecondary Education
1024 Capital Center Drive
Suite 250
Frankfort, KY 40601

502-573-5114
800-928-7323
Fax: 502-573-5436
TTY: 502-573-5114
www.kyae.ky.gov
ginny.sullivan@ky.gov

Ginny Sullivan, Executive Secretary
To provide a responsive and innovative adult education system that enables students to acheive and prosper.

1623 Kentucky Client Assistance Program
275 East Main Street
2nd Floor, Mail Stop 2EJ
Frankfort, KY 40601

502-564-8035
800-633-6283
Fax: 502-564-1566
http://kycap.ky.gov
vickil.staggs@ky.gov

Vicki Staggs, Contact
Provides advocacy for persons with disabilities who are clients or applicants of the Office of Vocational Rehabilitation or the Office for the Blind and are having problems receiving services.

1624 Kentucky Department of Corrections
Health Services Building
275 East Main Street
P.O. Box 2400
Frankfort, KY 40602-2400

502-564-4726
Fax: 502-564-5037
www.corrections.ky.gov

LaDonna H. Thompson, Commissioner
Kimberly Potter Blair, Deputy Commissioner
Paula Holden, Deputy Commissioner
To protect the citizens of the Commonwealth and to provide a safe, secure and human environment for staff and offenders in carrying out the mandates of the legislative and judicial processes; and to provide opportunities for offenders to acquire skills which facilitate non-criminal behavior.

1625 Kentucky Department of Education
Capital Plaza Tower
500 Mero St.
Frankfort, KY 40601

502-564-4770
Fax: 502-564-7749
TTY: 502-564-4970
www.education.ky.gov
melissa.terrell@education.ky.gov

Ken Draut, Commissioner

1626 Kentucky Protection and Advocacy
100 Fair Oaks Lane
Frankfort, KY 40601

502-564-2967
800-372-2988
Fax: 502-564-0848
www.kypa.net

Marsha Hockensmith, Executive Director
An independent state agency that was designated by the Governor as the protection and advocacy agency for Kentucky. To protect and promote the rights of Kentuckians with disabilities through legally based individuals and systemic advocacy, and education.

1627 Learning Disabilities Association of Kentucky
2210 Goldsmith Lane
#118
Louisville, KY 40218

502-473-1256
877-587-1256
Fax: 502-473-4695
www.ldaofky.org
Info@LDAofKy.org

Tim Woods, Executive Director

Louisiana

1628 Client Assistance Program (CAP): Louisiana HDQS Division of Persons with Disabilities
Advocacy Center
8325 Oak Street
New Orleans, LA 70118

504-522-2337
800-960-7705
Fax: 504-522-5507
TTY: 855-861-3577
www.advocacyla.org
AdvocacyCenter@AdvocacyLA.org

John Felt, Chief Information Officer
Lois Simpson, Executive Director
Charles Tubre, Program Director
Advocacy services to applicants and clients of Louisiana Rehabilitation Services (LRS) and American Indian Rehabilitation Services (AIRS). No fee. Committed to the belief in the dignity of every life and the freedom of everyone to experience the highest degree of self-determination. Exists to protect and advocate for human and legal rights of the elderly and disabled. Umbrella organization for Advocacy Centers in Baton Rouge, Lafayette, Shreveport, Monroe, Pineville, Jackson, and Mandeville.

1629 Client Assistance Program (CAP): Shreveport Division of Persons with Disabilities
Advocacy Center
2620 Centenary Blvd.
Bldg. 2, Suite 248
Shreveport, LA 71104   318-227-6186
                               800-960-7705
                          Fax: 318-227-1841
                          www.advocacyla.org
                          dmirvis@advocacyla.org
John Felt, Chief Information Officer
Lois Simpson, Executive Director
Charles Tubre, Program Director
Advocacy services for applicants and clients of Louisiana Rehabilitation Services (LRS) and American Indian Rehabilitation Services (AIRS). No fee.

1630 Correctional Education
Louisiana Department of Education
P.O.Box 94064
Baton Rouge, LA 70804-9064   225-383-4761
                                     877-453-2721
                                Fax: 225-342-0193
                                www.doe.state.la.us
George Nelson, President
Cosby Joiner, Director
Promotes quality correctional education.

1631 Louisiana Assistive Technology Access Network
3042 Old Forge Drive, Suite D
PO Box 14115
Baton Rouge, LA 70898   225-925-9500
                                800-270-6185
                           Fax: 225-925-9560
                           www.latan.org
                           cpourciau@latan.org
Julie Nesbit, ATP, President/CEO
Clara Pourciau, VP
Maria Yiannopoulos, Public Information Officer
Assists individuals with disabilities to achieve a higher quality of life and greater independence through increased access to assistive technology as part of their daily lives.

1632 State Department of Education
Department of Education
P.O.Box 94064
Baton Rouge, LA 70804-9064   225-383-4761
                                     877-453-2721
                                Fax: 225-342-0193
                                www.louisianabelieves.com
                                customerservice@la.gov
George Nelson, President
Cosby Joiner, Director
Paul G Pastorek, Superintendent

1633 State GED Administration
Louisiana Department of Education
P.O.Box 94604
Baton Rouge, LA 70804-9064   225-383-4761
                                     877-453-2721
                                Fax: 225-342-0193
                                www.doe.state.la.us
George Nelson, President
Cosby Joiner, Director
Debi K Faucette, Director
Promotes quality education.

Maine

1634 Adult Education Team
Maine Department of Education
23 State House Station
Augusta, ME 04333-0023   207-624-6752
                            Fax: 207-624-6821
                            www.maine.gov
                            jeff.fantine@maine.gov

Paul R. LePage, Governor
Joseph Ponte, Commissioner
Jonathan P. Labonte, Director

1635 Bureau of Rehabilitation Services
Department of Labor
150 State House Station
Augusta, ME 04333-0150   800-698-4440
                            Fax: 207-287-5292
                            TTY: 888-755-0023
                            www.maine.gov
Paul R. LePage, Governor
Joseph Ponte, Commissioner
Jonathan P. Labonte, Director
Works to bring about full access to employment, independence and community integration for people with disabilities.

1636 Client Assistance Program (CAP) C.A.R.E.S., Inc.
CARES
134 Main St
Suite 2C
Winthrop, ME 04364   207-377-7055
                             800-773-7055
                        Fax: 207-377-7057
                        www.caresinc.org
                        steve.beam@caresinc.com
Stephen Beam, Executive Director
Kathy Despres, Program Director
Jenny Ardito, Advocate
A federally funded program that provides information, assistance and advocacy to people with disabilities who are applying for or receiving services under the Rehabilitation Act.

1637 Developmental Disabilities Council
225 Western Avenue
Suite 4
Augusta, ME 04330   207-287-4213
                            800-244-3990
                       Fax: 207-287-8001
                       www.maineddc.org
                       nancy.e.cronin@maine.gov
Nancy Cronin, Executive Director
Rachel Dyer, Associate Director
Erin Howes, Office Manager
A partnership of people with developmental disabilities, family memebers, and state and local agencies and organizations. The purpose is to assure that individuals with disabilities and their families participate in the design of, and have access to needed community services, individualized supports, and other forms of assistance thqat promote-self determination, independence, productivity, integration, and inclusion in all facets of family and community life.

1638 Maine Human Rights Commission
#51 State House Station
19 Union Street
Augusta, ME 04330   207-624-6290
                       Fax: 207-624-8729
                       TTY: 888-577-6690
                       www.maine.gov/mhrc
                       amy.sneirson@mhrc.maine.gov
Amy Sneirson, Executtive Director
Barbara Archer Hirsch, Commission Counsel
Victoria Ternig, Chief Investigator
Holds the responsibility of enforcing Maine's anti-discrimination laws. The Commission investigates complaints of unlawful discrimination in employmen, housing, education, access to public accommodatoins, extension of credit, and offensive names.

1639 Protection & Advocacy Agency
Disability Rights Center
24 Stone Street
Suite 24
Augusta, ME 04330

207-626-2774
800-452-1948
Fax: 207-621-1419
TTY: 800-452-1948
www.drcme.org
advocate@drcme.org

Kim Moody, Executive Director
Rick Langley, Advocacy Director
Peter M. Rice, Esq., Legal Director
The Disability Rights Center is Maine's protection and advocacy agency for people with disabilities. To enhance and promote the equality, self-determination, independence, productivity, integratio, and inclusion of people with disabilities through education, strategoc advocacy and legal intervention.

1640 Security and Employment Service Center
Dept of Administrative and Financial Services
23 State House Station
Augusta, ME 04333-0023

207-624-6752
Fax: 207-624-6821
TTY: 800-794-1110
www.maine.gov

Paul R. LePage, Governor
Joseph Ponte, Commissioner
Jonathan P. Labonte, Director
Provides financial and human resource services to the Departments of Defense, Veterans, and Emergency Management; Labor; Professional and Financial REgulation; and, Public Safety.

Maryland

1641 Client Assistance Program (CAP) Maryland Division of Rehabilitation Services
2301 Argonne Drive
Baltimore, MD 21218

410-554-9442
888-554-0334
Fax: 410-554-9362
TDD: 410-554-9411
TTY: 410-554-9411
www.dors.state.md.us
dors@dors.state.md.us

Thomas Laverty, Director
Helps individuals who have concerns or difficulties when applying or receiving rehabiliation services funded under the Rehabilitation Act.

1642 Correctional Education
Division of Career Technology & Adult Learning
200 West Baltimore Street
Baltimore, MD 21201-2595

410-767-0100
888-246-0016
Fax: 410-333-6033
www.marylandpublicschools.org
mmechlinski@msde.state.md.us

Mark Mechlinski, Director
Provides educational programs and library services to residents of the Division of Correction and the Patuxent Institution.

1643 Disability Law Center
1500 Union Avenue
Suite 2000
Baltimore, MD 21211

410-727-6352
800-233-7201
Fax: 410-727-6389
TTY: 410-235-5387
www.mdlclaw.org
feedback@mdlclaw.org

Virginia Knowlton Marcus, Executive Director
Meghan Marsh, Director of Operations
Charmaine Glass, Director of Finance

A provate, non-profit organization staffed by attorneys and paralegals. MDLC is the Protection and Advocacy organization for Maryland. MDLC's mission is to endure that people with disabilities are accorded the full rights and entitlements afforded to them by state and federal law.

1644 Maryland Developmental Disabilities Council
217 E. Redwood Street
Suite 1300
Baltimore, MD 21202

410-767-3670
800-305-6441
Fax: 410-333-3686
www.md-council.org
BrianC@md-council.org

Brian Cox, Executive Director
Catherine Lyle, Deputy Director
Angela Castillo Epps, Director of Communications
A public policy organization comprised of people with disabilities and family memebers who are joined by state officials, service providers an dother designated partners. Also an independent, self-governing organization that represents the interests of people with developmental disabilities and their families.

1645 Maryland Technology Assistance Program
Rm T-17
2301 Argonne Dr
Baltimore, MD 21218-1628

410-554-9361
800-832-4827
Fax: 410-554-9237
TTY: 866-881-7488
www.mdtap.org
mdtap@mdtap.org

Beth Lash, Executive Director
Provides tools to help people who are disabled or elderly enjoy the same rights and opportunities as other citizens.

1646 State Department of Education
200 West Baltimore Street
Baltimore, MD 21201-2595

410-767-0100
888-246-0016
Fax: 410-333-2275
TDD: 410-333-6442
www.marylandpublicschools.org
mmechlinski@msde.state.md.us

Nancy Grasmick, State Superintendent
To provide leadership, support, and accountability for effective systems of public education, library services, and rehabilitation services.

Massachusetts

1647 Autism Support Center: Northshore Arc
6 Southside Road
Danvers, MA 01923

978-777-9135
800-728-8476
Fax: 978-762-3980
http://www2.shore.net/~nsarc
asc@nsarc.org

Susan Gilroy, Director
Jerry Carthy, Executive Director
Created to support parents and professionals who expressed a need for assistance finding information and support about autism, pervasive developmental disorder (PDD) and Asperger's Disorder. Empowers families who have a member with autism or related disorder by providing current, accurate, and unbiased information about autism, services, referrals, resources and research trends.

1648 Department of Corrections
50 Maple Street
Suite 3
Milford, MA 01757-3698

508-422-3300
Fax: 508-422-3386
www.mass.gov

Harold Clark, Commissioner

Promote public safety by incarcerating offenders while providing opportunities for participation in effective programs.

1649 Massachusetts Commission Against Discrimination
One Ashburton Place
13thFloor, Room 1301
Boston, MA 02108   617-727-3200
Fax: 617-727-5732
TTY: 617-994-6196
www.mass.gov
DPSInfo@state.ma.us
Malcolm Medley, Chairman
The state's chief civil rights agency that works to eliminate discrimination on a variety of bases and areas, and strives to advance the civil rights of the people of the Commonwealth through law enforcement, outreach and training.

1650 Massachusetts General Education Development (GED)
MA Department of Elementary & Secondary Education
75 Pleasant Street
Malden, MA 02148-4906   781-338-3000
800-439 2370
www.doe.mass.edu
rmechem@doe.mass.edu
Tom Mechem, State GED Chief Examiner
Brian O'Dwyer, Operations
James O'Riordan, Operations
Thirty-two test centers operate state-wide to serve the needs of the adult population in need of a high school credential.

1651 Massachusetts Office on Disability
One Ashburton Place
13thFloor, Room 1301
Boston, MA 02108   617-727-3200
800-322-2020
Fax: 617-727-5732
TTY: 617-994-6196
www.mass.gov
Myra Berloff, Director
To bring about full and equal participation of people with disabilities in all aspects of life. It works to assure the advancement of legal rights and for the promotion of maximum opportunities, supportive services, accommodations and accessibility in a manner which fosters dignity and self determination.

1652 Massachusetts Rehabilitation Commission
600 Washington Street
Boston, MA 02211-1616   617-204-3600
800-245-6543
Fax: 617-727-1354
www.mass.gov/mrc
commissioner@mrc.state.ma.us
Charles Carr, Commissioner
Promotes dignity for individuals with disabilities through employment and independent living in the community.

1653 Office of Civil Rights: Massachusetts
US Department of Education
400 Maryland Avenue, SW
Washington, DC 20202   202-245-7488
800-872-5327
Fax: 303-844-4303
TDD: 877-521-2172
www.ed.gov
ocr.boston@ed.gov
Emma Vadehra, Chief of Staff
Eric Waldo, Senior Advisor
John Easton, Director
This office covers the states of Connecticut, Maine, Massachusetts, New Hampshire, Rhode Island and Vermont.

1654 Office of Federal Contract Compliance: Boston District Office
US Department of Labor
200 Constitution Ave. NW
Washington, DC 20210   312-596-7010
866-4-USA-DO
Fax: 312-596-7044
TDD: 617-565-9869
www.dol.gov
beatty.reba@dol.gov
Thomas E. Perez, Secretary of Labor
Christopher Lu, Deputy Secretary of Labor
Matthew Colangelo, Chief of Staff
Enforces laws prohibiting employment discrimination on the basis of disability.

1655 Protection & Advocacy Agency
Disability Law Center
11 Beacon Street
Suite 925
Boston, MA 02108   617-723-8455
800-872-9992
Fax: 617-723-9125
TTY: 617-227-9464
www.dlc-ma.org
mail@dlc-ma.org
Robert Whitney, President
A private, non-profit organization responsible for providing protection and advocacy for the rights of Massachusetts residents with disabilities.Provides legal advocacy on disability issues that promote the fundamental rights of all pepole with disabilities to participate fully and equally in the social and economic life of Massachusetts.

1656 Region I: Office for Civil Rights
US Department Health & Human Services
200 Independence Avenue, S.W.
Washington, DC 20201   877-696-6775
877-696-6775
Fax: 877-696-6775
www.hhs.gov
brian.golden@hhs.gov
Kathleen Falk, Regional Director
Kim Gillan, Regional Director
Stephene Moore, Regional Director

1657 Region I: US Small Business Administration
Massachusetts District Office
10 Causeway Street
Room 265
Boston, MA 02222   617-565-5590
www.sba.gov
Robert H Nelson, District Director
Anne Hunt, Deputy District Director
Maria Contreras Sweet, SBA Administrator
These regional offices of agencies enforce laws prohibiting employment discrimination on the basis of disability.

1658 State Department of Adult Education
Adult and Community Learning Services
75 Pleasant Street
Malden, MA 02148-4906   781-338-3000
800-439 2370
Fax: 781-388-3394
www.doe.mass.edu/acls/#
acls@doe.mass.edu
Tom Mechem, State GED Chief Examiner
Brian O'Dwyer, Operations
James O'Riordan, Operations
Adult and Community Learning Services, a unit at the MA Department of Education, oversees and improves no-cost basic educational services (ABE) for adults in Masssachusetts. ACLS's mission is to provide each and every adult with opportunities to develop literacy skills needed to qualify for further education, job training, and better employment, and to reach his/her full potential as a family member, productive worker, and citizen.

Michigan

1659 Client Assistance Program (CAP): Michigan Department of Persons with Disabilities
4095 Legacy Pkwy
Suite 500
Lansing, MI 48911-4264
517-487-1755
800-288-5923
Fax: 517-487-0827
TTY: 800-288-5923
www.mpas.org
molson@mpas.org
Kate Pew Wolters, President, Grand Rapids
Thomas Landry, First VP, Highland
Elmer L. Cerano, Executive Director
Assists people who are seeking or receiving services from Michigan Rehabilitation Services, Consumer Choice Programs, Michigan Commission for the Blind, Centers for Independent Living, and Supported Employment and Transition Programs.

1660 Michigan Correctional Educational Division
Department of Corrections: Prisoner Education Prog
206 E. Michigan Ave., Grandview Pla
PO Box 30003
Lansing, MI 48909
517-335-1426
Fax: 517-335-0045
www.michigan.gov/corrections
spencede@state.mi.us
Daniel H. Heyns, Director
The goal of the Michigan Department of Corrections is to provide the greatest amount of protection while making the most efficient use of the State's resources.

1661 Michigan Department of Community Health
201 Townsend Street
Capitol View Building
Lansing, MI 48913
517-373-3740
877-932-6424
www.michigan.gov
adulted@michigan.gov
James K. Haveman, Director
Nick Lyon, Deputy Director
Matthew Davis, M.D., Chief Medical Executive
An advocacy organization that engages in advocacy, capacity building and systemic change activities that promote self-determination, independence, productivity, integration and inclusion in all facets of community life for people with developmental disabilities.

1662 Michigan Protection and Advocacy Service
4095 Legacy Pkwy
Suite 500
Lansing, MI 48911-4264
517-487-1755
800-288-5923
Fax: 517-487-0827
TTY: 800-288-5923
www.mpas.org
molson@mpas.org
Kate Pew Wolters, President, Grand Rapids
Thomas Landry, First VP, Highland
Elmer L. Cerano, Executive Director
Advocates for people with disabilities and gives information and advice about their rights as a person with disabilities.

1663 State Department of Adult Education
Michigan Department of Labor & Economic Growth
201 N. Washington Square
5th Floor
Lansing, MI 48913
517-373-8800
877-932-6424
Fax: 517-335-3630
www.michigan.gov
adulted@michigan.gov
Dianne Duthie, Director
Promotes quality adult education.

1664 State GED Administration
DELEG
201 N. Washington Square
5th Floor
Lansing, MI 48913
517-373-1692
Fax: 517-335-3461
www.michigan.gov
heckmana@michigan.gov
Dianne Duthie, GED State Administrator
Amy Heckman, Department Analyst
Jeannie Flak, Department Technician
Promotes adult education.

Minnesota

1665 Health Services Minneapolis
University of St Thomas
Ste 110
1000 Lasalle Ave
Minneapolis, MN 55403-2025
651-962-4763
www.stthomas.edu
lifework@stthomas.edu
Brian D Dusbiber, Director
Steve Fritz, Athletic Director
Gene McGivern, Sports Information Director
Provides special services and resources to meet the unique needs of graduate students, education students (both graduate and undergraduate), and alumni/ae.

1666 Minnesota Department of Children, Families & Learning
Department of Education
1500 Highway36 West
Roseville, MN 55113
651-582-8200
Fax: 651-582-8202
www.education.state.mn.us
alice.seagren@state.mn.us
Dr. Brenda Cassellius, Commissioner
Jessie Montano, Deputy Commissioner
Charlene Briner, Chief of Staff
To improve educational achievement by establishing clear standards, measuring performance, assisting educators and increasing opportunities for life long learning.

1667 Minnesota Department of Human Rights
625 Robert Street North
Freeman Building
Saint Paul, MN 55155
651-539-1100
800-657-3704
Fax: 651-296-9042
TTY: 651-296-1283
www.humanrights.state.mn.us
Info.MDHR@state.mn.us
Kevin M. Lindsey, Commissioner
Christine Dufour, Communications
Kristi Streff, Human Resources
To make Minnesota discrimination free.

1668 Minnesota Governor's Council on Developmental Disabilities
658 Cedar Street
370 Centennial Office Building
Saint Paul, MN 55155
651-296-4018
877-348-0505
Fax: 651-297-7200
TTY: 800-627-3529
www.mnddd.org
admin.dd@state.mn.us
Colleen Wieck PhD, Executive Director
Mary Hauff, Council Member
Pamela Hoopes, Council Member
To provide information, education, and training to build knowledge, develop skills, and change attitudes that will lead to increased independence, productivit, self determination, integration and inclusion for all people with developmental disabilities and their families.

1669 Minnesota's Assistive Technology Act Program
Minnesota STAR Program
658 Cedar Street
358 Centennial Office Building
Saint Paul, MN 55155 651-201-2640
888-234-1267
Fax: 651-282-6671
www.starprogram.state.mn.us
star.program@state.mn.us
Jo Erbes, Executive Director
Jennie Delisi, Program Staff
Joan Gillum, Program Staff
STAR's mission is to help all Minnesotans with disabilities
gain access to and acquire the assistive technology they need
to live, learn, work and play. The Minnesota STAR Program
is federally funded by the Rehabilitation Services Administration in assordance with the Assistive Technology Act of
1998.

1670 Protection & Advocacy Agency
Minnesota Disability Law Center
430 1st Avenue N
Suite 300
Minneapolis, MN 55401-1780 612-332-1441
800-292-4150
Fax: 612-334-5755
TDD: 612-332-4668
www.mndlc.org
mndlc@midmnlegal.org
Cathy Haukedahl, Executive Director
Lisa Cohen, Deputy Director for Operations
Andrea Kaufman, Director of Development
To advance the dignity, self-determination and equality of
individuals with disabilities.

1671 State Department of Adult Basic Education
Department of Education
1500 Highway36 West
Roseville, MN 55113 651-582-8200
Fax: 651-582-8202
http://education.state.mn.us
mde.abe@state.mn.us
Dr. Brenda Cassellius, Commissioner
Jessie Montano, Deputy Commissioner
Charlene Briner, Chief of Staff
Offered through Minnesota's public school system, pro-
vides opportunities to obtain academic, interpersonal and
problem-solving skills necessary to live self-sufficient
lives.

Mississippi

1672 Mississippi Department of Corrections
723 N President St
Jackson, MS 39202-3021 601-359-5600
Fax: 601-359-5680
www.mdoc.state.ms.us
cepps@mdoc.state.ms.us
Christopher Epps, Commissioner
Phil Bryant, Governor
Archie Longley, Deputy Commissioner
To provide and promote public safety through efficient and
effective offender custody, care, control and treatment consistent with sound correctional prinicpals and constitutional standards.

1673 Mississippi Department of Employment Security
1235 Echelon Parkway
P.O. Box 1699
Jackson, MS 39215-1699 601-321-6000
www.mdes.ms.gov
comments@mdes.ms.gov
Tommye Dale Favre, Executive Director
Brings people and jobs together.

1674 Mississippi Project START
2550 Peachtree Street
P.O. Box 1698
Jackson, MS 39216 601-987-4872
800-852-8328
Fax: 601-364-2349
www.msprojectstart.org
contactus@msprojectstart.org
Patsy Galtelli, Project Director
Nekeba Simmons, Administrative Assistant
Jason Mac McMaster, Repair Specialist
To ensure the provision of appropriate Technology-Related
services for Mississippians with disabilities by increasing
the awareness of and access to Assistive Technology and by
helping the existing service systems to become more consumer repsonsive so that all Mississippians with disabilities
will receive appropriate Technology-related services and
devices.

1675 State Department of Adult Education
359 North West Street
P.O. Box 771
Jackson, MS 39205-0771 601-359-3513
Fax: 601-359-2198
www.mde.k12.s.us/special_education
eburnham@mdek12.state.ms.us
Ann Moore, State Director
Ellen Davis Burnham, Bureau Director, Data/Fiscal Mgt
Promotes adult education.

1676 State Department of Education
359 North West Street
P.O. Box 771
Jackson, MS 39205-0771 601-359-3513
www.mde.k12.ms.us
Dr. O. Wayne Gann, Chair
Howell Gage, Vice-Chair
Kami Bumgarner, Board of Director
Promotes quality education.

Missouri

1677 Assistive Technology
1501 NW Jefferson Street
Blue Springs, MO 64015 816-655-6700
800-647-8557
Fax: 816-655-6710
TTY: 816-655-6711
www.at.mo.gov
MoAT1501@att.net
C. Marty Exline, Director
David Baker, Program Coordinator
Eileen Belton, Program Coordinator
To increase access to assistive technology for Missourians
with all types of disabilities, of all ages.

1678 Assistive Technology Project
University of Missouri-Kansas City
5100 Rockhill Road
Kansas City, MO 64110 816-235-1000
Fax: 816-235-2662
www.umkc.edu
Murray Blackwelder, President
Carol Hintz, Assoc. Vice Chancellor
Curt Crespino, Vice Chancellor - Advancement
Promotes independent living through technology.

1679 EEOC St. Louis District Office
Robert A Young Federal Building
1222 Spruce St.
Rm 8.100
Saint Louis, MO 63103 800-669-4000
Fax: 314-539-7894
TTY: 800-669-6820
www.eeoc.gov

James R Neely Jr, Director
Jacqueline A Berrien, Chair
Barbara Seely, Regional Attorney
These regional offices of agencies enforce laws prohibiting employment discrimination on the basis of disability.

1680 Great Plains Disability and Business Technical Assistance Center (DBTAC)
100 Corporate Lake Dr
100 Corporate Lake Dr
Columbia, MO 65203-7170

573-882-3600
800-949-4232
Fax: 573-884-4925
TTY: 573-882-3600
www.adaproject.org
ada@missouri.edu

Jim De Jong, Director
Julie Brinkhoff, Assistant Director
Troy Balthazor, Information Specialist
To provide information, materials and technical assistance to individuals and entities that are covered by the Americans with Disabilities Act. In addition to the ADA, Great Plains ADA Center provides the ADA and disability-related legislation such as the Family Medical Leave Act, Workforce Investment Act and the Telecommunications Act.

1681 Missouri Protection & Advocacy Services
925 S Country Club Dr
Ste 3
Jefferson City, MO 65109

573-893-3333
866-777-7199
Fax: 573-893-4231
www.moadvocacy.org
mopasjc@embarqmail.com

Joe Wrinkle, Chair, Independence
Barbara H. French, Vice Chair, Beulah
Susan Pritchard Green, Secretary/Treasurer
A federally mandated system in the state of Missouri which provides protection of the rights of persons with disabilities through leagally-based avocacy

1682 Office of Civil Rights: Missouri
US Department of Education
400 Maryland Avenue, SW
Washington, DC 20202

202-245-7488
800-872-5327
Fax: 303-844-4303
TDD: 877-521-2172
www.ed.gov
ocr.kansascity@ed.gov

Emma Vadehra, Chief of Staff
Eric Waldo, Senior Advisor
John Easton, Director
This office covers the states of Kansas, Missouri, Nebraska, Oklahoma and South Dakota.

1683 Protection & Advocacy Agency
925 South Country Club Dr.
Jefferson City, MO 65109

573-893-3333
866-777-7199
Fax: 573-893-4231
www.moadvocacy.org
mopasjc@embarqmail.com

Joe Wrinkle, Chair, Independence
Barbara H. French, Vice Chair, Beulah
Susan Pritchard Green, Secretary/Treasurer
Protects the rights of individuals with disabilities by providing advocacy and legal services.

1684 Region VII: US Department of Health and Human Services
Office For Civil Rights
200 Independence Avenue, S.W.
Washington, DC 20201

877-696-6775
877-696-6775
Fax: 877-696-6775
TDD: 816-426-7065
www.hhs.gov/region7
frank.campbell@hhs.gov

Kathleen Falk, Regional Director
Kim Gillan, Regional Director
Stephene Moore, Regional Director

Montana

1685 Assistive Technology Project
University of Montana Rural Institute
52 Corbin Hall
University of Montana
Missoula, MT 59812

406-243-5467
800-732-0323
Fax: 406-243-4730
TTY: 800-732-0323
www.ruralinstitute.umt.edu
rural@ruralinstitute.umt.edu

Perry J. Brown, Ph.D., Provost
R. Timm Vogelsberg, Ph.D., Executive Director
Martin Blair, Executive Director
This statewide program at the University of Montana promotes assistive devices and services for persons of all ages with disabilities.

1686 Correctional Education
Montana Department of Corrections
PO Box 200113
Helena, MT 59620-0113

406-444-2511
Fax: 406-444-2701
TTY: 406-444-1421
http://mt.gov/statejobs/pocontacts.mcpx

Mike Ferriter, Director

1687 Montana Council on Developmental Disabilities (MCDD)
2714 Billings Avenue
Helena, MT 59601

406-443-4332
866-443-4332
Fax: 406-443-4192
www.mtcdd.org
deborah@mtcdd.org

Deborah Swingley, CEO
Dee Burrell, Contract Manager
The goal of the Council is to increase the indpendence, productivity, inclusion and integration into the community of people with developmental disabilities through systemic change, capacity building and advocacy activities.

1688 Montana Department of Labor & Industry
PO Box 1728
Helena, MT 59624-1728

406-444-2840
Fax: 406-444-1419
TTY: 406-444-0532
http://dli.mt.gov
dliquestions@mt.gov

Pam Bucy, Commissioner
Dore Schwinden, Deputy Commissioner
George Parisot, Office of Information Technology
Promotes the well-being of Montana's workers, employers, an dcitixens, and upholds their rights and responsibilities. Committed to being responsive to communities and businesses at the local level.

1689 Montana Office of Public Instruction
PO Box 202501
Helena, MT 59620-2501

406-444-3095
888-231-9393
http://opi.mt.gov
opisupt@mt.gov

Denise Juneau, Superintendent
Supports schools so that students acheive high standards.

1690 Office of Adult Basic and Literacy Education
Montana Office of Public Instruction
PO Box 202501
Helena, MT 59620-2501

406-444-3095
888-231-9393
http://opi.mt.gov

Denise Juneau, Superintendent
Adult education programs include basic literacy, workplace literacy, family literacy, preparation for GED, English as a Second Language and other services that provide adults and out of school youth opportunities at enhancing skills, improving parenting, and youth assistance related to employment and self-sufficiency.

1691   University of Montana's Rural Institute - MonTECH
700 SW Higgins Ave.
Suite 200
Missoula, MT 59803   406-243-5751
                                       877-243-5511
http://montech.ruralinstitute.umt.edu
montech@ruralinstitute.umt.edu
Kathy Laurin PhD, Program Director
A program of the University of Montana Rural Institute: Center for Excellence in Disability, Education, Research and Service. Specialize in Assistive Technology and oversee a variety of AT related grants and contracts. The overall goal is to develop a comprehensive, statewide system of assistive technology related assistance.

Nebraska

1692   Answers4Families: Center on Children, Families and the Law
206 South 13th Street
Suite 1000
Lincoln, NE 68588-0227   402-472-0844
                                       800-746-8420
www.answers4families.org
jwilliam@answers4families.org
Charlotte Lewis, Director
A project of the Center on Children, Families and Law at University of Nebraska. Mission is to provide info, opportunities, education and support to Nebraskans through Internet resources. The Center serves individuals with special needs and mental health disorders, foster families, caregivers, assisted living, and school nurses.

1693   Assistive Technology Partnership
3901 N 27th Street
Suite 5
Lincoln, NE 68521   402-471-0734
                                       888-806-6287
                                  Fax: 402-471-6052
http://atp.ne.gov
mark.schultz@atp.state.ne.us
Leslie Novacek, Director
Nancy Coffman, Advisory Council Chair
Greg Anderson, Advisory Council Member
Dedicated to helping Nebraskan's with disabilities, their families and professionals obtain assistive technology devices and services.

1694   Client Assistance Program (CAP): Nebraska Division of Persons with Disabilities
Nebraska Department of Education
301 Centennial Mall South
Box 94987
Lincoln, NE 68509   402-471-3656
                                       800-742-7594
                                  Fax: 402-471-0117
                                  TTY: 800-742-7594
www.cap.state.ne.us
victoria.rasmussen@cap.ne.gov
Frank Lloyd, Executive Director
The Client Assistance Program helps individuals who have concerns or difficulties when applying for or receiving rehabilitation services funded under the Rehabilitation Act.

1695   Nebraska Advocacy Services
Center for Disability Rights, Law & Advocacy
134 South 13th Street
Suite 600
Lincoln, NE 68508   402-474-3183
                                       800-422-6691
                                  Fax: 402-474-3274
www.disabilityrightsnebraska.org
info@disabilityrightsnebraska.org
Timothy F Shaw, CEO
Eric Evans, Chief Operating Officer
Tania Diaz, Legal Services Director
Created to assist individuals with disabilities and their families in protecting and advocating for their rights. From its beginning, NAS has promoted the principles of equality, self-determination, and dignity of persons with disabilities.

1696   Nebraska Department of Labor
550 S 16th St
Lincoln, NE 58508   402-471-9000
                                       800-833-7352
                                  Fax: 402-471-2318
www.dol.nebraska.gov
lmi_ne@nebraska.gov
Phillip Baker, Administrator

1697   Nebraska Equal Opportunity Commission
301 Centennial Mall South, 5th Floo
PO Box 94934
Lincoln, NE 68509-4934   402-471-2024
                                       800-642-6112
                                  Fax: 402-471-4059
www.neoc.ne.gov.
Barbara Albers, Executive Director
A state agency that investigates complaints of discrimination in employment, housing and public accomodations.

1698   State Department of Education
PO Box 94987
Lincoln, NE 68509-4987   402-471-2295
                                  Fax: 402-471-8127
www.nde.state.ne.us
vicki.l.bauer@nebraska.gov
Douglas D Christensen, Commissioner
Vicki L Bauer, Director
Organized into teams that interact to operate the agency and carry out the duties assigned by state and federal statutes and the policy directions of the State Board of Education.

1699   State GED Administration: Nebraska
Nebraska Department of Education
PO Box 94987
Lincoln, NE 68509-4987   402-471-4807
                                  Fax: 402-471-8127
www.nde.state.ne.us
vicki.l.bauer@nebraska.gov
Vicki L Bauer, Director
Douglas D Christensen, Commissioner
To provide educational opportunities for adults to improve their literacy skills to a level requisite for effective citizenship and productive employment. This includes preparation for and successful completion of the high school equivalency program.

1700   Vocational Rehabilitation
Nebraska Department of Education
203 E Stolley Park Rd
Suite B
Grand Island, NE 68801   308-385-6200
                                       800-632-3382
                                  Fax: 308-385-6104
www.vocrehab.state.ne.us
vr.grandisland@vr.ne.gov
Frank C Lloyd, Asst Commissioner of Education
The Nebraska Rehabilitation Program has people with disabilities join the workforce. Our team of experts provides direct services for employers and people with disabilities that lead to employment.

Nevada

1701 Assistive Technology
Office of Disability Services
3656 Research Way
Suite 32
Carson City, NV 89706-7932

775-687-4452
Fax: 775-687-3292
TTY: 775-687-3388
www.dhhs.nv.gov
jrosenlund@dhhs.nv.gov
John Rosenlund, NV Asst Tech Coll Proj Dir
Todd Butterworth, Bureau Chief
Promotes independent living through technology.

1702 Client Assistance Program (CAP): Nevada Division of Persons with Disability
Dpt of Employment, Training and Rehabilitation
2800 E. St. Louis Ave.
Las Vegas, NV 89104

702-486-6688
800-633-9879
Fax: 702-486-6691
TTY: 702-486-1018
www.detr.state.nv.us
detrcap@nvdetr.org

Dennis Perea, Deputy Director
Renee Olson, Administrator
Shelley Hendren, Administrator
To assist and advocate for clients and applicants in their relationships with projects, programs, and community rehabilitation programs that provide services under the Act. The program is also responsible for informing individuals with disabilities in Nevada, of the services and benefits available to them.

1703 Correctional Education and Vocational Training
Bldg 17
5500 Snyder Ave
Carson City, NV 89701-6752

775-887-3285
Fax: 775-687-6715
www.doc.nc.gov
mhall@doc.nv.gov

Jackie Crawford, Director
Marta Hall, Education Coordinator
To continue and expand an educational training program which contains literacy, ESL, numeracy, community outreach, and vocational training that will provide long-term benefits to both inmates and the Nevada community in general.

1704 Department of Employment, Training and Rehabilitation
2800 E. St. Louis Ave.
Las Vegas, NV 89104

702-486-6688
800-633-9879
Fax: 702-486-6691
TTY: 702-486-1018
www.detr.state.nv.us

Dennis Perea, Deputy Director
Renee Olson, Administrator
Shelley Hendren, Administrator
Comprised of four divisions with numerous bureaus programs, and services housed in offices throughout Nevada to provide citizens the state's premier source of employment, training, and rehabilitative programs.

1705 Nevada Bureau of Disability Adjudication
Ste 300
1050 E William St
Carson City, NV 89701-3102

775-687-4430
Fax: 775-886-0101
http://detr.state.nv.us/rehab
detrvr@nvdetr.org

Sandra Kelley, Manager
Evaluates applications from individuals with permanent disabilities to determine if they are eligible for federal Supplemental Security Income or Social Security Disability Insurance (SSDI).

1706 Nevada Disability and Law Center
6039 Eldora Ave
#C-3
Las Vegas, NV 89146

702-257-8150
888-349-3843
Fax: 702-257-8170
TTY: 702-257-8160
www.ndalc.org
lasvegas@ndalc.org

Jack Mayes, Executive Director
William Heaivilin, Supervising Rights Attorney
A private, nonprofit organization and serves as Nevada's federally mandated protection and advocacy system for the human, legal, and service rights of individuals with disabilities.

1707 Nevada Equal Rights Commission
2800 E. St. Louis Ave.
Las Vegas, NV 89104

702-486-6688
800-633-9879
Fax: 702-486-6691
TTY: 702-486-1018
www.nvdetr.org
detrnerc@nvdetr.org

Dennis Perea, Deputy Director
Renee Olson, Administrator
Shelley Hendren, Administrator
To foster the rights of all persons to seek, obtain and maintain employment, and to access services in places of public accomodation without discrimination, distinction, exclusion or restriction because of race, religion creed, color, age, sex (gender and/or orientation), disability, national origin, or ancestry.

1708 Nevada Governor's Council on Developmental Disabilities
896 W. Nye Lane
Suite 202
Carson City, NV 89703

775-684-8619
Fax: 775-684-8626
www.nevadaddcouncil.org
smanning@dhhs.nv.gov

Sherry Manning, Executive Director
Kari Horn, Projects Manager
Diana Peachay, Executive Assistant
To provide resources at the community level which promote equal opportunity and life choices for people with disabilities through which they may positively contribute to Nevada society.

1709 Nevada State Rehabilitation Council
Nevada Rehabilitation Division
2800 E. St. Louis Ave.
Las Vegas, NV 89104

702-486-6688
800-633-9879
Fax: 702-486-6691
TTY: 702-486-1018
www.detr.state.nv.su
pjjune@nvdetr.org

Dennis Perea, Deputy Director
Renee Olson, Administrator
Shelley Hendren, Administrator
To help insure vocational rehabilitation programs are consumer oriented, driven and result in employment outcomes for Nevadans with disabilities. Funding for innovation and expansions grants

1710 State Department of Adult Education
Nevada Department of Education
700 E. Fifth Street
Carson City, NV 89701

775-687-9200
Fax: 775-687-9101
http://nde.doe.nv.gov
mailto:rfitzpatrick@doe.nv.gov

Dena Durish, Director
Mindy Martini, Deputy Superintendent
Steve Canavero, Ph.D., Deputy Superintendent

To provide leadership and resources to enable all learners to gain knowledge and skills needed to achieve career and employment goals, meet civic duties and accomplish educational objective.

1711 State Department of Education

700 E. Fifth Street
Carson City, NV 89701

775-687-9200
Fax: 775-687-9101
www.doe.nv.gov

Dena Durish, Director
Mindy Martini, Deputy Superintendent
Steve Canavero, Ph.D., Deputy Superintendent
The Nevada State Board of Education acts as an advocate and visionary for all children and sets the policy that allows every child equal access to educational services, provides the vision for a premier educational system and works in partnership with other stakeholders to ensure high levels of success for all in terms of job readiness, graduation, ability to be lifelong learners, problem solvers, citizens able to adapt to a changing world and contributing members of a society.

New Hampshire

1712 Disability Rights Center

18 Low Avenue Concord
Concord, NH 03301-4971

603-228-0432
800-834-1721
Fax: 603-225-2077
TTY: 800-834-1721
www.drcnh.org
advocacy@drcnh.org

Richard Cohen, Executive Director
Amy Messer, Legal Director
Julia Freeman-Woolpert, Outreach Advocacy Director
Dedicated to eliminating barriers existing in New Hampshire to the full an dequal enjoyment of civil and other legal rights by people with disabilities.

1713 Granite State Independent Living

21 Chenell Drive
Concord, NH 03301

603-228-9680
800-826-3700
Fax: 603-225-3304
TTY: 888-396-3459
www.gsil.org
info@gsil.org

Clyde E. Terry, JD, Chief Executive Officer
Debora Krider, Ed.D, Chief Operating Officer
Mara Olisky, VP, Human Resources
A statewide non-profit, service and advocacy organization that provides tools for living life on your terms. To promote life with independence for people with disabilities through the four core services of advocacy, information, education and support.

1714 Institute on Disability

University of New Hampshire
10 West Edge Drive
Suite 101
Durham, NH 03824

603-862-4320
Fax: 603-862-0555
www.iod.unh.edu
contact.iod@unh.edu

Charles E. Drum, Director & Professor
Susan Fox, Associate Director
Andrew Houtenville, Director of Research
Established to provide a coherent university-based focus for the improvement of knowledge, policies, and practices related to the lives of persons with disabilities and their families. Also advances policies and systems changes, promising practices, education, and research that strengthen communities and ensure full access, equal opportunities, and participation for all persons.

1715 New Hampshire Commission for Human Rights

2 Chenell Drive
Unit 2
Concord, NH 03301-8501

603-271-2767
Fax: 603-271-6339
TDD: 800-735-2964
www.nh.gov/hrc
humanrights@nhsa.state.nh.us

Joni N. Esperian, Executive Director
Roxanne Juliano, Assistant Director
Deborah Evans, Administrative Secretary
Enforcement of RSA 354-A, the Law Against Discrimination and the ADA Title I, Employment, and Housing. Private School/Pre-and After School program enrollees, not public school. All employees covered regardless of public/private distinction if 6 or more employees (NH) 15 or more (Federal).

1716 New Hampshire Developmental Disabilities Council

21 South Fruit Street, Walker Build
Suite 22
Concord, NH 03301-2451

603-271-3236
800-852-3345
Fax: 603-271-1156
TDD: 800-735-2964
www.nhddc.org
Carol.M.Stamatakis@ddc.nh.gov

Carol Stamatakis, Executive Director
David Ouellette, Project Manager
Chris Rueggeberg, Policy Director
A federally funded agency that supports public policies and initiative that remoce barriers and promote opportunities in all areas of life.

1717 New Hampshire Employment Security

64 South Street
Concord, NH 03301

603-224-3311
800-852-3400
Fax: 603-228-4145
TDD: 800-852-3400
www.nh.gov
webmaster@nhes.state.nh.us

Maggie Hassan, Commissioner
Darrell Gates, Deputy Commissioner
Refers individuals with disabilities to organizations and agencies that assist people with disabilities without charge.

1718 New Hampshire Governor's Commission on Disability

64 South Street
Concord, NH 03301

603-271-2773
800-852-3405
Fax: 603-271-2837
TTY: 603-271-2774
www.nh.gov
Disability@nh.gov

Maggie Hassan, Commissioner
Jillian Shedd, Accessibility Coordinator
Gayle Baird, Accountant I
To remove barriers, architectural or attitudinal, which bar persons with disabilities from participating in the mainstream of society.

1719 Parent Information Center

54 Old Suncook Road
Concord, NH 03301

603-224-7005
800-947-7005
Fax: 603-224-4365
TDD: 800-947-7005
www.parentinformationcenter.org

Michelle Lewis, Executive Director
Sylvia Abbott, Administrative Supervisor
James Butterfield, Accountant
A recognized leader in building strong family/school partnerships. PIC provides information, support, and educational programs for parents, family members, educators, and the community. PIC is a pioneer in promoting effective parent involvment in the special education process.

1720 ServiceLink
64 South Street
Concord, NH 03301

603-644-2240
866-634-9412
Fax: 603-644-2361
www.nh.gov
Disability@nh.gov

Maggie Hassan, Commissioner
Jillian Shedd, Accessibility Coordinator
Gayle Baird, Accountant I
Provides community supportive information and referral assistance to Edlers, their families and Adults with Disabilities in accessing services for caregivee support, financial and legal concerns, home care services, housing information and assistance, recreational and social events, information about applying for Medicaid and Medicaid programs such as Choices For Independence program.

1721 State Department of Education: Division of Career Technology & Adult Learning-Vocational Rehab
101 Pleasant Street
Concord, NH 03301-3860

603-271-3494
800-299-1647
Fax: 603-271-1953
www.ed.state.nh.us
Lori.Temple@doe.nh.gov

Paul K Leather, Deputy Commissioner
Lisa Danley, CTE State Director
Judy Fillion, Director
Provides services to both individuals with disabilities and employers. People with disabilities can work and take advantage of the opportunities available to the citizens of New Hampshire. A joint State/Federal program that seeks to empower people to make informed choices, build viable careers, and live more independently in the community.

New Jersey

1722 Assistive Technology Center (ATAC)
Disability Rights New Jersey
210 South Broad Street
3rd Floor
Trenton, NJ 08608

609-292-9742
800-922-7233
Fax: 609-777-0187
TTY: 609-633-7106
www.drnj.org
advocate@drnj.org

Joseph B. Young, Executive Director
Curtis Edmonds, AT Program Director
Ellen Catanese, Director of Administration
Assists individuals in overcoming barriers in the system and making assistive technology more accessible to individuals with disabilities throughout the state.

1723 New Jersey Department of Law and Public Safety
New Jersey Division on Civil Rights
PO Box 46001
Newark, NJ 07101-8003

973-648-2700
Fax: 973-648-4405
TTY: 973-648-4678
www.nj.gov/

Chris Christie, Governor
J Frank Vespa-Papaleo Esq, Director
The Division on Civil Rights enforces the New Jersey Law Against Discrimination which prohibits discrimination in employment, housing and public accommodations because of race, creed, color, national origin, ancestry, sex, affectional and sexual orientation, marital status, nationality or handicap.

1724 New Jersey Department of Special Education
New Jersey Department of Education
PO Box 500
Trenton, NJ 08625

609-292-0147
Fax: 609-984-8422
www.state.nj.us

Chris Christie, Governor
Roberta Wohle, Director
The office is resonsible for administering all federal funds received for educating people with disabilities ages 3 through 21. Also monitors the delivery of special education programs operated under state authority, provides mediation services to parents and school districts, processes hearings and conducts complaint investigations. Also funds four learning resource centers (LRCs) that provide information, circulate materials, offer technical assistance/consultation and production services.

1725 New Jersey Programs for Infants and Toddlers with Disabilities: Early Intervention System
New Jersey Department of Health
50 E State St
P.O. Box 360
Trenton, NJ 08625-0360

609-777-7734
888-653-4463
Fax: 609-777-7739
www.state.nj.us/health/fhs/eiphome.htm
terry.harrison@ddn.state.nj.us

Terri Harrison, M.Ed., Part C Coordinator
Theresa Goeke, SICC Secretary
The New Jersey Early Intervention System provides a comprehensive system of services for children, birth to age three, with developmental delays or disabilities and their families.

1726 Protection & Advocacy Agency (NJP&A)
210 South Broad Street
3rd Floor
Trenton, NJ 08608

609-292-9742
800-922-7233
Fax: 609-777-0187
TTY: 609-633-7106
www.drnj.org
advocate@drnj.org

Joseph B. Young, Executive Director
Curtis Edmonds, AT Program Director
Ellen Catanese, Director of Administration
To protect, advocate for and advance the rights of persons with disabilites in pursuit of a society in which persons with disabilities exercise self-determination and choice, and are treated with dignity.

1727 State Department of Adult Education
Department of Education
PO Box 001
Trenton, NJ 08625

609-292-6000
Fax: 609-633-9825
www.state.nj.us/education

Arlene Roth, Director Adult Education
Alfred Murray, Executive Director

1728 State GED Administration: Office of Specialized Populations
New Jersey Department of Education
PO Box 001
Trenton, NJ 08625

609-292-6000
Fax: 609-633-9825
www.state.nj.us/education

Arlene Roth, Director Adult Education
Alfred Murray, Executive Director

New Mexico

1729 Client Assistance Program (CAP): New Mexico Protection and Advocacy System
1720 Louisiana Blvd. NE
Suite 204
Albuquerque, NM 87110-7070

505-256-3100
800-432-4682
Fax: 505-256-3184
TTY: 505-256-3100
www.drnm.org
info@drnm.org

Adam Carrasco, President
Deanna DeVore, Vice President
Jonathan Toledo, Secretary Treasurer
Helps persons with disabilities who have concerns about agencies in New Mexico that provide rehabilitation or independent living services. The kind of help may be information or advocacy. For questions about Division of Vocational Rehabilitation, Commission for the Blind, Independent Living Centers and Preojects With Industsry CAP can help.

1730 New Mexico Department of Workforce Solutions: Workforce Transition Services Division
401 Broadway NE
Albuquerque, NM 87102   505-841-8405
Fax: 505-841-8491
www.dws.state.nm.us
Currently composed of two bureaus and under the supervision of a Division Director responsible for the design, administration, management and implementation of the Workforce Investment Act in New Mexico and any successor legislation. Within this capacity, the Division serves on behalf of the Governor with respect to statewide oversight and compliance, and as the principle support staff to the State Workforce Development Board.

1731 New Mexico Human Rights Commission Education Bureau
Ste 103
1596 Pacheco St
Santa Fe, NM 87505-3960   505-827-6817
Fax: 505-827-9676
www.dws.state.nm.us/LaborRelation
Francie Cordova, Executive Director

1732 New Mexico Public Education Department
300 Don Gaspar Ave
Santa Fe, NM 87501-2744   505-827-5800
www.ped.state.nm.us
join.ped@state.nm.us
Dr Veronica Garcia, Secretary
Lisa G Salazar, GED Administrator
Andrew Winnegar, Project Director
To provide leadership, technical assistance and quality assurance to improve student performance and close the achievement gap.

1733 New Mexico State GED Testing Program
New Mexico Public Education Department
300 Don Gaspar Ave
Santa Fe, NM 87501-2744   505-827-5800
www.ped.state.nm.us
join.ped@state.nm.us
Lisa G Salazar, GED Administrator
Dr Veronica Garcia, Secretary
Andrew Winnegar, Project Director
The primary aid of the GED testing program in New Mexico is to proive a second opportunity for individuals to obtain their high school diplomas.

1734 New Mexico Technology-Related Assistance Program
Department of Education
300 Don Gaspar Ave
Santa Fe, NM 87501   505-827-5800
www.ped.state.nm.us
join.ped@state.nm.us
Andrew Winnegar, Project Director
Lisa G Salazar, GED Administrator
Dr Veronica Garcia, Secretary

1735 State Department of Adult Education
Department of Education
300 Don Gaspar Ave
Santa Fe, NM 87501-2744   505-827-5800
www.ped.state.nm.us
join.ped@state.nm.us
Patricia Chavez, Contact
Lisa G Salazar, GED Administrator
Dr Veronica Garcia, Secretary

New York

1736 DBTAC: Northeast ADA Center
Cornell University
201 Ives Hall
Ithaca, NY 14853   607-255-7816
800-949-4232
Fax: 607-255-2358
www.ilr.cornell.edu
dbtacnortheast@cornell.edu
Wendy Strobel, Project Director
Susanne Bruyere, Principal Investigator
Provides information, referrals, resources, and raining on equal opportunity for people with disabilities and on the Americans with Disabilities Act. Serve businesses, employers, government entities, individuals with disabilities, and the media in NY, NJ, PR, and the US Virgin Islands.

1737 Department of Correctional Services
1220 Washington Ave
Bldg 2
Albany, NY 12226-2050   518-457-8126
www.doccs.ny.gov
Andrew M. Cuomo, Governor
Brian Fischer, Commissioner
To provide for public protection by administering a network of correctional facilities that: retain inmates in safe custody until released by law; offer inmates an opportunity to improve their rmployment potential and their ability to function in a non-criminal fashion; offer staff a variety of opportunities for career enrichment and advancement; and, offer stable and humane community environments in which all participants, staff anf inmates can perform their required tasks.

1738 NYS Commission on Quality of Care/TRAID Program
401 State St
Schenectady, NY 12305-2303   518-388-2892
800-624-4143
Fax: 518-388-2890
TTY: 800-624-4143
www.cqcapd.state.ny.us
lisa.rosano@cqcapd.state.ny.us
Andrew M. Cuomo, Governor
Roger Bearden, Chair
Bruce Blower, Member
A statewide systems advocacy program promoting assistive technology devices and services to persons of all ages with all disabilities.

1739 NYS Developmental Disabilities Planning Council
99 Washington Avenue, 12th Floor
Suite 1230
Albany, NY 12210-2329   518-486-7505
800-395-3372
Fax: 518-402-3505
http://ddpc.ny.gov
ddpc.sm.pio@ddpc.ny.gov
Andrew M. Cuomo, Governor
Rose Marie Toscano, Chairperson
Shiela M. Carey, Executive Director
In partnership with individuals with developmental disabilities, their families and communities provides leadership by promoting policies, plans and practices.

1740 New York Department of Labor: Division of Employment and Workforce Solutions
W.A. Harriman Campus
Building 12
Albany, NY 12240   518-457-9000
888-469-7365
Fax: 518-457-9526
TDD: 800-662-1220
www.labor.ny.gov
nysdol@labor.state.ny.us
Andrew M. Cuomo, Governor
Peter M. Rivera, Commissioner
Karen Coleman, Division Director

1741 New York State Commission on Quality Care and Advocacy for Persons with Disabilities (CQCAPD)
401 State St
Schenectady, NY 12305-2303   518-388-2892
                                    800-624-4143
                              Fax: 518-388-2890
                              TTY: 800-624-4143
                              www.cqcapd.state.ny.us
                  rosemary.lamb@cqcapd.state.ny.us

Andrew M. Cuomo, Governor
Rose Marie Toscano, Chairperson
Shiela M. Carey, Executive Director
Our mission is to improve the quality of life for persons with disabilities, to protect their rights, and to advocate needed changes by promoting the development of laws, policies and practices that advance the inclusion of all persons with disabilities into the rich fabric of our society.

1742 New York State Office of Vocational & Educational Services for Individuals with Disabilities
89 Washington Ave.
Room 580 EBA
Albany, NY 12234-1000   518-465-2492
                                  800-222-5627
                              www.vesid.nysed.gov
                        accesadm@mail.nysed.gov

Michael Irwin, Chairman
LaWanda Cook, Co-Chair
Philip Larocque, Deputy Commissioner
To promote educational equity and excellence for students with disabilities while ensuring that they receive the rights and protection to which they are entitles; assure appropriate continuity between the child and adult services systems; and provide the highest quality vocational rehabilitation and independent living services to all eligible persons as quickly as those services are required to enable them to work and live independent, self-directed lives.

1743 Office of Civil Rights: New York
US Department of Education
32 Old Slip
25th Floor
New York, NY 10005-3534   646-428-3906
                              Fax: 646-428-3904
                              TDD: 877-521-2172
                                   www.ed.gov.
                              ocr.newyork@ed.gov

Kathleen S. Tighe, Inspector General
Teresa Clark, Chief of Staff
Patrick Howard, Assistant Inspector General
This office covers the states of New Jersey and New York.

1744 Office of Curriculum & Instructional Support
New York State Department of Education
89 Washington Ave
Rm 319
Albany, NY 12234-1000   518-474-3852
                              Fax: 518-474-0319
                              www.p12.nysed.gov
                        hgoldsmi@mail.nysed.gov

Merryl H. Tisch, Chancellor
Anthony S. Bottar, Vice Chancellor
Robert M. Bennett, Chancellor Emeritus
Support quality curriculum, instruction, career and technical education, adult and famiy literacy, middle-level education, professional development for teachers, and promote workforce development.

1745 Programs for Children with Special Health Care Needs
Bureau of Child & Adolescent Health Dept of Health
Corning Tower Building
Room 208
Albany, NY 12237   518-474-2084
                              Fax: 518-474-5445
                              www.health.state.ny.us
                        cak03@health.state.ny.us

Andrew M. Cuomo, Governor
Nirav R. Shah, M.D., M.P.H., Commissioner

Our mission is to achieve a statewide system of care for CSHCN and their families that links them to appropriate health and related services, identifies gaps and barriers and assists in their resolution, and assures access to quality health care.

1746 Programs for Infants and Toddlers with Disabilities
Bureau of Early Intervention
Corning Tower Building
Room 287
Albany, NY 12237   518-473-7016
                                  800-577-2229
                              Fax: 518-486-1090
                              www.health.state.ny.us
                        blm01@health.state.ny.us

Andrew M. Cuomo, Governor
Nirav R. Shah, M.D., M.P.H., Commissioner
The Early Intervention Program offers a variety of therapeutic and support services to eligible infants and toddlers with disabilities and their families.

1747 Protection & Advocacy Agency
NY Commission on Quality of Care
Ste 1002
99 Washington Ave
Albany, NY 12210-2822   518-487-7708
                              Fax: 518-487-7777
                              http://ddpc.ny.gov
                        ddpc.sm.pio@ddpc.ny.gov

Andrew M. Cuomo, Governor
Rose Marie Toscano, Chairperson
Shiela M. Carey, Executive Director

1748 Region II: US Department of Health and Human Services
26 Federal Plz
New York, NY 10278-0004   212-264-4600
                              Fax: 212-264-3620
                                   www.hhs.gov
                        jaime.torres@hhs.gov

Sylvia M. Burwell, Secretary
Bill Corr, Deputy Secretary
E.J. Holland,Jr, Assistant Secretary
The United States government's principal agency for protecting the health of all Americans and providing essential human services, especially for those who are least able to help themselves.

1749 State GED Administration
State Department of Education
89 Washington Ave
PO Box 7348
Albany, NY 12234   518-474-3852
                              Fax: 518-474-3041
                              www.p12.nysed.gov
                        ged@mail.nysed.gov

Merryl H. Tisch, Chancellor
Anthony S. Bottar, Vice Chancellor
Robert M. Bennett, Chancellor Emeritus
Instruction and testing for those over the age of 16 to earn the General Educational Development diploma.

North Carolina

1750 Assistive Technology Program
1110 Navaho Dr
Raleigh, NC 27609-7352   919-872-2298
                              Fax: 919-850-2792
                              TTY: 919-850-2787
                                   www.ncatp.org
                              ldeese@ncatp.org

A Lynne Deese MA ATP, Assistive Technologist
Tammy Koger, Director
Sonya Clark, Information Specialist
A state and federally funded program that provides assistive technology services statewide to people of all ages and abilities.

1751 Client Assistance Program (CAP): North Carolina Division of Vocational Rehabilitation Services
2806 Mail Service Ctr
Raleigh, NC 27699-2800 919-855-3600
800-215-7227
Fax: 919-715-2456
www.ncdhhs.gov/dvrs
kathy.brack@ncmail.net
Gloria Sims, Director
Tami Andrews, Administrative Assistant
The Client Assistance Program helps people understand and use rehabilitation services.

1752 North Carolina Council on Developmental Disabilities
3125 Poplarwood Court
Suite 200
Raleigh, NC 27604 919-850-2901
800-357-6916
Fax: 919-850-2915
TTY: 919-850-2901
www.nc-ddc.org
info@nccdd.org
Ronald Reeve, Council Chairperson
Chris Egan, Executive Director
Kelly Bohlander, Assistant Director
To ensure that people with developmental disabilities and their families participate in the design of and have access to culturally competent services and supports, as well as other assistance and opportunities, which promote inclusive communities.

1753 North Carolina Division of Vocational Rehabilitation
2801 Mail Service Ctr
Raleigh, NC 27699-2801 919-324-1500
800-689-9090
Fax: 919-733-7968
TTY: 919-855-3579
www.ncdhhs.gov/dvrs
dvr.info@ncmail.net
Linda Harrington, Director
To promote employment and independence for people with disabilities through customer partnership and community leadership.

1754 North Carolina Division of Workforce Services
301 North Wilmington Street
Ste 12
Raleigh, NC 27601-1058 919-733-4151
800-228-8443
Fax: 919-662-4770
www.nccommerce.com
Sharon Allred Decker, Secretary of Commerce
John Hoomani, General Counsel/Chief of Staff
Dale Folwell, Assistant Secretary

1755 North Carolina Employment Security Commission
700 Wade Avenue
P.O. Box 25903
Raleigh, NC 27605 919-733-7522
888-737-0259
Fax: 919-250-4315
http://desncc.com/deshome
assistantsecretary@nccommerce.com
Pat McCrory, Governor
Sharon Allred Decker, Secretary of Commerce
Dale Folwell, Assistant Secretary

1756 North Carolina Office of Administrative Hearings: Civil Rights Division
1711 New Hope Church Road
Raleigh, NC 27609 919-431-3000
Fax: 919-733-4866
www.oah.state.nc.us
oah.postmaster@oah.nc.gov
Julian Mann, III, Director
Gene Cella, General Counsel
Margaret Reader, Human Resource Director

Responsible for charges alleging discrimination in the basis of race, color, sex, religion, age, national origin or disability in employment, or charges alleging retaliation for opposition to such discrimination brought by previous and current state employees or applicants for employment for positions covered by the State Personnel Act, including county government employees.

1757 State Department of Adult Education
North Carolina Community College
200 West Jones Street
Raleigh, NC 27603 919-807-7100
Fax: 919-807-7164
www.nccommunitycolleges.edu
whitfieldr@nccommunitycolleges.edu
Hilda Pinnix-Ragland, Chair
Dr. Stuart Fountain, Vice Chair

North Dakota

1758 Client Assistance Program (CAP): North Dakota
Wells Fargo Bank Building
400 East Suite 409
Bismarck, ND 58501-4071 701-328-2950
800-472-2670
Fax: 701-328-3934
www.nd.gov/cap
panda@nd.gov
David Boeck, Director of Legal Services
Corinne Hofmann, Director of Policy and Operation
Teresa Larsen, Executive Director
Assists clients and client applicants of North Dakota Vocational Rehabilitation services, Tribal Vocational Rehabilitation, or Independent Living services.

1759 North Dakota Department of Human Services
600 E Boulevard Ave
Dept 325
Bismarck, ND 58505-250 701-328-2310
800-472-2622
Fax: 701-328-2359
TTY: 800-366-6888
www.nd.gov/dhs
dhseo@nd.gov
Maggie Anderson, Interim Executive Director
To provide quality, efficient, and effective human services, which improve the lives of people.

1760 North Dakota Department of Labor: Fair Employment Practice Agency
600 E Boulevard Ave
Department 406
Bismarck, ND 58505-340 701-328-2660
800-582-8032
Fax: 701-328-2031
TTY: 800-366-6888
www.nd.gov/labor
labor@nd.gov; humanrights@nd.gov
Tony Weiler, Commissioner of Labor
Kathy Kulesa, Human Rights Director
Robin Bosch, Business Manager
Provides information and enforces laws related to labor standards and discrimination in employment, housing, public services, public accommodations and lending. The department also issues sub minimum wage certificates, verifies independent contractor status and licenses employment agencies.

1761 North Dakota Department of Public Instruction
600 E Boulevard Ave
Department 201
Bismarck, ND 58505-440 701-328-2660
Fax: 701-328-1717
www.dpi.state.nd.us
dpi@nd.gov

Jerry Coleman, Director - School Finance
Valerie Fischer, Director - Coordinated School
Greg Gallagher, Director - Standards
To ensure a uniform, statewide system for effective learning.

1762 North Dakota State Council on Developmental Disabilities
ND Department of Human Services
600 E Boulevard Ave
Bismarck, ND 58505
701-328-2372
Fax: 701-328-4727
www.ndhealth.gov
asmith@nd.gov

Arvy Smith, Deputy State Health Officer
Darin Meschke, Director
Terry Dwelle, M.D., M.P.H.T., State Health Officer

Ohio

1763 Assistive Technology
Area 1700
1314 Kinnear Rd.
Columbus, OH 43212
614-293-9134
800-784-3425
TTY: 614-293-0767
www.atohio.org
atohio@osu.edu

William T Darling PhD, Director
Eric Rathburn, Public Policy Director
Gaye Spetka, ATP, Program Manager
To help Ohioans with disabilities acquire assistive technology. Offer several programs and services to achieve that goal. Also keep up with current legislative activity that affects persons with disabilities.

1764 Client Assistance Program (CAP)
Ohio Legal Rights Service
50 W Broad St
Suite 1400
Columbus, OH 43215-5923
614-466-7264
800-282-9181
Fax: 614-728-3749
TTY: 614-728-2553
www.disabilityrightsohio.org
webmaster@olrs.state.oh.us

Kalpana Yalamanchili, Chair
William Crum, Member
Elena Lidrbauch, Member
Advocates for and protects the rights of individuals with disabilities who are applying for or receiving rehabilitation services from the Ohio BUreau of Vocational Rehabilitation (BVR) or the Ohio Bureau of Services for the Visually Impaired (BSVI).

1765 Correctional Education
Department of Rehabilitation & Correction
770 W Broad St
Columbus, OH 43222-1419
614-752-1159
Fax: 614-752-0900
www.drc.ohio.gov
drc.publicinfo@odrc.state.oh.us

Gary C. Mohr, Director
Stephen J. Huffman, Assistant Director
Linda Janes, Chief of Staff
Protects and supports Ohioans by ensuring that adult felony offenders are effectively supervised in environments that are safe, humane, and appropriately secure.

1766 Office of Civil Rights: Ohio
US Department of Education
600 Superior Ave E
Suite 750
Cleveland, OH 44114-2602
216-522-4970
Fax: 216-522-2573
TDD: 877-521-2172
www.ed.gov
ocr.cleveland@ed.gov

Arne Duncan, Secretary of Education
Tony Miller, Deputy Secretary
Russlynn Ali, Assistant Secretary
This office covers the states of Michigan and Ohio.

1767 Ohio Adult Basic and Literacy Education
25 S Front St
Columbus, OH 43215-4183
614-995-1545
877-644-6338
Fax: 614-728-8470
TTY: 888-886-0181
http://education.ohio.gov
contact.center@education.ohio.gov

John R. Kasich, Governor
Debe Terhar, President
Richard A. Ross, Superintendent
Provides quality leadership for the establishment, improvement an dexpansion of lifelong learning opportunities for adults in their family, community and work roles.

1768 Ohio Civil Rights Commission
30 E Broad St
5th Floor
Columbus, OH 43215-3414
614-466-2785
888-278-7101
Fax: 614-644-8776
http://crc.ohio.gov
paytonm@ocrc.state.oh.us

G. Michael Payton, Executive Director
Keith P. McNeil, Esq., Director Regional Operations
Stephanie Bostos-Demers, Chief Legal Counsel
To enforce state laws against discrimination. OCRC receives and investigates charges of discrimination in employment, public accommodations, housing, credit and higher education on the bases of race, colo, religion, sex, national origin, disability, age, ancestry or familial status.

1769 Ohio Developmental Disabilities Council
899 E Broad St
Ste 203
Columbus, OH 43205
614-466-5205
800-766-7426
Fax: 614-466-0298
http://ddc.ohio.gov
carolyn.knight@dodd.ohio.gov

Renee Wood, Chairman
Mark Greenblatt, Vice Chairman
Carolyn Knight, Executive Director
To create change that improves independence, productivity and inclusion for people with developmental disabilities and their families in community life.

1770 Ohio Office of Workforce Development
Ohio Department of Job & Family Services
Fl 32
30 E Broad St
Columbus, OH 43215-3414
614-752-3091
Fax: 614-995-1298
http://jfs.ohio.gov
workforce@jfs.ohio.gov

Michael B. Colbert, Director
Roxanne Ward, Executive Assistant
Sonnetta Sturkey, Chief Operations Officer
The role of OWD is to work in partnership with the U.S. Department of Labor, Governor's Office and a variety of stakeholders in order to provide administration and operational management for several federal programs and to offer specific services in support of the programs. OWD's primary responsibility is to promote job creation and to advance Ohio's workforce.

1771 Protection & Advocacy Agency
Ohio Legal Rights Service
50 W Broad St
Suite 1400
Columbus, OH 43215-5923
614-466-7264
800-282-9181
Fax: 614-728-3749
TTY: 614-728-2553
www.disabilityrightsohio.org
webmaster@olrs.state.oh.us
Michael B. Colbert, Director
Roxanne Ward, Executive Assistant
Sonnetta Sturkey, Chief Operations Officer
To protect and advocate, in partnership with people with disabilities, for their human, civil and legal rights.

1772 State Department of Education
25 S Front St
Columbus, OH 43215-4183
614-995-1545
877-644-6338
Fax: 614-728-8470
TTY: 888-886-0181
http://education.ohio.gov
contact.center@education.ohio.gov
John R. Kasich, Governor
Debe Terhar, President
Richard A. Ross, Superintendent

1773 State GED Administration
State Department of Education
25 S Front St
Rm 309
Columbus, OH 43215-4176
614-466-8872
Fax: 614-995-7544
http://education.ohio.gov
contact.center@education.ohio.gov
John R. Kasich, Governor
Debe Terhar, President
Richard A. Ross, Superintendent

Oklahoma

1774 Assistive Technology
Seretean OSU-Wellness Center
1514 W Hall of Fame
Stillwater, OK 74078
405-744-9748
800-257-1705
Fax: 405-744-2487
TDD: 888-885-5588
www.ok.gov/abletech/
linda.jaco@okstate.edu
Linda Jaco, Director of Sponsored Programs
Milissa Gofourth, Program Manager
Brenda Dawes, Program Manager

1775 Client Assistance Program (CAP): Oklahoma Division
Office of Handicapped Concerns
2401 NW 23rd St
Suite 90
Oklahoma City, OK 73107-2431
405-521-3756
800-522-8224
Fax: 405-522-6695
TDD: 405-522-6706
www.ohc.state.ok.us
steven.stokes@ohc.state.ok.us
Steve Stokes, Director
The purpose of this program is to advise and inform clients and client applicants of all services and benefits available to them through programs authorized under the Rehabilitation Act of 1973. Assist and advocates for clients and client applicants in their relationships with projects, programs, and community rehabilitation programs providing services under the Act.

1776 Correctional Education
Department of Corrections
PO Box 11400
Oklahoma City, OK 73136
405-425-2500
Fax: 405-425-2500
www.doc.state.ok.us
justin.jones@doc.state.ok.us
Justin Jones, Director
Ed Evans, Associate Director
Linda Parrish, Deputy Director, Administrative

1777 Oklahoma State Department of Education
2500 N Lincoln Blvd
Oklahoma City, OK 73105-4596
405-521-3301
Fax: 405-521-6938
www.ok.gov/sde/
sdeservicedesk@sde.ok.gov
Joyce DeFehr, Executive Director
Janet Barresi, State Superintendent
Liz Young, Executive Assistant
Improve student success through: service to schools, parents and students; leadership for education reform; and regulation/deregulation of state and federal laws to provide accountability while removing any barriers to student success.

1778 Protection & Advocacy Agency
Disability Law Center
2915 Classen Blvd.
300 Cameron Building
Oklahoma City, OK 73106
405-525-7755
800-880-7755
Fax: 405-525-7759
www.redlands-partners.org
kayla@okdlc.org
Kayla Bower, Executive Director
Valerie Williams, Director
Anne Trudgeon, Director
Helps people with disabilities achieve equality, inclusion in society and personal independence without regard to disabling conditions.

1779 State Department of Adult Education
Department of Education
2500 N Lincoln Blvd
Oklahoma City, OK 73105-4596
405-521-3301
800-405-0355
Fax: 405-521-6938
www.ok.gov/sde/
sdeservicedesk@sde.ok.gov
Joyce DeFehr, Executive Director
Janet Barresi, State Superintendent
Liz Young, Executive Assistant

1780 State GED Administration
State Department of Education
2500 N Lincoln Blvd
Oklahoma City, OK 73105-4596
405-521-3301
800-405-0355
Fax: 405-521-6938
www.ok.gov/sde/
sdeservicedesk@sde.ok.gov
Joyce DeFehr, Executive Director
Janet Barresi, State Superintendent
Liz Young, Executive Assistant

Oregon

1781 Assistive Technology Program
Access Technologies
2225 Lancaster Drive NE
Salem, OR 97305-1396
503-361-1201
800-677-7512
Fax: 503-370-4530
www.accesstechnologiesinc.org
info@accesstechnologiesinc.org
Laurie Brooks, President
Phyllis Petteys, Center Director
Davey Hulse, Chair

A statewide program promoting services and assistive devices for people with disabilities.

1782 Department of Community Colleges and Workforce Development
255 Capitol St NE
Salem, OR 97310-1300
503-378-8648
Fax: 503-378-8434
www.oregon.gov
ccwd.info@odccwd.state.or.us

John Kitzhaber, Governor
Kate Brown, Secretary of State
Ted Wheeler, State Treasurer
Contribute leadership and resources to increase skills, knowledge and carrier opportunities.

1783 Disability Rights Oregon
610 SW Broadway
Suite 200
Portland, OR 97205
503-243-2081
800-452-1694
Fax: 503-243-1738
www.disabilityrightsoregon.org

Evelyn Lowry, Chair
Daniel Bartz, Vice Chair
Bob Joondeph, Executive Director
An independent non-profit organization which provides legal advocacy services for people with disabilities anywhere in Oregon. OAC offers free legal assistance and other advocacy services to individuals who are considered to have physical or mental disabilities. OAC works only on legal problems which relate directly to the disability.

1784 Office of Vocational Rehabilitation Services
Department of Human Services
500 Summer St NE E-87
Salem, OR 97301-1120
503-945-5880
877-277-0513
Fax: 503-947-5010
TTY: 866-801-0130
www.oregon.gov
vr.info@state.or.us

Stephanie Taylor, Administrator
Helps Oregonians with disabilities to prepare for, finad and retain jobs.

1785 Oregon Bureau of Labor and Industry: Fair Employment Practice Agency
800 NE Oregon St
Suite 1045
Portland, OR 97232-2162
971-673-0761
Fax: 971-673-0762
www.oregon.gov/BOLI/
mailb@boli.state.or.us

Brad Avakian, Commissioner

1786 Oregon Council on Developmental Disabilities
540 24th Pl NE
Salem, OR 97301-4517
503-945-9941
800-292-4154
Fax: 503-945-9947
www.ocdd.org
ocdd@ocdd.org

Jamie Daignault, Executive Director
Josiah Barber, Self Advocate Coordinator
Laura Bronson, Comm and Projects Coordinator
To create change that improves the lives of Oregonians with developmental disabilities.

1787 Oregon Department of Education: School-to-Work
255 Capitol St NE
Salem, OR 97310-203
503-947-5600
Fax: 503-378-5156
TDD: 503-378-3825
www.ode.state.or.us
ode.frontdesk@ode.state.or.us

Katy Coba, Executive Director
Patrick Burk, Education Policy Deputy Director

School-to-Work is a federally funded initiative that provides funding for state and local implementation of the Oregon Educational Act for the 21st Century.

1788 Oregon Department of Human Services: Children, Adults & Families Division
500 Summer St NE
E15
Salem, OR 97301-1097
503-945-5600
Fax: 503-378-2897
www.dhs.state.or.us
dhs.info@state.or.us

Bruce Goldberg, Interim Director
This group is responsible for administering self-sufficiency and child-protective programs. These include Jobs, Temporary Assistance for Needy Families, Employment Related Day Care, Food Stamps, child-abuse investigation and intervention, foster care and adoptions.

1789 Oregon Employment Department
875 Union St NE
Salem, OR 97311
877-517-5627
800-237-3710
Fax: 503-947-1472
www.oregon.gov/EMPLOY/
findit.emp.state.or.us/write-us/

Laurie Warner, Director
Supports economic stability for Oregonians and communities during times of unemployment through the payment of unemployment benefits. Serves businesses by recruiting and referring the best qualified applicants to jobs, and provides resources to diverse job seekers in support of their employment needs.

Pennsylvania

1790 Bureau of Adult Basic & Literacy Education
12th Floor
333 Market St
Harrisburg, PA 17126
717-772-3737
Fax: 717-783-0583
http://www1.whsd.net/admin/Special_Educa
rosbrandt@state.pa.us

Cheryl Keenan, Director
Pedro Cortes, Manager

1791 Client Assistance Program (CAP): Pennsylvania Division
1515 Market Street
Suite 1300
Philadelphia, PA 19102
215-557-7112
888-745-2357
Fax: 215-557-7602
TDD: 215-577-7112
www.equalemployment.org
info@equalemployment.org

Stephen S. Pennington, Executive Director
Jamie C. Ray-Leonetti, Co-Director
Margaret Passio-McKenna, Senior Advocate
CAP is an advocacy program for people with disabilities administered by the Center for Disability Law and Policy. CAP helps people who are seeking services from the Office of Vocational Rehabilitation, Blindness and Visual Services, Centers for Independent Living and other programs funded under federal law. CAP services are provided at no charge.

1792 Disability Rights Network of Pennsylvania
1414 N Cameron St
Second Floor
Harrisburg, PA 17103-1049
717-236-8110
800-692-7443
Fax: 717-236-0192
TDD: 877-375-7139
TTY: 800-692-7443
http://drnpa.org
ldo@drnpa.org

Ken Oakes, Chair
Nicole Turman, Vice Chair
Peri Jude Radecic, Chief Executive Officer
A statewide, non-profit corporation designated as the federally-mandated organization to advance and protect the civil rights of adults and children with disabilities. DRN works with people with disabilities and their families, their organizations, and their advocates to ensure their rights to live in their communities with the services they need, to receive a full and inclusive education, to live free of discrimination, abuse and neglect.

1793 Office of Civil Rights: Pennsylvania
US Department of Education
100 Penn Sq E
Suite 515
Philadelphia, PA 19107   215-656-8541
                                      Fax: 215-656-8605
                                      TDD: 877-521-2172
                                               www.ed.gov
                              ocr_philadelphia@ed.gov
Bernard Tadley, Regional IG for Audit
Steven Anderson, Special Agent In Charge
Russlynn Ali, Assistant Secretary
This office covers the states of Delaware, Kentucky, Maryland, Pennsylvania and West Virginia.

1794 Pennsylvania Department of Corrections
1920 Technology Parkway
Mechanicsburg, PA 17050   717-728-2573
                                      Fax: 717-975-2242
                                         www.cor.state.pa.us
                                    ra-contactdoc@pa.gov
John E. Wetzel, Secretary
Harry Jones, Director
Theron Perez, Chief Counsel
To protect the public by confining persons committed to our custody in safe, secure facilities, and to provide opportunities for inmates to acquire the skills and values necessary to become productive law-abiding citizens; while respecting the rights of crime victims.

1795 Pennsylvania Developmental Disabilities Council
605 South Dr
Room 561 Forum Building
Harrisburg, PA 17120   717-787-6057
                                             877-685-4452
                                      TTY: 717-705-0819
                                            www.paddc.org
Tom Corbett, Governor
Nancy Richey, Council Chairperson
Graham Mulholland, Executive Director
Engages in advocacy, systems change and capacity building for people with disabilities and their families in order to: support people with disabilities in taking control of their own lives; ensure access to goods, services, and supports; build inclusive communities; pursue a cross-disability agenda; and to change negative societal attitudes towards people with disabilities.

1796 Pennsylvania Human Rights Commission
301 Chestnut St
Ste 300
Harrisburg, PA 17101-2702   717-787-4412
                                      Fax: 717-787-0420
                                      TTY: 717-787-4087
                              http://hfloyd@state.pa.us
Homer Floyd, Executive Director
To administer and enforce the PHRAct and the PFEOA of the Commonwealth of the Pennsylvania for the identification and elimination of discrimination and the providing of equal opportunity for all persons.

1797 Pennsylvania's Initiative on Assistive Technology
1755 N 13th St
Student Center, Rm 411 S
Philadelphia, PA 19122-6024   215-204-1356
                                             800-204-7428
                                      Fax: 215-204-6336
                                      TTY: 215-204-1805
                              http://disabilities.temple.edu
                                          iod@temple.edu
Celia Feinstein, Co-Executive Director
Amy Goldman, Co-Executive Director
Ann Marie White, Deputy Director
Strives to enhance the lives of Pennsylvanians with disabilities, older Pennsylvanians, and their families, through access to and acquisition of assitive technology devices and services, which allow for choice, control and independence at home, work, school, play and in their neighborhoods.

1798 Region III: US Department of Health and Human Services Civil Rights Office
US Department of Health & Human Services
105 S Independence Mall W
Suite 436
Philadelphia, PA 19106   215-861-4633
                                      Fax: 215-861-4625
                                               www.hhs.gov
                              gordon.woodrow@hhs.gov
Sylvia M. Burwell, Secretary
Bill Corr, Deputy Secretary
E.J. Holland, Jr, Assistant Secretary

1799 State Department of Education
333 Market St
Harrisburg, PA 17126   717-783-6788
                                      TTY: 717-783-8445
                                        www.pdeinfo.state.pa.us
                                    ra-edwebmaster@pa.gov
Tom Corbett, Governor
Carolyn C. Dumaresq, Acting Secretary
To lead and serve the educational community to enable each individual to grow into an inspired, productive, fulfilled lifelong learner.

1800 State GED Administration
Pennsylvania Department of Education
333 Market St
Harrisburg, PA 17126   717-783-6788
                                      Fax: 717-783-0583
                    http://www1.whsd.net/admin/Special_Educa
Janice Wessell, Director

Rhode Island

1801 Correctional Education
Rhode Island Department of Corrections
40 Howard Avenue
PO Box 8312
Cranston, RI 02920   401-462-1000
                                      Fax: 401-464-2509
                                      TDD: 401-462-5180
                                      TTY: 401-462-5180
                                               www.doc.ri.gov
                                     director@doc.ri.gov
Ashbel T. Wall, II, Director
Susan Lamkins, Programming Services Officer
Kathleen Kelly, Chief Legal Counsel

1802 Protection & Advocacy Agency
Rhode Island Disability Law Center
275 Westminster St
Suite 401
Providence, RI 02903-3434   401-831-3150
                                             800-733-5332
                                      Fax: 401-274-5568
                                      TTY: 401-831-5335
                                               www.ridlc.org
                                          info@ridlc.org

Raymond Bandusky, Executive Director
To assist people with differing abilities in their efforts to achieve full inclusion in society and to exercise their civil and human rights through the provision of legal advocacy.

1803 Rhode Island Commission for Human Rights

180 Westminster St
3rd Floor
Providence, RI 02903-1918   401-222-2661
                                    Fax: 401-222-2616
                                    TTY: 402-222-2664
                                    www.richr.ri.gov

John B. Susa, Ph.D., Chairperson
Michael Evora, Executive Director
Cynthia M. Hiatt, Legal Counsel
A state agency that enforces civil rights law.

1804 Rhode Island Department of Elementary and Secondary Education

Rhode Island Department of Education
255 Westminster St
Providence, RI 02903-3400   401-222-4600
                                    Fax: 401-222-5106
                                    www.ride.ri.gov

Eva-Marie Mancuso, Chairman
Deborah A. Gist, Commissioner
David V. Abbott, Deputy Commissioner

1805 Rhode Island Department of Labor & Training

1511 Pontiac Ave
Cranston, RI 02920-4407   401-462-8000
                                  Fax: 401-462-8872
                                  TDD: 401-462-8006
                                  www.dlt.state.ri.us
                                  mmadonna@dlt.ri.gov

Sandra Powell, Director
Providing workforce protection and development services with courtesy, responsiveness and effectiveness.

1806 Rhode Island Developmental Disabilities Council

400 Bald Hill Rd
Suite 515
Warwick, RI 02886-1692   401-737-1238
                                 Fax: 401-737-3395
                                 TDD: 401-732-1238
                                 www.riddc.org
                                 riddc@riddc.org

Mary Okero, Executive Director
Kevin Nerney, Associate Director
Sue Babin, Special Projects Coordinator
Promotes the ideas that will enhance the lives of people with developmental disabilities.

1807 State Department of Adult Education

255 Westminster St
Providence, RI 02903-3400   401-222-4600
                                    Fax: 401-222-5106
                                    www.ride.ri.gov

Eva-Marie Mancuso, Chairman
Deborah A. Gist, Commissioner
David V. Abbott, Deputy Commissioner
Administer grant funded programs in Adult Basic Education, GED, and English for Speakers of Other Languages. Promote stronger families, upward mobility, and active citizenship through effective adult basic education services. The classes support adults who wish to advance their education towards a high school credential, training, and/or post secondary degrees.

South Carolina

1808 Assistive Technology Program

South Carolina Developmental Disabilities Council
1205 Pendleton St
Suite 461
Columbia, SC 29201-3756   803-734-0465
                                  TTY: 803-734-1147
                                  www.scddc.state.sc.us
                                  vbishop@oepp.sc.gov

Valarie Bishop, Executive Director
Cheryl English, Program Information Coordinator
Esther Williams, Administrative Support Specialis
A statewide project established to provide an opportunity for individuals with disabilities to lead the fullest, most productive lives possible.

1809 Protection & Advocacy for People with Disabilities

3710 Landmark Dr
Ste 208
Columbia, SC 29204-4034   803-782-0639
                                  866-275-7273
                                  Fax: 803-790-1946
                                  TTY: 866-232-4525
                                  www.pandasc.org
                                  info@pandasc.org

Travis Dayhuff, Chairman
Dana Lang, Vice Chairman
Gloria Prevost, Executive Director
To protect the legal, civil, and human rights of people with disabilities in South Carolina by enabling individuals to advocate for themselves, speaking in their behalf when they have been discriminated against or denied a services to which they are entitled, and promoting policies and services which respect their choices.

1810 South Carolina Developmental Disabilities Council

1205 Pendleton St
Suite 461
Columbia, SC 29201-3756   803-734-0465
                                  TTY: 803-734-1147
                                  www.scddc.state.sc.us
                                  vbishop@oepp.sc.gov

Valarie Bishop, Executive Director
Cheryl English, Program Information Coordinator
Esther Williams, Administrative Support
To provide leadership in advocating, funding and implementing initiatives which recognize the inherent dignity of each individual, and promote independence, productivity, respect and inclusion for all persons with disabilities and their families.

1811 South Carolina Employment Security Commission

1550 Gadsden Street
PO Box 995
Columbia, SC 29202   803-737-2400
                             800-436-8190
                             Fax: 803-737-0140
                             www.sces.org
                             aturner@dew.sc.gov

Major Genera Turner, Executive Director
Joseph Lowder, Chief of Staff
Laura W. Robinson, Assistant Executive Director

1812 South Carolina Employment Services and Job Training Services

1550 Gadsden Street
PO Box 995
Columbia, SC 29202   803-737-2400
                             800-436-8190
                             Fax: 803-737-0140
                             www.sces.org
                             aturner@dew.sc.gov

Major Genera Turner, Executive Director
Joseph Lowder, Chief of Staff
Laura W. Robinson, Assistant Executive Director

1813 South Carolina Human Affairs Commission

1026 Sumter Street
Suite 200
Columbia, SC 29201-2379
803-737-7800
800-521-0725
Fax: 803-253-4191
TDD: 803-253-4125
www.state.sc.us/schac/
information@schac.state.sc.us

Raymond Buxton, Commissioner
John A. Oakland, Chair
Rev. Willie Albert Thompson, Vice Chair
To eliminate and prevent unlawful discrimination in: employment on the basis of race, color, national origin, religion, sex, age and disability; housing on the basis of race, color, national origin, religion, sex, familial status and disability; and public accommodations on the basis of race, color, national origin and religion.

1814 State Department of Adult Education

South Carolina Department of Education
1429 Senate St
Ste 402
Columbia, SC 29201-3730
803-734-8500
Fax: 803-734-3643
http://ed.sc.gov
info@ed.sc.gov

John Cooley, CFO
Don Cantrell, CIO
Scott English, COO
Provides the opportunity for adults with low literacy skills (less than eighth grade level), to work with materials to be taught in an environment conducive to their level, and to improve their reading, math, and writing skills.

1815 State GED Administration

South Carolina Department of Education
1429 Senate St
Ste 105
Columbia, SC 29201-3730
803-734-8500
Fax: 803-734-8336
http://ed.sc.gov
info@ed.sc.gov

John Cooley, CFO
Don Cantrell, CIO
Scott English, COO

South Dakota

1816 Client Assistance Program (CAP): South Dakota Division

South Dakota Advocacy Services
221 S Central Ave
Suite 38
Pierre, SD 57501-2479
605-224-8294
800-658-4782
Fax: 605-224-5125
TTY: 800-658-4782
www.sdadvocacy.com
sdas@sdadvocacy.com

Robert J. Kean, Executive Director
Provides free services to eligible consumers and applicants for projects, programs and facilities funded under the rehabilitation act.

1817 Department of Correction: Education Coordinator

4904 S Quail Run Ave
Sioux Falls, SD 57108-2962
605-332-8335
Fax: 605-332-8335
www.state.sd.us

Tim Reisch, Secretary
Dennis Daugaard, Governor
To protect the citizens of South Dakota by providing safe and secure facilities for juvenile and adult offenders committed to our custody by the courts, to provide effective community supervision upon their release.

1818 Easter Seals - South Dakota

1351 N Harrison Ave
Pierre, SD 57501-2373
605-224-5879
Fax: 605-224-133
http://sd.easterseals.com

Richard W. Davidson, Chairman
Sandra L. Bouwman, 1st Vice Chairman
Joseph G. Kern, 2nd Vice Chairman
Creates solutions that change the lives of children, adults and families with disabilities or other needs; to promote disability prevention and awareness.

1819 South Dakota Advocacy Services

221 S Central Ave
Suite 38
Pierre, SD 57501-2479
605-224-8294
800-658-4782
Fax: 605-224-5125
TTY: 800-658-4782
www.sdadvocacy.com
sdas@sdadvocacy.com

Robert J. Kean, Executive Director
To protect and advocate the rights of South Dakotans with disabilities through legal, administrative, and other remedies.

1820 South Dakota Council on Developmental Disabilities

Department of Human Services
500 E Capitol Ave
Pierre, SD 57501-5007
605-773-5990
800-265-9684
Fax: 605-773-5483
TTY: 605-773-6412
http://dhs.sd.gov
infoddc@state.sd.us

Arlene Poncelet, Director
The SD Council is authorized under federal law to address the unmet needs of people with developmental disabilities through advocacy, capacity building and systems change activities. The mission is to assist people with developmental disabilities and their families in achieving the quality of life they desire.

1821 South Dakota Department of Labor: Employment Services & Job Training

711 E. Wells Avenue
Pierre, SD 57501-2291
605-773-5422
800-872-6190
Fax: 605-773-4211
TTY: 605-773-3101
www.sdreadytowork.com
goedinfo@state.sd.us

Dennis Daugaard, Governor
Pat Costello, Commissioner
Aaron Scheibe, Deputy Commissioner
Job training programs provide an important framework for developing public-private sector partnerships. We help prepare South Dakotans of all ages for entry or re-entry into the labor force.

1822 South Dakota Division of Human Rights

711 E. Wells Avenue
Pierre, SD 57501-2291
605-773-3681
800-872-6190
Fax: 605-773-4211
www.sdreadytowork.com
goedinfo@state.sd.us

Dennis Daugaard, Governor
Pat Costello, Commissioner
Aaron Scheibe, Deputy Commissioner
To promote equal opportunity through the administration and enforcement of the Human Relations Act of 1972. The act is designed to protect the public from discrimination because of race, color, creed, religion, sex, disability, ancestry or national origin.

1823 South Dakota Division of Special Education
Department of Education
711 E. Wells Avenue
Pierre, SD 57501-2291

605-773-3678
800-872-6190
Fax: 605-773-3782
www.sdreadytowork.com
goedinfo@state.sd.us

Dennis Daugaard, Governor
Pat Costello, Commissioner
Aaron Scheibe, Deputy Commissioner
The Office of Special Education advocates for the availability of the full range of personnel, programming, and placement options, including early intervention and transition services, required to assure that all individuals with disabilities are able to achieve maximum independence upon exiting from school.

1824 State GED Administration
Department of Labor
700 Governors Dr
Pierre, SD 57501-2291

605-773-3101
Fax: 605-773-6184
www.sdjobs.org
barb.unruh@state.sd.us

Marcia Hultman, Labor Secretary
Lyle Harter, Director
Bret Afdahl, Director

Tennessee

1825 Department of Human Services: Division of Rehabilitation Services
400 Deaderick St
15th Floor
Nashville, TN 37243-1403

615-313-4700
Fax: 615-741-4165
www.tennessee.gov/humanserv
Human-Services.Webmaster@tn.gov
Raquel Hatter, Commissioner
Bill Haslam, Governor
To improve the well-being of economically disadvantaged, disabled or vulnerable Tennesseans through a network of financial, employment, rehabilitative and protective services.

1826 State Department of Education
6th Floor
Andrew Johnson Tower
Nashville, TN 37243

615-532-1617
www.state.tn.us
education.comments@state.tn.us
John Sharp, Director
Amy Sharp, Director
Debbie Crews, Supervisor
The department provides many services, and it is our responsibility to ensure equal, safe, and quality learning opportunities for all students, pre-kindergartern through 12th grade.

1827 State GED Administration
TDLWFD/Adult Education
220 French Landing Dr
Nashville, TN 37243

615-741-2731
800-531-1515
Fax: 615-532-4899
www.state.tn.us

Phil White, Administrator

1828 Tennessee Council on Developmental Disabilities
500 James Robertson Pkwy
Ste 130
Nashville, TN 37243-0001

615-532-6615
Fax: 615-532-6964
TTY: 615-741-4562
www.tn.gov/cdd
tnddc@tn.gov

Wanda Willis, Executive Director

A State office that promotes public policies to increase and support the inclusion of individuals with developmental disabilities in their communities.

1829 Tennessee Technology Access Project
400 Deadrick St
15th Floor
Nashville, TN 37243-1403

615-313-4700
800-732-5059
Fax: 615-741-4165
TTY: 615-313-5695
www.tn.gov/humanserv/rehab/ttap.html
tn.ttap@tn.gov

Raquel Hatter, Commissioner
Shalonda Cawthon, Deputy Commissioner
Sandy Troope, Executive Assistant
A statewide program designed to increase access to, and acquisition of, assisitve technology devices and services.

Texas

1830 Advocacy
2222 West Braker Lane
Ste 171E
Austin, TX 78758-1097

512-454-4816
800-252-9108
Fax: 512-323-0902
www.disabilityrightstx.org
infoai@advocacyinc.org
Mary Faithful, Executive Director
Nonprofit legal organization that provides services and advances the rights of people with disabilities.

1831 Learning Disabilities Association
PO Box 831392
Richardson, TX 75083-1392

512-458-8234
800-604-7500
Fax: 512-458-3826
www.ldat.org
contact@ldat.org

Jean Kueker, President
Ann Robinson, State Coordinator
Promotes the educational and general welfare of individuals with learning disabilities.

1832 Office of Civil Rights: Texas
US Department of Education
1999 Bryan St
Suite 1620
Dallas, TX 75201-6817

214-661-9540
Fax: 214-661-9587
TDD: 877-521-2172
www.ed.gov
ocr.dallas@ed.gov

Keith M. Maddox, Regional IG for Audit
Thomas Utz Jr., Special Agent In Charge
Russlynn Ali, Assistant Secretary
The Dallas office covers the states of Alabama, Arkansas, Louisiana, Mississippi and Texas.

1833 Southwest Texas Disability & Business Technical Assistance Center: Region VI
1333 Moursund
#1000
Houston, TX 77030-7019

713-520-0232
800-949-4232
Fax: 713-520-5785
TTY: 713-520-0232
www.swdbtac.org
swdbtac@ilru.org

Laurie Redd, Executive Director
Wendy Wilkinson, Project Director
One of ten DBTACs funded by the National Institute on Disability and Rehabilitation Research. The DBTAC serves a wide range of audiences who are interested in or impacted by these laws, including employers, businesses, government agencies, schools and people with disabilities.

1834 State GED Administration
Texas Education Agency
1701 Congress Ave
Austin, TX 78701-1402   512-463-9292
                               Fax: 512-305-9493
                               www.tea.state.tx.us
                               ged@tea.state.tx.us
G Paris Ealy, GED State Program Administrator
Bill Abasolo, Staff
Kim Ackermann, Staff
To build capacity for consistent testing services throughout
the state in order that all eligible candidates may have an
pooporunity to earn high school equivalency credentials
based on the General Educational Development (GED)
Tests.

1835 Texas Council for Developmental Disabilities
6201 E Oltorf St
Suite 600
Austin, TX 78741-7509   512-437-5432
                               800-262-0334
                               Fax: 512-437-5434
                               http://tcdd.texas.gov
                               tcdd@tcdd.texas.gov
Roger Webb, Executive Director
Martha Cantu, Operations Director
Jessica Ramos, Public Policy Director
To create change so that all people with disabilities are fully
included in their communities and exercise control over
their own lives.

1836 Texas Department of Assistive and Rehabilitative Services
4800 N Lamar Blvd
Austin, TX 78756-3106   512-377-0500
                               800-628-5115
                               Fax: 512-424-4730
                               TTY: 866-581-9328
                               www.dars.state.tx.us
                               dars.inquiries@dars.state.tx.us
Veronda L. Durden, Commissioner
Glenn Neal, Deputy Commissioner
Karin Hill, Director
To work in partnership with Texans with disabilities and
families with children who have developmental delays to
improve the quality of their lives and to enable their full par-
ticipation in society.

1837 Texas Department of Criminal Justice
PO Box 99
Huntsville, TX 77342-99   936-295-6371
                               Fax: 512-305-9398
                               www.tdcj.state.tx.us
Brad Livingston, Executive Director
To provide public safety, promote positive change in of-
fender behavior, reintegrate offenders into society, and as-
sist victims of crime.

1838 Texas Education Agency
1701 N Congress Ave
Austin, TX 78701-1494   512-463-9734
                               Fax: 512-463-9838
                               www.tea.state.tx.us
                               commissioner@tea.state.tx.us
David A. Anderson, General Counsel
Joanie Allen, General Counsel
Andrew Allen, General Counsel
To provide leadership, guidance, and resources to help
schools meet the educational needs of all students.

1839 Texas Workforce Commission: Civil Rights Division
101 E 15th St
Rm 665
Austin, TX 78778-0001   512-463-2236
                               800-711-2989
                               Fax: 512-463-2643
                               TTY: 800-735-2989
                               www.twc.state.tx.us
                               ombudsman@twc.state.tx.us
Andres Alcantar, Chairman
Ronald G. Congleton, Commissioner
Hope Andrade, Commissioner
Enforces the Texas Commission on Human Rights Act and
the Texas Fair Housing Act. The Human Rights Act prohib-
its employment discrimination based on race, color, religion, sex, age, national origin, disability and retaliation. The
Fair Housing Act prohibits housing discrimination based on
race, color, religion, sex, national origin, mental or physical
disability, familial status and retaliation.

1840 Texas Workforce Commission: Workforce Development Division
PO Box 12728
Austin, TX 78711-2728   512-936-0697
                               www.twc.state.tx.us
                               ombudsman@twc.state.tx.us
Andres Alcantar, Chairman
Ronald G. Congleton, Commissioner
Hope Andrade, Commissioner
Provides oversight, coordination, guidance, planning, technical assistance and implementation of employment and
training activities with a focus on meeting the needs of employers throughout the state of Texas. Also supports work
conducted in local workforce development areas, provides
assistance to boards in the achievement of performance
goals, evaluates education and training providers, and promotes and develops partnerships with other agencies and
institutions.

Utah

1841 Assistive Technology Center
1595 W 500 S
Salt Lake City, UT 84104-5238   801-887-9380
                                     800-866-5550
                                     www.usor.utah.gov/ucat
Kent Remund, Director
Lynn Marcoux, Executive Secretary
Craig Boogaard, Manager
To enhance human potential through facilitating the applica-
tion of assistive technologies for persons with disabilities.

1842 Assistive Technology Program
6588 Old Main Hill
6855 Old Main Hill
Logan, UT 84322-6855   435-797-3824
                                     800-524-5152
                                     Fax: 435-797-2355
                                     www.uatpat.org
Sachin Pavithran, Program Director
Marilyn Hammond, UATF Director
Lois Summers, Staff Assistant
Serve individuals with disabilities of all ages in Utah and the
intermountain region. Provide AT devices and services, and
train university students, parents, children with disabilities
and professional services providers about AT. Also coordinate the services with community organizations and others
who provide independence-related support to individuals
with disabilities.

1843 Center for Persons with Disabilities
Utah State University
6800 Old Main Hl
Logan, UT 84322-6800   435-797-1981
                                     866-284-2821
                                     Fax: 435-797-3944
                                     www.cpdusu.org

M Bryce Fifield PhD, Executive Director
Cynthia Rowland, Associate Director
Julie Williams, Front Office Receptionist
Utah's University Center for excellence in developmental disabilities education, research, and services. We collaborate with partners to strengthen families and individuals across the lifespan through education, policy, research and services.

1844 Department of Workforce Services

P.O. Box 143245
Salt Lake City, UT 84145-3245   801-526-9675
877-837-3247
Fax: 801-526-9500
http://jobs.utah.gov
dwscontactus@utah.gov
Kristen Cox, Executive Director
Provides employment and support services for our customers to improve their economic opportunities.

1845 Disability Law Center

205 N 400 W
Salt Lake City, UT 84103-1125   801-363-1347
800-662-9080
Fax: 801-363-1437
TTY: 800-500-4182
www.disabilitylawcenter.org
mattknotts@disabilitylawcenter.org
Bryce Fifield PhD, President
Jared Fields, Vice President
Barbara M. Campbell, Treasurer
A private non-profit organization designated as the Protection and Advocacy agency for the state of Utah to protect the rights of people with disabilities in Utah. To enforce and strengthen laws that protect the opportunities, choices and legal rights of people with disabilities in Utah.

1846 Utah Antidiscrimination and Labor Division

Utah Labor Commission
160 East 300 South
3rd Floor
Salt Lake City, UT 84114-6600   801-530-6801
800-222-1238
Fax: 801-530-7609
www.laborcommission.utah.gov
laborcom@utah.gov
Sherrie M Hayashi, Commissioner
Jaceson Maughan, Deputy Commissioner
Pete Hackford, Director
Investigates and resolves employment and housing discrimination complaints and enforces Utah's minimum wage, wage payment requirements, laws which protect youth in employment and the requirement that private employemnt agencies be licensed. The Division also conducts public awareness and educational presentations.

1847 Utah Developmental Disabilities Council

155 S 300 W
Suite 100
Salt Lake City, UT 84101-1288   801-533-3965
Fax: 801-533-3968
www.utahddcouncil.org
Deborah Bowman, Chair
Eric Stoker, Vice Chair
Dustin Erekson, Treasurer
The mission of the Utah DD council is to be the states leading source of critical innovative and progressive knowledge, advocacy, leadership and collaboration to enhance the life of individuals with developmental disabilities.

1848 Utah State Office of Education

250 East 500 South
PO Box 144200
Salt Lake City, UT 84114-4200   801-538-7821
Fax: 801-538-7882
www.utahged.org
marty.kelly@schools.utah.gov
Marty Kelly, State GED Administrator
Kellie Tyrrell, Score Reports

Promotes adult education and GED Testing in Utah.

Vermont

1849 Vermont Department of Children & Families

103 South Main Street
2 & 3 North
Waterbury, VT 05671-5500   802-241-3110
800-649-2642
http://dcf.vermont.gov
kim.keiser@ahs.state.vt.us
Dave Yacovone, Commissioner
To promote the social, emotional, physical and economic well being and the safety of Vermont's children and families.

1850 Vermont Department of Education

120 State St
Montpelier, VT 05620-2501   802-479-1030
www.education.vermont.gov
doe-edinfo@state.vt.us
Kate Nicolet, Director of Adult Education
Sharon Parker, Assistant Director
Donna McAllister, Health Education Consultant
Provide leadership and support to help all Vermont students achieve excellence.

1851 Vermont Department of Labor

5 Green Mountain Drive
PO Box 488
Montpelier, VT 05601-488   802-828-4000
Fax: 802-828-4022
TDD: 802-828-4203
www.labor.vermont.gov
pat.moulton.powden@state.vt.us
Annie Noonan, Commissioner
Rose Lucenti, Director
Steve Monahan, Director of Workers' Comp
To improve and enhance services to the public by combining under one department: employment security, employment-related services, labor market information, safety and training for Vermont workers, and employers, workers compensation, and wage and hour.

1852 Vermont Developmental Disabilities Council

103 S Main St
One North,Suite117
Waterbury, VT 05671-0206   802-828-1310
888-317-2006
Fax: 802-828-1321
www.ddc.vermont.gov
vtddc@state.vt.us
Karen Schwartz, Executive Director
Statewide board that works to increase public awareness about critical issues affecting Vermonters with developmental disabilities and their families. 13 of the 21 board members are people with developmental disabilities or family members.

1853 Vermont Governor's Office

109 State St
Pavilion
Montpelier, VT 05609   802-828-3333
800 649-6825
Fax: 802-828-3339
TTY: 800-649-6825
www.governor.vermont.gov
Peter Shumlin, Governor
Jeb Spaulding, Secretary
Chuck Ross, Secretary

1854 Vermont Protection and Advocacy Agency
Ste 7
141 Main St
Montpelier, VT 05602-2916
802-229-1355
877-805-9624
Fax: 802-229-1359
www.vtpa.org
ed.paquin@vtpa.org
Ed Paquin, Executive Director
Dedicated to addressing problems, questions and complaints brought to it by Vermonters with disabilities. Mission is to promote the equality, dignity, and self-determination of people with disabilities. Provides information, referral and advocacy services, including legal representation when appropriate, to individuals with disabilities throughout Vermont. Also advocates to promote positive systematic responses to issues affecting people with disabilities.

1855 Vermont Special Education
Vermont Department of Education
219 North Main Street
Suite 402
Barre, VT 05641-2501
(802) 479-10
http://education.vermont.gov
AOE.EdInfo@state.vt.us
Kate Nicolet, Director of Adult Education
Sharon Parker, Assistant Director
Donna McAllister, Health Education Consultant
Provides technical assistance to schols and other organization to help ensure that schools understand and comply with federal and state laws and regulations related to providing special education services.

Virginia

1856 Assistive Technology System
8004 Franklin Farms Dr
Richmond, VA 23229
804-662-9990
800-435-8490
Fax: 804-622-9478
www.vats.org
kathryn.hayfield@drs.virginia.gov
Elizabeth Flaherty, Chairperson
Kelly Lum, Vice-Chair
Peggy Fields, Council Secretary
To ensure that Virginians of all ages and abilities can acquire the appropriate, affordable assistive and information technologies and services they need to participate in society as active citizens.

1857 Department of Correctional Education
PO Box 26963
Richmond, VA 23261-6963
804-674-3000
Fax: 804-225-3255
TDD: 804-371-8647
http://dce.virginia.gov
docmail@vadoc.virginia.gov
Debra Gardner, Chief Deputy Director
Harold W. Clarke, Director
A. David Robinson, Chief of Corrections Operations
Provides quality educational programs that enable incarcerated youth and adults to become responsible, productive, tax-paying members of their community.

1858 Office of Adult Education and Literacy
Virginia Department of Education
PO Box 2120
Richmond, VA 23218
804-225-2075
Fax: 804-225-3352
www.doe.virginia.gov
Christisn N. Barunlich, President
Winsome E. Sears, Vice President
Diane T. Atkinson, Board Member
Operates as the designated agency to coordinate all secondary adult education and literacy services in the commonwealth.

1859 State Department of Education
Office of Adult Education and Literacy
PO Box 2120
Richmond, VA 23218
804-225-2075
Fax: 804-225-3352
www.doe.virginia.gov
Christisn N. Barunlich, President
Winsome E. Sears, Vice President
Diane T. Atkinson, Board Member
Promotes quality education.

1860 State GED Administration
Office of Adult Education and Literacy
PO Box 2120
Richmond, VA 23218
804-225-2075
Fax: 804-225-3352
www.doe.virginia.gov
Christisn N. Barunlich, President
Winsome E. Sears, Vice President
Diane T. Atkinson, Board Member
Promotes quality education for adults.

1861 Virginia Board for People with Disabilities
1100 Bank Street
7th Floor
Richmond, VA 23219
804-786-0016
800-845-4464
Fax: 804-786-1118
TTY: 800-845-4464
www.vaboard.org
katherine.lawson@vbpd.virginia.gov
Korinda Rusinyak, Chair
Charles Meacham, Vice Chair
Heidi Lawyer, Director
To enrich the lives of Virginians with disabilities by providing a voice for their concerns.

1862 Virginia Office for Protection & Advocacy Agency
1910 Byrd Ave
Suite 5
Richmond, VA 23230
804-225-2042
800-552-3962
Fax: 804-662-7057
TTY: 800-552-3962
www.vopa.state.va.us
general.vopa@vopa.virginia.gov
CW Tillman, President
Angela MW Thanyachareon, Vice President
Donald Price, Treasurer
Through zealous and effective advocacy and legal representation to: protect and advance legal, human, and civil rights of persons with disabilities; combat and prevent abuse, neglect, and discrimination; and to promote independence, choice, and self determination by persons with disabilities.

Washington

1863 Correctional Education
Department of Corrections
PO Box 41100
Mail Stop 41100
Olympia, WA 98504-1100
360-725-8213
Fax: 360-586-6582
www.doc.wa.gov
doccorrespondence@doc1.wa.gov
Lynne Delano, Chair
Peter Dawson, Chief of Staff
Sarian Scott, Director
The Department of Corrections, in collaboration with its criminal justice partners, will contribute to staff and community safety and hold offenders accountable through administration of criminal sanctions and effective re-entry programs.

1864 Department of Personnel & Human Services
619 Division St
Port Orchard, WA 98366 360-337-5777
Fax: 360-337-7187
www.kitsapgov.com
appserv@co.kitsap.wa.us
Robert Gelder, Commissioner
Charlotte Garrido, Commissioner
Linda Streissguth, Commissioner
Exists to serve the needs of elected County Officials, appointed department heads, County employees and the entire community through a variety of programs and processes. The employees of this department perform work in a wide variety of specialized areas, providing programs and services vital to the community and to Kitsap County as a unit of local government.

1865 Disability Rights Washington
315-5th Ave S
Suite 850
Seattle, WA 98104 206-324-1521
800-562-2702
Fax: 206-957-0729
TTY: 206-957-0728
www.disabilityrightswa.org
info@dr-wa.org
Mark Stroh, Executive Director
Andrea Kadlec, Director of Community Relations
David Carlson, Director of Legal Advocacy
A private non-profit organization that protects the rights of people with disabilities statewide. To advance the dignity, equality, and self-determination of people with disabilities. Also work to pursue justice on matters related to human and legal rights.

1866 Region X: Office of Federal Contract Compliance
US Department of Labor
200 Constitution Ave NW
Washington, DC 20210 202-693-0103
800-397-6251
Fax: 415-625-7799
TTY: 877-889-5627
www.dol.gov/ofccp
OFCCP-Public@dol.gov
Thomas E. Perez, Secretary of Labor
Matthew Colangelo, Chief of Staff
Elizabeth Kim, Executive Secretariat Director
Administers Federal Law requiring recipients of Federal Contract dollars to uphold affirmative action and equal employment pooprtunity for all workers, including but not limited to minorities, women, veterans and disabled employees.

1867 Region X: US Department of Education Office for Civil Rights
US Department of Education
Room 3362
915 2nd Ave
Seattle, WA 98174-1009 206-220-7900
Fax: 206-220-7887
TDD: 877-521-2172
www.ed.gov
ocr.seattle@ed.gov
Arne Duncan, Secretary of Education
Tony Miller, Deputy Secretary
Russlynn Ali, Assistant Secretary
This office covers the states of Alaska, Hawaii, Idaho, Montana, Nevada, Oregon, and Washington.

1868 Region X: US Department of Health and Human Services, Office of Civil Rights
US Department of Health & Human Services
200 Independence Avenue, S.W.
Washington, DC 20201 206-615-2010
Fax: 206-615-2087
www.hhs.gov
susan.johnson@hhs.gov
Sylvia M. Burwell, Secretary
Bill Corr, Deputy Secretary
E.J. Holland, Asst. Secretary for Admin

1869 WA State Board for Community and Technical Colleges
PO Box 42495
1300 Quince Street SE
Olympia, WA 98504-2495 360-704-4400
Fax: 360-704-4415
www.sbctc.ctc.edu
bgordon@sbctc.edu
Beth Willis, Chair
Shaunta Hyde, Vice Chair
Marty Brown, Executive Director
Promotes adult education.

1870 Washington Human Rights Commission
PO Box 42490
711 S. Capitol Way, Suite 402
Olympia, WA 98504-2490 360-753-6770
800-233-3247
Fax: 360-586-2282
TTY: 800-300-7525
www.hum.wa.gov
Sharon Ortiz, Executive Director
Steve Hunt, Commission Chair
Shawn Murinko, Commissioner
The Washington State Human Rights Commission enforces the Washington Law Against Discrimination, the broadest civil rights statute in the United States. It provides technical assistance and training. It also does studies and writes white papers on issues of social justice.

1871 Washington State Board for Community and Technical Colleges
Office of Adult Basic Education
PO Box 42495
1300 Quince Street SE
Olympia, WA 98504-2495 360-704-4400
Fax: 360-704-4415
www.sbctc.ctc.edu/
imendoza@sbctc.edu
Beth Willis, Chair
Shaunta Hyde, Vice Chair
Marty Brown, Executive Director
Promotes the quality of adult education.

1872 Washington State Client Assistance Program
2531 Rainier Avenue South
Seattle, WA 98144 206-721-5999
800-544-2121
Fax: 206-721-4537
TTY: 888-721-6072
www.washingtoncap.org
info@washingtoncap.org
Jerry Johnsen, Director
Bob Huven, Rehabilitation Coordinator
Provides information and advocacy for persons seeking services from the Department of Services for the Blind and the Division of Vocational Rehabilitation. Approximately 25 percent of cases involve assistive technology issues.

1873 Washington State Developmental Disabilities Council
PO Box 48314
Olympia, WA 98504-8314 360-586-3560
800-634-4473
Fax: 360-586-2424
www.ddc.wa.gov
Ed.Holen@ddc.wa.gov
Ed Holen, Executive Director
Laurie Bahr, Budget Director
Donna Patrick, Public Policy Director
Holds that individuals with developmental disabilities, including those with the most severe disabilities, have the right to achieve independence, productivity, integration and inclusion into the community.

1874 Washington State Governor's Committee on Disability Issues & Employment
PO Box 9046
Olympia, WA 98507
360-902-9500
800-318-6022
Fax: 866-610-9225
TTY: 800-833-6388
www.esd.wa.gov
Uitelecenters@Esd.wa.gov
Sheryl Hutchison, Communications Director
Bill Tarrow, Deputy Communications Director
Joe Elling, Chief Labor Economist
Information about disability rights programs and services.

West Virginia

1875 Client Assistance Program (CAP): West Virginia Division
West Virginia Advocates
1207 Quarrier St
Suite 400
Charleston, WV 25301
304-346-0847
800-950-5250
Fax: 304-346-0867
www.wvadvocates.org
contact@wvadvocates.org
Terry Dilcher, President
John Galloway, Treasurer
Don Neurman, Secretary
Mandated in 1984, to provide advocacy to individuals seeking services under the federal Rehabilitation Act (such as services from the West Virginia Division of Rehabilitation Services, Centers for Independent Living, supported employment programs and sheltered workshops).

1876 Office of Institutional Education
State Department of Education
Building 6, Room 728
1900 Kanawha Blvd East
Charleston, WV 25305-0330
304-558-7881
Fax: 304-558-5042
http://wvde.state.wv.us/institutional/
fwarsing@access.k12.wv.us
Dr Fran Warsing, Superintendent
Rhonda Mahan, Secretary
Jacob C. Green, Assistant Director
Provides educational services to over 6,000 institutionalized juveniles and adults. It protects the constitutional rights of institutionalized persons by providing programs and services that help change their lives.

1877 State Department of Education
1900 Kanawha Blvd E
Building 6
Charleston, WV 25305-0330
304-558-2681
Fax: 304-558-0048
http://wvde.state.wv.us
dvermill@access.k12.wv.us
Jorea M Marple, State Superintendent
Charles Heinlein, Deputy Superintendant
Promotes quality education.

1878 State GED Administration
1900 Kanawha Blvd E
Charleston, WV 25305-0009
304-558-6315
Fax: 304-558-4874
www.wvabe.org/ged/
dkimbler@access.k12.wv.us
Debra Kimbler, GED Administrator
Our organization's goal is to provide reasonable accommodations to qualifying GED candidates.

1879 West Virginia Adult Basic Education
West Virginia Department of Education
1900 Kanawha Blvd E
Rm 6
Charleston, WV 25305-0001
304-558-0280
800-642-2670
Fax: 304-558-3946
http://wvde.state.wv.us
dvarner@access.k12.wv.us
Dr Debra L Frazier Varner, Executive Director
To enable adult learners to be literate, productive, and successful in the workplace, home and community by delivering responsive adult education programs and services.

1880 West Virginia Assistive Technology System
959 Hartman Run Rd
Morgantown, WV 26505
304-293-4692
800-841-8436
Fax: 304-293-7294
TTY: 800-518-1448
http://wvats.cedwvu.org
wvats@hsc.wvu.edu
Monica G. Andis, Program Manager
Debra S. Cain, Administrative Secretary
Martha Ankney, Accountant
Provides access to Assistive Technology through information and referral, technical assistance training, device demonstration, loan & exchange.

Wisconsin

1881 Department of Public Instruction
PO Box 7841
125 S. Webster Street
Madison, WI 53707-7841
608-266-3390
800-441-4563
http://dpi.wi.gov
webadmin@dpi.wi.gov
Tony Evers, State Superintendent
Michael Thompson, Deputy State Superintendent
Jessica Justman, Chief of Staff
Promotes quality education.

1882 Disability Rights Wisconsin
Suite 700
131 W Wilson Street
Madison, WI 53703-3263
608-267-0214
800-928-8778
Fax: 608-267-0368
TTY: 888-758-6049
www.disabilityrightswi.org
Tom Masseau, Executive Director
DRW challenges systems and society to achieve positive changes in the lives of people with disabilities and their families.

1883 State GED Administration
Department of Public Instruction
PO Box 7841
125 S. Webster Street
Madison, WI 53707-7841
608-266-3390
800-441-4563
Fax: 608-267-9275
http://dpi.wi.gov
beth.lewis@dpi.wi.gov
Tony Evers, State Superintendent
Michael Thompson, Deputy State Superintendent
Jessica Justman, Chief of Staff
Promotes quality adult education.

1884 Wisconsin Board for People with Developmental Disabilities
101 East Wilson Street
Room 219
Madison, WI 53703

608-266-7826
888-332-1677
Fax: 608-267-3906
TDD: 608-266-6660
TTY: 602-266-6660
www.wi-bpdd.org
bpddhelp@wi-bpdd.org

Kevin Fech, Chair
Beth Swedeen, Executive Director
James Giese, Director of Communications
Established to advocate on behalf of individuals with developmental disabilities, foster welcoming and inclusive communities, and improve the disability service system. To help people with developmental disabilities become independent, productive, and included in all facets of community life.

1885 Wisconsin Department of Workforce Development
PO Box 7946
Madison, WI 53707-7946

608-266-3131
Fax: 608-266-1784
TTY: 608-267-0477
http://dwd.wisconsin.gov/
reggie.newson@dwd.wisconsin.gov

Reggie Newson, Department Secretary
Jonathan Barry, Deputy Secretary
Kathleen Reed, Administrator
A state agency charged with building and strengthening Wisconsin's workforce in the 21st century and beyond. The Departmen's primary responsibilities include providing job services, training and employment assistance to people looking for work, at the same time as it works with employers on finding the necessary workers to fill current job openings.

1886 Wisconsin Equal Rights Division
201 E. Washington Ave.
Madison, WI 53703

608-266-3131
Fax: 608-266-1784
TTY: 608-264-8752
www.dwd.wisconsin.gov/er
Jim Chiolino@dwd. wisconsin.gov

Reggie Newson, Department Secretary
Jonathan Barry, Deputy Secretary
Kathleen Reed, Administrator
To protect the rights of all people in Wisconsin under the civil rights and labor standards laws we administer; to achieve compliance through education, outreach, and enforcement by empowered and committed employees; and to perform our responsibilities with reasonableness, efficiency, and fairness.

1887 Wisconsin Governor's Committee for People with Disabilities
1 W. Wilson Street
Madison, WI 53703

608-266-1865
Fax: 608-266-3386
TTY: 888-701-1251
http://dhs.wisconsin.gov
DHSwebmaster@wisconsin.gov

Jean O'Leary, Northeast Region
Tamara Feest, Northern Region
Emily Campbell, Southern Region
Established to improve employment opportunities for people with disabilities.

Wyoming

1888 Adult Basic Education
Wyoming Community College Commission
2300 Capitol Ave, 5th Floor
Suite B
Cheyenne, WY 82002

307-777-7763
Fax: 307-777-6567
http://communitycolleges.wy.edu
mhess@commission.wu.edu

Dr. Jim Rose, Executive Director
Larry Atwell, Commissioner
Charlene Bodine, Commissioner
Focuses on strengthening basic reading, writing, and math skills for adults.

1889 Client Assistance Program (CAP): Wyoming
7344 Stockmann Street
Cheyenne, WY 82009

307-632-3496
Fax: 307-638-0815
www.wypanda.com
wypanda@wypanda.com

Tori Rosenthal, President
Jeanne A. Thobro, CEO
Provides free services to consumers and applicants for projects, programs and facilities funded under the rehabilitation act.

1890 Correctional Education: Wyoming Women's Center
1934 Wyott Drive
Suite 100
Cheyenne, WY 82002

307-777-7208
Fax: 307-777-7846
http://corrections.wy.gov/institutions/wwc/educ
chris.thayer@wyo.gov

Phil Myer, Warden
Martha Decker, Associate Warden
The Wyoming Women's Center is a full service, secure correctional facility for female offenders and the sole adult female facility in the State of Wyoming. In October 2000, WWC opened a self-contained 16 bed intensive addiction treatment unit, a is highly structured long term 7-9 month program based upon the therapeutic community treatment model. It is tailored to provide gender specific services and is funded with a combination of state and federal resources.

1891 Protection & Advocacy System
7344 Stockmann Street
Cheyenne, WY 82009

307-632-3496
Fax: 307-638-0815
www.wypanda.com
wypanda@wypanda.com

Tori Rosenthal, President
Jeanne A. Thobro, CEO
It is the goal of Wyoming's Protection & Advocacy System, Inc. to ensure that all of its web resources are accessible to all who use this website. The pages reflect this process.

1892 State Department of Education
1 Research Park
Inwood, WV 25428-9733

304-229-0100
800-325-7759
Fax: 304-229-0295
www.youseemore.com
info@TLCdelivers.com

Annette Harwood, Chairman/President/ CEO
Calvin Whittington, Director of Finance & Admin
Bradley Cole, Sales Director

1893 State GED Administration
State Department of Education
2300 Capitol Ave
Hathaway Building, 2nd Floor
Cheyenne, WY 82002-2060

307-777-7673
Fax: 307-777-6234
www.k12.wy.us

Cindy Hill, Superintendent
Deb Lindsey, Assesment
Tiffany Dobler, Special Programs
Promotes quality adult education.

1894   Wyoming Department of Workforce Services

1510 East Pershing Blvd
Cheyenne, WY 82002   307-777-3700
                                         866-804-3678
                                    Fax: 307-777-5870
                              www.wyomingworkforce.org
                                joan.evans@wyo.gov

Joan K. Evans, Director
Lisa M. Osvold, Deputy Director
Employment training for persons working in Wyoming.

National Programs

1895 Academic Institute
2495 140th Ave NE
Suite D-210
Bellevue, WA 98005
425-401-6844
Fax: 425-556-6972
www.academicinstitute.com
sherrill@academicinstitute.com
Sherrill O'Shaughnessy, Founder/Executive Director
To prepare students for success in college and their lives beyond by helping them cultivate: a sense of capability, determination, resilience, self-advocacy and a love of learning.

1896 American Association for Adult and Continuing Education
10111 Martin Luther King Jr Hwy
Ste 200C
Bowie, MD 20720
301-459-6261
Fax: 301-459-6241
www.aaace.org
office@aaace.org
Steven Schmidt, President
Jonathan Taylor, Secretary
Jim Berger, Treasurer
Provides leadership for the field of adult and continuing education by expanding opportunities for adult growth and development; unifying adult educators; fostering the development and dissemination of theory, research, informaiton and best practices; promoting identity and standards for the profession; and advocating relevant public policy and social change initiatives.

1897 American Literacy Council
1441 Mariposa Avenue
Boulder, CO 80302
303-440-7385
www.americanliteracy.com
presidentalc3@americanliteracy.com
Alan Mole, President
Roberta Mahoney, Vice President
Joe Little, Director
Conveys information on new solutions, innovative technologies and tools for engaging more boldly in the battle for literacy.

1898 Association of Educational Therapists
7044 S. 13th St.
Oak Creek, WI 53154
414-908-4949
800-286-4267
Fax: 414-768-8001
www.aetonline.org
aet@aetonline.org
Jane Utley Adelizzi, Chair
Jeanette Rivera, MA, BCET, President
Judith Brennan, Director
Dedicated to defining the professional practice of educational therapy, setting standards for ethical practice, and promoting state-of-the-art service delivery through on-going professional development and training programs.

1899 Association on Higher Education and Disability
107 Commerce Center Drive
Ste 204
Huntersville, NC 28078
704-947-7779
Fax: 704-948-7779
TTY: 617-287-3882
www.ahead.org
ahead@ahead.org
Bea Awoniyi, President
Stephan Hamlin-Smith, Executive Director
Kristie Orr, Director
A professional membership organization for individuals involved in the development of policy and in the provision of quality services to meet the needs of persons with disabilities involved in all areas of higher education.

1900 Career College Association (CCA)
1101 Connecticut Ave NW
Ste 900
Washington, DC 20036
202-336-6700
866-711-8574
Fax: 202-336-6828
www.career.org
cca@career.org
Robert Herzog, Chair
Jeffery Cooper, Vice Chair
Steve Gunderson, President and CEO
A voluntary membership organization of accredited, private, postsecondary schools, institutes, colleges and universities that provide career-specific educational programs.
1,400 members

1901 Center for the Improvement of Early Reading Achievement (CIERA)
University of Michigan School of Education
610 E University Ave
Rm 2002 SEB
Ann Arbor, MI 48109-1259
734-647-6940
Fax: 734-615-4858
www.ciera.org
ciera@umich.edu
Karen Wixon, Former Director
Joanne Carlisle, Former Co-Director
Deanna Birdyshaw, Former Associate Director
To improve the reading achievement of America's youth by generating and disseminating theoretical, empirical, and practical solutions to the learning and teaching of beginning reading.

1902 Council for Educational Diagnostic Services
Council for Exceptional Children
2900 Crystal Drive
Suite 1000
Arlington, VA 22202-3557
888-232-7733
888-232-7733
Fax: 703-264-9494
TTY: 866-915-5000
www.cec.sped.org
Robin D. Brewer, President
Alexander T. Graham, Secretary
Benjamin White, Student Member
Ensures the highest quality of diagnostic and prescriptive procedures involved in the education of individuals with disabilities and/or who are gifted.

1903 Distance Education and Training Council (DETC)
1601 18th St NW
Ste 2
Washington, DC 20009
202-234-5100
Fax: 202-332-1386
www.detc.org
detc@detc.org
Leah K. Matthews, Executive Director
Charles Baldwin, CFO
Sally R. Welch, Associate Director
A voluntary, non-governmental, educational organization that operates a nationally recognized accrediting association. Fosters and preserves high quality, educationally sound and widely accepted distance education and independent learning solutions.
1926

1904 Division for Children's Communication Development
Council for Exceptional Children
2900 Crystal Drive
Suite 1000
Arlington, VA 22202-3557
888-232-7733
888-232-7733
Fax: 703-265-9494
TTY: 866-915-5000
www.cec.sped.org
service@cec.sped.org
Robin D. Brewer, President
Alexander T. Graham, Secretary
Benjamin White, Student Member

Dedicated to improving the education of children with communication delays and disorders and hearing loss. Members include professionals serving individuals with hearing, speech and language disorders in the areas of receptive and expressive, verbal and nonverbal spoken, written and sign communication. Members receive a quarterly journal and newsletter three times a year.

1905 Division for Culturally and Linguistically Diverse Learners
Council for Exceptional Children
2900 Crystal Drive
Suite 1000
Arlington, VA 22202-3557   888-232-7733
                                 888-232-7733
                          Fax: 703-264-9494
                          TTY: 866-915-5000
                          www.cec.sped.org

Robin D. Brewer, President
Alexander T. Graham, Secretary
Benjamin White, Student Member
Advances educational opportunities for culturally and linguistically diverse learners with disabilities and/or who are gifted, their families and the professionals who serve them.

1906 Division for Research
Council for Exceptional Children
2900 Crystal Drive
Suite 1000
Arlington, VA 22202-3557   888-232-7733
                                 888-232-7733
                          Fax: 703-264-9494
                          TTY: 866-915-5000
                          www.cec.sped.org

Robin D. Brewer, President
Alexander T. Graham, Secretary
Benjamin White, Student Member
Devoted to the advancement of research related to the education of individuals with disabilities and/or who are gifted.

1907 Educational Advisory Group
2222 Eastlake Ave E
Seattle, WA 98102-3419   206-323-1838
                          Fax: 206-267-1325
                          www.eduadvisory.com

Yvonne Jones, Director
Specializes in matching children with the learning environments that are best for them and works with families to help them identify concerns and establish priorities about their child's education.

1908 Institute for Educational Leadership
4301 Connecticut Avenue
Suite 100
Washington, DC 20008-2304   202-822-8405
                          Fax: 202-872-4050
                          www.iel.org
                          iel@iel.org

S. Decker Anstrom, Chair
Eileen Fox, Director of Finance and Budget
S. Kwesi Rollins, Director, Leadership Programs
To improve education and the lives of children and their families through positive and visionary change.

1909 Institute for Human Centered Design
200 Portland St
Boston, MA 02114   617-695-1225
                          Fax: 617-482-8099
                          TTY: 617-695-1225
                          www.adaptiveenvironments.org
                          info@IHCDesign.org

Ralph Jackson, President
Chris Pilkington, Vice President
Valerie Fletcher, Executive Director
Founded as Adaptive Environments, committed to advancing the role of design in expanding opportunity and enhancing experience for people of all ages and abilities through excellence in design.

1910 Institute for the Study of Adult Literacy
Pennsylvania State Univ. College of Education
226 Chambers Building
University Park, PA 16802   814-865-0488
                          Fax: 814-863-6108
                          www.ed.psu.edu/isal
                          isal@psu.edu

David H. Monk, Co-Director
Emily Martell, Finance Office
Suzanne Wayne, Public Relations
Experienced staff assista providers with: program design and delivery; customized instructional materials and assessment development; professional development (including distance learning); and program evaluations.

1911 International Dyslexia Association
40 York Rd
4th Fl
Baltimore, MD 21204   410-296-0232
                          Fax: 410-321-5069
                          www.interdys.org
                          lisa@barbclapp.com

Kristen Penczek, Interim Executive Director
David. Holste, Director of Operations
Stacy Friedman, Manager of Operations
Nonprofit, scientific and educational organization dedicated to the study and treatment of dyslexia.

1912 Learning Resource Network
PO Box 9
River Falls, WI   715-426-9777
                          800-678-5376
                          Fax: 888-234-8633
                          www.lern.org
                          info@lern.org

Cathy Noonan, Chair
Kim Becicka, Treasurer
William A Draves, President
An international association of lifelong learning programming, offering information and resources to providers of lifelong learning programs.

1913 National Adult Education Professional Development Consortium
444 N Capital St NW
Ste 422
Washington, DC 20001   202-624-5250
                          Fax: 202-624-1947
                          www.naepdc.org
                          lmclendon@naepdc.org

Jennifer Foster, Chair
Dr Lennox McLendon, Executive Director
Dr. Gene Sofer, Govt. Relations Director
Advances the leadership of state staff in adult education throughout the states and territories so that every program will be of quality and excellence as we together increase literacy and prepare adults for success as contributing members of the society through work, community and family; and, will be the leading voice in adult education for the nation.

1914 National Adult Literacy & Learning Disabilities Center (NALLD)
FHI360
359 Blackwell Street
Suite 200
Durham, NC 27701   919-544-7040
                          Fax: 919-544-7262
                          www.fhi360.org
                          media@fhi360.org

Parick c. Fine, Chief Executive Officer
Robert S. Murphy, CFO
Deborah Kennedy, COO
The center is a national resource for information on learning disabilities in adults and on the relationship between learning disabilities and low-level literacy skills.

1915 **National Association for Adults with Special Learning Needs**

c/o KOC Member Services
1143 Tidewater Court
Westerville, OH 43082　　　　　888-562-2756
　　　　　　　　　　　　　　Fax: 614-392-1559
　　　　　　　　　　　　　　www.naasln.org

Richard Cooper, President
Joan Hudson-Miller, Co-President
Frances A. Holthaus, Vice President
An association for those who serve adults with special learning needs. Members include educators, trainers, employers and human service providers. The goal is to ensure that adults with special learning needs have opportunities necessary to become successful lifelong learners.

1916 **National Association of Private Special Education Centers**

601 Pennsylvania Ave NW
Ste 900, South Bldg
Washington, DC 20004　　　　　202-434-8225
　　　　　　　　　　　　　　Fax: 202-434-8224
　　　　　　　　　　　　　　www.napsec.org
　　　　　　　　　　　　　　napsec@aol.com
The indispensable voice and premier resource for the private special education community. Represents early intervention services, school, residential therapeutic centers, postsecondary college experience programs and adult living services.
1971

1917 **National Center for Family Literacy**

325 W Main St
Ste 300
Louisville, KY 40202　　　　　502-584-1133
　　　　　　　　　　　　　　Fax: 502-584-0172
　　　　　　　　　　　　　　www.famlit.org
　　　　　　　　　　notify@familieslearning.org
George Siemens, Board Member
Sharon Darling, Board Member
Jason Falls, Board Member
Mission is to not only provide every family with the opportunity to learn, but the ability to learn anf grow together. Ensures the cycle of learning and progress passes from generation to generation.

1918 **National Center for Learning Disabilities (NCLD)**

381 Park Ave S
Suite 1401
New York, NY 10016　　　　　212-545-7510
　　　　　　　　　　　　　　888-575-7373
　　　　　　　　　　　　　　Fax: 212-545-9665
　　　　　　　　　　　　　　www.ncld.org
Frederic M. Poses, Chair
Mary Kalikow, Vice Chair
William Haney, Secretary
To ensure that the nation's 15 million children, adolescents, and adults with learning disabilities have every opportunity to succeed in school, work and life.

1919 **National Center for the Study of Adult Learning & Literacy**

Harvard Graduate School of Education
Appian Way
Cambridge, MA 02138　　　　　617-495-3414
　　　　　　　　　　　　　　Fax: 617-495-4811
　　　　　　　　　　　　　　www.gse.harvard.edu
　　　　　　　　　　webedltor@gse.harvard.edu
James E. Ryan, Dean
The National Center for the Study of Adult Learning & Literacy both informs and learns from practice. Its rigorous, high quality research increases knowledge and gives those teaching, managing, and setting policy in adult literacy education a sound basis for making decisions.

1920 **National Center on Adult Literacy (NCAL)**

University of Pennsylvania
3700 Walnut Street
Philadelphia, PA 19104-6216　　　215-898-9803
　　　　　　　　　　　　　　Fax: 215-573-2115
　　　　　　　　　　　　　　www.literacy.org/
　　　　　　　　　　boyle@literacy.upenn.edu
Daniel A. Wagner, Founder and Director
Mohamed Maamouri, Associate Director
Ruth Boyle, Administrative Assistant
NCAL's mission incorporates three primary goals: to improve understanding of youth and adult learning; to foster innovation and increase effectiveness in youth and adult basic education and literacy work; and to expand access to information and build capacity for literacy and basic skills service.
1990

1921 **National Education Association (NEA)**

1201 - 16th St NW
Washington, DC 20036-3290　　　202-833-4000
　　　　　　　　　　　　　　Fax: 202-822-7974
　　　　　　　　　　　　　　www.nea.org
Lily Eskelsen García, President
Becky Pringle, Vice-President
John C. Stocks, Executive Director
Advocates for education professionals and seeks to unite members and the nation to fulfill the promise of public education to prepare every student to succeed in a diverse and interdependent world.

1922 **National Lekotek Center**

2001 N Clybourn
Chicago, IL 60614　　　　　773-528-5766
　　　　　　　　　　　　　　Fax: 773-537-2992
　　　　　　　　　　　　　　TTY: 773-973-2180
　　　　　　　　　　　　　　www.lekotek.org
　　　　　　　　　　　　　　lekotek@lekotek.org
Elaine D. Cottey, Chair
Kevin Limbeck, President & CEO
Carol Neiger, Secretary
The central source on toys and play for children with special needs.

1923 **Office of Special Education Programs**

US Department of Education
400 Maryland Avenue, SW
Washington, DC 20202　　　　　202-208-5815
　　　　　　　　　　　　　　800-872-5327
　　　　　　　　　　　　　　http://www2.ed.gov
Melody Musgrove, Director
Dedicated to improving results for infants, toddlers, children and youth with disabilities ages birth through 21 by providing leadership and financial support to assist states and local districts.

1924 **ProLiteracy**

104 Marcellus Street
Syracuse, NY 13204　　　　　315-422-9121
　　　　　　　　　　　　　　888-528-2224
　　　　　　　　　　　　　　Fax: 315-422-6369
　　　　　　　　　　　　　　www.proliteracy.org
　　　　　　　　　　　　　　info@proliteracy.org
John Ward, Chair
Nikki Zollar, Vice Chair
Kevin Morgan, President/CEO
Champions the power of literacy to improve the lives of adults and their families, communities, and societies. Works with its members and partners, and the adult learners they serve, along with local, national, and international organizations. Helps build the capacity and quality of programs that are teaching adults to read, write, compute, use technology and learn English as a new language.

1925 Thinking and Learning Connection
Parents Helping Parents
1400 Parkmoor Avenue
Suite 100
San Jose, CA 95126
408-727-5775
855-727-5775
Fax: 408-286-1116
www.php.com

Hitesh Shah, Chair
Mary Ellen Peterson, Executive Director/CEO, PHP
Paul Schutz, CFO
A group of independent associates committed to teaching learning different students. The primary focus is working with dyslexia and dyscalculia. The individualized education programs utilize extensive multisensory approaches to teach reading, spelling, handwriting, composition, comprehension and mathematics.

Alabama

1926 Alabama Commission on Higher Education
PO Box 302000
Montgomery, AL 36130-2000
334-242-1998
Fax: 334-242-0268
www.ache.state.al.us

Gregory G Fitch PhD, Executive Director
Jacinta Whitehurst, Administrative Assistant
Margaret Gunter, Director
Ths state agency responsible for the overall statewide planning and coordination of higher education in Alabama. Seeks to provide reasonable access to quality collegiate and university education for the citizens of Alabama.

1927 South Baldwin Literacy Council
21441 U.S. Hwy 98 East
Foley, AL 36535
251-943-7323
Fax: 251-970-3578
www.southbaldwinliteracycouncil.org/
literacy@gulftel.com

Keith Cardwell, President
Jan Taylor, Vice President
Rosalie Wolfe, Treasurer
Provides instruction by trained volunteer tutors in a one-on-one or small group setting to residents of South Baldwin County. Instruction is centered around the learners' individual goals and capabilities and is designed to improve basic reading, writing and life skills.

1928 The Literacy Council
2301 1st Ave N
Ste 102
Birmingham, AL 35203
205-326-1925
888-448-7323
www.literacy-council.org
info@literacy-council.org

Leigh Hancock, Chairman
Jordan DeMoss, Vice Chair
Beth Wilder, President & Executive Director
A non-profit organization which serves a five-county area, is dedicated to reducing literacy. Efforts include providing resources and referrals by maintaining a toll-free literacy helpline which serves as a primary point of contact for individuals seeking literacy assistance.

Alaska

1929 Alaska Adult Basic Education
SERRC
210 Ferry Eay
Juneau, AK 99801
907-586-6806
Fax: 907-463-3811
www.serrc.org
info@serrc.org

Eugene Avey, Board Member
Robert Boyle, Board Member
Steve Bradshaw, Board Member

The mission of the Adult Basic Education program is to provide instruction in the basic skills of reading, writing, and mathematics to adult learners in order to prepare them for transitioning into the labor market or higher academic or vocational training.

1930 Anchorage Literacy Project
Ste 104
1345 Rudakof Cir
Anchorage, AK 99508
907-337-1981
Fax: 907-338-3105
www.alaskaliteracyprogram.org
akliteracy@alaskaliteracyprogram.org

Linda Gerwin, President
Anne Newell, Vice President
Polly Smith, Executive Director
Dedicated to improving the lives of adults and their families by helping to build their literacy skills. Offer direct literacy skills for adults-native born citizens and recent immigrants alike-through on-site classes and one-on-one tutoring.

1931 Literacy Council of Alaska
517 Gaffney Rd
Fairbanks, AK 99701
907-456-6212
Fax: 907-456-4302
www.literacycouncilofalaska.org
lca@literacycouncilofalaska.org

Lisa Baker, Chairman
Mike Kolsa, Executive Director
Becky Magowan, Business Manager
Promotes literacy for people of all ages in Fairbanks and the Interior. The goals are to help community members achieve individual educational goals and to raise public awareness about literacy.

Arizona

1932 Chandler Public Library Adult Basic Education
PO Box 4008
Mail Stop 601
Chandler, AZ 85244-4008
480-782-2800
www.chandlerlibrary.org
marybeth.gardner@chandleraz.gov

Dolly Franco, President
Chris Loschiavo, Secretary
Marybeth Gardner, Library Development
Provides adult basic education classes for learners who need to improve their basic skills in reading, writing, and math. Gives GED preparation classes to help students prepare to take the GED exam.

1933 Literacy Volunteers of Maricopa County
1616 East Indian School Road
Suite 200
Phoenix, AZ 85016
602-274-3430
Fax: 602-274-6831
www.literacyvolunteers-maricopa.org
lvmc@lvmc.net

John Faulds, President
Jesus Love, Vice President
Brenda Church, Secretary
A non-profit organization dedicated to teaching adults 16 years and older how to read, write, speak English and prepare for the GED. Also offer computer literacy which includes the basics of using a computer, accessing the Internet and using basic Microsoft programs.

1934 Literacy Volunteers of Tucson A Program of Literacy Connects
200 E. Yavapai Road
Tucson, AZ 85705
520-882-8006
www.literacyconnects.org
info@literacyconnects.org

Sylvia Lee, Chairman
Cliff Bowman, Vice Chair
Betty Stauffer, Executive Director

Recruits, trains and matches tutors with adults (age 16 and up) in need of basic literacy (reading and writing) skills and/or English Language Acquisition for Adults (ELAA). Provides a friendly non-threatening environment that appeals to adult learners in all walks of life.

1935 Yuma Reading Council

2951 S. 21st Dr.
Yuma, AZ 85364-3846
928-782-1871
Fax: 928-782-9420
www.yumalibrary.org
greg.ferguson@yumacountyaz.go
Gregory Ferguson, Chairman
Brian D. Ewing, President
Provides one to one tutoring for basic literacy and english as a second language, and converstaion classes for beginning, intermediate and advanced levels for English as a second language students.

Arkansas

1936 Arkansas Adult Learning Resource Center

3905 Cooperative Way
Ste D
Little Rock, AR 72209
877-963-4433
Fax: 501-907-2492
www.aalrc.org/
info@aalrc.org
Marsha Talyor, Director
The Arkansas Adult Learning Resource Center was established in 1990 to provide a source for identification, evaluation, and dissemination of materials and information to adult education/literacy programs within the state.

1937 Arkansas Literacy Council

801 South Louisiana Street
Little Rock, AR 72201
501-907-2490
800-264-7323
Fax: 501-907-2492
www.arkansasliteracy.org
info@arkansasliteracy.org
Barbara Hanley, Chairman
Joe Burkett, Vice Chair
Nancy Leonhardt, Executive Director
Provides structure to a network of local literacy councils. These councils recruit and train volunteers to tutor adults who either need help with basic reading, writing, and math skills, or who want to learn English as a Second Language

1938 Drew County Literacy Council

801 South Louisiana Street
Little Rock, AR 72201
501-907-2490
800-264-7323
Fax: 501-907-2492
www.arkansasliteracy.org
info@arkansasliteracy.org
Barbara Hanley, Chairman
Joe Burkett, Vice Chair
Nancy Leonhardt, Executive Director
Formed by citizens that were concerned about the adult illiteracy rate reported in the 1980 census. Strives to recruit, train and match volunteer tutors with illiterate adults in the county using The Laubach Way to Reading and Laubach Way to English.

1939 Faulkner County Literacy Council

615 E Robins St
PO Box 2106
Conway, AR 72033
501-329-7323
www.faulknercoliteracy.org
fclc@conwaycorp.net
Emily Maggion, Executive Director
Provides free instruction through trained volunteers to adults in Faulkner County who lack basic reading, writing, mathematics, English as a second language and life skills.

1940 Literacy Action of Central Arkansas

P.O. Box 900
Little Rock, AR 72203
501-372-7323
Fax: 501-371-9888
www.literacylittlerock.org
ca@literacylittlerock.org
Dan Boland, President
Lee Hartz, Vice President
Bill Foster, Treasurer
A non-profit organization that teaches reading skills to adults and English skills to non-native adults.
1986

1941 Literacy Council of Arkansas County

801 South Louisiana Street
Little Rock, AR 72201
501-907-2490
800-264-7323
Fax: 501-907-2492
www.arkansasliteracy.org
info@arkansasliteracy.org
Barbara Hanley, Chairman
Joe Burkett, Vice Chair
Nancy Leonhardt, Executive Director

1942 Literacy Council of Benton County

205 NW A St
Bentonville, AR 72712
479-273-3486
Fax: 479-273-7545
http://goliteracy.org
readlcbc@sbcgloabl.net
Andy Gottman, President
Martha Walsh, Vice President
Vicki Ronald, Executive Director
A non-profit agency that increases Adult English literacy by developing volunteer tutors to teach students because Literacy Changes Lives. Empowers people to improve their wuality of lives within the community we all share by increasing adult English Literacy.

1943 Literacy Council of Crittenden County

2000 W Broadway St
West Memphis, AR 72301
870-733-6760
Fax: 870-733-6737
www.arkansasliteracy.org
jkfluker@midsouthcc.edu
Kim Fluker, Director

1944 Literacy Council of Garland County

119 Hobson Ave
Hot Springs, AR 71901
501-624-7323
Fax: 501-624-2994
www.arkansasliteracy.org
literacylady@sbcglobal.net
Pat McClaran, Director

1945 Literacy Council of Grant County

201 S Rose St
PO Box 432
Sheridan, AR 72150
870-942-5711
Fax: 870-942-7228
www.arkansasliteracy.org
literacy@windstream.net
Jo Ann Click, Director

1946 Literacy Council of Hot Spring County

122 E Page
PO Box 1485
Malvern, AR 72104
501-304-6679
Fax: 501-332-4043
www.readhelp.com
readhelp@sbcglobal.net
Jane Goodwin, Director
Offers a variety of educational services at no charge that range from literacy for adults to peer-tutoring for children; English as a second language to Learning Differences screening.

1947 Literacy Council of Jefferson County
402 E 5th
PO Box 7066
Pine Bluff, AR 71611   920-675-0500
                              Fax: 870-850-0984
                              www.jclc.us/
                              Karyn at kcable@jclc.us
Lynn Forseth, Executive Director

1948 Literacy Council of Lonoke County
306 N Center
PO Box 234
Lonoke, AR 72086   501-676-7478
                          Fax: 501-676-7478
                          www.arkansasliteracy.org
                          lonokeliteracy@sbcglobal.net
Claire Rogers, Director

1949 Literacy Council of Monroe County
234 W Cedar St
Brinkley, AR 72021   870-734-3333
                            Fax: 870-734-3333
                            www.arkansasliteracy.org
                            lcmc1992@gmail.com
Martha Pineda, Director

1950 Literacy Council of North Central Arkansas
PO Box 187
Leslie, AR 72645   870-447-3241
                          800-264-7323
                          Fax: 870-447-3241
                          www.arkansasliteracy.org
                          pogocatwoman26@gmail.com
Susan Vorwald, Director

1951 Literacy Council of Western Arkansas
PO Box 423
Fort Smith, AR 72902   479-783-2665
                              Fax: 479-783-5332
                              www.arkansasliteracy.org
                              helptoread@sbcglobal.net
Bruce Singleton, Director

1952 Literacy League of Craighead County
324 W Huntington Ave
PO Box 9251
Jonesboro, AR 72403   870-910-6511
                             Fax: 870-910-0552
                             www.arkansasliteracy.org
                             acbutts2006@yahoo.com
Amy Butts, Director

1953 Ozark Literacy Council
2596 Keystone Crossing
Fayetteville, AR 72703   479-521-8250
                                Fax: 479-582-0846
                                www.ozarkliteracy.org
                                info@ozarkliteracy.org
Don Moore, Chairman
Margot Jackson, Executive Director
Mina Phebus, Progarm Director
Provides quality basic literacy and language instruction enabling people to learn and communicate effectively.

1954 Pope County Literacy Council
1000 S Arkansas Ave
PO Box 1276
Russellville, AR 72811   479-967-7323
                                Fax: 479-968-6248
                                www.arkansasliteracy.org
                                popecoliteracy@centurytel.net
Jennifer Merkey, Director

1955 St. John's ESL Program
583 W Grand Ave
Hot Springs, AR 71901   501-624-3171
                               Fax: 501-624-3171
                               www.sjshs.org
                               aisaacs@sjshs.org
Angela Issacs, Principal
Jamie Cardenas, President
Lori Hinson, Secretary

1956 Twin Lakes Literacy Council
1318 Bradley Dr
Ste 14
Mountain Home, AR 72653   870-425-7323
                                 Fax: 870-424-3646
                                 www.twinlakesliteracycouncil.org
                                 twinlakeslc@yahoo.com
Nancy Tester, Executive Director
To promote and enhance literacy efforts and to encourage volunteers to participate in all phases of this endeavor.

1957 Van Buren County Literacy Council
Clinton, AR 72031   501-745-6440
                           Fax: 501-745-6440
                           www.arkansasliteracy.org
                           dogwood@artelco.com
Brenda Wood, Director

California

1958 Butte County Library Adult Reading Program
25 County Center Dr.
Suite 200
Oroville, CA 95965   530-538-7631
                            888-538-7198
                            Fax: 530-538-7120
                            www.buttecounty.net
                            literacy@buttecounty.net
Paul Hahn, CAO/Clerk of the Board
Kathleen Sweeney, Assistant Clerk of the Board
Tutoring at no charge in reading, writing and math. Participants will learn the basics and more with one-on-one tutoring. A volunteer tutor will meet with participants at any branch library in Butte County.

1959 California Association of Special Education & Services
CASES Executive Office
520 Capitol Mall
Ste 280
Sacramento, CA 95814   916-447-7061
                              Fax: 916-447-1320
                              www.capses.com
                              director@capses.com
Wayne K Miyamoto MEd, Public/Governmental Affairs Dir
Janeth Rodriguez MA, Communications/Operations Dir
A statewide professional association of nonpublic schools, agencies, organizations and individuals who specialize in the delivery of quality special education programs to students with special education needs.

1960 California Department of Education
Office of the Secretary for Education
1430 N Street
Sacramento, CA 95814   916-323-0611
                              Fax: 916-323-3753
                              www.cde.ca.gov/
Tom Torlakson, State Superintendent
The Office of the Secretary for Education is responsible for advising and making policy recommendations to the Governor on education issues.

1961 California Literacy
PO Box 70916
Pasadena, CA 91117-7916
626-395-9989
Fax: 626-356-9327
www.caliteracy.org
office@caliteracy.org

Archana Carey, Director
California Literacy was founded in 1956 and is the nation's oldest and largest statewide adult volunteer literacy organization. Its purpose is to establish literacy programs and to support them through tutor training, consulting, and ongoing education.

1962 Lake County Literacy Coalition
1425 N High St
Lakeport, CA 95453
707-263-8817
Fax: 707-263-6796
www.co.lake.ca.us

Jim Comstock, 1st District
Jeff Smith, 2nd District
Denise Rushing, 3rd District
A non-profit volunteer organization that sponsors and supports the Adult Literacy Program of Lake County Library. Also offer special training sessions on specific topics, such as ESL, learning disabilities and teaching grammar.

1963 Literacy Program: County of Los Angeles Public Library
Rm 208
7400 E. Imperial Hwy
Downey, CA 90242-3375
562-940-8400
www.colapublib.org
mdtodd@library.lacounty.gov

William T Fujioka, CEO
J. Tyler McCauley, Auditor/Controller
The Literacy Centers of the County of Los Angeles Public Library offer a variety of literacy services for adults and families at no charge. Literacy services include one-to-one basic literacy tutoring, English as a Second Language group instruction, Family Literacy and self-help instruction on audio cassettes, videocassettes and computer-based training. The literacy program is an affiliate of Literacy Volunteers of America, Inc.

1964 Literacy Volunteers of America: Willits Public Library
501 Low Gap Road
Ukiah, CA 95482
707-459-5908
www.mendolibrary.org
lvawillits@pacific.net

Carre Brown, 1st District
John McCowen, 2nd District
John Pinches, 3rd District
The Literacy program offers one-on-one reading, writing and tutoring for adults in the area.

1965 Marin Literacy Program
San Rafael Public Library
1100 E St
San Rafael, CA 94901
415-485-3318
Fax: 415-485-3112
www.marinliteracy.org
readandwrite@marinliteracy.org

Paul Cummins, President
Robin Carpenter, Executive Director
David Sason, Secretary
Provides Marin County adults with free student-centered instruction in reading, writing, and speaking to help them reach their full potential at work, at home, and in the community.

1966 Merced Adult School
3430 A Street
Atwater, CA 95301
209-385-6400
Fax: 209-385-6442
www.muhsd.k12.ca.us
dglass@muhsd.k12.ca.us

Sam Spangler, President
Dave Honey, Vice President
William G. Snyder, Clerk
To empower adult students to discover their own unique, productive places in our dynamic world and encourage them to be lifelong learners.

1967 Metropolitan Adult Education Program
760 Hillsdale Ave
San Jose, CA 95136
408-723-6400
www.metroed.net

Daniel Bobay, President
Matthew Dean, Vice President
Lan Nguyen, Clerk
A unit of the Metropolitan Education and offers adult education classes for free or at a very low-cost. Classes are convenient, accessible, and have flexible schedules to meet the family and work needs of adults. Courses range from basic skills in math, reading and writing, ESL Citizenship, 50+ Program to Career Technical (Vocational) certificate programs.

1968 Mid City Adult Learning Center
Belmont Community Adult School
1510 Cambria St
Los Angeles, CA 90017
213-483-5256
Fax: 213-413-1356
www.literacynet.org/slrc/la/home.html
midcity@otan.dni.us

Judy Griffin, Resource Manager
Fernando Dejo, Technical Assistant
Elanie Svensson, ESL Resource Teacher
Provides adult education on ESL, basic reading, language and literacy programs.

1969 Newport Beach Public Library Literacy Services
1000 Avocado Ave
Newport Beach, CA 92660
949-717-3800
Fax: 949-640-5681
www.newportbeachlibrary.org/literacy

Robyn Grant, Chair
John Prichard, Vice Chair
Eleanor M. Palk, Secretary
Provides free literacy instruction to adults who live or work in the Newport Beach area.

1970 Sacramento Public Library Literacy Service
828 I St
Sacramento, CA 95814
916-264-2920
800-561-4636
www.saclibrary.org
director@saclibrary.org

Mary Ellen Shay, President
April Butcher, Executive Director
Yolanda Torrecillas, Development Manager
The Literacy Service is committed to helping adults attain the skills they need to achieve their goals and develop their knowledge and potential. Free one-on-one tutoring is provided to English speaking adults who want to improve their basic reading and writing skills.

1971 Sweetwater State Literacy Regional Resource Center
Adult Resource Center
458 Moss St
Chula Vista, CA 91911-1726
619-691-5791
Fax: 619-425-8728
www.literacynet.org/slrc/sweetwater/home
hurley@otan.dni.us

Alice Hurley, Director
The Sweetwater State Literacy Resource Center is located at the Adult and Continuing Education Division of the Sweetwater Union High School District. The Division is the fourth largest adult education program in the State of California, serving over 32,000 adult learners yearly.

1972 **Vision Literacy of California**
Pro Literacy Worldwide
540 Valley Way
Bldg 4
Milpitas, CA 95035
408-676-7323
Fax: 408-956-9384
www.visionliteracy.org
info@visionliteracy.org

Steven C. Toy, President
Candace Levers, Secretary
Kathleen Campbell, Treasurer
Vision Literacy is dedicated to enriching the community in which we live by helping adults improve their literacy skills.

Colorado

1973 **Adult Literacy Program**
PO Box 4856
Basalt, CO 81621
970-963-9200
Fax: 970-963-9200
www.englishinaction.org
info@englishinaction.org

Julie Fox-Rubin, Founder
Lara Beaulieu, Executive Director
Viviana Gonzalez, Program Coordinator/Case Manager
Building community through language and leadership development.

1974 **Archuleta County Education Center**
P.O.Box 1079
Pagosa Springs, CO 81147-1079
970-264-2835
www.archuletacountyeducationcenter.com

Lynell Wiggers, Adult Education Program Director
A non-profit organization, that through fundraising, grants and strategic partnerships with other organizations and agencies, provides a wide variety of learning experiences and services for children, youth and adults as well as providing a fundamental infrastructure asset that supports the economic development priorities of the communities it serves.

1975 **Colorado Adult Education and Family Literacy**
Colorado Department of Education
201 E Colfax Ave
Denver, CO 80203
303-866-6600
Fax: 303-866-6599
www.cde.state.co.us

Margaret Kirkpatrick, State Director
To assist adults to become literate in English and obtain the knowledge and skills necessary for employment and self-sufficiency.

1976 **Durango Adult Education Center**
701 Camino del Rio
Suite 301
Durango, CO 81301
970-385-4354
Fax: 970-385-7968
www.durangoaec.org
info@durangoedcenter.org

Lon Erwin, President
Teresa Malone, Executive Director
Christine Imming, Director, Finance
A private, non-profit organization that has been dedicated to providing educational resources for adults, seniors and youth in the duragno area.

1977 **Learning Source**
455 South Pierce Street
Lakewood, CO 80226
303-922-4683
Fax: 303-742-9929
www.coloradoliteracy.org
info@thelearningsource.org

Joshua Evans, Executive Director
Harry Chan, Family Literacy Program Manager
Daun Miller Barr, Assistant to Executive Director

Provides opportunities for motivated adult learners and families to attain their educational goals through adult and family literacy, GED preparation and English Language instruction.

1978 **Pine River Community Learning Center**
535 Candelaria Dr
Ignacio, CO 81137
970-563-0681
www.prclc.org
lowen@prclc.org

Susan Visser, Executive Director
Cathy Calderwood, Director
Tish Nelson, Education Coordinator
A nonprofit educational organization dedicated to the principle that life is learning, to the unparalleled welath of cultures in the rural Southwest and the unique gifts of its people.

Connecticut

1979 **Connecticut Literacy Resource Center**
111 Charter Oak Avenue
Hartford, CT 06106
860-247-2732
Fax: 860-246-3304
www.crec.org
tjohnsonsmith@crec.org

Sandy Cruz Serrano, COO, Interim CFO
Dr. Bruce E. Douglas, Ph.D., Executive Director
Mason Thrall, Director of Operations
The Literacy Center offers services that foster literacy development from early childhood to adult. Technical assistance and training are available in the following areas: School Readiness; k-12; and Family Literacy.

1980 **LEARN: Regional Educational Service Center**
44 Hatchetts Hill Road
Old Lyme, CT 06371
860-434-4800
Fax: 860-434-4837
www.learn.k12.ct.us
ehowley@learn.k12.ct.us

Eileen S. Howley, Executive Director
Doreen Marvin, Director of Development
Jean Paul LeBlanc, Director of Business/Finance
LEARN initiates, supports and provides a wide range of programs and services that enhance the quality and expand the opportunities for learning in the educational community.

1981 **Literacy Center of Milford**
Fannie Beach Community Center
16 Dixon Street
Milford, CT 06460
203-878-4800
Fax: 203-878-1080
www.literacycenterofmilford.com
director@literacycenterofmilford.com

Martin O'Neill, President
Sheila Hageman, VP
Pam Reiss, Treasurer
Serves people from other countries who want to learn the English language and it helps people in need of mastering basic reading, writing and math skills. Provides a quality program where people can find the help and support they require to meet their basic literacy needs.

1982 **Literacy Volunteers of Central Connecticut**
20 High Street
New Britain, CT 06051
860-229-7323
Fax: 860-223-6729
www.literacycentral.org
lvcctraining@gmail.com

Cassandra Crowal, President
Sumakshi Vali, VP
Lynne Prairie, Associate Director
Provides small group and one-on-one literacy tutoring to over 350 adults with flexible hours, individual attention, student centered learning, and high quality, caring volunteer tutors. Provide free, high quality training to adults who would like to become Literacy Volunteers.

1983 **Literacy Volunteers of Eastern Connecticut**
106 Truman Street
OIC Building - 3rd Floor
New London, CT 06320   860-443-4800
                                Fax: 860-443-4880
                                www.englishhelp.org
                                office@englishhelp.org
Jerold A. Sinnamon, President
Edward G. Perkins, VP
Terrence Hickey, Treasurer
A not-for-profit, volunteer-based organization whose mission is to help people communicate in English and thrive in American culture, as consumers and as workers.

1984 **Literacy Volunteers of Greater Hartford**
30 Arbor Street
First Floor South Building
Hartford, CT 06106   860-233-3853
                                Fax: 860-838-6442
                                www.lvgh.org
                                cj.hauss@lvgh.org
Carol DeVido Hauss, Executive Director
Mark Briggs, Program Development Director
Shannon Houston, Assistant Director
Improves the ability of Greater Hartford adults to read, write and speak English. Trains volunteers to provide English literacy instruction to over 600 Hartford area adults per year.

1985 **Literacy Volunteers of Greater New Haven**
4 Science Park
New Haven, CT 06511   203-776-5899
                                Fax: 203-745-4629
                                www.lvagnh.org
                                info@lvagnh.org
Bernadette Holodak, VP
Nicholas Iwanec, CPA, Treasurer
Doss Venema, Executive Director
A non-profit educational organization that trains and supports volunteer tutors who provide free literacy tutoring for adults who need to improve their reading, writing, and oral communication skills.

1986 **Literacy Volunteers of Northern Connecticut**
Asnuntuck CC B-131
1010 Enfield Street
Enfield, CT 06082-3873   860-253-3038
                http://connecticut.networkofcare.org
Brain J Mc Cartney, Executive Director

1987 **Literacy Volunteers-Valley Shore**
61 Goodspeed Drive
Westbrook, CT 06498   860-399-0280
                                Fax: 860-767-1038
                                www.vsliteracy.org
                                info@vsliteracy.org
Gina Calabro, President
Sharon Colvin, VP
John Ferrara, Executive Director

1988 **Literacy Volunteers: Stamford/Greenwich**
60 Palmer's Hill Road
Stamford, CT 06902   203-324-3167
                                Fax: 203-358-2327
                                www.lvsg.org
                                barnold@familycenters.org
Bob Arnold, President, CEO
Carole Elias, EVP
Bob Short, VP
A community-based organization that utilizes the services of trained volunteers to provide free, high-quality reading, writing and English language programs to adults, both American and foreign born, for the purpose of enabling them to acquire the literacy skills necessary to achieve personal and occupational goals.

1989 **Mercy Learning Center**
637 Park Avenue
Bridgeport, CT 06604   203-334-6699
                                Fax: 203-332-6852
                                www.mercylearningcenter.org
                                info@mercylearningcenter.org
Jane E Ferreira, President/CEO
Nicole Cassidy, Development Director
Cathy Alfandre, Vocational Counselor
Provides basic literacy and life skills training to low-income women using a holistic approach within a compassionate, supportive environment.

Delaware

1990 **Delaware Department of Education: Adult Community Education**
Department of Public Instruction
401 Federal Street
John G. Townsend Building
Dover, DE 19901   302-735-4000
                                Fax: 302-739-4654
                                www.doe.k12.de.us
Jack Markell, Governor
Mike Barlow, Chief of Staff
James Collins, Deputy Chief of Staff
Provides students with opportunities to develop skills needed to qualify for further education, job training, and better employment.

1991 **Literacy Council of Prince George's County**
17527 Nassau Commons
Suite 213
LewesHyattsville, DE 19958   302-645-7177
                                Fax: 301-699-9707
                                www.technogoober.com
                                info@technogoober.com
Frank Payton, Uber Goober
Nathan Bradshaw, Code Goober
Chad Lane, Network Gobber
The primary non-profit organization for the advocacy and implementation of literacy programs in the county. Provides services for adult learners in acquiring, improving and applying basic literacy skills includinf reading, writing, math and oral communication.

1992 **Literacy Volunteers Serving Adults: Northern Delaware**
PO Box 2083
Wilmington, DE 19899-2083   302-658-5624
                                Fax: 302-654-9132
                                www.litvolunteers.org
                                c.shermeyer@verizon.net
Bob Hurka, Chair
Cynthia E. Shermeyer, Executive Director
Alyssa Almond, Program Coordinator
Helps adults improve literacy skills and thereby realize their potential to be confident, self sufficient and productive employees and community members. Deliver services and programs in reading, writing, English language, math, workplace and computer skills.

1993 **Literacy Volunteers of America: Wilmington Library**
10 E 10th Street
Wilmington, DE 19801   302-571-7400
                                Fax: 302-654-9132
                                www.wilmlib.org
                                wilmref@lib.de.us
H. Rodney Scott, President
Samuel A. Nolen, VP
John R. Matlusky, Chief of Staff
An organization of volunteers that provide a variety of services locally to enable people to achieve personal goals through literacy programs.

1994 NEW START Adult Learning Program
115 High Street
Odessa, DE 19730   302-378-8838
                                Fax: 302-378-7803
                                http://corbitlibrary.org
                                corbitlibrary@gmail.com
Susan Menei, Coordinator
A non-profit educational organization whose mission is to enable adults to acquire the listening, speaking, reading, writing, mathematics and technology skills they need to solve problems they encounter in daily life.

1995 State of Delaware Adult and Community Education Network
516 W. Loockerman St.
Dover, DE 19904   302-739-7080
                                     800-464-4357
                                Fax: 302-739-5565
                                www.acenetwork.org
Joanne Heaphy, Director
The ACE Network is a service agency that supports adult education and literacy providers through training and resource development.

District of Columbia

1996 Academy of Hope
601 Edgewood St NE
Suite 25
Washington, DC 20017   202-269-6623
                                Fax: 202-269-6632
                                www.aohdc.org
Brian McNamee, COO
Lecester Johnson, Executive Director
Adriana Kao, Senior Director, Development
Changes lives and improves community by providing high-quality adult education in a supportive and empowering environment.

1997 Carlos Rosario International Public Charter School
1100 Harvard St NW
Washington, DC 20009   202-797-4700
                                Fax: 202-232-6442
                                www.carlosrosario.org
                                info@carlosrosario.org
Sonia Gutierrez, President, Emeritus
Allison R. Kokkoros, CEO, Executive Director
Dr. Ryan Monroe, Principal, Harvard Campus
Offers an array of classes integrated within award-winning adult education programs which are considered models at the national and international level.

1998 District of Columbia Public Schools
1200 First Street NE
Washington, DC 20002   202-442-5885
                                Fax: 202-442-5026
                                http://dcps.dc.gov
Kaya Henderson, Chancellor
The public school system is committed to constant improvements in the achievement of all students today in preparation for their world tomorrow.

1999 Literacy Volunteers of the National Capital Area
635 Edgewood Street NE
Washington, DC 20017   202-387-1772
                                Fax: 202-588-0714
                                www.lvanca.org
                                info@lvanca.org
Patricia Evans, President
LaMar Hortman, Treasurer
Rita Daniels, Executive Director
Empowers adults and families by providing literacy instruction and skills-based education, thereby enriching all aspects of their personal and professional lives.

2000 U.S. Department Of Education
400 Maryland Avenue, SW
Washington, DC 20202   202-842-0973
                                     800-872-5327
                                Fax: 202-205-8748
                                www.ed.gov
                                ovae@ed.gov
Emma Vadehra, Chief of Staff
Eric Waldo, Senior Advisor
John Easton, Director
To help all people achieve the knowledge and skills to be lifelong learners, to be successful in their chosen careers, and to be effective citizens.

2001 Washington Literacy Council
1918 18th St NW
Ste B2
Washington, DC 20009-1794   202-387-9029
                                Fax: 202-387-0271
                                www.washingtonliteracycouncil.org
                                info@washlit.org
Terry Algire, Executive Director
The Washinton Literacy Council trains volunteers to use reading redmediation approaches when tutoring and leading small groups.

Florida

2002 Adult Literacy League
345 W. Michigan Street
Suite 100
Orlando, FL 32806   407-422-1540
                                Fax: 407-422-1529
                                www.adultliteracyleague.org
                                info@adultliteracyleague.org
Joyce Whidden, Executive Director
Gina Solomon, Director of Adult Education
Jennifer Grozio, Development Director
Develops readers to build a strong and literate community. Serves as the premier literacy resource providing education, training and information in Central Florida.

2003 Advocacy Center for Persons with Disabilities
National Disability Rights Network
2728 Centerview Drive
Ste 102
Tallahassee, FL 32301   850-488-9071
                                     800-342-0823
                                Fax: 850-488-8640
                                TDD: 800-346-4127
                                www.advocacycenter.org
Hubert Grissom, President
To advance the quality of life, dignity, equality, and freedom of choice of persons with disabilities through collaboration, education, advocacy, as well as legal and legislative strategies.

2004 Florida Coalition
250 N. Orange Avenue
Suite 1110
Orlando, FL 32801   407-246-7110
                                     800-237-5113
                                Fax: 407-246-7104
                                www.floridaliteracy.org
                                info@floridaliteracy.org
Gregory Smith, Executive Director
Annie Schmidt, Resource Specialist
Jessica Ward, Education &Training Coordinator
A nonprofit organization funded through private and corporate donations, state of Florida grants, and a diverse membership.

2005 Florida Literacy Resource Center
283 Trojan Trail
Tallahassee, FL 32311
850-922-5343
Fax: 850-922-5352
www.ace-leon.org
aceinfo@leonschools.net
Regina Browning, Principal
As part of the State Library, the State Resource Center provides electronic and print resources.

2006 Florida Vocational Rehabilitation Agency: Division of Vocational Rehabilitation
4070 Esplanade Way
Tallahassee, FL 32399-7016
850-245-3399
800-451-4327
TDD: 800-451-4327
www.rehabworks.org
Aleisa McKinlay, Division Director
Patrick Cannon, Council Member
Don Chester, Council Member
A federal state program that works with people who have physical or mental disabilities to prepare for, gain or retain employment.

2007 Learn to Read
303 N. Laura St.
P.O. Box 2178
Jacksonville, FL 32202
904-399-8894
Fax: 904-399-2508
www.learntoreadinc.org
learntoread.jax@gmail.com
Judy Bradshaw, Executive Director
Sherri Jackson, Literacy Program Manager
Alicia Harris, Literacy Program Coordinator
Dedicated to improving adult literacy in Duval County. Serves adults 16 years of age and older in Northeats Florida who want to improve reading skills or learn to read.

2008 Learning Disabilities Association of Florida
7100 W. Camino Real
Suite 215
Boca Raton, FL 33433
561-247-0221
Fax: 561-327-2633
www.lda-florida.org
cathyeldafl@gmail.com
Mark Halpert, Co-President
Cathy Einhorn, Co-President
Dale King, Board Member
The Learning Disabilities Association of Florida is a non-profit volunteer organization of parents, professionals and LD adults.

2009 Literacy Florida
2981 South Lookout Blvd
Port St Lucie, FL 34984
www.aflo.freeservers.com/whats_new.htm
havenpsl@adelphia.net
Jim Wilder, President
Sandy Newell, VP
Glenda Norvell, Secretary
Supports Florida's adult literacy volunteers and their programs. Provides information and services to literacy volunteers and providers in communications and networking, technical assistance and training, public affairs, advocacy, and student leadership.

Georgia

2010 Gainesville Hall County Alliance for Literacy
4-1/2 Stallworth Street
Gainesville, GA 30501
770-531-4337
Fax: 770-531-6406
http://allianceforliteracy.org
all4lit@bellsouth.net
Dorothy W. Shinafelt, Executive Director

Serves as the Umbrella agency for all literacy concerns in the community. Provides free educational programs for adults 16 years and older who have not graduated from high school or whose native language is not English.

2011 Georgia Department of Education
Department of Technical & Adult Education
Ste 400
1800 Century Pl NE
Atlanta, GA 30345-4304
404-679-1625
Fax: 404-679-1630
www.dtae.org
mdelaney@dtae.org
Ron Jackson, Director
To oversee the state's system of technical colleges, the adult literacy program, and a host of economic workforce development programs.

2012 Georgia Department of Technical & Adult Education
Ste 400
1800 Century Pl NE
Atlanta, GA 30345-4304
404-679-1625
Fax: 404-679-1630
www.dtae.org
mdelaney@dtae.org
Ron Jackson, Director
The Georgia Department of Technical and Adult Education oversees the state's system of technical colleges, the adult literacy program, and a host of economic and workforce development programs

2013 Georgia Literacy Resource Center: Office of Adult Literacy
Ste 400
1800 Century Pl NE
Atlanta, GA 30345-4304
404-679-1625
Fax: 404-679-1630
www.dtae.org
mdelaney@dtae.org
Ron Jackson, Director
The mission of the adult literacy programs is to enable every adult learner in Georgia to acquire the necessary basic skills in reading, writing, computation, speaking, and listening to compete successfully in today's workplace, strengthen family foundations, and exercise full citizenship.

2014 Literacy Volunteers of America: Forsyth County
PO Box 1097
Cumming, GA 30028-1097
770-887-0074
www.litreacyforsyth.org
focolit@sellsouth.net
Eddith DeVeau, Executive Director
Dianne Anth, Director
Dedicated to teaching adults to read in the Forsyth County region.

2015 Literacy Volunteers of Atlanta
246 Sycamore Street
Suite 110
Decatur, GA 30030
404-377-7323
Fax: 404-377-8662
www.lvama.org
kprovence@literacyaction.org
Michele Henry, Executive Director
Kelley Provence, Site Director
Angela Green, Basic Literacy Coordinator
To increase adult and family literacy primarily through volunteer tutoring. The goal is to provide all of the literacy skills crucial for more productive, prosperous and confident lives, thus improving the quality of life of all Georgians.

2016 Newton County Reads
8134 Geiger St
Box 5
Covington, GA 30014
678-342-7943
Fax: 678-342-7964
www.newtonreads.org
newtoncountyreads@earthlink.net

Renee' Jones, Director
Helps adults improve their literacy skills and/or earn a GED certificate through an active volunteer tutoring program; maintain an ever-expanding list of literacy resources available in Newton County; helps adults find and get started in the literacy programs that most effectively meet their needs.

2017   North Georgia Technical College Adult Education
1500 Hwy 197 N
PO Box 65
Clarkesville, GA 30523   706-754-7700
                              Fax: 706-754-7777
                        www.northgatech.edu/adulted
                           info@northgatech.edu
Steve Dougherty, President
Designed for adults who have different needs, backgrounds, and skill levels. Provide a full range of services for adults who need to acquire or improve basic reading, math, and/or written communication skills in order to prepare them to enter or succeed in the workplace or postsecondary educational programs.

2018   Okefenokee Regional Library System
401 Lee Avenue
Waycross, GA 31501   912-287-4978
                              Fax: 912-284-2533
                                 www.okrls.org
                              ikeaton@okrls.org
Pat Prevatt, Chair
Charles Eames, Vice Chair
John Miller, Manager
Public library

2019   Toccoa/Stephens County Literacy Council
P.O.Box 63
Toccoa, GA 30577-1400   706-886-6082
                              Fax: 706-282-7633
                           mwalters3@yahoo.com
Michelle Austin, Director

2020   Volunteers for Literacy of Habersham County
555 Monroe St.
Unit 20
Clarkesville, GA 30523   706-839-0200
                              Fax: 706-754-1014
                              www.habershamga.com

Hawaii

2021   CALC/Hilo Public Library
300 Waianuenue Ave
Hilo, HI 96720-2447   808-933-8893
                              Fax: 808-933-8895
                         http://literacynet.org
                            calchilo@gte.net
Kit Holz, Project Manager
Mission is to provide access to learning resources and tutoring services to help adults acquire and/or improve their skills in reading, writing, math, English as a Second Language and computer use.

2022   Hawaii Literacy
245 N. Kukui St.
Suite 202
Honolulu, HI 96817   808-537-6706
                              Fax: 808-528-1690
                           www.hawaiiliteracy.org
                           info@hawaiiliteracy.org
R. Scott Simon, President
Brandon Kurisu, VP
Suzanne Skjold, Executive Director
Helps people gain knowledge and skills by providing literacy and lifelong learning services.

2023   Hui Malama Learning Center
375 Mahalani Street
Wailuku, HI 96793   808-244-5911
                              Fax: 808-242-0762
                                 www.mauihui.org
                           huimalama@mauihui.org
Pualani Enos, J.D., Executive Director
Deanna Kramer, Finance & HR Manager
Robyn Delima, Operations Manager
Provides middle school, high-school, and GED-preparation programs, as well as tutoring and educational enrichment programs to public and private school students grades K-12.

Idaho

2024   ABE:College of Southern Idaho
Adult Basic Education
315 Falls Ave
P.O. Box 1238
Twin Falls, ID 83303   208-732-6221
                                      800-680-0274
                              Fax: 208-736-4705
                                 www.csi.edu
                                 info@csi.edu
Dr. Jeff Fox, President
Dr. Todd Schwarz, EVP, Chief Academic Officer
Mike Mason, VP, Administration
Designed to improve the educational level of adults, out-of-school youth and non-English speaking persons in our eight-county service area.

2025   Idaho Adult Education Office
650 West State Street
P.O. Box 83720
Boise, ID 83720-0027   208-332-6800
                                      800-432-4601
                              Fax: 208-334-2228
                              www.sde.idaho.gov
                           MRMcGrath@sde.idaho.gov
Tom Luna, State Superintendant
Luci Willits, Chief of Staff
Melissa McGrath, Public Information officer

2026   Idaho Coalition for Adult Literacy
325 W State St
Boise, ID 83702   208-334-2150
                                      800-458-3271
                              Fax: 208-334-4016
                                 www.lili.org
                           lili@libraries.idaho.gov
Ann Joslin, Coordinator
An nonprofit organization which raise public awareness about the importance of a literate society.

2027   Idaho State Library
325 W State St
Boise, ID 83702   208-334-2150
                                      800-458-3271
                              Fax: 208-334-4016
                                 www.lili.org
                           lili@isl.state.id.us
Ann Joslin, Director
Offers a history of pioneering new frontiers in library services.

2028   Learning Lab
308 E 36th St
Garden City, ID 83714   208-344-1335
                              Fax: 208-344-1171
                           www.learninglabinc.org
                           info@learninglabinc.org
Ann Heilman, Executive Director
Monique Smith, Education Director
Martha Strong, Adult Education Coordinator

A computer-assisted learning center for adults and families with birth to six-year-old children. Students receive basic skills instruction including mathematics, reading, writing, spelling, GED preparation and workplace skills in a comfortable, confidential environment.

Illinois

2029 Adult Literacy at People's Resource Center

201 S Naperville Rd
Wheaton, IL 60187

630-682-5402
Fax: 630-682-5412
www.peoplesrc.org

Mark Demich, President
Henry Davis, Jr., VP
Kim Perez, Executive Director
Exists to respond to basic human needs, promote dignity and justice, and create a future of hope and opportunity for the residents of DuPage County, IL through discovering and sharing personal and community resources.

2030 Aquinas Literacy Center

3540 S Hermitage Ave
Chicago, IL 60609

773-927-0512
Fax: 773-927-8980
www.aquinasliteracycenter.org
aquinaslit@aol.com

Alison Altmeyer, Executive Director
Meg Green, Program Director
Lori Rogers, Volunteer Coordinator
A nonprofit, community-based literacy center serving the residents of McKinley Park and other south and southwest side Chicago neighborhoods. Offers individualized English language instruction, group conversation classes, and group computer classes at not cost to students.

2031 C.E.F.S. Literacy Program

1805 S Banker
PO Box 928
Effingham, IL 62401-0928

217-342-2193
Fax: 217-342-4701
www.cefseoc.org
learningcenter@cefseoc.org

Helps adults and families meet their literacy goals in reading, writing, math and English language skills and to promote education and lifelong learning as the key to personal, economic, and social success.

2032 Carl Sandburg College Literacy Coalition

2400 Tom L. Wilson Blvd.
Galesburg, IL 61401

309-344-2518
855-468-6272
Fax: 309-344-1395
www.sandburg.edu
kavalos@sandburg.edu

Improves the reading and basic math skills of adults and their families by offering one-on-one and small group tutoring services.

2033 Common Place Family Learning Center

514 S Shelley St
Peoria, IL 61605

309-674-3315
Fax: 309-674-0627
www.commonplacepeoria.org
commonplace@sbcglobal.net

Cheryl Dawson, Chair
Connie Voss, Executive Director
Wayne Cannon, Director of Adult Programs
A non-profit, social service agency located on the south side of Peoria, IL. Strive to eliminate poverty and injustice through education. The youth and adult programs are based on education and literacy.

2034 Dominican Literacy Center

260 Vermont Avenue
Aurora, IL 60505

630-898-4636
Fax: 630-898-4636
www.dominicanliteracycenter.org
domlitctr@sbcglobal.net

David Cox, Advisory Board
Laura Martinez, Advisory Board
Mary Kennedy, Advisory Board
Helps women learn to read, write and speak English within an atmosphere of mutual respect and dignity.

2035 Equip for Equality

20 North Michigan Ave.
Suite 300
Chicago, IL 60602

312-341-0022
800-537-2632
Fax: 312-541-7544
TTY: 800-610-2779
www.equipforequality.org
contactus@equipforequality.org

Duane C. Quaini, Chairperson
Jeannine M. Cordero, Vice Chairperson
Zena Naiditch, President/CEO
Advances the human and civil rights of children and adults with physical and mental disabilities in Illinois. The only statewide, cross-disability, comprehensive advocacy organization prodiving self-advocacy assistance, legal services, and disability rights education while also engaging in public policy and legislative advocacy and conducting abuse investigations and other oversight activities.

2036 Equip for Equality: Carbondale

300 East Main Street
Suite 18
Carbondale, IL 62901

618-457-7930
800-758-0559
Fax: 618-457-7985
TTY: 800-610-2779
www.equipforequality.org
contactus@equipforequality.org

Duane C. Quaini, Chairperson
Jeannine M. Cordero, Vice Chairperson
Zena Naiditch, President/CEO
Independent, private, not-for-profit organization that provides free legal services and self advocacy assistance to people with disabilities in the areas of discrimination, assistive technology, special education, guardianship defense, abuse and neglect, and community integration.

2037 Equip for Equality: Moline

1515 Fifth Avenue
Suite 420
Moline, IL 61265

309-786-6868
800-758-6869
Fax: 309-797-8710
TTY: 800-610-2779
www.equipforequality.org
contactus@equipforequality.org

Duane C. Quaini, Chairperson
Jeannine M. Cordero, Vice Chairperson
Zena Naiditch, President/CEO
Independent, private, not-for-profit organization that provides free legal services and self advocacy assistance to people with disabilities in the areas of discrimination, assistive technology, special education, guardianship defense, abuse and neglect, and community integration.

2038 Equip for Equality: Springfield

1 West Old State Capitol Plaza
Suite 816
Springfield, IL 62701

217-544-0464
800-758-0464
Fax: 217-523-0720
TTY: 800-610-2779
www.equipforequality.org
contactus@equipforequality.org

Duane C. Quaini, Chairperson
Jeannine M. Cordero, Vice Chairperson
Zena Naiditch, President/CEO
Independent, private, not-for-profit organization that provides free legal services and self advocacy assistance to people with disabilities in the areas of discrimination, assistive technology, special education, guardianship defense, abuse and neglect, and community integration.

2039 Illinois Library Association
33 West Grand Avenue
Suite 401
Chicago, IL 60654-6799 312-644-1896
Fax: 312-644-1899
www.ila.org
ila@ila.org
Jeannie Dilger, President
Betsy Adamowski, Vice President/President-Elect
Leora Siegel, Treasurer
The Illinois Library Association is the voice for Illinois Libraries and the millions who depend on them. It provides leadership for the development, promotion, and improvement of library services in Illinois and for the library community.

2040 Illinois Literacy Resource Development Center
209 W Clark St
Ste 15
Champaign, IL 61820-4640 217-355-6068
Fax: 217-355-6347
www.champaign.illinoiscircle.com/c-15597
Suzanne Knell, Executive Director
The Illinois Literacy Resource Development Center is dedicated to improving literacy policy and practice at the local, state, and national levels. It is a nonprofit organization supporting literacy and adult education efforts throughout Illinois and the nation. One key to its success has been its ability to build partnerships among the organizations, individuals and agencies working in the literacy arena from the local to the national level.

2041 Illinois Office of Rehabilitation Services
Illinois Department of Human Services
100 South Grand Avenue East
Springfield, IL 62762 217-557-1601
800-843-6154
TTY: 217-557-2134
www.dhs.state.il.us
Carol Kraus, CFO, Operations
Grace Hong Duffin, Chief of Staff
Tom Green, Director, Communications
DHS' Office of Rehabilitation Services is the state's lead agency serving individuals with disabilities.

2042 Literacy Chicago
17 North State Street
Suite 1010
Chicago, IL 60602 312-870-1100
Fax: 312-870-4488
www.literacychicago.org
info@literacychicago.org
Richard Dominguez, Executive Director
June C. Porter, Director of Adult Literacy
John Mosman, Administrative Assistant
A nonprofit organization that empowers individuals to achieve greater self sufficiency through language and literacy instruction.

2043 Literacy Connection
270 North Grove Ave.
Elgin, IL 60120 847-742-6565
Fax: 847-742-6599
www.elginliteracy.org
info@elginliteracy.org
Chris Awe, President
Deborah Giardina, VP
Karen Oswald, Executive Director

A non-profit, community-based organization helping individuals acquire fundamental literacy skills and learn to read, write, speak and understand English.

2044 Literacy Council
982 N Main St
Rockford, IL 61103 815-963-7323
Fax: 815-963-7347
www.theliteracycouncil.org
read@theliteracycouncil.org
Cindy Waddick, Executive Director
Heather Tucker, Finance Director
Debra Lindley, Program Director
Provides literacy instruction to individuals and families to strengthen communities.

2045 Literacy Volunteers of America: Illinois
30 East Adams Street
Suite 1130
Chicago, IL 60603 312-857-1582
Fax: 312-857-1586
www.literacyvolunteersillinois.org
info@lvillinois.org
Dorothy M Miaso, Executive Director
Chamala Travis, Program Coordinator
Trudye Connolly, Program Associate
A statewide organization committed to developing and supporting volunteer literacy programs that help families, adults and out-of-school teens increase their literacy skills.

2046 Literacy Volunteers of DuPage
24W500 Maple Ave
Ste 217
Naperville, IL 60540-6057 630-416-6699
Fax: 630-416-9465
www.literacyvolunteersdupage.org
info@literacydupage.org
Rick Lochner, President
Bernie Steiger, Executive Director
Carol Garcia, Program Director
A nonprofit, community-based organization that provides accessible and customized tutoring in reading, writing, speaking, and understanding English to help adults achieve independence.

2047 Literacy Volunteers of Fox Valley
One South Sixth Avenue
Saint Charles, IL 60174 630-584-2811
Fax: 630-584-3448
www.lvfv.org
info@lvfv.org
Peg Coker, Executive Director
Maureen Powelson, Program Coordinator
Angelo Cobo, Office Assistant
Helps individuals in the region acquire and validate the literacy skills that they need to function more effectively in contemporary U.S. society.

2048 Literacy Volunteers of Lake County
128 N County St
Waukegan, IL 60085 847-623-2041
Fax: 847-623-2092
www.adultlearningconnection.org
Mission is to extend educational opportunities to Lake COunty adult students and their families.

2049 Literacy Volunteers of Western Cook County
1010 West Lake Street, Suite 603B
PO Box 4502
Oak Park, IL 60301 708-848-8499
Fax: 708-848-9564
www.lvwcc.org
info@lvwcc.org
Esther Chase, President, Acting Exe. Director
Mario K. Medina, Treasurer
Jasmine Brown, Partnerships Specialist
Helps adults reach their literacy goals through customized one-on-one tutoring by trained volunteers.

2050 Project CARE
Morton College
3801 S Central Ave
Cicero, IL 60804

708-656-8000
Fax: 708-656-3186
www.morton.edu
projectcare@morton.edu

Dr. Dana A. Grove, President
Marlena A. Thompson, Director, Student Development
Kenneth Stock, SPHR, Director, HR
A volunteer adult literacy program that uses trained tutors to teach adult students seeking assistance with reading and writing, and/or adults who are learning English as a second language.

2051 Project READ
5800 Godfrey Road
Benjamin Godfrey Campus
Godfrey, IL 62035

618-468-7000
800-YES-LCCC
Fax: 618-468-7820
www.lc.cc.il.us
lartis@lc.edu

Robert Watson, Chairman
Brenda W. McCain, Vice Chairman
Walter S. Ahlemeyer, Secretary
Goal is to increase literacy throughout the area with one-on-one tutoring. Project READ Community Service Coordinators are available to provide information to community groups, arrange free training for volunteers and distribute materials and support to tutor-learner pairs.

Indiana

2052 Adult Literacy Program of Gibson County
232 W Broadway
P.O. Box 1134
Princeton, IN 47670

812-386-9100
www.gibsonadultliteracy.org
literacy@gibsoncounty.net

Sharen Buyher, President
Cynthia Schrodt, Secretary
Ruth Jones, Board Member
Provides an opportunity for any adult in Gibson County to attain basic English Language literacy skills.

2053 Indy Reads: Indianapolis/Marion County Public Library
PO Box 211
Indianapolis, IN 46206-0211

317-275-4100
www.imcpl.org
jimlingenfelter@five2fivedesign.com

Dorothy R. Crenshaw, President
Dr. David W. Wantz, VP
Jackie Nytes, Library's CEO
Indy Reads, a nationally recognized not-for-profit affiliate of the Indianapolis-Marion County Public Library, exists to improve the reading and writing skills of adults in Marion County who read at or below the sixth grade level.

2054 Literacy Alliance
709 Clay St
Ste 100
Fort Wayne, IN 46802-2019

260-426-7323
Fax: 260-424-0371
www.tria.org
trlafw@yahoo.com

Judith Stabelli, Executive Director
Adult education

2055 Morrisson/Reeves Library Literacy Resource Center
80 North 6th Street
Richmond, IN 47374

765-966-8291
Fax: 765-962-1318
www.mrlinfo.org
library@mrlinfo.org

Paris Pegg, Library Director
Sue King, Adult Services Manager
Sarah Morey, Technical Services Manager
The Literacy Resource Center provides free training for volunteers to tutor adults in Wayne County who want to learn to read, write and do basic math.

2056 Steuben County Literacy Coalition
1208 S Wayne St
Angola, IN 46703

260-665-1414
Fax: 260-665-3357
www.steubenliteracy.org

Dolores Tichenor, President
Lon Keyes, President-Elect
Breann Fink, Executive Director
Mission shall be to foster lifelong leraning and improved literacy through high quality and accessible educational opportunities for children and adults in Steuben County.

Iowa

2057 Adult Basic Education and Adult Literacy Program
Kirkwood Community College
6301 Kirkwood Blvd SW
Cedar Rapids, IA 52404

319-398-5411
800-332-2055
www.kirkwood.edu
ask@kirkwood.edu

Dr. Mick Starcevich, President
Bill Lamb, VP, Academic Affairs
John Henik, Associate VP, Academic Affairs
Provides instruction to enable adults to increase self-sufficiency, improve employability, prepare for continued learning and better meet their responsibilities. Recruits volunteers, trains them in literacy teaching techniques and matches them with adults wanting instruction in reading skills development.

2058 Iowa Department of Education: Iowa Literacy Council Programs
400 E 14th Street
Grimes State Office Buliding
Des Moines, IA 50319-0146

515-281-5294
Fax: 515-242-5988
www.educateiowa.gov
jason.glass@iowa.gov

Brad Buck, Director
Nicole Proesch, Legal Director
Ryan Wise, Deputy Director, Policy
Helps adults and families develop their potential through improved literacy, education, and training.

2059 Iowa Literacy Resource Center
415 Commercial St
Waterloo, IA 50701-1317

319-233-1200
800-772-2023
Fax: 319-233-1964
www.readiowa.org
riesberg@neilsa.org

Eunice Riefberg, Director
The Center provides a link to resource materials in Iowa and at a regional and national level for adult literacy practitioners and students. These resources are available in many formats: including print, audio, video and online.

2060 Iowa Vocational Rehabilitation Agency
Department of Education
510 East 12th Street
Jessie Parker Building
Des Moines, IA 50319-0240

515-281-4211
Fax: 515-281-7645
TTY: 515-281-4211
www.ivrs.iowa.gov
David.Mitchell@iowa.gov

David Mitchell, Administrator

2061   Iowa Workforce Investment Act
200 East Grand Avenue
Des Moines, IA 50309
515-725-3000
Fax: 515-725-3010
www.iowaeconomicdevelopment.com
info@iowa.gov
Debi Durham, Director
Tina Hoffman, Media
Job placement and training services. Especially for those workers who have been laid off, or have other barriers to steady employment.

2062   Learning Disabilities Association of Iowa
5665 Greendale Rd
Ste D
Johnston, IA 50131
515-280-8558
888-690-5324
Fax: 515-243-1902
www.lda-ia.org
kathylda@askresource.org
Vicki Goshon, President
Kim Miller, 1st VP
Patty Beyer, 2nd VP
Dedicated to identifying causes and promoting prevention of learning disabilities and to enhancing the quality of life for all individuals with learning disabilities and their families.

2063   Library Literacy Programs: State Library of Iowa
1112 E Grand Ave
Miller Building
Des Moines, IA 50319
515-281-4105
800-248-4483
Fax: 515-281-6191
www.statelibraryofiowa.org
helpdesk@silo.lib.ia.us
Mary Wegner, Director/State Librarian

2064   Southeastern Community College:Literacy Program
200 North Main
Mt Pleasant, IA 52641
319-385-8012
www.scciowa.edu
jcouch@scciowa.edu
Dr. Michael Ash, President
Dr. Carole Richardson, VP, Academic Affairs
Jeff Ebbing, Director, Marketing & Comm.
Provides information to students who need to get their GED, and helps them to read and write.

2065   Western Iowa Tech Community College
4647 Stone Avenue
P.O. Box 5199
Sioux City, IA 51102-5199
712-274-6400
800-352-4649
www.witcc.edu
info@witcc.edu
Dr. Robert Rasmus, Board President
Russell Wray, Board VP
Neal Adler, District I
Recruits volunteer mentors and adult learners throughout the year, and arranges for them to meet and work together.

Kansas

2066   Arkansas City Literacy Council
Arkansas City Public Library
120 E 5th Ave
Arkansas City, KS 67005
620-442-1280
www.arkcity.org
literacy@acpl.org
Lianne Flax, Adult Services Director
A non-profit, volunteer organization that provides literacy and English language tutoring to adults and older youth so they may gain the listening, speaking, and reading skills needed to be successful in life.

2067   Butler Community College Adult Education
901 S. Haverhill Rd
El Dorado, KS 67042
316-321-2222
Fax: 316-322-8450
www.butlercc.edu
kallen2@butlercc.edu
Kimberley Krull, President
Kirsten Allen, Director, Admissions
Todd Carter, Athletic Director
Mission is to produce students who make measurable gains in educational skill, workplace readiness, and technology skills.

2068   Emporia Literacy Program
3301 West 18th Avenue
Flint Hills Technical College
Emporia, KS 66801
620-343-4600
800-711-6947
Fax: 620-343-4610
www.fhtc.edu
askus@fhtc.edu
Mary Beth Voorhees, Chair
Mark Remmert, Vice Chair
Dr. Dean Hollenbeck, President

2069   Hutchinson Public Library: Literacy Resources
901 N Main St
Hutchinson, KS 67501
620-663-5441
Fax: 620-663-1583
www.hutchpl.org
info@hutchpl.org
Sandra Gustafson, Coordinator
Dianne Brown, Head of Circulation
Ruth Heidebrecht, Head of Collection Development
Provides staff to help adults improve their reading, writing and language skills.

2070   Kansas Adult Education Association
Barton County Community College
Barton Community College
245 NE 30 Rd
Great Bend, KS 67530
620-792-2701
800-748-7594
www.bartonccc.edu
quinnp@bartonccc.edu
Dr. Penny Quinn, VP, Student Services
Mike Johnson, Trustee
Marsha Miller, Assistant to the Vice President
The Kansas Adult Education Association has been the professional association for adult educators at community colleges, school districts, and non-profit organizations.

2071   Kansas Correctional Education
714 SW Jackson
Suite 300
Topeka, KS 66603
785-296-3317
888-317-8204
www.doc.ks.gov
kdocpub@doc.ks.gov
Keith Bradshaw, Director, Fiscal Services
Jan Clausing, Director of Human Resources
Ray Roberts, Secretary of Corrections
The provision of correctional education programming to inmates.

2072   Kansas Department of Corrections
714 SW Jackson
Suite 300
Topeka, KS 66603
785-296-3317
888-317-8204
Fax: 785-296-0014
www.doc.ks.gov
kdocpub@doc.ks.gov
Keith Bradshaw, Director, Fiscal Services
Jan Clausing, Director of Human Resources
Ray Roberts, Secretary of Corrections
State corrections agency/department.

2073 Kansas Department of Social & Rehabilitation Services
915 SW Harrison St
Topeka, KS 66612-1505

785-296-3959
888-369-4777
Fax: 785-296-2173
TTY: 785-296-1491
www.dcf.ks.gov

Phyllis Gilmore, Secretary
Wm. Jeff Kahrs, Chief of Staff
Angela de Rocha, Communications Director
To assist people with disabilities achieve suitable employment and independence.

2074 Kansas Literacy Resource Center
1000 SW Jackson St
Ste 520
Topeka, KS 66612-1368

785-296-3421
Fax: 785-296-0983
www.kansasregents.org
dglass@ksbor.org

Andy Tompkins, President & CEO
Connie Bollig, Executive Assistant
Julene Miller, General Counsel
Enhances systems, both public and private, which provide basic skills education across Kansas. The Center serves as the catalyst for collaborative efforts that address the needs of undereducated adults in Kansas.

2075 Kansas State Department of Adult Education
900 SW Jackson Street
Topeka, KS 66612-1212

785-296-3201
Fax: 785-296-7933
www.ksde.org
contact@ksde.org

Lori Adams, Education Program Consultant
Kayeri Akweks, Education Program Consultant
Evelyn Alden, Web editor
To assist adults to become literate and obtain the knowledge and skills necessary for employment and self-sufficiency.

2076 Kansas State Literacy Resource Center: Kansas State Department of Education
1000 SW Jackson St
Ste 520
Topeka, KS 66612-1368

785-296-3421
Fax: 785-296-0983
www.kansasregents.org
dglass@ksbor.org

Andy Tompkins, President & CEO
Connie Bollig, Executive Assistant
Julene Miller, General Counsel
The State Literacy Resource Center can assist adult education practitioners across the nation in locating and accessing the most current materials in their issue area.

2077 Preparing for the Future: Adult Learning Services
230 W 7th St
Junction City, KS 66441-3097

785-238-4311
Fax: 785-238-7873
www.jclib.org
jclibrary@jclib.org

Susan Moyer, Director
Cheryl Jorgensen, Assistant Director
Sarah Jones, Head of Circulation

Kentucky

2078 Ashland Adult Education
Ashland Community & Technical College
1400 College Drive
Ashland, KY 41101-3617

606-326-2000
800-928-4256
http://ashland.kctcs.edu
joan.flanery@kctcs.edu

Kay Adkins, President and CEO
Richard Adams, Custodial Worker II
Linda Adkins, Office Support Asst

Provides education services that prepare adults with the essential skills they need to function as workers, citizens and family members of the 21st century. The program enables them to develop essential skills for living and wage earning and to better their self-concepts.

2079 Kentucky Laubach Literacy Action
1024 Capital Center Dr
Suite 250
Frankfort, KY 40601-7514

502-573-5114
800-928-7323
Fax: 502-573-5436
TTY: 800-928-7323
http://kyae.ky.gov
dvislisel@mail.state.ky.us

Elizabeth Arauz, Business Specialist
D.J. Begley, Senior Associate
Gayle Box, Senior Associate
Dedicated to helping adults of all ages improve their lives and their communities by learning reading, writing, match and problem-solving skills.

2080 Kentucky Literacy Volunteers of America
1024 Capital Center Dr
Suite 250
Frankfort, KY 40601-7514

502-573-5114
800-928-7323
Fax: 502-573-5436
TTY: 800-928-7323
http://kyae.ky.gov
dvislsel@mail.state.ky.us

Elizabeth Arauz, Business Specialist
D.J. Begley, Senior Associate
Gayle Box, Senior Associate
Promotes literacy for people of all ages.

2081 Operation Read
470 Copper Drive
Lexington, KY 40507-0235

859-254-9964
866-774-4872
Fax: 859-254-5834
http://bluegrass.kctcs.edu
opread@gx.net

Nicholas Mueller, Executive Director
Helping adults learn to read to help imrove their lives, the lives of their children and the lives in their community.

2082 Simpson County Literacy Council
231 S College St
Franklin, KY 42134-1809

270-586-7234
Fax: 270-598-0906
www.readtobefree.org
read@readtobefree.org

Debra Thompson, Director
A private, non-profit organization that provides a variety of services to enable people to achieve personal goals through literacy, basic reading & math, GED prep, computer classes, math & reading for college and more.

2083 Winchester Adult Education Center
52 N Maple St
Winchester, KY 40391

859-744-1975
Fax: 859-744-1424
www.winchesteradulteducation.org
mwells_cae@roadrunner.com

Victor Brown, Staff
Bill Baber, Staff
Deckie Denton, Staff
For those 16 years of age and older and out of school, provides facilities, materials, and services in order to improve lifelong learning skills leading to economic independence and quality of life.

Louisiana

2084 Adult Literacy Advocates of Baton Rouge
460 North 11th Street
Baton Rouge, LA 70802-4607   225-383-1090
                              Fax: 225-387-5999
                    www.adultliteracyadvocates.org
                    info@adultliteracyadvocates.org
Pam Creighton, Executive Director

2085 Literacy Council of Southwest Louisiana
Central School Arts & Humanities Center
809 Kirby St
Ste 126
Lake Charles, LA 70601   337-494-7000
                          Fax: 337-494-7915
                    www.literacyswla.org
                    info@literacyswla.org
Vicky Hand, President
Tommeka Semien, Executive Director
Alvin Joseph, President-Elect
A community-based, non-profit organization that provides
instructional programs to improve educational skill levels in
Southwest Louisiana and works to increase public aware-
ness of literacy-related issues.

2086 Literacy Volunteers Centenary College
2911 Centenary Boulevard
PO Box 41188
Shreveport, LA 71134-1188   318-869-2411
                              Fax: 318-869-2474
                    www.literacyconnections.com
                    lvecent@bellsouth.net
Sue Lee, Executive Director

2087 VITA (Volunteer Instructors Teaching Adults)
905 Jefferson St
Ste 404
Lafayette, LA 70501-7913   337-234-4600
                          Fax: 337-234-4672
                    www.vitalaf.org
                    vitala@bellsouth.net
Bill Bowers, President
Jeff Ackermann, Vice -Chairman
Gene Cole, Secretary
Specially trained volunteers learn to teach reading and writing using easy to follow manuals and to also provide
goal-oriented, one on one or in small group. VITA provides
the professional training, materials, and support that enable
the volunteers to assist adults in acquiring basic reading and
writing skills.

Maine

2088 Biddeford Adult Education
64 West Street
PO Box 624
Biddeford, ME 04005   207-282-3883
                          Fax: 207-286-9581
                    http://biddeford.maineadulted.org
                    adulted@biddefordschooldepartment.org
Paulette Bonneau, Director
Sue De Cesare, Community Adult Education Leader
Anne Beaulieu, Administrative Assistant

**2089 Center for Adult Learning and Literacy: University of
Maine**
Pro Literacy Worldwide
5749 Merrill Hall
Orono, ME 04469-5749   207-581-1865
                              877-486-2364
                          Fax: 207-581-1517
                    www.umaine.edu
                    president@umaine.edu
Paul W. Ferguson, President

The Center for Adult Learning and Literacy offers quality,
research-based professional development and resources,
based on funded initiatives to improve the quality of services
within the Maine Adult Education System.

2090 Literacy Volunteers of Androscoggin
15 Sacred Heart Place
Auburn, ME 04210   207-333-4785
                    www.literacyvolunteersandro.org
                    literacy@literacyvolunteersandro.org
Tahlia Chamberlain, Executive Director
Providing free one-on-one tutoring and other educational
services to help adults in Androscoggin County acquire the
basic reading, writing and math skills they need to enhance
their lives and achieve their personal goals.

2091 Literacy Volunteers of Aroostook County
Caribou Learning Center
75 Bennett Drive
Caribou, ME 04736   207-325-3490
                          Fax: 207-325-8916
                    http://rsu39.maineadulted.org
                    lvaroostook@gmail.com
Lyn Michaud, Director
Provides free, confidential services to any Aroostokk
COunty adult with the desire to increase their literacy skill.

2092 Literacy Volunteers of Bangor
200 Hogan Rd
Bangor, ME 04401-5604   207-947-8451
                              Fax: 207-942-1391
                          http://lvbangor.org
                          admin@lvbangor.org

Audrey Braccio, President
Brendan Trainor, Vice President
Tina Dowling, Treasurer
A group of people who are dedicated to improving literacy in
the community one person at a time. Many of the volunteers
choose to become a tutor and teach another adult to read or
speak English.

2093 Literacy Volunteers of Greater Augusta
12 Spruce St
Ste 2
Augusta, ME 04330   207-626-3440
                          Fax: 207-626-3440
                    www.lva-augusta.org
                    info@lva-augusta.org

Mark Flight, Chairperson
Lori Gray, Vice-Chairperson
Virginia Marriner, Affiliate Director
Promote and foster increased literacy for adults who have
low literacy skills or those for whom English is not their na-
tive language through volunteer tutoring.

2094 Literacy Volunteers of Greater Portland
PO Box 8585
Portland, ME 04104   207-775-0105
                          Fax: 207-780-1701
                    www.lvaportland.org
                    lvportland@learningworks.me
Kristen Stevens, Executive Director
Offers, free, confidential, student-centered, individual and
small group tutoring to adults seeking to develop the literacy
skills they need to reach important life goals like reading
their first books, obtaining citizenship, helping their children with homework, taking care of personal bills and
finding employment.

2095 Literacy Volunteers of Greater Saco/Biddeford
841 North Road
Dover Foxcroft, ME 04426   207-283-2954
                    www.maineadulted.org
                    info@maineadulted.org
Brenda Gagne, Director
Bernadette Farrar, Asst. Director
Lisa Robertson, ABE Coordinator

Trains volunteers to provide educational programs and services that improve reading, writing and related literacy skills, and to empower adults by enhancing their life skills in the area of family, work, health and community.

2096 **Literacy Volunteers of Greater Sanford**
883 Main St
Ste 4
Sanford, ME 04073
207-324-2486
Fax: 207-324-2486
www.sanfordliteracy.org
lvgsanford@gmail.com
Kimberley Moran, Executive Director
Supports the literacy needs of local adults with free, confidential, one-on-one tutoring and small group instruction in reading, math, computers, studying for the GED, licenses, and other life skills by trained adult volunteers.

2097 **Literacy Volunteers of Maine**
142 High St
Ste 526
Portland, ME 04101
207-773-3191
Fax: 207-221-1123
www.lvmaine.org
info@lvmaine.org
Chip Brewer, Co-President
Benjamin Smith, Co-President
Dedicated to providing increased access to literacy services for Maine adults who wish to acquire or improve their literacy skills.

2098 **Literacy Volunteers of Mid-Coast Maine**
28 Lincoln St
Rockland, ME 04841
207-594-5154
Fax: 207-594-5154
http://lvmidcoast.maineadulted.org
bgifford@msad5.org
Beth A Gifford, Program Director
Dedicated to improving the literacy skills of adults in our community. Deliver instruction using a dedicated corps of well trained volunteer tutors.

2099 **Literacy Volunteers of Waldo County**
5 Stephenson Ln
Belfast, ME 04915
207-338-2200
Fax: 207-338-1652
www.broadreachmaine.org
info@brmaine.org
Kate Quinn Finlay, Executive Director
Karla Edney, Financial Director
Deborah Schilder, Director of Development
Helps children and families to develop the skills they need to lead healthy and productive lives. Share the knowledge and experience with child-and-family serving organizations across the state and nation.

2100 **Maine Literacy Resource Center**
University of Maine
5749 Merrill Hall
Orono, ME 04469-5749
207-581-1865
877-486-2364
Fax: 207-581-1517
www.umaine.edu
president@umaine.edu
Susan J. Hunter, President
Jeffery Hecker, EVP
Jake Ward, VP
As part of the State Library, the State Resource Center provides electronic and print resources.

2101 **Tri-County Literacy**
2 Sheridan Rd
Bath, ME 04530
207-443-6384
877-885-7441
www.tricountyliteracy.org
tricountyliteracy@tricountyliteracy.org
Darlene Marciniak, Executive Director

A non-profit organization dedicated to improving people's lives through three literacy programs; Adult Literacy, Read With Me (Family Literacy), and Reading For Better Business.

Maryland

2102 **Anne Arundel County Literacy Council**
80 W St
Ste A, P.O. Box 1303
Annapolis, MD 21401-2401
410-269-4465
Fax: 410-974-2023
www.icanread.org
programdirector@aaclc.org
Lisa Vernon, President
Joann Cook, Student coordinator
Anita Ewing, Tutor Coordinator
A volunteer, non-profit organization dedicated to serving the needs of functionally illiterate adults in Anne Arundel County. Provides free, personalized one-on-one training to adults who read at a 5th grade level or lower.

2103 **Calvert County Literacy Council**
37600 New Market Road
P.O. Box 459
Charlotte, MD 20622-2508
301-934-9442
Fax: 301-884-0438
http://smrla.org
calvertliteracy@somd.lib.md.us
Maria Isle Birnkammer, Director
Provides volunteers to help with one-on-one tutoring or small group tutoring.

2104 **Center for Adult and Family Literacy: Community College of Baltimore County**
7200 Sollers Point Rd
Building E, Ste 104
Baltimore, MD 21222-4649
443-840-3692
www.ccbcmd.edu
abonner@ccbcmd.edu
Sandra Kurtinitis, President
Classes to provide training and instruction for adults with literacy problems.

2105 **Charles County Literacy Council**
United Way Bldg
10250 La Plata Rd
La Plata, MD 20646
301-934-6488
Fax: 301-392-9286
www.charlescountyliteracy.org
charlescountyliteracy@comcast.net
Valerie Kettner, President
Lisa Hackley, Vice President
Kathy Joy, Treasurer
A not-for-profit organization, provides free community-based one-on-one adult literacy tutoring to ensure that all adults have the access to quality education needed to fully realize their potential as individuals, parents and citizens

2106 **Howard University School of Continuing Education**
2400 Sixth Street, NW
Suite 440
Washington, DC 20059-5603
202-806-6100
Fax: 301-585-8911
www.howard.edu
csnell@howard.edu
Stacey J. Mobley, Chairman
Wayne A.I. Frederick, President
Larkin Arnold, Founder
Howard University Continuing Education was established in April 1986 to meet the education and training needs of professionals, administrators, entrepreneurs, technical personnel, paraprofessionals and other adults on an individual or group basis.

2107 Literacy Council of Frederick County
110 E Patrick St
Frederick, MD 21701 301-600-2066
www.frederickliteracy.org
info@frederickliteracy.org
Caroline Gaver, President
Beth Lowe, 1st Vice President
Sandy Doggett, 2nd Vice President
A non-profit, non-secretarian, educational organization
dedicated to helping non-literate and semi-literate adult residents in the county improve their language skills through
one-on-one tutoring.

2108 Literacy Council of Montgomery County
21 Maryland Ave
Ste 320
Rockville, MD 20850 301-610-0030
Fax: 301-610-0034
www.literacycouncilmcmd.org
info@literacycouncilmcmd.org
Marty Stephens, Executive Director
Danielle Verbiest, Deputy Director
Patrick Salami, Development Director
A non-profit organization founded to help adults living or
working in the county who want to achieve functional levels
of reading, writing, and speaking English so that they may
improve the quality of their life and their ability to participate in the community.

2109 Maryland Adult Literacy Resource Center
UMBC, Department of Education
1000 Hilltop Circle
Baltimore, MD 21250-2029 410-455-6725
888-464-3346
Fax: 410-455-1139
www.umbc.edu
ira@umbc.edu
Freeman A. Hrabowski, President
As part of the State Library, the State Resource Center provides resources and information for adult literacy providers
and students in Maryland.

Massachusetts

2110 A Legacy for Literacy
330 Homer St
Newton Center, MA 02459 617-796-1360
TTY: 617-552-7154
www.newtonfreelibrary.net
legacyforliteracy@yahoo.com
Barbara Lietzke, President
Robert Klivans, Treasurer
Audrey Cooper, Trustee
Provides free tutoring services for adults of limited English
proficiency.

2111 Adult Center at PAL
Curry College
1071 Blue Hill Ave
Milton, MA 02186 617-333-0500
Fax: 617-333-2114
www.curry.edu
lhubbard@curry.edu
Kennet K. Quigley, President
Offers adults with learning disabilities or attention deficits a
safe, supportive place to work on developing their strengths.
Serves adult students enrolled in courses at Curry College or
at other institutions of higher education.

2112 ESL Center
43 Amity St
Amherst, MA 01002 413-259-3090
Fax: 413-256-4096
www.joneslibrary.org
esl@joneslibrary.org
Austin Sarat, President
Chris Hoffmann, Vice President
Tamson Ely, Secretary
Provides volunteer tutors, tutoring space, study materials,
computer-assisted instruction, citizenship classes, English
classes and referrals to adult immigrants in the Amherst
area.

2113 Eastern Massachusetts Literacy Council
English at Large
800 West Cummings Park
Suite 5550
Woburn, MA 01801-3608 781-395-2374
TTY: 781-395-2374
www.englishatlarge.org
info@englishatlarge.org
Catherine Corliss, President
Laura Henry, Vice President
Evan Fitzpatrick, Treasurer
The Eastern Massachusetts Literacy Council is a private
non-profit affiliate of ProLiteracy Worldwide, the largest
nonprofit volunteer adult literacy organization in the world.
The EMLC trains volunteers to assist adults who are learning
English as another language and adults who wish to
strengthen their basic reading skills.

**2114 JOBS Program: Massachusetts Employment Services
Program**
19 Staniford St
Charles F. Hurley Building
Boston, MA 02114-1704 617-626-5300
Fax: 617-348-5191
www.mass.gov
DCSCustomerfeedback@detma.org
Deval Patrick, Governer
Glen Shor, Secretary
Matthew H. Malone, Secretary of Education
The Employment Services Program is a joint federal and
state funded program whose primary goal is to provide a way
to self-sufficiency for TAFDC families ESP is an employ-
ment-oriented program that is based on a work-first
approach.

2115 Literacy Network of South Berkshire
100 Main St
Lee, MA 01238-1614 413-243-0471
Fax: 413-243-6754
www.litnetsb.org
info@litnetsb.org
Lucy Prashker, President
Bill Dunlaevy, Treasurer
Laura Qualliotine, Executive Director
Serving the 15 towns of Southern Berkshire County in Massachusetts. Providing free one-on-one tutoring to adults in
reading, GED preparation, ESL, and citizenship
preparation.

2116 Literacy Volunteers of Greater Worcester
3 Salem Sq
Rm 332
Worcester, MA 01608 508-754-8056
Fax: 508-754-8056
www.lvgw.org
info@lvgw.org
Hank Stolz, President
Harold Jones, Vice President
Lionel Carbonneau, Trasurer
Provides confidential, free, individualized, year-round tu-
toring in either basic reading or English for speakers of other
languages.

2117 Literacy Volunteers of Massachusetts
8 Faneuil Hall Marketplace
3rd floor
Boston, MA 02108 617-367-1313
Fax: 617-367-8894
TTY: 888-466-1313
www.lvm.org
kgriffiths@lvm.org

Kristin Griffiths, Director
Literacy Volunteers of Massachusetts helps adults learn to read and write or speak English by matching them with trained volunteer tutors.

2118 Literacy Volunteers of Methuen
305 Broadway
Methuen, MA 01844-6806   978-686-4080
Fax: 978-686-8669
www.nevinslibrary.org
litvolmeth@gmail.com

James H. Smith, Chairman
Ralph Prolman, Vice chairman
Kritika McLeod, Director
Brings free, private, flexible, individualized instruction to adults in the community who are struggling everyday with basic reading and language problems.

2119 Literacy Volunteers of the Montachusett Area
610 Main St
Fitchburg, MA 01420   978-343-8184
Fax: 978-343-4680
www.literacyvolunteersmontachusett.org
literacy26@aol.com

Shirley Shirley, President
Gloria Maybury, Program Coordinator
Laura Beauregard, Secretary
Promotes and fosters increased literacy in the Montachusett Area through trained volunteer tutoring and to empower adults for whom English is a second language. Encourage and aid individuals, groups or organizations desiring to increase literacy through voluntary programs.

2120 Massachusetts Correctional Education: Inmate Training & Education
PO Box 71
Hodder House, Two Merchant Road
Framingham, MA 01704   508-935-0901
Fax: 508-935-0907
www.mass.gov
cvicari@doc.state.ma.us

Carolyn J. Vicari, Director
To establish departmental policy regarding inmates' involvement in academic and vocational training programs.

2121 Massachusetts Family Literacy Consortium
MA Dept of Elementary & Secondary Education
75 Pleasant St
Malden, MA 02148   781-338-3102
Fax: 781-338-3770
www.doe.mass.edu
boe@doe.mass.edu

Maura o. Banta, Chairman
Donald Willyard, Chairman
Vanessa Calderon Rosado, Cheif Executive officer
A statewide initiative with the mission of forging effective partnerships among state agencies, community organizations, and other interested parties to expand and strengthen family literacy and support.

2122 Massachusetts GED Administration: Massachusetts Department of Education
75 Pleasant St
Malden, MA 02148   781-338-3102
Fax: 781-338-3770
www.doe.mass.edu
boe@doe.mass.edu

Maura o. Banta, Chairman
Donald Willyard, Chairman
Vanessa Calderon Rosado, Cheif Executive officer
Thirty-three test centers operate state-wide to serve the needs of the adult population in need of a high school credential.

2123 Massachusetts Job Training Partnership Act: Department of Employment & Training
19 Staniford St
Boston, MA 02114-2502   617-626-5400
Fax: 617-570-8581
www.detma.org
mstonge@detma.org

Edward Malmberg, Executive Director
Supplies information on the local labor market and assists companies in locating employees.

2124 Pollard Memorial Library Adult Literacy Program
401 Merrimack St
Lowell, MA 01850-5999   978-970-4120
Fax: 978-970-4117
TDD: 978-970-4129
www.pollardml.org

Victoria Woodley, Director
Susan Fougstedt, Assistant Director
Molly Hancock, Coordinator of Youth Services
Offers free, confidential, private and flexibly scheduled tutoring to adults with little or no reading or writing skills, and those who wish to become more fluent English speakers, readers or writers.

Michigan

2125 Capital Area Literacy Coalition
1028 E Saginaw
Lansing, MI 48906-5518   517-485-4949
Fax: 517-485-1924
www.thereadingpeople.org
mail@thereadingpeople.org

Lois Bader, Executive Director
Di Clark, Assistant Director
Sarah Crockett, Administrative Assistant
The Capital Area Literacy Coalition helps children and adults learn to read, write and speak English with an ultimate goal of helping individuals achieve self-sufficiency.

2126 Kent County Literacy Council
111 Library St NE
Grand Rapids, MI 49503-3268   616-459-5151
Fax: 616-245-8069
www.kentliteracy.org
info@kentliteracy.org

Susan Ledy, Executive Director
A non-profit organization founded in 1986 that provides literacy services to over 1,000 adults in reading and english communication. In addition to the adult tutoring programs, we also serve area counties through the Customized Workplace English Program providing fee-based customized Workplace English Language, accent modification, and multicultrual training to area companies; and the Family Literacy Program which offers literacy and ESL instruction, workshops, and events.

2127 Michigan Assistive Technology: Michigan Rehabilitation Services
119 Pere Marquette Dr
Suite 1C
Lansing, MI 48912-1231   517-485-4477
Fax: 517-485-4488
www.publicpolicy.com
ppa@publicpolicy.com

Jeffrey D. Padden, President
Nancy Hewat, Executive Director
Chris Andrews, Senior Communications Consultant
Solves information and policy-development problems for clients.

2128 Michigan Libraries and Adult Literacy
PO Box 30007
702 W. Kalamazoo St.
Lansing, MI 48909-7507

517-373-1300
877-479-0021
Fax: 517-373-5700
TDD: 517-373-1592
www.michigan.gov
librarian@michigan.gov

Nancy Robertson, Director
Rick Snyder, Governor
Allison Scott, Exe Director to the Governor

2129 Michigan Workforce Investment Act
119 Pere Marquette Dr
Suite 1C
Lansing, MI 48912-1231

517-485-4477
Fax: 517-485-4488
www.publicpolicy.com
ppa@publicpolicy.com

Jeff Padden, President
Colleen E. Graber, Director
Dr. Paul Elam, Dirctor of Safety and Justice

Minnesota

2130 Adult Basic Education
Minnesota Department of Education
1500 Highway 36 W
Roseville, MN 55113

651-582-8200
Fax: 651-634-5154
www.education.state.mn.us

Alice Seagren, Commissioner
Barry Shaffer, Director
Mark Dayton, Office of Governor
Available statewide at no cost to adult learners and is administered through the Minnesota Department of Education. To be eligible for ABE services, a person must be 16 years old or older, not enrolled in K-12 public or private school and lack basic academic skills in one or more of the following areas: reading, writing, speaking and mathematics.

2131 Alexandria Literacy Project
1204 Hwy 27 W
Room 907
Alexandria, MN 56308

320-762-3312
Fax: 320-762-3313
www.thealp.org
rfinke@alexandria.k12.mn.us

Rollie Finke, Coordinator
Purpose is to recruit and tutor adults who want to improve their basic reading, writing, spelling and/or math skills; to tutor adults originally from other countries who want to improve their English listening, speaking, reading and writing skills; to train volunteer tutors and literacy leaders; to promote and encourage this teaching and training.

2132 English Learning Center
Our Saviour's Outreach Ministries
2315 Chicago Ave S
Minneapolis, MN 55404

612-871-5900
Fax: 612-871-0017
www.osom-mn.org

Michael Kuchta, Chairman
Colleen Whalen, Vice-Chairman
Justin Kappel, Secretary
Educationally empowering immigrant and refugee adults and their families towards self-determination.

2133 LDA Minnesota Learning Disability Association
6100 Golden Valley Rd
Golden Valley, MN 55422

952-582-6000
Fax: 952-582-6031
www.ldaminnesota.org
info@ldaminnesota.org

Willie J. Johnson, President
W. Brooks Donald, Vice President
Jeff Fox, Secretary
A non-profit agency providing programs and services for learners of all ages, specializing in learning disabilities or other learning difficulties such as ADHD.

2134 Minnesota Department of Employment and Economic Development
Minnesota Workforce Center
332 Minnesota St
Suite E-200
Saint Paul, MN 55101-1351

651-259-7114
800-657-3858
TTY: 651-296-3900
http://mn.gov/deed
deed.lmi@state.mn.us

Mark R. Phillips, Commisioner
Bonnie Elsey, Director
The Department of Employment and Economic Development is Minnesota's principal economic development agency, with programs promoting business expansion and retention, workforce development, international trade, community development and tourism.

2135 Minnesota LINCS: Literacy Council
700 Raymond Avenue
Suite 180
Saint Paul, MN 55114

651-645-2277
800-225-7323
Fax: 651-645-2272
www.mnliteracy.org
email@mnliteracy.org

Jewelie Grape, President
Rudy Brynolfson, Treasurer
Carla Engstrom, Executive Committee Chair
Makes information available to literacy and other educators throughout Minnesota. The system is a result of cooperation between numerous agencies and organizations in Minnesota that realize the benefit of using the internet to provide information to the public. The system allows literacy and other educators to locate information at one central site or follow links to connect to wherever the information resides.

2136 Minnesota Life Work Center
University of St Thomas
1000 LaSalle Ave
Ste 110
Minneapolis, MN 55403

651-962-4763
www.stthomas.edu/lifeworkcenter
lifework@stthomas.edu

Provides special services and resources to meet the needs of all students, especially those on the Minneapolis campus.

2137 Minnesota Literacy Training Network
University of St Thomas
2115 Summit Avenue
Minneapolis, MN 55105-2025

651-962-5000
800-328-6819
Fax: 651-962-4014
www.stthomas.edu
webmaster@stthomas.edu

Julie H. Sullivan, Ph.D., President
Deborah Simmons, Director
Literacy Training Network offers noncredit learning opportunities for adult basic education and literacy training staff in Minnesota.

2138 Minnesota Vocational Rehabilitation Services
332 Minnesota St
Ste E-200
Saint Paul, MN 55101-1805

651-259-7366
800-328-9095
Fax: 651-297-5159
TTY: 651-296-3900
http://mn.gov/deed
deed.lmi@state.mn.us

Kimberley Pack, Director

Provides basic vocational rehabilitation services to consumers including vocational counseling, planning, guidance and placement, as well as certain special services based on individual circumstances.

Mississippi

2139 Corinth-Alcorn Literacy Council
1023 N Fillmore St
Corinth, MS 38834-4100   662-286-9759
                               Fax: 662-286-8010
                               www.alcornliteracy.com
                               literacy38834@yahoo.com

Cheryl Meints, President
Tommy Hardwick, Treasurer
Becky Williams, Secretary

Missouri

2140 Joplin NALA Read
ProLiteracy America
123 S. Main Street
Joplin, MO 64801-0447   417-782-2646
                               Fax: 417-782-2648
                               www.joplinnala.org
                               joplinnala@123mail.org

Marj Boudreaux, Director
Joan Doner, Program Coordinator
Gail Brown, Administrative Assistant
An adult literacy council, serving adults 17 years and older in the areas of Math, ESL, and reading. Trains volunteers to tutor and furnish all books for the tutors and students. A not-for-profit organization, that receives funding from United Way and the state Adult Education & Literacy department.

2141 LIFT: St. Louis
815 Olive St
Ste 22
Saint Louis, MO 63101   314-678-4443
                               800-729-4443
                               Fax: 314-678-2938
                               www.lift-missouri.org
                               todea@webster.edu

Dawn Kitchell, President
Doug Crews, Vice President
Del Doss Hemsley, Trasurer
Serves as Missouri's Literacy Resource Center, provides training, technical assistance, and materials for educators and family literacy programs.

2142 Literacy Kansas City
211 W Armour Blvd
Third Fl
Kansas City, MO 64111   816-333-9332
                               Fax: 816-444-6628
                               www.literacykc.org
                               info@literacykc.org

Lynne O'Connell, Vice President
Judy Pfannenstiel, Secretary
Julee Fox, Trasurer
To advance literacy through direct services, advocacy and collaboration.

2143 Literacy Roundtable
YMCA Literacy Council
2635 Gravois Ave
Saint Louis, MO 63118   314-776-7102
                               Fax: 314-776-6872
                               www.literacyroundtable.org
                               cmithcell@ymcastlouis.org

Caroline Mitchell, Coordinator
A consortium of literacy providers throughout the St. Louis-Metro East area whose mission is to support literacy efforts in the Missouri and Illinois bi-state region.

2144 MVCAA Adult/Family Literacy
1415 S Odell Ave
Marshall, MO 65340-3144   660-886-7476
                               Fax: 660-886-5868
                               www.mvcaa.net
                               info@mvcaa.net

Pam LaFrenz, Executive Director
Peggy McGaugh, Vice -Chairman

2145 Parkway Area Adult Education and Literacy
13157 N Olive Spur
Saint Louis, MO 63141   314-415-4940
                               Fax: 314-415-4938
                               www.edline.net
                               pkwyael@yahoo.com

Sally Sandy, Director
Adult basic skills, literacy, GED prep, work readiness, transition to post-secondary, ESL, citizenship, TOFEL prep for those 17 years of age and no longer enrolled in school.

2146 St Louis Public Schools Adult Education and Literacy
801 N. 11th Street
Saint Louis, MO 63101   314-231-3720
                               Fax: 314-367-3057
                               www.slps.org
                               Supt@slps.org

Dr. Kevin Adams, Superintendent
Dr. Nicole Williams, Chief Academics Officer
Provides opportunities for adults to participate in the GED; ESOL; Workforce Development; Life Skills; Literacy Enhancement and Family Literacy programs.

Montana

2147 LVA Richland County
121 3rd Ave NW
Sidney, MT 59270   406-480-1971
                               www.richlandlva.org
                               info@richlandlva.org

Sue Zimmerman, Program Coordinator
A non-profit, community-based organization working to help adults improve their basic literacy skills, and learn other skills needed for today's modern life.

2148 Montana Literacy Resource Center
1515 E 6th Avenue
PO Box 201800
Helena, MT 59620-1800   406-444-3115
                               800-338-5087
                               Fax: 406-444-0266
                               TDD: 406-444-4799
                               TTY: 406-444-4799
                               www.msl.mt.gov
                               msl@mt.gov

Jennie Stapp, State Librarian
Kris Schmitz, Central Service Manager
Stacy Bruhn, GIS Web Developer
A state-wide literacy support network.

Nebraska

2149 Answers4Families: Center on Children, Families, Law
206 S 13th St
Ste 1000
Lincoln, NE 68508-0227   402-472-0844
                               800-746-8420
                               Fax: 402-472-8412
                               www.answers4families.org
A project of the Center on Children, Families and Law at University of Nebraska. Mission is to provide info, opportunities, education and support to Nebraskans through Internet resources. The Center serves individuals with special needs and mental health disorders, foster families, caregivers, assisted living, and school nurses.

2150   Client Assistance Program (CAP): Nebraska Division of Persons with Disabilities
301 Centennial Mall S
Box 94987
Lincoln, NE 68509   402-471-3656
                                            800-742-7594
                                        Fax: 402-471-0117
                                    www.cap.state.ne.us
                        victoria.rasmussen@nebraska.gov
Frank Lloyd, Executive Director
The Client Assistance Program helps individuals who have concerns or difficulties when applying for or receiving rehabilitation services funded under the Rehabilitation Act.

2151   Lincoln Literacy Council
745 S 9th St
Lincoln, NE 68508   402-476-7323
                                        Fax: 402-476-2122
                                    www.lincolnliteracy.org
                                    info@lincolnliteracy.org
David Bargen, President
Cynthia Martinez, First Vice President
Kelly Neil, Second Vice President
To assist people of all cultures and strengthen the community by teaching English language and literacy skills.

2152   Literacy Center for the Midlands
1823 Harney St
Ste 204
Omaha, NE 68102   402-342-7323
                                        Fax: 402-345-9045
                                    www.midlandsliteracy.org
                                btodd@midlandsliteracy.org
Beverly Todd, Executive Director
To empower adults and families by helping them acquire the literacy skills and practices to be active and contributing members of their communities.

2153   Platte Valley Literacy Association
P.O. Box 159
Columbus, NE 68602   402-562-5904
                                        Fax: 402- 564-944
                                    www.megavision.net
                                literacy@megavision.com
Jolene Hake, Executive Director
Organization that collaborates with Central Community College Adult Basic Education to respond to the educational needs of our community.

Nevada

2154   Nevada Department of Adult Education
755 N Roop St
Carson City, NV 89701   775-687-7289
                                        Fax: 775-687-8636
                                    http://nde.doe.nv.gov
Brad Deeds, ABE/ESL/GED Programs
provides adult basic education and literacy services in order to assist adults to become literate and obtain the knowledge and skills necessary for employment and self-sufficiency; to assist adults who are parents to obtain the educational skills necessary to become full partners in the education of their children; and to assist adults in the completion of a secondary school education.

2155   Nevada Economic Opportunity Board: Community Action Partnership
330 W. Washington Ave
Suite 7
Las Vegas, NV 89106   702-647-3307
                                        Fax: 702-647-0803
                                    www.eobccnv.org
                                    Info@eobccnv.org
Lawrence Weekly, President
Aaron Ford, Secretary
Fred Haron, Treasurer

Located in one of the fastest growing and most diverse communities in the United States, the Economic Opportunity Board of Clark County is a highly innovative Community Action Agency. Our mission is to eliminate poverty by providing programs, resources, services, and advocacy for self-sufficiency and economic empowerment.

2156   Nevada Literacy Coalition: State Literacy Resource Center
100 N Stewart St
Carson City, NV 89701-4285   775-885-1010
                                            800-445-9673
                                        Fax: 775-684-3344
                                    www.nevadaculture.org
                                    sfgraf@clan.lib.nv.us
Claudia Vechio, Director
Larry Friedman, Deputy Director
Greg Fine, Marketing and Advertising
The Nevada State Literacy Resource Center has books, newsletters and a wide variety of multi-media resources such as videos, audiotapes and games for literacy instruction and programs for literacy students, trainers and tutors.

2157   Northern Nevada Literacy Council
1400 Wedekind Rd
Reno, NV 89512-2465   775-356-1007
                                        Fax: 775-356-1009
                                    www.nnlc.org
                                    director@nnlc.org
Susan Robinson, Executive Director
Mike Benson, Data Manager
Katie Plaz, Bookkepper and Office Manager
Provides English as a second language, adult basic skills, and GED preparatory instructions for adults, 18 years of age and over, who lack a high school diploma or GED or essential basic skills to function successfully in the workplace.

New Hampshire

2158   New Hampshire Literacy Volunteers of America
405 Pine St
Manchester, NH 03104-6106   603-624-6550
                                        Fax: 603-624-6559
                                    www.manchesternh.gov
Mark Brewer, Director
Robert Gagne, Chairman
Wesley Anderson, Director
This program is the only nationally accredited adult literacy program in New Hampshire. Provides free confidential one-to-one tutoring for adults who want to learn to write and read for lifelong learning.

2159   New Hampshire Second Start Adult Education
17 Knight St
Concord, NH 03301   603-228-1341
                                        Fax: 603-228-3852
                                    www.second-start.org
                                    abe@second-start.org
Frank Lamay, Director
Deb Shea, Director
Linda Vincent, Diector
Provides instruction in basic reading, writing and math.

New Jersey

2160   Jersey City Library Literacy Program
472 Jersey Ave
Jersey City, NJ 07302-3456   201-547-4526
                                        Fax: 201-435-5746
                                    www.jclibrary.org
                                    literacy@jclibrary.org
Sondra E. Buesing Riley, President
John A. Mehos, Treasurer
Esther Wintner, Secretary

Provides free one-on-one basic reading instruction for Jersey City residents aged sixteen and older. Work with students ranging from non-readers through the fifth grade level. Offers small conversation group classes for immigrants striving to learn to speak, read and write English.

2161 Literacy Volunteers in Mercer County
224 Main St.
Ste 104
Metuchen, NJ 08840   732-906-5456
                                       800- 848-004
                                   Fax: 609-587-6137
                                   http://literacynj.org
                                   lvmercer@verizon.net
Perrine Robinson Geller, President
Elizabeth Gloeggler, CEO
Jessica Tomkins, COO
Trains, coordinates and supports the efforts of a dedicated group of volunteer literacy tutors. Volunteers provide free, confidential literacy tutoring services to adult residents in Mercer COunty at a variety of locations including the public libraries, workplace sites, churches and retirement homes.

2162 Literacy Volunteers of America Essex/Passaic County
Passaic Public Library
195 Gregory Ave
Passaic, NJ 07005   973-470-0039
                                   Fax: 973-470-0098
                                   www.lvanewark.org
                                   lvanewark@verizon.net
Sally Rice, President
Kathy Mollica, Vice President
Jordan Fried, Treasury
Provides free literacy services to adults who have been identified as needing instruction in reading and/or English conversation; and to families who are experiencing literacy and/or learning difficulties.

2163 Literacy Volunteers of Camden County
203 Laurel Rd
3rdfloor
Voorhees, NJ 08043-2349   856-772-1636
                                   Fax: 856-772-2761
                                   http://lva.camden.lib.nj.us
                                   literacy@camdencountylibrary.org
Denise Weinberg, Director
An adult literacy organization that tutors Camden County, NJ adults (18 years or over) residents who are at the lowest levels of literacy and who need help speaking or understanding English (ESL) or who need help with elementary reading or math skills.

2164 Literacy Volunteers of Cape-Atlantic
743 N Main St
Pleasantville, NJ 08232-1541   609-383-3377
                                   Fax: 609-383-0234
                                   www.lvacapeatlantic.com
                                   literacyvolunteers@comcast.net
Pamela Grites, Executive Director
Katherine Micale, Program Director
Patrica Epps, Administrative Assistant
Helps individuals in Atlantic and Cape May Counties improve their English language skills so they can participate more fully in family, workplace and community life.

2165 Literacy Volunteers of Englewood Library
31 Engle St
Englewood, NJ 07631-2903   201-568-2215
                                   Fax: 201-568-6895
                                   www.englewoodlibrary.org
                                   ctaylor@bccls.org
Katharine Glynn, President
Frank Huttle, Mayor
Catherine Wolverton, Library Director
Offers three tutor-training workshops each year with an extensive collection of books, workbooks, and cassettes for tutors and students to borrow with a current library card.

2166 Literacy Volunteers of Gloucester County
PO Box 1106
Turnersville, NJ 08012   856-218-4743
                                   www.literacyvgc.org
                                   info@literacyvgc.org
Trudy Lawrence, Executive Director
Providing free, one-on-one adult tutoring to those with the lowest level of literacy - below a 5th grade level.

2167 Literacy Volunteers of Middlesex
Suite F
380 Washington Road
Sayreville, NJ 08872   732-432-8000
                                   Fax: 732-432-8189
                                   www.lpnj.org
                                   info@lpnj.org
Mary Ellen Firestone, President
Christine Sienkielewski, Director
Trained volunteers that provide free tutoring services to adults with limited literacy skills, enabling them to achieve their personal goals and to enhance their contributions to the community.

2168 Literacy Volunteers of Monmouth County
213 Broadway
Long Branch, NJ 07740   732-571-0209
                                   Fax: 732-571-2474
                                   www.lvmonmouthnj.org
                                   lvmonmouth@brookdalecc.edu
Chris Vecere, President
Manuel J. Alarez, Vice President
Thomas J. White, Secretary
Mission is to promote increased literacy for adults in Monmouth County through the effetive use of volunteers and in collaboration with individuals, groups and organizations desiring to foster increased literacy.

2169 Literacy Volunteers of Morris County
10 Pine St
Morristown, NJ 07960   973-984-1998
                                   Fax: 973-971-0291
                                   www.lvamorris.org
                                   lvamorris@yahoo.com
Debbie Leon, Director
Promotes increased literacy and fluency in English for adult learners in this area through the effective use of volunteers, the provisions of support services for volunteers and learners, and through collaboration with individuals, groups and any organization desirous of fostering increased literacy.

2170 Literacy Volunteers of Plainfield Public Library
800 Park Ave
Plainfield, NJ 07060-2517   908-757-1111
                                   Fax: 908-754-0063
                                   www.plainfieldlibrary.info
                                   literacy@plfdpl.info
Joseph Hugh Da Rold, Director
Mary Ellen Rogan, Assistant Director
Scott Kuchinsky, Coordinator
Mission is to develop the literacy skills of adults with minimum reading skills.

2171 Literacy Volunteers of Somerset County
120 Finderne Ave
Box 7
Bridgewater, NJ 08807   908-725-5430
                                   Fax: 908-707-2077
                                   www.literacysomerset.org
                                   info@literacysomerset.org
Martha Davis, President
Phil Areminio, Vice President
Steve Cummins, Trasurer
Promotes literacy through a network of community volunteers.

2172 Literacy Volunteers of Union County
224 Main St.
Metuchen, NJ 08840
732-906-5456
Fax: 800-848-0048
http://literacynj.org
literacyinfo@lvaunion.org
Perrine Robinson Geller, President
Elizabeth Gloeggler, CEO
Jessica Tomkins, COO
A non-profit organization that improves the lives of adults in
the county by teaching them to read, write and speak English
so they can participate more fully in family, workplace and
community life.

2173 People Care Center
120 Finderne Avenue
Bridgewater, NJ 08807
908-725-2299
Fax: 908-725-2607
www.peoplecarecenter.org
info@peoplecarecenter.org
Joseph Antico, President
Jay Perantoni, VP
Marie Hughes, Executive Director

New Mexico

**2174 Adult Basic Education Division of Dona Ana Commu-
nity College**
2800 N. Sonoma Ranch Blvd
Las Cruces, NM 88011
575-527-7500
800-903-7503
Fax: 575-528-7300
http://dabcc-www.nmsu.edu
sdegiuli@nmsu.edu
Renay Scott, President
Andrew Burke, VP, Business & Finance
Monica Torres, Interim VP, Academic Affairs

2175 Carlsbad Literacy Program
Ann Wood Literacy Center
511 N 12th Street
P.O. Box 3112
Carlsbad, NM 88221
575-885-1752
Fax: 575-885-7980
www.carlsbadliteracyprogram.com
literacy1@valornet.com
Delora Elizondo, Coordinator
Provides opportunities for adult community members to
learn to read and to improve their reading and writing abilities.

2176 Curry County Literacy Council
Clovis Community College
417 Schepps Blvd
Rm 171
Clovis, NM 88101
575-769-2811
800-769-1409
Fax: 575-769-4190
www.clovis.edu
curry.literacy@clovis.edu
Dr. Becky Rowley, President
Dr. Robin Jones, VP
Tom Drake, VP, Administration
Goal is to provide one with a sense of security to gain em-
ployment, have life skills, and assist in language develop-
ment.

2177 Deming Literacy Program
PO Box 1932
2301 South Tin St.
Deming, NM 88031-1932
575-546-7571
Fax: 505-546-1356
www.centerfornonprofitexcellence.org
dlpdeming@gmail.com
Marisol D. Perez, Director

The Literacy Home Mentoring and After School Project will
encourage parents to read to their children at home, as well
as provide mentors to help children with their reading skills
after school.

2178 Literacy Volunteers of America: Dona Ana County
MSC 3DA
P.O. Box 30001
Las Cruces, NM 88003-8001
575-527-7544
800-903-7540
Fax: 575-528-7065
www.readwritenow.org
sdegiuli@nmsu.edu
Linda Coshenet, Chair
Anita C. Hernandez, Ph.D., Vice Chair
Jackie Kiefer, Treasurer, Secretary
The Literacy Volunteers of America is designed to help peo-
ple who cannot read or write the English language. This pro-
gram gives adults a new opportunity to learn reading through
the sixth-grade level.

2179 Literacy Volunteers of America: Las Vegas, San Miguel
Box 9000
Las Vegas, NM 87701
505-425-7511
877-850-9064
www.nmhu.edu
president_office@nmhu.edu
James Fries, President
Gilbert D. Rivera, Vice President
Darlene Chavez, Development Finance Officer
Las Vegas/San Miguel Literacy Volunteers are a part of the
national non-profit organization Literacy Volunteers of
America, which is dedicated to promoting literacy through-
out the country.

2180 Literacy Volunteers of America: Socorro County
PO Box 1431
Socorro, NM 87801-1431
505-835-4659
Fax: 505-835-1182
www.volunteermatch.org
lva_socorro@hotmail.com
Joyce Aguilar, Executive Director
Promotes literacy for people of Socorro County.

2181 Literacy Volunteers of Santa Fe
6401 Richards Avenue
Room 514A
Santa Fe, NM 87508
505-428-1353
Fax: 505-428-1338
www.lvsf.org
lvsf@sfcc.edu
Letty Naranjo, Executive Director
Israel Garcia, Program Assistant
Dedicated to providing free tutoring and encouragement for
adults and their families who want to read, write and speak
English.

2182 New Mexico Coalition for Literacy
3209 Mercantile Ct
Suite B
Santa Fe, NM 87507
505-982-3997
800-233-7587
Fax: 505-982-4095
www.nmcl.org
info@nmcl.org
Heather Heunermund, Executive Director
Encourages and supports community-based literacy programs and is the New Mexico affiliate and coordinator for
the national program of ProLiteracy America, overseeing
certification and coordination of its volunteer, tutor trainers.

2183 Read West
2900 Grande Blvd
PO Box 44508
Rio Rancho, NM 87124
505-892-1131
Fax: 505-896-3780
www.readwest.org
readwest@readwest.org

Linda Stokes, President
Kitty McMahon, VP
Gwenevere Johnson, Treasurer
Targets adults with low literacy or whose first language is not English. Provides free, customized, one-to-one, tutoring to help adults improve. their reading, writing and English language.
1989

2184 Roswell Literacy Council

609 West 10th Street
Roswell, NM 88201

575-625-1369
Fax: 575-622-8280
www.roswell-literacy.org
literacy@dfn.com

Andrae England, Director
Dedicated to adult learning in Chaves County.

2185 Valencia County Literacy Council

280 La Entrada
Los Lunas, NM 87031

505-925-8926
Fax: 505-925-8924
www.valencialiteracy.org
joglesby@valencialiteracy.org

Dolores Padilla, President
Roberta Scott, VP
Paul Baca, Executive Director
To enable adults to achieve personal goals and very young children to achieve pre-literacy skills through literacy services provided to families free of charge.

New York

2186 Literacy Volunteers of America: Middletown

70 Fulton Street
Middletown, NY 10940

845-341-5460
Fax: 845-343-7191
www.literacyorangeny.org
info@LiteracyOrangeNY.com

Christine Rolando, Executive Director
An organization of volunteers that provides a variety of services to enable people to achieve personal goals through literacy. Their belief is that the ability to read is critical to personal freedom and maintenance of a democratic society. These beliefs have led to the following commitments: the personal growth of their students; the effective use of their volunteers; the improvement of society and strengthening and improving the organization.

2187 Literacy Volunteers of Oswego County

45 E. Schuyler Street
Bldg. 31, Fort Ontario
Oswego, NY 13126

315-342-8839
Fax: 315-342-3489
www.lvoswego.org
lvoswego@oco.org

Jane Murphy, Executive Director
Beth Kazel, Director of Education Services
Meg Henderson, Program Coordinator
A non-profit community-based educational organization that provides quality tutoring in basic literacy skills and conversational English.

2188 Literacy Volunteers of Otsego & Delaware Counties

Oneonta Adult Education
31 Center Street
Oneonta, NY 13820-3510

607-433-3645
800-782-3858
http://oneontaadulteducation.org
lvodc@oneonta.edu

To change lives of courageous, motivated adults who do not possess functional skills needed to perform ordinary, everyday tasks in an ever-changing global society.

2189 New York Literacy Assistance Center

39 Broadway
Suite 1250
New York, NY 10006

212-803-3300
Fax: 212-785-3685
www.lacnyc.org
elyser@lacnyc.org

Elizabeth Horton, Chair
John Gordon, Associate VP, Programs
J. David Nelson, Chief Operating Officer
A nonprofit organization dedicated to supporting and promoting the expansion of quality literacy services in New York.

2190 New York Literacy Resource Center

State University of New York
1400 Washington Ave
Albany, NY 12222

518-442-3300
800-331-0931
Fax: 518-442-5383
www.albany.edu

Robert J. Jones, President
Miriam Trementozzi, Associate VP
Daniel Butterworth, Program Director
State Literacy Resource Center is a statewide literacy information network throughout the state.

2191 New York Literacy Volunteers of America

149 Central Ave.
Lancaster, NY 14086

716-651-0465
Fax: 716-651-0542
http://literacynewyork.org
info@literacynewyork.org

Janice Cuddahee, Executive Director
Kathy Houghton, Director of Program Services
Chip Carlin, Associate Executive Director
Provides technical program, and training assistance and workshops to a network of 36 local, community-based affiliates who annually provide over 400,000 hours of reading and basic skills instruction to adult learners.

2192 Resources for Children with Special Needs

116 E. 16th Street
5th Floor
New York, NY 10003

212-677-4650
Fax: 212-254-4070
www.resourcesnyc.org
info@resourcesnyc.org

Rachel Howard, Executive Director
Stephen Stern, Director, Finance
Todd Dorman, Director, Communications
Independent nonprofit organization that works for families and children with all special needs, across all boroughs, to understand, navigate, and access the services needed to ensure that all children have the opportunity to develop their full potential.

North Carolina

2193 Blue Ridge Literacy Council

PO Box 1728
Hendersonville, NC 28793

828-696-3811
Fax: 828-696-3887
www.litcouncil.org
skirkland@litcouncil.org

Judy Hansen, President
Rickey Parker, Vice President
Steve Kirkland, Executive Director
Provides adults in Henderson County the English communication and literacy skills they need to reach their full potential as individuals, parents, workers and citizens.

2194   Durham Literacy Center

1905 Chapel Hill Road
P.O. Box 52209
Durham, NC 27707

919-489-8383
Fax: 919-489-7637
www.durhamliteracy.org
info@durhamliteracy.org

Reginald Hodges, Executive Director
Shondra Brewer, Administrative Assistant
Gardy Perard, Coordinator
Works to assist Durham County teenagers and adults achieve personal goals and experience positive life change through increased literacy. Helps teenagers and adults gain the reading and writing skills, English language skills, and educational credentials (GED) needed to earn a living wage.

2195   Gaston Literacy Council

116 South Marietta Street
Gastonia, NC 28052

704-868-4815
Fax: 704-867-7796
www.gastonliteracy.org
literacy@gastonliteracy.org

Gayle Kersh, Chair
Tim Efird, Vice Chair
Kaye Gribble, Executive Director
A progressive organization dedicated to helping individuals improve their reading, writing, mathematics, listening, speaking, and technology skills.

2196   Literacy Council Of Buncombe County

31 College Place
Suite B-221
Asheville, NC 28801

828-254-3442
Fax: 828-254-1742
www.litcouncil.com
info@litcouncil.com

Ashley Lasher, Executive Director
Brantlee Eisenman, Development Director
Erin Sebelius, ESOL Director
Promotes increased adult literacy in Buncombe County through effective use of trained tutors; to provide support services for tutors and learners; and to collaborate with individuals, groups, or other community organizations desiring to foster increased adult literacy.

2197   Literacy Volunteers of America: Pitt County

3107 S Evans Street
Suite E
Greenville, NC 27858

252-353-6578
Fax: 252-353-6868
www.pittliteracy.org
info@pittliteracy.org

Lynn Pischke, Executive Director
To promote literacy in Pitt County through trained volunteer tutors who provide one on one and small group tutoring to adults with limited reading, writing or English speaking/literacy skills.

2198   North Carolina Literacy Resource Center

North Carolina Community College
200 West Jones Street
Raleigh, NC 27603

919-807-7100
Fax: 919-807-7165
www.nccommunitycolleges.edu
allenb@ncccs.cc.nc.us

Dr. R. Scott Ralls, President
Lisa Tolley, Program Manager
North Carolina Community College Literacy Resource Center collects and disseminates information about literacy resources and organizations.

2199   Reading Connections of North Carolina

122 N. Elm Street
Suite 920
Greensboro, NC 27401

336-230-2223
Fax: 336-230-2203
www.readingconnections.org
info@readingconnections.org

Jennifer Gore, Executive Director
Roberta Hawthorne, Program Manager
Alexana Garcia, ABE Coordinator
To provide and advocate for free, individualized adult literacy services to promote life changes for Guilford County residents and surrounding communities.

North Dakota

2200   North Dakota Adult Education and Literacy Resource Center

600 E. Boulevard Avenue
Dept. 201, Floors 9, 10, and 11
Bismarck, ND 58505-0440

701-328-2260
Fax: 701-328-2461
www.dpi.state.nd.us
dpi@nd.gov

Kirsten Baesler, State Superintendent
Valerie Fischer, State Director
Jolli Marcellais, Administrative Assistant
Promotes and supports free programs that help adults over the age of 16 obtain the basic academic and educational skills they need to be productive workers, family members, and citizens.

2201   North Dakota Department of Career and Technical Education

State Capitol 15th Floor
600 E Boulevard Ave
Bismarck, ND 58505

701-328-3180
Fax: 701-328-1255
www.nd.gov
cte@nd.us

Wayne Kutzer, Director
The mission of the Board for Vocational and Technical Education is to work with others to provide all North Dakota citizens with the technical skills, knowledge, and attitudes necessary for successful performance in a globally competitive workplace.

2202   North Dakota Department of Human Services: Welfare & Public Assistance

600 East Boulevard Avenue
Dept. 325
Bismarck, ND 58505-0250

701-328-2310
800-472-2622
Fax: 701-328-2359
TTY: 800-366-6888
www.nd.gov/dhs
dhseo@nd.gov

Carol K Olson, Executive Director
To provide services and support for poor, disabled, ill, elderly or juvenile clients in North Dakota.

2203   North Dakota Department of Public Instruction

600 E. Boulevard Avenue
Dept. 201, Floors 9, 10, and 11
Bismarck, ND 58505-0440

701-328-2260
Fax: 701-328-2461
www.dpi.state.nd.us
dpi@nd.gov

Kirsten Baesler, State Superintendent
Valerie Fischer, State Director
Jolli Marcellais, Administrative Assistant
This unit provides funding and technical assistance to local programs and monitors progress of each funded project. This unit is also responsible for the administration of the GED Testing Program.

2204   North Dakota Reading Association

2420 2nd Ave SW
Minot, ND 58701-3332

701-857-4642
Fax: 701-857-8761
http://ndreadon.utma.com
Paula.Rogers@sendit.nodak.edu

Joyce Hinman, State Coordinator

To provide a variety of professional development opportunities; to increase the building of partnerships with other organizations; to actively promote literacy locally and globally; to assist in the strengthening of local councils and their services to members; and to promote writing with young authors.

2205 North Dakota Workforce Development Council

1600 E Century Ave, Suite 2
P.O. Box 2057
Bismarck, ND 58503   701-328-5300
                                  Fax: 701-328-5320
                                  TTY: 800-366-6888
                                  www.commerce.nd.gov
                                  commerce@nd.gov
Al Anderson, Commissioner, Dept. of Commerce
Paul Lucy, Director, Finance
Wayde Sick, Director, Workforce Development
The role of the North Dakota Workforce Development Council is to advise the Governor and the Public concerning the nature and extent of workforce development in the context of North Dakota's economic development needs, and how to meet these needs effectively while maximizing the efficient use of available resources and avoiding unnecessary duplication of effort.

Ohio

2206 Central/Southeast ABLE Resource Center

Ohio University
338 McCracken Hall
Athens, OH 45701   740-593-4419
                                       800-753-1519
                                  Fax: 740-593-2834
                                  www.ouliteracycenter.org
                                  literacy@ohio.edu
Sharon Reynolds, Director
Committed to the development of literacy in southeastern Ohio and to research in all areas of literacy.

2207 Clark County Literacy Coalition

137 East High Street
Springfield, OH 45502-1215   937-323-8617
                                  Fax: 937-328-6911
                                  www.clarkcountyliteracy.org
                                  david.smiddy@clarkcountyliteracy.org
Lisa Holmes, President
Dedicated to increasing the level of functional literacy and self-sufficiency among the people in Clark County.

2208 Columbus Literacy Council

195 N Grant Ave
Columbus, OH 43215-2607   614-221-5013
                                  Fax: 614-221-5892
                                  www.columbusliteracy.com
                                  jwatson@columbusliteracy.org
Joy D Watson, Executive Director
A volunteer-based organization dedicated to increasing the level of functional literacy of adults in Central Ohio through teaching the English language skills of listening, speaking, reading and writing.

2209 Literacy Council of Clermont/Brown Counties

745 Center Street
Suite 300
Milford, OH 45150   513-831-7323
                                  Fax: 513-943-3002
                                  www.clermontbrownliteracy.org
                                  susan.vilardo@clermontbrownliteracy.org
Rose M. Tepe, President
Meredith Delaney, Vice President
Susan Vilardo, Executive Director
Offers one-on-one volunteer tutor education in reading, writing, spelling and comprehension to adults 19 years of age and older who cannot read and adults who are ESL/ESOL.

2210 Miami Valley Literacy Council

333 West First St
Ste 130
Dayton, OH 45402   937-223-4922
                                  Fax: 937-223-0271
                                  www.discoverliteracy.org
                                  rgilmore@discoverliteracy.org
Russ Gilmore, Executive Director
Offers classes, one-to-one tutoring, and independent study options to adults in the Miami Valley who have low-level literacy of English language skills. Also works with school-aged children and teens below grade level in reading and math in the after-school program The Learning Club.

2211 Ohio Literacy Network

6161 Busch Blvd
Ste 84
Columbus, OH 43229   614-505-0716
                                       800-228-7323
                                  Fax: 614-505-0718
                                  www.ohioliteracynetwork.org
                                  atoops@ohioliteracynetworking.org
Allen Toops, Executive Director
Mission is to build Ohio's workforce by strengthening adult and family literacy education accomplished by connecting learners, educators and volunteers to a wide variety of educational resources.

2212 Ohio Literacy Resource Center

Kent State University
Research 1-1100 Summit Street, Kent
PO Box 5190
Kent, OH 44242-0001   330-672-2007
                                       800-765-2897
                                  Fax: 330-672-4841
                                  http://literacy.kent.edu
                                  olrc@literacy.kent.edu
Marty Ropog, Director
Tim Ponder, LINCS coordinator
Susie Lockhart, Office Manager
The OLRC Mission is to stimulate joint planning and coordination of literacy services at the local, regional and state levels, and to enhance the capacity of state and local organizations and services delivery systems.

2213 Project LEARN of Summit County

60 South High Street
Akron, OH 44326   330-434-9461
                                       866-934-7323
                                  Fax: 330-643-9195
                                  www.projectlearnsummit.org
                                  info@projectlearnsummit.org
Rick Mc Intosh, Executive Director
Stephanie Norris, Admissions Assistant
Rose Austin, Data Manager
Project LEARN is a nonprofit, community-based organization providing Summit County's nonreading adult population with free, confidential, small group classes and tutoring. Helps adults reach their goals of self-sufficiency, independence and job retention.

2214 Project LITE

6th And Reid Ave
Lorain, OH 44052   440-244-1192
                                       800-322-READ
                                  Fax: 440-244-1733
                                  www.lorain.lib.oh.us
                                  contact lite@lorain.lib.oh.us
Linda Pierce, Director

2215 Project: LEARN

105 W. Liberty Street
Medina, OH 44256   330-723-1314
                                  www.projectlearnmedina.org
                                  projectlearn.medina@gmail.com
Linda Smalley, Executive Director
Provides one-on-one tutoring to adults in reading, math and English as a second language.

2216 Seeds of Literacy Project: St Colman Family Learning Center
3104 W. 25th Street
3rd Floor
Cleveland, OH 44109   216-661-7950
Fax: 216-661-7952
www.seedsofliteracy.org
bonnieentler@seedsofliteracy.org
Bonnie Entler, Executive Director
Rachel Cotton, Site Coordinator
Daniel McLaughlin, Program Officer
Helping adults in need of assistance in reading, writing and mathematical skills and to improve their ability to function, compete, and advance in society in an atmosphere of Christian care and compassion.

Oklahoma

2217 Center for Study of Literacy
Northeastern State University
2400 W. Shawnee
PO Box 549
Muskogee, OK 74401   918-683-0040
Fax: 918-781-5425
www.nsuok.edu
mcelroyt@nsuok.edu
Dr. Steve Turner, President
Dr. Laura Boren, VP, Student Affairs
David Koehn, VP, Finance & Business
Provides the illiterate or undereducated adult with training; provides instructional support for the Northeastern State University's faculty and pre-service teachers participate in computer literacy training to gain an understanding of computer assisted instruction; to serve as a reesource unit for other social agencies, teachers, administrators and public school students; to serve as the clearinghouse for literacy for the state of Oklahoma; to initiate research on literacy.

2218 Community Literacy Center
5131 N. Classen Circle
Suite 204
Oklahoma City, OK 73118-4420   405-524-7323
Fax: 405-608-0533
www.communityliteracy.com
okcread@caol.com
Becky O'Dell, Executive Director
Laura Taylor, Coordinator
Tara Beall, Communications Coordinator
A private, non-profit organization dedicated to teaching adults to read.

2219 Creek County Literacy Program
27 W Dewey Ave
Sapulpa, OK 74066-3909   918-224-9647
Fax: 918-224-3546
www.creeklit.okpls.org
creeklit@yahoo.com
Barbara Belk, Executive Director
Provides free reading instruction to functionally illiterate adults who live or work in Creek County, to prepare families to manage their health care needs and to be effectively involved in the education of their children, to tutor children/youth who may have different learning styles, and to provide reading improvement programs county-wide

2220 Great Plains Literacy Council
Southern Prairie Library System
421 North Hudson
Altus, OK 73521   580-477-2890
888-302-9053
Fax: 580-477-3626
www.spls.lib.ok.us
literacy1@spls.lib.ok.us
Ida Fay Winters, Director

Helps to increase the awareness of the illiteracy problem and offers a viable solution. Recruits dedicated, tutors who help to motivate those who are considered illiterate and give them the opportunity to become contributing members of the community.

2221 Guthrie Literacy Program
201 N Division Street
Guthrie, OK 73044   405-282-0050
Fax: 405-282-2804
www.guthrie.okpls.org
co@cityofguthrie.com
Linda Gens, Library Services Director
Utilizes curriculum that focuses on the individual student's interests and needs, then tutors help the student set the goals and work with them to achieve those goals.

2222 Junior League of Oklahoma City
1001 NW Grand Boulevard
Oklahoma City, OK 73118   405-843-5668
Fax: 405-843-0994
www.jloc.org
info@jloc.org
Kristi Leonard, President
Nazette Zuhdi, President Elect
Jenifer Randle, Administrative VP
Organization of women committed to promoting volunteerism, developing the potential of women and to improving the community through the effective action and leadership of trained volunteers. The purpose is exclusively educational and charitable.

2223 Literacy & Evangelism International
1800 S Jackson Ave
Tulsa, OK 74107   918-585-3826
Fax: 918-585-3224
www.literacyevangelism.org
general@literacyevangelism.org
A missionary fellowship desiring to see the Church in every nation effectively reaching the illiterate, bringing them the Living Word Jesus Christ, through enabling them to read the written Word of God.

2224 Literacy Volunteers of America: Tulsa City County Library
400 Civic Center
Tulsa, OK 74103   918-549-7323
Fax: 918-596-7907
www.tulsalibrary.org
jgreb@tccl.lib.ok.us
Linda Saferite, Executive Director
Sally Frasier, Commission Member
Rebecca Marks, Commission Member
We offer one-on-one tutoring to adults and young adults who wish to improve their reading and writing skills.

2225 Muskogee Area Literacy Council
801 West Okmulgee
Muskogee, OK 74401-6840   918-682-6657
888-291-8152
Fax: 918-682-9466
www.eok.lib.ok.us
muskpublib@eodls.org
Penny Chastain, Coordinator
Jan Bryant, Head of Muskogee Public Library
Debbie Goodwin, Head of Circulation

2226 Northwest Oklahoma Literacy Council
1500 Main St
Woodward, OK 73801-3044   580-254-8582
Fax: 580-254-8546
nwoklitcouncil@woodward.lib.ok.us
Cathy Johnson, Director
Mission is to break the intergenerational cycle of illiteracy by broadening the learner and service base to include family members. Services include literacy and parenting instruction, as a compliment to ESL, adult basic education, and learning disabilities programs.

2227 Oklahoma Literacy Council
300 Park Ave
Oklahoma City, OK 73102-3600   405-232-3780
Fax: 405-606-3722
www.literacyokc.org
director@literacyokc.org
Millonn Lamb, Executive Director
Promotes literacy in adults who are in need of improving literacy skills to function successfully in society.

2228 Oklahoma Literacy Resource Center
200 N.E. 18th St.
Oklahoma City, OK 73105   405-521-2502
800-522-8116
Fax: 405-525-7804
www.odl.state.ok.us
lgelders@oltn.state.ok.us
Leslie Gelders, Literacy Administrator
Susan C. McVey, Director
Vicki Sullivan, Deputy Director
Provides leadership, resources, training, and information to Oklahoma;s library and community-based literacy network.

2229 Opportunities Industrialization Center of Oklahoma County
400 N Walnut Ave
Oklahoma City, OK 73104-2207   405-235-2651
Fax: 405-235-2653
http://oicofoklahomacounty.org
oicoc@sbcglobal.net
Jerry Day, Chairman
Monique Jackson, Vice Chairman
Patricia Kelly, Executive Director
Empowers individuals through Academic and Career education to become more productive citizens in the community.

Oregon

2230 Oregon Department of Human Resource Adult & Family Services Division
500 Summer St NE
Salem, OR 97301   503-945-5944
Fax: 503-378-2897
TTY: 503-945-6214
www.oregon.gov
dhr.info@state.or.us
John Kitzhaber, Governor
Carolyn Ross, Director
Ellen F. Rosenblum, Attorney General
This group combines programs from the former Adult & Family Services Division and the State Office for Services to Children and Families.

2231 Oregon Employment Department
875 Union St NE
Salem, OR 97311   877-517-5627
800-237-3710
Fax: 503-947-1472
www.workinginoregon.org
Laurie Warner, Director
Supports economic stability for Oregonians and communities during times of unemployment through the payment of unemployment benefits. Serves businesses by recruiting and referring the best qualified applicants to jobs, and provides resources to diverse job seekers in support of their employment needs.

2232 Oregon GED Administrator: Office of Community College Services
255 Capitol St NE
Salem, OR 97310-1300   503-378-8648
Fax: 503-378-3365
www.oregon.gov
sharlene.walker@state.or.us
John Kitzhaber, Governor
Carolyn Ross, Director
Ellen F. Rosenblum, Attorney General

Mission is to contribute leadership and resources to increase the skills, knowledge and career opportunities of Oregonians.

2233 Oregon State Library
250 Winter St NE
Salem, OR 97301-3950   503-378-4243
Fax: 503-585-8059
www.oregon.gov
leann.bromeland@state.or.us
John Kitzhaber, Governor
Carolyn Ross, Director
Ellen F. Rosenblum, Attorney General
Mission is to provide quality information services to Oregon state government, to provide reading materials to blind and print-disabled Oregonians, and to provide leadership, grants, and other assistance to improve local library service for all Oregonians.

Pennsylvania

2234 Delaware County Literacy Council
2217 Providence Avenue
Chester, PA 19013   610-876-4811
Fax: 610-876-5414
www.delcoliteracy.org
khyzer@delcoliteracy.org
Kate Hyzer, Executive Director
Susan Keller, Comm & Technology Specialist
Deb Charley, Adult Education Coordinator
Dedicated to providing free, individual and small group literacy instruction to non-and low-reading adults residing in Delaware County, through a county-wide network of trained volunteer tutors and instructors.

2235 Learning Disabilities Association of Pennsylvania
4751 Lindle Rd
Ste 114
Harrisburg, PA 17111   717-939-3731
888-775-3272
www.ldapa.org
ldapaininfo@aol.com
Deborah Rodes, President
An advocacy organization dedicated to helping children and adults with learning disabilities and other related neurological disorders.

2236 Literacy Council of Lancaster/Lebanon
24South Queen Street
Lancaster, PA 17603   717-295-5523
Fax: 717-295-5342
www.adultlit.org
info@adultlit.org
Cheryl Hiester, Executive Director
Jenny Bair, Program Director
Bobbi Hurst, Student Coordinator, Lancaster
A private, non-profit education agency that provides high quality basic education to adults in Lancaster and Lebanon Counties. Promotes literacy and help adults reach their reading, writing, math and English communication goalsthrough personalized instruction.

2237 Pennsylvania Literacy Resource Center
12th Floor
333 Market St
Harrisburg, PA 17126   717-783-6788
800-992-2283
Fax: 717-783-5420
TTY: 717-783-8445
www.portal.state.pa.us
alubrecht@pa.gov
Alice Lubrecht, Director
As part of the State Library, the State Resource Center provides electronic and print resources.

2238 York County Literacy Council
800 E King St
York, PA 17403
717-845-8719
Fax: 717-699-5620
www.yorkliteracy.org
exec.dir@yorkliteracy.org

Bobbi Anne DeLeo, Executive Director
Rita Hewitt, Community Relations Manager
Lezlie Phillips, Adult Reading Coordinator
Dedicated to advancing adult literacy in York County. Client services are provided confidentially and free of charge to York County residents

Rhode Island

2239 Literacy Volunteers of America: Rhode Island
Ste 106
260 W Exchange St
Providence, RI 02903
401-861-0815
Fax: 401-861-0863
www.literacyvolunteers.org
lvaricindy@aol.com

Yvette Kenner, Executive Director
The mission of LVA-RI is to advance adult literacy in Rhode Island by: providing training and support services to local LVA-RI affiliates, volunteer tutors and adult literacy services; providing the state with information about adult literacy and with appropriate referral services; collaborating with other organizations to promote adult literacy in Rhode Island.

2240 Literacy Volunteers of Kent County
1672 Flat River Road
Route 117
Coventry, RI 02816
401-822-9100
Fax: 401-822-9133
www.coventrylibrary.org
AskReference@coventrylibrary.org

John Ball, Chair
Patricia Pare, VP
Colleen Duffy-Golec, Secretary
Receive intensive tutor training through a series of workshops that will prepare you to teach one-on-one or in small groups.

2241 Literacy Volunteers of Providence County
P.O.Box 72611
Providence, RI 02907-0611
401-351-0511
www.lvari.org
chris@lvari.org

Christine Hedenberg, Executive Director
Provides critical support services to local literacy volunteer affiliates, volunteer tutors and adult literacy students; collaborating with organizations to promote adult literacy in Rhode Island; partnering with companies and employers to improve workforce literacy skills; and acting as a state-wide resource for awareness and information about adult literacy, and for adult learner referrals to educational programs.

2242 Literacy Volunteers of South County
1935 Kingstown Rd
Wakefield, RI 02879
401-225-1068
www.211ri.org
info@uwri.org

David Henley, President
Volunteer-based literacy agent that provides services in Narragansett, North Kingstown and South Kingstown. Provides free, one-on-one tutoring to sdults who request Basic English Skills or English as a Second Language.

2243 Literacy Volunteers of Washington County
93 Tower Street
Units 25 & 26
Westerly, RI 02891
401-596-9411
www.literacywashingtoncounty.org
litwashcty@verizon.net

Ramon Garcia, President
Terence J. Malaghan, CPA, Treasurer
Ruth Tureckova, Executive Director
Assists adults interested in improving their literacy skills through free programs based on a participant's individual goals.

2244 Literary Resources Rhode Island
Brown University
PO Box 1974
Providence, RI 02912
401-863-1000
Fax: 401-863-3094
www.brown.edu
president@brown.edu

Christina H. Paxson, President
Elizabeth Huidekoper, EVP, Finance & Administration
David Savitz, VP, Research
Literacy Resources Rhode Island was established in 1997. Its goals include: expand existing professional capacity within the state's adult education community; increase educator and learner capacity to use and interact with online technology; and assist in improving delivery of services to adult learners, thereby strengthening adult education provision across the state.

2245 Rhode Island Human Resource Investment Council
1511 Pontiac Avenue
Building 72-2
Cranston, RI 02920
401-462-8860
Fax: 401-462-8865
www.rihric.com
rbrooks@dlt.ri.gov

Constance Howes, Chair
Rick Brooks, Executive Director
Amelia Anne Roberts, Office Manager

2246 Rhode Island Vocational and Rehabilitation Agency
40 Fountain Street
Providence, RI 02903
401-421-7005
Fax: 401-421-9259
TDD: 401-421-7016
www.ors.ri.gov
rcarroll@ors.state.ri.us

John Microulis, Administrator
Ronald Racine, Acting Associate Director
Roberta Greene Whittemore, Assistant Administrator of VR
Assists people with disabilities to become employed and to live independently in the community. In order to achieve this goal, we work in partnership with the State Rehabilitation Council, our customers, staff and community.

2247 Rhode Island Workforce Literacy Collaborative
260 W Exchange St
Ste 201
Providence, RI 02903-1047
401-861-0815
Fax: 401-861-0863
www.riwlc.org

Yvette Kenner, Executive Director
A group of non-profit agencies and other companies funded by the Human Resource Investment Council to provide workforce or worksite literacy services to adults in Rhode Island. These services are designed to upgrade the skills of those who are employed or seeking employment, in order to help Rhode Island achieve a high-performance workforce.

South Carolina

2248 Greater Columbia Literacy Council Turning Pages Adult Literacy
4840 Forest Dr
Ste 6-B, PMB 267
Columbia, SC 29206-2412
803-240-2441
Fax: 803-782-1210
www.literacycolumbia.org
literacycolumbia@earthlink.net

Deborah W Yoho, Executive Director

Mission is to enable adults, through customized learning programs, to improve English language and reading skills.

2249 Greenville Literacy Association
225 S Pleasantburg Dr
Ste C-10
Greenville, SC 29607-2533
864-467-3456
Fax: 864-467-3558
www.greenvilleliteracy.org
thomas@greenvilleliteracy.org
Jane Thomas, Executive Director
Leah Clark, ABE Training
Cheryl Bentley, Book Sale
To empower adults to participate more effectively in the community by providing quality instruction in reading, writing, math and speaking English

2250 Greenwood Literacy Council
1855 Calhoun Road
P.O. Box 248
Greenwood, SC 29648-0248
864-941-5400
Fax: 864-941-5427
www.gwd50.org
kjennings12@gwd50.org
Kathy Jennings, Director
Ken Cobb, Board Member
Claude Wright, Board Member
Provides ongoing, comprehensive adult literacy programs in Greenwood, for illiterate adults and their families.

2251 Literacy Volunteers of the Lowcountry
Pro Literacy America
1-B Kittie's Landing Way
P.O. Box 3725
Bluffton, SC 29910
843-815-6616
Fax: 843-686-6949
www.lowcountryliteracy.org
nwilliams@lowcountryliteracy.org
Jean Heyduck, Executive Director
Marie Lewis, Program Manager
Phil Lindstrom, Finance Director
To increase adult literacy in the greater Beaufort County area by providing leadership, creating awareness, and offering quality instructional services.

2252 Oconee Adult Education
414 South Pine Street
Walhalla, SC 29691
864-886-4429
Fax: 864-886-4430
www.oconee.k12.sc.us
mthorsland@oconee.k12.sc.us
Dr. Michael Thorsland, Superintendent
Maxine Pettit, Administrative Assistant
Deb Wickliffe, Communications Specialist
To assist adults in becoming literate, to assist adults in the completion of a secondary school education, and to assist adults in improving their knowledge and skills relating to employment and parenting.

2253 South Carolina Adult Literacy Educators
297 Pascallas Street
Blackville, SC 29817
803-284-5605
Fax: 803-284-4417
www.barnwell19.k12.sc.us
leah.bias@barnwell19.k12.sc.us
Teresa L. Pope, Superintendent
Rebecca Grubbs, Director, Finance
Leah Bias, Director, Special Education

2254 South Carolina Department of Education
1429 Senate Street
Columbia, SC 29201
803-734-8500
Fax: 803-734-4426
www.ed.sc.gov
sc.supfed@ed.sc.gov
Mick Zais, State Superintendent
Scott English, Chief Operating Officer
Mr. Don Cantrell, Chief Information Officer

Provides people of all ages and backgrounds who are blind, visually impaired or reading disabled with free books, magazines, and special publications in Braille, Large Print and Audio formats.

2255 South Carolina Literacy Resource Center
1722 Main Street
Suite 104
Columbia, SC 29201
803-929-2563
800-277-7323
Fax: 803-929-2571
http://www2.ed.gov/pubs/TeachersGuide/slrc.html
SCLRC@aol.com
Peggy May, Director
The mission of the South Carolina Resource Center is to provide leadership in literacy to South Carolina's adults and their families, in conjunction with state and local public and private nonprofit efforts. The Center serves as a site for training for adult literacy providers, as a reciprocal link with the National Institute for Literacy for the purpose of sharing information to service providers, and as a clearinghouse for state-of-the-art literacy materials and technology.

2256 Trident Literacy Association
5416-B Rivers Avenue
North Charleston, SC 29406
843-747-2223
Fax: 843-744-2970
www.tridentlit.org
echepenik@tridentlit.org
Eileen Chepenik, Executive Director
Stella Necker, Program Director
Judianne Schmenk, Development Director
To increase literacy in Charleston, Berkeley, and Dorchester counties by offering instruction, using a self-paced, individualized curriculum in reading, writing, mathematics, English as a second language, GED preparation, and basic computer use.

South Dakota

2257 Adult Education and Literacy Program
South Dakota Department of Labor
Kneip Bldg
700 Governors Dr
Pierre, SD 57501
605-773-3101
Fax: 605-773-6185
www.state.sd.us
marcia.hess@state.sd.us
Marcia Hess, State Administrator
Adult Education & Literacy instruction is designed to teach persons 16 years of age or older to read and write English and to substantially raise their educational level. The purpose of the program is to expand the educational opportunities for adults and to establish programs that will enable all adults to acquire basic skills necessary to function in society and allow them to continue their education to at least the level of completion of secondary school.

2258 South Dakota Literacy Council
816 Samara Ave
Volga, SD 57071
605-627-5138
Fax: 605-627-5138
www.readsd.org
jberglund@blackhills.com
John Berglund, President
Alma McClanahan, VP
Betty VanderZee, Treasurer
Goal is to help people receive educational help in a confidential setting.

2259 South Dakota Literacy Resource Center
700 Governors Drive
Pierre, SD 57501
605-773-3101
800-423-6665
Fax: 605-773-6184
http://wdcrobcolp01.ed.gov/programs/EROD
marcia.hess@state.sd.us

Marcia Hess, State Administrator
The mission of the SD Literary Resource Center is to establish a state wide on-line computer catalog of all existing literacy materials within South Dakota and a South Dakota Literacy Resource Center home page with links to other literacy sites within South Dakota, regionally and nationally.

Tennessee

2260 Adult Education Foundation of Blount County
1500 Jett Rd
Maryville, TN 37804-3359   865-982-8998
Fax: 865-983-8848
www.blountk12.org/adult_ed/index.htm
blountliteracy@gmail.com
Carol Ergenbright, Coordinator
Serving as an advocate for adult literacy by partnering with Adult Education programs and staff; promoting community involvement and providing assistance with funding.

2261 Center for Literary Studies
University of Tennessee
600 Henley St
Suite 312
Knoxville, TN 37996   865-974-4109
Fax: 865-974-3857
www.cls.utk.edu
Geri Mulligan, Director
Aaron Kohring, Interim Director
Gail Cope, Program Coordinator
To support and advance literacy education across the lifespan. Works with providers of literacy edcuation to strengthen their capacity to help individuals build knowledge and improve skills needed to be life-long learners and active members of families, communities, and workplaces.

2262 Claiborne County Adult Reading Experience
Claiborne County Schools
1403 Tazewell Road
P.O. Box 179
Tazewell, TN 37879   423-626-3543
Fax: 423-626-5945
www.claibornecountyschools.com
swilliams3@k12tn.net
Michelle Huddleston, Chairman
Tim Duncan, Vice Chairman
Connie Holdway, Director of Schools

2263 Collierville Literacy Council
167 Washington Street
Collierville, TN 38017   901-854-0288
www.colliervilleliteracy.org
colliervilleliteracy@earthlink.net
John Barrios, President
Annette Key, Immediate Past President
Wanda Chism, Secretary
A non-profit organization dedicated to providing opportunities for adults to attain educational goals that enhance individual growth and benefit families, the work place and the community.

2264 Learning Center for Adults and Families
833 N Ocoee St
Cleveland, TN 37311-2254   423-478-1117
Fax: 423-478-1153
www.learningcenter.ws
clewis@learningcenter.ws
Candace Lewis, Executive Director

2265 Literacy Council of Kingsport
326 Commerce Street
Kingsport, TN 37660   423-392-4643
www.literacycouncilofkingsport.org
admin@literacycouncilofkingsport.org
Nada J. Weekley, Executive Director
Pat Mattingly, Program/Volunteer Coordinator

A non-profit organization dedicated to serving citizens in Kingsport and Sullivan County. Offers free, one-on-one tutoring for adults and qualified children who want to learn to read or to improve their reading skills.

2266 Literacy Council of Sumner County
260 W Main Street
City Square Shopping Center
Hendersonville, TN 37075   615-822-8112
Fax: 615-822-3665
www.literacysumner.org
info@literacysumner.org
Margie Anderson, Director
To provide resources, counseling, and tutoring to children, youth, and adults to enhance their skills in all academic areas.

2267 Literacy Mid-South
2158 Union Ave., Suite 515
P.O. Box 111229
Memphis, TN 38104   901-327-6000
Fax: 901-458-4969
www.literacymidsouth.org
kdean@literacymidsouth.org
Kevin Dean, Executive Director
Jeff Rhodin, Director, Collaborative Action
Heather Nordtvedt, Director of Development

2268 Nashville Adult Literacy Council
Cohn Adult Learning Center
4805 Park Ave
Suite 305
Nashville, TN 37209   615-298-8060
Fax: 615-298-8444
www.nashvilleliteracy.org
info@nashvilleliteracy.org
Meg Nugent, Director
Jill Mora, Marketing Director
Patty Swartzbaugh, Program Manager
Teaches reading to U.S.-born adults and English skills to adult immigrants.

2269 Read To Succeed
200 East Main Street
PO Box 12161
Murfreesboro, TN 37130   615-738-7323
www.readtosucceed.org
info@readtosucceed.org
Steve Daniel, President
Brian Coleman, VP
Lisa Mitchell, Executive Director
The community literacy collaborative in Rutherford County, will promote reading, with an emphasis on family literacy. This non-profit initiative supports literacy programs and fosters awareness of the importance of reading.

2270 Tennessee Department of Education
710 James Robertson Parkway
Andrew Johnson Tower, 6th Floor
Nashville, TN 37243-0382   615-741-2731
800-531-1515
www.state.tn.us
education.comments@tn.gov
Timothy K Webb, Commissioner
Mission is to take Tennessee to the top in education. Guides administration of the state's K-12 public schools.

2271 Tennessee School-to-Work Office
14th Floor, Citizens Plaza State Of
400 Deaderick Street
Nashville, TN 37243   615-313-4981
www.state.tn.us
maryjane.ware@tn.gov
Bill Haslam, Governor

Texas

2272 Commerce Library Literacy Program
1210 Park Street
Commerce, TX 75429   903-886-6858
                                   Fax: 903-886-7239
                          www.commercepubliclibrary.org
                              commerce@koyote.com
Pricilla Donovan, Director

2273 Greater Orange Area Literacy Services
PO Box 221
520 W Decatur Ave
Orange, TX 77631   409-886-4311
                                   Fax: 409-886-0149
                           goalsliteracy@sbcglobal.net
Sharon LeBlanc, Executive Director
Adult literacy program

2274 Irving Public Library Literacy Program
825 W Irving Blvd
PO Box 152288
Irving, TX 75060   972-721-2411
                                   Fax: 972-721-3733
                               http://cityofirving.org
                    Customer-Service@cityofirving.org
Tracy Bearden, Manager
Charles Anderson, City Attorney
Promotes literacy among people of all ages.

2275 Literacy Austin
2222 Rosewood Ave
Austin, TX 78702   512-478-7323
                                   Fax: 512-479-7323
                                   TDD: 512-478-7323
                                www.literacyaustin.org
                               info@literacyaustin.org
Gail Harmon, Program Director
Melinda Mitchiner, Program Services Coordinator
Mission is to provide instruction for basic literacy and English as a Second Language (ESL) to adults, age 17 and older, who read below the fifth-grade leve. Vision is to improve the quality of an adult's life through improved literacy skills.

2276 Literacy Center of Marshall: Harrison County
700 W. Houston Street
P.O. Box 148
Marshall, TX 75670   903-935-0962
                               www.marshallliteracy.org
                             kdeluca23@gmail.com
Karla DeLuca, Executive Director

2277 Literacy Volunteers of America: Bastrop
1201 Church St
Bastrop, TX 78602-2909   512-321-6686
                           www.main.org/lva-bastrop/
                              suemunster@aol.com
Sue Steinbring, Director
Provides literacy training and pre-GED for students, English as a Second Language, tutoring and tutor training.

2278 Literacy Volunteers of America: Bay City Matagorda County
PO Box 1596
Bay City, TX 77404-1596   979-244-9544
                                   Fax: 979-244-9566
                                 www.literacymc.org
                               lva_mc@yahoo.com
Linda Brown, Director
Sandy Thomas, Program Coordinator
Promotes literacy for people of all ages.

2279 Literacy Volunteers of America: Laredo
P 10 Fort McIntosh
LCC Main Campus
Laredo, TX 78040   956-724-5207
                                   Fax: 956-725-4253
                                    www.lvalaredo.org
                           lvlaredo@grandecom.net
Doroteo Sandoval, Executive Director
Promotes literacy for people of all ages.

2280 Literacy Volunteers of America: Montgomery County
412 W. Phillips, Suite 125
P.O. Box 2704
Conroe, TX 77305-2704   936-494-0635
                                         888-878-9400
                                      http://lvamc.org
                            literacymc@yahoo.com
Linda Ricketts, Director
Laura Davis, Program Manager
Ranak Amin, Office Volunteer
As part of the national literacy organization, combats illiteracy in Montgomery County through volunteer tutoring.

2281 Literacy Volunteers of America: Port Arthur Literacy Support
4615 9th Avenue
Port Arthur, TX 77642-5818   409-985-8838
                                   Fax: 409-985-5969
                                    www.pap.lib.tx.us
                          jmartine@paplibrary.org
Jose Martinez, Director
Debra Lawrence, Administrative Assistant
LaTrice Gallow, Senior Library Clerk
A library based umbrella group which works with three primary programs: ono-on-one tutoring for those who cannot read or read at a very low level; GED Computer Lab assistance for adults who are striving to get their General Equivalency Diploma - in cooperation with Port Arthur Independent School District; and English-as-a-Second Language (ESL) in cooperation with the Port Arthur Independent School District.

2282 Literacy Volunteers of America: Wimberley Area
14100 Ranch Road 12
P.O. Box 12
Wimberley, TX 78676   512-847-2201
                                   Fax: 701-254-4313
                                   www.wimberley.org
                           trailsend@anvilcom.com
Linda Mueller, Director
Nonprofit, volunteer organization which exists to improve the reading, writing, speaking, cultural and life skills of adults reading at or below the sixth grade level and/or those for whom English is not their native language. Provides GED instruction. All services are free.

2283 Texas Families and Literacy
1006 C, Junction Hwy.
Kerrville, TX 78028   830-896-8787
                                   Fax: 830-896-3639
                             www.familiesandliteracy.org
                               famandlit1@hctc.net
Mike Hunter, Executive Director
Annette Kurtz, Operations Coordinator
Anita Rios, Administrative Assistant

2284 Texas Family Literacy Center
601 University Drive
College of Education, EDU Room 2112
San Marcos, TX 78666   512-245-9600
                                   Fax: 512-245-8151
                        www.tei.education.txstate.edu/famlit
                               yr01@txstate.edu
Ysabel Ramirez, Grant Directror
Gloria Rodriguez, Grant Secretary
Dr. Emily Miller Payne, Director

Mission is to strengthen family literacy programs and enhance the knowledge skills, instructional practices and resources available to family literacy educators statewide.

2285 Victoria Adult Literacy
802 E. Crestwood Drive
Victoria, TX 77901
361-582-4273
Fax: 361-582-4348
www.victorialiteracycouncil.org
valcsm@yahoo.com
Stacey Milberger, Executive Director
Eden Casal, VALC Program Coordinator
Dani Clowers, Program Assistant

2286 Weslaco Public Library
525 S Kansas Ave
Weslaco, TX 78596
956-968-4533
Fax: 956-968-8922
www.weslaco.lib.tx.us
webmaster@weslaco.lib.tx.us
Michael Fisher, Executive Director

Utah

2287 Bridgerland Literacy
1301 N 600 W
Logan, UT 84321
435-750-3262
www.bridgerlandliteracy.org
bridgerland.literacy@gmail.com
Alex Stoddard, Director
Linda Fretwell, Student Coordinator
Melissa Allen, Outreach Coordinator

2288 Project Read
550 N University Avenue
Suite 215
Provo, UT 84601
801-852-6654
Fax: 801-852-7663
www.project-read.com
projectreadutah@gmail.com
Shauna K Brown, Director
Chelsea Hansen, Program Coordinator
Seeks to prevent and alleviate adult illiteracy in Utah County. Provides one-on-one tutoring services to help improve reading and writing skills sufficiently to meet personal goals, function well in society, and become more productive citizens.

2289 Utah Literacy Action Center
3595 South Main Street
Salt Lake City, UT 84115-4434
801-265-9081
Fax: 801-265-9643
www.literacyactioncenter.org
lac@literacyactioncenter.org
Margaret Griffin, Treasurer
Deborah Young, Ed.D., Executive Director
Charles Curtin, Secretary
Transforms English-speaking adults, who enter the program with limited reading, writing, or math skills, into skilled, passionate, habitual, critical readers, writers, and mathematicians.

Vermont

2290 ABE Career and Lifelong Learning: Vermont Department of Education
120 State St
Montpelier, VT 05620-2501
802-828-3135
800-881-1561
Fax: 802-828-3146
http://women.vermont.gov/resource-directory/edu
srobinson@doe.state.vt.us
Cary Brown, Executive Director
Lilly Talbert, Coordinator
Claire Greene, Executive Staff Assistant

Promotes quality education.

2291 Central Vermont Adult Basic Education
46 Washington Street
Suite 100
Barre, VT 05641
802-476-4588
Fax: 802-476-5860
www.cvabe.org
info@cvabe.org
Sydney Lea, President, Treasurer
Jon Bourgo, VP
Carol Shults-Perkins, Executive Director
Provides free adult education and literacy instruction for adults, out of school youth, and immigrants and refugees in the belief that a person who is literate has the essential key for self understanding and for full and active membership in the world.

2292 Tutorial Center
208 Pleasant Street
Bennington, VT 05201
802-447-0111
Fax: 802-447-7607
http://tutoringvermont.org
Jack Glade, Executive Director
Provides tutoring to improve success for 200 children; prevents 20 teenagers at risk of dropping out from doing so; helps 80 high school dropouts to earn a high school diploma or GED; builds literacy skills of 400 adults; helps 20 adults transition into college or post-secondary career paths; and transforms 50 computer-illiterate adults into competent computer users.

2293 Vermont Assistive Technology Project: Dept of Aging and Disabilities
103 South Main Street
Weeks Building
Waterbury, VT 05671-1601
802-241-2620
800-750-6355
Fax: 802-241-2174
TTY: 802-241-1464
http://dail.vermont.gov
julie.tucker@ahs.state.vt.us
Julie L Tucker, Program Director
Provides information and referrals, training for service providers and others, equipment and software demonstrations, tryouts, and technical assistance.

2294 Vermont Division of Vocational Rehabilitation
VocRehab Of Vermont
103 South Main Street
Weeks 1A
Waterbury, VT 05671-2303
866-879-6757
TTY: 802-241-1455
www.vocrehab.vermont.gov
jana.sherman@ahs.state.vt.us
Diane Dalmasse, Director of VocRehab Division
VocRehab's mission is to assist Vermonters with disabilities, find and maintain meaningful employment in their communities. VocRehab Vermont works in close partnership with the Vermont Association of Business, Industry and Rehabilitation. Contact local VocRehab office for information about services.

2295 Vermont Literacy Resource Center: Dept of Education
120 State St
Montpelier, VT 05602-2703
802-828-5148
Fax: 802-828-0573
www.state.vt.us
wross@doe.state.vt.us
Wendy Ross, Director
The Vermont Literacy Resource Center links Vermont to national, regional, and state literacy organizations, provides staff development and serves as a clearinghouse for the literacy community. The Vermont Literacy Resource Center is located at the Vermont Department of Education.

Virginia

2296 Adult Learning Center
4160 Virginia Beach Blvd
Virginia Beach, VA 23452
757-648-6050
Fax: 757-306-0999
www.adultlearning.vbschools.com
ppalombo@vbschools.com
Paul Palombo, Director
Heather Lamb, Coordinator
Joseph Panchik, Coordinator
To respond to the needs of the adult population by offering a comprehensive educational program to the community.

2297 Charlotte County Literacy Program
395 Thomas Jefferson Hwy, Suite B
P.O. Box 286
Charlotte Court House, VA 23923
434-542-5782
www.charlotte-learning.org
charlit@pure.net
Tonya Pulliam, Director
Offers basic and family literacy programs, ESL and computer, parenting and work skills.

2298 Citizens for Adult Literacy & Learning
PO Box 123
Monroe, VA 24574
434-929-2630
www.callamherst.org
marcia.swain@callamherst.org
Marcia Swain, Program Coordinator
Aim is to help adults improve their quality of life by mastering basic reading, writing and math skills.

2299 Eastern Shore Literacy Council
29300 Lankford Highway
White Building
Melfa, VA 23410
757-789-1761
Fax: 757-442-6517
www.shoreliteracy.org
esliteracy@gmail.com
Laura Chuquin-Naylor, Executive Director
Janet Booth, Director
Renee Beall, Program Coordinator
Providing literacy tutoring without charge to adult residents of the Eastern Shore so they may acquire the skills needed to improve their particiaption in society and enrich their lives.

2300 Highlands Educational Literacy Program
13168 Meadowview Square
Meadowview, VA
276-944-5144
Fax: 276-676-0677
www.helpliteracyofwc.org
helplit2@gmail.com
Christy Hicks, Chairperson
Beth Hilton, Executive Director
Tina Mitchell, Volunteer Coordinator
To provide basic literacy instruction for adults in Washington County, changing lives one word at a time.

2301 Literacy Council of Northern Virginia
2855 Annandale Road
Falls Church, VA 22042
703-237-0866
Fax: 703-237-2863
www.lcnv.org
info@lcnv.org
Patricia Donnelly, Executive Director
Carole Vinograd Bausell, Director of Tutoring Programs
Nathan Caruso, Program Assistant
To teach adults the basic skills of reading, writing, speaking and understanding English in order to empower them to participate more fully and confidently in their communities.

2302 Literacy Volunteers of America: Nelson County
PO Box 422
Lovingston, VA 22949
434-996-0485
www.nelsoncountyliteracy.org
nanamump@aol.com

Charles Strauss, Director

2303 Literacy Volunteers of America: New River Valley
195 West Main Street
Christiansburg, VA 24073
540-382-7262
Fax: 540-382-7262
www.lvnrv.org
lvnrv@verizon.net
Dr. Toni Cox, President
C. Barry Anderson, President Elect
Janet Kester, Program Coordinator
The empowerment of every adult in the New River Valley through the provision of opportunities to achieve independence through literacy.

2304 Literacy Volunteers of America: Prince William
4326 Dale Blvd
Suite 6
Woodbridge, VA 22193
703-670-5702
Fax: 703-583-0703
www.lvapw.org
lvapw@aol.com
Ken Ikeda, President
Vicki Gross, Executive Director
Deborah Abbott, Program Director
Mission is to teach adults to read. Takes volunteers from the community, train them to be tutors and then match them with adults with low literacy skills. Provides the professional training, materials, and support that enable the volunteers to be effective tutors.

2305 Literacy Volunteers of America: Shenandoah County
PO Box 303
Woodstock, VA 22664
540-459-2446
www.lv-sc.org
inquiries@lv-sc.org
Paula Gould, Director

2306 Literacy Volunteers of Charlottesville/Albemarle
233 4th Street NW
PO Box 1156
Charlottesville, VA 22903
434-977-3838
http://literacyforall.org
info@literacyforall.org
Jean Kollar, President
Mary Jane King, VP
Ellen Moore Osborne, Executive Director
Provides one-on-one, confidential tutoring in basic literacy and English as a second language to adults living ot working in Charlottesville and Albemarle County.

2307 Literacy Volunteers of Roanoke Valley
706 S Jefferson St
Roanoke, VA 24016-5104
540-265-9339
877-582-7323
Fax: 540-265-4814
www.lvarv.org
info@lvarv.org
Annette Loschert, Executive Director
To teach English literacy skills to adults and to raise literacy awareness throughout the Roanoke Valley.

2308 Literacy Volunteers: Campbell County Public Library
PO Box 310
Rustburg, VA 24588-0310
434-332-9561
Fax: 434-332-9697
www.campbellcountylibraries.org
lpwheeler@co.campbell.va.us
Nan Carmack, Program Manager
Provides free, confidential instruction for adults who live or work in Campbell COunty, VA. Adult Basic Education and English for Speakers of other languages.

2309 **Loudoun Literacy Council**
17 Royal Street SW
Leesburg, VA 20175 703-777-2205
Fax: 703-777-7260
www.loudounliteracy.org
info@loudounliteracy.org
Sean Jordan, President
David Bruce, VP
Leslie Mazeska, Executive Director
A community-based, nonprofit, educational organization dedicated to improving literacy throughout Loudoun County. Recruit and train volunteers to teach adults, both native-speakers and speakers of other languages, to read, speak, write and understand English. Also provides early literacy enrichment for at-risk preschool children and children who reside in local homeless shelters, while supporting their parents as their child's first teacher.

2310 **READ Center Reading & Education for Adult Development**
2000 Bremo Road
Suite 102
Richmond, VA 23226 804-288-9930
Fax: 804-288-9915
www.readcenter.org
frontdesk@readcenter.org
Helps low-level reading adults develop basic reading and communication skills through one-to-one tutoring so they can fulfill their goals and their roles as citizens, workers and family members.

2311 **Skyline Literacy Coalition**
975 S. High Street
Harrisonburg, VA 22801 540-433-0505
Fax: 540-433-0955
http://skylineliteracy.org
skylineliteracy@gmail.com
Laura Zarrugh, President
Charlette McQuilkin, VP
Elizabeth Girvan, Executive Director
A nonprofit organization dedicated to promoting learning and literacy throughout the Shenandoah Valley.

2312 **Virginia Adult Learning Resource Center**
3600 W Broad St, Suite 112
PO Box 842037
Richmond, VA 23230-4930 804-828-6521
800-237-0178
Fax: 804-828-7539
www.valrc.org
vdesk@vcu.edu
Barbara Gibson, Manager
Katie Bratisax, Technology & Support Specialist
Hillary Major, Communications Specialist
To equip the field of adult education and literacy with essential skills and resources by delivering innovative and effective training, publications, curriculum design, and prgram development.

2313 **Virginia Council of Administrators of Special Education**
1110 N Glebe Rd
Ste 300
Arlington, VA 22201-5704 703-264-9454
800-224-6830
Fax: 703-264-9494
www.vcase.org
marylwall@aol.com
Jim Gallagher, President
Dr. Jessica McClung, Secretary
Leorie K Mallory, Treasurer
A professional organization that promotes professional leadership through the provision of collegial support and current information on recommended instructional practices as well as local, state and national trends in Special Education for professionals who serve students with disabilities in order to improve the quality and delivery of special education services in Virginia's public schools.

2314 **Virginia Literacy Foundation**
413 Stuart Circle
Executive Suite 303
Richmond, VA 23220 804-237-8909
Fax: 804-237-8901
www.virginialiteracy.org
vlilv@earthlink.net
Jeannie P Baliles, Founder/Chairperson
Mark E Emblidge, Ph.D., Founding Director
Jane Bassett Spilman, Vice Chairperson
Provides funding and technical cupport to private, volunteer literacy organizations throughout Virginia via challenge grants, training and direct consulting.

Washington

2315 **Division of Vocational Rehabilitation**
PO Box 45340
Olympia, WA 98504-5340 360-725-3636
800-367-5621
Fax: 360-407-8007
www.dshs.wa.gov
Serves people with disabilities who want to work but face a substantial barrier to finding or keeping a job. Provides individualized employment services and counseling to people with disabilites and also provides technical assistance and training to employers about the employment of people with disabilities.

2316 **Literacy Council of Kitsap**
616 5th Street
Bremerton, WA 98337-1416 360-373-1539
Fax: 360-373-6859
www.kitsapliteracy.org
info@kitsapliteracy.org
Carol Rainey, Chair
Terry Schroeder, Treasurer
Winnie Flores-Logan, Board Member
Dedicated to Adult Basic Education (ABE) and GED testing preparation, along with English as a Second Language. Promote and provide literacy services to the residents of Kitsap County.

2317 **Literacy Council of Seattle**
8500 14th Ave NW
Crown Hill UMC
Seattle, WA 98117 206-233-9720
www.literacyseattle.org
info@literacyseattle.org
Kristen Holway, President
Jennifer Collins-Friedrichs, Executive Director
Valerie Margulis, Treasurer
Volunteers teach adults the English skills they need to be successful in their jobs, families, and the community.

2318 **Literacy Source: Community Learning Center**
720 N 35th St
Suite # 103
Seattle, WA 98103 206-782-2050
Fax: 206-781-2583
www.literacy-source.org
info@literacy-source.org
Jack Kuester, President
Theresa Verwey, Vice President
Ann Dalton, Secretary
Builds a literate community and promote self-sufficiency by providing learner-centered instruction to adults in English literacy and basic life skills.

2319 **Sound Learning of Mason & Thurston County**
133 W Railroad Ave
P.O. Box 2529
Shelton, WA 98584 360-426-9733
Fax: 360-426-9789
www.masoncountyliteracy.org

Pamela Farr, Chair
Toby Kevin, Vice Chair
Ross Wiggins, Secretary
Provides free instruction to adults to improve reading, writing and math skills, study for a GED, or learn English as a second language.

2320 St. James ESL Program
St. James Cathedral
804 Ninth Avenue
Seattle, WA 98104-1265   206-622-3559
                              Fax: 206-622-5303
                        www.stjames-cathedral.org
                        esl@stjames-cathedral.org
Chris Koehler, Director
Helping adult refugees and immigrants learn English and become U.S. citizens.

2321 Whatcom Literacy Council
3028 Lindbergh Ave
Building A
Bellingham, WA 98225   360-752-8678
                              Fax: 360-752-6770
                          www.whatcomliteracy.org
                          info@whatcomliteracy.org
Valerie Lagen, President
Mike Henniger, Vice President
Joyce Eschliman, Treasurer
Helping adults in Whatcom County improve their literacy skills or learn to use English as a second language. Through customized, individual tutoring, students learn critical skills needed to become self-sufficient.

West Virginia

2322 Division of Technical & Adult Education Services: West Virginia
1900 Kanawha Boulevard East
Charleston, WV 25305   304-558-2000
                              Fax: 304-342-7025
                       http://careertech.k12.wv.us
                        gparsons@access.k12.wv.us
Kathy D'Antoni EdD, Asst State Superintendent
Gigi Parsons, Division Secretary
Better prepare students for the world of work and higher education through education programs and training offered at the career and technical education sites throughout the state.

2323 W Virginia Regional Education Services
501 22nd St
Dunbar, WV 25064-1711   304-766-7655
                                      800-642-2670
                              Fax: 304-766-2824
Chuck Nichols, Executive Director
Offers services for literacy and adult basic education including literacy hotline, networks newsletter, resources for English as a second language, beginning literacy, learning disabilities and other special learning needs.

2324 West Virginia Department of Education
1900 Kanawha Blvd E
Bldg 6, Rm 351
Charleston, WV 25305-0330   304-558-3660
                                      800-642-2670
                              Fax: 304-558-0198
                            http://wvde.state.wv.us

Wisconsin

2325 ADVOCAP Literacy Services
W911 State Highway 44
Markesan, WI 53946   920-398-3907
                                      800-631-6617
                              Fax: 920-398-2103
                               www.advocap.org
                              mikeb@advocap.org
Michael Bonertz, Executive Director
Tony Beregszazi, Deputy Director
Tanya Marcoe, Finance Director

2326 Fox Valley Literacy Coalition
103 E Washington St
Appleton, WI 54911   920-991-9840
                              Fax: 920-991-1012
                                 www.fvlc.net
                           foxvalleylit@tds.net
Terry Dawson, Chair
Julia Drobeck, Vice Chair
Karen E Probst, Secretary
Provides English literacy education to adults with the help of trained volunteers. To improve people's lives and build community by providing and coordinating literacy services.

2327 Jefferson County Literacy Council
112 S Main St
Jefferson, WI 53549   920-675-0500
                              Fax: 920-675-0510
                                 www.jclc.us
                              jottow@jclc.us
Lynn Forseth, Executive Director
Karyn Cable, Operations Manager
Jessica Hellenbrand, Educational Coordinator
Committed to building communities that are strong in literacy, language and cultural understandings through information and resource sharing, referral, assessment and instructional services.

2328 Literacy Council of Greater Waukesha
217 Wisconsin Ave
Ste 16
Waukesha, WI 53186   262-547-7323
                          www.waukeshaliteracy.org
                       drunning@waukeshaliteracy.org
Debra Running, Executive Director
Cathy Kozlowicz, Program Coordinator
Provides, confidential, one-on-one tutoring and mentoring services to individuals who need help with reading, writing, spelling, math and English as a second language.

2329 Literacy Network
1118 South Park Street
Madison, WI 53715-1755   608-244-3911
                              Fax: 608-244-3899
                         www.madisonarealiteracy.org
                            info@litnetwork.org
Maureen Miner, President
Rich Birrenkot, Vice President
Jessica Jackson, Secretary
Teaches reading, writing, and speaking skills to Dane County adults and families so they can achieve financial independence, good health and greater involvement in the community.

2330 Literacy Services of Wisconsin
2724 W Wells St
Milwaukee, WI 53208-3597   414-344-5878
                              Fax: 414-344-1061
                           www.literacyservices.org
                          india@literacyservices.org
David Hanson, President
Ginger Duivon, Executive Director
Mary Tobin, Treasurer

Provides literacy education motivated adults through the efforts of dedicated volunteers, the support of th ecommunity and the use of specialized curriculum to meet the individual and community needs.

2331 Literacy Volunteers of America: Chippewa Valley

770 Scheidler Rd
Chippewa Falls, WI 54729   715-738-3857
                                     Fax: 715-967-2445
                                          www.lvcv.org

Paul Kulig, President
Laurie Klinkhammer, Vice President
Greta Heike, Treasurer
A community-based literacy program that trains and supports volunteers to educate adults and their families, helping them acquire the skills necessary to achieve economic self-sufficiency and function effectively in their roles as citizens, workers, and family members.

2332 Literacy Volunteers of America: Eau Claire

800 Wisconsin St #70
Bldg D02, Ste 301
Eau Claire, WI 54703   715-834-0222
                                     Fax: 715-834-2546
                                          www.lvcv.org

Paul Kulig, President
Laurie Klinkhammer, Vice President
Greta Heike, Treasurer
A community-based literacy program that trains and supports volunteers to educate adults and their families, helping them acquire the skills necessary to achieve economic self-sufficiency and function effectively in their roles as citizens, workers, and family members.

2333 Literacy Volunteers of America: Marquette County

PO Box 671
Montello, WI 53949-0671   608-297-8900
                                     Fax: 608-297-2673
                                         www.mcreads.org
                                   literacyvmc@yahoo.com

Vicki Huffman, President
Luann Zieman, Vice President
Mary Faltz, Secretary
Promotes literacy for people of all ages.

2334 Marathon County Literacy Council

300 1st St
Wausau, WI 54403   715-261-7292
                                     Fax: 715-261-7232
                                   http://wvls.lib.wi.us
                                    info@mcliteracy.us

Tom Bobrofsky, President
Douglas Lay, Vice President
Michael Otten, Treasurer
A nonprofit organization dedicated to improving literacy throughout Marathon County. Offers tutoring services for all Marathon County adults in need of assistance.

2335 Milwaukee Achiever Literacy Services

5566 N 69th St
Milwaukee, WI 53218   414-463-7389
                                     Fax: 414-463-9484
                             http://milwaukeeachiever.org
                            ssterling@milwaukeeachiever.org

Tracy Loken Webber, President
Dan Berton, Chair
Brenda Thompson, Secretary
Provides education, life skills training and workforce development instruction for adult learners in an atmosphere of mutual acceptance and respect.

2336 Racine Literacy Council

734 Lake Ave
Racine, WI 53403   262-632-9495
                                     Fax: 262-632-9502
                                    www.racineliteracy.com
                                 kgregor@racineliteracy.com

Don Cress, President
Sandy Brosseau, Secretary
Mary Biesack, Treasurer
A volunteer-based organization whose mission is to provide adult literacy programs in Racine County and to bring awareness to the community about the importance and impact of literacy.

2337 Walworth County Literacy Council

1000 E Centralia St
Elkhorn, WI 53121   262-957-0142
                                     Fax: 262-741-5275
                                www.walworthcoliteracy.com
                                wclc@walworthcoliteracy.com

Abby Baker, Coordinator
Provides student-centered instruction in basic literacy skills and English as a second language. Promotes awareness of literacy issues and seeks support from the community to develop literacy programs.

2338 Winnebago County Literacy Council

106 Washington Ave
Oshkosh, WI 54901-4985   920-236-5185
                                     Fax: 920-236-5227
                                          www.winlit.org
                                      traska@winlit.org

Natalie Johnson, President
Donna Altepeter, Vice President
Becky Srubas, Secretary
To increase literacy skills of adults and families so they can make informed decisions in order to function effectively in society.

2339 Wisconsin Literacy Resource Center

211 S Paterson St
Ste 310
Madison, WI 53703   608-257-1655
                                     Fax: 608-661-0208
                                www.wisconsinliteracy.orgs
                                info@wisconsinliteracy.org

Dave Endres, President
Greg Simmons, Vice President
Lorie Zantow, Treasurer
A statewide agency that was formed as a coalition of adult, family and workplace literacy providers for the purpose of supporting one another through resource development, information and referrals, training and advocacy.

Wyoming

2340 Pomona Public Library Literacy Services

2300 Capitol Ave
Hathaway Building, 2nd Floor
Cheyenne, WY 82002-2060   307-777-7690
                                     Fax: 307-777-6234
                                     TTY: 307-777-7744
                                          www.k12.wy.us

Cindy Hill, State Superintendant
Deb Lindsey, Assesment
Tiffany Dobler, Special Programs
The Pomona Literacy Service provides free adult literacy services to the City of Pomona. Volunteers provide tutorial programs to adults (16 years and older) who do not have basic literacy skills or whose literacy skills are so limited that they are not able to function independently in daily life or acquire employment or higher education.

2341 Teton Literacy Program

1715 High School Rd, Ste 260
PO Box 465
Jackson, WY 83001   307-733-9242
                                     Fax: 307-733-9086
                                       www.tetonliteracy.org
                                    info@tetonliteracy.org

Bill Maloney, President
Jim Thorburn, Vice President
Petria Fossel, Secretary

Serves Teton County with educational resources to better reading, writing, and language skills of the diverse community.

Adults

2342 A Mind At A Time
Simon & Schuster
1230 Avenue of the Americas
New York, NY 10020-1513   212-698-7000
                              www.simonandschuster.biz
                              shop.feedback@simonsays.com
Mel Levine, Author
Written by Melvin Levine, and published in 2003. It shows
parents and others how to identify the individual learning
patterns, explaining how to strenghten a child's abilities and
either bypasss or overcome the child's weakness, producing
positive results instead of reapeated frustration and failure.
$15.00
352 pages
ISBN 0-743202-23-6

2343 A Miracle to Believe In
Option Indigo Press
2080 S Undermountain Rd
Sheffield, MA 01257-9643   413-229-8727
                                  800-714-2779
                              Fax: 413-229-8727
                              www.optionindigo.com
                              indigo@bcn.net
Barry Neil Kaufman, Author
A group of people from all walks of life come together and
are transformed as they reach out, under the direction of
Kaufman, to help a little boy the medical world had given up
as hopeless. This heartwarming journey of loving a child
back to life will not only inspire, but presents a compelling
new way to deal with life's traumas and difficulties. *$7.99*
388 pages Yearly

**2344 All Kinds of Minds: Young Student's Book About
Learning Disabilities & Disorders**
Educators Publishing Service
PO Box 9031
Cambridge, MA 02139-9031   617-547-6706
                                  800-225-5750
                              Fax: 888-440-2665
                          http://eps.schoolspecialty.com/
                      CustomerService.EPS@schoolspecialty.com
Melvin Levine, Author
Alana Trisler, Author
Carol Einstein, Author
Written by Melvin Levine, and published in 1992. Helps
children with learning disabilities to come to terms with it.
Shows them how to get around or just work out any problems
with their disabilities.
283 pages paperback
ISBN 0-838820-90-5

**2345 Closer Look: Perspectives & Reflections on College Stu-
dents with LD**
Curry College Bookstore
1071 Blue Hill Ave
Milton, MA 02186-2302   617-333-0500
                              Fax: 617-333-6860
                              www.curry.edu
                              dgoss@curry.edu
Diane Goss, Editor/Author
Jane Adelizzi, Co-Author
This book is a collection of personal accounts by teachers
and learners. It's a sensitive portrayal of the real world of
teaching and learning, particularly as it impacts on those
with learning differences. Topics include connections between theory and practice, emotions and learning disabilities, classroom trauma, learning disabilities and social
deficits, metacognitive development, ESL and learning disabilities, models for inclusion and practical strategies.
$24.95
241 pages paperback
ISBN 0-964975-20-3

**2346 Diverse Learners in the Mainstream Classroom: Strate-
gies for Supporting ALL Students Across Areas**
Heinemann
PO Box 6926
Portsmouth, NH 03802-6926   603-431-7894
                                  800-225-5800
                              Fax: 877-231-6980
                              www.heinemann.com
                              custserv@heinemann.com
Yvonne S Freeman, Author
Davide E Freeman, Co-Author
Reynaldo Ramirez, Co-Author
A comprehensive book offering strategies and practices
teachers can use from PreK-through high school. Provides
everything from the big picture to the everyday details
teachers want. *$27.00*
272 pages
ISBN 0-325013-13-8

2347 Dyslexia in Adults: Taking Charge of Your Life
Taylor Publishing
7211 Circle S Road
Austin, TX 78745   512-444-0571
                          800-225-3687
                      Fax: 512-440-2160
                      www.balfour.com
                      Rings@balfour.com
Kathleen Nosek, Author
Adult dyslexics are experts at hiding reading, writing, and
spelling difficulties long after high school. Dyslexia in
Adults is a perfect guidebook for adult dyslexias to use in
coping with day-to-day problems that are complicated by
their learning disability. *$12.95*
206 pages Paperback
ISBN 0-878339-48-5

2348 Faking It: A Look into the Mind of a Creative Learner
Heinemann
PO Box 6926
Portsmouth, NH 03802-6926   603-431-7894
                                  800-225-5800
                              Fax: 877-231-6980
                              www.heinemann.com
                              custserv@heinemann.com
Christopher Lee, Author
Rosemary Jackson, Co-Author
Engage in professional dialog with Heinemann's celebrated
authors and colleagues! *$17.95*
200 pages paperback
ISBN 0-867092-96-3

**2349 From Disability to Possibility: The Powerof Inclusive
Classrooms**
Heinemann
PO Box 6926
Portsmouth, NH 03802-6926   603-431-7894
                                  800-225-5800
                              Fax: 877-231-6980
                              www.heinemann.com
                              custserv@heinemann.com
Patrick Schwarz, Author
Offers a meaningful, practical and doable alternative to tra-
ditional special education practice both during the school
years and after. *$15.00*
112 pages
ISBN 0-325009-93-3

2350 How to Get Services by Being Assertive
Family Resource Center on Disabilities
Room 300
20 E Jackson Blvd
Chicago, IL 60604-2265   312-939-3513
                              800-952-4199
                          Fax: 312-854-8980
                          TDD: 312-939-3519
                              www.frcd.org
                              info@frcd.org

Charlotte Jardins, Author
Myra Christian, Contact
Gloria Mikucki, Contact
A 100 page manual that demonstrates positive assertiveness techniques. Price includes postage and handling. *$12.00*
100 pages

2351 Inclusion-Classroom Problem Solver; Structures and Supports to Serve ALL Learners
Heinemann
PO Box 6926
Portsmouth, NH 03802-6926

603-431-7894
800-225-5800
Fax: 877-231-6980
www.heinemann.com
custserv@heinemann.com

Constance McGrath, Author
Provides proven ways to create a classroom that replaces frustrating temporary accommodations with and inclusive, joyous environment designed to work for every student. *$17.50*
144 pages
ISBN 0-325012-70-4

2352 Kids Behind the Label: An Inside at ADHD for Classroom Teachers
Heinemann
PO Box 6926
Portsmouth, NH 03802-6926

603-431-7894
800-225-5800
Fax: 877-231-6980
www.heinemann.com
custserv@heinemann.com

Trudy Knowles, Author
Students with Attention-Deficit/Hyperactivity Disorder (ADHD) tell you what they experience coming to class each day. Their descriptions will forever change how you approach ADHD students, allowing you to contrast their frustrating in-school behavior with the frustration they feel trying to complete their work and make sense of their world. *$18.50*
160 pages
ISBN 0-325009-67-4

2353 Myth of Laziness
Simon & Schuster
1230 Avenue of the Americas
New York, NY 10020-1513

212-698-7000
www.simonandschuster.biz
shop.feedback@simonsays.com

Mel Levine, Author
Written by Melvin Levine and published in 2003. It shows parents how to nurture their children's strength's and improve their classroom productivity. Also, it shows how correcting these problems early will help children live a fulfilling and productive adult life.
288 pages
ISBN 0-743213-68-8

2354 New Horizons Information for the Air Traveler with a Disability
Office of Aviation Enforcement and Proceedings
1200 New Jersey Ave SE
Washington, DC 20590

www.dot.gov/airconsumer
This guide is designed to offer travelers with disabilities a brief but authoritative source of information about Air Carrier Access rules; the accommodations, facilities, and services that are now required to be available.

2355 No Easy Answer
Bantam Partners
1745 Broadway
New York, NY 10019-4305

212-782-9000
www.randomhouse.com
bdpublicity@randomhouse.com

Rob Meritt, Author
Brooker Brown, Co-Author

Parents and teachers of learning disabled children have turned to No Easy Answer for information, advice, and comfort. This completely updated edition contains new chapters on Attention Deficit Disorder and Attention Deficit Hyperactivity Disorder, and on the public laws that guarantee an equal education for learning disabled children. *$23.00*
416 pages paperback
ISBN 0-553354-50-7

2356 Out of Darkness
Connecticut Assoc for Children and Adults with LD
Ste 15-5
25 Van Zant St
Norwalk, CT 06855-1729

203-838-5010
Fax: 203-866-6108
www.cacld.org
cacld@optonline.net

Russell Freedman, Author
Article by an adult who discovers at age 30 that he has ADD. *$1.00*
4 pages

2357 Painting the Joy of the Soul
Learning Disabilities Association of America
4156 Library Rd
Pittsburgh, PA 15234-1349

412-341-1515
Fax: 412-344-0224
www.ldanatl.org
info@LDAAmerica.org

Peter Rippe, Author
P Buckley Moss, Co-Author
The first comprehensively researched and written book on the art and life of America's beloved artist, P. Buckley Moss, whose passion for painting is equal only to her passion for people, especially those with learning disabilities. Inspirational book about a woman who succeeded not in spite of her disability, but because of it. Contains 168 full color pages, over 100 art images. *$50.00*
168 pages
ISBN 0-964687-09-7

2358 Rethinking the Education of Deaf Students: Theory and Practice from a Teacher's Perspective
Heinemann
PO Box 6926
Portsmouth, NH 03802-6926

603-431-7894
800-225-5800
Fax: 877-231-6980
www.heinemann.com
custserv@heinemann.com

Sue Livingston, Author
Offers alternatives and demonstrates how American Sign Language (ASL) and English can coexist in the same classroom, embedded in the context of what is being taught. *$23.00*
180 pages
ISBN 0-435072-36-0

2359 Son-Rise: The Miracle Continues
Option Indigo Press
2080 S Undermountain Rd
Sheffield, MA 01257-9643

413-229-2100
800-714-2779
Fax: 413-229-8727
www.optionindigo.com
indigo@bcn.net

Barry Neil Kaufman, Author
Raun Kaufman, Co-Author
This book documents Raun Kaufman's astonishing development from a lifeless, autistic, retarded child into a highly verbal, lovable youngster with no traces of his former condition. It includes details of Raun's extraordinary progress from the age of four into young adulthood. It also shares moving accounts of five families that successfully used the Son-Rise Program to reach their own special children. An awe-inspiring reminder that love moves mountains. *$14.95*
372 pages
ISBN 0-915811-61-8

2360 The Eight Ball Club: Ocean of Fire
ESOL Publishing LLC
10305 Colony View Dr
Fairfax, VA 22032-3222 703-250-7097
www.theeightballclub.com
esolpublishing@cox.net; mcpuginrodas@aol.com
MC Pugin-Roads, Author
Publisher of novels designed for Special Ed and ESL students and activity books that go with the novel. These novels can be enjoyed by mainstream students as well. The Eight Ball Club: Ocean of Fire has vocac words in bold print, photographic illustrations, academic science terms, and a glossary. It's a teen-interest, easy reading adventure. *$18.95*
144 pages

2361 What About Me? Strategies for Teaching Misunderstood Learners
Heinemann
PO Box 6926
Portsmouth, NH 03802-6926 603-431-7894
800-225-5800
Fax: 877-231-6980
www.heinemann.com
custserv@heinemann.com
Christopher Lee, Author
Rosemary Jackson, Co-Author
A practical yet personal book on how to help special learners grow into self-sufficient responsible adults who can recognize their strengths and manage their weeknesses. *$19.50*
166 pages
ISBN 0-325003-48-1

2362 You're Welcome: 30 Innovative Ideas for the Inclusive Classroom
Heinemann
PO Box 6926
Portsmouth, NH 03802-6926 603-431-7894
800-225-5800
Fax: 877-231-6980
www.heinemann.com
custserv@heinemann.com
Patrick Schwarz, Author
Paula Kluth, Co-Author
Three handbooks; 30 key ideas-all the information you need to start making inclusion work effectively. *$18.00*
ISBN 0-325012-04-9

Children

2363 An Alphabet of Animal Signs
Harris Communications
15155 Technology Dr
Eden Prairie, MN 55344-2273 952-906-1180
800-825-6758
Fax: 952-906-1099
TDD: 952-906-1198
TTY: 800-825-9187
www.harriscomm.com
info@harriscomm.com
S Harold Collins, Author
Darla Hudson, Customer Service
A fun sign language starter book that presents an animal sign for each letter of the alphabet. Part #B816. *$4.95*
16 pages Paperback
ISBN 0-931993-65-2

2364 Basic Vocabulary: American Sign Language Basic Vocabulary: American Sign Language for Parents
Harris Communications
15155 Technology Dr
Eden Prairie, MN 55344-2273 952-906-1180
800-825-6758
Fax: 952-906-1099
TDD: 952-906-1198
TTY: 800-825-9187
www.harriscomm.com
info@harriscomm.com

Terrance K O'Rourke, Author
Darla Hudson, Customer Service
A child's first dictionary of signs. Arranged alphabetically, this book incorporates developmental lists helpful to both deaf and hearing children with over 1,000 clear illustrations. Part #B294. *$8.95*
228 pages Paperback
ISBN 0-932666-00-0

2365 Beginning Signing Primer
Harris Communications
15155 Technology Dr
Eden Prairie, MN 55344-2273 952-906-1180
800-825-6758
Fax: 952-906-1099
TDD: 952-906-1198
TTY: 800-825-9187
www.harriscomm.com
info@harriscomm.com
Darla Hudson, Customer Service
A set of 100 cards designed especially for beginning signers. The cards present seven topics with words and signs. The topics: Color; Creatures; Family; Months; Days; Time and Weather. Part #B398. *$7.95*

2366 Christmas Bear
Teddy Bear Press
Suite 67
3703 S. Edmunds Street
Seattle, WA 98118 206-402-6947
866-870-7323
Fax: 866-870-7323
www.teddybearpress.net
fparker@teddybearpress.net
Fran Parker, President/Author
An 11x17 big book with color illustrations and a large print format uses the same simple sentence structure fount in I Can Read and Reading Is Fun programs. This story adds seasonal words to the developing sight vocabulary found in our reading programs. *$19.95*
12 pages
ISBN 1-928876-11-0

2367 Don't Give Up Kid
Verbal Images Press
46 Duncott Rd.
Fairport, NY 14450-8602 585-746-7239
Fax: 585-264-1448
http://verbalimagespress.com
jeanne@verbalimagespress.com
Victoria Harmison, Marketing Director
Jeanne Gehret MA, Author
Like a river overflowing its banks, Ben wreaks havoc until he learns to recognize his Attention Deficit Disorder (ADD). By the end of this tale, Ben's family wonders how they could have gotten along without his specia way of seeing the world. *$9.95*
40 pages Paperback
ISBN 1-884281-10-9

2368 Fischer Decoding Mastery Test
Oxton House Publishers
124 Main Street
Suite 203
Farmington, ME 04938 207-779-1923
800-539-7323
Fax: 207-779-0623
www.oxtonhouse.com
info@oxtonhouse.com
William Berlinghoff PhD, Managing Editor
Cheryl Martin, Marketing
Debra Richards, Office Manager
This powerful, flexible diagnostic tool tells you precisely which decoding skills have been mastered (don't need to be taught), which skills are in transition (need some attention), and which skills need to be taught from scratch. Based on more than 40 years of clinical experience, it is a highly reliable way to pinpoint each beginning reader's exact needs and to measure progress against previous performance.

2369 Fundamentals of Autism
Slosson Educational Publications
PO Box 280
538 Buffalo Road
East Aurora, NY 14052 888-756-7766
Fax: 800-655-3840
www.slosson.com
slosson@slosson.com

Steven Slosson, President
Georgina Moynihan, TTFM
A handbook for those who work with children diagnosed as autistic.

2370 Funny Bunny and Sunny Bunny
Teddy Bear Press
Suite 67
3703 S. Edmunds Street
Seattle, WA 98118 206-402-6947
866-870-7323
Fax: 866-870-7323
www.teddybearpress.net
fparker@teddybearpress.net

Fran Parker, President/Author
An 11x17 big book with color illustrations and a large print format uses the same simple sentence structure fount in I Can Read and Reading Is Fun programs. This story adds seasonal words to the developing sight vocabulary found in our reading programs. *$19.95*
17 pages
ISBN 1-928876-14-5

2371 Halloween Bear
Teddy Bear Press
Suite 67
3703 S. Edmunds Street
Seattle, WA 98118 206-402-6947
866-870-7323
Fax: 866-870-7323
www.teddybearpress.net
fparker@teddybearpress.net

Fran Parker, President/Author
An 11x17 big book with color illustrations and a large print format uses the same simple sentence structure fount in I Can Read and Reading Is Fun programs. This story adds seasonal words to the developing sight vocabulary found in our reading programs. *$19.95*
13 pages
ISBN 1-928876-15-3

2372 Handmade Alphabet
Harris Communications
15155 Technology Dr
Eden Prairie, MN 55344-2273 952-906-1180
800-825-6758
Fax: 952-906-1099
TDD: 952-906-1198
TTY: 800-825-9187
www.harriscomm.com
info@harriscomm.com

Laura Rankin, Author
Darla Hudson, Customer Service
An alphabet book which celebrates the beauty of the manual alphabet. Each illustration consists of the manual representation of the letter linked with an item beginning with that letter. Part #B310SC. *$6.99*
32 pages Paperback
ISBN 0-803709-74-9

2373 I Can Read Charts
Teddy Bear Press
Suite 67
3703 S. Edmunds Street
Seattle, WA 98118 206-402-6947
866-870-7323
Fax: 866-870-7323
www.teddybearpress.net
fparker@teddybearpress.net

Frank Babaloni, President/Author

Designed to accompany the I Can Read program is an 11x17 big book containing 54 charts which can be used to assist in introducing new words to students. These charts also provide review for previously taught words with either individual student or a small group. *$59.95*
54 pages

2374 I Can Sign My ABC's
Harris Communications
15155 Technology Dr
Eden Prairie, MN 55344-2273 952-906-1180
800-825-6758
Fax: 952-906-1099
TDD: 952-906-1198
TTY: 800-825-9187
www.harriscomm.com
info@harriscomm.com

Darla Hudson, Customer Service
The Sign with Me alphabet book is a book for all children. It is designed to teach the 26 letters of the alphabet and the corresponding manual alphabet in sign language. The book provides early exposure to letter recognition plus a unique opportunity to introduce sign language to young children. Part #B132. *$11.95*
52 pages Hardcover
ISBN 0-939849-00-3

2375 Jumpin' Johnny Get Back to Work: A Child's Guide to ADHD/Hyperactivity
Connecticut Assoc for Children and Adults with LD
Ste 15-5
25 Van Zant St
Norwalk, CT 06855-1729 203-838-5010
Fax: 203-866-6108
www.CACLD.org
cacld@juno.com

Michael Gordon PhD, Author
Written primarily for elementary age youngsters with ADHD, this book helps them to understand their disability. Also valuable as an educational tool for parents, siblings, friends and classmates. The author's text reflects his sensitivity toward children with ADHD. *$12.50*
24 pages

2376 Leo the Late Bloomer
Connecticut Assoc for Children and Adults with LD
Ste 15-5
25 Van Zant St
Norwalk, CT 06855-1729 203-838-5010
Fax: 203-866-6108
www.CACLD.org
cacld@juno.com

Beryl Kaufman, Executive Director
Robert Kraus, Author
A wonderful book for the young child who is having problems learning. Children follow along with Leo as he finally blooms. *$6.50*

2377 My First Book of Sign
Harris Communications
15155 Technology Dr
Eden Prairie, MN 55344-2273 952-906-1180
800-825-6758
Fax: 952-906-1099
TDD: 952-906-1198
TTY: 800-825-9187
www.harriscomm.com
info@harriscomm.com

Pamela J Baker, Author
Darla Hudson, Customer Service

This book is an excellent source to teach children and even adults sign language. The illustrations are accurate in their representation of sign. It is colorful and visually attractive which makes it easy to read. The black and white manual alphabet, the fingerspelling, and aspects of sign provide exellent directions and pointers to signing correctly. The sign descriptions are a great supplement to the illustrations. Part #B147. *$22.95*
76 pages Hardcover
ISBN 0-930323-20-3

2378 My Signing Book of Numbers
Harris Communications
15155 Technology Dr
Eden Prairie, MN 55344-2273
952-906-1180
800-825-6758
Fax: 952-906-1099
TDD: 952-906-1198
TTY: 800-825-9187
www.harriscomm.com
info@harriscomm.com
Patricia Bellan Gillen, Author
Darla Hudson, Customer Service
Learn signs for numbers 0 through 20, and 30 through 100 by tens. *$22.95*
56 pages Hardcover
ISBN 0-930323-37-8

2379 Rosey: The Imperfect Angel
Special Needs Project
Ste H
324 State St
Santa Barbara, CA 93101-2364
818-718-9900
800-333-6867
Fax: 818-349-2027
www.specialneeds.com
books@specialneeds.com
Sandra Lee Peckinpah, Author
Rosie, an angel with a cleft palate, works hard in her heavenly garden after the Boss Angel declares her disfigured mouth as lovely as a rose petal. Her reward is to be born on earth, as a baby with a cleft. *$15.95*
28 pages
ISBN 0-962780-60-8

2380 Scare Bear
Teddy Bear Press
3703 S. Edmunds Street
Suite 67
Seattle, WA 98118
206-402-6947
866-870-7323
Fax: 866-870-7323
www.teddybearpress.net
fparker@teddybearpress.net
Fran Parker, President/Author
An 11x17 big book with color illustrations and a large print format uses the same simple sentence structure fount in I Can Read and Reading Is Fun programs. This story adds seasonal words to the developing sight vocabulary found in our reading programs. *$19.95*
13 pages
ISBN 1-928876-16-1

2381 Signing is Fun: A Child's Introduction to the Basics of Sign Language
Harris Communications
15155 Technology Dr
Eden Prairie, MN 55344-2273
952-906-1180
800-825-6758
Fax: 952-906-1099
TDD: 952-906-1198
TTY: 800-825-9187
www.harriscomm.com
info@harriscomm.com
Mickey Flodin, Author
Darla Hudson, Customer Service

The author of Signing for Kids offers children their first glimpse at a whole new world. Starting with the alphabet and working up to everyday phrases, this volume uses clear instructions on how to begin using American Sign Language and features an informative introduction to signing and its importance. One hundred and fifty illustrations. Part #B496 *$9.00*
95 pages Paperback
ISBN 0-613720-18-0

2382 Sixth Grade Can Really Kill You
Penquin Putnam Publishing Group
375 Hudson St
New York, NY 10014-3658
212-366-2000
800-847-5515
Fax: 212-366-2666
www.penguingroup.com
ecommerce@us.penguingroup.com
Barthe DeClements, Author
Helen's learning difficulties cause her to act up and are threatening to keep her from passing sixth grade.
160 pages Paperback
ISBN 0-142413-80-1

2383 Snowbear
Teddy Bear Press
Suite 67
3703 S. Edmunds Street
Seattle, WA 98118
206-402-6947
866-870-7323
Fax: 866-870-7323
www.teddybearpress.net
fparker@teddybearpress.net
Fran Parker, President/Author
An 11x17 big book with color illustrations and a large print format uses the same simple sentence structure fount in I Can Read and Reading Is Fun programs. This story adds seasonal words to the developing sight vocabulary found in our reading programs. *$19.95*
13 pages
ISBN 1-928876-12-9

2384 Someone Special, Just Like You
Special Needs Project
Ste H
324 State St
Santa Barbara, CA 93101-2364
818-718-9900
800-333-6867
Fax: 818-349-2027
www.specialneeds.com
books@specialneeds.com
Tricia Brown, Author
A handsome photo-essay including a range of youngsters with disabilities at four preschools in the San Francisco Bay area. *$7.95*
64 pages

2385 Study Skills: A Landmark School Student Guide
429 Hale St
Prides Crossing
Prides Crossing, MA 01965
978-236-3216
Fax: 978-927-7268
www.landmarkoutreach.org
outreach@landmarkschool.org
Robert Broudo, Principal

2386 Unicorns Are Real!
Learning Disabilities Association of America
4156 Library Rd
Pittsburgh, PA 15234-1349
412-341-1515
Fax: 412-344-0224
www.ldanatl.org
ldanatl@usaor.net
Barbara Meister Vitale, Author

This mega best-seller provides 65 practical, easy-to-follow-lessons to develop the much ignored right brain tendencies of children. These simple yet dramatically effective ideas and activities have helped thousands with learning difficulties. Includes an easy-to-administer screening checklist to determine hemisphere dominance, engaging instructional activities that draw on the intuitive, nonverbal abilities of the right brain, a list of skills associated with each brain hemisphere and more. *$14.95*
174 pages
ISBN 0-446323-40-3

2387 Valentine Bear
Teddy Bear Press
Suite 67
3703 S. Edmunds Street
Seattle, WA 98118   206-402-6947
                                        866-870-7323
                                Fax: 866-870-7323
                                www.teddybearpress.net
                        fparker@teddybearpress.net
Fran Parker, President/Author
An 11x17 big book with color illustrations and a large print format uses the same simple sentence structure fount in I Can Read and Reading Is Fun programs. This story adds seasonal words to the developing sight vocabulary found in our reading programs. *$19.95*
13 pages
ISBN 1-928876-13-7

2388 Visual Perception and Attention Workbook
Therapro
225 Arlington St
Framingham, MA 01702-8723   508-872-9494
                                        800-257-5376
                                Fax: 508-875-2062
                                www.therapro.com
                                info@therapro.com
Karen Conrad, Owner
Kathleen Anderson MS CCC-SP, Author
Pamela Crow Miller, Co-Author
Simple mazes, visual discrimination and visual form constancy task, telling time and much more.

Law

2389 ADA Quiz Book
DBTAC: Rocky Mountain ADA Center
Ste 103
3630 Sinton Rd
Colorado Springs, CO 80907-5072   719-444-0268
                                        800-949-4232
                                Fax: 719-444-0269
                                TTY: 719-444-0268
                                www.adainformation.org
                        publications@mtc-inc.com
Jana Copeland, Editor
Bob Cook, Religious Leader
Candice Brandt, Training Coordinator
A collection of puzzles, quizzes, questions and case studies on the Americans with Disabilities Act of 1990 and accessible information technology. Features sections on ADA basics, employment, state and local governments, public accommodations, architectural accessibility, disability etiquette, effective communication, and electronic and information technology. *$9.95*
81 pages 4.00 shipping

2390 Discipline
Special Education Resource Center
25 Industrial Park Rd
Middletown, CT 06457-1516   860-632-1485
                                Fax: 860-632-8870
                                www.ctserc.org
                                info@ctserc.org
Mary Ann Kirner, Executive Director

A general analysis of the problems encountered in the discipline of students with disabilities. Discussion of the legal principles of discipline that have evolved pursuant to Public Law 94-142.

2391 Dispute Resolution Journal
American Arbitration Association
Fl 10
1633 Broadway
New York, NY 10019-6708   212-716-5800
                                        800-778-7879
                                Fax: 212-716-5905
                                www.adr.org
                                zuckermans@adr.org
William K Slate Ii, CEO
Susan Zuckerman, Author
Provides information on mediation, arbitration and other dispute resolution alternatives. *$150.00*
96 pages Quarterly

2392 Education of the Handicapped: Laws
William Hein & Company
1285 Main St
Buffalo, NY 14209-1987   716-882-2600
                                        800-828-7571
                                Fax: 716-883-8100
                                www.wshein.com
                                mail@wshein.com
Kevin Marmion, President
Bernard D Reams Jr, Author
Focuses on elementary and secondary Education Act of 1965 and its amendment, Education For All Handicapped Children Act of 1975 and its amendments and acts providing services for the disabled.
ISBN 0-899411-57-6

2393 Ethical and Legal Issues in School Counseling
American School Counselor Association
Ste 625
1101 King St
Alexandria, VA 22314-2957   703-683-2722
                                        800-306-4722
                                Fax: 703-683-1619
                                www.schoolcounselor.org
                                asca@schoolcounselor.org
Wayne C Huey, Author
Theodore Phant Remley, Editor
Perhaps the increase in litigation involving educators and mental health practitioners is a factor. Certainly the laws are changing or at least are being interpreted differently, requiring counselors to stay up-to-date. The process of decision-making and some of the more complex issues in ethical and legal areas are summarized in this digest. *$40.50*
341 pages
ISBN 1-556200-55-2

2394 Individuals with Disabilities: Implementing the Newest Laws
Corwin Press
2455 Teller Rd
Thousand Oaks, CA 91320-2218   805-499-9734
                                        800-233-9936
                                Fax: 805-499-5323
                                www.corwin.com
                                order@corwin.com
Joan L Curcio, Author
Patricia F First, Co-Author
Aimed at school administrators, this highly readable book covers the three major pieces of legislation: Americans with Disabilities Act of 1990; Individuals with Disabilities Education Act; and the Rehabilitation Act of 1973. Suitable for lay public use, anyone needing an overview of the laws affecting education and disabilities. *$12.95*
64 pages
ISBN 0-803960-55-7

2395 Learning Disabilities and the Law in Higher Education and Employment
JKL Communications
Ste 707
2700 Virginia Ave NW
Washington, DC 20037-1909 202-321-4100
Fax: 850-233-3350
lathamlaw@gmail.com
Peter S Latham JD, Director
Patricia Horan Latham JD, Director
Deals with issues in education and employment. Covers: Section 504, the IDEA, and ADA. Reviews court cases. *$15.00*
ISBN 1-883560-13-6

2396 Least Restrictive Environment
Special Education Resource Center
25 Industrial Park Rd
Middletown, CT 06457-1516 860-632-1485
Fax: 860-632-8870
www.ctserc.org
info@ctserc.org
Mary Ann Kirner, Executive Director
A general discussion and analysis of the mandate to educate students with disabilities to the maximum extent appropriate with nondisabled students.

2397 Legal Notes for Education
Oakstone Business Publishing
136 Madison Avenue
8th Floor
New York, NY 10016 212-209-0500
Fax: 212-209-0501
www.haightscross.com
info@haightscross.com
Steven B. Epstein, Chairman
Summaries of court decisions dealing with education law. *$122.00*

2398 Legal Rights of Persons with Disabilities: An Analysis of Federal Law
LRP Publications
360 Hiatt Drive
Palm Beach Gardens
Florida, FL 33418 800-341-7874
Fax: 561-622-2423
www.lrp.com
custserv@lrp.com
Bonnie P Tucker, Author
This book will provide professionals working with the disabled a comprehensive analysis of the rights accorded individuals with disabilities under federal law. *$185.00*
2226 pages
ISBN 0-934753-46-6

2399 New Directions
Association of State Mental Health Program Direct
113 Oronoco St
Alexandria, VA 22314-2015 703-683-4202
Fax: 703-683-8773
www.nasddds.org
ksnyder@nasddds.org
Robert Glover, Executive Director
A newsletter offering information on laws, amendments, and legislation affecting the disabled. *$55.00*

2400 New IDEA Amendments: Assistive Technology Devices and Services
Special Education Resource Center
25 Industrial Park Rd
Middletown, CT 06457-1516 860-632-1485
Fax: 860-632-8870
www.ctserc.org
info@ctserc.org
Mary Ann Kirner, Executive Director

A discussion of new mandates created by the 1990 Amendments to Public Law 94-142. An overview of the requirement for the provision of assistive technology devices and services as well as a discussion on the transition services that are to be provided to disabled adolescents.

2401 Numbers that add up to Educational Rights for Children with Disabilities
Children's Defense Fund
25 E Street N.W.
Washington, DC 20001-1522 202-628-8787
800-233-1200
www.childrensdefense.org
cdfinfo@childrensdefense.org
Ellen Mancuso, Author
Information on the laws 94-142 and 504. *$4.75*
68 pages
ISBN 0-938008-73-0

2402 Parent's Guide to the Social Security Administration
The Eden Family of Services
2 Merwick Rd
Princeton, NJ 08540-5711 609-987-0099
Fax: 609-987-0243
www.edenautism.org
info@edenau.orgtism
Tom Mc Cool, President
A parents' guide to the Social Security Administration and Social Security Work Incentive Programs. *$16.00*

2403 Procedural Due Process
Special Education Resource Center
25 Industrial Park Rd
Middletown, CT 06457-1516 860-632-1485
Fax: 860-632-8870
www.ctserc.org
www.ctserc.org
Mary Ann Kirner, Executive Director
Analyzes the importance of the procedural safeguards afforded to parents and their children with disabilities by the Public Law 94-142. Safeguards are discussed and possible legal implications are addressed.

2404 Public Law 94-142: An Overview
Special Education Resource Center
25 Industrial Park Rd
Middletown, CT 06457-1516 860-632-1485
Fax: 860-632-8870
www.ctserc.org
info@ctserc.org
Mary Ann Kirner, Executive Director
An overview of the general provisions of the Individuals with Disabilities Education Act, commonly referred to as Public Law 94-142. Designed to provide the less-experienced viewer with a fundamental understanding of the Public Law and its significance.

2405 Purposeful Integration: Inherently Equal
Federation for Children with Special Needs
Suite 1102
529 Main Street
Boston, MA 02109 617-236-7210
800-331-0688
Fax: 617-241-0330
www.fcsn.org
fcsninfo@fcsn.org
James F. Whalen, President
Michael Weiner, Treasurer
This publication covers integration, mainstreaming, and least restrictive environments. *$8.00*
55 pages

2406 Section 504 of the Rehabilitation Act
Special Education Resource Center
25 Industrial Park Rd
Middletown, CT 06457-1516 860-632-1485
Fax: 860-632-8870
www.ctserc.org
info@ctserc.org

Mary Ann Kirner, Executive Director
A general overview of the legal implications of the Rehabilitation Act and its implementing regulations, a law that is often forgotten in the process of appropriately educating children with disabilities.

2407 Section 504: Help for the Learning Disabled College Student
Connecticut Assoc for Children and Adults with LD
Ste 15-5
25 Van Zant St
Norwalk, CT 06855-1729

203-838-5010
Fax: 203-866-6108
www.cacld.org
cacld@juno.com

Beryl Kaufman, Executive Director
Joan Sedita, Author
Provides a review of Section 504 of the Vocational Rehabilitation Act as it relates specifically to the learning disabled. *$3.25*

2408 So You're Going to a Hearing: Preparing for Public Law 94-142
Learning Disabilities Association of America
4156 Library Rd
Pittsburgh, PA 15234-1349

412-341-1515
Fax: 412-344-0224
www.ldanatl.org
ldanatl@usaor.net

A public informational source offering legal advice to children and youth with learning disabilities. *$5.50*

2409 Special Education Law Update
Data Research
Ste 3100
4635 Nicols Rd
Eagan, MN 55122-3337

651-452-8267
800-365-4900
Fax: 651-452-8694
www.dataresearchinc.com

Monthly newsletter service. Cases, legislation, administrative regulations and law review articles dealing with special education law. Annual index and binder included. *$159.00*

2410 Special Education in Juvenile Corrections
Council for Exceptional Children
Suite 1000
2900 Crystal Drive
Arlington, VA 22202-3557

703-620-3660
866-509-0218
Fax: 703-264-9494
TTY: 866-915-5000
www.cec.sped.org
service@cec.sped.org

Margaret J. McLaughin, President
James P. Heiden, Treasurer
This topic is of increasing concern. This book describes the demographics of incarcerated youth and suggests some promising practices that are being used. *$8.90*
25 pages
ISBN 0-865862-03-6

2411 Special Law for Special People
Gray,Rust, St. Amand, Moffett & Brieske LLP
950 E Paces Ferry Rd NE
1700 Atlanta Plaza
Atlanta, GA 30326-1180

404-870-7373
Fax: 404-870-7374
www.grsmb.com

James T. Brieske, Attorney
Matthew A. Ericksen, Attorney
A ten-tape video series that is designed to assist in educating regular education personnel as to the legal requirements of IDEA and Section 504. *$5.95*

2412 Statutes, Regulations and Case Law
Center for Education and Employment Law
PO Box 3008
Malvern, PA 19355

800-365-4900
Fax: 610-647-8089
www.ceelonline.com
curt_brown@pbp.com

Curt Brown Esq, Group Publisher
Steve McEllistrem Esq, Senior Editor
Provides summaries of recent court cases impacting disability issues as well as reports on legislation and administrative regulations that are of importance to you. *$259.00*
Monthly

2413 Stories Behind Special Education Case Law
Special Needs Project
Ste H
324 State St
Santa Barbara, CA 93101-2364

818-718-9900
800-333-6867
Fax: 818-349-2027
www.specialneeds.com
books@specialneeds.com

Reed Martin, Author
The personal stories behind ten leading court cases that shaped the basic principles of special education law. *$12.95*
119 pages Paperback
ISBN 0-878223-32-0

2414 Students with Disabilities and Special Education
Center for Education and Employment Law
PO Box 3008
Malvern, PA 19355

800-365-4900
Fax: 610-647-8089
www.ceelonline.com
curt_brown@pbp.com

Curt Brown Esq, Group Publisher
Steve McEllistrem Esq, Senior Editor
A desk reference that helps you determine if your program conforms to IDEA statutes and regulations in a comprehensive and concise format. We bring you analyses of recent court cases across the country that will help you safeguard your legal rights, and educate your colleagues in the law so they too are better qualified to identify and deal with developing legal issues. *$294.00*
500+ pages
ISBN 0-939675-44-7

2415 Technology, Curriculum, and Professional Development
Corwin Press
2455 Teller Rd
Thousand Oaks, CA 91320-2218

805-499-9734
800-233-9936
Fax: 805-499-5323
www.corwin.com
order@corwin.com

John Woodward, Author/Editor
Larry Cuban, Co-Author/Editor
Adapting schools to meet the needs of students with disabilities. The history of special education technologies, the requirements of IDEA '97, and the successes and obstacles for special education technology implementation. *$76.95*
264 pages
ISBN 0-761977-42-2

2416 Testing Students with Disabilities
Corwin Press
2455 Teller Rd
Thousand Oaks, CA 91320-2218

805-499-9734
800-233-9936
Fax: 805-499-5323
www.corwin.com
order@corwin.com

Martha Thurlow, Author
James Ysseldyke, Co-Author
Judy Elliot, Co-Author

Practical strategies for complying with district and state requirements. Helps translate the issues surrounding state and district testing of students with disabilities, including IDEA, into what educators need to know and do. *$80.95*
344 pages
ISBN 0-761938-08-7

2417 US Department of Justice: Disabilities Rights Section
950 Pennsylvania Ave NW
Washington, DC 20530

202-307-0663
800-514-0301
Fax: 202-307-1197
TTY: 800-514-0383
www.ada.gov
askdoj@usdoj.gov

Rebecca B. Bond, Chief
Zita Jhonson Betts, Deputy Chief
Roberta Kirkendall, Special Councel
Information concerning the rights people with learning disabilities have under the Americans with Disabilities Act.

2418 US Department of Justice: Disability Rights Section
950 Pennsylvania Ave NW
Washington, DC 20530

202-307-0663
800-514-0301
Fax: 202-307-1197
TTY: 800-514-0383
www.ada.gov
askdoj@usdoj.gov

Rebecca B. Bond, Chief
Zita Jhonson Betts, Deputy Chief
Roberta Kirkendall, Special Councel
The primary goal of the Disability Rights Section is to achieve equal opportunity for people with disabilities in the United States by implementing the Americans with Disabilities Act (ADA).

Parents & Professionals

2419 125 Brain Games for Babies
Therapro
225 Arlington St
Framingham, MA 01702-8723

508-872-9494
800-257-5376
Fax: 508-875-2062
www.therapro.com
info@therapro.com

Jackie Silberg, uthor
Packed with everyday opportunities to enhance brain development of children from birth to 12 months. Each game includes notes on recent brain research in practical terms. *$14.95*
143 pages
ISBN 0-876591-99-3

2420 A Miracle to Believe In
Option Indigo Press
2080 S Undermountain Rd
Sheffield, MA 01257-9643

413-229-8727
800-562-7171
Fax: 413-229-8727
www.optionindigo.com
indigo@bcn.net

Barry Kausman, Author
A group of people from all walks of life come together and are transformed as they reach out, under the direction of Kaufman, to help a little boy the medical world had given up as hopeless. This heartwarming journey of loving a child back to life will not only inspire, but presents a compelling new way to deal with life's traumas and difficulties. *$7.99*
388 pages
ISBN 0-449201-08-2

2421 A Practical Parent's Handbook on Teaching Children with Learning Disabilities
Charles C Thomas
2600 S 1st St
Springfield, IL 62704-4730

217-789-8980
800-258-8980
Fax: 217-789-9130
www.ccthomas.com
books@ccthomas.com

Shelby Holley, Author
Publisher of Education and Special Education books.
308 pages
ISBN 0-398061-50-5

2422 ADHD in Adolescents: Diagnosis and Treatment
Guilford Publications
72 Spring St
New York, NY 10012-4019

212-431-9800
800-365-7006
Fax: 212-966-6708
www.guilford.com
info@guilford.com

Arthur L Robin, Author
Here Dr. Robin teaches us not only about the facts of the disorder, but also about its nature and the proper means of clinically evaluating it. Includes numerous reproducible forms for clinicians and clients, among them rating scales and detailed checklists for psychological testing, interviewing, treatment planning, and school and family interventions. *$35.00*
461 pages Paperback
ISBN 1-572303-91-3

2423 About Dyslexia: Unraveling the Myth
Connecticut Assoc for Children and Adults with LD
Ste 15-5
25 Van Zant St
Norwalk, CT 06855-1729

203-838-5010
Fax: 203-866-6108
www.cacld.org
cacld@optonline.net

Beryl Kaufman, Executive Director
Priscilla Vail, Author
This book focuses on the communication patterns of strength and weaknesses in dyslexic people from early childhood through adulthood. *$7.95*
49 pages
ISBN 1-864010-55-8

2424 Absurdities of Special Education: The Best of Ants...Flying...and Logs
Corwin Press
2455 Teller Rd
Thousand Oaks, CA 91320-2218

805-499-9734
800-233-9936
Fax: 805-499-5323
www.corwin.com
order@corwin.com

Kevin Ruelle, Editor
Michael F Giangreco, Author
Now available in this full color edition. Create beautiful transperances or use in PowerPoint presentations for staff development. Also a great gift for parents of educators. *$30.95*
114 pages Paperback
ISBN 1-890455-40-7

2425 Access Aware: Extending Your Reach to People with Disabilities
Alliance for Technology Access
1119 Old Humboldt Road
Jackson, TN 38305

731-554-5282
1-800-914-30
Fax: 731-554-5283
TTY: 731-554-5284
www.ataccess.org
atainfo@ataccess.org

Allegra Wilson, Administrative Assistant
Todd Plummer, Development Manager

This easy-to-use manual is designed to help any organization become more accessible for people with disabilities.
$45.00
219 pages
ISBN 0-897933-00-1

2426 Activities for a Diverse Classroom
PEAK Parent Center
Ste 200
611 N Weber St
Colorado Springs, CO 80903-1072
719-531-9400
800-284-0251
Fax: 719-531-9452
www.peakparent.org
info@peakparent.org

Leah Katz, Author
Caren Sax, Co-Author
Douglas Fisher, Co-Author
A valuable resource for elementary teachers, this book helps begin the sometimes difficult conversation about diversity in the classroom. With the 18 fun, enriching, and do-it-tomorrow activities outlined in this text, teachers can help create a sense of community in the classroom as they introduce students to new ways of thinking about the need for friendships and the acceptance of others. *$11.00*
68 pages
ISBN 1-884720-07-2

2427 Activity Schedules for Children with Autism: A Guide for Parents and Professionals
Woodbine House
6510 Bells Mill Rd
Bethesda, MD 20817-1636
301-897-3570
800-843-7323
Fax: 301-897-5838
www.woodbinehouse.com
info@woodbinehouse.com

Lynn E McClannahan PhD, Author
Patricia J Krantz PhD, Author
Detailed instructions and examples help parents prepare their child's first activity schedule, then progress to more varied and sophisticated schedules. The goal of this system is for children with autism to make effective use of unstructured time, handle changes in routine, and help them choose among an established set of home, school, and leisure activities independently. *$14.95*
117 pages Paperback
ISBN 0-933149-93-X

2428 Alternate Assessments for Students with Disabilities
Corwin Press
2455 Teller Rd
Thousand Oaks, CA 91320-2218
805-499-9734
800-233-9936
Fax: 805-499-5323
www.corwin.com
order@corwin.com

Robb Clouse, Editorial Director
Sandra Thompson, Author
Martha Lurlow, Co-Author
Distinguished group of experts in a landmark book, co-published with the Council for Exceptional Children show you how to shift to high expectations for all learners, improve schooling for all. *$30.95*
168 pages Paperback
ISBN 0-761977-74-0

2429 American Sign Language Concise Dictionary
Harris Communications
15155 Technology Dr
Eden Prairie, MN 55344-2273
952-906-1180
800-825-6758
Fax: 866-870-7323
TDD: 952-906-1198
TTY: 800-825-9187
www.harriscomm.com
info@harriscomm.com

Martin Sternberg, Author
Darla Hudson, Customer Service

A portable version containing 2,000 of the most commonly used words and phrases in ASL. Illustrated with easy-to-follow hand, arm and facial movements. Part #B104. *$11.95*
737 pages Paperback

2430 American Sign Language Dictionary: A Comprehensive Abridgement
Harris Communications
15155 Technology Dr
Eden Prairie, MN 55344-2273
952-906-1180
800-825-6758
Fax: 866-870-7323
TDD: 952-906-1198
TTY: 800-825-9187
www.harriscomm.com
info@harriscomm.com

Martin Sternberg, Author
Darla Hudson, Customer Service
An abridged version of American Sign Language. A comprehensive dictionary with 4,400 illustrated signs. It has 500 new signs and 1,500 new illustrations. Third edition. Part #B103HC, and B103SC. *$24.00*
772 pages Paperback

2431 Another Door to Learning
Independent Publishers Group
814 N Franklin St
Chicago, IL 60610-3813
312-337-0747
800-888-4741
Fax: 312-337-5985
www.ipgbook.com
frontdesk@ipgbook.com

Judy Schwartz, Author
Stories of eleven atypical learners who got the help they needed to make a lasting difference in their lives.
ISBN 0-824513-85-1

2432 Ants in His Pants: Absurdities and Realities of Special Education
Corwin Press
2455 Teller Rd
Thousand Oaks, CA 91320-2218
805-499-9734
800-233-9936
Fax: 805-499-5323
www.corwin.com
order@corwin.com

Michael F Giangreco, Author
Kevin Ruelle, Editor
With wit, humor, and profound one liners, this book will transform your thinking as you take a lighter look at the often comical and occasionally harsh truth in the field of special education. This carefully crafted collection of 101 cartoons can be made into transparencies for staff development and training. *$20.95*
128 pages
ISBN 1-890455-42-3

2433 Attention-Deficit Hyperactivity Disorder
slosson Educational Publications
PO Box 544
538 Buffalo Road
East Aurora, NY 14052
716-652-0930
888-756-7766
Fax: 800-655-3840
www.slosson.com
slosson@slosson.com

Steve Slosson, President
Sue Larson, Author
The book addresses issues of theory and practice quickly, with compassion and practicality and, most importantly, is very effective. Well-grounded answers and suggestions which would facilitate behavior, learning, social-emotional functioning, and other factors in preschool and adolescence are discussed.

2434 Attention-Deficit Hyperactivity Disorder: A Handbook for Diagnosis and Treatment
Guilford Publications
72 Spring St
New York, NY 10012-4019   212-431-9800
                                 800-365-7006
                             Fax: 212-966-6708
                             www.guilford.com
                             info@guilford.com
Russell A Barkley, Author
Incorporates the latest findings on the nature, diagnosis, assessment, and treatment of ADHD. Clinicians, researchers, and students will find practical and richly referenced information on nearly every aspect of the disorder. *$55.00*
628 pages

2435 Autism and the Family: Problems, Prospects and Coping with the Disorder
Charles C Thomas Publisher
PO Box 19265
Springfield, IL 62794-9265   217-789-8980
                                    800-258-8980
                                Fax: 217-789-9130
                                www.ccthomas.com
                                books@ccthomas.com
David E Gray, Author
Publisher of Education and Special Education books. *$52.95*
198 pages Hardcover
ISBN 0-398068-43-7

2436 Backyards & Butterflies: Ways to Include Children with Disabilities
Brookline Books
Suite B-001
8 Trumbull Rd
Northampton, MA 01060   413-584-0184
                               800-666-2665
                           Fax: 413-5846184
                           www.brooklinebooks.com
                           brbooks@yahoo.com
Doreen Greenstein PhD, Author
This colorful, profusely illustrated book shows parents and others who work with disabled children how to design and build simple, inexpensive assistive technology devices that open up the world of outdoor experiences for these children. *$14.95*
72 pages Paperback
ISBN 1-571290-11-7

2437 Behavior Technology Guide Book
The Eden Family of Services
2 Merwick Rd
Princeton, NJ 08540-5711   609-987-0099
                              Fax: 609-987-0243
                              www.edenautism.org
                              info@edenau.orgtism
Peter H. Bell, President
Jennifer Bizub, COO
John Inzilla, CFO
Techniques for increasing and decreasing behavior using the principles of applied behavior analysis and related teaching strategies — discrete trial, shaping, task analysis and chaining.

2438 Children with Cerebral Palsy: A Parent's Guide
Therapro
225 Arlington St
Framingham, MA 01702-8723   508-872-9494
                                   800-257-5376
                               Fax: 508-875-2062
                               www.therapro.com
                               info@therapro.com
Elaine Geralis, Editor
This book explains what cerebral palsy is, and discusses its diagnosis and treatment. It also offers information and advice concerning daily care, early intervention, therapy, educational options and family life. *$18.95*
481 pages
ISBN 0-933149-82-4

2439 Children with Special Needs: A Resource Guide for Parents, Educators, Social Worker
Charles C Thomas
PO Box 19265
Springfield, IL 62794-9265   217-789-8980
                                    800-258-8980
                                Fax: 217-789-9130
                                www.ccthomas.com
                                books@ccthomas.com
Michael P Thomas, President
Publisher of Education and Special Education books. *$57.95*
234 pages Cloth
ISBN 0-398069-33-6

2440 Children with Tourette Syndrome
Woodbine House
6510 Bells Mill Rd
Bethesda, MD 20817-1636   301-897-3570
                                 800-843-7323
                             Fax: 301-897-5838
                             www.woodbinehouse.com
                             info@Woodbinehouse.com
Tracy Haerle, Editor
A guide for parents of children and teenagers with Tourette syndrome. Covers medical, educational, legal, family life, daily care, and emotional issues, as well as explanations of related conditions. *$14.95*
352 pages Paperback
ISBN 0-933149-39-5

2441 Classroom Success for the LD and ADHD Child
Therapro
225 Arlington St
Framingham, MA 01702-8723   508-872-9494
                                   800-257-5376
                               Fax: 508-875-2062
                               www.therapro.com
                               info@therapro.com
Suzanne H Stevens, Author
Helpful book for parents and therapists who work with children with learning disabilities. It addresses specific issues such as organization, homework and concentration. Stevens offers practical suggestions on adjusting teaching techniques, adapting texts, adjusting classroom management procedures and testing and grading fairly. *$13.95*
342 pages Revised
ISBN 0-895871-59-9

2442 Common Ground: Whole Language & Phonics Working Together
Educators Publishing Service
PO Box 9031
Cambridge, MA 02139-9031   800-225-5750
                              Fax: 888-440-2665
                              http://eps.schoolspecialty.com
                              customer_service@epsbooks.com
Priscilla L Vail, Author
Offers guidelines for reading instruction in the primary grades that combines whole language with multisensory phonics instruction. *$8.95*
88 pages
ISBN 0-838852-11-4

2443 Common Sense About Dyslexia
Special Needs Project
Ste H
324 State St
Santa Barbara, CA 93101-2364   818-718-9900
                                      800-333-6867
                                  Fax: 818-349-2027
                                  www.specialneeds.com
                                  books@specialneeds.com
Ann Marshall Huston, Author
Offers important, need-to-know information about dyslexia. *$26.50*
284 pages Hardcover
ISBN 0-819163-23-6

2444 Complete IEP Guide: How to Advocate for Your Special Ed Child
NOLO
950 Parker St
Berkeley, CA 94710-2524　　　　　　800-728-3555
　　　　　　　　　　　　　　　　　Fax: 800-645-0895
　　　　　　　　　　　　　　　　　www.nolo.com

Lawrence M Siegel, Author
This book has all the plain-English suggestions, strategies, resources and forms to develop an effective IEP. *$34.99*
402 pages paperback
ISBN 1-413305-10-5

2445 Complete Learning Disabilities Resource Library
Slosson Educational Publications
PO Box 544
538 Buffalo Road
East Aurora, NY 14052　　　　　　716-652-0930
　　　　　　　　　　　　　　　　　888-756-7766
　　　　　　　　　　　　　　　　　Fax: 800-655-3840
　　　　　　　　　　　　　　　　　www.slosson.com
　　　　　　　　　　　　　　　　　slosson@slosson.com

Joan M Harwell, Author
These volumes provide easy-to-use tips, techniques, and activities to help students with learning disabilities at all grade levels. *$29.95*
320 pages Paperback
ISBN 0-787972-32-0

2446 Computer & Web Resources for People with Disabilities: A Guide to...
Alliance for Technology Access
1119 Old Humboldt Road
Jackson, TN 38305　　　　　　　731-554-5282
　　　　　　　　　　　　　　　　　800-914-3017
　　　　　　　　　　　　　　　　　Fax: 731-554-5283
　　　　　　　　　　　　　　　　　TTY: 731-554-5284
　　　　　　　　　　　　　　　　　www.ataccess.org
　　　　　　　　　　　　　　　　　atainfo@ataccess.org

James Allison, President
Bob Van der Linde, VP
Mike Hewirr, Treasurer
This highly acclaimed book includes detailed descriptions of software, hardware and communication aids, plus a gold mine of published and online resources. *$20.75*
364 pages

2447 Conducting Individualized Education Program Meetings that Withstand Due Process
Charles C Thomas Publisher
PO Box 19265
Springfield, IL 62794-9265　　　　217-789-8980
　　　　　　　　　　　　　　　　　800-258-8980
　　　　　　　　　　　　　　　　　Fax: 217-789-9130
　　　　　　　　　　　　　　　　　www.ccthomas.com
　　　　　　　　　　　　　　　　　books@ccthomas.com

James N Hollis, Author
Publisher of Education and Special Education books. *$41.95*
171 pages Hardcover
ISBN 0-398068-46-1

2448 Connecting Students: A Guide to Thoughtful Friendship Facilitation
PEAK Parent Center
Ste 200
611 N Weber St
Colorado Springs, CO 80903-1072　　719-531-9400
　　　　　　　　　　　　　　　　　800-284-0251
　　　　　　　　　　　　　　　　　Fax: 719-531-9452
　　　　　　　　　　　　　　　　　www.peakparent.org
　　　　　　　　　　　　　　　　　info@peakparent.org

C Beth Schaffner, Author
Barbara Buswell, Co-Author

Offers real-life examples of how friendship facilitation can be implemented in natural ways in schools, neighborhoods, and communities. Perfect for anyone working to build classrooms and schools that ensure caring, acceptance and belonging for ALL students. *$11.00*
48 pages Paperback
ISBN 1-884720-01-3

2449 Contemporary Intellectual Assessment: Theories, Tests and Issues
Guilford Publications
72 Spring St
New York, NY 10012-4019　　　　212-431-9800
　　　　　　　　　　　　　　　　　800-365-7006
　　　　　　　　　　　　　　　　　Fax: 212-966-6708
　　　　　　　　　　　　　　　　　www.guilford.com
　　　　　　　　　　　　　　　　　info@guilford.com

Patti L Harrison, Editor
Judy L Genshaft, Editor
This unique volume provides a comprehensive conceptual and practical overview of the current state of the art of intellectual assessment. The book covers major theories of intelligence, methods of assessing human cognitive abilities, and issues related to the validity of current intelligence test batteries. *$75.00*
667 pages Hardcover
ISBN 1-593851-25-1

2450 Deciding What to Teach and How to Teach It Connecting Students through Curriculum and Instruction
PEAK Parent Center
Ste 200
611 N Weber St
Colorado Springs, CO 80903-1072　　719-531-9400
　　　　　　　　　　　　　　　　　800-284-0251
　　　　　　　　　　　　　　　　　Fax: 719-531-9452
　　　　　　　　　　　　　　　　　www.peakparent.org
　　　　　　　　　　　　　　　　　info@peakparent.org

Elizabeth Castagnera, Author
Douglas Fisher, Co-Author
Karen Rodifer, Co-Author
Provides exciting and practical resource tips to ensure that all students participate and learn successfully in secondary general education classrooms. Leads the reader through a step-by-step process for accessing general curriculum, making accommodations and modifications, and providing appropriate supports. Planning grids and concrete strategies make this an essential tool for both secondary educators and families. Support strategies are enhanced in this second edition *$14.00*
48 pages
ISBN 1-884720-19-6

2451 Defiant Children
Guilford Publications
72 Spring St
New York, NY 10012-4019　　　　212-431-9800
　　　　　　　　　　　　　　　　　800-365-7006
　　　　　　　　　　　　　　　　　Fax: 212-966-6708
　　　　　　　　　　　　　　　　　www.guilford.com
　　　　　　　　　　　　　　　　　info@guilford.com

Russell A Barkley, Author
Christine M Benton, Co-Author
This book is written expressly for parents who are struggling with an unyielding or combative child, helping them understand what causes defiance, when it becomes a problem, and how it can be resolved. Its clear eight-step program stresses consistency and cooperation, promoting changes through a system of praise, rewards, and mild punishment. Filled with helpful sidebars, charts, and checklists. *$39.00*
264 pages Paperback
ISBN 1-572301-23-6

2452 Developing Fine and Gross Motor Skills
Therapro
225 Arlington St
Framingham, MA 01702-8723
508-872-9494
800-257-5376
Fax: 508-875-2062
www.therapro.com
info@therapro.com

Donna Staisiunas Hurley, Author
This new home exercise program has dozens of beautifully illustrated, reproducible handouts for the parent, therapists, health care and child care workers. Each interval of 3 to 6 months in the child's development is divided into a fine motor and a gross motor section. Each section has several exercise sheets that guide parents in ways to develop specific motor skills that typically occur at that age level. Also includes practical information on how to guide parents when doing the exerecises.
157 pages
ISBN 0-890799-43-1

2453 Diamonds in the Rough
Slosson Educational Publications
PO Box 544
538 Buffalo Road
East Aurora, NY 14052
716-652-0930
888-756-7766
Fax: 800-655-3840
www.slosson.com
slosson@slosson.com

Peggy Strass Dias, Author
An invaluable multidisciplinary reference guide to learning disabilities. It is an indispensable resource for educators, health specialists, parents and librarians. The author has printed a clear picture of the archetypical learner with a step-by-step view of the learning disabled child. *$53.00*
156 pages Spiral-Bound
ISBN 0-970379-90-0

2454 Dictionary of Special Education & Rehabilitation
Love Publishing Company
Ste 2200
9101 E Kenyon Ave
Denver, CO 80237-1854
303-221-7333
Fax: 303-221-7444
www.lovepublishing.com
lpc@lovepublishing.com

Glenn A Vergason, Author
M L Anderegg, Co-Author
This updated edition of one of the most valuable resources in the field is over six years in the making incorporates hundreds of additions. It provides clear, understandable definitions of more than 2,000 terms unique to special education and rehabilitation. *$34.95*
210 pages Paperback
ISBN 0-891082-43-3

2455 Early Childhood Special Education: Birth to Three
Connecticut Assoc for Children and Adults with LD
Ste 15-5
25 Van Zant St
Norwalk, CT 06855-1729
203-838-5010
Fax: 203-866-6108
www.cacld.org
cacld@optonline.net

J B Jordan, Author
Beryl Kaufman, Executive Director
Resources on early childhood education. *$34.00*
262 pages Paperback
ISBN 0-865861-79-X

2456 Educating Deaf Children Bilingually
Harris Communications
15155 Technology Dr
Eden Prairie, MN 55344-2273
952-906-1180
800-825-9187
Fax: 866-870-7323
TDD: 952-906-1198
TTY: 800-825-9187
www.harriscomm.com
info@harriscomm.com

Darla Hudson, Customer Service
Shawn Neal Mahshie, Author
Perspectives and practices in educating deaf children with the goal of grade-level achievement in fluency in the languages of the deaf community, general society and of the home are discussed in this book. Part #B442. *$16.95*
262 pages

2457 Educating Students Who Have Visual Impairments with Other Disabilities
Brookes Publishing Company
PO Box 10624
Baltimore, MD 21285
410-337-9580
800-638-3775
Fax: 410-337-8539
www.brookespublishing.com
custserv@brookespublishing.com

Sharon Z Sacks PhD, Editor
Rosanne K Silberman EdD, Editor
This text provides techniques for facilitating functional learning in students with a wide range of visual impairments and multiple disabilities. *$49.95*
552 pages Paperback
ISBN 1-557662-80-0

2458 Effective Teaching Methods for Autistic Children
Charles C Thomas
PO Box 19265
Springfield, IL 62794-9265
217-789-8980
800-258-8980
Fax: 217-789-9130
www.ccthomas.com
books@ccthomas.com

Rosalind C Oppenheim, Author
Publisher of Education and Special Education books. *$21.25*
116 pages Hardcover
ISBN 0-398028-58-3

2459 Emergence: Labeled Autistic
Academic Therapy Publications
20 Commercial Blvd
Novato, CA 94949-6120
415-883-3314
800-422-7249
Fax: 888-287-9975
www.academictherapy.com
books@ccthomas.com

Jim Arena, President
Joanne Urban, Manager
An autistic individual shares her history, and includes her own suggestions for parents and professionals. Technical Appendix, which overviews recent treatment methods and more.

2460 Essential ASL: The Fun, Fast, and Simple Way to Learn American Sign Language
Harris Communications
15155 Technology Dr
Eden Prairie, MN 55344-2273
952-906-1180
800-825-6758
Fax: 866-870-7323
TDD: 952-906-1198
TTY: 800-825-9187
www.harriscomm.com
info@harriscomm.com

Darla Hudson, Customer Service
This pocket version contains more than 700 frequently used signs with 2,000 easy-to-follow illustrations. Also, 50 common phrases. Part #B511. *$7.95*
322 pages Paperback

2461 Family Guide to Assistive Technology
Federation for Children with Special Needs
Suite 1102
529 Main Street
Boston, MA 02109

617-236-7210
800-331-0688
Fax: 617-241-0330
www.fcsn.org
fcsninfo@fcsn.org

Katherine A Kelker, Author
Roger Holt, Co-Author
John Sullivan, Co-Author
This guide is intended to help parents learn more about assistive technology and how it can help their children. Includes tips for getting started, ideas about how and where to look for funding and contact information for software and equipment. *$15.95*
160 pages Paperback
ISBN 1-571290-74-5

2462 Family Place in Cyberspace
Alliance for Technology Access
1119 Old Humboldt Road
Jackson, TN 38305

731-554-5282
800-914-3017
Fax: 731-554-5283
TTY: 731-554-5284
www.ataccess.org
atainfo@ataccess.org

Allegra Wilson, Administrative Assistant
Todd Plummer, Development Manager
Includes We Can Play, a variety of suggestions and ideas for making play activities accessible to all. Available in English and Spanish. Access in Transition. Information and resources for students with disabilities who are facing the transition from public school to the next stage in life. Includes links and resources. Assistive Technology in K-12 Schools gives a range of information about integrating assistive technology into schools.

2463 Fine Motor Skills in Children with Downs Syndrome: A Guide for Parents and Professionals
Therapro
225 Arlington St
Framingham, MA 01702-8773

508-872-9494
800-257-5376
Fax: 508-875-2062
www.theraproducts.com
info@theraproducts.com

Maryanne Bruni, Author
Fine motor skills are the hand skills that allow us to do the things like hold a pencil, cut with scissors, eat with a fork, and use a computer. This practical guide shows parents and professionals how to help children with Downs syndrome from infancy to 12 years improve fine motor functioning. Includes many age appropriate activities for home or school, with step by step instructions and photos. Invaluable for families and professionals. *$19.95*
241 pages Paperback
ISBN 1-890627-67-4

2464 Fine Motor Skills in the Classroom: Screening & Remediation Strategies
Therapro
225 Arlington St
Framingham, MA 01702-8773

508-620-0022
800-257-5376
Fax: 508-620-0023
www.theraproducts.com
info@theraproducts.com

Arthur Berry, Author

The Give Yourself a Hand program, revised. Developed as a tool to facilitate consultation in the classroom. The manual consists of training modules, a screening to administer to an entire class, report formats for teachers and parents, and classroom and home remediation activities. The program is designed to include everyone involved in the education process and to make them aware of the opportunites offered by occupational therapy in the classroom.
96 pages

2465 Flying By the Seat of Your Pants: More Absurdities and Realities of Special Education
Corwin Press
2455 Teller Rd
Thousand Oaks, CA 91320-2218

805-499-9734
800-233-9936
Fax: 805-499-5323
www.corwin.com
order@corwin.com

Michael F Giangreco, Author
Kevin Ruelle, Co-Author
In the sequel to Ants in His Pants, Giangreco continues to stimulate the reader to think differently about some of our current educational practices and raise questions about specific issues surrounding special education. Whether an educator, parent or advocate for persons with disabilities, you will smile, laugh aloud and ponder the hidden truths playfully captured in these carefully crafted cartoons. Transparencies may be created directly from the book. *$20.95*
112 pages Paperback
ISBN 1-890455-41-5

2466 Gross Motor Skills Children with Down Syndrome: A Guide For Parents and Professionals
Therapro
225 Arlington St
Framingham, MA 01702-8723

508-872-9494
800-257-5376
Fax: 508-875-2062
www.therapro.com
info@therapro.com

Patricia C Winders, Author
Children with Down syndrome master basic gross motor skills, everything from rolling over to running, just as their peers do, but may need additional help. This guide describes and illustrates more than 100 easy to follow activities for parents and professionals to practice with infants and children from birth to age six. Checklists and statistics allow readers to track, plan and maximize a child's progress. *$18.95*
236 pages
ISBN 0-933149-81-6

2467 Guide for Parents on Hyperactivity in Children Fact Sheet
Learning Disabilities Association of America
4156 Library Rd
Pittsburgh, PA 15234-1349

412-341-1515
Fax: 412-344-0224
www.ldanatl.org
ldanatl@usaor.net

Klaus K Minde, Author
Describes difficulties faced by a child with ADHD. Elaborates on types of management and ends with a section called 'A Day With a Hyperactive Child: Possible Problems'. *$2.00*
23 pages

2468 Guide to Private Special Education
Porter Sargent Handbooks
2 LAN Drive
Suite 100
Westford, MA 01886

978-692-9708
Fax: 978-692-2304
www.portersargent.com
info@portersargent.com

Daniel P. McKeever, Senior Editor
Leslie Weston, Manager

Lists and describes educational programs for families and consultants looking to place elementary and secondary students with special needs in the best possible learning environments. *$75.00*
1152 pages Triannual
ISBN 0-875581-50-1

2469 Guidelines and Recommended Practices for Individualized Family Service Plan
Education Resources Information Center
Suite 500
655 15th St. NW
Washington, DC 20005
800-538-3742
www.eric.ed.gov
Mary J McGonigel, Author
Presents a growing consensus about best practices for comprehensive family-centered early intervention services as required by Part H of the Individuals with Disabilities Education Act. *$15.00*
208 pages

2470 Handbook for Implementing Workshops for Siblings of Special Needs Children
Special Needs Project
Ste H
324 State St
Santa Barbara, CA 93101-2364
818-718-9900
800-333-6867
Fax: 818-349-2027
www.specialneeds.com
books@specialneeds.com
Donald Meyer, Author
Based on three years of professional experience working with siblings ages 8 through 13 and their parents, this handbook provides guidelines and technologies for those who wish to start and conduct workshops for siblings. *$40.00*
65 pages

2471 Handbook of Research in Emotional and Behavioral Disorders
Guilford Publications
72 Spring St
New York, NY 10012-4019
212-431-9800
800-365-7006
Fax: 212-966-6708
www.guilford.com
info@guilford.com
Robert B Rutherford Jr, Author
Mary Magee Quinn, Co-Author
Sarup R Mathur, Editor
Integrates current knowledge on emotional and behavioral disorders in the school setting. Also, emphasizes the importance of interdisciplinary collaboration in service provision and delineates best-practice guidelines for research. *$38.00*
622 pages Paperback
ISBN 1-593854-71-4

2472 Handling the Young Child with Cerebral Palsy at Home
Therapro
225 Arlington St
Framingham, MA 01702-8723
508-872-9494
800-257-5376
Fax: 508-875-2062
www.therapro.com
info@therapro.com
Nancie R Finnie, Author
This guide for parents remains a classic book on handling their cerebral palsied child during all activities of daily living. It has been said that its message is so important that it should be read by all those caring for such children including doctors, therapists, teachers and nurses. Many simple line drawings illustrate handling problems and solutions. *$55.95*
320 pages paperback
ISBN 0-750605-79-0

2473 Help Build a Brighter Future: Children at Risk for LD in Child Care Centers
Learning Disabilities Association of America
4156 Library Rd
Pittsburgh, PA 15234-1349
412-341-1515
Fax: 412-344-0224
www.ldanatl.org
ldanatl@usaor.net
Offers information for parents and professionals caring for the learning disabled child. *$3.00*

2474 Help Me to Help My Child
Hachette Book Group
3 Center Plz
Boston, MA 02108-2003
800-759-0190
Fax: 800-331-1664
www.hachettebookgroup.com
customer.service@hbgusa.com
Jill Bloom, Author
Contains nontechnical information on testing, advocacy, legal issues, instructional practices, and social-emotional development, as well as a resource list and bibliography.
324 pages Hardcover
ISBN 0-316099-81-3

2475 Help for the Hyperactive Child: A Good Sense Guide for Parents
Learning Disabilities Association of America
4156 Library Rd
Pittsburgh, PA 15234-1349
412-341-1515
Fax: 412-344-0224
www.ldanatl.org
ldanatl@usaor.net
William G Crook, Author
A practical guide; offering parents of ADHD children alternatives to Ritalin. *$16.95*
245 pages
ISBN 0-933478-18-6

2476 Help for the Learning Disabled Child
Slosson Educational Publications
PO Box 544
538 Buffalo Road
East Aurora, NY 14052
716-652-0930
888-756-7766
Fax: 800-655-3840
www.slosson.com
slosson@slosson.com
Lou Stewart, Author
An easy-to-read text describes observable behaviors, offers remediation techniques, materials, and specific test to assist in further diagnosis.

2477 Helping Your Child with Attention-Deficit Hyperactivity Disorder
Learning Disabilities Association of America
4156 Library Rd
Pittsburgh, PA 15234-1349
412-341-1515
Fax: 412-344-0224
www.ldanatl.org
ldanatl@usaor.net
M Fowler, Author

2478 Helping Your Hyperactive Child
Connecticut Assoc for Children and Adults with LD
Ste 15-5
25 Van Zant St
Norwalk, CT 06855-1729
203-838-5010
Fax: 203-866-6108
www.cacld.org
cacld@optonline.net
Beryl Kaufman, Executive Director
John Taylor, Author

A large, comprehensive book for parents, covering everything from techniques pertaining to sibling rivalry to coping with marital stresses. Contains thorough discussions of various treatments: nutritional, medical and educational. Also is an excellent source of advice and information for parents of kids with ADHD.
496 pages Hardcover
ISBN 1-559580-13-5

2479 **How the Special Needs Brain Learns**
Corwin Press
2455 Teller Rd
Thousand Oaks, CA 91320-2218   805-499-9734
                                          800-233-9936
                                     Fax: 805-499-5323
                                          www.corwin.com
                                          order@corwin.com

David A Sousa, Author
Research on the brain function of students with various learning challenges. Practical classroom activities and strategies, such as how to build self-esteem, how to work in groups, and strategies for engagement and retention. Focuses on the most commmon challenges to learning for many students. *$35.95*
248 pages Paperback
ISBN 1-412949-87-4

2480 **How to Get Services by Being Assertive**
Family Resource Center on Disabilities
Room 300
20 E Jackson Blvd
Chicago, IL 60604-2265   312-939-3513
                                           800-952-4199
                                      Fax: 312-854-8980
                                      TDD: 312-939-3519
                                           www.frcd.org
                                           info@frcd.org

Charlotte Jardins, Executive Director
Myra Christian, Contact
Gloria Mikucki, Contact
A 100 page manual that demonstrates positive assertiveness techniques. Price includes postage and handling. *$12.00*

2481 **How to Organize Your Child and Save Your Sanity**
Learning Disabilities Association of America
4156 Library Rd
Pittsburgh, PA 15234-1349   412-341-1515
                                      Fax: 412-344-0224
                                           www.ldanatl.org
                                           ldanatl@usaor.net

Ruth Brown, Author
13 pages $3.00

2482 **How to Organize an Effective Parent-Advocacy Group and Move Bureaucracies**
Family Resource Center on Disabilities
Room 300
20 E Jackson Blvd
Chicago, IL 60604-2265   312-939-3513
                                           800-952-4199
                                      Fax: 312-854-8980
                                      TDD: 312-939-3519
                                           www.frcd.org
                                           info@frcd.org

Charlotte Jardins, Executive Director
Myra Christian, Contact
Gloria Mikucki, Contact
A 100-page handbook that gives step-by-step directions for organizing parent support groups from scratch. *$12.00*

2483 **How to Own and Operate an Attention Deficit Disorder**
Learning Disabilities Association of America
4156 Library Rd
Pittsburgh, PA 15234-1349   412-341-1515
                                      Fax: 412-344-0224
                                           www.ldanatl.org
                                           ldanatl@usaor.net

Debra W Maxey, Author

Clear, informative and sensitive introduction to ADHD. Packed with practical things to do at home and school, the author offers her insight as a professional and mother of a son with ADHD. *$8.95*
43 pages

2484 **Hyperactive Children Grown Up**
Guilford Publications
72 Spring St
New York, NY 10012-4019   212-431-9800
                                           800-365-7006
                                      Fax: 212-966-6708
                                           www.guilford.com
                                           info@guilford.com

Gabrielle Weiss, Author
Long considered a standard in the field, this book explores what happens to hyperactive children when they grow into adulthood. Updated and expanded, this second edition describes new developments in ADHD, current psychological treatments of ADHD, contemporary perspectives on the use of medications, and assessment, diagnosis and treatment of ADHD adults. *$35.00*
473 pages Paperback
ISBN 0-898625-96-3

2485 **If it is to Be, It is Up to Me to Do it!**
AVKO Educational Research Foundation
Ste W
3084 Willard Rd
Birch Run, MI 48415-9404   810-686-9283
                                           866-285-6612
                                      Fax: 810-686-1101
                                           www.avko.org
                                           webmaster@avko.org

Don Mc Cabe, Research Director/Author
This is a tutors' book that can be used by anyone who can read this paragraph. It also contains the student's response pages. It is especially good to use to help an older child or adult. It uses the same basic format as Sequential Spelling I except it has the sentences to be read along with the word to be spelled. The students get to correct their own mistakes immediately. This way they quickly learn that mistakes are opportunities to learn. *$19.95*
96 pages
ISBN 1-564007-42-1

2486 **In Their Own Way: Discovering and Encouraging Your Child's Learning**
Special Needs Project
Ste H
324 State St
Santa Barbara, CA 93101-2364   818-718-9900
                                           800-333-6867
                                      Fax: 818-349-2027
                                           www.specialneeds.com
                                           books@specialneeds.com

Dr Thomas Armstrong, Author
An unconventional teacher has written a very popular book for a wide audience. It's customary to be categorical about youngsters who learn conventionally/are normal/are OK — and those who don't/who need special ed/are learning disabled. *$8.37*
224 pages Paperback
ISBN 0-791716-67-8

2487 **In Time and with Love**
Special Needs Project
Ste H
324 State St
Santa Barbara, CA 93101-2364   818-718-9900
                                           800-333-6867
                                      Fax: 818-349-2027
                                           www.specialneeds.com
                                           books@specialneeds.com

Marilyn Segal, Author
Wendy Masi, Co-Author
Roni Leiderman, Co-Author

Play and parenting techniques for children with disabilities.
$18.95
256 pages Paperback

2488 In the Mind's Eye
Prometheus Books
59 John Glenn Drive
Amherst, NY 14228-2197

716-691-0133
800-421-0351
Fax: 716-691-0137
www.prometheusbooks.com
marketing@prometheusbooks.com

Thomas West, Author
The second edition will review a number of recent developments, which support and extend the ideas and perspectives originally set forth in the first edition. Among these will be brief profiles of two dyslexic scientists known for their ability to generate, in quite different fields, powerful but unexpected innovations and discoveries. *$25.98*
440 pages
ISBN 1-591027-00-3

2489 Inclusion: A Practical Guide for Parents
Corwin Press
2455 Teller Rd
Thousand Oaks, CA 91320-2218

805-499-9734
800-233-9936
Fax: 805-499-5323
www.corwin.com
order@corwin.com

Lorraine O Moore, Author
This comprehensive resource answers parent questions related to inclusive education and provides the tools to promote and enhance their child's learning. This publication includes practical strategies, exercises, questionnaires and do-it-yourself graphs to assist parents with their child's learning. Beneficial for parents, psychologists, social workers, and educators. *$28.95*
152 pages
ISBN 1-890455-44-6

2490 Inclusion: Strategies for Working with Young Children
Corwin Press
2455 Teller Rd
Thousand Oaks, CA 91320-2218

805-499-9734
800-233-9936
Fax: 805-499-5323
www.corwin.com
order@corwin.com

Lorraine O Moore, Author
Developed for early childhood through grade two educators and parents, this comprehensive developmentally focused publication focuses on the whole child. Hundreds of developmentally-based strategies help young children learn about feelings, empathy, resolving conflicts, communication, large/small motor development, prereading, writing and math strategies are included, plus much more. Excellent training tool. *$28.95*
146 pages
ISBN 1-890455-33-4

2491 Inclusive Elementary Schools
PEAK Parent Center
Ste 200
611 N Weber St
Colorado Springs, CO 80903-1072

719-531-9400
800-284-0251
Fax: 719-531-9452
www.peakparent.org
info@peakparent.org

Douglas Fisher, Author
Nancy Frey, Co-Author
Caren Sax, Co-Author

Walks readers through a state of the art, step-by-step process to determine what and how to teach elementary school students with disabilities in general education classrooms. Highlights strategies for accommodating and modifying assignments and activities by using core curriculum. Complete with user-friendly sample forms and creative support strategies, this is an essential text for elementary educators and parents. *$13.00*
45 pages Paperback
ISBN 1-884720-21-8

2492 Innovations in Family Support for People with Learning Disabilities
Brookes Publishing Company
PO Box 10624
Baltimore, MD 21285

410-337-9580
800-638-3775
Fax: 410-337-8539
www.brookespublishing.com
custserv@pbrookes.com

Barbara Coyne Cutler, Author
272 pages Paperback $22.00
ISBN 1-870335-15-5

2493 Interventions for ADHD: Treatment in Developmental Context
Guilford Publications
72 Spring St
New York, NY 10012-4019

212-431-9800
800-365-7006
Fax: 212-966-6708
www.guilford.com
info@guilford.com

Phyllis Anne Teeter, Author
This book takes a lifespan perspective on ADHD, dispelling the notion that it is only a disorder of childhood and enabling clinicians to develop effective and appropriate interventions for preschoolers, school-age children, adolescents, and adults. The author reviews empirically-and clinically-based treatment interventions including psychopharmacology, behavior management, parent/teacher training, and self-management techniques. *$40.00*
378 pages Hardcover
ISBN 1-572303-84-0

2494 Invisible Disability: Understanding Learning Disabilities in the Context of Health & Edu.
Learning Disabilities Association of America
4156 Library Rd
Pittsburgh, PA 15234-1349

412-341-1515
Fax: 412-344-0224
www.ldanatl.org
ldanatl@usaor.net

Pasquale Accardo, Author
50 pages Paperback $9.00
ISBN 0-937846-39-2

2495 It's Your Turn Now
Harris Communications
15155 Technology Dr
Eden Prairie, MN 55344-2273

952-906-1180
800-825-6758
Fax: 866-870-7323
TDD: 952-906-1198
TTY: 800-825-9187
www.harriscomm.com
info@harriscomm.com

Darla Hudson, Customer Service
Using dialogue journals with deaf students help the students learn to enjoy communicating ideas, information, and feelings through reading and writing. The book reviews teacher's questions and answers, frustrations and successes. Part #B584. *$14.95*
130 pages

2496 Key Concepts in Personal Development
Marsh Media
PO Box 8082
Shawnee Mission
Kansas City, MO 66208

800-821-3303
Fax: 866-333-7421
www.marshmedia.com
info@marshmedia.com

Puberty Education for Students with Special Needs. Comprehensive, gender-specific kits and supplemental parent packets address human sexuality education for children with mild to moderate developmental disabilities. *$19.95*

2497 Ladders to Literacy: A Kindergarten Activity Book
Brookes Publishing Company
PO Box 10624
Baltimore, MD 21285

410-337-9580
800-638-3775
Fax: 410-337-8539
www.brookespublishing.com
custserv@brookspublishing.com

Rollanda E O'Connor, Author
Angela Notari Syverson, Co-Author
Patricia F Vadasy, Co-Author
The kindergarten activities are designed for higher developmental levels, focusing on preacademic skills, early literacy development, and early reading development. Goals and scaffolding are more intense as children learn to recognize letters, match sounds with letters, and develop phonological awareness and the alphabetic principle. *$49.95*
337 pages Spiral bound
ISBN 1-557668-32-9

2498 Ladders to Literacy: A Preschool Activity Book
Brookes Publishing Company
PO Box 10624
Baltimore, MD 21285

410-337-9580
800-638-3775
Fax: 410-337-8539
www.brookespublishing.com
custserv@brookespublishing.com

Rollanda E O'Connor, Author
Angela Notari Syverson, Co-Author
The preschool activity book targets basic preliteracy skills such as orienting children toward printed materials and teaching letter sounds. It also provides professionals (and parents) with developmentally appropriate and ecologically valid assessment procedures — informal observation guidelines, structured performance samples, and a checklist — for measuring children's learning. *$49.95*
486 pages Spiral bound
ISBN 1-557669-13-9

2499 Landmark School's Language-Based Teaching Guides
Landmark School
429 Hale St
PO Box 227
Prides Crossing, MA 01965

978-236-3216
Fax: 978-927-7268
www.landmarkoutreach.org
outreach@landmarkschool.org

Robert Broudo, Author
Landmark School's Language-Based Teaching Guides provide research-based practical teaching strategies for teachers and parents working with students who have learning disabilities. Topics inlcude study skills, expressive langage skills, writing, mathematics. *$30.00*
104 pages Paperback
ISBN 0-962411-96-1

2500 Language and Literacy Learning in Schools
Guilford Publications
72 Spring St
New York, NY 10012-4019

212-431-9800
800-365-7006
Fax: 212-966-6708
www.guilford.com
info@guilford.com

Elaine R Stillman, Author
Louise C Wilkinson, Co-Author
Interweaves the voices of classroom teachers, speech-language pathologists whos children learning to become literate in English as a first or second language, and researchers from multiple disciplines. *$27.00*
366 pages Hardcover
ISBN 1-593854-69-2

2501 Language-Related Learning Disabilities
Brookes Publishing Company
PO Box 10624
Baltimore, MD 21285

410-337-9580
800-638-3775
Fax: 410-337-8539
www.brookespublishing.com
custserv@pbrookes.com

Adele Gerber, Author
416 pages Hardcover $47.00
ISBN 1-557660-53-0

2502 Learning Disabilities & ADHD: A Family Guide to Living and Learning Together
John Wiley & Sons Inc
111 River Street
Hoboken, NJ 07030-5774

201-748-6000
Fax: 201-748-6088
www.wiley.com
info@wiley.com

Betty Osman, Author
228 pages paperback $14.95
ISBN 0-471155-10-1

2503 Learning Disabilities A to Z
Simon and Schuster
1230 Avenue of the Americas
New York, NY 10020-1513

212-698-7000
800-233-2336
www.simonandschuster.biz
shop.feedback@simonsays.com

Corinne Smith, Author
Lisa Strick, Co-Author
Brings the best of recent research and educational experience to parents, teachers and caregivers who are responsible for children with information processing problems. Corinne Smith and Lisa Strick provide a comprehensive guide to the causes, indentification and treatment of learning disabilities. You will learn how these subtle neurological disorders can have a major impact on a child's development, both in and out of school. *$17.00*
416 pages Paperback
ISBN 0-684844-68-0

2504 Learning Disabilities: Lifelong Issues
Brookes Publishing Company
PO Box 10624
Baltimore, MD 21285

410-337-9580
800-638-3775
Fax: 410-337-8539
www.brookespublishing.com
custserv@brookespublishing.com

Shirley C Cramer, Author
William Ellis, Editor
Based on the diverse, representative viewpoints of educators, practitioners, policy makers, and adults with learning disabilities, this volume sets forth an agenda for improving the educational and ultimately, social and economic, futures of people with learning disabilities. *$36.00*
310 pages Paperback
ISBN 1-557662-40-1

2505 Learning Disabilities: Literacy, and Adult Education
Brookes Publishing Company
PO Box 10624
Baltimore, MD 21285

410-337-9580
800-638-3775
Fax: 410-337-8539
www.brookespublishing.com
custserv@pbrookes.com

Susan A Vogel PhD, Author
Stephen Reder PhD, Editor
This book focuses on adults with severe learning disabilities and the educators who work with them. *$49.95*
377 pages Paperback
ISBN 1-557663-47-5

2506 Learning Disabilities: Theories, Diagnosis and Teaching Strategies
Houghton Mifflin
222 Berkeley St
Boston, MA 02116-3748   617-351-5000
                                  Fax: 617-351-1119
                       www.houghtonmifflinbooks.com
                  TradeCustomerService@hmhpub.com
J Lerner, Author
Theories on learning disabilities.
ISBN 0-395794-86-2

2507 Learning Outside The Lines: Two Ivy League Students with Learning Disabilities and ADHD
Fireside
1230 Avenue of the Americas
New York, NY 10020-1513   212-698-7000
                                      800-233-2336
                         www.simonandschuster.biz
                    shop.feedback@simonsays.com
Edward M Hallowell, Author
Jonathan Mooney, Co-Author
David Cole, Co-Author
Takes you on a personal empowerment and profound educational change, proving once again that rules sometimes need to be broken. *$14.00*
288 pages
ISBN 0-684865-98-X

2508 Legacy of the Blue Heron: Living with Learning Disabilities
Oxton House Publishers
124 Main Street
Suite 203
Farmington, ME 04938   207-779-1923
                                      800-539-7323
                                 Fax: 207-779-0623
                            www.oxtonhouse.com
                            info@oxtonhouse.com
William Berlinghoff PhD, Managing Editor
Cheryl Martin, Marketing
Debra Richards, Office Manager
This book is available in soft cover or as a six-cassette audiobook. It is an engaging personal account by a severe dyslexic who became a successful engineer, business man, boat builder, and president of the Learning Disabilities Association of America. Drawing on his life experiences, the author presents a rich array of wise, common-sense advice for dealing with learning disabilities.
256 pages Paperback
ISBN 1-881929-20-5

2509 Let's Learn About Deafness
Harris Communications
15155 Technology Dr
Eden Prairie, MN 55344-2273   952-906-1180
                                      800-825-6758
                                 Fax: 866-870-7323
                                 TDD: 952-906-1198
                                 TTY: 800-825-9187
                              www.harriscomm.com
                              info@harriscomm.com
Darla Hudson, Customer Service
Hands-on activities, games, bulletin board displays, surveys, quizzes, craft projects, and skits used to help teachers and their students become more aware of deafness and its implications are included in this book. Part #B253. *$16.95*
82 pages

2510 Life Beyond the Classroom: Transition Strategies for Young People with Disabilities
Brookes Publishing Company
PO Box 10624
Baltimore, MD 21285   410-337-9580
                                      800-638-3775
                                 Fax: 410-337-8539
                         www.brookespublishing.com
                  custserv@brookespublishing.com
Paul Wehman, Author
Community living, leisure activities, personal relationships as well as employment. Planning with community, individualized, state and local governments, curriculum for transition, job development and placement, independent living plans for people with mild MR, severe disabilities, LD, physical and health impairments, and traumatic brain injury. *$74.95*
719 pages Hardcover
ISBN 1-557667-52-7

2511 Living with a Learning Disability
Southern Illinois University Press
1915 University Press Dr
Carbondale, IL 62901-4323   618-453-2281
                                      800-621-2736
                                 Fax: 800-453-1221
                              www.siupress.com
                  custserv@press.uchicago.edu
Barbara Martin, Director
Amy Etcheson, Marketing and Sales Manager
This book presents the kinds of adaptations needed for educating, communicating with, and parenting the child, the adolescent, and the young adult with learning disabilities. Deals with such issues as relationships, the legal process, implications for the professional, juvenile delinquency, and the future.
17.5 pages
ISBN 0-809316-68-4

2512 Making the Writing Process Work: Strategies for Composition & Self-Regulation
Brookline Books
Suite B-001
8 Trumbull Rd
Northampton, MA 01060   413-584-0184
                                      800-666-2665
                                 Fax: 413-5846184
                           www.brooklinebooks.com
                           brbooks@yahoo.com
Karen R Harris, Author
Steve Graham, Co-Author
Presents cognitive strategies for writing sequences of specific steps which make the writing process clearer and enable students to organize their thoughts about the writing task. *$24.95*
239 pages Paperback
ISBN 1-571290-10-9

2513 McGraw Hill Companies
PO Box 182604
Columbus, OH 43272-2604   877-833-5524
                                 Fax: 614-759-3749
                              www.mcgraw-hill.com
                  customer.service@mcgraw-hill.com
Henry Hirschberg, President
Corrective reading program, helps students master the essential decoding and comprehension skills.

2514 Me! A Curriculum for Teaching Self-Esteem Through an Interest Center
Connecticut Assoc for Children and Adults with LD
Ste 15-5
25 Van Zant St
Norwalk, CT 06855-1729   203-838-5010
                                 Fax: 203-866-6108
                                 www.cacld.org
                                 cacld@optonline.com
Beryl Kaufman, Executive Director
A curriculum for the professional. *$18.50*

2515 Meeting the Needs of Students of ALL Abilities
Corwin Press
2455 Teller Rd
Thousand Oaks, CA 91320-2218   805-499-9734
                                                                 800-233-9936
                                                   Fax: 805-499-5323
                                                   www.corwin.com
                                                   order@corwin.com

Colleen Capper, Author
Elise Fattura, Co-Author
Maureen Keyes, Co-Author
Step-by-step handbook offers practical strategies for administrators, teachers, policymakers and parents who want to shift from costly special learning programs for a few students, to excellent educational services for all students and teachers, and adapting curriculum and instruction. *$75.95*
224 pages Hardcover
ISBN 0-761975-00-4

2516 Misunderstood Child
Connecticut Assoc for Children and Adults with LD
Ste 15-5
25 Van Zant St
Norwalk, CT 06855-1729   203-838-5010
                                                   Fax: 203-866-6108
                                                   www.cacld.org
                                                   cacld@optonline.net
Beryl Kaufman, Executive Director
A guide for parents of learning disabled children. *$14.95*
448 pages Paperback
ISBN 0-307338-63-0

2517 Negotiating the Special Education Maze
Woodbine House
6510 Bells Mill Rd
Bethesda, MD 20817-1636   301-897-3570
                                                   800-843-7323
                                                   Fax: 301-897-5838
                                                   www.woodbinehouse.com
                                                   info@woodbinehouse.com
Stephen Chitwood, Author
Deidre Hayden, Co-Author
Now in its fourth edition, Negotiating the Special Education Maze is one of the best tools available to parents and teachers for developing an effective special education program for their child or student. Every step is explained, from eligibility and evaluation to the Individualized Education Program and beyond. *$16.95*
264 pages Paperback
ISBN 0-933149-72-7

2518 New Language of Toys
Woodbine House
6510 Bells Mill Rd
Bethesda, MD 20817-1636   301-897-3570
                                                   800-843-7323
                                                   Fax: 301-897-5838
                                                   www.woodbinehouse.com
                                                   info@woodbinehouse.com
Sue Schwartz PhD, Author
This revised and updated edition presents a fun, hands-on approach to developing communication skills in children with disabilities using everyday toys. There's a fresh assortment of toys and books, as well as newe chapters on computer technology and language learning, videotapes and television. *$16.95*
289 pages Paperback 7x10
ISBN 0-933149-73-5

2519 No One to Play with: The Social Side of Learning Disabilities
Connecticut Assoc for Children and Adults with LD
Ste 15-5
25 Van Zant St
Norwalk, CT 06855-1729   203-838-4353
                                                   Fax: 203-866-6108
                                                   www.cacld.org
                                                   cacld@juno.com

Marie Armstrong, Information Specialist
Beryl Kaufman, Executive Director
Your child suffers from a learning disability and you have read reams on how to improve on her academic skills and now want to address his or her social needs. *$13.00*

2520 Nobody's Perfect: Living and Growing with Children who Have Special Needs
Brookes Publishing Company
PO Box 10624
Baltimore, MD 21285   410-337-9580
                                                   800-638-3775
                                                   Fax: 410-337-8539
                                                   www.brookespublishing.com
                                                   custserv@brookespublishing.com
Paul H Brookes, President
Melissa A Behm, VP
Study of four families with children who have special needs. How they all adapted in surviving, how they care for the child, family, parents and siblings. How families react and relate. What it is like in community and extended family? Basic issues dicussed: self-esteem, separating parent from the adult with special needs and other issues. *$23.00*
352 pages Paperback
ISBN 1-557661-43-X

2521 Opening Doors: Connecting Students to Curriculum, Classmate, and Learning, Second Edition
PEAK Parent Center
Ste 200
611 N Weber St
Colorado Springs, CO 80903-1072   719-531-9400
                                                   800-284-0251
                                                   Fax: 719-531-9452
                                                   www.peakparent.org
                                                   info@peakparent.org
Barbara Buswell, Author
Beth Schaffner, Co-Author
Alison B Seyler, Co-Author
This innovative text contains practical how-to's for including and supporting students with disabilities in the general education classroom. It explores the processes, thinking, and approaches that successful implementers of inclusion have used. Written for educators and parents of both elementary and secondary students, topics include instructional strategies, curriculum modifications, behavior, standards, literacy, and providing support. *$13.00*
ISBN 0-884720-12-9

2522 Optimizing Special Education: How Parents Can Make a Difference
Insight Books
233 Spring St
New York, NY 10013-1522   212-460-1500
                                                   800-221-9369
                                                   Fax: 212-647-1898
                                                   www.springer.com
                                                   info@springer.com
Rudiger Gebauer, Owner
The author shows families how to use education laws to increase services or change services to suit a child's needs. Book contains personal anecdotes and balanced viewpoint of parent and professional relationships. *$26.50*
300 pages
ISBN 0-306443-23-6

2523 Out of Sync Child: Recognizing and Coping with Sensory Integration Dysfunction
Therapro
225 Arlington St
Framingham, MA 01702-8723   508-872-9494
                                                   800-257-5376
                                                   Fax: 508-875-2062
                                                   www.therapro.com
                                                   info@therapro.com
Karen Conrad, Owner

Finally, a parent-friendly book about sensory integration (SI) clearly written to explain SI dysfunction from the perspective of a teacher who has worked extensively with an OT. Part I deals with recognizing SI dysfunction. Part II addresses coping with SI dysfunction.

2524 Out of the Mouths of Babes: Discovering the Developmental Significance of the Mouth
Therapro
225 Arlington St
Framingham, MA 01702-8723

508-872-9494
800-257-5376
Fax: 508-875-2062
www.therapro.com
info@therapro.com

Karen Conrad, Owner
Help children who have difficulty with focusing, staying alert, or being calm with these simple techniqes and activities. Learn how behavior is affected by suck/swallow/breathe (SSB) synchrony with suggestions for correcting specific problems. This informal writing style and many illustrations make it a great resource for parents, teachers and therapists.

2525 Parent Manual
Federation for Children with Special Needs
Suite 1102
529 Main Street
Boston, MA 02109

617-236-7210
800-331-0688
Fax: 617-241-0330
TDD: 617-236-7210
www.fcsn.org
fcsninfo@fcsn.org

Rich Robison, President
Outlines parents' and children's rights in special education as guaranteed by Chapter 766, the Massachusetts special education law, and the Individuals with Disabilities Education Act (IDEA), the federal special education law *$25.00*
75 pages

2526 Play Therapy
Books on Special Children
PO Box 3378
Amherst, MA 01004-3378

413-256-8164
Fax: 413-256-8896
www.boscbooks.com
irene@boscbooks.com

Irene Slovak, Founder
Kevin John O'Connor, Author
Leading authorities present various theoretical models of play therapy treatment and application. Case studies on how various treatments are applied. *$44.95*
350 pages Hardcover
ISBN 0-471106-38-0

2527 Positive Self-Talk for Children
PO Box 305
Congers, NY 10920

845-638-1236
Fax: 845-638-0847
www.boscbooks.com/
irene@boscbooks.com

D Bloch, Author
This book teaches positive talk and ideas to achieve positive self-esteem. Use this as a refererence in specific situations: ie: fears on 1st day of school, doctor's visit. Covers cases, includes specific dialogue.

2528 Practical Parent's Handbook on Teaching Children with Learning Disabilities
Charles C Thomas
PO Box 19265
Springfield, IL 62794-9265

217-789-8980
800-258-8980
Fax: 217-789-9130
www.ccthomas.com
books@ccthomas.com

Michael P Thomas, President

Publisher of Education and Special Education books. *$65.95*
308 pages Cloth
ISBN 0-398059-03-9

2529 Raising Your Child to be Gifted: Successful Parents
Brookline Books
Suite B-001
8 Trumbull Rd
Northampton, MA 01060

413-584-0184
800-666-2665
Fax: 413-5846184
www.brooklinebooks.com
brbooks@yahoo.com

James R Campbell PhD, Author
Moving beyond the usual genetic eplanations for giftedness, Dr. James Campbell presents powerful evidence that it is parental involvement- very specific methods of working with and nurturing a child which increases the child's chances of being gifted. *$21.95*
275 pages Paperback
ISBN 1-571290-94-X

2530 Right from the Start: Behavioral Intervention for Young Children with Autism: A Guide
Therapro
225 Arlington St
Framingham, MA 01702-8723

508-872-9494
800-257-5376
Fax: 508-875-2062
www.therapro.com
info@therapro.com

Karen Conrad, Owner
This informative and user-friendly guide helps parents and service providers explore programs that use early intensive behavioral intervention for young children with autism and related disorders. Within these programs, many children improve in intellectual, social and adaptive functioning, enabling them to move on to regular elementary and preschools. Benefits all children, but primarily useful for children age five and younger.
215 pages

2531 SMARTS: A Study Skills Resource Guide
Connecticut Assoc. for Children and Adults with LD
Ste 15-5
25 Van Zant St
Norwalk, CT 06855-1729

203-838-5010
Fax: 203-866-6108
www.cacld.org
cacld@juno.com

Marie Armstrong, Information Specialist
Beryl Kaufman, Executive Director
A comprehensive teachers handbook of activities to help students develop study skills. *$20.50*

2532 School-Based Home Developmental PE Program
Therapro
225 Arlington St
Framingham, MA 01702-8723

508-872-9494
800-257-5376
Fax: 508-875-2062
www.therapro.com
info@therapro.com

Karen Conrad, Owner
A wire bound flip book. Comprehensive developmental physical education program indentifies and improves motor ability right down to the specific sensory and perceptual motor areas for children. Has what you need: assessment; parent involvement; understandable directions; examples; and sample letters to parents. Includes fun sheets that parents/professionals can use with children. Activities are for vestibular integration, body awareness, eye-hand coordination, and fine motor manipulation.

2533 **Seeing Clearly**
Therapro
225 Arlington St
Framingham, MA 01702-8773
508-872-9494
800-257-5376
Fax: 508-875-2062
www.theraproducts.com
info@theraproducts.com
Karen Conrad, Owner
This booklet is chock-full of great information regarding vision and visual perceptual problems and activities designed to improve visual skills of both adults and children. Begins with an overview of the development of vision with a checklist of warning signs of vision problems. 25 eye game activities are divided into those for Eye Movements, Suspended Ball, Chalkboard and Visualization (e.g. Pictures in your Mind, Spelling Comprehension, etc.)

2534 **Self-Perception: Organizing Functional Information Workbook**
Therapro
225 Arlington St
Framingham, MA 01702-8773
508-872-9494
800-257-5376
Fax: 508-875-2062
www.therapro.com
info@theraproducts.com
Karen Conrad, Owner
Kathleen Anderson MS CCC-SP, Author
Pamela Crow Miller, Co-Author
Recognizing human and animal body parts, discriminating between right and left, and exploring attitudes, emotions, humor and personal problem-solving.

2535 **Sensory Integration and the Child: Understanding Hidden Sensory Challenges**
Therapro
225 Arlington St
Framingham, MA 01702-8773
508-872-9494
800-257-5376
Fax: 508-875-2062
www.therapro.com
info@theraproducts.com
Karen Conrad, Owner
Designed to educate parents, students, and beginning therapists in sensory integration treatment.

2536 **Sensory Integration: Theory and Practice**
Therapro
225 Arlington St
Framingham, MA 01702-8773
508-872-9494
800-257-5376
Fax: 508-875-2062
www.therapro.com
info@theraproducts.com
Karen Conrad, Owner
This is the very latest in sensory integration theory and practice. The entire volume achieves an admirable balance between theory and practice, covering sensory integration theory, various kinds of sensory integrative dysfunction and comprehensive discussions of assessment, direct treatment, consultation and continuing research issues.

2537 **Siblings of Children with Autism: A Guide for Families**
Therapro
225 Arlington St
Framingham, MA 01702-8773
508-872-9494
800-257-5376
Fax: 508-875-2062
www.therapro.com
info@theraproducts.com
Karen Conrad, Owner
An invaluable guide to understanding sibling relationships, how they are affected by autism, and what families can do to support their other children while coping with the intensive needs of the child with autism.

2538 **Simple Steps: Developmental Activities for Infants, Toddlers & Two Year Olds**
Therapro
225 Arlington St
Framingham, MA 01702-8773
508-872-9494
800-257-5376
Fax: 508-875-2062
www.therapro.com
info@theraproducts.com
Karen Conrad, Owner
300 activites linked to the latest research in brain development. Outlines a typical developmental sequence in 10 domains: social/emotional, fine motor, gross motor, language, cognition, sensory, nature, music & movement, creativity and dramatic play. Chapters on curriculum development and learning environment also included.

2539 **Social Perception of People with Disabilities in History**
4156 Library Rd
Pittsburgh, PA 15234-1349
412-341-1515
Fax: 412-344-0224
www.ldanatl.org
ldanatl@usaor.net
Herbert C Covey, Author
Patrica H. Latham, President
Sharon Bloechle, Secretary
Shows how historical factors shape some of our current perceptions about disability. Of interest to special educators, historians, students of the humanities and social scientists.

2540 **Son Rise: The Miracle Continues**
Option Indigo Press
2080 S Undermountain Rd
Sheffield, MA 01257-9643
413-229-2100
800-562-7171
Fax: 413-229-8727
www.optionindio.com
indigo@bcn.net
Barry Neil Kaufman, Author
This book documents Raun Kaufman's astonishing develpment from a lifeless, autistic, retarded child into a highly verbal, lovable youngster with no traces of his former condition. It details Raun's extraordinary progress from the age of four into young adulthood. It also shares moving accounts of five families that successfully used the Son-Rise Program to reach their own special children. An awe-inspiring reminder that love moves mountains. A must for any parent, professional or teacher.-OUT OF *$14.95*
346 pages Bi-Annually
ISBN 0-915811-61-8

2541 **Study Skills: A Landmark School Teaching Guide**
Landmark School
429 Hale St
Prides Crossing, MA 01965
978-236-3216
Fax: 978-927-7268
www.landmarkoutreach.org
outreach@landmarkschool.org
Dan Ahearn, Program Director
Trish Newhall, Associate Director
Designed to help all students learn to comprehend and organize the information they must learn in school, Study Skills: A Landmark School Student Guide offers instruction in how to apply specific comprehension and study skills including multiple exercises to practice each skill. Intended for reading levels of middle school and beyond. *$25.00*
104 pages
ISBN 0-962411-96-5

2542 **Stuttering and Your Child: Questions and Answers**
Stuttering Foundation of America
PO Box 11749
Memphis, TN 38111
901-452-7343
800-992-9392
Fax: 901-761-0484
www.stutteringhelp.org
info@stutteringhelp.org
Jane Fraser, President

Provides help, information, and resources to those who stutter, their families, schools day care centers, and all others who need help for a stuttering problem. *$2.00*
64 pages
ISBN 0-933388-43-8

2543 **Substance Use Among Children and Adolescents**
John Wiley & Sons Inc
10475 Crosspoint Blvd
Indianapolis, IN 46256-3386   877-762-2974
                                     Fax: 800-597-3299
                                     www.wiley.com

Stephen M. Smith, President/CEO
Anne Marie Pagliaro, Author
Peter B. Wiley, Chairman
Exposure and use among infants, children and adolescents. Impact on mental and physical health. Ingestion of substances during pregnancy and effects on fetus and neonate. Drug abuse effects on learning, memory.. Preventing and treating children and adolescents. Available only as a print on demand title. *$132.00*
416 pages Hardcover
ISBN 0-471580-42-2

2544 **Success with Struggling Readers: The Benchmark School Approach**
Guilford Publications
72 Spring St
New York, NY 10012-4019   212-431-9800
                                 800-365-7006
                                 Fax: 212-966-6708
                                 www.guilford.com
                                 info@guilford.com
Irene West Gaskins, Author
Presents a proven approach for helping struggling students become fully engaged readers, learners, thinkers, and problem solvers. Demonstrates ways to teach effective strategies for decoding words and understanding concepts, and to give students the skills to apply these strategies across the curriculum based on their individual cognitive styles and the specific demands of the task at hand. *$30.00*
264 pages
ISBN 1-593851-69-3

2545 **Supporting Children with Communication Difficulties In Inclusive Settings**
Special Needs Project
Ste H
324 State St
Santa Barbara, CA 93101-2364   818-718-9900
                                      800-333-6867
                                      Fax: 818-349-2027
                                      www.specialneeds.com
                                      editor@specialneeds.com
Hod Gray, Founder/President
Linda McCormick, Author
Diane Frome Loeb, Co-Author
A collaboration of professionals and parents can achieve language communication competence in classroom and other settings. Essential background material, assessment and intervention and needs of special populations are discussed. Contains sectional headings and marginal comments, chapter summary. *$75.00*
530 pages Paperback
ISBN 0-023792-72-8

2546 **Tactics for Improving Parenting Skills (TIPS)**
Sopris West
4093 Specialty Pl
Longmont, CO 80504-5400   303-651-2829
                                 800-547-6747
                                 Fax: 303-776-5934
                                 www.soprislearning.com.
Bob Algozzine, Author
Jim Ysseldyke, Author

Perhaps best described as a compliation of one-page parenting brochures, this helpful resource represents volumes of ideas and suggestions on topics of concern in today's families.OUT OF BUSINESS
202 pages
ISBN 1-570350-35-3

2547 **Teach Me Language**
Slosson Educational Publications
PO Box 280
East Aurora, NY 14052   716-652-0930
                               800-828-4800
                               Fax: 800-655-3840
                               www.slosson.com
                               slosson@slosson.com
Steven Slosson, President
Teach Me Language is designed for teachers, therapists, and parents, and includes a step-by-step how to manual with 400 pages of instructions, explanations, examples, and games and cards to attack language weaknesses common to children with pervasive developmental disorders. *$29.95*

2548 **Teaching Developmentally Disabled Children**
Slosson Educational Publications
PO Box 280
East Aurora, NY 14052   716-652-0930
                               800-828-4800
                               Fax: 800-655-3840
                               www.slosson.com
                               slosson@slosson.com
Steven Slosson, President
This instructional program for teachers, nurses, and parents is clear and concisely shows how to help children who are developmentally disabled function more normally at home, in school, and in the community. *$34.00*
250 pages

2549 **Teaching Reading to Children with Down Syndrome**
Woodbine House
6510 Bells Mill Rd
Bethesda, MD 20817-1636   301-897-3570
                                 800-843-7323
                                 Fax: 301-897-5838
                                 www.woodbinehouse.com
                                 info@woodbinehouse.com
Patricia Logan Oelwin, Author
Teach your child with Down syndrome to read using the author's nationally recognized, proven method. From introducing the alphabet to writing and spelling, the lessons are easy to follow. The many pictures and flash cards included appeal to visual learners and are easy to photocopy! *$16.95*
392 pages Paperback
ISBN 0-933149-55-7

2550 **Teaching of Reading: A Continuum from Kindergarten through College**
AVKO Educational Research Foundation
Ste W
3084 Willard Rd
Birch Run, MI 48415-9404   810-686-9283
                                  866-285-6612
                                  Fax: 810-686-1101
                                  www.avko.org
                                  avkoemail@aol.com
Don Mc Cabe, Research Director/Author
Barry Chute, President
Gloria Goldsmith, Secretary
This book covers concepts, techniques, and practical diagnostic tests not normally taught in regular college courses on reading. It is designed to be used by teachers, parents, tutors, and college reading instructors willing to try new approaches to old problems. *$49.95*
364 pages
ISBN 1-564006-50-6

2551 Teaching the Dyslexic Child
Slosson Educational Publications
PO Box 280
East Aurora, NY 14052
716-652-0930
800-828-4800
Fax: 800-655-3840
www.slosson.com
slosson@slosson.com

Steven Slosson, President
Teaching the Dyslexic Child talks about the frustrations that the dyslexic youngsters and their parents encounter in the day to day collisions with life's demand. *$12.00*
128 pages

2552 Understanding Learning Disabilities: A Parent Guide and Workbook, Third Edition
York Press
P.O.Box 504
Timonium, MD 21094-0504
410-560-1557
800-962-2763
Fax: 410-560-6758
www.yorkpress.com
york@abs.net

Elinor Hartwig, President
An invaluable resource for parents who are new to the field of learning disabilities. Easy to read and overflowing with helpful information and advice. *$25.00*
380 pages
ISBN 0-912752-67-X

2553 Understanding and Teaching Children with Autism
John Wiley & Sons Inc
10475 Crosspoint Blvd
Indianapolis, IN 46256-3386
317-572-3000
Fax: 317-572-4000
www.wiley.com

Stephen M. Smith, President/CEO
Rita Jordan, Author
Stuart Powell, Co-Author
The triad of impairment: social, language and communication and thought behavior aspects of development discussed. Difficulties in interacting, transfer of learning and bizarre behaviors are syndome. Many LD are associated with autism. *$175.00*
188 pages Hardcover
ISBN 0-471958-88-3

2554 What to Expect: The Toddler Years
Workman Publishing
225 Varick St
New York, NY 10014-4304
212-254-5900
800-722-7202
Fax: 212-254-8098
www.workman.com
Info@workman.com

Peter Workman, President
Jenny Mandel, Special Markets Director
They guided you through pregnancy, they guided you through baby's first year, and now they'll guide you through the toddler years. In a direct continuation of What to Expect When You're Expecting and What to Expect the Frist Year, American's bestselling pregnancy and childcare authors turn their uniquely comprehensive, lively, and reassuring coverage to years two and three. *$15.95*
928 pages Paperback

Young Adults

2555 Assertive Option: Your Rights and Responsibilities
Research Press
PO Box 9177
Champaign, IL 61826-9177
217-352-3273
800-519-2707
Fax: 217-352-1221
www.researchpress.com
rp@researchpress.com

Russell Pence, President
Albert Ellis, Author

A self instructional assertiveness book, with many exercises and self tests. *$24.95*
348 pages
ISBN 0-878221-92-1

2556 Behavior Survival Guide for Kids
Free Spirit Publishing
Ste 200
217 5th Ave N
Minneapolis, MN 55401-1299
612-338-2068
866-703-7322
Fax: 612-337-5050
www.freespirit.com
help4kids@freespirit.com

Judy Galbraith, President
Offers up-to-date information, practical strategies, and sound advice for kids with diagnosed behavior problems (BD, ED, EBD) and those with general behavior problems so they can help themselves. *$14.95*
176 pages
ISBN 1-575421-32-1

2557 Delivered form Distraction: Getting the Most out of Life with Attention Deficit Disorder
Ballantine Books
1745 Broad way
New york, NY 10019
FAX 212-572-6066
www.randomhouse.com
BBDPublicity@randomhouse.com

Edward M Hallowell, Author
John J Ratey, Co-Author
Random House has long been committed to publishing the best literature by writers both in the United States and abroad. In addition to their commercial success, books published by Random House, Inc. have won an unrivalled number of Nobel and Pulitzer Prizes. *$25.95*
416 pages
ISBN 0-345442-30-X

2558 Education of Students with Disabilities: Where Do We Stand?
National Council on Disability
Suite 1050
1331 F St NW
Washington, DC 20004
202-272-2004
Fax: 202-272-2022
TTY: 202-272-2074
www.ncd.gov
mquigley@ncd.ogv

Ethel D Briggs, Acting Executive Director
Brenda Bratton, Executive Secretary
The council reviews the education of students with disabilities as a critical priority. Success in education is a predictor of success in adult life. For students with disabilities, a good education can be the difference between a life of dependence and nonproductivity and a life of independence and productivity.

2559 HEATH Resource Directory: Clearinghouseon Postsecondary Edu for Individuals with Disabilities
George Washington University
2134 G St NW
Washington, DC 20052
202-973-0904
800-544-3284
Fax: 202-973-0908
www.heath.gwu.edu
askheath@gwu.edu

Donna Martinez, Director
Jessica Queener, Project Director
Reina Guartico, Principal Investigator
The HEATH Resource Center is an online clearinghouse on postsecondary education for individuals with disabilities. The HEATH Resource Center Clearinghouse has information for students with disabilities on educational disability support services, policies, procedures, adaptations, accessing college or university campuses, career-technical schools, and other postsecondary training entities.

2560 Keeping Ahead in School: A Students Book About Learning Disabilities & Learning Disorders
Educators Publishing Service
PO Box 9031
Cambridge, MA 02139-9031

617-547-6706
800-225-5750
Fax: 617-547-0412
www.epsbooks.com
eps@epsbooks.com

Gunnar Voltz, President
Alana Trisler, Author
Written for students 9 to 15 years of age with learning disorders. This book helps students gain important insights into their problems by combining realism with justifiable optimism. *$24.75*
ISBN 0-838820-09-7

2561 Modern Consumer Education: You and the Law
Triumph Learning
PO Box 1270
Northborough, MA 01460-4270

800-338-6519
Fax: 866-805-5723
www.triumphlearning.com
customerservice@triumphlearning.com

Buz Traugot, Sales Representative
An instructional program to teach independent living, with emphasis on legal resources and survival skills. *$59.00*

2562 Phonemic Awareness: Lessons, Activities & Games
Sage/Corwin Press
2455 Teller Rd
Thousand Oaks, CA 91320-2218

805-499-9734
Fax: 805-499-5323
www.corwinpress.com
order@corwin.com

Mike Soules, President
Lisa Shaw, Executive Director
Help struggling readers with Phonemic Awareness training. This all inclusive book iuncludes 48 scripted lessons. May be used as a prerequisite to reading or for stuggling students. Includes 49 reproducible masters. May be used with individual students or with groups. *$27.95*
176 pages

2563 Reading Is Fun
Teddy Bear Press
3703 S. Edmunds Street
Suite B-182
Seattle, WA 98118

858-560-8718
Fax: 866-870-7323
www.teddybearpress.net
fparker@teddybearpress.net

Fran Parker, President
Introduces 55 primer level words in six reading books and accompaning activity sheets. This easy to use reading program provides repition, visual motor, visual discrimination and word comprehension excersies. The manual and placement test. *$85.00*
ISBN 1-928876-01-3

2564 Reading and Writing Workbook
Therapro
225 Arlington St
Framingham, MA 01702-8773

508-872-9494
800-257-5376
Fax: 508-875-2062
www.theraproducts.com
info@theraproducts.com

Karen Conrad, Owner
Kathleen Anderson MS CCC-SP, Author
Pamela Crow Miller, Co-Author
Writing checks and balancing a checkbook, copying words and sentences, and writing messages and notes. Helps with recognition and understanding of calenders, phone books and much more.

2565 Survival Guide for Kids with ADD or ADHD
Free Spirit Publishing
Ste 200
217 5th Ave N
Minneapolis, MN 55401-1299

612-338-2068
866-703-7322
Fax: 612-337-5050
www.freespirit.com
help4kids@freespirit.com

Judy Galbraith, President
Explains how kids diagnosed with ADD and ADHD can help themselves succeed in school, get along better at home, and form healthy, enjoyable relationships with peers. In kid-friendly language and a format that welcomes reluctant and easily distracted readers, this book helps kids know they're not alone and offers practical strategies for taking care or oneself, modifying behavior, enjoying school, having fun, and dealing with doctos, counselors, and medication. Includes scenarios and quizzes. *$13.95*
128 pages
ISBN 1-575421-95-X

2566 Survival Guide for Kids with LD Learning Differences
Free Spirit Publishing
Ste 200
217 5th Ave N
Minneapolis, MN 55401-1299

612-338-2068
866-703-7322
Fax: 612-337-5050
www.freespirit.com
help4kids@freespirit.com

Judy Galbraith, President
Answers the many questions young people have, like 'Why is it hard for kids with LD to learn?' and 'What happens when you grow up?' It explains what LD means (and doesn't mean); defines different kinds of LD; describes what happens in LD programs; helps kids deal with sad, hurt, and angry feelings; suggests ways to get along better in school and at home; and inspires young people to set goals and plan for the future. Also includes resources for parents and teachers. *$10.95*
112 pages
ISBN 1-575421-19-4

2567 Survival Guide for Teenagers with LD Learning Differences
Free Spirit Publishing
Ste 200
217 5th Ave N
Minneapolis, MN 55401-1299

612-338-2068
866-703-7322
Fax: 612-337-5050
www.freespirit.com
help4kids@freespirit.com

Judy Galbraith, President
This guide helps young people with LD succeed in school and prepare for life as adults. It explains what LD is and how kids get into LD programs, clarifies readers' legal rights and responsibilities, and covers other vital topics including assertiveness, jobs, friends, dating, self-sufficiency, and responsible citizenship. *$12.95*
200 pages
ISBN 0-915793-51-2

2568 Who I Can Be Is Up To Me: Lessons in Self-Exploration and Self-Determination
Research Press
2612 N. Mattis Ave PO Box 9177
Champaign, IL 61822-9177

217-352-3273
800-519-2707
Fax: 217-352-1221
www.researchpress.com
rp@researchpress.com

Gloria D Campbell-Whatley, Author
Robert W. Parkinson, Founder
127 pages $24.95
ISBN 0-878224-84-X

2569 **Winning at Math: Your Guide to Learning Mathematics Through Successful Study Skills**
Academic Success Press
6023 26th St W
Bradenton, FL 34207-4402   941-746-1645
                                             800-444-2524
                                        Fax: 941-753-2882
                                 www.academicsuccess.com
                                        pnolting@ad.com
Paul Nolting, Owner
A guide that helps people with learning disabilities learn math easier. *$24.95*

2570 **Winning the Study Game**
Sage/Corwin Press
2455 Teller Rd
Thousand Oaks, CA 91320-2218   805-499-9734
                                        Fax: 805-499-9734
                                   www.corwinpress.com
                                     order@corwin.com
Peggy Hammeken, President
Kevin Ruelle, Illustrator
A comprehensive study skills program for students with learning differences in grades 6-11. The student book has 16 units which will help students learn to study better, take notes, advance their thinking skills while stregthening their reading and writing. The student version is available in a re-producible or consumable format. Teachers guide sold separately. *$34.95*
2500 pages
ISBN 1-890455-48-2

General

2571 A Student's Guide to Jobs
NICHCY
1825 Connecticut Ave NW c/o FHI360
Suite 700
Washington, DC 20009
202-884-8200
800-695-0285
Fax: 202-884-8441
TDD: 800-695-0285
www.nichcy.org
nichcy@fhi360.org

Susan Ripley, Director
Young people with intellectual and developmental disabilities speak freely about their job-related experiences. *$2.00*
8 pages

2572 A Student's Guide to the IEP
NICHCY
1825 Connecticut Ave
Washington, DC 20009
202-884-8200
800-695-0285
Fax: 202-884-8441
www.nichcy.org
nichcy@fhi360.org

Susan Ripley, Director
A guide for students that features other students discussing their experiences as active members on their IEP team. *$2.00*
12 pages

2573 Accessing Parent Groups
NICHCY
1825 Connecticut Ave NW
Suite 700
Washington, DC 20009
202-884-8200
800-695-0285
Fax: 202-884-8441
www.nichcy.org
nichcy@fhi360.org

Susan Ripley, Director
Helps parents locate support groups where they can share information, give and receive emotional support, and address common concerns. *$2.00*
12 pages

2574 Accessing Programs for Infants, Toddlers and Pre-schoolers
NICHCY
1825 Connecticut Ave NW
Suite 700
Washington, DC 20009
202-884-8200
800-695-0285
Fax: 202-884-8441
www.nichcy.org
nichcy@fhi360.org

Susan Ripley, Director
This guide helps locate intervention services for infants and toddlers with disabilities. Also answers questions about educational programs for preschoolers. *$2.00*
20 pages

2575 Advocacy Services for Families of Children in Special Education
Arizona Department of Education
1535 W Jefferson St
Phoenix, AZ 85007-3209
1-800-352-45
800-352-4558
Fax: 602-542-5440
www.ade.state.az.us
ADE@ade.az.gov

Robert Plummer, Manager
Art Heikkila, Auditor
Information provided to families that have children in special education.

2576 Assessing Children for the Presence of a Disability
NICHCY
1825 Connecticut Ave NW
Suite 700
Washington, DC 20009
202-884-8200
800-695-0285
Fax: 202-884-8441
www.nichcy.org
nichcy@fhi360.org

Susan Ripley, Director
Describes the criteria and process preformed by school systems to determine if a child has a learning disabilty. *$4.00*
28 pages

2577 Assessing the ERIC Resource Collection
NICHCY
1825 Connecticut Ave NW
Suite 700
Washington, DC 20009
202-884-8200
800-695-0285
Fax: 202-884-8441
www.nichcy.org
nichcy@fhi360.org

Susan Ripley, Director
A nationwide network that gives access to education literature, this document explains how to search and retrieve documents from ERIC. Also explains how to find information about children with disabilites. *$2.00*
8 pages

2578 Complete Set of State Resource Sheets
NICHCY
1825 Connecticut Ave NW
Suite 700
Washington, DC 20009
202-884-8200
800-695-0285
Fax: 202-884-8441
www.nichcy.org
nichcy@fhi360.org

Susan Ripley, Director
Provides a sheet for every state and territory in the United States. *$10.00*
200 pages

2579 Directory of Organizations
NICHCY
1825 Connecticut Ave NW
Suite 700
Washington, DC 20009
202-884-8200
800-695-0285
Fax: 202-884-8441
www.nichcy.org
nichcy@fhi360.org

Susan Ripley, Director
Lists many organizations and services *$4.00*
28 pages

2580 Education of Children and Youth with Special Needs: What do the Laws Say?
NICHCY
1825 Connecticut Ave NW
Suite 700
Washington, DC 20009
202-884-8200
800-695-0285
Fax: 202-884-8441
www.nichcy.org
nichcy@fhi360.org

Susan Ripley, Director
Provides an overview of 3 laws that aid disabled children; 1. Section 504 of the Rehabilitation Act of 1973, 2. the Individuals with Disabilities Education Act, and 3. the Carl P. Perkins Vocational Educational Act. *$4.00*
16 pages

2581 Ethical and Legal Issues in School Counseling
American School Counselor Association
Ste 625
1101 King St
Alexandria, VA 22314-2957   703-683-2722
                                    800-306-4722
                                Fax: 703-683-1619
                                www.schoolcounselor.org
                                asca@schoolcounselor.org
Richard Wong, Executive Director
Stephanie Will, Office Manager
Jill Cook, Assistant Director
Contains answers to many of the most controversial and
challenging questions school counselors face every day.
$40.50
ISBN 1-556200-55-2

2582 Fact Sheet: Attention Deficit Hyperactivity Disorder
Learning Disabilities Association of America
4156 Library Rd
Pittsburgh, PA 15234-1349   412-341-1515
                                Fax: 412-344-0224
                                www.ldanatl.org
                                ldanatl@usaor.net
Patrica H. Latham, President
Sharon Bloechle, Secretary
Ed Schlitt, Treasurer
A pamphlet offering factual information on ADHD.

2583 Fundamentals of Autism
Slosson Educational Publications
PO Box 280
East Aurora, NY 14052   716-652-0930
                                800-828-4800
                            Fax: 800-655-3840
                            www.slosson.com
                            slosson@slosson.com
Steven Slosson, President
John Slosson, Vice President
Provides a quick, user friendly effective and accurate approach to help in identifying and developing educationally
related program objectives for children diagnosed as Autistic. These materials have been designed to be easily and
functionally used by teachers, therapists, special educa-
tion/learning disability resource specialists, psychologists,
and others who work with children diagnosed with similar
disabilites.

2584 General Information about Autism
NICHCY
1825 Connecticut Ave NW
Suite 700
Washington, DC 20009   202-884-8200
                                800-695-0285
                            Fax: 202-884-8441
                            www.nichcy.org
                            nichcy@fhi360.org
Susan Ripley, Director
Offers information about autism.

2585 General Information about Disabilities
NICHCY
1825 Connecticut Ave NW
Suite 700
Washington, DC 20009   202-884-8200
                                800-695-0285
                            Fax: 202-884-8441
                            www.nichcy.org
                            nichcy@fhi360.org
Susan Ripley, Director
A fact sheet offering information on the Education of the
Handicapped Act.
2 pages

**2586 General Information about Speech and Language Disor-
ders**
NICHCY
1825 Connecticut Ave NW
Suite 700
Washington, DC 20009   202-884-8200
                            Fax: 202-884-8441
                            www.nichcy.org
                            nichcy@fhi360.org
Susan Ripley, Director
Offers characteristics, educational implications and associ-
ations in the area of speech and language disorders.

2587 IDEA Amendments
NICHCY
1825 Connecticut Ave NW
Suite 700
Washington, DC 20009   202-884-8200
                                800-695-0285
                            Fax: 202-884-8441
                            www.nichcy.org
                            nichcy@fhi360.org
Susan Ripley, Director
Examines the important changes that have occured in the In-
dividuals Education Act, amended in June of 1997. *$4.00*
40 pages

2588 If Your Child Stutters: A Guide for Parents
Stuttering Foundation of America
PO Box 11749
Memphis, TN 38111   901-452-7343
                                800-992-9392
                            Fax: 901-452-3931
                            www.stutteringhelp.org
                            info@stutteringhelp.org
Jane Fraser, President
A guide that enables parents to provide appropriate help to
children who stutter. *$1.00*

2589 Individualized Education Programs
NICHCY
1825 Connecticut Ave NW
Suite 700
Washington, DC 20009   202-884-8200
                                800-695-0285
                            Fax: 202-884-8441
                            www.nichcy.org
                            nichcy@fhi360.org
Susan Ripley, Director
Provides guidance regarding the legal requirement for be-
ginning a student's IEP. *$2.00*
32 pages

2590 Interventions for Students with Learning Disabilities
NICHCY
1825 Connecticut Ave NW
Suite 700
Washington, DC 20009   202-884-8200
                                800-695-0285
                            Fax: 202-884-8441
                            www.nichcy.org
                            nichcy@fhi360.org
Susan Ripley, Director
A document that examines 2 different interventions for stu-
dents who have learning disabilities; the first deals with
strategies and the second with phonological awareness.
$4.00
10 pages

2591 National Resources
NICHCY
1825 Connecticut Ave NW
Suite 700
Washington, DC 20009   202-884-8200
                                800-695-0285
                            Fax: 202-884-8441
                            www.nichcy.org
                            nichcy@fhi360.org

Susan Ripley, Director
Lists different organizations that provide information about different disabilities.
6 pages

2592 National Toll-free Numbers
NICHCY
1825 Connecticut Ave NW
Suite 700
Washington, DC 20009

202-884-8200
800-695-0285
Fax: 202-884-8441
www.nichcy.org
nichcy@fhi360.org

Susan Ripley, Director
Gives the names of organizations with toll-free numbers who specialize in different disabilities.
6 pages

2593 Parenting a Child with Special Needs: A Guide to Reading and Resources
NICHCY
1825 Connecticut Ave NW
Suite 700
Washington, DC 20009

202-884-8200
800-695-0285
Fax: 202-884-8441
www.nichcy.org
nichcy@fhi360.org

Susan Ripley, Director
Provides information to families whose child has been diagnosed with a disability. Also gives insight on how disabilities can in turn affect the family. *$4.00*
24 pages

2594 Parents Guide
NICHCY
1825 Connecticut Ave NW
Suite 700
Washington, DC 20009

202-884-8200
800-695-0285
Fax: 202-884-8441
www.nichcy.org
nichcy@fhi360.org

Lisa Kupper, Editor
Susan Ripley, Manager
Talks directly to parents about specific disability issues.

2595 Planning a Move: Mapping Your Strategy
NICHCY
1825 Connecticut Ave NW
Suite 700
Washington, DC 20009

202-884-8200
800-695-0285
Fax: 202-884-8441
www.nichcy.org
nichcy@fhi360.org

Susan Ripley, Director
This guide helps to make moving to a new place easier for parents and their children by listing available services in the new area and compiling educational and medical records. *$2.00*
12 pages

2596 Planning for Inclusion: News Digest
NICHCY
1825 Connecticut Ave NW
Suite 700
Washington, DC 20009

202-884-8200
800-695-0285
Fax: 202-884-8441
www.nichcy.org
nichcy@fhi360.org

Susan Ripley, Director
Provides a general guide to raising children with learning disabilities in an educational setting. *$4.00*
32 pages

2597 Promising Practices and Future Directions for Special Education
NICHCY
1825 Connecticut Ave NW
Suite 700
Washington, DC 20009

202-884-8200
800-695-0285
Fax: 202-884-8441
www.nichcy.org
nichcy@fhi360.org

Susan Ripley, Director
Examines different research regarding the educational methods for children with learning disabilities. *$4.00*
24 pages

2598 Public Agencies Fact Sheet
NICHCY
1825 Connecticut Ave NW
Suite 700
Washington, DC 20009

202-884-8200
800-695-0285
Fax: 202-884-8441
www.nichcy.org
nichcy@fhi360.org

Susan Ripley, Director
General information on public agencies that serve the disabled individual.
2 pages

2599 Questions Often Asked about Special Education Services
NICHCY
1825 Connecticut Ave NW
Suite 700
Washington, DC 20009

202-884-8200
800-695-0285
Fax: 202-884-8441
www.nichcy.org
nichcy@fhi360.org

Susan Ripley, Director
Offers information regarding special education.

2600 Questions Often Asked by Parents About Special Education Services
NICHCY
1825 Connecticut Ave NW
Suite 700
Washington, DC 20009

202-884-8200
800-695-0285
Fax: 202-884-8441
www.nichcy.org
nichcy@fhi360.org

Susan Ripley, Director
A publication to help parents learn about the Individuals with Disabilities Education Act. Also discusses how student access special education and other related services.
12 pages

2601 Questions and Answers About the IDEA News Digest
NICHCY
1825 Connecticut Ave NW
Suite 700
Washington, DC 20009

202-884-8200
800-695-0285
Fax: 202-884-8441
www.nichcy.org
nichcy@fhi360.org

Susan Ripley, Director
Covers the more commonly asked questions from families and professionals about the IDEA. *$4.00*
28 pages

2602 **Related Services for School-Aged Children with Disabilities**
NICHCY
1825 Connecticut Ave NW
Suite 700
Washington, DC 20009   202-884-8200
                                         800-695-0285
                                    Fax: 202-884-8441
                                         www.nichcy.org
                                         nichcy@fhi360.org

Susan Ripley, Director
Examines the different services offered to children with disabilities such as speech-language pathology, transportation, occupational and physical therapy and special health services. *$4.00*
24 pages

2603 **Resources for Adults with Disabilities**
NICHCY
1825 Connecticut Ave NW
Suite 700
Washington, DC 20009   202-884-8200
                                         800-695-0285
                                    Fax: 202-884-8441
                                         www.nichcy.org
                                         nichcy@fhi360.org

Susan Ripley, Director
Helps adults with disabilities find organizations that will help them find employment, education, recreation and independent living. *$2.00*
16 pages

2604 **Serving on Boards and Committees**
NICHCY
1825 Connecticut Ave NW
Suite 700
Washington, DC 20009   202-884-8200
                                         800-695-0285
                                    Fax: 202-884-8441
                                         www.nichcy.org
                                         nichcy@fhi360.org

Susan Ripley, Director
Part of the Parent's Guide series, this publication examines the different boards and committees on which parents of children with disabilities often serve. Also suggests ways to go about becoming involved with such organizations. *$2.00*
8 pages

2605 **Special Education and Related Services: Communicating Through Letterwriting**
NICHCY
1825 Connecticut Ave NW
Suite 700
Washington, DC 20009   202-884-8200
                                         800-695-0285
                                    Fax: 202-884-8441
                                         www.nichcy.org
                                         nichcy@fhi360.org

Susan Ripley, Director
Identifies the rights of parents and their children with disabilities and explains when and how to notify the school in writing about such conditions. *$2.00*
20 pages

2606 **State Resource Sheet**
NICHCY
1825 Connecticut Ave NW
Suite 700
Washington, DC 20009-1492   202-884-8200
                                         800-695-0285
                                    Fax: 202-884-8441
                                         www.nichcy.org
                                         nichcy@fhi360.org

Susan Ripley, Director
List numbers of different organizations that deal with disabilities by state.

2607 **Underachieving Gifted**
Council for Exceptional Children
2900 Crystal drive
Suite 1000
Arlington, VA 22202-3557   703-264-9454
                                         888-232-7733
                                    Fax: 703-264-9494
                                    TTY: 866-915-5000
                                         www.cec.sped.org/
                                         service@cec.sped.org

Michael George, Director
A collection of annotated references from the ERIC and Exceptional Child Evaluation Resources (171 abstracts). Note: Abstracts only. Not the complete research. *$1.00*

2608 **What Every Parent Should Know about Learning Disabilities**
Connecticut Assoc. for Children and Adults with LD
Ste 15-5
25 Van Zant St
Norwalk, CT 06855-1729   203-838-5010
                                    Fax: 203-866-6108
                                         www.CACLD.org

Beryl Kaufman, Executive Director
What to do with a child with a learning disability.

2609 **Who's Teaching Our Children with Disabilities?**
NICHCY
1825 Connecticut Ave NW
Suite 700
Washington, DC 20009-1492   202-884-8200
                                         800-695-0285
                                    Fax: 202-884-8441
                                         www.nichcy.org
                                         nichcy@fhi360.org

Susan Ripley, Director
Takes a detailed look at the people who are teaching children with disabilities. *$4.00*
24 pages

2610 **Your Child's Evaluation**
NICHCY
1825 Connecticut Ave NW
Suite 700
Washington, DC 20009-1492   202-884-8200
                                         800-695-0285
                                    Fax: 202-884-8441
                                         www.nichcy.org
                                         nichcy@fhi360.org

Susan Ripley, Director
This document describes the steps that the school system will use to determine if you child has a learning disability. *$2.00*
4 pages

Adults

2611 International Dyslexia Association: Illinois Branch Newsletter
Bldg 7
751 Roosevelt Rd
Glen Ellyn, IL 60137-5904
630-469-6900
Fax: 630-469-6810
www.readibida.org
info@readibida.org.

Jo Ann Paldo, President
Kathleen L Wagner, Executive Director

2612 NICHCY News Digest
NICHCY
1825 Connecticut Ave NW
Suite 700
Washington, DC 20009-1492
202-884-8200
800-695-0285
Fax: 202-884-8441
www.nichcy.org
nichcy@fhi360.org

Lisa Kupper, Editor
Susan Ripley, Director
Addresses a single disability issue in depth.

2613 Volta Voices
Alexander Graham Bell Association
3417 Volta Pl NW
Washington, DC 20007-2737
202-337-5220
Fax: 202-337-8314
TTY: 202-337-5221
www.agbell.org
info@agbell.org

Melody Felzein, Production/Editing Manager
Harrison Judy, Director
Covers a wide variety of topics, including hearing aid and cochlear implants, early intervention and education, professional guidance, legislative updates and perspectives from individuals from across the United States and around the world.

Children

2614 Calliope
Cobblestone Publishing
Ste C
30 Grove St
Peterborough, NH 03458-1453
603-924-7209
800-821-0115
Fax: 603-924-7380
www.cobblestonepub.com
cobbfeedback@caruspub.com

Rosalie Baker, Editor
Kid's world history magazine, written for kids ages 9 to 14, goes beyond the facts to explore provoactive issues. *$29.95*
52 pages 9 times anually
ISSN 1050-7086

2615 KIND News
NAHEE
Washington, DC 02000
202-452-1100
Fax: 860-434-9579
www.kidsnews.org
membership@humanesociety.org

Wayne Pacelle, President
Laura Maloney, COO
Andrew Rowman, CIO
Four-page color newspaper with games, puzzles and entertaining, informative articles designed to install kindness to people, animals, and the enviroment and to make reading fun. *$30.00*
4 pages 9x school year
ISSN 1050-9542

2616 KIND News Jr: Kids in Nature's Defense
Kind News
2100 L St., NW
Washington, DC 02000
202-452-1101
Fax: 860-434-6282
www.kindnews.org
membership@humanesociety.org

Wayne Pacelle, President
Laura Maloney, COO
Andrew Rowman, CIO
Short, easy-to-read items on the environment and animal world with puzzles, contests and cartoons. Many illustrations, pictures.

2617 KIND News Primary: Kids in Nature's Defense
Kind News
2101 L St., NW
Washington, DC 02000
202-452-1102
Fax: 860-434-6282
www.kindnews.org
membership@humanesociety.org

Wayne Pacelle, President
Laura Maloney, COO
Andrew Rowman, CIO
Short, easy-to-read items on the environment and animal world with puzzles, pictures to color and cartoons. Many illustrations, pictures.

2618 KIND News Sr: Kids in Nature's Defense
NAHEE
2102 L St., NW
Washington, DC 02000
202-452-1103
Fax: 860-434-6282
www.kindnews.org
membership@humanesociety.org

Wayne Pacelle, President
Laura Maloney, COO
Lona Rowman, CIO
Publication put out by the National Association for Humane and Environmental Education, KIND News Sr. is intended for children between grades 5 through 6. The magazine covers different pet issues such as how to care for,feed and play with pets.

2619 Let's Find Out
Scholastic
555 Broadway
New York, NY 10012-3919
212-625-0778

Jamie Martillo, Editor
Richard Robinson, CEO
Get your PreK and K classes off to a great start with Free-trail copies of Let's Find Out, and bring all this to your teaching program: monthly seasonal themes in 32 colorful weekly issues, activity pages to develop early reading and math skills. *$4.25*

2620 National Association for Humane and Environmental Education
2100L St.,NW
Washington, DC 02000
202-452-1100
Fax: 860-434-6282
www.kidsnews.org
membership@humanesociety.org

Wayne Pacelle, President
Laura Maloney, COO
Andrew Rowman, CIO

2621 Ranger Rick
National Wildlife Foundation/Membership Services
989 Avenue of Americans
Suite 400
New York, NY 10018
212-730-1700
800-822-9919
Fax: 212-730-1823
www.nuf.org
info@nuf.com

Gerry Bishop, Editor
Mark Putten, CEO
Anthony Winn, Director,PSLDI

A magazine for children ages 6-12 that is dedicated to helping students gain a greater understanding and appreciation of nature. *$15.00*

2622 Stone Soup, The Magazine by Young Writers& Artists
Children's Art Foundation
PO Box 83
Santa Cruz, CA 95063

831-426-5557
800-447-4569
www.stonesoup.com
editor@stonesoup.com

Gerry Mandel, Editor
William Rubel, Editor
A literary magazine publishing fiction, poetry, book reviews and art by children through age 13. ISSN: 0094 579X. *$34.00*
48 pages 6x/year

Parents & Professionals

2623 Association of Higher Education Facilities Officers Newsletter
1643 Prince St
Alexandria, VA 22314-2818

703-684-1446
Fax: 703-549-2772
www.appa.org
webmaster@appa.org

Randolph Hare, President
Peter Strazdas, Vice President
Jerry Carlson, Secretary
A newsletter whose purpose is to promote excellence in the administration, care, operation, planning, and development of higher education facilities.

2624 Children and Families
National Head Start Association
1651 Prince St
Alexandria, VA 22314-2818

703-739-0875
Fax: 703-739-0878
www.nhsa.org
mmcgrady@nhsa.com

Vanessa Rich, Chairman
Alvin Jones, Vice Chairperson
Mary Cose Rox, Secretary
The magazine of the National Head Start Association.

2625 Connections: A Journal of Adult Literacy
Adult Literacy Resource Institute
100 William T Morrissey Blvd
Dorchester, MA 2125-3300

617-782-8956
Fax: 617-782-9011
TTY: 617-782-9011
www.alri.org

Connections is primarily intended to provide an opportunity for adult educators in the Boston area to communicate with colleagues.

2626 Council for Exceptional Children
2900 Crystal Drive
Ste 1000
Arlington, VA 22202

703-243-0446
888-232-7733
Fax: 703-264-9494
TTY: 703-264-9446
www.cec.sped.org
service@cec.sped.org

Robin D. Brewer, President
Mikki Garcia, Executive Director
John H. Hess, Consultant
The Council for Exceptional Children (CEC) is the largest international professional organization dedicated to improving the educational success of individuals with disabilities and/or gifts and talents. CEC advocates for appropriate governmental policies, sets professional standards, provides professional development, advocates for individuals with exceptionalities, and helps professionals obtain conditions and resources necessary for effective professional practice.

2627 Education Funding News
Education Funding Research Council
1725 K St NW
Washington, DC 20006-1401

202-872-4000
800-876-0226
Fax: 800-926-2012
www.grantsandfunding.com

Emily Lechy, Editor
Phil Gabel, CEO
Provides the latest details on funding opportunities in education. *$298.00*
50 pages

2628 Exceptional Children
Council for Exceptional Children
2900 Crystal Drive
Ste 1000
Arlington, VA 22202

703-264-9454
888-232-7733
Fax: 703-264-9494
TTY: 703-264-9446
www.cec.sped.org
service@cec.sped.org

Robin D. Brewer, President
Mikki Garcia, Executive Director
John H. Hess, Consultant
Peer review journal publishing original research on the education and development of toddlers, infants, children and youth with exceptionality and articles on professional issues of concern to special educators. Published quarterly.

2629 Exceptional Parent Magazine
551 Main St
Johnstown, PA 15901-2032

877-372-7368
www.eparent.com
webmaster@eparent.com

Joseph M. Valenzano, President/CEO
Rick Rader, Editor in Chief
Ron Peterson, Webmaster
EP is the magazine for exceptional parents with exceptional children. Each month EP provides a forum to network with others who are providing a richer life for themselves and for their children. ISSN: 0046-9157. *$39.95*
92 pages Monthly

2630 Federation for Children with Special Needs Newsletter
529 Main St
Ste 1M3 Boston
Boston, MA 2129

617-236-7210
800-331-0688
Fax: 617-241-0330
www.fcsn.org
fcsninfo@fcsn.org

James F. Whalen, President/CEO
Michael Weiner, Treasurer
Miryam Wiley, Clerk
The mission of the Federation is to provide information, support, and assistance to parents of children with disabilities, their professional partners, and their communities. Major services are information and referrals and parent and professional training.

2631 International Dyslexia Association Quarterly Newsletter: Perspectives
4th Fl
40 York Rd
Baltimore, MD 21204-5243

410-296-0232
800 ABC D123
Fax: 410-321-5069
www.interdys.org
jdallam@interdys.org

Hal Malchow, President
Ben Shifrin, Vice President
Suzzane Carreker, Secretary

Leading resource for individuals with dyslexia, their families, teachers, and educational professionals around the world. A non-profit organization dedicates to the study and treatment of dyslexia, we encourage you to join our mission and become a member. You will receive regular information about managing dyslexia, access to an international network of professionals in the field, discounts on conference fees and publications, quarterly and biannual publications
50-56 pages Free to Members

2632 International Dyslexia Association: Illinois Branch Newsletter
Bldg 7
751 Roosevelt Rd
Glen Ellyn, IL 60137-5904   630-469-6900
                                          Fax: 630-469-6810
                                          www.readibida.org
                                          info@readibida.org
Dr.Suzzane O'Brien, President
Julia Nelson, Vice President
John Bloomfield, Treasurer
The Illinois Branch, serving the entire state of Illinois and founded in 1978, is dedicated to the study and remediation of dyslexia and to the support and encouragement of individuals with dyslexia and their families.

2633 International Dyslexia Association: Philadelphia Branch Newsletter
P.O.Box 251
Bryn Mawr, PA 19010-251   610-527-1548
                                       Fax: 610-527-5011
Jann Glider, President
Amy Ress, Manager
An international 501 (c) (3) nonprofit, scientific and educational organization dedicated to the study and treatment of dyslexia. All branches hold at least one public meeting, workshop or conference per year.

2634 International Reading Association Newspaper: Reading Today
PO Box 8139
800 Barksdale Rd.
Newark, DE 19714-8139   302-731-1600
                                       800-336-7323
                                       Fax: 302-731-1057
                                       www.reading.org
                              customerservice@reading.org
Jill Lewis-Spector, President
Diane Barone, Vice President
Marcie Craig Post, Executive Director
The International Reading Association is a professional membership organization dedicated to promoting high levels of literacy for all by improving the quality of reading instruction, disseminating research and information about reading, and encouraging the lifetime reading habit. Our members include classroom teachers, reading specialistsss, consultants, administrators, supervisors, university faculty, researchers, psychologists, librarians, media specialists, and parents.
Bi-monthly

2635 Journal of Physical Education, Recreation and Dance
1900 Association Dr
Reston, VA 20191-1502   703-476-3400
                                       800-213-7193
                                       Fax: 703-476-9527
                                       www.shapeamerica.org
Dolly D. Lambdin, President
E.Paul Roetert, CEO
Gale Wiedow, Past President
Most frequently published, and most wide-ranging periodical reaching over 20,000 members and providing information on a greater variety of HPERD issues than any other publication. ISSN NUMBER: 0730-3084 *$9.00*
80 pages monthly

2636 LDA Alabama Newsletter
Learning Disabilities Association Alabama
P.O.Box 11588
Montgomery, AL 36111-588   334-277-9151
                                       Fax: 334-284-9357
                                       www.ldaal.org
                                       alabama@ldaal.org
Tamara Massey-Garrett, President
Jenida Grisett, Secretary
Linda Graham, Treasurer
Educational, support, and advocacy group for individuals with learning disabilities and ADD.

2637 LDA Illinois Newsletter
Learning Disabilities Association Illinois
Ste 106
10101 S Roberts Rd
Palos Hills, IL 60465-1556   708-430-7532
                                       Fax: 708-430-7592
                                       www.idanatl.org/illinois
Sharon Schussler, Manager
A non profit organization dedicated to the advancement of the education and general welfare of children and youth of normal or potentially normal intelligence who have perceptual, conceptual, coordinative or related learning disabilities.

2638 Link Newsletter
Parent Information Center of Delaware
5570 Kirkwood Hwy
Wilmington, DE 19808-5002   302-366-0152
                                       888-547-4412
                                       Fax: 302-999-7637
                                       www.glrppr.org
                                       l-barnes@illinois.edu
Laura Barnes, Executive Director
GLRPPR is a professional organization dedicated to promoting information exchange and networking to P2 professionals in the Great Lakes regions of the United States and Canada. *$12.00*
20 pages quarterly

2639 OSERS Magazine
Office of Special Education & Rehabilitative Svcs.
303 C St SW
Washington, DC 20202   202-727-6436
                                       800-433-3243
                                       TTY: 202-205-8241
                                       www.ed.gov
Provides information, research and resources in the area of special learning needs.
Quarterly

2640 Resources in Education
US Government Printing Office
710 N Capitol St NW
Washington, DC 20401   202-512-0132
                                       Fax: 202-512-1355
                                       www.access.gpo.gov
                               Contactcenter@gpo.gov.in
Patricia Simmons, Manager
A monthly publication announcing education related documents.

2641 TESOL Journal
Teachers of English to Speakers of Other Languages
1925 Ballenger Avenue
Ste 500
Alexandria, VA 22314-4287   703-836-0774
                                       888-547-3369
                                       Fax: 703-836-7864
                                       www.tesol.org
                                       info@tesol.org
Rosa Aronson, Executive Director
Rita Gainer, Executive Assistant
Jim Trope, Director of Finance

TESOL Journal articles focus on teaching and classroom research for classroom practitioners. The journal includes articles about adult education and literacy in every volume year. Subscriptions available to members only.

2642 TESOL Newsletter
Teachers of English to Speakers of Other Languages
1925 Ballenger Avenue
Ste 500
Alexandria, VA 22314-4287   703-836-0774
                                        888-547-3369
                                   Fax: 703-836-7864
                                        www.tesol.org
                                        info@tesol.org

Rosa Aronson, Executive Director
Rita Gainer, Executive Assistant
Jim Trope, Director of Finance
TESOL produces the Adult Education Interest Section Newsletter and the Refugee Concerns Interest Section Newsletter. They provide news, ideas, and activities for ESL instructors. Subscriptions are available to members only.

2643 TESOL Quarterly
Teachers of English to Speakers of Other Languages
1925 Ballenger Avenue
Ste 500
Alexandria, VA 22314-4287   703-836-0774
                                        888-547-3369
                                   Fax: 703-836-7864
                                        www.tesol.org
                                        info@tesol.org

Rosa Aronson, Executive Director
Rita Gainer, Executive Assistant
Jim Trope, Director of Finance
TESOL Quarterly is a referred interdisciplinary journal teachers of English to speakers of other languages. Subscriptions available to members.

Young Adults

2644 Get Ready to Read!
National Center for Learning Disabilities
381 Park Ave S
New York, NY 10016-8806   212-545-7510
                                       888-575-7373
                                  Fax: 212-545-9665
                                       www.ld.org
                                       help@ncld.org

Frederic M. Poses, CEO
Mary Kalikow, Vice Chair
John R. Langeler, Treasurer
The National Center for Learning Disabilities (NCLD) works to ensure that the nation's 15 million children, adolescents, and adults with learning disabilities have every opportunity to succeed in school, work, and life.
Quarterly

2645 LD Advocate
National Center for Learning Disabilities
381 Park Ave S
New York, NY 10016-8806   212-545-7510
                                       888-575-7373
                                  Fax: 212-545-9665
                                       www.ld.org
                                       help@ncld.org

Frederic M. Poses, CEO
Mary Kalikow, Vice Chair
John R. Langeler, Treasurer
The National Center for Learning Disabilities (NCLD) works to ensure that the nation's 15 million children, adolescents, and adults with learning disabilities have every opportunity to succeed in school, work, and life.
Monthly

2646 LD News
National Center for Learning Disabilities
381 Park Ave S
New York, NY 10016-8806   212-545-7510
                                       888-575-7373
                                  Fax: 212-545-9665
                                       www.ld.org
                                       help@ncld.org

Frederic M. Poses, CEO
Mary Kalikow, Vice Chair
John R. Langeler, Treasurer
The National Center for Learning Disabilities (NCLD) works to ensure that the nation's 15 million children, adolescents, and adults with learning disabilities have every opportunity to succeed in school, work, and life.
Monthly

2647 Our World
National Center for Learning Disabilities
381 Park Ave S
New York, NY 10016-8806   212-545-7510
                                       888-575-7373
                                  Fax: 212-545-9665
                                       www.ld.org
                                       help@ncld.org

Frederic M. Poses, CEO
Mary Kalikow, Vice Chair
John R. Langeler, Treasurer
The National Center for Learning Disabilities (NCLD) works to ensure that the nation's 15 million children, adolescents, and adults with learning disabilities have every opportunity to succeed in school, work, and life.
Quarterly

General

2648 Academic Communication Associates
Educational Book Division
PO Box 4279
Oceanside, CA 92052-4279
760-758-9593
888-758-9558
Fax: 760-758-1604
www.acadcom.com
acom@acadcom.com
Larry Mattes, Founder/President
Publishes hundreds of speech and language products, educational books and assessment materials for children and adults with speech, language, and hearing disorders, learning disabilities, developmental disabilities, and special learning needs. Products include books, software programs, learning games, augmentative communication materials, bilingual/multicultural materials, and special education resources.

2649 Academic Success Press
6023 26th Street W
PO Box 132
Bradenton, FL 34206
888-822-6657
www.academicsuccess.com
info@academicsuccess.com
Paul D Nolting PhD, Learning Specialist
Kimberly Nolting, VP of Marketing & Research
Publishes books and materials in the interest of making the classroom learning experience less difficult, while improving student learning, to transform the classroom into a more successful environment where educators and students can use inventive learning techniques based on sound academic research.

2650 Academic Therapy Publications
20 Commercial Blvd
Novato, CA 94949-6191
415-883-3314
800-422-7249
Fax: 415-883-3720
www.academictherapy.com
sales@academictherapy.com
Jim Arena, President
Publishes supplementary education materials for people with reading, learning and communication disabilities; features professional texts and reference books, curriculum materials, teacher/parent resources, and visual/perceptual training aids.

2651 Active Parenting Publishers
1220 Kennestone
Ste 130
Marietta, GA 30066-6022
770-429-0565
800-825-0060
Fax: 770-429-0334
www.activeparenting.com
cservice@activeparenting.com
Michael Popkin PhD, President
Melody Popkin, Manager of Christian Resources
Virginia Murray, Marketing Manager
Provides parenting education curricula, including one for parents of ADD/ADHD children.

2652 Alexander Graham Bell Association for the Deaf and Hard of Hearing
3417 Volta Pl NW
Washington, DC 20007-2737
202-337-5220
866-37-5226
Fax: 202-337-8314
TTY: 202-337-5221
www.agbell.org
info@agbell.org
Meredith K. Sugar, President
Emilio Alonso-Mendoza, CEO
Ted A. Meyer, Secretary

Publishes and distributes books, brochures, instructional materials, videos, CDs and audiocassettes relating to hearing loss. *$62.00*
64 pages Bimonthly

2653 American Guidance Service
PO Box 99
Circle Pines, MN 55014
651-287-7220
800-328-2560
Fax: 800-471-8457
www.agsnet.com
agsmail@agsnet.com
Produces assessments, textbooks, and instructional materials for people with a wide range of needs; publishes individually administered tests to measure cognitive ability, achievement, behavior, speech and language skills, and personal and social adjustment.

2654 American Printing House for the Blind
1839 Frankfort Avenue
PO Box 6085
Louisville, KY 40206-0085
502-895-2405
800-233-1839
Fax: 502-899-2284
www.aph.org
info@aph.org
Tuck Tinsley, President
Marsha Overstreet, Customer Service Manager
Tony Grantz, Business Development Manager
Promotes independence of blind and visually impaired persons by providing specialized materials, products, and services needed for education and life.

2655 American Psychological Association
750 1st St NE
Washington, DC 20002-4242
202-336-5500
800-374-2722
Fax: 202-336-5518
www.apa.org/psycinfo
psycinfo@apa.org
Norman B Anderson, CEO
L.Michael Honaker, Deputy CEO
Ellen G. Garrison, Senior Advisor
Publishes periodicals, including PsycSCAN, a quarterly print abstract that provides citations to the journal literature on Learning Disorders and Mental Retardation, including theories, research, assessment, treatment, rehabilitation, and educational issues. Also publishes Psychological Abstracts, a monthly print reference tool containing summaries of journal articles, book chapters and books in the field of psychology and related disciplines.

2656 Associated Services for the Blind
919 Walnut St
Philadelphia, PA 19107-5287
215-627-5930
Fax: 215-922-0692
www.asb.org
asbinfo@asb.org
Patricia C Johnson, CEO
Lauren Scarpa, Public Relations Officer
Linda Gaffney, Coordinator
Promotes self-esteem, independence, and self determination in people who are blind or visually impaired. ASB accomplishes this by providing support through education, training and resources, as well as through community action and public education, serving as a voice for the rights of all people who are blind or visually impaired.

2657 Association on Higher Education and Disability
Ste 204
107 Commerce Centre Dr
Huntersville, NC 28078-5870
704-947-7779
Fax: 704-948-7779
www.ahead.org
information@ahead.org
Bea Awoniyi, President
Michael Johnson, Treasurer
Stephen Hamlin-Smith, Executive Director

A professional membership organization for individuals involved in the development of policy and in the provision of quality services to meet the needs of persons with disabilities involved in all areas of higher education.

2658   At-Risk Youth Resources
Sunburst Visual Media
PO Box 170
Farmingville, NY 11738   800-999-6884
                                       Fax: 800-262-1886
                                          www.at-risk.com
                         customerservice@guidance-group.com
Publisher of life-skills educational media for the K-12 market. In addition, we also produce science and social studies programs for students in grades K-8
78 pages

2659   Bethany House Publishers
6030 East Fulton Road
Ada, MI 49301   952-829-2500
                                            800-877-2665
                                       Fax: 952-829-2572
                                      www.bethanyhouse.com
                                     orders@bakerbooks.com
Gary Johnson, President
Teresa Fogarty, General Publicist
Publishes books in large-print format for the learning disabled.

2660   Blackwell Publishing
350 Main St
Malden, MA 2148-5020   781-870-1200
                                       Fax: 781-388-8255
                                  www.blackwellpublishing.com
                        dpeters@bos.blackwellpublishing.com
Lisa Bybee, President
Rene Olivieri, Chief Executive
Dawn Peters, Media Contact
Publishes books and journals for the higher education, research and professional markets, including several journals on topics relating to learning disabilities.

2661   Brookes Publishing Company
PO Box 10624
Baltimore, MD 21285   410-337-9580
                                            800-638-3775
                                       Fax: 410-337-8539
                                   www.brookespublishing.com
                            custserv@brookespublishing.com
Paul Brooks, Owner
Melissa Behm, Vice President
Publishes books, texts, curricula, videos, tools and a newsletter based on research in disabilities, education and child development, including learning disabilities, ADHD, communication and language, reading and literacy, and special education.

2662   Brookline Books/Lumen Editions
34 University Rd
Brookline, MA 2445-4533   617-734-6772
                                            800-666-2665
                                       Fax: 617-734-3952
                                    www.brooklinebooks.com
                                      brbooks@yahoo.com
Milton Budoff, Executive Director
Publishes books on education, learning and topics relating to disabilities.

2663   Charles C Thomas, Publisher, Ltd.
2600 S 1st St
Springfield, IL 62704-4730   217-789-8980
                                            800-258-8980
                                       Fax: 217-789-9130
                                         www.ccthomas.com
                                       books@ccthomas.com
Michael P Thomas, President

Publisher of titles in Criminal Justice and Police Science, the Behavioral Sciences, Education and Special Education, Biomedical Sciences.

2664   City Creek Press
PO Box 8415
Minneapolis, MN 55408   612-823-2500
                                            800-585-6059
                                       Fax: 877-286-1163
                                         www.citycreek.com
                                         info@citycreek.com
Judy Liautaud, Owner
Publishes books and products offering a literature-based method of learning, such as books, clue cards, posters, magnetic math story boards, workbooks and audio tapes; the program is multisensory, interactive, and appeals to the visual, auditory and tactile learning styles.

2665   Concept Phonics
Oxton House Publishers
P.O.Box 209
Farmington, ME 4938-209   207-779-1923
                                            800-539-7323
                                       Fax: 207-779-0623
                                        www.oxtonhouse.com
                                       info@oxtonhouse.com
William Burlinghoff, Owner
Bobby Brown, Marketing Director
Publisher of effective, economical educational materials for early reading and math. We pay special attention to materials that work well for students with dyslexia and other learning disabilities.

2666   Corwin Press
Sage Publications
2455 Teller Rd
Woodbury
Thousand Oaks, CA 91320-2218   805-499-0721
                                            800-818-7243
                                       Fax: 805-499-9774
                                        www.corwinpress.com
                                     webmaster@sagepub.com
Mike Soules, President
Lisa Shaw, Executive Director
Kristin Anderson, Director of Learning
Publishes books and products for all learners of all ages and their educators, including subjects such as classroom management, early childhood education, guidance and counseling, higher/adult education, inclusive education, exceptional students, student assessment, as well as behavior, motivation and discipline.

2667   Educators Publishing Service
PO Box 9031
Cambridge, MA 2139-9031   617-547-6706
                                            800-435-7728
                                       Fax: 617-547-0285
                                          www.epsbooks.com
                                      epsbooks@epsbooks.com
Gunnar Voltz, President
Publishes vocabulary, grammar and language arts materials for students from kindergarten through high school, and specializes in phonics and reading comprehension as well as materials for students with learning differences.

2668   Federation for Children with Special Needs
529 Main St
Ste 1M3 Boston
Boston, MA 2129   617-236-7210
                                            800-331-0688
                                       Fax: 617-241-0330
                                             www.fcsn.org
                                         fcsinfo@fcsn.org
James F. Whalen, President
Micheal Weiner, Treasurer
Miryam Wiley, Head Clerk

The mission of the Federation is to provide information, support, and assistance to parents of children with disabilities, their professional partners, and their communities. Major services are information and referrals and parent and professional training.

2669 Free Spirit Publishing
217 5th Ave N
Ste 200
Minneapolis, MN 55401-1299   612-338-2068
                                    800-735-7323
                                Fax: 866-419-5199
                                www.freespirit.com
                            help4kids@freespirit.com
Judy Galbraith, Owner
Publishes non-fiction materials which empower young people and promote self-esteem through improved social and learning skills. Topics include self-awareness, stress management, school success, creativity, friends and family, and special needs such as gifted and talented learners and children with learning differences.

2670 Gander Publishing
450 Front St
Avila Beach, CA 93424   805-541-5523
                                    800-554-1819
                                Fax: 805-782-0488
                                 www.ganderpub.com
Wendy Cook, Sales Director
Publisher and distributor of Lindamood-Bell Programs; Seeing Stars, Visualizing and Verbalizing, On Cloud Nine and Talkies.

2671 Gordon Systems & GSI Publications
PO Box 746
Syracuse, NY 13214-746   315-446-4849
                                    800-550-2343
                                Fax: 315-446-2012
                                  www.gsi-add.com
                                 info@gsi-add.com
Michael Gordon PhD, Founder
Books and videos for parents, teachers, children, siblings and adults re: ADHD and foster care. Gordon Diagnostic System is and FDA approved objective measure for use in evaluations of ADHD anf traumatic brain injury. Attention Training System is used in classroom with ADHD children.

2672 Grey House Publishing
4919 Route 22
Amenia, NY 12501   518-789-8700
                                    800-562-2139
                                Fax: 845-373-6360
                                www.greyhouse.com
                        customerservice@greyhouse.com
Richard Gottlieb, President
Leslie Mackenzie, Publisher
Laura Mars, Vice President, Editorial
Publisher of reference materials, especially directories and encyclopedias. Other Health titles include: The Complete Directory for People with Disabilities; The Complete Directory of Pediatric Disorders; The Chronic Illness Directory; The Mental Health Directory; Older Americans Information Directory; The Directory of Hospital Personnel; The HMO/PPO Directory; and The Medical Device Register.

2673 Guilford Publications
72 Spring St
New York, NY 10012-4068   212-431-9800
                                    800-365-7006
                                Fax: 212-966-6708
                                  www.guilford.com
                                 info@guilford.com
Bob Matloff, President
Chris Jennison, Senior Editor Education
Publishes books for education on the subjects of literacy, general education, school psychology and special education. Also offers books, videos, audio cassettes and software, as well as journals, newsletters, and AD/HD resources.

2674 Hazelden Publishing
PO Box 11
Center City, MN 55012   651-213-4200
                                    800-257-7810
                                Fax: 651-213-4411
                                  www.hazelden.org
                                 info@hazelden.org
Sharon Birnbaum, Corporate Director
James A Blaha, CFO
Marvin D. Seppala, CMO
Hazelden a national nonprofit organization founded in 1949,helps people reclaim their lives from the disease of addiction.Built on decades of knowledge and exsperience,Hazelden offers a comprehensive approach to addiction that addresses the full range of patient,family, and professional needs, including treatment and continuing care for youth and adults,research,higher education, piblic education and advocacy,and publishing.

2675 Heinemann-Boynton/Cook
361 Hanover St
Portsmouth, NH 3802-6926   603-431-7894
                                    800-225-5800
                                Fax: 603-431-7840
                                www.boyntoncook.com
                            custserv@heinemann.com
Lesa Scott, VP Human Resources
Publishes professional resources and provides educational services for teachers, and offers nearly 100 titles related to learning disabilities.

2676 High Noon Books
20 Commercial Blvd
Novato, CA 94949-6120   6
                                    800-422-7249
                                Fax: 888-287-9975
                            www.academictherapy.com
                           sales@academictherapy.com
Jim Arena, President
Features over 35 sets of high-interest, low-level books written on a first through fourth grade reading level, for people with reading difficulties, ages nine and up.

2677 JKL Communications
Ste 707
2700 Virginia Ave NW
Washington, DC 20037-1909   202-333-1713
                                Fax: 202-333-1735
                                 www.lathamlaw.org
                               lathamlaw@gmail.com
Peter S Latham JD, Director
Patricia Horan Latham JD, Director
Publishes books and videos on learning disabilities and ADD with a focus on legal issues in school, higher education and employment.

2678 Jewish Braille Institute of America
110 E 30th St
New York, NY 10016-7393   212-889-2525
                                    800-433-1531
                                Fax: 212-689-3692
                                www.jewishbraille.org
                              eisler@jbilibrary.org
Dr. Ellen Isler, President
Israel Taub, Associate Director
Sandra Radinsky, Director of Development
Publishes magazines, a newsletter, and special resources available to the reading disabled who are themselves print-handicapped in varying degrees. Seeks the integration of Jews who are blind, visually impaired and reading disabled into the Jewish community and society.

2679 Learning Disabilities Association of America
4156 Library Rd
Pittsburgh, PA 15234-1349   412-341-1515
                                Fax: 412-344-0224
                                  www.ldanatl.org
                               info@ldaamerica.org

Nancie Payne, President
Beth Mcgaw, Secretary
Joanthan Jones, Treasurer
Maintains a large inventory of publications, videos and other materials related to learning disabilities, and publishes two periodicals available by subscription as well as various books, booklets, brochures, papers and pamphlets on topics related to learning disabilities.

2680 Learning Disabilities Resources
6 E Eagle Rd
Havertown, PA 19083-1424
610-446-6126
800-869-8336
Fax: 610-446-6129
www.learningdifferences.com
rcooper-ldr@comcast.net
Rich Cooper, Owner
Offers a variety of resources to help teach the learning disabled, including alternative ways to teach math, language, spelling, vocabulary, and also how to organize and study. Available in books, videos, and audio tapes.

2681 Library Reproduction Service
14214 S Figueroa St
Los Angeles, CA 90061-1034
310-354-2610
800-255-5002
Fax: 310-354-2601
www.lrs-largeprint.com
lrsprint@aol.com
Peter Jones, Owner
Offers large print reproductions to special needs students in first grade through post-secondary, as well as adult basic and continuing education programs; also produces an extensive collection of large print classics for all ages as well as children's literature.

2682 LinguiSystems
8700 Shoal Creek Blvd
Austin, TX 70757-6897
309-755-2300
800-897-3202
Fax: 800-397-7633
TDD: 800-933-8331
www.linguisystems.com
info@proedinc.com
Linda Bowers, CEO
Rosemary Huisingh, Co-Owner
Publishes a newsletter and speech-language materials for learning disabilities, ADD/ADHD, auditory processing and listening, language skills, fluency and voice, reading and comprehension, social skills and pragmatics, vocabulary and concepts, writing, spelling, punctuation and other specialized subjects.

2683 Love Publishing Company
Ste 2200
9101 E Kenyon Ave
Denver, CO 80237-1854
303-221-7333
Fax: 303-221-7444
www.lovepublishing.com
lpc@lovepublishing.com
Stan Love, Owner
Publishes titles for use in special education, counseling, social work, and individuals with learning differences.

2684 Magination Press
750 1st St NE
Washington, DC 20002-4241
202-336-5510
800-374-2721
Fax: 202-336-5500
www.apa.org
magination@apa.org
Norman B Anderson, CEO
L.Michael Honaker, Deputy CEO
Ellen G. Garrison, Senior Advisor
Publishes special books for children's special concerns, including starting school, learning disabilities, and other topics in psychology, development and mental health.

2685 Marsh Media
PO Box 8082
Kansas City, MO 66208-82
816-523-1059
800-821-3303
Fax: 866-333-7421
www.marshmedia.com
info@marshmedia.com
Joan Marsh, President
Puberty education for students with special needs curriculum. DVDs on personal safety and social skills.
1969

2686 Mindworks Press
4019 Westerly Pl
Ste 100
Newport Beach, CA 92660-2333
949-266-3700
Fax: 949-266-3770
http://amenclinics.com
contact@amenclinic.com
Daniel G Amen, Medical Director & CEO
Features books, audio, video, and CD-ROMs addressing a range of disorders, including anxiety, depression, obsessive-compulsiveness and ADD.

2687 National Association for Visually Handicapped
111 E 59th St
New York, NY 10022-1202
212-889-3141
Fax: 212-727-2931
www.lighthouse.org
staff@navh.org
Lorianie Marchi, CEO
Publishes information about sight and sight problems for adults and children. Offers a product line of low-vision aids, a collection of articles about eye conditions, causes and treatment modalities, and a newsletter issued four times a year with information to assist people in dealing with low vision.

2688 National Bible Association
488 Madison Ave
24 Floor
New York, NY 10022
917-371-0868
212-907-6427
Fax: 212-408-1360
www.nationalbible.org
nba@nationalbible.org
Richard Glickstein, President
Publishes Read it! A Journal for Bible Readers, which is issued three times a year. Also offers many versions of the Bible, including large-print editions and the easy-to-read Contemporary English Version.

2689 Northwest Media
326 W 12th Ave
Eugene, OR 97401-3449
541-343-6636
800-777-6636
Fax: 541-343-0177
www.sociallearning.com
nwm@northwestmedia.com
Lee White, President
Susan Larson, Marketing Director
Publishes material with a focus on independent living and foster care products. Training resources for parents: www.fosterparentcollege.com and for teens: www.vstreet.com.

2690 PEAK Parent Center
Ste 200
611 N Weber St
Colorado Springs, CO 80903-1072
719-531-9400
800-284-0251
Fax: 719-531-9452
www.peakparent.org
info@peakparent.org
Kent Wilis, President
Sarah Billerbeck, VP
Brandi Young, Secretary

A federally-designated Parent Traning and Information Center (PTI). As a PTI, PEAK supports and empowers parents, providing them with information and strategies to use when advocating for their children with disabilities by expanding knowledge of special education and offering new strategies for success.

2691 Performance Resource Press
Ste F
1270 Rankin Dr
Troy, MI 48083-2843 248-588-7733
800-453-7733
Fax: 248-588-6633
www.prponline.net
customerservice@prponline.net
George Watkins, President
Publishes over 600 products, including catalogs, journals, digests, newsletters, books, videos, posters and pamplets with a focus on behavioral health.

2692 Peytral Publications
PO Box 1162
Minnetonka, MN 55345 952-949-8707
877-739-8725
Fax: 952-906-9777
www.peytral.com
help@peytral.com
Peggy Hammeken, President
Publishes and distributes special education materials which promote success for all learners.

2693 Phillip Roy Catalog
Phillip Roy
PO Box 130
Largo, FL 33785 727-593-2700
800-255-9085
Fax: 727-595-2685
www.philliproy.com
info@philliproy.com
Phillip Roy, Owner
Ruth Bragman, President
Publishes educational materials written for students of any age with different learning abilities. Offers an alternative approach to traditional education. Free catalog upon request.

2694 Reader's Digest Partners for Sight Foundation
Reader's Digest Rd
Pleasantville, NY 10570 914-244-4900
800-877-5293
www.rd.com
partnersforsight@rd.com
Susan Olivo, VP/General Manager
Dianna Kelly-Naghizadeh, Program Manager
Thomas Ryder, CEO
Offers large type editions of select books and large print editions of Readers Digest Magazines, as well as a foundation newsletter, Sightlines, which is published in large format with large type.

2695 Research Press Publisher
PO Box 7886
Champaign, IL 61826-9177 217-352-3273
800-519-2707
Fax: 217-352-1221
www.researchpress.com
orders@researchpress.com
Gail ll Salyards, President
Dennis Wiziecki, Marketing
Research Press provides user-friendly research-based prevention and intervention materials.

2696 Riggs Institute
21106 479th Ave
White, SD 57276-6605 503-646-9459
800-200-4840
Fax: 503-644-5191
www.riggsinst.org
riggs@riggsinst.org

Myrna McCulloch, Founder/Director/Author
Publishes materials to help remedial students using the Orton method, a multisensory approach to learning. Offers a catalog of products, including teacher's editions, phonogram cards, audio CDs for students, student materials and classroom materials.

2697 Scholastic
557 Broadway
New York, NY 10012-3999 212-343-6100
800-246-2986
Fax: 212-343-6934
www.scholastic.com
Richard Robinson, CEO
Barbara A Marcus, VP/President Children's Books
Richard M Spaulding, Executive VP Marketing
Produces educational materials to assist and inspire students of all ages, including a range of special education books, software, and other products.

2698 Schwab Learning
201 Mission Strt
Ste 1960
San Francisco, CA 94105 415-795-4920
800-230-0988
Fax: 415-795-4921
www.schwabfoundation.org
info@schwabfoundation.org
Helen O. Schwab, President
Charles R. Schwab, Chairman
Nancy Bechtle, Director
Provides information, guidance, support and materials that address the emotional, social, practical and academic needs and concerns of children with learning difficulties, and their parents.

2699 Slosson Educational Publications
538 Buffalo Road
East Aurora, NY 14052-280 716-652-0930
888-756-7766
Fax: 716-655-3840
www.slosson.com
slossonprep@gmail.com
Steven Slosson, President
Publishes and distributes educational materials in the areas of intelligence, aptitude, developmental disabilities, school screening and achievement, speech-language and assessment therapy, emotional/behavior, and special needs. Offers a product line of testing and assessment materials, books, games, videos, cassettes and computer software intended for use by professionals, psychologists, teachers, counselors, students and parents.

2700 Teddy Bear Press
3703 S. Edmunds Street
Suite 67
Seattle, WA 98118 206-402-6947
Fax: 866-870-7323
www.teddybearpress.net
fparker@teddybearpress.net
Fran Parker, Author
Publishes books and reading materials designed with the beginning reader in mind, written and illustrated by a special education teacher specializing in elementary education, learning disabilities, and education for the emotionally and mentally challenged.

2701 Therapro
225 Arlington St
Framingham, MA 1702-8773 508-872-9494
800-257-5376
Fax: 508-875-2062
www.theraproducts.com
info@theraproducts.com
Karen Conrad, Owner

Offers specialty products and publications for all ages in the field of occupational therapy, including assistive technology, evaluations, handwriting programs, sensory-motor awareness and alerting products, oral motor products, early learning products, and perception, cognition and language resources.

2702 Thomas Nelson Publishers
PO Box 141000
Nashville, TN 37214-1000 615-248-2110
800-889-9000
Fax: 615-391-5225
www.thomasnelson.com
publicity@thomasnelson.com
Thomas Lewis Nelson, Owner
Michael S Hyatt, Executive VP/Group Publisher
Phil Stoner, Executive VP/Group Publisher
Publishes books and other resources for the learning disabled.

2703 Thorndike Press
295 Kennedy Memorial Dr
Waterville, ME 4901-4539 207-859-1000
800-223-1244
Fax: 207-859-1008
www.thorndike.gale.com
gale.printorders@cengage.com
Jamie Knobloch, Director Marketing
Jill Leckta, Publisher
Publishes and distributes over 900 new large-print editions per year, with an emphasis on bestsellers and genre fiction, as well as nonfiction titles.

2704 Ulverscroft Large Print Books
PO Box 1230
West Seneca, NY 14224-8230 716-674-4270
800-955-9659
Fax: 716-674-4195
www.ulverscroft.com
enquiries@ulverscroft.co.uk
Janice Gowan, Executive Director
Publishes large print books and audio products for people hard of seeing.

2705 Wadsworth Publishing Company
10 Davis Dr
Belmont, CA 94002-3002 650-598-9757
800-354-9706
Fax: 650-637-7544
www.wadworth.com
brian.joyner@cangage.com
Susan Badger, Acquisitions Editor
Publishes books on a wide range of topics in special education, including behavior modification, language disorders and development, and learning disabilities.

2706 Woodbine House
6510 Bells Mill Rd
Bethesda, MD 20817-1636 301-897-3570
800-843-7323
Fax: 301-897-5838
www.woodbinehouse.com
info@woodbinehouse.com
Irv Shapell, Owner
Specializes in books about children with special needs; publishes sixty-five titles within the Special Needs Collection, covering AD/HD, learning disabilities, special education, communication skills, and other disabilities, for use by parents, children, therapists, health care providers and teachers.

2707 Xavier Society for the Blind
154 E 23rd St
New York, NY 10010-4595 212-473-7800
www.xaviersocietyfortheblind.org
info@xaviersocietyfortheblind.org
Kathleen Lynch, Manager
Gina Ballero, Secretary to Director

Provides resources for the visually impaired, including large-print, braille, and audio products.

Classroom Resources

2708 Collaboration in the Schools: The Problem-Solving Process
Pro-Ed
8700 Shoal Creek Blvd
Austin, TX 78757-6897
512-451-3246
800-897-3202
Fax: 512-451-8542
www.proedinc.com
info@proedinc.com

Donald D Hammill, Owner
An inservice/preservice video that demonstrates the stages of the consultative/collaborative process, as well as many of the various communicative/interactive skills and collaborative problem solving skills. *$106.00*

2709 Educational Evaluation
Stern Center for Language and Learning
183 Talcott Road
Suite 101
Williston, VT 5495-9209
802-878-2332
800-544-4863
Fax: 802-878-0230
www.sterncenter.org
learning@sterncenter.org

Blanche Podhajski, President
Jane Nathan, Research Director
Michael Saphiro, CFO
The evaluation is an assessment of intelligence, academic achievement, language, and emotional and behavioral issues related to learning and includes pre- and post- evaluation conferences with parents and/ or students as well as an extensive written report detailing results and recommendations.

2710 Fundamentals of Reading Success
Educators Publishing Service
PO Box 9031
Cambridge, MA 2139-9031
617-547-6706
800-225-5750
Fax: 617-547-0412
www.epsbooks.com
eps@epsbooks.com

Arlene W Sonday, Author
This Orton-Gillingham-based video series teaches a phonic or code-emphasis approach to reading, spelling, and handwriting, and provides the foundation for a multisensory phonics curriculum. May be used by teachers and tutors. *$480.00*
ISBN 0-838872-52-2

2711 Individual Instruction
Stern Center for Language and Learning
135 Allen Brook Ln
Williston, VT 5495-9209
802-878-2332
800-544-4863
Fax: 802-878-0230
www.sterncenter.org
learning@sterncenter.org

Blanche Podhajski, President
Jane Nathan, Research Director
Michael Saphiro, CFO
Individualized instruction to help students develop literacy skills and achieve academic success, building on learning strengths and compensating for areas of difficulty.

2712 Instructional Strategies for Learning Disabled Community College Students
Graduate School and University Center
365 5th Ave
New York, NY 10016-4309
212-817-7000
Fax: 212-817-1503
www.gc.cuny.edu

Frances Degenhorowitz, President
For working with a cross-section of types of individuals with learning problems. *$47.50*

2713 Key Concepts in Personal Development
Marsh Media
PO Box 8082
Kansas City, MO 66208-82
816-523-1059
800-821-3303
Fax: 866-333-7421
www.marshmedia.com
info@marshmedia.com

Joan Marsh, President
Puberty Education for Children with Special Needs. Comprehensive, gender-specific kits and supplemental parent packets address human sexuality for children with miild to moderate developmental disabilities.

2714 Living With Attention Deficit Disorder
Aquarius Health Care Media
30 Forest Road
Millis, MA 20054
508-376-1244
888-440-2963
Fax: 508-376-1245
www.aquariusproductions.com
aquarius@aquariusproductions.com

Leslie Kussmann, President
Anne Baker, Billing and Accounting
This video presents tips for teachers and students how to deal with ADD, including how to adapt school structures and classes. *$125.00*
Video, 22 mins

2715 New Room Arrangement as a Teaching Strategy
Teaching Strategies
7101 Wisconsin Avenue
Suite 700
Bethesda, MD 20814
301-634-0818
800-637-3652
Fax: 301-657-0250
www.teachingstrategies.com
info@teachingstrategies.com

Andrea Valentine, President
Ron Davies, CEO
Amy Houser, CMO
A manual and video present the impact of the early childhood classroom environment on how children learn, how they relate to others and how teachers teach. *$35.00*

2716 Now You're Talking: Extend Conversation
Educational Productions
7101 Wisconsin Avenue
Suite 700
Bethesda, MD 20814
800-637-3652
Fax: 301-634-0826
www.teachingstrategies.com
info@teachingstrategies.com

Andrea Valentine, President
Ron Davies, CEO
Amy Houser, CMO
Video. Teachers in a language-based preschool and speech-language pathologists model effective techniques that focus and extend conversations of young children. *$295.00*

2717 Phonemic Awareness: Lessons, Activities and Games
Sage/Corwin Press
2455 Teller Rd
Thousand Oaks, CA 91320-2218
805-410-7408
Fax: 805-499-2692
www.corwinpress.com

Mike Soules, President
Lisa Shaw, Executive Director
Kristin Anderson, Director of Learning
Exceptional field tested guide to help educators who want to reach phonemic awareness as a prerequisite to reading, and/or to supplement the current curriculum. Special educators and speech clinicians will find this practical guide especially helpful as research indicates that deficits in phonemic awareness is often a major contributor to reading disabilities. This book or video contains fifty-eight scripted lessons, forty-nine reproducible blackline master and progress charts.

2718 Professional Development
Stern Center for Language and Learning
183 Talcott Road
Suite 101
Williston, VT 5495-9209

802-878-2332
800-544-4863
Fax: 802-878-0230
www.sterncenter.org
learning@sterncenter.org

Blanche Podhajski, President
Jane Nathan, Research Director
Michael Saphiro, CFO
Staff development programs for preschool through grade 12 designed in response to requests from teachers and administrators for cutting-edge information about different kinds of learners and the teaching strategies most successful for them.

2719 Purdue University Speech-Language Clinic
100 N University St
West Lafayette, IN 47907-2098

765-494-3663
800-359-2968
Fax: 765-494-3660
www.cla.purdue.edu

Irwin Weiser, Dean
The Speech-Language Clinic provides opportunities for individuals with communication problems to receive individual and group diagnostic evaluations, screenings and therapy services. The clinic provide services for children and adults with mild to severe speech sound problems and/or impaired oral-motor control, language problems associated with autism, language-learning disabilities, hearing impairment, stuttering, and voice problems. *$81.00*

2720 Restructuring America's Schools
Association for Supervision/Curriculum Development
1703 N Beauregard St
Alexandria, VA 22311-1746

703-578-9600
Fax: 703-549-3891
www.ascd.org

Nancy Gibson, President
Marie Adair, Executive Director
Jon Chapman, Chief Strategy Officer
A leader's guide and videotape designed for administrators, teachers, parents, school board members, and community leaders.

2721 Skillstreaming Video: How to Teach Students Prosocial Skills
Research Press
PO Box 9177
Champaign, IL 61826-9177

217-352-3273
800-519-2707
Fax: 217-352-1221
www.researchpress.com
rp@researchpress.com

Russell Pence, President
A video and two books providing an overview of a training procedure for teaching elementary and secondary level students the skills they need for coping with typical social and interpersonal problems. *$365.00*

2722 Spelling Workbook Video
Learning Disabilities Resources
PO Box 716
Arlington, VA 22206

610-525-8336
800-869-8336
Fax: 703-998-2060
www.ldonline.org

An instructional video which works through the spelling workbooks for teachers and students. *$16.00*

2723 Strategic Planning and Leadership
Association for Supervision/Curriculum Development
1703 N Beauregard St
Alexandria, VA 22311-1714

703-578-9600
800-933-2723
Fax: 703-575-5400
www.ascd.org

Nancy Gibson, President
Marie Adair, Executive Director
Jon Chapman, Chief Strategy Officer
Designed to explain and illustrate effective approaches to dealing with change through strategic planning.

2724 Teaching Adults with Learning Disabilities
Stern Center for Language and Learning
183 Talcott Road
Suite 101
Williston, VT 5495-9209

802-878-2332
800-544-4863
Fax: 802-878-0230
www.sterncenter.org
bpodhajski@sterncenter.org

Blanche Podhajski, President
Jane Nathan, Research Director
Michael Saphiro, CFO
A videotape training program and companion guide designed to help adult literacy teachers identify and instruct adults with learning disabilities. The focus of this five hour video series is on teaching basic reading and spelling skills. *$199.95*

2725 Teaching Math
Learning Disabilities Resources
2775 S. Quincy St
Arlington, VA 22206

610-525-8336
800-869-8336
Fax: 610-525-8337
www.ldonline.org
ldonline@weta.org

Neol Gunther, Executive Director
Susannah Harris, Senior Manager
A video for educational professionals teaching math to disabled children. *$12.00*

2726 Teaching People with Developmental Disabilities
Research Press
PO Box 9177
Champaign, IL 61826-9177

217-352-3273
800-519-2707
Fax: 217-352-1221
www.researchpress.com
rp@researchpress.com

Russell Pence, President
A set of four videotapes and accompanying participant workbooks designed to help teachers, staff, volunteers, or family members master task analysis, prompting, reinforcement and error correction. *$595.00*

2727 Teaching Strategies Library: Research Based Strategies for Teachers
Association for Supervision/Curriculum Development
1703 N Beauregard St
Alexandria, VA 22311-1714

703-548-9600
Fax: 703-575-5400
www.ascd.org

Nancy Gibson, President
Marie Adair, Executive Director
Jon Chapman, Chief Strategy Officer
A trainer's manual and five videotapes designed for inservice education of teachers K-12 focusing on four different types of learning expected of students: mastery, understanding, synthesis and involvement.

2728 Teaching Students Through Their Individual Learning Styles
St. John's University, Learning Styles Network
PO Box 417
Henrietta, NY 14467

888-887-7552
Fax: 256-740-0310
www.learningstyles.net

James Benson, Executive Director
A set of six videotapes introducing the Dunn and Dunn learning styles model. Explains the environmental, emotional, sociological, physical and psychological elements of style.

2729 Telling Tales
KET, The Kentucky Network Enterprise Division
600 Cooper Dr
Lexington, KY 40502-1669   859-258-7000
                                  800-354-9067
                              Fax: 859-258-7396
                              www.tellingtales.org
                              info@tellingtales.org
Susan Jasper, Founder
Resource for teachers,librarians and drama departments at
all levels of instruction. Telling Tales can be used to encourage creativity and self expression and help students understand their cultural and language arts skills, and develop
openess to diverse cultures, build self confidence and leadership skills, improve communication and language arts
skills and develop oral history projects. *$30.00*

2730 Word Feathers
KET, The Kentucky Network Enterprise Division
600 Cooper Dr
Lexington, KY 40502-1669   859-258-7000
                                  800-354-9067
                              Fax: 859-258-7396
                              www.tellingtales.org
                              info@tellingtales.org
Susan Jasper, Founder
An activity-oriented language arts video series.

Parents & Professionals

2731 3 R'S for Special Education: Rights, Resources, Results
Brookes Publishing Company
PO Box 10624
Baltimore, MD 21285   410-337-9580
                                 800-638-3775
                             Fax: 410-337-8539
                             www.pbrookes.com
                             custserv@pbrookes.com
Paul H Brooks, Owner
This video helps parents navigate the steps of the special ed-
ucation system and work towards securing the best educa-
tion and services for their children. *$49.95*
Video

2732 A Child's First Words
Orange County Learning Disabilities Association
PO Box 25772
Santa Ana, CA 92799-5772   714-547-4206
                             www.oclda.org
                             info@oclda.org
Shows the importance of not waiting until your child is older
to worry about their speech. *$20.00*
Catalog #7353

2733 A Culture Undiscovered
Fanlight Productions
32 Court St
21 Floor
Brooklyn, NY 11201   718-488-8900
                                 800-876-1710
                             Fax: 718-488-8642
                             www.fanlight.com
                             fanlight@fanlight.com
Ben Achtenberg, Owner
Nicole Johnson, Publicity Coordinator
Explores the needs and experiences of college students,
from diverse racial and/or ethnic backgrounds, who have
learning disabilities.
Video, 36 min

2734 A Mind of Your Own
Fanlight Productions
32 Court St
21 Floor
Brooklyn, NY 11201   718-488-8900
                                 800-876-1710
                             Fax: 718-488-8642
                             www.fanlight.com
                             fanlight@fanlight.com
Ben Achtenberg, Owner
Nicole Johnson, Publicity Coordinator
New video on learning disabilities from the National Film
Board of Canada, follows four learning disabled students
through their struggles academically and socially as well as
their successes in learning to cope with their disabilities and
develop their own unique talents. Amtec Award of Merit. 37
minutes. *$199.00*
Rental $60/day
ISSN DD29-0

2735 ABC's of Learning Disabilities
American Federation of Teachers
555 New Jersey Ave NW
Washington, DC 20001-2029   202-879-4400
                             Fax: 202-879-4597
                             www.aft.org
                             online@aft.org
Sandra Feldman, President
This film illustrates the case histories of four learning dis-
abled students with various learning disabilities.

2736 ADHD
Brookes Publishing Company
PO Box 10624
Baltimore, MD 21285   800-638-3775
                             Fax: 410-337-8539
                             www.pbrookes.com
                             custserv@pbrookes.com
Paul H Brooks, President
Melissa A Behm, Executive Vice President
George Stamathis, Vice President/Publisher
This video shows methods for helping students who have
ADHD increase attention to tasks, improve listening skills,
become better organized, and boost work production. *$99.00*
Video
ISBN 1-557661-15-4

2737 ADHD in Adults
Guilford Publications
72 Spring St
New York, NY 10012-4019   212-431-9800
                                 800-365-7006
                             Fax: 212-966-6708
                             www.guilford.com
                             info@guilford.com
Bob Matloff, President
Jody Falco, Editor in Chief
This program integrates information on ADHD with the actual experiences of four adults who suffer from the disorder.
Representing a range of professions, from a lawyer to a
mother working at home, each candidly discusses the impact
of ADHD on his or her daily life. These interviews are
qugmented by comments from family members and other
clinicians who treat adults with ADHD *$95.00*
36-min VHS

2738 ADHD in the Classroom: Strategies for Teachers
Guilford Publications
72 Spring St
New York, NY 10012-4019   212-431-9800
                                 800-365-7006
                             Fax: 212-966-6708
                             www.guilford.com
                             info@guilford.com
Bob Matloff, President
Jody Falco, Editor in Chief

Viewers see the problems teachers encounter with children who suffer with ADHD, as well as instructive demonstrations of effective behavior management techbiques including color charts and signs, point system, token economy, and turtle-control technique. Also includes a Leader's Guide and a 42-page Manual. *$95.00*
36-min. VHS

2739   ADHD: What Can We Do?
Guilford Publications
72 Spring St
New York, NY   10012-4019   212-431-9800
                                   800-365-7006
                              Fax: 212-966-6708
                              www.guilford.com
                              info@guilford.com
Bob Matloff, President
Jody Falco, Editor in Chief
A video program that introduces teachers and parents to a variety of the most effective techniques for managing ADHD in the classroom, at home, and on gamily outings. Includes Leader's Guide and 30-page Manual. *$95.00*
ISBN 0-898629-72-1

2740   ADHD: What Do We Know?
Guilford Publications
72 Spring St
New York, NY   10012-4019   212-431-9800
                                   800-365-7006
                              Fax: 212-966-6708
                              www.guilford.com
                              info@guilford.com
Bob Matloff, President
Jody Falco, Editor in Chief
An introduction for teachers and special education practitioners, school psychologists and parents of ADHD children. Topics outlined in this videoinclude the causes and prevalence of ADHD, ways children with ADHD behave, otherconditions that may accompany ADHD and long-term prospects for children with ADHD. *$95.00*
Video

2741   Adapting to Your Child's Personality
Aquarius Health Media Care
30 Forest Road
Millis, MA   20054-1066   508-376-1244
                                    888-440-2963
                               Fax: 508-376-1245
                          www.aquarisproductions.com
                          aquarius@aquarisproductions.com
Leslie Kussmann, President
Anne Baker, Billing and Accounting
Join a child behavioral specialist, two moms and their toddlers (with different personalities!) to find out how to mold your own responses so that you can more effectively influence your child. VHS: A-KIDSPERSONAL also on DVD. *$145.00*
Video, 30 mins

2742   Adults with Learning Problems
Learning Disabilities Resources
2775 S. Quincy St
Arlington, VA   22206   610-525-8336
                                    800-869-8336
                               Fax: 703-998-2060
                               www.ldonline.org
                               ldonline@weta.org
Neol Gunther, Executive Director
Susannah Harris, Senior Manager
Educational materials for adults with a learning disability.

2743   All Children Learn Differently
Orange County Learning Disabilities Association
PO Box 25772
Santa Ana, CA   92799-5772   714-547-7206
                               www.oclda.org
                               info@oclda.org

Covers cognitive, perceptual, nutritional, optometric, speech and language motor aspects. *$29.95*
Catalog #6812

2744   American Sign Language Phrase Book Videotape Series
Harris Communications
15155 Technology Dr
Eden Prairie, MN   55344-2273   952-906-1180
                                    800-825-6758
                               Fax: 952-906-1099
                               TDD: 952-906-1198
                               TTY: 800-825-9187
                               www.harriscomm.com
                               info@harriscomm.com
Darla Hudson, Customer Service
Includes book and three videotapes, each 60 minutes long. In Volume 1 you will find everyday expressions, signing and deafness, getting acquainted, health and water; in Volume 2 you will find family, school, food and drink, clothing, sports and recreation; and in Volume 3 you will find travel, animal, colors, civics, religion, numbers, time, dates and money. Set of books and videos. Part #BVT141. *$134.95*

2745   Andreas: Outcomes of Inclusion
Center on Disability and Community Inclusion
208 Colchester Avenue
3rd Floor
Burlington, VT   5405   802-656-3131
                               Fax: 802-656-1357
                               TTY: 802-656-4031
                          www.uvm.edu/zvapvt/timfox
                               syuan@uvm.edu
Tom Sullivan, President
Video portrays the academic, occupational, and social inclusion of a high school student with severe disabilities. Includes commentary of parents, administrators, teachers, support personnel, classmates.

2746   Around the Clock: Parenting the Delayed ADHD Child
Guilford Publications
72 Spring St
New York, NY   10012-4019   212-431-9800
                                   800-365-7006
                              Fax: 212-966-6708
                              www.guilford.com
                              info@guilford.com
Bob Matloff, President
Jody Falco, Editor in Chief
This videotape provides both professionals and parents a helpful look at how the difficulties facing parents of ADHD children can be handled. *$150.00*
45-min. VHS

2747   Art of Communication
United Learning
Ste 100
1560 Sherman Ave
Evanston, IL   60201-4817   847-328-6700
                                    800-424-0362
                               Fax: 847-328-6706
                               www.unitedlearning.com
                               info@unitedlearning.com
Ronald Reed, Vice President
Designed for parents and professionals, this video focuses on: effective parent-child communication; nonverbal communication in children; effective listening; effects of negative and critical messages; and deterrents limiting child/parent communication. *$99.00*

2748   Attention Deficit Disorder
Pro-Ed
8700 Shoal Creek Blvd
Austin, TX   78757-6816   512-451-3246
                                    800-897-3202
                               Fax: 512-451-8542
                               www.proedinc.com
                               info@proedinc.com
Donald D Hammill, Owner
DR Jordan, Author

A video and book providing helpful suggestions for both home and classroom management of students with attention deficit disorder. *$60.00*
Yearly

2749 Augmentative Communication Without Limitations
Prentke Romich Company (PRC)
1022 Heyl Rd
Wooster, OH 44691-9786 330-262-1984
800-262-1984
Fax: 330-263-4829
www.prentrom.com
David L Moffatt, President
Cherie Weaver, Marketing Coordinator
Prentke Romich Company (PRC) is a worldwide leader in the development and manufacture of augmentative communication devices, computer access products, and other assistive technology for people with severe disabilities.

2750 Autism
Aquarius Health Media Care
30 Forest Road
Millis, MA 20054-1066 508-376-1244
888-440-2963
Fax: 508-376-1245
www.aquariusproductions.com
orders@aquariusproductions.com
Leslie Kussmann, President/Producer
Through therapeutic horseback riding a young boy emerges from his isolated world. He finds a connection with his horse when he isn't able to talk to adults. A teenage girl gains social confidence as she leads her llama at a local fair. This film explores the power animals can have on helping someone with autism to connect. This film is great for anyone working the autistic and their families. VHS: A-DISHWAA also on DVD. *$125.00*
Video, 30 mins

2751 Behind the Glass Door: Hannah's Story
32 Court St
21 Floor
Brooklyn, NY 11201 718-488-8900
800-876-1710
Fax: 718-488-8642
www.fanlight.com
fanlight@fanlight.com
Karen Pascal, Producer
Ben Achtenberg, Owner
New video, produced in association with Vision TV, follows the Shepard family through five years of struggle, hardship and bittersweet success in raising their child, Hannah, who was diagnosed with autism. Offers insight into the stress families and educators face as they tackle this mysterious disorder. Offers hope and inspiration to parents. Recipient of Silver Screen Award; US International Film and Video Festival.

2752 Beyond the ADD Myth
Brookes Publishing Company
PO Box 10624
Baltimore, MD 21285 410-337-9580
800-638-3775
Fax: 410-337-8539
www.pbrookes.com
custerv@pbrookes.com
Paul H Brooks, President
Melissa A Behm, Executive VP
George Stamthis, VP/Publisher
This video builds on the theory that many of the behaviors associated with attention deficit disorder are not solely due to neurological dysfunction but actually result from a wide range of social, psychological, and educational causes. *$22.00*
Video
ISBN 1-557661-15-4

2753 Child Who Appears Aloof: Module 5
Educational Productions
7101 Wisconsin Avenue
Suite 700
Bethesda, MD 20814 503-297-6393
800-637-3652
Fax: 503-297-6395
www.teachingstrategies.com
info@teachingstrategies.com
Andrea Valentine, President
Ron Davies, CEO
Amy Houser, CMO
A 30 minute video and 60 page facilitation packet focusing on children who pull back, who avoid social contact. Teaches strategies to understand and support these children. Part of the Hand-in-Hand Series. *$295.00*

2754 Child Who Appears Anxious: Module 4
Educational Productions
7101 Wisconsin Avenue
Suite 700
Bethesda, MD 20814 503-297-6393
800-637-3652
Fax: 503-297-6395
www.teachingstrategies.com
info@teachingstrategies.com
Andrea Valentine, President
Ron Davies, CEO
Amy Houser, CMO
A 35 minute video and 60 page training facilitation packet examining the issues of anxious children and how a supporting adult can help bring them into play. Part of the Hand-in-Hand Series. *$295.00*

2755 Child Who Dabbles: Module 3
Educational Productions
7101 Wisconsin Avenue
Suite 700
Bethesda, MD 20814 503-297-6393
800-637-3652
Fax: 503-297-6395
www.teachingstrategies.com
info@teachingstrategies.com
Andrea Valentine, President
Ron Davies, CEO
Amy Houser, CMO
A 30-minute video and 60-page training facilitation guide that compares dabbling to quality, invested play and offers various strategies for adults to help children build play skills. Part of Hand-in-Hand Series. *$295.00*

2756 Child Who Wanders: Module 2
Educational Productions
7101 Wisconsin Avenue
Suite 700
Bethesda, MD 20814 503-297-6393
800-637-3652
Fax: 503-297-6395
www.teachingstrategies.com
info@teachingstrategies.com
Andrea Valentine, President
Ron Davies, CEO
Amy Houser, CMO
A 30-minute video and 67-page training facilitation packet showing how to identify children who cannot engage in play so wander about the room. Shows creative interventions to help teach new skills. Part of Hand-in-Hand Series.

2757 Child Who is Ignored: Module 6
Educational Productions
7101 Wisconsin Avenue
Suite 700
Bethesda, MD 20814 503-644-7000
800-637-3652
Fax: 503-350-7000
www.teachingstrategies.com
info@teachingstrategies.com
Andrea Valentine, President
Ron Davies, CEO
Amy Houser, CMO

A 30 minute video and 60 page facilitation guide illustrating the children who are ignored by others and offering several interventions for them to learn social skills. Part of the Hand-in-Hand Series. *$295.00*

2758 Child Who is Rejected: Module 7
Educational Productions
7101 Wisconsin Avenue
Suite 700
Bethesda, MD 20814   503-297-6393
                                     800-637-3652
                                Fax: 503-297-6395
                              www.teachingstrategies.com
                              info@teachingstrategies.com
Andrea Valentine, President
Ron Davies, CEO
Amy Houser, CMO
A 35-minute video and 60-page facilitation packet with strategies to help children whose behavior and/or appearance causes them to be rejected by other children. Part of Hand-in-Hand Series.

2759 Concentration Video
Center for Alternative Learning
6 E Eagle Rd
Havertown, PA 19083-1424   610-446-6126
                                     800-204-7667
                                Fax: 610-446-6129
                              www.learningdifferences.com
                              rcooper-ldr@comcast.net
Rich Cooper, Director/Founder/Author
A 53 minute instructional video provides an optimistic perspective about attention problems ADD. Dr. Cooper discusses different types of attention problems causes and solutions. The second part of the video contains concentration exercises to help children and adults with attention problems. *$16.00*
53 Mins/Video

2760 Degrees of Success: Conversations with College Students with LD
4th Fl
240 Greene St
New York, NY 10003-6675   212-387-8205
                                Fax: 212-995-4114
                              www.nyu.edu/osl/csd
A new video which features college students with learning disabilities speaking in their own words about: making the decision to attend college, developing effective learning strategies, coping with frustrations and utilizing college support services. Includes resource packet with suggested discussion questions and list of other resources.

2761 Developing Minds: Parent's Pack
Learning Disabilities Resources
2775 S. Quincy St
Arlington, VA 22206   610-525-8336
                                     800-869-8336
                                Fax: 703-998-2060
                              www.ldonline.org
                              ldonline@weta.com
Dr. Mel Levine, Author
Lia Salza, Editorial Associate
Created especially for parents, this video set provides an overview of why some children struggle with learning. The programs offer strategies for supporting kids' learning differences, based on the work of Dr. Mel Levin and his neurodevelopmental view on how to help children and adolescents become successful learners. *$59.90*
2 Videos

2762 Developing Minds: Teacher's Pack
Learning Disabilities Resources
2775 S. Quincy St
Arlington, VA 22206   610-525-8336
                                     800-869-8336
                                Fax: 703-998-2060
                              www.ldonline.org
                              ldonline@weta.com

Dr. Mel Levine, Author
Lia Salza, Editorial Associate
Created especially for educators, this video set provides an overview of why some children struggle with learning. The programs offer strategies for supporting kids' learning differences, based on the work of Dr. Mel Levin and his neurodevelopmental view on how to help children and adolescents become successful learners. *$59.90*
2 Videos

2763 Dyslexia: A Different Kind of Learning
Aquarius Health Media Care
18 N Main St
Millis, MA 20054-1066   508-376-1244
                                     888-440-2963
                                Fax: 508-376-1245
                              www.aquarisproductions.com
                              aquarius@aquarisproductions.com
Leslie Kussmann, President
Part of the Prescription for Learning Series. This programs shows us what it's like to grow up with dyslexia and the challenge people with dyslexia face in school. The video presents tips for teachers and students on how to deal with it, including how to adapt school structures and classes. VHS: A-TISDYSLEXIA *$125.00*
Video, 24 mins

2764 FAT City
Connecticut Assoc. for Children and Adults with LD
Ste 15-5
25 Van Zant St
Norwalk, CT 6855-1713   203-838-5010
                                Fax: 203-866-6108
                              www.CACLD.org
                              cacld@juno.com
Beryl Kaufman, Executive Director
Marie Armstrong, Information Specialist
Nationally acclaimed video designed to sensitize adults to the frustration, anxiety and tension that the learning disabled child experiences daily. Add $5.00 for shipping and handling. *$49.95*

2765 First Steps Series: Supporting Early Language Development
Educational Productions
7101 Wisconsin Avenue
Suite 700
Bethesda, MD 20814   503-297-6393
                                     800-637-3652
                                Fax: 503-297-6395
                              www.teachingstrategies.com
                              info@teachingstrategies.com
Andrea Valentine, President
Ron Davies, CEO
Amy Houser, CMO
Four 20-minute videos used in early intervention efforts for training staff and parents. Teach how to support language acquisition and model responsive, connected adult-child relationships foundational for all development and learning

2766 Getting Started With Facilitated Communication
Syracuse Univ./Facilitated Communication Institute
370 Huntington Hall
Syracuse, NY 13244-2324   315-443-9379
                                Fax: 315-443-9218
                              www.soeweb.syr.edu/thefci
                              fcstaff@syr.edu
Annegret Schubert, Author
Douglas Biklen, Ph.D., Director
Details on the getting started process, including discussion of candidacy, facilitator attitude, materials and equipment, and the components involved in a first session. Several first sessions are excerpted, showing a child, a teenager, a person with challenging behavior, and a child with significant but not fully functional speech.
14-min/Video

2767 Getting Started with Facilitated Communication
Syracuse University, Institute on Communication
370 Huntington Hall
Syracuse, NY 13244 · · · · · · · · · · · · · · · 315-443-9657
Fax: 315-443-2274
www.soeweb.syr.edu/thefci
fcstaff@syr.edu
Annegret Schubert, Author
Douglas Biklen, Ph.D., Director
This videotape describes the details of the getting started
process, including discussion of candidacy, facilitator attitude, materials and equipment, and the components involved
in a first session.

2768 Help! This Kid's Driving Me Crazy!
Pro-Ed
8700 Shoal Creek Blvd
Austin, TX 78757-6816 · · · · · · · · · · · · · 512-451-3246
800-897-3202
Fax: 512-451-8542
www.proedinc.com
info@proedinc.com
Donald D Hammill, Owner
Designed for parents and professionals working with children up to five years old, this videotape and booklet offers
information about the nature, special needs, and typical behavioral characteristics for young children with attention
deficit disorder. *$5.00*

2769 How Difficult Can This Be?
Learning Disabilities Resources
2775 S. Quincy St
Arlington, VA 22206 · · · · · · · · · · · · · · · 610-525-8336
800-869-8336
Fax: 703-998-2060
www.ldonline.org
ldonline@weta.com
Richard Lavoie, Author
Lia Salza, Editorial Associate
This program looks at the world through the eyes of a child
with learning disabilities by taking you to a unique workshop attended by parents, educators, psychologists, and social workers. There they join in a series of classroom
activities that cause frustration, anxiety and tension - emotions all too familiar to the student with a learning disability.
$49.95
70 mins/Video

2770 I Want My Little Boy Back
BBC - Autism Treatment Center of America
2080 S Undermountain Rd
Sheffield, MA 1257-9643 · · · · · · · · · · · · 413-229-2100
877-766-7473
Fax: 413-229-8931
www.autismtreatment.com
autism@option.org
Tracy Baisden, Marketing Associate
This BBC documentary follows an English family with a
child with autism before, during, and after their time at the
Son-Rise Program. It uniquely captures the heart of the
Son-Rise Program and is extremely useful in understanding
its techniques. *$20.00*

2771 I'm Not Stupid
Learning Disabilities Association of America
4156 Library Rd
Pittsburgh, PA 15234-1349 · · · · · · · · · · 412-341-1515
Fax: 412-344-0224
www.ldanatl.org
ldanatl@usaor.net
This video depicts the constant battle of the learning disabled child in school. *$22.00*

2772 Identifying Learning Problems
Center for Alternative Learning
6 E Eagle Rd
Havertown, PA 19083-1424 · · · · · · · · · · 610-446-6126
800-204-7667
Fax: 610-446-6129
www.learningdifferences.com
rcooper-ldr@comcast.net
Rich Cooper, Director/Founder/Author
A presentation made to adult educators and volunteer tutors
discusses what to look for in a student who has difficulty
learning. The red flags (common behaviors and errors) are
described. *$16.00*
1hr 40mins

2773 Inclusion Series
Comforty Mediaconcepts
2145 Pioneer Rd
Evanston, IL 60201-2564 · · · · · · · · · · · · 847-475-0791
Fax: 847-475-0793
comforty@comforty.com
Jacky Comforty, Owner
A series of video programs on inclusive education and community life. Titles include: Choices, providing instruction
for all audiences to the inclusion process; Inclusion: Issues
for Educators, focusing on particular teachers and administrators in Illinois schools; Families, Friends, Futures, emphasizing the need for early inclusion; and Together We're
Better, providing an overview of this comprehensive
program. Videos available separately or as a set.

**2774 International Professional Development Training
Catalog**
Center for Alternative Learning
6 E Eagle Rd
Havertown, PA 19083-1424 · · · · · · · · · · 610-446-6126
800-204-7667
Fax: 610-446-6129
www.learningdifferences.com
scooper-ldr@comcast.net
Rich Cooper, Director
Training session details how individuals with learning dif-
ferences, problems and disabilities think and learn.

2775 Latest Technology for Young Children
Western Illinois University: Macomb Projects
27 Horrabin Hall
Macomb, IL 61455 · · · · · · · · · · · · · · · · · 309-298-1955
Fax: 309-298-2305
www.mprojects.wiu.edu
PL-Hutinger@wiu.edu
Patricia Hutinger EdD, Director
Joyce Johanson, Coordinator
Amanda Silberer, Manager
This 25 minute videotape focuses on the Macintosh LC and
adaptations for young children and includes a discussion of
the features and advantages of the Macintosh LC, software
demonstrations, footage of child applications, and ideas for
off-computer activities. Videotape and written materials
available.OUT OF BUSINESS *$40.00*
16-20 pages

**2776 Learning Disabilities and Discipline: Rick Lavoie's
Guide to Improving Children's Behavior**
Connecticut Assoc. for Children and Adults with LD
Ste 15-5
25 Van Zant St
Norwalk, CT 6855-1713 · · · · · · · · · · · · · 203-838-5010
Fax: 203-866-6108
www.CACLD.org
cacld@juno.com
Beryl Kaufman, Executive Director
In this video, Richard Lavoie, a nationally known expert on
learning disabilities, offers practical advice on dealing with
behavioral problems quickly and effectively. Shows how
preventive discipline can anticipate many problems before
they start. Explains how teachers and parents can create stable, predictable environments in which children with learning disabilities can flourish. 62 minutes. *$49.95*

2777 **Learning Disabilities and Self-Esteem**
Connecticut Assoc. for Children and Adults with LD
Ste 15-5
25 Van Zant St
Norwalk, CT 6855-1713   203-838-5010
                               Fax: 203-866-6108
                               www.CACLD.org
                               cacld@juno.com
Beryl Kaufman, Executive Director
The 60 minute Teacher video contains program material for building self-esteem in the classroom. The 60 minute Parent video contains program material for building self-esteem in the home. A 16 page Program Guide accompanies each video. Dr. Robert Brooks, a clinical psychologist, renowned speaker and nationally known expert on learning disabilities, is on the faculty at Harvard Medical School and is the author of The Self-Esteem Teacher. *$49.95*

2778 **Learning Disabilities and Social Skills: Last One Picked..First One Picked On**
Connecticut Assoc. for Children and Adults with LD
Ste 15-5
25 Van Zant St
Norwalk, CT 6855-1713   203-838-5010
                               Fax: 203-866-6108
                               www.CACLD.org
                               cacld@juno.com
Beryl Kaufman, Executive Director
Nationally recognized expert on learning disabilities, Richard Lavoie, gives examples on how to help LD children succeed in everyday social situations. Lavoie helps students dissect their social errors to learn correct behavior. Mistakes are seen as opportunities for learning. Available in parent (62 min.) or teacher (68 min.) version. *$49.95*

2779 **Learning Disabilities: A Complex Journey**
Aquarius Health Media Care
18 N Main St
Millis, MA 20054-2324   508-376-1244
                               888-440-2963
                               Fax: 508-376-1245
                               www.aquariusproductions.com
                               orders@aquariusproductions.com
Leslie Kussmann, President/Producer
Does your child have trouble reading? Does your daughter seem to have more difficulty with schoolwork than you would expect, even though she's trying her hardest? Is your son avoiding school, claiming illness a little to often, insisitng that he's stupid when you know that's not really true? If so, your child may have a learning disability— a neurological problem processing information that he's actually smart enough to understand. How do you find out? VHS: A-KIDSLD also on DVD. *$125.00*
Video, 26 mins

2780 **Learning Problems in Language**
Center for Alternative
6 E Eagle Rd
Havertown, PA 19083-1424   610-446-6126
                               800-204-7667
                               Fax: 610-446-6129
                               www.learningdifferences.com
                               rcooper-ldr@comcast.net
Rich Cooper, Founder/Director/Author
This video was recorded at the National Laubach Conference in 1992 for reading tutors and teachers. In the video, Dr. Cooper discusses ideas for teaching reading and other academic skills to adults. *$16.00*
2hr, 50 mins

2781 **Legacy of the Blue Heron: Living with Learning Disabilities**
Oxton House Publishers
PO Box 209
Farmington, ME 4938   207-779-1923
                               800-539-7323
                               Fax: 207-779-0623
                               www.oxtonhouse.com
                               info@oxtonhouse.com

William Berlinghoff PhD, Managing Editor
Cheryl Martin, Marketing
Debra Richards, Office Manager
Thi book is available in soft cover or as a six-cassette audiobook. It is an engaging personal account by a servere dyslexic who became a successful engineer, business man, boat builder, and prcsidcnt of thc Lcarning Disabilities Association of America. Drawing on his life experiences, the author presents a rich array of wise, common-sense advice for dealing with learning disabilities.

2782 **Letting Go: Views on Integration**
Iowa University Affiliated Programs
300 CMAB
Iowa City, IA 52242-1016   319-353-6390
                               800-272-7713
                               Fax: 319-356-8284
                               www.healthcare.uiowa.edu
                               disability-library@uiowa.edu
Three parents share their thoughts regarding the struggle between protecting their children with disabilities verses allowing the same freedom as other children. *$25.00*
19 mins/Video

2783 **Lily Videos : A Longitudinel View of Lily with Down Syndrome**
Davidson Films
Ste 210
735 Tank Farm Rd
San Luis Obispo, CA 93401-7073   805-594-0422
                               888-437-4200
                               Fax: 805-594-0532
                               www.davidsonfilms.com
                               dfi@davidsonfilms.com
Elaine Taunt, Manager
Fran Davidson, Owner
1. Lily: A Story About a Girl Like Me 2. Lily: A Sequal 3. Lily: At Thirty.

2784 **Making Sense of Sensory Integration**
Therapro
225 Arlington St
Framingham, MA 1702-8773   508-872-9494
                               800-257-5376
                               Fax: 508-875-2062
                               www.theraproducts.com
                               info@theraproducts.com
Karen Conrad, Owner
A discussion for parents and caregivers about sensory integration (SI), how it affects children throughout their lives, how diagnosis is made, appropriate treatment, recognizing red flags, and how SI difficulties affect child and family in their everyday lives. Informative 33 page book included. 75 minute CD. *$17.95*
31 pages Audio CD
ISBN 1-931615-14-4

2785 **Motivation to Learn: How Parents and Teachers Can Help**
Association for Supervision/Curriculum Development
1703 N Beauregard St
Alexandria, VA 22311-1746   703-578-9600
                               800-933-2723
                               Fax: 703-575-5400
                               www.ascd.org
Nancy Gibson, President
Marie Adair, Executive Director
Two videos intended for all those concerned about how educators and families can develop student motivation to learn, solve motivational problems, and effectively participate in parent-teacher conferences.

2786 Normal Growth and Development: Performance Prediction
Love Publishing Company
9101 East Kenyon Ave
Ste 2200
Denver, CO 80237   303-221-7333
                                Fax: 303-221-7444
                                www.lovepublishing.com
                        lovepublishing@compuserve.com
Dan Love, Director
Stan Love, Owner
Teaches the age at which skills are normally achieved by children ages 0 to 48 months. *$140.00*
Video

2787 Oh Say What They See: Language Stimulation
Educational Productions
9000 SW Gemini Dr
Beaverton, OR 97008-7151   503-644-7000
                                     800-950-4949
                                Fax: 503-350-7000
                                www.edpro.com
                                custserv@edpro.com
Linda Freedman, Owner
Molly Krumm, Marketing Director
A complete video training program illustrating indirect language stimulation techniques to teachers, parents, students, child care staff, and other adult caregivers working with children.

2788 Parent Teacher Meeting
Learning Disabilities Resources
2775 S. Quincy St
Arlington, VA 22206   610-525-8336
                                     800-869-8336
                                Fax: 703-998-2060
                                www.ldonline.org
                                ldonline@weta.org
Discusses learning differences and instructional techniques. *$12.00*

2789 Phonemic Awareness: The Sounds of Reading
Sage/Corwin Press
2455 Teller Rd
Thousand Oaks, CA 91320-2218   805-410-7408
                                Fax: 805-499-2692
                                www.corwinpress.com
                                order@corwin.com
Mike Soules, President
Lisa Shaw, Executive Director
Kristin Anderson, Director of Learning
This staff development video may be used with paraprofessionals and teachers to learn the techniques of teaching pnomemic awareness. *$59.95*
Video
ISBN 1-890455-29-6

2790 Puberty Education for Students with Special Needs
Marsh Media
PO Box 8082
Shawnee Mission, KS 66208   802-821-3303
                                Fax: 866-333-7421
                                www.marshmedia.com
                                info@marshmedia.com
Liz Smith, Author
Liz Sweeney, Co-Author
Two gender-specific kits include an instructional video, a comprehensive teaching guide and packets of 10 student booklets. These reassuring titles are clear, practical and positive and are intended for the following special populations: Students with developmental disabilities or delays, Intrusive behavior or mental illness, Down Syndrome, Autism Spectrum Disorder, Learning disabilities, Behavioral disabilities, Communicative disorders.
36 pages

2791 Regular Lives
WETA-TV, Department of Educational Activities
Ste 440
2775 S Quincy St
Arlington, VA 22206   610-525-8336
                                     800-869-8336
                                Fax: 703-998-2060
                                www.weta.com
                                info@weta.com
Sharon P Rockefeller, President
Designed to show the successful integration of handicapped students in school, work and community settings. Demonstrates that sharing the ordinary routines of learning and living is essential for people with disabilities.

2792 STEP/Teen: Systematic Training for Effective Parenting of Teens
AGS
PO Box 99
Circle Pines, MN 55014   763-786-4343
                                     800-328-2560
                                Fax: 763-786-9077
                                www.agsnet.com
                                agsmail@agsnet.com
Kevin Brueggeman, Manager
A parent training program designed to help parents of teenagers in the following areas: understanding misbehavior; improving communication and family relationships; understanding and expressing emotions and feelings and discipline. *$229.50*

2793 Speech Therapy: Look Who's Not Talking
Aquarius Health Media Care
18 N Main St
Sherborn, MA 1770-1066   508-650-1616
                                     888-440-2963
                                Fax: 508-650-1665
                                www.aquariusproductions.com
                        aquarius@aquarisproductions.com
Leslie Kussmann, President
A Keeping Kids Healthy Series. Your child is old enough to be talking - other children are by this age - but for some reason, your child just can't put the words together. When should you step in to help? And what, exactly, can you do? VHS: A-KIDSSPEECH. Also available on DVD. *$125.00*
Video, 14 mins

2794 Student Directed Learning: Teaching Self Determination Skills
Beech Center on Disability, University of Kansas
1200 Sunnyside Ave
Lawrence, KS 0   785-864-7600
                                Fax: 785-864-7605
                                www.beachcenter.org
                                wehmeyer@ku.edu
Mike Wehmeyer, Associate Director
Written for educators and service providers who seek a comprehensive understanding of the process of helping students develop self-determination skills. The text follows academic principles and clearly is geared to professionals rather than to families. An educator seeking to understand technical self-determination concepts will find this organizational structure effective. *$73.00*
ISBN 0-534159-42-7

2795 Study Skills: How to Manage Your Time
Guidance Associates
31 Pine View Rd
Mount Kisco, NY 10549-3425   914-244-1055
                                     800-431-1242
                                Fax: 914-244-1056
                                www.guidanceassociates.com
                                info@guidanceassociates.com
Fred Gaston Jr, Owner
Describes how to create a personal schedule that will help users get more accomplished each day and waste less time. *$61.00*
Video

2796 The Power of Positive Communication
Educational Productions
7101 Wisconsin Avenue
Suite 700
Bethesda, MD 20814

503-297-6393
800-637-3652
Fax: 503-297-6395
www.teachingstrategies.com
info@teachingstrategies.com

Andrea Valentine, President
Ron Davies, CEO
Amy Houser, CMO
A complete three-session training on CD-ROM teaches how and why to use clear, positive language to help children to follow expectations and learn. Emphasizes strategies that assist both children with special needs and English language learners.

2797 Time Together: Adults Supporting Play
Educational Productions
7101 Wisconsin Avenue
Suite 700
Bethesda, MD 20814

503-297-6393
800-637-3652
Fax: 503-297-6395
www.teachingstrategies.com
info@teachingstrategies.com

Andrea Valentine, President
Ron Davies, CEO
Amy Houser, CMO
A complete video training program for beginning childhood teachers, aides and parents illustrating when to join a child's play, how to enhance and extend the play, and when to step back.

2798 Tools for Students
Therapro
225 Arlington St
Framingham, MA 1702-8773

508-872-9494
800-257-5376
Fax: 508-875-2062
www.theraproducts.com
info@theraproducts.com

Karen Conrad, Owner
This is a 30 minute fun and participatory 'how-to' presentation which provides solutions to the problems indentified in the Tools for Teachers Video. It can be used by teachers in the classroom and by parents at home. There are 25 sensory tools for movement, proprioception, mouth and hand fidgets, calming and recess. Pencil-holding and hand games to develop hand manipulation skills are also demonstrated. *$25.95*
Video

2799 Tools for Teachers
Therapro
225 Arlington St
Framingham, MA 1702-8773

508-872-9494
800-257-5376
Fax: 508-875-2062
www.theraproducts.com
info@theraproducts.com

Karen Conrad, Owner
Provides a logical approach to sensory integration and hand skill strategies for anyone to use, is ideal for in-services. Within 20 minutes, you'll learn how to help students calm down, focus, and increase their self-awareness. This is a great tool for teachers and therapists (it shows how to inplement sensory diet, into classroom), administrators and parents. *$25.95*
Video

2800 TrainerVision: Inclusion, Focus on Toddlers and Pre-K
Educational Productions
PO Box 957
Hillsboro, OR 97123

503-297-6393
800-950-4949
Fax: 503-297-6395
www.edpro.com
custserv@edpro.com

Linda Freedman, Owner
Instructive video clips focus on non-typically developing toddlers and pre-K children. Shows how to gently support skill building, independence and social competence. The clips are ideal to enrich training, classes and online courses.

2801 Treatment of Children's Grammatical Impairments in Naturalistic Context
Purdue University Continuing Education
1586 Stewart Ctr
West Lafayette, IN 47907

765-494-7231
800-830-0269
Fax: 765-494-0567
www.continuinged.purdue.edu/media/speech

Marc Fey, Presenter
The basic assumption is challenged that language intervention which takes place in naturalistic settings will be more effective than intervention that occurs in settings that are more heavily constrained by a clinician or other intervention agent. The concept of naturalness will be described as a continuum that is influenced by a number of factors that can be manipulated by clinicians. Several effective intervention approaches that reflect different levels of naturalness are presented. *$50.00*
1hr:42 mins

2802 Understanding Attention Deficit Disorder
Connecticut Assoc. for Children and Adults with LD
Ste 15-5
25 Van Zant St
Norwalk, CT 6855-1713

203-838-5010
Fax: 203-866-6108
www.CACLD.org
cacld@juno.com

Beryl Kaufman, Executive Director
A video in an interview format for parents and professionals providing the history, symptoms, methods of diagnosis and three approaches used to ease the effects of attention deficit disorder. A comprehensive general introduction to ADHD. 45 minutes. *$20.00*
Video

2803 United Learning
Ste 100
1560 Sherman Ave
Evanston, IL 60201-4817

847-328-6700
888-892-3494
Fax: 847-328-6706
www.unitedlearning.com
crechner@unitedlearning.com

Ronald Reed, President
Joel Altschul, Vice President
Coni Rechner, Vice President
United Learning is a provider of audio-visual materials that inform and educate people of all ages. It helps teachers teach more effectively and to help students learn more efficiently. Offering videos, cd's, dvd's, and now delivery of video clips and text via the internet.

2804 What Every Teacher Should Know About ADD
United Learning
Ste 100
1560 Sherman Ave
Evanston, IL 60201-4817

847-328-6700
888-892-3484
Fax: 847-328-6706
www.unitedlearning.com
info@unitedlearning.com

Ronald Reed, President
Mark Zinselmeier, Operations VP/General Manager
Coni Rechner, Marketing VP
This program is for teachers, paraprofessionals, administrators, and special educators because it separates clearly fact from fiction and is written specifically for and about educators who deal with disruptive, inattentive, and hyperactive pre-school and elementary age children on a daily basis. *$79.00*
28-min. video

2805 **When a Child Doesn't Play: Module 1**
Educational Productions
PO Box 957
Hillsboro, OR 97123

800-950-4949
Fax: 503-297-6395
www.edpro.com
custserv@edpro.com

Linda Freedman, Owner
A 30 minute video with 100 pages of facilitation materials presentsdramatic footage of children with play problems and how they miss critical opportunities to learn. Illustrates supportive strategies for adults. Foundation program for Hand-in-Hand Series. *$350.00*

Vocational

2806 **Different Way of Learning**
Brookes Publishing Company
PO Box 10624
Baltimore, MD 21285

800-638-3775
Fax: 410-337-8539
www.pbrookes.com
custserv@pbrookes.com

Paul H Brooks, President
Melissa A Behn, Executive Vice President
George Stamthis, Vice President/Publisher
This video prepares students with learning disabilities for the transition from school to the workplace. *$49.00*
Video
ISBN 1-557663-49-1

2807 **Employment Initiatives Model: Job Coach Training Manual and Tape**
Young Adult Institute
460 W 34th St
New York, NY 10001-2320

212-273-6100
Fax: 212-268-1083
www.yai.org
ahorowitz@yai.org

Philip Levy, Manager
Thomas A Dern, Assoc. Executive Director
Aimee Horowitz, Project Specialist
Video and manual providing an overview and orientation for staff members involved in transition services to ensure that they are well-grounded inthe concepts, responsibilities, and activities that are required to provide quality supported employment services.

2808 **First Jobs: Entering the Job World**
Triumph Learning
PO Box 1270
Littleton, MA 1460-4270

800-338-6519
Fax: 212-675-8922
www.triumphlearning.com
customerservice@triumphlearning.com
Career/vocational education with emphasis on job search skills, job interviews and survival skills. *$139.00*

2809 **How Not to Contact Employers**
Nat'l Clearinghouse of Rehab. Training Materials
6524 Old Main Hil
Logan, UT 84322-6524

435-797-7537
Fax: 866-821-5355
http://https://ncrtm.org/
ncrtm@usu.edu

Sara P. Johnston, M.S, Director
Jennifer Robinson, Official Assistant
A single vignette of what not to do when visiting perspective employers to secure positions for clients. *$10.00*

2810 **KET Basic Skills Series**
KET, The Kentucky Network Enterprise Division
600 Cooper Dr
Lexington, KY 40502-2296

859-258-7000
800-354-9067
Fax: 859-258-7399
www.ket.org
feedback@ket.org

Barbra Ledford, President
Offers an independent learning system for workers who need retraining or help with basic skills

2811 **KET Foundation Series**
KET, The Kentucky Network Enterprise Division
600 Cooper Dr
Lexington, KY 40502-2296

859-258-7000
800-354-9067
Fax: 859-258-7399
www.ket.org
feedback@ket.org

Barbra Ledford, President
A highly effective basic skills series that is tailor-made for the needs of proprietary and vocational schools.

2812 **KET/GED Series**
KET, The Kentucky Network Enterprise Division
600 Cooper Dr
Lexington, KY 40502-1669

859-258-7000
800-354-9067
Fax: 859-258-7399
www.ket.org
feedback@ket.org

Barbra Ledford, President
This nationally acclaimed instructional series helps adults prepare for the GED test.

2813 **KET/GED Series Transitional Spanish Edition**
KET, The Kentucky Network Enterprise Division
600 Cooper Dr
Lexington, KY 40502-1669

859-258-7000
800-354-9067
Fax: 859-258-7399
www.ket.org
feedback@ket.org

Barbra Ledford, President
This award-winning series offers ESL students effective preparation for the GED test.

2814 **Life After High School for Students with Moderate and Severe Disabilities**
Beech Center on Disability, University of Kansas
3111 Haworth Hall
Lawrence, MA 0

785-864-7600
Fax: 785-864-7605
www.beachcenter.org
beachcenter@ku.edu

Shonda Anderson, Project Coordinator
A set of three videotapes and a participant handbook document, and a teleconference in which family members, people with disabilities, teachers, rehabilitation specialists, program administrators and policy makers focus on improving the quality of services in high school and supported employment programs.

2815 **On Our Own Transition Series**
Young Adult Institute
460 W 34th St
New York, NY 10001-2320

212-273-6100
Fax: 212-268-1083
www.yai.org
ahorowitz@yai.org

Thomas A Dern, Assoc. Executive Director
Aimee Horowitz, Project Specialist
Designed for parents and professionals, this series of 15 videotapes examines innovative transitional approaches that help create marketable skills, instill self-esteem and facilitate successful transition for individuals with developmental disabilities.

General

2816 **www.HealthCentral.com**
Former Surgeon-General Dr. C Everett Koop
Information on health and conditions that affect learning, particularly heavy on the ADHD side.

2817 **www.ala.org**
American Library Association
Run by the American Library Association, this site works to raise public awareness about learning disabilities.

2818 **www.allaboutvision.com**
All About Vision
Vision information and resources, including articles on learning-related vision problems.

2819 **www.apa.org/psycinfo**
American Psychological Association
An online abstract database that provides access to citations to the international serial literature in psychology and related disciplines from 1887 to present. Available via PsycINFO Direct at www.psycinfo.com.

2820 **www.autismtreatment.com**
Autism Treatment Center of America
Since 1983, the Autism Treatment Center of America, has provided innovative training programs for parents and professionals caring for children challenged by Autism, Autism Spectrum Disorders, Pervasive Developmental Disorders (PDD) and other developmental difficulties. The Son-Rise Program teaches a specific yet comprehensive system of treatment and education designed to help families and caregivers enable their children to dramatically improve in all areas of learning.

2821 **www.childdevelopmentinfo.com**
Child Development Institute
Provides online information on child development, psychology, parenting, learning, health and safety as well as childhood disorders such as attention deficit disorder, dyslexia and autism. Provides comprehensive resources and practical suggestions for parents.

2822 **www.disabilityinfo.gov**
DisabilityInfo.gov
Provides one-stop online access to resources, services, and information available throughout the federal government to Americans with disabilities, their families, employers and service providers; also promotes awareness of disability issues to the general public.

2823 **www.disabilityresources.org**
Disability Resources
A guide to internet resources available with information and recommendations for disability assistance.

2824 **www.doleta.gov/programs/**
O'Net: Department of Labor's Occ. Information
Employment assistance, descriptions, and articles about learning disabled employees and government resources.

2825 **www.dyslexia.com**
Davis Dyslexia Association International
Links to internet resources for learning. Includes dyslexia, Autism and Asperger's Syndrome, ADD/ADHD and other learning disabilities.

2826 **www.familyvillage.wisc.edu**
University of Wisconsin-Madison
A global community that integrates information, resources and communication opportunities on the Internet for all those involved with cognitive and other disabilities.

2827 **www.funbrain.com**
Quiz Lab
Internet education site for teachers and kids. Access thousands of assessment quizzes online. Assign paperless quizzes that are graded automatically by email. Teaching tools are free and easy to use.

2828 **www.health.disovery.com**
Discovery Health
Information on conditions that impact learning.

2829 **www.healthanswers.com**
Health Answers Education
Health information, including learning disabilities, etc.

2830 **www.healthatoz.com**
Medical Network
Health information, including ADD, ADHD, etc.

2831 **www.healthcentral.com**
HealthCentral Network
Information and products for a healthier life. Includes conditions that impact learning.

2832 **www.healthymind.com**
HealthyMind.com
Information on ADD and learning disabilities.

2833 **www.hood.edu/seri/serihome.htm**
Special Education Resources on the Internet
Contains links to information about definitions, legal issues, and teaching and learning related to learning disabilities.

2834 **www.icpac.indiana.edu/infoseries/is-50.htm**
Finding Your Career: Holland Interest Inventory
Includes information on self-assessing one's skills and matching them to careers.

2835 **www.intelihealth.com**
Aetna InteliHealth
Includes information on learning disabilities.

2836 **www.irsc.org**
Internet Research for Special Children
Attention deficit and hyperactivity disorder help website, created so information, support and ADD coaching are available without having to pour over all 531,136 links that come up on a net search.

2837 **www.jobhunt.org/slocareers/resources.html**
Online Career Resources
Contains assessment tools, tutorials, labor market information, etc.

2838 **www.ld-add.com**
Attention Deficit Disorder (ADD or ADHD)
Do you think that you or your child has ADHD with or without learning disabilities? If the answer is yes, this webpage is for you.

2839 **www.ldonline.org**
Learning Project at WETA
Learning disabilities information and resources.

2840 **www.ldpride.net**
LD Pride Online
Inspired by Deaf Pride, a site developed as an interactive community resource for youth and adults with learning disabilities and ADD.

2841 **www.ldteens.org**
Study Skills Web Site
Run by the New York State Chapter of the International Dyslexia Association; a site for students, created by students; provides helpful tips and links.

2842 www.marriottfoundation.org
Marriott Foundation
Provides information on job opportunities for teenagers and young adults with disabilities.

2843 www.my.webmd.com
Web MD Health
Medical website with information which includes learning disabilities, ADD/ADHD, etc.

2844 www.ntis.gov
National Techinical Information Service
A worldwide database for research, development and engineering reports on a range of topics, including architectural barrier removal, employing individuals with disabilities, alternative testing formats, job accommodations, school-to-work transition for students with disabilities, rehabilitation engineering, disability law and transportation.

2845 www.ocde.K12.ca.us/PAL/index2.html
Peer Assistance Leadership (PAL)
A California-based outreach program for elementary, intermediate and high school students.

2846 www.oneaddplace.com
One A D D Place
A virtual neighborhood of information and resources relating to ADD, ADHD and learning disorders.

2847 www.optimums.com
JR Mills, MS, MEd
Information on learning disabilities.

2848 www.pacer.org
Does My Child Have An Emotional Disorder
Our mission is to expand opportunities and enhance the quality of life of children and young adults with disabilities and their families, based on the concept of parents helping parents.

2849 www.parentpals.com
Ameri-Corp Speech and Hearing
Offers parents and professionals special education support, teaching ideas and tips, special education continuing education, disability-specific information and more.

2850 www.peer.ca/peer.html
Peer Resources Network
A Canadian organization that offers training, educational resources, and consultation to those interested in peer helping and education. Their resources section has information on books, articles and videos.

2851 www.petersons.com
Peterson's Education and Career Center
Contains postings for full-and part-time jobs as well as summer job opportunities.

2852 www.specialchild.com
Resource Foundation for Children with Challenges
Variety of information for parents of children with disabilities, including actual stories, family and legal issues, diagnosis search, etc.

2853 www.specialneeds.com
Special Needs Project
A place to get books about disabilities.

2854 www.wrightlaw.com
Wrightslaw
Provides information about advocacy.

Counseling & Psychology

2855 American Psychologist
American Psychological Association
750 1st St NE
Washington, DC 20002-4242

202-336-5500
800-374-2721
Fax: 202-336-5518
TDD: 202-336-6123
TTY: 202-336-6123
www.apa.org
journals@apa.org

Norman B Anderson, Editor
Contains archivel documents and articles covering current issues in psychology, the science and practice of psychology, and psychology's contribution to public policy.
9 times x year
ISSN 0003-066X

2856 Educational Therapist Journal
Association of Educational Therapists
7044 S. 13th Street
Oak Creek, WI 53154

414-908-4949
Fax: 414-768-8001
www.aetonline.org
aet@aetonline.org

Jeanette Rivera, President
A multidisciplinary publication, that publishes articles and reviews on clinical practice, research, and theory. In addition, it serves to inform the reader of AET activities and business and presents issues relevant to the practice of educational therapy. *$40.00*
Quarterly

2857 Journal of Social and Clinical Psychology
Guilford Press
72 Spring Street
New York, NY 10012-4019

800-365-7006
Fax: 212-966-6708
www.guilford.com
info@guilford.com

Thomas E Joiner PhD, Editor
Discusses theory, research and research methodology from personality and social psychology toward the goal of enhancing the understanding of human well-being and adjustment. Also covers a wide range of areas, including intimate relationships, attributions, stereotyping, social skills, depression research, coping strategies, and more. It fosters interdisciplinary communication and scholarship among students and practitioners of social/personality and clinical/counseling/health psychology. *$165.00*
128 pages 10x a year
ISSN 0736-7236

2858 Learning Disabilities Research & Practice
Blackwell Publishing
350 Main St
Malden, MA 2148-5089

781-388-8200
Fax: 781-388-8210
www.blackwellpublishing.com

Charles Hughes, Editor
Because learning disabilities is a multidisciplinary field of study, this important journal publishes articles addressing the nature and characteristics of learning disabled students, promising research, program development, assessment practices, and teaching methodologies from different disciplines. In so doing, LDRP provides information of great value to professionals involved in a variety of different disciplines including school psychology, counseling, reading and medicine. *$68.00*
Quarterly
ISSN 0938-8982

2859 School Psychology Quarterly
American Psychological Association
750 1st St NE
Washington, DC 20002-4241

202-336-5500
800-374-2721
Fax: 202-336-5518
TDD: 202-336-6123
TTY: 202-336-6123
www.apa.org
journals@apa.org

Norman B Anderson, Editor
This journal advances the latest research, theory, and practice and features a new book review section. Strengthening the relationship between school psychology and broad-based psychological science. *$57.00*
Quarterly
ISSN 1045-3830

General

2860 ASCD Express
Association for Supervision/Curriculum Development
1703 N Beauregard St
Alexandria, VA 22311-1714

703-578-9600
800-933-2723
Fax: 703-575-5400
www.ascd.org
express@ascd.org

Rick Allen, Editor
Willona Sloan, Editor
This newsletter highlights articles on research-based teaching practices and provides you with quick links to these articles, relevant resources, and multimedia clips. *$29.00*
Bi-weekly

2861 American Journal of Occupational Therapy
American Occupational Therapy Association
4720 Montgomery Lane
Bethesda, MD 20814

301-652-2682
800-729-2682
Fax: 301-652-7711
TDD: 800-377-8555
www.aota.org
ajoteditor@cox.net

Mary A Corcoran PhD, Editor
An official publication of the American Occupational Therapy Association, inc. This peer reviewed journal focuses on research, practice, and health care issues in the field of occupational therapy. Also publishes articles that are theoretical and conceptual and that represent theory-based research, research reviews, and applied research realted to innovative program approaches, educational activities, and professional trends. *$50.00*
6x a year

2862 American School Board Journal
National School Boards Association
1680 Duke St
Alexandria, VA 22314-3474

703-838-6722
703-838-6722
Fax: 703-549-6719
www.asbj.com

Marilee C Rist, Publisher
Glenn Cook, Editor
American School Board Journal chronicles change, interprets issues, and offers readers — some 40,000 school board members and school administrators — practical advice on a broad range of topics pertinent to school go9vernance and management, policy making, student achievement, and the art of school leadership. In addition, regular departments cover education news, school law, research, and new books. *$54.00*
Monthly

2863 Annals of Otology, Rhinology and Laryngology
Annals Publishing Company
4507 Laclede Ave
Saint Louis, MO 63108-2103
314-367-4987
Fax: 314-367-4988
www.annals.com
manager@annals.com

Ken Cooper, President
Richard J. H Smith, Managing Director
Offers original manuscripts of clinical and research importance in otolaryngology - head and neck surgery, audiology, speech pathology, head and neck oncology and surgery, and related specialties. All papers are peer-reviewed *$179.00*
112 pages Monthly
ISSN 0003-4894

2864 Autism Research Review International
Autism Research Institute
4182 Adams Ave
San Diego, CA 92116-2599
619-281-7165
Fax: 619-563-6840
www.autism.com

Steve Edelson, Editor
Janet Johnson, Managing Director
Covering biomedical and educational advances in autism research. *$18.00*
Quarterly

2865 CABE Journal
Connecticut Association of Boards of Education
81 Wolcott Hill Rd
Wethersfield, CT 6109-1286
860-571-7446
800-317-0033
Fax: 860-571-7452
www.cabe.org
bcarney@cabe.org

Robert Rader, Executive Director
Patrice McCarthy, Deputy Director
Reaches virtually all board members, superintendents and business managers in Connecticut. It's the only publication which does so on a regular basis. It is designed to encompass all material in an easy-to-read fashion. Readers if the journal find a wide range of topics covered in each issue.
11x a year

2866 CEC Today
Council for Exceptional Children
Ste 300
1110 N Glebe Rd
Arlington, VA 22201-5704
703-245-0600
888-232-7733
Fax: 703-264-9494
TTY: 866-915-5000
www.cec.sped.org
service@cec.sped.org

Lynda Voyles, Editor
Drew Albritten M.D., President
Bruce Ramirez, Manager
An online member newsletter that keeps you up-to-date on professional and legal developments.
4x per year

2867 Disability Compliance for Higher Education
LRP Publications
PO Box 24668
West Palm beach
Palm Beach Gardens, FL 33418-7106
561-622-6520
800-341-7874
Fax: 561-622-0757
www.lrp.com
webmaster@lrp.com

Kenneth Kahn, CEO
Virginia Charleston, Product Group Manager
Cynthia Gomez, Author
Combines insightful analyses of disability laws with details of innovative accomodations for your students and staff. *$198.00*
12 issues/yr

2868 Education Digest
Prakken Publications
PO Box 8623
Ann Arbor, MI 48107-8623
734-975-2800
Fax: 734-975-2787
www.eddigest.com
pam@eddigest.com

Pam Moore, Editor
The Education Digest reviews recent periodicals and reports on education to produce 12 or more condensations for quick, easy reading, along with the regular monthly columns and features. *$32.00*
9 Issues

2869 Education Week
Editorial Projects in Education
Ste 100
6935 Arlington Rd
Bethesda, MD 20814-5287
301-280-3100
800-346-1834
Fax: 301-280-3200
www.edweek.org

Virginia Edwards, Editor
Offers articles of interest to educators, teachers, professionals and special educators on the latest developments, laws, issues and more in the various fields of education. *$74.94*

2870 Educational Leadership
Association for Supervision/Curriculum Development
1703 N Beauregard St
Alexandria, VA 22311-1746
703-578-9600
800-933-2722
Fax: 703-575-5400
www.ascd.org
edleadership@ascd.org

Marge Scherer, Editor
RICHARD J. H. SMITH
8x a year

2871 Educational Researcher
American Educational Research Association
1430 17th St NW
Washington, DC 20036
202-238-3200
Fax: 202-238-3250
www.aera.net
pubs@aera.net

Patricia B Elmore, Editor
Gregory Camilli, Editor
Received by all members of AERA, contains scholarly articles that come from a wide range of dosciplines and are of general significance to the education research community.
9x a year
ISSN 0013-189X

2872 Educational Technology
Educational Technology Publications
700 E Palisade Ave
Englewood Cliffs, NJ 7632-3060
201-871-4007
800-952-BOOK
Fax: 201-871-4009
www.asianvu.com/bookstoread/etp
edtecpubs@aol.com

Lawrence Lipsitz, Editor
The world's leading periodical publication covering the entire field of educational technology, an area pioneered by the magazine's editors in the early 1960s. *$179.00*
6x annually

2873 Gifted Child Today
Prufrock Press
Ste 220
5926 Balcones Dr
Austin, TX 78731-4263
512-300-2220
Fax: 512-300-2221
www.prufrock.com
info@prufrock.com

Susan K Johnsen PhD, Editor
Sarah Morrison, Editor

Offers teachers information about teaching gifted children. Offers parents information about raising a gifted child, how to tell if your child is gofted, and effective strategies for parenting a gifted child. *$40.00*
Quarterly

2874 Journal of Learning Disabilities
Sage Publications
2455 Teller Rd
Thousand Oaks, CA 91320-2218

805-499-9774
800-818-7243
Fax: 805-499-0871
www.sagepub.com
journals@sagepub.com

H Lee Swanson, Editor
Recognized internationally as the oldest and most authoritative journal in the area of learning disabilities. The editorial board reflects the international, multidisciplinary nature of JLD, comprising researchers and practitioners in numerous fields, including education, psychology, neurology, medicine, law and counseling. *$69.00*
Bimonthly
ISSN 0022-2194

2875 Journal of Postsecondary Education and Disability
Association on Higher Education and Disability
Ste 204
107 Commerce Centre Dr
Huntersville, NC 28078-5870

704-947-7779
Fax: 704-948-7779
www.ahead.org
ahead@ahead.org

James Martin PhD, Editor
Serves as a resource to members and other professionals dedicated to the advancement of full participation in higher education for persons with disabilities. Is also the leading forum for scholarship in the field of postsecondary disability support services.

2876 Journal of Rehabilitation
National Rehabilitation Association
PO Box 150235
Alexandria, VA 22314-4109

703-836-0850
888-258-4295
Fax: 703-836-0848
www.nationalrehab.org
info@nationalrehab.org

Daniel C Lustig, Editor
David R Strauser, Editor
Sara Sundeen, President
The Journal of Rehabilitation publishes articles by leaders in the fields of rehabilitation. The articles are written for rehabilitation professionals and students studying in the fields of rehabilitation *$65.00*
Quarterly
ISSN 0022-4154

2877 Journal of School Health
Blackwell Publishing
350 Main St
Malden, MA 2148-5089

781-388-8200
Fax: 781-388-8210
www.blackwellpublishing.com
customerservices@blackwellpublishing.com

James H Price, Editor
Committed to communicating information regarding the role of schools and school personnel in facilitating the development and growth of healthy youth and healthy school environments.
Monthly
ISSN 0022-4391

2878 Journal of Special Education Technology
Council for Exceptional Children
2900 Crystal Drive
Ste 1000
Arlington, VA 22202-3557

703-245-0600
888-232-7733
Fax: 703-264-9494
www.cec.sped.org
service@cec.sped.org

J Emmett Gardner, Editor
The Journal of Special Education Technology (JSET) is a refereed professional journal that presents up-to-date information and opinions about issues, research, policy, and practice related to the use of technology in the field of special education. The publication is sent to subscribers and members of the Technology and Media Division of the Council for Exceptional Children. *$60.00*
Quarterly

2879 LDA Alabama Newsletter
Learning Disabilities Association of Alabama
PO Box 11588
Montgomery, AL 36111

334-277-9151
Fax: 334-284-9357
www.ldaal.org

Debbie Gibson, President
Dr. Jendia Grissett, Secretary
Educational support and advocacy for those with learning disabilities and Attention Deficit Disorder.

2880 LDA Rhode Island Newsletter
Learning Disabilities Association of Rhode Island
4156 Library Road
Pittsburgh, PA 15234-1349

412-341-1515
Fax: 412-344-0224
TDD: 401-946-6968
www.ldanatl.org
info@ldaamerica.org

Mary Clare Reynolds, Interim Executive Director
Frank Kline PhD, Editor
A nonprofit, volunteer organization whose members give their time and support to children with learning disabilities as well as share information with other parents, professionals and individuals with learning disabilities.

2881 Learning Disabilities Quarterly
Council for Learning Disabilities
PO Box 405
Overland Park, KS 66201

913-491-1011
Fax: 913-941-1012
www.cldinternational.org
ldq@bc.edu

David Scanlon, Editor
Presents scientifically-based research, and includes articles by nationally known authors.
4x a year

2882 Learning Disabilities: A Multidisciplinary Journal
Learning Disabilities Association of America
4156 Library Rd
Pittsburgh, PA 15234-1349

412-341-1515
Fax: 412-344-0224
www.LDAAmerica.org
info@ldaamerica.org

Steve Russell, Editor
A technical publication oriented toward professionals in the field of learning disabilities. *$30.00*
Quarterly

2883 Learning and Individual Differences
Elsevier
6277 Sea Harbor Dr
Orlando, FL 32887

407-563-6022
877-839-7126
Fax: 407-363-1354
TDD: 301-657-4155
www.elsevier.com
journalcustomerservice-usa@elsevier.com

E L Grigorenko, Editor

A multidisciplinary journal in education.
ISSN 1041-6080

2884 National Organization on Disability
77 Water ST
Ste 204
New York, NY 10005

646-505-1191
800-248-2253
Fax: 202-293-7999
TTY: 202-293-5968
www.nod.org
info@nod.org

H.W. Bush, President
Website offering information and articles on the organization.

2885 OT Practice
American Occupational Therapy Association
PO Box 31220
Bethesda, MD 20824-1220

301-652-2682
800-SAY-AOTA
Fax: 301-652-7711
TDD: 800-377-8555
www.aota.org
otpractice@aota.org

Laura Collins, Editor
Frederick P Somers, Executive Director
The clinical and professional magazone of the AOTA. It serves as a comprehensive, authoritative source for practical information to help occupational therapists and occupational therapy assistants to succeed professionally. Provides professional news and information on all aspects of practice and encourages a dialogue among AOTA members on professional concerns and views.
64 pages

2886 Occupational Outlook Quarterly
US Department of Labor
200 Constitution Ave
Washington, DC 20212

202-693-5000
Fax: 202-693-6111
www.dol.gov

Olivia Crosby, Editor
Information on new educational and training opportunities, emerging jobs, prospects for change in the work world and the latest research findings.

2887 Publications from HEATH
HEATH Resource Center
2134 G St NW
Washington, DC 20052

202-973-0904
Fax: 202-994-3365
www.heath.gwu.edu
askheath@gwu.edu

Donna Martinez, Director
Dr. Lynda West, Principal Investigator
A newsletter offering information on postsecondary education for individuals with disabilities.

2888 Teaching Exceptional Children
Council for Exceptional Children
2900 Crystal Drive
Ste 1000
Arlington, VA 22202-3557

888-232-7733
Fax: 703-264-9494
TTY: 866-915-5000
www.cec.sped.org/
service@cec.sped.org

Drew Albritten MD, President
Bruce Ramirez, Manager
Published specifically for teachers and administrators of children who are gifted. Features practical articles that present methods and materials for classroom use as well as current issues in special education teaching and learning. Brings together its readers the latest data on technology, assistive technology, and procedures and techniques with applications to students with exceptionalities. The focus of its practical content is on immediate application.
6x per year

2889 Texas Key
Learning Disabilities Association of Texas
PO Box 831392
Richardson, TX 75083-1392

800-604-7500
Fax: 512-458-3826
www.ldat.org
contact@ldat.org

Ann Robinson, Editor
Jean Kueker, President
Quarterly newsletter providing information of intrest to parents and professionals in the field of learning.
16-24 pages

Language Arts

2890 ASHA Leader
American Speech-Language-Hearing Association
2200 Research Blvd
Rockville, MD 20850-3289

301-296-5700
800-498-2071
Fax: 301-296-8580
www.asha.org
leader@asha.org

Susan Boswell, Editor
Pertains to the professional and administrative activities in the fields of speech-language pathology, audiology and the American Speech-Language-Hearing Association.
16X/year

2891 American Journal of Speech-Language Pathology: A Journal of Clinical Practice
American Speech-Language-Hearing Association
2200 Research Blvd
Rockville, MD 20850-3289

301-296-5700
800-498-2071
Fax: 301-296-8580
www.asha.org
subscribe@asha.org

Laura Justice, Editor
The journal pertains to all aspects of clinical practice in speech-language pathology. Articles address screening, assessment, and treatment techniques; prevention; professional issues; supervision; and administration, and may appear in the form of clinical forums, clinical reviews, letters to the editor, or research reports that emphasize clinical practice.
Quarterly
ISSN 1058-0360

2892 Communication Outlook
Michigan State University Artificial Language Lab
405 Computer Ctr
East Lansing, MI 48824-1042

517-353-0870
Fax: 517-353-4766
www.msu.edu
artlang@pilot.msu.edu

Rebecca Ann Baird, Editor
Quarterly journal which focuses on communication aids and techniques. Provides information also for blind and visually impaired persons. *$18.00*
Quarterly

2893 Journal of Speech, Language, and Hearing Research
American Speech-Language-Hearing Association
2200 Research Blvd
Rockville, MD 20850-3289

301-296-5700
888-498-2071
Fax: 301-296-8580
www.asha.org
subscribe@asha.org

Katherine Verdolini, Editor
Karla K McGregor, Editor
Robert Slauch, Editor

Pertains broadly to the studies of the processes and disorders of hearing, language, and speech and to the diagnosis and treatment of such disorders. Articles may take any of the following forms: reports of original research, including single-study experiments; theoretical, tutorial, or review pieces; research notes; and letters to the editor.
Bi-Monthly
ISSN 1092-4388

2894   Kaleidoscope, Exploring the Experience of Disability Through Literature and Fine Arts
United Disability Services
701 S Main St
Akron, OH 44311-1019   330-762-9755
                                            Fax: 330-762-0912
                                            www.udsakron.org
                                      kaleidoscope@udsakron.org
Gail Willmott, Editor
Creatively focuses on the experience of disability through diverse forms of literature and the fine arts. An award-winning magazine unique to the field of disability studies, it is open to writers with or without disabilities. KALEIDO-SCOPE strives to express how disability does or does not affect society and individuals feelings and reactions to disability. Its portrayals of disability reflect a conscious effort to challenge and overcome stereotypical and patronizing attitudes. *$6.00*
64 pages $10.00/year

2895   Language Arts
National Council of Teachers of English
1111 W Kenyon Rd
Urbana, IL 61801-1010   217-328-3870
                                                877-369-6283
                                            Fax: 217-328-9645
                                                www.ncte.org
                                        public_info@ncte.org
Patricia Enciso, Editor
Laurie Katz, Editor
Barbara Kiefer, Editor
Language Arts provides a forum for discussions on all aspects of language arts learning and teaching, primarily as they relate to children in pre-kindergarten through the eighth grade. Articles discuss both theory and classroom practice, highlight current research, and review children's and young adolescent literature, as well as classroom and professional resources of interest to language arts educators. *$25.00*
Bi-monthly

College Guides

2896 **NACE Journal**
National Association of Colleges and Employers
62 Highland Ave
Bethlehem, PA 18017-9481

610-868-1421
800-544-5272
Fax: 610-868-0208
www.naceweb.org
callen@naceweb.org

Marilyn Mackes, Editor
Gives hard data on practitioners, budgets, the college relations and recruitment function, entry-level hiring, on-campus recruitment, new hires and much much more. *$70.00*
100+ pages Quarterly

Counseling & Psychology

2897 **Accommodations in Higher Education under the Americans with Disabilities Act (ADA)**
Guilford Press
72 Spring St
New York, NY 10012-4019

800-365-7006
Fax: 212-966-6708
www.guilford.com
info@guilford.com

Michael Gordon, Editor
Shelby Keiser, Editor
This practical manual offers essential information and guidance for anyone involved with ADA issues in higher education settings. Fundamental principals and actual clinical and administrative procedures are outlined for evaluating, documenting, and accommodating a wide range of mental and physical impairments. *$29.00*
245 pages
ISBN 1-572303-23-9

2898 **Affect and Creativity**
Routledge
7625 Empire Drive
Florence, KY 41042-2919

212-216-7800
800-634-7064
Fax: 212-563-2269
www.routledge.com
book.orders@tandf.co.uk

Sandra Walker Russ, Author
This volume offers information on the role of affect and play in the creative process. Designed as a required or supplemental text in graduate level courses in creativity, children's play, child development, affective/cognitive development and psychodynamic theory. *$39.95*
160 pages
ISBN 0-805809-86-4

2899 **Best Practice Occupational Therapy: In Community Service with Children and Families**
Therapro
225 Arlington St
Framingham, MA 1702-8773

508-872-9494
800-257-5376
Fax: 508-875-2062
www.theraproducts.com
info@theraproducts.com

Winnie Dunn PhD OTR FAOTA, Author
An invaluable resource for sudents and practitioners interested in working with children and families in early intervention programs and public schools. Includes screening, pre-assessment, the referral process, best practice assessments, designing best paractice services and examples of IEPs and IFSPs. Many of the forms (screenings, checklists for teachers, referral forms assessment planning guide, etc.) are reproducible. The case studies give good examples of reports. *$55.00*

2900 **Cognitive-Behavioral Therapy for Impulsive Children**
Guilford Press
72 Spring St
New York, NY 10012-4019

800-365-7006
Fax: 212-966-6708
www.guilford.com
info@guilford.com

Philip C Kendall, Author
Lauren Braswell, Co-Author
The first edition of this book has been used successfully by thousands of clinicians to help children reduce impulsivity and improve their self-control. Building on the procedures reviewers call powerful tools and of great value to professionals who work with children. This second edition includes treatments, assessment issues and procedures and information on working with parents, teachers and groups of children. *$39.00*
239 pages
ISBN 0-898620-13-9

2901 **Curriculum Based Activities in Occupational Therapy: An Inclusion Resource**
Therapro
225 Arlington St
Framingham, MA 1702-8773

508-872-9494
800-257-5376
Fax: 508-875-2062
www.theraproducts.com
info@theraproducts.com

Lisa Loiselle, Author
Susan Shea, Co-Author
This book is a comprehensive guide to classroom based occupational therapy. The authors have compiled over 162 classroom activities developed to provide a strong linkage between educational and therapeutic goals. Each structured activity is categorized into standard curriculum subsections (reading, math, written language, etc.). Designed for a 3rd and 4th grade classroom, it can be modified for use in lower grades. *$35.00*
225 pages

2902 **Emotional Disorders & Learning Disabilities in the Elementary Classroom**
Corwin Press
2455 Teller Rd
Thousand Oaks, CA 91320-2218

805-499-9734
800-233-9936
Fax: 805-499-5323
www.corwinpress.com
order@corwinpress.com

Jean Cheng Gorman, Author
This unique book focuses on the interaction between learning disabilities and emotional disorders, fostering an understanding of how learning problems affect emotional well-being and vice-versa. This resource and practical classroom guide for all elementary school teachers includes an overview of common learning disabilities and emotional problems and a classroom-tested, research-based list of classroom interactions and interventions. *$30.95*
160 pages
ISBN 0-761976-20-2

2903 **Emotionally Abused & Neglected Child: Identification, Assessment & Intervention**
John Wiley & Sons Inc
111 River St
Hoboken, NJ 7030-5773

201-748-6000
Fax: 201-748-6088
www.wiley.com
info@wiley.com

Dorota Iwaniec, Author
Describes emotional abuse and neglect and how it affects child's growth, development and well-being. Diagnosis, assessment and issues that should be addressed. *$60.00*
424 pages Paperback
ISBN 0-470011-01-7

2904 **Ethical Principles of Psychologists and Code of Conduct**
American Psychological Association
750 1st St NE
Washington, DC 20002-4241
202-336-5500
800-374-2722
Fax: 202-336-5633
TDD: 202-336-6123
www.apa.org
psycinfo@apa.org

Marion Harrell, Deport Manager
Norman Anderson, CEO
General ethical principles of psychologists and enforceable ethical standards.

2905 **General Guidelines for Providers of Psychological Services**
American Psychological Association
750 1st St NE
Washington, DC 20002-4241
202-336-5500
800-374-2722
Fax: 202-336-5633
TDD: 202-336-6123
www.apa.org
psycinfo@apa.org

Marion Harrell, Deport Manager
Norman Anderson, CEO
Offers information for the professional in the area of psychology.

2906 **HELP...at Home**
Therapro
225 Arlington St
Framingham, MA 1702-8773
508-872-9494
800-257-5376
Fax: 508-875-2062
www.theraproducts.com
info@theraproducts.com

Stephanie Parks MA, Author
Practical and convenient format covers the 650 assesment skills from the Hawaii Early Learning Profile, with each page formatted as a separate, reproducible activity sheet. Therapist annotates, copies and hands out directly to parents to facilitate their involvement. *$112.50*

2907 **Handbook of Psychological and Educational Assessment of Children**
Guilford Press
72 Spring St
New York, NY 10012-4019
800-365-7006
Fax: 212-966-6708
www.guilford.com
info@guilford.com

Cecil R Reynolds, Editor
Randy W Kamphaus, Editor
Provides practitioners, researchers, professors, and students with an invaluable resource, this unique volume covers assessment of intelligence, learning styles, learning strategies, academic skills, and special populations, and discusses special topics in mental testing. Chapter contributions are by eminent psychologists and educators in the field of assessment with special expertise in research or practice in their topic areas. *$89.00*
718 pages

2908 **Helping Students Become Strategic Learners: Guidelines for Teaching**
Brookline Books
8 Trumbull Rd
Suite B-001
Northampton, MA 1060
413 584 0184
Fax: 413-584-6184
www.brooklinebooks.com
brbooks@yahoo.com

Karen Schneid, Author

A practical book that helps the beginning or experienced teacher translate skill-specific strategy methods into their classroom teaching. The author demonstrates how teachers can implement cognitive strategy instruction in their own classrooms. Each chapter includes an introduction to the principles of a given teaching strategy and a review of the skill area in question—namely reading, writing and mathematics. *$27.95*
Paperback
ISBN 0-914797-85-9

2909 **Overcoming Dyslexia in Children, Adolescents and Adults**
Pro-Ed
8700 Shoal Creek Blvd
Austin, TX 78757-6897
512-451-3246
800-397-7633
Fax: 512-451-8542
www.proedinc.com
info@proedinc.com

Dale R Jordan, Author
This book describes some forms of dyslexia in detail and then relates those problems to the social, emotional and personal development of dyslexic individuals. *$42.00*
417 pages

2910 **Pathways to Change: Brief Therapy Solutions with Difficult Adolescents**
Guilford Press
72 Spring St
New York, NY 10012-4019
800-365-7006
Fax: 212-966-6708
www.guilford.com
info@guilford.com

Matthew D Selekman, Author
This innovative, practical guide presents an effective brief therapy model for working with challenging adolescents and their families. The solution-oriented techniques and strategies so skillfullly presented in the original volume are now augmented by ideas and findings from other therapeutics traditions, with a heightened focus on engagement and relationship building. *$44.00*
292 pages
ISBN 1-572309-59-8

2911 **Practitioner's Guide to Dynamic Assessment**
Guilford Press
72 Spring St
New York, NY 10012-4019
800-365-7006
Fax: 212-966-6708
www.guilford.com
info@guilford.com

Carol S Lidz, Author
A hands-on guide that is degined specifically for practitioners who engage in diagnostic assessment related to the functioning of children in school. It reviews and critiques current models of dynamic assessment and presents the research available on these existing models. *$25.00*
210 pages Paperback
ISBN 0-898622-42-5

2912 **Reading and Learning Disability: A Neuropsychological Approach to Evaluation & Instruction**
Charles C Thomas
2600 S 1st St
Springfield, IL 62704-4730
217-789-8980
800-258-8980
Fax: 217-789-9130
www.ccthomas.com
books@ccthomas.com

Estelle L Fryburg, Author
Publisher of Education and Special Education books. *$74.95*
398 pages Paper
ISBN 0-398067-45-8

2913 Revels in Madness: Insanity in Medicine and Literature
University of Michigan Press
839 Greene St
Ann Arbor, MI 48104-3209
734-764-4388
Fax: 734-615-1540
www.press.umich.edu
ump.webmaster@umich.edu
Allen Thiher, Author
Karen Hill, Interim Director
Kelly Sippell, Assistant Director
Revels in Madness offers a history of western culture's shifting understanding of insanity as evidenced in its literature and as influenced by medical knowledge. *$75.00*
368 pages Cloth
ISBN 0-472110-35-3

2914 Teaching Students with Learning and Behavior Problems
Pro-Ed
8700 Shoal Creek Blvd
Austin, TX 78757-6816
512-451-3246
800-897-3202
Fax: 512-451-8542
www.proedinc.com
info@proedinc.com
Donald D Hammill, Author
Nettie R Bartel, Co-Author
Provides teachers with a comprehensive overview of the best practices in informal assessment and adaptive instruction. With the current trend both regular and exceptional students will find this text a useful resource. *$63.00*

2915 Treating Troubled Children and Their Families
Guilford Press
72 Spring St
New York, NY 10012-4019
800-365-7006
Fax: 212-966-6708
www.guilford.com
info@guilford.com
Ellen F Wachtel, Author
Integrating systemic, psychodynamic, and cognitive-behavioral perspectives, this acclaimed book presents an innovative framework for therapeutic work. Shows how parents and children all too often get entangled in patterns that cause grief to both generations, and demonstrates ho to help being about change with a combinations of family-focused interventions. *$30.00*
320 pages Paperback
ISBN 1-593850-72-7

General

2916 A History of Disability
University of Michigan Press
839 Greene St
Ann Arbor, MI 48104-3209
734-764-4388
Fax: 734-615-1540
www.press.umich.edu
ump.webmaster@umich.edu
Henri Jacques Stiker, Author
A bold analysis of the evolution of western attitudes toward disability. The book traces the history of western cultural responses to disability, from ancient times to the present. *$23.95*
264 pages Paper
ISBN 0-472086-26-9

2917 A Human Development View of Learning Disabilities: From Theory to Practice
Charles C Thomas, 2nd Ed.
2600 S 1st St
Springfield, IL 62704-4730
217-789-8980
800-258-8980
Fax: 217-789-9130
www.ccthomas.com
books@ccthomas.com
Corraine E Kass, Author
Cleborne D Maddux, Co-Author

Publisher of Education and Special Education books. 252 pp (7x10), 5 tables, ISBN 978-0-398-07565-1 (paper) $39.95 Published 2005 *$35.95*
252 pages Paper
ISBN 0-398075-65-1

2918 Academic Skills Problems Workbook
Guilford Press
72 Spring St
New York, NY 10012-4019
800-365-7006
Fax: 212-966-6708
www.guilford.com
info@guilford.com
Edward S Shapiro, Author
This user-friendly workbook offers numerous opportunities for practicing and mastering direct assessment and intervention procedures. The workbook also includes teacher and student interview forms; a complete guide to using the Behavioral Observation of Students in Schools (BOSS) Observation code, exercises on administering assessments and scoring, interpreting, and graphing the results; and much more. *$30.00*
147 pages
ISBN 1-572309-68-7

2919 Academic Skills Problems: Direct Assessment and Intervention
Guilford Press
72 Spring St
New York, NY 10012-4019
800-365-7006
Fax: 212-966-6708
www.guilford.com
info@guilford.com
Edward S Shapiro, Author
Provides comprehensive framework for the direct assessment of academic skills. Presented is a readily applicable, four-step approach for working with students experiencing a range of difficulties with reading, spelling, written language, or math. *$45.00*
370 pages
ISBN 1-572309-77-6

2920 Adapted Physical Education for Students with Autism
Charles C Thomas, Publisher, Ltd.
2600 S 1st St
Springfield, IL 62704-4730
217-789-8980
800-258-8980
Fax: 217-789-9130
www.ccthomas.com
books@ccthomas.com
Kimberly Davis, Author
Publisher of Education and Special Education books. 142 pp. (7x10), 10 il. ISBN 978-0-398-06085-5 (paper) $29.95. Published 1990. *$27.95*
142 pages Paper
ISBN 0-398060-85-5

2921 Adapting Curriculum & Instruction in Inclusive Early Childhood Settings
Indiana Institute on Disability and Community
2853 E 10th St
Bloomington, IN 47408-2601
812-855-9396
Fax: 812-855-9630
TTY: 812-855-9396
www.iidc.indiana.edu
iidc@indiana.edu
David Mank, Director
Offers ideas and strategies that will be beneficial to all young children, including children with identified disabilities, children who are at risk, and students who need enriched curricular options. This is also an excellent resource for preservice training as well as inservice training for independent child care providers, center, and schools. *$11.00*

2922 Annals of Dyslexia
International Dyslexia Association
4th Fl
40 York Rd
Baltimore, MD 21204-5243

410-296-0232
Fax: 410-321-5069
www.interdys.org
subscriptions@springer.com

Rob Hott, Editor
Chris Schatschneider PhD, Editor
Lee Grossman, Executive Director
The Society's scholarly journal contains updates on current research and selected proceedings from talks given at each ODS international conference. Issues of Annals are available from 1982 through the present year. *$15.00*
2X / year

2923 Art for All the Children: Approaches to Art Therapy for Children with Disabilities, 2nd Ed.
Charles C Thomas, Publisher, Ltd.
2600 S 1st St
Springfield, IL 62704-4730

217-789-8980
800-258-8980
Fax: 217-789-9130
www.ccthomas.com
books@ccthomas.com

Frances E Anderson, Author
Publisher of Education and Special Education books. *$56.95*
398 pages Paper
ISBN 0-398060-07-7

2924 Art-Centered Education & Therapy for Children with Disabilities
Charles C Thomas, Publisher, Ltd.
2600 S 1st St
Springfield, IL 62704-4730

217-789-8980
800-258-8980
Fax: 217-789-9130
www.ccthomas.com
books@ccthomas.com

Frances E Anderson, Author
Publisher of Education and Special Education books. 284 pp (6-3/4x9), 100 il, 14 tables. ISBN 978-0-398-06006-0 (paper) $42.95. Published 1994. *$41.95*
284 pages Cloth
ISBN 0-398058-96-2

2925 Atypical Cognitive Deficits in Developmental Disorders: Implications for Brain Function
Routledge
7625 Empire Drive
Florence, KY 41042-2919

212-216-7800
Fax: 212-563-2269
www.routledge.com
book.orders@tandf.co.uk

Sarah H Broman, Editor
Jordan Grafman, Editor
This volume is based on a conference held to examine what was known about cognitive behaviors and brain structure and function in three syndromes. *$99.95*
360 pages
ISBN 0-805811-80-0

2926 Auditory Processes
Academic Therapy Publications
20 Commercial Blvd
Novato, CA 94949-6120

415-883-3314
800-422-7249
Fax: 888-287-9975
www.academictherapy.com
sales@academictherapy.com

Jim Arena, President
Joanne Urban, Manager
Pamela Gillet PhD, Author

Explains how teachers, educational consultants and parents can identify auditory processing problems, understand their impact and implement appropriate instructional strategies to enhance learning. *$15.00*
120 pages
ISBN 0-878790-94-2

2927 Body and Physical Difference: Discourses of Disability
University of Michigan Press
839 Greene St
Ann Arbor, MI 48104-3209

734-764-4388
Fax: 734-615-1540
www.press.umich.edu
ump.webmaster@umich.edu

David T Mitchell, Editor
Sharon L Synder, Editor
Karen Hill, Executive Director
For years the subject of human disability has engaged those in the biological, social and cognitive sciences, while at the same time, it has been curiously neglected within the humanites. The Body and Physical Difference seeks to introduce the field of disability studies into the humanities by exploring the fantasies and fictons that have crystallized around conceptions of physical and cognitive difference. *$65.00*
320 pages cloth
ISBN 0-472066-59-9

2928 Brief Intervention for School Problems: Outcome-Informed Strategies
Guilford Press
72 Spring St
New York, NY 10012-4019

800-365-7006
Fax: 212-966-6708
www.guilford.com
info@guilford.com

John J Murphy, Author
Barry L Duncan, Co-Author
This practical guide provides innovative strategies for resolving academic and behavioral difficulties by enlisting the strengths and resources of students, parents, and teachers. *$30.00*
210 pages
ISBN 1-593854-92-7

2929 Cognitive Strategy Instruction That Really Improves Children's Performance
Brookline Books
PO Box 1209
Brookline, MA 2446

617-734-6772
800-666-2665
Fax: 413-584-6184
www.brooklinebooks.com
brbooks@yahoo.com

Michael Pressley, Author
A concise and focused work that summarily presents the few procedures for teaching strategies that aid academic subject matter learning that are empirically validated and fit well with the elementary school curriculum. *$27.95*
203 pages
ISBN 0-914797-66-2

2930 Competencies for Teachers of Students with Learning Disabilities
Council for Exceptional Children
Ste 300
1110 N Glebe Rd
Arlington, VA 22201-5704

703-245-0600
888-232-7733
Fax: 703-264-9494
TTY: 703-264-9446
www.cec.sped.org/
service@cec.sped.org

Amme Graves, Author
Mary Landers, Author
Bruce Ramirez, Manager

Lists 209 specific professional competencies needed by teachers of students with learning disabilities and provides a conceptual framework for the ten areas in which the competencies are organized. *$5.00*
25 pages

2931 Cooperative Learning and Strategies for Inclusion
Brookes Publishing Company
PO Box 10624
Baltimore, MD 21285
410-337-9580
800-638-3775
Fax: 410-337-8539
www.brookspublishing.com
custserv@brookespublishing.com
JoAnne Putnam PhD, Editor
This book supplies educators, classroom support personnel, and administrators with numerous tools for creating positive, inclusive classroom environments for students from preschool through high school. *$32.95*
288 pages Paperback
ISBN 1-557663-46-7

2932 Creative Curriculum for Preschool
Teaching Strategies
7101 Wisconsin Avenue
Suite 700
Bethesda, MD 20814
301-634-0818
800-637-3652
Fax: 301-657-0250
www.teachingstrategies.com
info@teachingstrategies.com
Andrea Valentine, President
Ron Davies, CEO
Amy Houser, CMO
Focuses on the developmentally appropriate program in early childhood education. Illustrates how preschool and kindergarten teachers set the stage for learning, and how children and teachers interact and learn in various interest areas. *$44.95*
540 pages
ISBN 1-879537-43-5

2933 Curriculum Development for Students with Mild Disabilities
Charles C Thomas, Publisher, Ltd.
2600 S 1st St
Springfield, IL 62704-4730
217-789-8980
800-258-8980
Fax: 217-789-9130
www.ccthomas.com
books@ccthomas.com
Carroll J Jones, Author
Publisher of Education and Special Education books. 454 pp. ISBN 978-0-398-079911-6, $69.95. Published 2010. *$38.95*
258 pages Spiral (paper)
ISBN 0-398707-18-2

2934 Curriculum-Based Assessment: A Primer, 3rd Ed.
Charles C Thomas
2600 S 1st St
Springfield, IL 62704-4730
217-789-8980
800-258-8980
Fax: 217-789-9130
www.ccthomas.com
books@ccthomas.com
Charles H Hargis, Author
Publisher of Education and Special Education books. 210 pp (8-1/2x11), 59 tables, ISBN 978-0-398-07815-7 (spiral) $39.95. Published 2008. *$33.95*
174 pages Paperback
ISBN 0-398075-52-1

2935 Curriculum-Based Assessment: The Easy Way to Determine Response-to-Intervention, 2nd Ed.
Charles C Thomas
2600 S 1st St
Springfield, IL 62704-4730
217-789-8980
800-258-8980
Fax: 217-789-9130
www.ccthomas.com
books@ccthomas.com
Carroll J Jones, Author
Publisher of Education and Special Education books. 210 pp, (8-1/2x11), 59 tables, ISBN 978-0-398-07815-7 (spiral) $39.95. Published 2008. *$33.95*
174 pages Spiral (paper)

2936 Defects: Engendering the Modern Body
University of Michigan Press
839 Greene St
Ann Arbor, MI 48104-3209
734-764-4388
Fax: 734-615-1540
www.press.umich.edu
ump.webmaster@umich.edu
Charles Watkinson, Director
Aaron McCollough, Director of Editorial
Defects brings together essays on the emergence of the concept of monstrosity in the eighteenth century and the ways it paralleled the emergence of notions of sexual difference. *$27.95*
344 pages Paper
ISBN 0-472066-98-8

2937 Developmental Variation and Learning Disorders
Educators Publishing Service
PO Box 9031
Cambridge, MA 2139-9031
800-435-7228
Fax: 888-440-2665
www.epsbooks.com
eps@epsbooks.com
Melvin D Levine MD FAAP, Author
The Second Edition of this useful reference includes completely revised on attention, memory, and language, with significant modifications of the remaining chapters. Sections on educational skills have been expanded and updated; the chapter on causes and complications of learning disorders has been updated to include recent references and ongoing reserach efforts. *$61.80*
ISBN 0-838819-92-3

2938 Dictionary of Special Education and Rehabilitation
Love Publishing Company
Ste 2200
9101 E Kenyon Ave
Denver, CO 80237-1854
303-221-7333
Fax: 303-221-7444
www.lovepublishing.com
lpc@lovepublishing.com
Glenn A Vergason, Author
M L Anderegg, Co-Author
This updated edition of one of the most valuable resources in the field is over six years in the making and incorporates hundreds of additions. It provides clear, understandable definitions of more than 2,000 terms unique to special education and rehabilitation. It also provides listing of professional organizations and resources, includes latest terms, and is a critical reference for anyone in the special education field. *$34.95*
210 pages Paperback
ISBN 0-891802-43-3

2939 Directory for Exceptional Children
Porter Sargent Handbooks
2 Lan Drive Ste 100 Westford
Boston, MA 1886
978-842-2812
800-342-7870
Fax: 978-692-2304
www.portersargent.com
info@portersargent.com

Daniel McKeever, Editor
John Yonce, Director
Leslie Weston, Production Editor
A comprehensive survey of 3000 schools, facilities, and organizations across the USA. Serving children and young adults with developmental, physical, medical, and emotional disabilities. Aide to parents, consultants, educators, and other professionals. *$75.00*
1152 pages
ISBN 0-875581-31-5

2940   Eden Family of Services Curriculum Series:
Eden Services
One Eden Way
Princeton, NJ 8540-5711   609-987-0099
                                      Fax: 609-987-0243
                                      www.edenservices.org
                                      info@edenservices.org
Tom Mc Cool, President
This volume contains teaching programs for students ages three through adult in the area of cognitive skills; self-care and domestics; vocational skills; speech and languages and physcial education, recreation and leisure. Complete series $700; individual volumes $150-200

2941   Educating All Students Together
Corwin Press
2455 Teller Rd
Thousand Oaks, CA 91320-2218   805-499-9734
                                           800-233-9936
                                      Fax: 805-499-5323
                                      www.corwinpress.com
                                      order@corwinpress.com
Mike Soules, President
Lisa Shaw, Executive Director
Kristin Anderson, Director of Learning
A plan for unifying the separate and parallel systems of special and general education. Key concepts include: schools embracing special services personnel; the role of the community; program evaluation and incentives; brain and holographic design; collaboration between school administrators and teachers; and adapting curriculum; and instruction. *$33.95*
264 pages
ISBN 0-761976-98-1

2942   Educating Children with Multiple Disabilities: A Collaborative Approach
Brookes Publishing Company
PO Box 10624
Baltimore, MD 21285   410-337-9580
                                           800-638-3775
                                      Fax: 410-337-8539
                                      www.brookespublishing.com
                                      custserv@brookespublishing.com
Fred P Orelove PhD, Editor
Dick Sobsey EdD, Editor
Rosanne K Silberman EdD, Editor
Gives undergraduate and graduate students up-to-the-minute research and strategies for educating children with severe and multiple disabilities. *$49.00*
672 pages Paperback
ISBN 1-557667-10-1

2943   Ending Discrimination in Special Education
Charles C Thomas
2600 South 1st Street
Springfield, IL 62704-4730   217-789-8980
                                           800-258-8980
                                      Fax: 217-789-9130
                                      www.ccthomas.com
                                      books@ccthomas.com
Herbert Grossman, Author
Charles C. Thomas, Publisher
Publisher of Education and Special Education books. *$23.95*
142 pages Paper
ISBN 0-398073-04-6

2944   Exceptional Teacher's Handbook: First Year Special Education Teacher's Guide for Success
Corwin Press
2455 Teller Rd
Thousand Oaks, CA 91320-2218   805-499-9734
                                           800-233-9936
                                      Fax: 805-499-5323
                                      www.corwinpress.com
                                      order@corwinpress.com
Mike Soules, President
Lisa Shaw, Executive Director Editorial
Elena Nikitina, Executive Director, Marketing
Provides a step-by-step management approach complete with planning checklists and other ready-to-use forms. Arranged sequentially, the book guides new teachers through the entire school year, from preplanning to post planning. *$35.95*
240 pages
ISBN 0-761931-96-6

2945   Focus on Exceptional Children
Love Publishing Company
9101 E Kenyon Ave
Suite 2200
Denver, CO 80237-1854   303-221-7333
                                      Fax: 303-221-7444
                                      www.lovepublishing.com
                                      lpc@lovepublishing.com
Edwin S Ellis, Editor
Timothy J Lewis, Editor
Chriss S Thomas, Editor
Published monthly except June, July, and August, get a constant flow of fresh teaching ideas-and keep up with the latest research- with this monthly newsletter that translates theory into strategies for action. Each issue focuses in depth on a single topic, such as assessment, cooperative learning, attention deficit disorders, inclusion, classroom management, discipline, and ohter timely issues. *$36.00*
ISSN 0015-511X

2946   Frames of Reference for the Assessment of Learning Disabilities
Brookes Publishing Company
PO Box 10624
Baltimore, MD 21285-0624   410-337-9580
                                           800-638-3775
                                      Fax: 410-337-8539
                                      www.brookespublishing.com
                                      custserv@brookespublishing.com
Lauren Rohe, Regional Sales Consultant
Cary Gold, Educational Sales Representative
Paul Kelly, College/University Sales Manager
This valuable reference offers an in-depth look at the fundamental concerns facing those who work with children with learning disabilities — assessment and identification. *$59.95*
672 pages Hardcover
ISBN 1-557661-38-3

2947   HELP Activity Guide
Therapro
225 Arlington Street
Framingham, MA 01702-8723   508-872-9494
                                           800-257-5376
                                      Fax: 508-875-2062
                                      www.theraproducts.com
                                      info@theraproducts.com
Karen Conrad, Owner
Setan Furuno PhD, Author
Takes you easily beyond assesment to offer the important next step, thousands of practical, task-analyzed curriculum activities and intervention strategies indexed by the 650 HELP skills. With up to ten activities and strategies per skill, this valuable resource includes definitions for each skill, illustrations, cross-references to skills in other developmental areas and a glossary. *$40.00*
190 pages

2948 **HELP for Preschoolers Assessment and Curriculum Guide**
Therapro
225 Arlington Street
Framingham, MA 01702-8723   508-872-9494
                                    800-257-5376
                                    Fax: 508-875-2062
                                    www.theraproducts.com
                                    info@theraproducts.com
Karen Conrad, Owner
Setan Furuns PhD, Author
Assessment procedure and instructional activities in one easy to use reference. Offers 6 sections of key information for each of the 622 skills: Definition, Materials, Assesment Procedures, Adaptions, Instructional Materials, and Instructional Activities.

2949 **Hidden Youth: Dropouts from Special Education**
Council for Exceptional Children
2900 Crystal Drive
Suite 1000
Arlington, VA 22202-3557   888-232-7733
                                    Fax: 703-264-9494
                                    TTY: 866-915-5000
                                    www.cec.sped.org/
                                    service@cec.sped.org
Donald L MacMillan, Author
Robin D. Brewer, President
James P. Heiden, President Elect
Christy A. Chambers, Immediate Past President
Examines the characteristics of students and schools that place students at risk for early school leaving. Discusses the accounting procedures used by different agencies for estimating graduation and dropout rates and cautions educators about using these rates as indicators of educational quality. *$8.90*
37 pages
ISBN 0-865862-11-7

2950 **How Difficult Can This Be?**
CT Association for Children and Adults with LD
Ste 15-5
25 Van Zant St
Norwalk, CT 06855-1713   203-838-5010
                                  Fax: 203-866-6108
                                  www.cacld.org
                                  caccld@optonline.net
Richard Lavoie, Producer
FAT City Workshop video and discussion guide. Looks at the world through the eyes of a learning disabled child. Features a unique workshop attended by educators, psychologists, social workers, parents, siblings and a student with LD. They participate in a series of classroom activities which cause Frustration, Anxiety, and Tension-emotions all too familiar to the student with a learning disability. A discussion of topics ranging from school/home communication to social skills follows. *$49.95*

2951 **How Does Your Engine Run? A Leaders Guide to the Alert Program for Self Regulation**
Therapro
225 Arlington Street
Framingham, MA 01702-8723   508-872-9494
                                    800-257-5376
                                    Fax: 508-875-2062
                                    www.theraproducts.com
                                    info@theraproducts.com
Karen Conrad, Owner
Mary Sue Williams OTR, Author
Sherry Schellenberge OTR, Co-Author
Introduces the entire Alert Program. Explains how we regulate our arousal states and describes the use of sensorimotor strategies to manage levels of alertness. This program is fun for students and the adults working with them, and translates easily into real life.

2952 **How to Write an IEP**
Academic Therapy Publications
20 Leveroni Court
Novato, CA 94949-5746   415-883-3314
                                 800-422-7249
                                 Fax: 888-287-9975
                                 www.academictherapy.com
                                 sales@academictherapy.com
Jim Arena, President
Joanne Urban, Manager
This practical guide for teachers and parents contains the latest updates to the 2004 Individuals with Disabilities Education Act (IDEA). *$19.00*
168 pages
ISBN 1-571284-43-5

2953 **IEP Success Video**
Sopris West
17855 Dallas Parkway
Suite 400
Dallas, TX 75287-3520   303-651-2829
                                 800-547-6747
                                 www.voyagersopris.com
                                 customerservice@sopriswest.com
Barbara D Baterman JD PhD, Author
Explains the five underlying principles of the individualized education program (IEP) process: evaluation and identification, IEPs and related services, placement, funding, and procedural safeguards. *$98.95*

2954 **Implementing Cognitive Strategy Instruction Across the School: The Benchmark Manual for Teachers**
Brookline Books
8 Trumbull Rd
Suite B-001
Northampton, MA 01060   413-584-0184
                                 800-666-2665
                                 Fax: 413-584-6184
                                 www.brooklinebooks.com
                                 brbooks@yahoo.com
Irene Gaskins, Author
Thorne Elliot, Author
Describes a classroom based program planned and executed by teachers to focus and guide students with serious reading problems to be goal oriented, planful, strategic and self-assessing. *$24.95*
Paperback
ISBN 0-914797-75-1

2955 **Improving Test Performance of Students with Disabilities in the Classroom**
Corwin Press
2455 Teller Rd
Thousand Oaks, CA 91320-2218   805-499-9734
                                        800-233-9936
                                        Fax: 805-499-5323
                                        www.corwinpress.com
                                        order@corwinpress.com
Mike Soules, President
Lisa Shaw, Executive Director Editorial
Elena Nikitina, Executive Director, Marketing
Elliott and Thurlow, long-time colleagues at the National Center on Educational Outcomes build on their highly respected work in accountability and assessment of students with disabilities to focus now on improving test performance — with an emphasis throughout on practical application. Common learning disabilities and emotional problems and a classroom-tested, research-based list of classroom interventions. *$35.95*
232 pages Paperback
ISBN 1-412917-28-X

2956 **Including Students with Severe and Multiple Disabilities in Typical Classrooms**
Brookes Publishing Company
PO Box 10624
Baltimore, MD 21285-0624 410-337-9580
800-638-3775
Fax: 410-337-8539
www.brookespublishing.com
custserv@brookespublishing.com
Lauren Rohe, Regional Sales Consultant
Cary Gold, Educational Sales Representative
Paul Kelly, College/University Sales Manager
This straightforward and jargon-free resource gives instructors the guidance needed to educate learners who have one or more sensory impairments in addition to cognitive and physical disabilities. *$44.95*
352 pages Paperback
ISBN 1-557669-08-2

2957 **Inclusion: 450 Strategies for Success**
Corwin Press
2455 Teller Rd
Thousand Oaks, CA 91320-2218 805-499-9734
800-233-9936
Fax: 805-499-5323
www.corwinpress.com
order@corwinpress.com
Mike Soules, President
Lisa Shaw, Executive Director Editorial
Elena Nikitina, Executive Director, Marketing
Commences with step-by-step guidelines to help develop, expand and improve the existing inclusive education setting. Hundreds of practical teacher tested ideas and accommodations are conveniently listed by topic and numbered for quick, easy reference. *$33.95*
192 pages Educators
ISBN 1-890455-25-3

2958 **Inclusion: An Essential Guide for the Paraprofessional**
Corwin Press
2455 Teller Rd
Thousand Oaks, CA 91320-2218 805-499-9734
800-233-9936
Fax: 805-499-5323
www.corwinpress.com
order@corwinpress.com
Mike Soules, President
Lisa Shaw, Executive Director Editorial
Elena Nikitina, Executive Director, Marketing
This best-selling publication is developed specifically for paraprofessionals and classroom assistants. The book commences with a simplified introduction to inclusive education, handicapping conditions, due process, communication, collaboration, confidentiality and types of adaptations. Used by many schools and universities as a training tool for staff development. *$35.95*
224 pages
ISBN 1-890455-34-2

2959 **Inclusive Elementary Schools**
PEAK Parent Center
611 North Weber Street
Suite 200
Colorado Springs, CO 80903-1072 719-531-9400
800-284-0251
Fax: 719-531-9452
www.peakparent.org
info@peakparent.org
Barbara Buswell, Executive Director
Kent Willis, President
Sarah Billerbeck, Vice President
Walks readers through a state of the art, step-by-step process to determine what and how to teach elementary school students with disabilities in general education classrooms. Highlights strategies for accommodating and modifying assignments and activities by using core curriculum. Complete with user-friendly sample forms and creative support strategies, this is an essential text for elementary educators and parents. *$13.00*

2960 **Instructional Methods for Secondary Students with Learning & Behavior Problems**
Allyn & Bacon
75 Arlington St
Suite 300
Boston, MA 02116-3988 800-848-9500
Fax: 877-260-2530
http://home.pearsonhighered.com
Patrick J Schloss, Author
Maureen A Schloss, Co-Author
Cynthia N Schloss, Co-Author
This book presents teaching principles useful to general high school educators and special educators working with students demonstrating a variety of academic, behavioral, and social needs in secondary schools. *$120.00*
432 pages
ISBN 0-205442-36-6

2961 **Intervention in School and Clinic**
Sage Publications
2455 Teller Rd
Thousand Oaks, CA 91320-2218 805-499-0721
800-818-7243
Fax: 805-583-2665
www.sagepub.com
journals@sagepub.com
Blaise R. Simqu, President
Tracey A. Ozmina, Executive VP/COO
Gretchen Bataille, Director
Equips teachers and clinicians with hands-on tips, techniques, methods and ideas for improving assessment, instruction, and management for individuals with learning disabilities or behavior disorders. Articles focus on curricular, instructional, social, behavioral, assessment, and vocational strategies and techniques that have a direct application to the classroom setting. This innovative and readable periodical provides educational information ready for immediate implementation
5 times a year
ISSN 1053-4512

2962 **KDES Health Curriculum Guide**
Harris Communications
15155 Technology Dr
Eden Prairie, MN 55344-2273 800-825-6758
800-825-9187
Fax: 952-906-1099
TTY: 800-825-9187
www.harriscomm.com
info@harriscomm.com
Sara Gillespie, Author
Doris Schwartz, Co-Author
Darla Hudson, Customer Service
This guide provides students with the information they need to make wise choices for healthy living. Divided into age-appropriate sections; preschool through middle school; the units cover four main areas: Health and Fitness, Safety and First Aid, Drugs, and Life. Asspendices provide resource lists and information on topics such as hygiene, street safety, teaching health. Part #B568. *$9.95*
125 pages

2963 **Making School Inclusion Work: A Guide to Everyday Practices**
Brookline Books
8 Trumbull Rd
Suite B-001
Northampton, MA 01060 413-584-0184
800-666-2665
Fax: 413-584-6184
www.brooklinebooks.com
brbooks@yahoo.com
Katie Blenk, Author
Doris Fine, Author

Tells the reader how to conduct a truly inclusive school program that educates a diverse student body together, regardless of ethnic or racial background, economic level, or physical or cognitive ability. Indication given on what is ment by true inclusion, what inclusion is not, and who should not be conducting an inclusive program. *$24.95*
264 pages Paperback
ISBN 0-914797-96-4

2964 Mentoring Students at Risk: An Underutilized Alternative Education Strategy for K-12 Teachers
Charles C Thomas
2600 South 1st Street
Springfield, IL 62704-4730   217-789-8980
                                     800-258-8980
                                Fax: 217-789-9130
                                www.ccthomas.com
                                books@ccthomas.com
Gary Reglin, Author
Charles C. Thomas, Publisher
Publisher of Education and Special Education books. *$20.95*
110 pages Paper
ISBN 0-398068-33-2

2965 Myofascial Release and Its Application to Neuro-Developmental Treatment
Therapro
225 Arlington Street
Framingham, MA 01702-8723   508-872-9494
                                     800-257-5376
                                Fax: 508-875-2062
                                www.theraproducts.com
                                info@theraproducts.com
Karen Conrad, Owner
Regi Boehme OTF, Author
This fully illustrated resource provides the therapist with techniques to approach myofascial restrictions which are secondary to tonal dysfunction in children and adults with neurological deficits. The Neuro-Developmental Treatment approach is included in the illustrated treatment rationale.

2966 Narrative Prosthesis: Disability and the Dependencies of Discourse
University of Michigan Press
839 Greene Street
Ann Arbor, MI 48104-3209   734-764-4388
                              Fax: 734-615-1540
                              www.press.umich.edu
                              dshafer@umich.edu
Charles Watkinson, Director
Ellen Bauerle, Executive Editor
Gabriela Beres, Business Manager
This book develops a narrative theory of the pervasive use of disability as a device of characterization in literature and film. It argues that, while other marginalized identities have suffered cultural exclusion due to dearth of images reflecting their experience, the marginality of disabled people has occurred in the midst of the perpetual circulation of images of disability in print and visual media. *$65.00*
264 pages Cloth
ISBN 0-472097-48-7

2967 Points of Contact: Disability, Art, and Culture
University of Michigan Press
839 Greene Street
Ann Arbor, MI 48104-3209   734-764-4388
                              Fax: 734-615-1540
                              www.press.umich.edu
                              dshafer@umich.edu
Charles Watkinson, Director
Ellen Bauerle, Executive Editor
Gabriela Beres, Business Manager

A richly diverse collection of essays, memoir, poetry and photography on aspects of disability and its representation in art. Brings together contributions by leading writers, artists, scholars, and critics to provide a remarkably broad and consistently engaging look at the intersection of disability and the arts. *$60.00*
312 pages Cloth
ISBN 0-472097-11-1

2968 Prescriptions for Children with Learning and Adjustment Problems: A Consultant's Desk Reference
Charles C Thomas
2600 South 1st Street
Springfield, IL 62704-4730   217-789-8980
                                     800-258-8980
                                Fax: 217-789-9130
                                www.ccthomas.com
                                books@ccthomas.com
Ralph F Blanco, Author
Charles C. Thomas, Publisher
Publisher of Education and Special Education books. *$35.95*
264 pages Paper

2969 Preventing Academic Failure
Educators Publishing Service
PO Box 9031
Cambridge, MA 02139-9031   617-547-6706
                                    800-225-5750
                               Fax: 888-440-2665
                               www.epsbooks.com
                          Feedback.EPS@schoolspecialty.com
Rick Holden, President
Phyllis Bertin, Author
Eileen Perlman, Co-Author
This multisensory curriculum meets the needs of children with learning disabilities in regular classrooms by providing a four-year sequence of written language skills (reading, writing and spelling). PAF has a handwriting and numerical program. *$42.00*
ISBN 0-838852-71-8

2970 Resourcing: Handbook for Special Education RES Teachers
Council for Exceptional Children
2900 Crystal Drive
Suite 1000
Arlington, VA 22202-3557   888-232-7733
                                    888-232-7733
                               Fax: 703-264-9494
                               TTY: 866-915-5000
                               www.cec.sped.org
                               service@cec.sped.org
Mary Yeomans Jackson, Author
Robin D. Brewer, President
James P. Heiden, President Elect
Christy A. Chambers, Immediate Past President
Be prepared to function at your best as a member of a school-based team. Resourcing wil help you take a leadership role as you work in collaboration with general classroom teachers and other practitioners. Assess your personal readiness for being a resource professional within your school. Includes many useful forms and checklists for conducting meetings and organizing your workday. *$12.00*
64 pages
ISBN 0-865862-19-2

2971 School-Home Notes: Promoting Children's Classroom Success
Guilford Press
72 Spring Street
New York, NY 10012-4019   800-365-7006
                              Fax: 212-966-6708
                              www.guilford.com
                              info@guilford.com
Seymour Weingarten, Editor-in-Chief
Jim Nageotte, Senior Editor
Jody Falco, Managing Editor

Describes common obstacles to parent and teacher communication and clearly explicates how these obstacles can be overcome. It provides a critical appraisal of the relevant literature on parent-and-teacher managed contingency systems and factors influencing the efficacy of the procedure. *$28.00*
198 pages Paperback
ISBN 0-898622-35-2

2972 Segregated and Second-Rate: Special Education in New York
Advocates for Children of New York
151 West 30th St
5th Floor
New York, NY 10001-4024

212-947-9779
866-427-6033
Fax: 212-947-9790
www.advocatesforchildren.org
info@advocatesforchildren.org

Eric F. Grossman, President
Harriet Chan King, Secretary
Paul D. Becker, Treasurer
Highlights the fact that New York rates last among all states in inclusive education.

2973 Sensory Integration: Theory and Practice
Therapro
225 Arlington Street
Framingham, MA 01702-8723

508-872-9494
800-257-5376
Fax: 508-875-2062
www.theraproducts.com
info@theraproducts.com

Karen Conrad, Owner
Anne Fisher, Author
Elizabeth Murray, Co-Author
The very latest in sensory integration theory and practice.
$60.00
481 pages

2974 Strangest Song: One Father's Quest to Help His Daughter Find Her Voice
Prometheus Books
59 John Glenn Drive
Amherst, NY 14228-2197

716-691-0133
800-421-0351
Fax: 716-691-0137
www.prometheusbooks.com
marketing@prometheusbooks.com

Jill Maxick, Vice President of Marketing
Lisa Michalski, Senior Publicist
Mary A Read, Permissions Manager
The first book to tell the story of Williams syndrome and the extraordinary musicality of many of the people who have it. An inspiring blend of human interest and breakthrough science, offers startling insights into the mysteries of the brain and hope that science can find new ways to help the handicapped. *$24.00*
296 pages
ISBN 1-591024-78-1

2975 Take Part Art
CT Association for Children and Adults with LD
Ste 15-5
25 Van Zant St
Norwalk, CT 06855-1713

203-838-5010
www.cacld.org
cacld@optonline.net

Bob Gregson, Author
Offers information on art therapies and their inclusion in learning disabled environments. *$19.50*

2976 Teachers Ask About Sensory Integration
Therapro
225 Arlington Street
Framingham, MA 01702-8723

508-872-9494
800-257-5376
Fax: 508-875-2062
www.theraproducts.com
info@theraproducts.com

Karen Conrad, Owner
Carol Kranowitz, Author
Stacey Szkult, Co-Author
A narration and discussion for teachers and school professionals about how to teach children with sensory integration problems. 60 page book included, filled with checklists, idea sheets, sensory profiles and resorces. 86 minute audio tape.
Audio Tape

2977 Teaching Gifted Kids in the Regular Classroom CD-ROM
Free Spirit Publishing
217 5th Ave North
Suite 200
Minneapolis, MN 55401-1299

612-338-2068
800-735-7323
Fax: 612-337-5050
www.freespirit.com
help4kids@freespirit.com

Judy Galbraith, President
Judy Galbrai
Includes all of the forms from the book, plus many additional extension menus, ready to customize and print for classroom use. Macintosh and Windows compatible. *$17.95*
ISBN 1-575421-01-4

2978 Teaching Gifted Kids in the Regular Classroom
Free Spirit Publishing
217 5th Ave North
Suite 200
Minneapolis, MN 55401-1299

612-338-2068
800-735-7323
Fax: 612-337-5050
www.freespirit.com
help4kids@freespirit.com

Judy Galbraith, President
The definitive guide to meeting the learning needs of gifted students, as well as those labeled slow, remedial, or LD, in the mixed-abilities classroom, without losing control, causing resentment, or spending hours preparing extra materials. The updated edition includes more than 50 reproducible forms and handouts for all grades. *$34.95*
256 pages
ISBN 1-575420-89-9

2979 Teaching Students Ways to Remember: Strategies for Learning Mnemonically
Brookline Books
8 Trumbull Rd
Suite B-001
Northampton, MA 01060

413-584-0184
800-666-2665
Fax: 413-584-6184
www.brooklinebooks.com
brbooks@yahoo.com

Margo Mastropieri MD, Author
This book was written in response to the enormous interest in mnemonic instruction by teachers and administrators, telling them how it can be used with their students. *$21.95*
ISBN 0-398074-77-7

2980 Teaching Visually Impaired Children, 3rd Ed.
Charles C Thomas
2600 South 1st Street
Springfield, IL 62704-4730

217-789-8980
800-258-8980
Fax: 217-789-9130
www.ccthomas.com
books@ccthomas.com

Virginia E Bishop, Author
Charles C. Thomas, Publisher

Publisher of Education and Special Education books. *$49.95*
352 pages Paper
ISBN 0-398065-95-0

2981 To Teach a Dyslexic
AVKO Educational Research Foundation
3084 Willard Rd
Birch Run, MI 48415-9404

810-686-9283
866-285-6612
Fax: 810-686-1101
www.avko.org
webmaster@avko.org

Don McCabe, President
Linda Heck, Vice President
Michael Lane, Treasurer
Just as it takes a thief to catch a thief, this is an autobiography of a dyslexic who discovered how to teach dyslexics. Common sense, logical approach, valuable to all who teach in our nation's classrooms. *$14.95*
288 pages
ISBN 1-564000-04-4

2982 Understanding & Management of Health Problems in Schools: Resource Manual
Temeron Books
PO Box 896
Bellingham, WA 98227

FAX 360-738-4016
www.temerondetselig.com
temeron@telusplanet.net

H Moghadam, Author
Intended as a supplement to information given by parents and physicians, this book is a valuable aid to teachers and other school personnel in regards to some of the primary health issues that affect children and adolescents. *$13.95*
152 pages
ISBN 1-550591-21-5

2983 Understanding and Managing Vision Deficits
Therapro
225 Arlington Street
Framingham, MA 01702-8723

508-872-9494
800-257-5376
Fax: 508-875-2062
www.theraproducts.com
info@theraproducts.com

Mitchell Scheiman, OD, Author
Karen Conrad, Owner
This book is a unique and comprehensive collaboration from OT's and optometrists developed to increase the understanding of vision. Learn to screen for common visual deficits and effectively manage patients with vision disorders. Provides recommendations for direct intervention techniques for a variety of vision problems and supportive and compensatory stratagies for visual field deficits and visual neglect.

2984 Working with Visually Impaired Young Students: A Curriculum Guide for 3 to 5 Year-Olds
Charles C Thomas
2600 South 1st Street
Springfield, IL 62704-4730

217-789-8980
800-258-8980
Fax: 217-789-9130
www.ccthomas.com
books@ccthomas.com

Ellen Trief, Editor
Charles C Thomas, Publisher
Publisher of Education and Special Education books. *$42.95*
208 pages Spiral Paper
ISBN 0-398068-75-2

Language Arts

2985 Communication Skills for Visually Impaired Learners, 2nd Ed.
Charles C Thomas, Publisher, Ltd.
2600 South 1st Street
Springfield, IL 62704-4730

217-789-8980
800-258-8980
Fax: 217-789-9130
www.ccthomas.com
books@ccthomas.com

Randall K Harley, Author
Charles C Thomas, Publisher
LaRhea D Sanford, Co-Author
Publisher of Education and Special Education books. 322 pp. (7x10), 39 il, $59.95 (paper) ISBN 978-0-398-06693-2 *$57.95*
322 pages Paper
ISBN 0-398066-93-2

2986 First Start in Sign Language
Harris Communications
15155 Technology Dr
Eden Prairie, MN 55344-2273

800-825-6758
800-825-9187
Fax: 952-906-1099
TTY: 800-825-9187
www.harriscomm.com
info@harriscomm.com

Amy J Strommer, Author
Darla Hudson, Customer Service
Fun pictures, stories, and activities are all included in this introduction to American Sign Language. Students first learn to sign words for people, animals, objects and actions. Then they learn to produce simple sentences and to sign stories. Reproducible activity pages are included throughout the book. For students in kindergarten through sixth grade. Part #B469. *$32.00*
190 pages Paperback

2987 From Talking to Writing: Strategies for Scaffolding Expository Expression
Landmark School
429 Hale Street
P.O. Box 227
Prides Crossing, MA 01965

978-236-3216
Fax: 978-927-7268
www.landmarkoutreach.org
outreach@landmarkschool.org

Dan Ahearn, Director
Terrill M Jennings, Author
Charles W Haynes, Co-Author
Designed for teachers who work with students who have difficulty with writing and/or expressive language skills, this book provides practical strategies for teaching expository expression at the word, sentence, paragraph, and short essay levels. *$25.00*
191 pages

2988 Language Learning Everywhere We Go
Academic Communication Associates
PO Box 4279
Oceanside, CA 92052-4279

760-722-9593
888-758-9558
Fax: 760-722-1625
TDD: 952-906-1198
TTY: 800-825-9187
www.acadcom.com
acom@acadcom.com

Cecilia Casas, Author
Patricia Portillo, Co-Author
Students learn the vocabulary associated with each situation that they encounter on their travels with Bernardo Bear. Questions and vocabulary lists are included in English and Spanish for each picture. The 103 situational pictures may all be reproduced. *$34.00*
209 pages Paperback

2989 Making the Writing Process Work: Strategies for Composition & Self-Regulation
Brookline Books
8 Trumbull Rd
Suite B-001
Northampton, MA 01060
413-584-0184
800-666-2665
Fax: 413-584-6184
www.brooklinebooks.com
brbooks@yahoo.com
Karen R Harris, Author
Steve Graham, Co-Author
Presents cognitive strategies for writing sequences of specific steps which make the writing process clearer and enable students to organize their thoughts about the writing task. The strategies help students know how to turn thoughts into writing products. This is especially important for students having difficulty producing acceptable writing products, but all students benefit from learning these procedures. *$24.95*
ISBN 1-571290-10-9

2990 Multisensory Teaching Approach
MTS Publications
415 N McGraw St
Forney, TX 75126-8661
972-564-6960
877-552-1090
Fax: 972-552-9889
www.mtsedmar.com
msmith@mtsedmar.com
Margaret Smith, Author
Margaret T. Smith, Executive Director
MTA is a comprehensive, multisensory program in reading, spelling, cursive handwriting, and alphabet and dictionary skills for both regular and remedial instruction. Ungraded, MTA is based on the Orton-Gillingham techniques and Alphabetic Phonics. *$192.99*

2991 Signs of the Times
Harris Communications
15155 Technology Dr
Eden Prairie, MN 55344-2273
800-825-6758
800-825-9187
Fax: 952-906-1099
TTY: 800-825-9187
www.harriscomm.com
info@harriscomm.com
Edgar H Shroyer, Author
Darla Hudson, Customer Service
Containing 1,185 signs in 41 lessons, this classroom text is an excellent beginning Pidgin or Contact Sign English book that fills the gap between sign language dictionaries and American Sign Language texts. Each lesson contains clearly illustrated vocabulary, English glosses and synonyms, sample sentences to defice vocabulary context, and sentences for practice. Part #B202. *$34.95*
433 pages Softcover

2992 Slingerland Multisensory Approach to Language Arts
Slingerland Institute for Literacy
12729 Northup Way
Suite 1
Bellevue, WA 98005-1935
425-453-1190
Fax: 425-635-7762
www.slingerland.org
mail@slingerland.com
Bonnie Meyer, Author
Beth H. Slingerland, Founder
This adaptation of the Orton-Gillingham approach for classroom teachers provides a phonetically structured introduction to reading, writing and spelling. Books 1 and 2 are for first and second grade, Book 3 for primary classrooms and older students. Numerous supplementary materials are available.

2993 Teaching Language Deficient Children: Theory and Application of the Association Method
Pro-Ed
8700 Shoal Creek Blvd
Austin, TX 78757-6897
512-451-3246
800-897-3202
Fax: 512-451-8542
www.proedinc.com
general@proedinc.com
N Etoile DuBard, Author
Maureen K Martin, Co-Author
This revised and expanded edition of Teaching Aphasics and Other Language Deficient Children offers information on its theory, implementation of the method and sample curriculum. *$52.00*
360 pages
ISBN 0-838823-40-8

2994 Visualizing and Verbalizing for Language Comprehension and Thinking
Lindamood Bell
416 Higuera St
San Luis Obispo, CA 93401-3833
805-541-3836
800-233-1819
Fax: 805-541-8756
www.lindamoodbell.com
Nanci Bell, Author
This book identifies the important sensory connection that imagery provides and teaches specific techniques. Specific steps and sample dialog are presented. Summary pages after each step make it easy to implement the program in the classroom.
284 pages
ISBN 0-945856-01-6

2995 Writing: A Landmark School Teaching Guide
Landmark School
429 Hale Street
P.O. Box 227
Prides Crossing, MA 01965
978-236-3216
Fax: 978-927-7268
www.landmarkoutreach.org
outreach@landmarkschool.org
Dan Ahearn, Director
Deborah Blanchard, Academic Dean
Jean Gudaitis Tarricone, Author
This book offers strategies for teaching writing at the paragraph and short essay levels. It emphasizees the integration of language and critical thinking skills within a five-step writing process. Sample templates and graphic organizers as well as exercises that teachers can use in their classrooms are included. *$25.00*
92 pages

Math

2996 Landmark Method for Teaching Arithmetic
Landmark School
429 Hale Street
P.O. Box 227
Prides Crossing, MA 01965
978-236-3216
Fax: 978-927-7268
www.landmarkoutreach.org
outreach@landmarkschool.org
Dan Ahearn, Director
Deborah Blanchard, Academic Dean
Christopher Woodin, Author
This book is written for teachers who work with students having difficulty learning math. It includes practical strategies for teaching multiplication, division, word problems, and math facts. It also introduces the reader to two learning tools developed at Landmark — Woodin Ladders and Woodmark Icons. Sample templates and exercises are included. *$25.00*
145 pages

2997 **Math and the Learning Disabled Student: A Practical Guide for Accommodations**
Academic Success Press
3547 53rd Ave. W.
PMB 132
Bradenton, FL 34210-4402

941-746-1645
888-822-6657
Fax: 941-753-2882
www.academicsuccess.com
info@academicsuccess.com

Paul D Nolting PhD, Author
Kim Ruble, Editor
Kimberly Nolting, MAT, VP for Marketing and Research
More and more learning disabled students are experiencing difficulty passing mathematics. The book is especially written for counselors and mathematics instructors of learning disabled students, and provides information on accommodations for students with different types of learning disabilities. *$49.95*
256 pages
ISBN 0-940287-23-4

2998 **Teaching Mathematics to Students with Learning Disabilities**
Pro-Ed
8700 Shoal Creek Blvd
Austin, TX 78757-6897

512-451-3246
800-897-3202
Fax: 512-451-8542
www.proedinc.com
general@proedinc.com

Nancy S Bley, Author
Carol A Thornton, Co-Author
Offers information on problem-solving, estimation and the use of computers in teaching mathematics to the child with learning disabilities. *$49.00*

Preschool

2999 **Access for All: Integrating Deaf, Hard of Hearing, and Hearing Preschoolers**
Harris Communications
15155 Technology Dr
Eden Prairie, MN 55344-2273

800-825-6758
800-825-9187
Fax: 952-906-1099
TTY: 800-825-9187
www.harriscomm.com
info@harriscomm.com

Gail Solit, Author
Maral Taylor, Co-Author
Darla Hudson, Customer Service
Covers basic information needed to establish a successful preschool program for deaf and hearing children; interagency cooperation, staff training, and parental involvement. Part #BUT103. *$29.95*
169 pages Video-90 min.

3000 **When Slow Is Fast Enough: Educating the Delayed Preschool Child**
Guilford Press
72 Spring Street
New York, NY 10012-4019

800-365-7006
Fax: 212-966-6708
www.guilford.com
info@guilford.com

Seymour Weingarten, Editor-in-Chief
Jim Nageotte, Senior Editor
Jody Falco, Managing Editor

This bold and controversial book asks what we are accomplishing in early intervention programs that attempt to accelerate development in delayed young children. She questions the value of such programs on educational, psychological, and moral grounds, suggesting that in pressuring these children to perform more, and sooner, we undermine their capacity for independent development and deprive them of the freedom we insist upon for the nondelayed. *$29.00*
306 pages Paperback
ISBN 0-898624-91-6

Reading

3001 **Gillingham Manual**
Educators Publishing Service
PO Box 9031
Cambridge, MA 02139-9031

617-547-6706
800-225-5750
Fax: 617-547-0412
www.epsbooks.com
Feedback.EPS@schoolspecialty.com

Rick Holden, President
Anna Gillingham, Author
Bessie W Stillman, Co-Author
This classic in the field of specific language disability has now been completely revised and updated. The manual covers reading, spelling, writing and dictionary technique. It may be used with individuals or small groups. *$74.15*
352 pages
ISBN 0-838802-00-1

3002 **Phonology and Reading Disability**
University of Michigan Press
839 Greene Street
Ann Arbor, MI 48104-3209

734-764-4388
Fax: 734-615-1540
www.press.umich.edu
dshafer@umich.edu

Charles Watkinson, Director
Ellen Bauerle, Executive Editor
Gabriela Beres, Business Manager
Discusses the importance to the learning process of the phonological structures of words. *$52.50*
184 pages Cloth
ISBN 0-472101-33-7

3003 **Preventing Reading Difficulties in Young Children**
National Academies Press
500 Fifth St NW
Washington, DC 20001

202-334-3313
888-624-8373
Fax: 202-334-2451
www.nap.edu
customer_service@nap.edu

Barbara Kline Pope, Director
Ann Merchant, Deputy Executive Director
Stephen Mautner, Executive Editor
Explores how to prevent reading difficulties in the context of social, historical, cultural, and biological factors. *$34.16*
448 pages Hardback
ISBN 0-309064-18-X

3004 **Readability Revisited: The New Dale-Chall Readability Formula**
Brookline Books
8 Trumbull Rd
Suite B-001
Northampton, MA 01060

413-584-0184
800-666-2665
Fax: 413-584-6184
www.brooklinebooks.com
brbooks@yahoo.com

Jeanne Chall, Author
Edgar Dale, Co-Author
Information is given on reading difficulties in children with learning disabilities and how to overcome them. *$29.95*
168 pages
ISBN 1-571290-08-7

3005 Reading Problems: Consultation and Remediation
Guilford Press
72 Spring Street
New York, NY 10012-4019   800-365-7006
                                Fax: 212-966-6708
                                www.guilford.com
                                info@guilford.com

Seymour Weingarten, Editor-in-Chief
Jim Nageotte, Senior Editor
Jody Falco, Managing Editor
Designed to both help school psychologists and reading specialists effectively assume the consultation role, this volume provides an overview of reading problems while serving as a guide to effective practice. *$42.00*
285 pages

3006 Reading Programs that Work: A Review of Programs from Pre-K to 4th Grade
Milken Family Foundation
1250 4th St
Santa Monica, CA 90401-1353   310-570-4800
                                     Fax: 310-570-4801
                                     www.mff.org
                                     media@mff.org

Lowell Milken, Chairman & Co Founder
Richard Sandler, Executive Vice President
Ralph Finerman, Senior Vice President
This publication tackles two questions, joining the research behind why children fail to read with research on effective solutions to reverse this failure. Included in the reading report are analyses of 35 different reading programs and their impact on student achievement.
72 pages

3007 Reading and Learning Disabilities: A Resource Guide
NICHCY
1825 Connecticut Ave NW
Suite 700
Washington, DC 20009   202-884-8200
                             800-695-0285
                             Fax: 202-884-8441
                             TDD: 800-695-0285
                             www.nichcy.org
                             emulligan@fhi360.org

Lisa Kupper, Editor
This publication describes some of the most common learning disabilities that can cause reading problems and provides information on organizations that can provide needed assistance.

3008 Reading and Learning Disability: A Neuropsychological Approach to Evaluation & Instruction
Charles C Thomas
2600 South 1st Street
Springfield, IL 62704-4730   217-789-8980
                                    800-258-8980
                                    Fax: 217-789-9130
                                    www.ccthomas.com
                                    books@ccthomas.com

Estelle L Fryburg, Author
Charles C. Thomas, Publisher
Publisher of Education and Special Education books. *$74.95*
398 pages Paper
ISBN 0-398067-45-8

3009 Starting Out Right: A Guide to Promoting Children's Reading Success
National Academies Press
500 Fifth St NW
Washington, DC 20001   202-334-3313
                             888-624-8373
                             Fax: 202-334-2451
                             www.nap.edu
                             customer_service@nap.edu

Barbara Kline Pope, Director
Ann Merchant, Deputy Executive Director
Stephen Mautner, Executive Editor

This book discusses how best to help children succeed in reading. This book also includes 55 activities yo do with children to help them become successful readers, a list of recommended children's books, and a guide to CD-ROMs and websites. A must read for specialists in primary education as well as pediatricians, childcare providers, tutors, literacy advocates, and parents. *$13.46*
192 pages
ISBN 0-309064-10-4

3010 Teaching Reading to Disabled and Handicapped Learners
Charles C Thomas
2600 South 1st Street
Springfield, IL 62704-4730   217-789-8980
                                    800-258-8980
                                    Fax: 217-789-9130
                                    www.ccthomas.com
                                    books@ccthomas.com

Harold D Love, Author
Charles C. Thomas, Publisher
Publisher of Education and Special Education books. *$43.95*
260 pages Paperback
ISBN 0-398062-48-4

3011 Textbooks and the Students Who Can't Read Them
Brookline Books
8 Trumbull Rd
Suite B-001
Northampton, MA 01060   413-584-0184
                              800-666-2665
                              Fax: 413-584-6184
                              www.brooklinebooks.com
                              brbooks@yahoo.com

Jean Ciborowski, Author
This book proposes how to involve low readers more effectively in textbook learning. It presents instructional techniques to improve students' willingness to work in mainstream textbooks. *$21.95*
Paperback
ISBN 0-914797-57-3

Social Skills

3012 ADHD in the Schools: Assessment and Intervention Strategies
Guilford Press
72 Spring Street
New York, NY 10012-4019   800-365-7006
                                Fax: 212-966-6708
                                www.guilford.com
                                info@guilford.com

Seymour Weingarten, Editor-in-Chief
Jim Nageotte, Senior Editor
Jody Falco, Managing Editor
This popular reference and text provides essential guidance for school-based professionals meeting the challenges of ADHD at any grade level. Comprehensive and practical, the book includes several reproducible assessment tools and handouts. *$30.00*
330 pages
ISBN 1-593850-89-1

3013 Behavior Change in the Classroom: Self-Management Interventions
Guilford Press
72 Spring Street
New York, NY 10012-4019   800-365-7006
                                Fax: 212-966-6708
                                www.guilford.com
                                info@guilford.com

Seymour Weingarten, Editor-in-Chief
Jim Nageotte, Senior Editor
Jody Falco, Managing Editor

This book presents practical approaches for designing and implementing self-management interventions in school settings. Rich with detailed instruction, the volume covers the conceptual foundation for the development of self-management from both contingency management and cognitive-behavioral perspectives. *$35.00*
204 pages
ISBN 0-898623-66-9

3014 **Group Activities to Include Students with Special Needs**
Corwin Press
2455 Teller Road
Thousand Oaks, CA 91320-2218   805-499-9734
                                                                 800-233-9936
                                                  Fax: 805-499-5323
                                                     www.corwin.com
                                                  order@corwin.com

Mike Soules, President
Lisa Shaw, Executive Director
Elena Nikitina, Executive Director
This hands-on resource offers 120 group activities emphasizing participation, cooperation, teamwork, mutual support, and improved self-esteem. This practical guide provides instant activities that can be used without preparation and incorporated into the daily routine with ease and confidence. Classroom games, gym and outdoor games, and ball games are designed to help your students gain the valuable skills they need to interact appropriately within the school setting. *$35.95*
240 pages
ISBN 0-761977-26-1

Publications

3015 Campus Opportunities for Students with Learning Differences
Octameron Associates
PO Box 2748
Alexandria, VA 22301-748
703-836-5480
Fax: 703-836-5650
www.octameron.com
Judith Crooker, Author
Stephen Crooker, Co-Author
A book about going to college for young adults with various learning disabilities. Details questions to ask in selecting a college and teaches how to be a self-advocate. *$5.00*
36 pages
ISBN 1-575090-52-X

3016 Career College and Technology School Databook
Chronicle Guidance Publications
66 Aurora Street
Moravia, NY 13118-3569
315-497-0330
800-622-7284
Fax: 315-497-0339
www.chronicleguidance.com
janet@chronicleguidance.com
Cheryl Fickeisen, President and CEO
Gary Fickeisen, Vice President
Christopher Fickeisen, Assistant Vice President
Offers information on occupational education programs currently available in the United States, Guam, and Puerto Rico. Programs consist of study or training leading to definite occupations. Prepares people for employment in recognized occupations, helps people make educated occupational choices, and upgrade and update their occupational skills. Includes data on vocational schools offering postsecondary occupational education. Accrediting associations are listed with contact information. *$25.46*
171 pages Annual
ISBN 1-556313-39-4

3017 Chronicle Financial Aid Guide
Chronicle Guidance Publications
66 Aurora Street
Moravia, NY 13118-3569
800-622-7284
Fax: 315-497-0339
www.chronicleguidance.com
janet@chronicleguidance.com
Cheryl Fickeisen, President and CEO
Gary Fickeisen, Vice President
Christopher Fickeisen, Assistant Vice President
Offers information on more than 1,950 financial aid programs, offering over 400,000 awards from current, verified sources. *$25.49*
434 pages Annual
ISBN 1-556313-40-0

3018 Colleges for Students with Learning Disabilities or ADD
Peterson's
2000 Lenox Drive
Lawrenceville, NJ 08648-2314
609-896-1800
800-338-3282
Fax: 609-896-4531
www.petersons.com
support@petersons.com
Charles Mangrum II, Author
Directs special-needs students to educational programs and services at 1,000 two-and four-year colleges and universities in the US and Canada. *$29.95*
560 pages Paperback
ISBN 0-768904-55-2

3019 Disabled Faculty and Staff in a Disabling Society: Multiple Identities in Higher Education
Association on Higher Education and Disability
107 Commerce Centre Drive
Suite 204
Huntersville, NC 28078-5870
704-947-7779
Fax: 704-948-7779
www.ahead.org
Bea Awoniyi, President
Srephan Hamlin Smith, Executive Director
Terra Beethe, Secretary
In this compelling anthology, 33 higher education professionals share personal stories, as well as relevant research associated with how they juggled both professional and personal needs. *$28.95*
300 pages

3020 Four-Year College Databook
Chronicle Guidance Publications
66 Aurora Street
Moravia, NY 13118-3569
315-497-0330
800-622-7284
Fax: 315-497-0339
www.chronicleguidance.com
janet@chronicleguidance.com
Cheryl Fickeisen, President and CEO
Gary Fickeisen, Vice President
Christopher Fickeisen, Assistant Vice President
Contains 2,160 institutions offering 790 four-year graduate and professional majors. *$25.48*
626 pages Annual
ISBN 1-556313-42-4

3021 From Legal Principle to Informed Practice
Association on Higher Education and Disability
107 Commerce Centre Drive
Suite 204
Huntersville, NC 28078-5870
704-947-7779
Fax: 704-948-7779
www.ahead.org
Bea Awoniyi, President
Srephan Hamlin Smith, Executive Director
Terra Beethe, Secretary
This must have resource for disability service providers in higher education demystifies the legal underpinnings of the work you do; offering valuable insight, discussion, and instruction on understanding the principles and premises of the legal framework that support the full participation of students with disabilities in higher education. *$75.00*
118 pages

3022 Going to College: Expanding Opportunities for People with Disabilities
Association on Higher Education and Disability
107 Commerce Centre Drive
Suite 204
Huntersville, NC 28078-5870
704-947-7779
Fax: 704-948-7779
www.ahead.org
Bea Awoniyi, President
Srephan Hamlin Smith, Executive Director
Terra Beethe, Secretary
An important textbook for DSS and other college professionals engaged in the transitoin of students with disabilities to college. *$34.95*
336 pages

3023 ISS Directory of International Schools
International Schools Services
15 Roszel Road
P.O. Box 5910
Princeton, NJ 08543-5910
609-452-0990
Fax: 609-452-2690
www.iss.edu
iss@iss.edu
Roger Hove, President
David Cobb, Executive Director
Kristin Evins, Chief Financial Officer

Comprehensive guide to over 550 American and international schools worldwide. *$49.95*
550 pages
ISBN 0-913663-24-7

3024 Learning Disabilities in Higher Educationand Beyond: An International Perspective
Association on Higher Education and Disability
107 Commerce Centre Drive
Suite 204
Huntersville, NC 28078-5870

704-947-7779
Fax: 704-948-7779
www.ahead.org

Bea Awoniyi, President
Srephan Hamlin Smith, Executive Director
Terra Beethe, Secretary
Builds upon an examination of the legal rights of people with learning disabilities in the United States, Canada, the United Kingdom, and Israel, then moves on to discuss assessment and diagnosis, programs, and support services, the social-emotional impact of learning disabilities, and how adults with learning disabilities fared after college. *$30.00*
384 pages

3025 Member Directory
NAPSEC
601 Pennsylvania Avenue
Suite 900
Washington, DC 20004-1202

202-434-8225
Fax: 202-434-8224
www.napsec.org
napsec@aol.com

Sherry Kolbe, Executive Director
A membership directory listing NAPSEC'S members, disabilities served, program descriptions, school profiles, admissions procedures and funding approval. *$32.00*
300 pages Bi-Annual

3026 Navigating College College Manual for Teaching the Portfolio
Association on Higher Education and Disability
107 Commerce Centre Drive
Suite 204
Huntersville, NC 28078-5870

704-947-7779
Fax: 704-948-7779
www.ahead.org

Bea Awoniyi, President
Srephan Hamlin Smith, Executive Director
Terra Beethe, Secretary
Provides in-class activity ideas for each chapter. As well, it provides suggestions to help students master the out of class assignments along with suggested grading rubrics. *$19.95*

3027 Navigating College: Strategy Manual for a Successful Voyage
Association on Higher Education and Disability
107 Commerce Centre Drive
Suite 204
Huntersville, NC 28078-5870

704-947-7779
Fax: 704-948-7779
www.ahead.org

Bea Awoniyi, President
Srephan Hamlin Smith, Executive Director
Terra Beethe, Secretary
A portfolio of readings and activities for new college students, all based in student persistance research. *$24.95*
131 pages

3028 Schoolsearch Guide to Colleges with Programs & Services for Students with LD
Schoolsearch
21 Starr Ridge Road
Needham, MA 02464-1146

617-899-3666
Fax: 781-444-0806
www.schoolsearch.com
mlipkin@schoolsearch.com

Midge Lipkin, Author
Midge Lipkin, Founder

Lists more than 600 colleges and universities that offer programs and services to high school graduates with learning disabilities. *$29.95*
706 pages
ISBN 0-962032-63-8

3029 Two-Year College Databook
Chronicle Guidance Publications
66 Aurora Street
Moravia, NY 13118-3569

315-497-0330
800-622-7284
Fax: 315-497-0339
www.chronicleguidance.com
janet@chronicleguidance.com

Cheryl Fickeisen, President and CEO
Gary Fickeisen, Vice President
Christopher Fickeisen, Assistant Vice President
Contains information on college majors, and on 2,432 institutions offering 760 occupational-career, associate, and transfer programs. *$25.47*
476 pages Annual
ISBN 1-556313-41-7

Alabama

3030 Auburn University
Program for Students with Disabilities
1244 Haley Ctr
Auburn, AL 36849

334-844-4000
Fax: 334-844-2099
www.auburn.edu
webmaster@auburn.edu

Sarah Colby Weaver PhD, Director
Provides reasonable accommodations and services for qualified students with documented disabilities who are attending Auburn University, enrolled in distance learning classes, or participating in programs sponsored by Auburn University.

3031 Auburn University at Montgomery
Center for Disability Services
PO Box 244023
Montgomery, AL 36124-4023

334-244-3000
800-227-2649
Fax: 334-244-3762
TDD: 334-244-3754
www.aum.edu
askaum@aum.edu

Tamara Massey-Garrett MS, Director
Robert Bentley, President
Grant Davis, Secretary
Offers a variety of services to students with disabilities including equipment, extended testing time, interpreting services, counseling services, and special accommodations.

3032 Birmingham-Southern College
900 Arkadelphia Rd
Birmingham, AL 35254-0002

205-226-4647
800-523-5793
Fax: 205-226-4627
www.bsc.edu
kleonard@bsc.edu

Sara Hoover, Director, Counselith/Health Svcs
Becky Baxter, Campus Visit Coordinator
Offers a variety of services to students with disabilities including notetakers, extended testing time, counseling services, and special accommodations.

3033 Chattahoochee Valley State Community College
2602 College Dr
Phenix City, AL 36869-7917

334-291-4900
Fax: 334-291-4944
www.cvcc.cc.al.us

Laurel M Blackwell, President
Jacquie Thacker, ADA Coordinator
Offers a variety of services to students with disabilities including note takers, extended testing time, counseling services and special accommodations.

3034 Churchill Academy

395 Ray Thorington Rd
Montgomery, AL 36117-8486
334-270-4225
Fax: 334-270-7805
www.churchillacademymontgomery.com
contact@ChurchillAcademyMontgomery.com
Lisa Hanlon Schroeder, Director
Kaye Pair, Student Service Co-ordinator
Pam Brown, Office Manager
A one-of-a-kind school for bright children with unique learning differences.

3035 Enterprise Ozark Community College

600 Plaza Drive
Enterprise, AL 36330-1300
334-347-2623
800-624-3438
Fax: 334-774-6399
www.escc.edu
Lizz Barton, Assistant
Dr. Nancy W. Chandler, President
A public two-year college with 15 special education students out of a total of 600. Certified by the Federal Aviation Administration, and offers the only comprehensive aviation maintenance training program in the state of Alabama, with instruction in airframe, powerplant and avionics.

3036 Horizons School

2018 15th Ave South
Birmingham, AL 35205-3812
205-322-6606
800-822-6242
Fax: 205-322-6605
www.horizonsschool.org
jcarter@horizonsschool.org
Jade K Carter, Director
Brian Geiger, Assistant Director
Don Lutomski, President
Offers a non-degree transition program specifically designed to facilitate personal, social and career independence for students with specific learning disabilities and other handicapping conditions.

3037 Jacksonville State University

Disability Support Services
700 Pelham Rd North
Jacksonville, AL 36265-1623
256-782-5781
800-231-5291
Fax: 256-782-5291
www.jsu.edu
info@jsu.edu
William A Meehan, Director
Bill Meehan, President
Pamela B. Stinson, Executive Secretary
Offers a variety of services to students with disabilities including notetakers, extended testing time, counseling services, and special accommodations.

3038 James H Faulkner State Community College

1900 Highway 31 South
Bay Minette, AL 36507-2698
251-580-2100
800-231-3752
Fax: 251-580-2236
www.faulknerstate.edu
bkennedy@faulknerstate.edu
Gary Branch, President
Adams Ken, Director
Elizabeth Thompson Day, Office & Legal Administration
A public two-year community college with approximately 125 students with disabilities out of a total student population of 4,350. Committed to the professional and cultural growth of each student without regard to race, color, qualified disability, gender, religion, creed, national origin, or age. Attempts to provide an educational environment that promotes development and learning through a wide variety of educational programs, adequate and comfortable facilities, and flexible scheduling.

3039 Troy State University Dothan

500 University Drive
Alabama, AL 36082
334-983-6556
800-414-5756
Fax: 334-983-6322
TTY: 800-414-5756
www.troy.edu
ask@troy.edu
Barbara Alford, President
Keith Seagle, Counseling Services Director
Offers a variety of services to students with disabilities including notetakers, extended testing time, counseling services, and special accommodations.

3040 University of Alabama

Office of Disability Services
PO Box 870132
Tuscaloosa, AL 35487
205-348-6010
Fax: 205-348-8377
www.ua.edu
intergradapply@aalan.ua.edu
Carl Bacon, President
Brenda F. Elliott, Treasurer
Cynthia Moore, Secretary
A public four-year college with approximately 650 students identified with disabilities out of a total of 19,200.

3041 University of Montevallo

Office of Disability Services
Palmer Hall, Station 6030
Montevallo, AL 35115
205-665-6000
800-292-4349
Fax: 205-665-6080
www.montevallo.edu
admissions@montevallo.edu
Dr. John W. Stewart III, President
Caroline Aderholt, Secretary
Dr. Michelle Johnston, Senior Vice President
Offers a variety of services to students with disabilities including notetakers, extended testing time, counseling services, and special accommodations.

3042 University of North Alabama

Office of Developmental Services
One Harrison Plaza
Florence, AL 35632
256-765-4608
800-825-5862
Fax: 256-765-6016
www.una.edu
jadams@unanov.una.edu
Jennifer S Adams, Director
Developmental services of UNA provides accommodation and supportive services to assist students with disabilities throughout their college expirence.

3043 University of South Alabama

Disabled Student Services
307 N University Blvd
Mobile, AL 36688
251-460-6101
Fax: 251-460-6080
www.usouthal.edu
aagnew@usouthal.edu
V Gordon Moulton, President
Dr. John W. Smith, Special Assistant
Offers a variety of services to students with disabilities including note takers, extended testing time, counseling services, and special accommodations.

3044 Wallace Community College Selma

3000 Earl Goodwin Parkway
Selma, AL 36702-2530
334-876-9227
Fax: 334-876-9250
www.wccs.edu
info@wccs.edu
Dr. James Mitchell, President
Robby Bennett, Director
Donitha Griffin, Dean of Students

Offers a variety of services to students with disabilities including note takers, extended testing time, counseling services and special accommodations.

Alaska

3045 Alaska Pacific University
Disabled Student Services
4101 University Drive
Anchorage, AK 99508-4647   907-564-8317
                                   Fax: 907-562-8248
                                   TTY: 800-252-7528
                                   www.alaskapacific.edu
                                   admissions@alaskapacific.edu
Bonnie Mehner, Chair
Roberta Graham, Vice Chair
Don Bantz, President
Four-year college offering special services to students that are learning disabled.

3046 Gateway School and Learning Center
900 W.Fireweed Lane
P.O.Box 113149
Anchorage, AK 99511-3149   907-522-2240
                                   Fax: 907-344-0304
                                   www.gatewayschoolak.com
                                   learning@gatewayschoolak.com
Beverly Lau, Principal
Provides specialized educational services for students grades 1-12 with dyslexia and other language-processing disorders.

3047 Juneau Campus: University of Alaska Southeast
11120 Glacier Hwy
Juneau, AK 99801-8699   907-796-6100
                                   877-465-4827
                                   Fax: 907-465-6365
                                   www.uas.alaska.edu
                                   uas.info@uas.alaska.edu
Patrick Gamble, President
Joel Milsat, Director
Fuller A. Cowell, Founder
Offers a variety of services to students with disabilities including notetakers, extended testing time, counseling services, and special accommodations.

3048 Ketchikan Campus: University of Alaska Southeast
2600 7th Ave
Ketchikan, AK 99901-5728   228-4511
                                   888-550-6177
                                   Fax: 225-3624
                                   TTY: 888-550-6177
                                   www.ketch.alaska.edu
                                   ketch.info@uas.alaska.edu
Kathleen Wiechelman, Assistant Professor
Laurie Williams, Administrative Assisstant
Offers a variety of services to students with disabilities including note takers, extended testing time, counseling services and special accommodations.

3049 University of Alaska Anchorage
Office of Disability Services
3211 Providence Drive
Anchorage, AK 99508-4645   907-786-1800
                                   Fax: 907-786-6123
                                   www.uaa.alaska.edu
                                   aydss@uaa.alaska.edu
Fran Ulmer, Director
Patrick Gamble, President
Provides equal opportunites for students who experience disabilities.

Arizona

3050 New Way Learning Academy
5048 E. Oak Street
Phoenix, AZ 85008-3776   602-629-6850
                                   Fax: 602-629-6851
                                   www.newwayacademy.org
                                   samantha@newwayacademy.org
Richard Schneider, Chairman
Diana Maudlin, Vice Chairman
Ann Brown, Secretary
Non-profit, private K-12 day school specializing in children with learning differences. We proudly and passionately serve students with dyslexia, AD/HD and other learning differences.

3051 SALT Center
University of Arizona
1010 North Highland Avenue
PO Box 210136
Tucson, AZ 85721-0136   520-621-1242
                                   Fax: 520-626-3260
                                   www.salt.arizona.edu
                                   saltnews@email.arizona.edu
Rudy M Molina, Director
Rhonda Burnett, Associate Director
Marsha Dean, Administrative Associate
An academic support program that provides a comprehensive range of fee-based services to University of Arizona students with learning and attention challenges.

3052 Upward Foundation
Special Education Program
6306 North 7th Street
Phoenix, AZ 85014-1549   602-279-5801
                                   Fax: 602-279-0033
                                   www.upwardaz.org
                                   Info@upwardaz.org
Sharon Graham, Executive Director
Jim Bissonett, President
Doug Carter, Chief Executive Officer
Improving the lives of children with severe disabilities and other special needs.

Arkansas

3053 Jones Learning Center
University of the Ozarks
415 N College Ave
Clarksville, AR 72830-2880   479-979-1403
                                   800-264-8636
                                   Fax: 479-979-1429
                                   www.ozarks.edu
                                   jlc@ozarks.edu
Julia Frost, Director
Dodi Pelts, Assistant Director
Richard L. Dunsworth, JD, President
Offers enhanced services to students who show potential for success in a competitive academic environment.

3054 Philander Smith College
Student Support Program (SPARK)
900 West Daisy Bates Drive
Little Rock, AR 72202-3717   501-370-5221
                                   800-446-6772
                                   Fax: 501-370-5277
                                   www.philander.edu
                                   administrator@philander.edu
Lloyd E. Hervey, Ed.D., President
Michael Hutchinson, Director for Public Relations
Anita Hatley, Administrative Assistant
Offers a variety of services to students with disabilities including notetakers, extended testing time, counseling services, and special accommodations.

3055 Southern Arkansas University
Disabled Student Programs and Services
100 East UniversityMagnolia
Magnolia, AR 71753-5000   870-235-5000
                                 Fax: 870-235-4133
                                 www.saumag.edu
                                 eewalker@saumag.edu

Eunice Walker, Director
Dr. David F Rankin phd CFA, President
Offers a variety of services to students with disabilities including notetakers, extended testing time, counseling services, and special accommodations.

3056 University of Arkansas
Center for Educational Access
Room 104 Arkansas Union
Fayetteville, AR 72701   479-575-2000
                                 800-377-8632
                                 Fax: 479-575-7445
                                 www.uark.edu
                                 ada@uark.edu

Annie Jannarone, Director
G David Gearhart, Chancellor
Offers a variety of services to students with disabilities including note takers, extended testing time, counseling services, and special accommodations.

California

3057 ACCESS Program
Moorpark College
7075 Campus Rd
Moorpark, CA 93021-1605   805-378-1400
                                 Fax: 805-378-1499
                                 TDD: 805-378-1461
                                 www.moorparkcollege.edu
                                 sdattile@vcccd.edu

Sherry D'Attile, Director
Dr. Bernard Luskin, President
Andrea Rambo, Executive Assistant
A public two-year college with 154 special education students out of a total of 12,414.

3058 Allan Hancock College
800 S College Dr
Santa Maria, CA 93454-6399   805-922-6966
                                 Fax: 805-928-7905
                                 www.hancockcollege.edu
                                 lap@hancockcollege.edu

Robert Parisi, Director
Students with mobility, visual, hearing and speech impairments, learning disabilities, acquired brain injury, developmental disabilities, psychological and other disabilities are eligible to receive special services which enable them to fully participate in the community college experience at Allan Hancock College.

3059 Antelope Valley College
Disabled Student Services Program
3041 W Avenue K
Lancaster, CA 93536-5426   661-722-6300
                                 Fax: 661-722-6333
                                 www.avc.edu
                                 llucero@avc.edu

Louis Lucero, Director
Edward Knudson, President
Patricia Harris, Senior Administrative Assistant
A public two-year college with 228 learning disabled students out of a total of 11,105.

3060 Aspen Education Group
17777 Center Court Dr N
Cerritos, CA 90703-9328   888-972-7736
                                 855-259-2288
                                 Fax: 562-402-7036
                                 www.aspeneducation.com

Elliot A Sainer, President

Provider of education programs for the struggling or underachieving young people. Offers professionals and families the opportunity to choose a setting that best meets a student's unique academic and emotional needs.

3061 Bakersfield College
Disabled Student Programs and Services
1801 Panorama Dr
Bakersfield, CA 93305-1299   661-565-0287
                                 Fax: 661-395-4079
                                 TTY: 661-395-4334
                                 www.2.bakersfieldcollege.edu
                                 david.riess@bakersfieldcollege.edu

Greg A Chamberlain, Director
A public two-year college with 207 special education students out of a total of 12,312.

3062 Barstow Community College
Disabled Student Programs and Services
2700 Barstow Rd
Barstow, CA 92311-6608   760-252-2411
                                 Fax: 760-252-1875
                                 TDD: 760-252-6759
                                 TTY: 760-252-6759
                                 www.barstow.edu
                                 nolson@barstow.edu

Dr. Debbie DiThomas, Superintendent /President
Michelle Henderson, Executive Assistant
Maureen Stokes, Director of Public Information
Educational support program for disabled students including special classes and support services for all disabled students.

3063 Bridge School
Educational Program
545 Eucalyptus Ave
Hillsborough, CA 94010-6404   650-696-7295
                                 Fax: 650-342-7598
                                 www.bridgeschool.org

Dr. Vicki Casella, Executive Director
Lorelei Garcia, Administrative Assistant
Mary Frances Allen, Executive Assistant
Our program is based on the principle of providing access to and participation in an age-appropriate curriculum adapted to the special needs of children with motor, sensory and speech impairments.

3064 Butte College
Disabled Student Programs and Services
3536 Butte Campus Dr
Oroville, CA 95965-8399   530-895-2511
                                 Fax: 530-895-2345
                                 TDD: 530-895-2308
                                 www.butte.edu
                                 dsps@butte.edu

Diana J Van Der Ploeg, Coordinator
Carol Oba-Winslow, Disabilities Specialist
Kimberly Perry, President
A public two-year college with 223 special education students out of a total of 12,848.

3065 Cabrillo College
Disabled Student Programs and Services
6500 Soquel Drive
Aptos, CA 95003   831-479-6100
                                 Fax: 831-477-5687
                                 TTY: 831-479-6421
                                 www.cabrillo.edu
                                 jonapoli@cabrillo.edu

Dr. Laurel Jones, Superintendent /President
Dr. Kathleen Welch, Vice President Instruction
Victoria Lewis, Vice President Administrative
A two-year college that offers services and programs to disabled students.

3066 California State University: East Bay
25800 Carlos Bee Blvd
Hayward, CA 94542-3001
510-885-3000
Fax: 510-885-2049
www.csuhayward.edu
sdrc@csueastbay.edu

Dr. Leroy Morishita, President
Brad Wells, Chief Financial Officer
Derek Atiken, Chief of Staff
Students with documented disabilities and functional limitations are eligible for accomodations designed to provide equivalent access to general campus and classroom programs and activities. The campus provides an SDRC - Student Disability Resource Center - with assistive technology and testing accomodations. They also offer Project Impact and the EXCEL Program, both of which serve their disabled student body.

3067 California State University: Fullerton
Disabled Student Services
800 N State College Blvd
PO Box 34080
Fullerton, CA 92831-3599
657-278-4444
Fax: 714-278-2408
TDD: 714-278-2786
www.fullerton.edu
dliverpool@fullerton.edu

Mildred Garcja, President
Danny C. Kim, Chief Financial Officer
Christopher Bugbee, Director of Media Relations
A public four-year college with 800 special education students out of a total of 75,000. The Office of Disabled Student Services aims to increase access and retention for students with permanent and temporary disabilities by ensuring equitable treatment in all aspects of campus life. Provides co-curricular and academically related services which empower students with disabilities to achieve academic and personal self-determination.

3068 California State University: Long Beach-Stephen Benson Program
Disabled Student Services
1250 N Bellflower Blvd
BH-377
Long Beach, CA 90840-0004
562-985-4430
Fax: 562-985-4529
www.csulb.edu/sbp
dss@csulb.edu

Jane Close Conoley, President
Brian Carey, Coordinator
Dominique Mota, Office Coordinator
Four-year college offers a program for the learning disabled.

3069 Chaffey Community College District
Disability Programs and Services
5885 Haven Avenue
Rancho Cucamonga, CA 91737-3002
909-652-8000
Fax: 909-652-6386
TTY: 909-466-2829
www.chaffey.edu
joe.jondreau@chaffey.edu

Joe Jondreau, Director
Lizza Napoli, Assistant
Henry D. Shannon, Ph.D, President
Chaffey College's Disabled Student Programs and Services (DSP&S) offer instruction and support services to students with developmental, learning, physical, psychological disabilities or aquired brain injury. Students can recieve a variety of services such as: test facilitation, note taking, tutoring, adaptive physical education, pre-vocational training, career preparation, and job placement.

3070 Charles Armstrong School
1405 Solana Drive
Belmont, CA 94002-3653
650-592-7570
Fax: 650-591-3114
www.charlesarmstrong.org
information@charlesarmstrong.org

David Evans, Chairman
David Obershaw, President
Audrey Fox, Vice-President
Serves students with language-based learning differences, such as dyslexia, by providing an appropriate educational experience which enables the students to acquire language skills, while instilling a joy of learning, enhancing self-worth, and allowing each student the right to identify, understand and fulfill personal potential.

3071 Chartwell School: Seaside
2511 Numa Watson Rd
Seaside, CA 93955-6774
831-394-3468
Fax: 831-394-6809
www.chartwell.org
info@chartwell.org

Mary Ann Leffel, President
Katrina Maestri, Vice President
Ralph Bailey, Treasurer
Our mission is to educate children with a wide range of language-related visual and auditory learning challenges in a way that provides them with the learning skills and self-esteem necessary to return successfully to mainstream education. Chartwell also helps individuals with specific learning challenges access their full potential by providing leading-edge education, research and community outreach.

3072 College of Alameda
Disabled Student Services
555 Ralph Appezzato Memorial Pkwy
Alameda, CA 94501-2109
510-522-7221
Fax: 510-748-2339
TTY: 510-748-2330
www.alameda.peralta.edu
hmaxwell@peralta.edu

Eric V. Gravenberg, Ph.D., President
Dr. Alexis S. Montevirgen, Ed.D., Vice President of Student
Tim Karas, Vice President of Instruction
Accommodations, assessment and special classes are provided for learning disabled students enrolled at College Alameda, a 2 year college located by San Francisco Bay.

3073 College of Marin
Disabled Students Program
835 College Ave
Kentfield, CA 94904-2590
415-457-8811
Fax: 415-457-4791
www.marin.cc.ca.us
WeListen@marin.edu

David Wain Coon, Ed.D., Superintendent/President
Eva Long, Ph.D., Vice President
Philip Kranenburg, Clerk
Offers a variety of services to students with disabilities including note takers, extended testing time, counseling services, and special accommodations. Also offers diagnostic testing and remedial classes for learning disabled students.

3074 College of the Canyons
Disabled Student Programs and Services
26455 Rockwell Canyon Rd
Santa Clarita, CA 91355-1899
661-259-7800
Fax: 661-259-8302
TTY: 661-255-7967
www.coc.cc.ca.us
jane.feuerhelm@canyons.edu

Dianne G Van Hook, President
A public two-year college with 45 special education students out of a total of 6,255.

3075 College of the Redwoods
Disabled Student Programs and Services
7351 Tompkins Hill Rd
Eureka, CA 95501-9300
707-476-4100
800-641-0400
Fax: 707-476-4400
TTY: 707-476-4284
www.redwoods.edu
kathy-smith@redwoods.edu

Jeff Marsee, Director
Kathryn Smith, President
Michelle Anderson, Assistant to the President
Mission is to assist individual students in the development of a realistic self-concept, assist in the development of educational interests and employment goals, provide the advice, counseling, and equipment necessary to facilitate success, starting with specialized assistance in the registration process.

3076   College of the Sequoias
Disability Resource Center
915 S. Mooney Blvd
Visalia, CA   93277   559-730-3700
                                                 Fax: 559-730-3803
                                                 TDD: 559-730-3913
                                                 TTY: 559-730-3913
                                                     www.cos.edu
                                               sharmeenl@cos.edu

David Maciel, Director
Stan A. Carrizosa, President
A public two-year college with approximately 600 special education students out of a total of 10,300.

3077   College of the Siskiyous
800 College Avenue
Weed, CA   96094-2899   530-938-5555
                                                       888-397-4339
                                                 Fax: 530-938-5378
                                                 www.siskiyous.edu
                                            dsps@siskiyous.edu

Sunny Greene, DSPS Director
Scotty Thomas, President
Offers services to learning and physically disabled students throught the DSPS - Disabled Students Programs & Services.

3078   Columbia College
11600 Columbia College Dr
Sonora, CA   95370-8580   209-588-5100
                                                 Fax: 209-588-5104
                                               www.gocolumbia.edu
                                            rodtsk@yosemite.edu

Karin Rodts, DSPS Coordinator/LD Specialist
Angela R. Fairchilds, Ph.D., President
Amy Nilson, Director of Development
Offers a variety of services to students with disabilities including note takers, extended testing time, counseling services and special accommodations.

3079   Cuesta College
Building 7400
Highway 1
San Luis Obispo, CA   93405-8106   805-546-3100
                                                 Fax: 805-546-3930
                                          http://academic.cuesta.edu
                                            dspsinfo@cuesta.edu

Patrick Schwab EdD, Director
A public, two-year community college, offering instruction and services to students with learning disabilities since 1973. A comprehensive set of services and special classes are available. Contact the program for further information.

3080   Disabled Students Programs & Services
Laney College
900 Fallon St
Oakland, CA   94607-4893   510-834-5740
                                                 Fax: 510-986-6913
                                                 TTY: 510-464-3400
                                               www.laney.peralta.edu
                                            rpruitt@peralta.edu

Elnora Webb, President
Provides services and instructional programs for students with disabilities.

3081   East Los Angeles College
1301 Avenida Cesar Chavez
Monterey Park, CA   91754-6099   323-265-8650
                                                 Fax: 323-265-8759
                                                 www.elac.cc.ca.us

Marvin Martinez, College President
Jeanette Gordon, Chief Financial Officer
Thomas Hall, Interim Executive Director
A public two-year college with 44 special education students out of a total of 14587. There is a an additional fee for the special education program in addition to the regular tuition.

3082   Excelsior Academy
Disabled Student Programs
7202 Princess View Dr
San Diego, CA   92120-1332   619-583-6762
                                                 Fax: 619-583-6762
                                           www.excelsioracademy.com
                                       nhallcy@excelsioracademy.com

Nance Maguire, Ed.D, Executive Director
Karina Arana, Director
Matthew Callaway, MA, Program Specialist
Provide a safe and nurturing environment wherein students become literate, thinking, independent, and productive citizens. Serving students in Grade 3-12 with unique learning profiles.

3083   Fresno City College
Disabled Student Programs and Services
1101 E University Ave
Fresno, CA   93741   559-442-4600
                                                       559-489-2281
                                                 Fax: 559-265-5777
                                                 TDD: 559-442-8237
                                         www.fresnocitycollege.edu
                             janice.emerzian@fresnocitycollege.edu

Cynthia Azari, District Director
Toni Cantu, President
Dr.Chris Willa, Vice President
A public two-year college with 259 special education students out of a total of 17,949.

3084   Frostig Center
Marianne Frostig Center of Educational Therapy
971 N Altadena Dr
Pasadena, CA   91107-1870   626-791-1255
                                                 Fax: 626-798-1801
                                                     www.frostig.org
                                               center@frostig.org

Phyllis Kochavi, Chair
Norm Solomon, Esq., Vice Chair
Susan Paciocco, Secretary
Dedicated to providing children with learning disabilities a quality academic program that also promotes their language, motor, social-emotional, and creative growth.

3085   Gavilan College
Disabled Student Programs and Services
5055 Santa Teresa Blvd
Gilroy, CA   95020-9599   408-848-4800
                                                       831-637-1158
                                                 Fax: 408-848-4801
                                                 TTY: 408-846-4924
                                                   www.gavilan.edu
                                               drc@gavilan.edu

Kent Child, President
Walt Glines, Vice-President
Susan Cheu, Chief Financial Officer
Offers a variety of services to students with disabilities including note takers, extended testing time, counseling services and special accommodations.

3086 Hartnell College
Disabled Student Programs and Services
411 Central Avenue
Salinas, CA 93901-1688   831-755-6700
                                   Fax: 831-755-6751
                                   TDD: 831-770-6199
                                    www.hartnell.edu

Phoebe K Helm, LD Specialist
Willard Clark Lewallen, Ph.D., Superintendent/President
Al Munoz, Vice President
A public two-year college with 72 special education students out of a total of 7,593.

3087 Institute for the Redesign of Learning
Transition and Adult Services
211 Pasadena Avenue
South Pasadena, CA 91030-2919   323-341-5632
                                        877-837-4332
                                   Fax: 323-341-5644
                            www.redesignlearning.org

Dr. Nancy J Lavelle, President
Jason D. Rubin, Managing Diredtor
Nita Moore MPA, Program Director
A full day school serving 100 boys and girls, at-risk infants and children. Vocational Program serves adults and includes Supported Employment Services and an Independent Living Program.

3088 Irvine Valley College
Disabled Student Programs and Services
5500 Irvine Center Drive
Irvine, CA 92618-300   949-451-5100
                                   TTY: 949-451-5785
                                        www.ivc.edu
                                     ivcdsps@ivc.edu

Glenn R. Roquemore, PhD, President
Craig Justice, PhD, Vice President of Instruction
Dr. Linda Fontanilla, Ed.D., VP Student Services
The goal is to effectivly provide assistance to all students with disabilities to achieve academic success while at Irvine Valley. The primary function is to accommodate a student's disability, whether it is a physical, communication, learning or psychological disability.

3089 Kayne Eras Center
Exceptional Children's Foundation
8740 Washington Boulevard
Culver City, CA 90232-8800   310-204-3300
                                   Fax: 310-845-8001
                                    www.kayneeras.org
                               jraffle@kayneeras.org

Scott Bowling, President
Philip G. Miller, Chairperson
Operates a state certified, non-public school for youth ages 5 to 22 who are having difficulty functioning in the public school system due to developmental delays, learning disabilities, emotional or behavior challenges, and/or health impairments.

3090 Long Beach City College: Liberal Arts Campus
Disabled Student Programs and Services
Rm A119
4901 E Carson St
Long Beach, CA 90808-1706   562-938-4111
                                   Fax: 562-938-4651
                                   TDD: 562-938-4833
                             www.dsps.lbcc.cc.ca.us
                               mmatsui@lbcc.edu

Eloy Oakley, President
Jeffrey Kellog, Vice President
Disabled Student Services (DSPS) is a program within Student Services at LBCC. DSPS provides many support services that enable students with disability related limitations to participate in the college's programs and activities. DSPS offers a wide range of services that compensate for a students limitations, like note taking assistance, interpretive services, alternative media, etc.

3091 Los Angeles Mission College
Disabled Student Programs and Services
13356 Eldridge Ave
Sylmar, CA 91342-3245   818-364-7600
                                   Fax: 818-364-7755
                                   TDD: 818-364-7861
                                    www.lamission.edu
                               scuderi@lamission.edu

Judith Valles, Director
Monte E. Perez. PhD, President
A support system that enables students to fully participate in the college's regular programs and activities. We provide a variety of services from academic and vocational support to assistance with finacial aid. All services are individulaized according to specific needs. They do not replace regular programs, but rather, accommodate students special requirements.

3092 Los Angeles Pierce College
Disabled Student Programs and Services
6201 Winnetka Ave
Woodland Hills, CA 91371   818-710-4100
                                   Fax: 818-710-9844
                                   TTY: 818-719-6430
                                  www.piercecollege.edu
                    special_services@piercecollege.edu

Robert M Garber, Director
Dr. Kathleen Burke, President
A public two-year college with 257 special education students out of a total of 19,207.

3093 Los Angeles Valley College Services for Students with Disabilities (SSD)
5800 Fulton Ave
Valley Glen, CA 91401-4096   818-947-2600
                                   Fax: 818-778-5775
                                   TDD: 818-947-2680
                                   TTY: 818-947-2680
                                       www.lavc.edu
                                    ssd@lavc.edu

Dr. Erika Endrijonas, President
Raul Castillo, Executive Director
Karen Daar, VP Academic Affairs
Provides specialized support services to students with disabilities which are in addition to the regular services provided to all students. Special accommodations and services are determined by the nature and extent of the disability related educational limitations of the student and are provided based upon the recommendation of DSPS.

3094 Monterey Peninsula College
Disabled Student Programs and Services
980 Fremont St
Monterey, CA 93940-4799   831-646-4000
                                   Fax: 831-646-4171
                                       www.mpc.edu
                                    ssandi@mpc.edu

Mr. Charles Brown, Chair
Dr. Loren Steck, Vice Chair
Mr. Maury Vasquez, Student Trustee
Supportive Services & Instruction program provides services and specialized instruction for enrolled students with disabilities.

3095 Mount San Antonio Community College
Disabled Student Programs and Services
1100 N Grand Ave
Walnut, CA 91789-1399   909-274-7500
                                   Fax: 909-594-7661
                                   TTY: 909-594-3447
                                       www.mtsac.edu
                                  ghanson@mtsac.edu

John S Nixon, Director
Dr.William T Scroggins, President
Jill Dolan, Director
A public two-year college with 1,500 students with disabilities who receive special services. Total population of students is approximately 40,000.

3096 **Napa Valley College**
Disabled Student Programs and Services
2277 Napa Valley Highway
Napa, CA 94558-7555
707-256-7000
800-826-1077
Fax: 707-259-8010
TTY: 707-253-3084
www.napavalley.edu
wmartinez@napavalley.edu
Dr. Ronald Kraft, President
Mr. Bruce Ketron, Board Chair
Mr. Dan Digardi, Vice President
Offers a variety of services to students with disabilities including note takers, extended testing time, counseling services and special accommodations.

3097 **Ohlone College**
Disabled Student Programs and Services
43600 Mission Blvd
Fremont, CA 94539-5847
510-659-6000
Fax: 510-659-6058
TTY: 510-659-6269
www.ohlone.edu
deafcenter@ohlone.edu
Gari Browning, President
Ronald Little, Vice President, Administrative
Paul Innaccone, Director
Special services are provided to meet the unique needs of Deaf, Hard of Hearing, and Disabled students and help them achieve a successful college career.

3098 **Orange Coast College**
Special Programs and Services
2701 Fairview Rd
Costa Mesa, CA 92626-5561
714-432-5072
Fax: 714-432-5739
www.orangecoastcollege.edu
omartinez@occ.cccd.edu
Robert Dees, Supervisor
Dennis Harkins, Ph.D., President
A public two-year college with 350 special education students out of a total of 27,960. There is a an additional fee for the special education program in addition to the regular tuition.

3099 **Park Century School**
3939 Landmark St
Culver City, CA 90232-2315
310-840-0500
Fax: 310-840-0590
www.parkcenturyschool.org
Sheila Cohn, Founder
Douglas E. Phelps, Head of School
A non-profit independent co-educational day school designed to meet the specific educational needs of bright children, ages 7 - 14 years, who have learning disabilities.

3100 **Prentice School**
18341 Lassen Drive
Santa Ana, CA 92705-2012
714-538-4511
800-479-4711
Fax: 714-538-5004
www.prentice.org
prenticeschool@prentice.org
Laura Khouri, President
Brian Sullivan, Vice President
Susan Konier, Secretary
The Prentice School is an independent, nonprofit, coeducational day school for children ages pre-k through 8th grade with language learning differences.

3101 **Raskob Learning Institute and Day School**
3520 Mountain Blvd
Oakland, CA 94619-1627
510-436-1275
Fax: 510-436-1106
www.raskobinstitute.org
raskobinstitute@hnu.edu
Edith Ben Ari, Executive Director
Jessica Baiocchi, Director of Admission
Stefani Wulkan, Assistant Director/Lead Teacher

A co-educational school for students from diverse cultural and economic backgrounds with language-based learning disabilities. Raskob seeks to recognize and nurture the talents and strengths of each student while remediating areas of academic weakness.

3102 **San Diego City College**
Disabled Student Programs and Services
1313 Park Blvd
San Diego, CA 92101-4787
619-388-3400
Fax: 619-388-3801
TTY: 619-388-3313
www.sdcity.edu
bmason@sdccd.edu
Harvey Marilyn, Director
Terrence Burgess, Coordinator
June E Richard, Co-Chairman
Offers a variety of services to students with disabilities including note takers, extended testing time, counseling services, and special accommodations.

3103 **San Diego Miramar College**
Disability Support Programs and Services
10440 Black Mountain Rd
San Diego, CA 92126-2999
616-536-7800
858-536-7800
Fax: 858-388-7901
TDD: 858-536-4301
www.sdmiramar.edu
kdoorly@sdccd.cc.ca.us
Patricia Hsieh, Ed.D., President
Gerald Ramsey, Vice President of Student
Brett Bell, VP, Admin Service
A public two-year college with 500 learning disabled students. These students receive services and accommodations appropriate for their success in college. Individual counseling, class advising and LD assessments are also available. Special classes are offered to support college courses.

3104 **San Diego State University**
Student Disability Services
5500 Campanile Drive
San Diego, CA 92182
619-594-5200
Fax: 619-594-5642
TDD: 619-594-2929
TTY: 619-594-2929
www.sa.sdsu.edu
marcomm@mail.sdsu.edu
Elliot Hirshman, President
Eric Rivera, Vice President
Dan Montoya, Development Officer
Program and Support services are available to students with certified visual limitations, hearing and communication impairments, learning disabilities, mobility, and other functional limitations.

3105 **Santa Monica College**
Center for Students with Disabilities
1900 Pico Boulevard
Santa Monica, CA 90405-1644
310-434-4000
Fax: 310-434-4272
TDD: 310-434-4273
www.smc.edu
schwartz_judy@smc.edu
Dr. Susan Aminoff, Chair
Rob Rader, Vice Chair
Dr. Chui L Tsang, Superintendent/President
Offers guidance and counseling on admissions requirements and procedures, as well as a number of special programs to help students with their academic, vocational, and career planning goals. In addition, the Center offers services such as tutoring, specialized equipment, test proctoring, among many other accommodations for students who are eligible.

3106 **Santa Rosa Junior College**
Adapted Physical Education
1501 Mendocino Ave
Santa Rosa, CA 95401-4395   707-527-4011
                                   Fax: 707-527-4967
                                   www.santarosa.edu
                                   disabilityinfo@santarosa.edu
Frank Chong, Ed.D, President
DON EDGAR,, Vice President
Robert F Agrella, Coordinator
Offers a variety of regular classes each semester for people
with disabilities.

3107 **Springall Academy**
Springall Program
6460 Boulder Lake Ave
San Diego, CA 92119-3142   619-460-5090
                                  Fax: 619-490-5091
                                  www.springall.org
                                  baker@springall.org
Arlene Baker, Executive Director
Heather Dierolf, School Director
Lanae Aquilera, Associate Director
Offers a variety of services to students with disabilities in-
cluding note takers, extended testing time, counseling ser-
vices, and special accommodations. The academy is a
nonprofit school for learning and behaviorally challenged
students.

3108 **Stanbridge Academy**
515 E Poplar Ave
San Mateo, CA 94401-1715   650-375-5860
                                  Fax: 650-375-5861
                                  www.stanbridgeacademy.org
                                  mainoffice@stanbridgeacademy.org
Jean-Louis Casabonne, Chairman
Linda Waissar, Vice Chairman
Pam Ehrlich, Secretary
A private, non-profit school for students with mild to moder-
ate learning differences, primary grades through high
school.

3109 **Stellar Academy for Dyslexics**
38325 Cedar Blvd
Newark, CA 94560-4801   510-797-2227
                               Fax: 510-797-2207
                               www.stellaracademy.org
                               stellaracademy@aol.com
Beth Mattsson-Boze, Director
Bonny Schleicher, Office Manager
Marlene Castillo, Office Administrator
To serve the needs of children with dyslexia using the
Slingerlandr approach.

3110 **Sterne School**
2690 Jackson Street
San Francisco, CA 94115-1123   415-922-6081
                                      Fax: 415-922-1598
                                      www.sterneschool.org
                                      jmcclave@sterneschool.org
Greg Hylton, SVP/Managing Director
Lee Schweichler, Managing Partner
Pascal Rigo, CEO/Owner
A private school serving students in 6-12 grade who have
specific learning disabilities.

3111 **Summit View School**
6455 Coldwater Canyon Ave
Valley Glen, CA 91606   818-623-6300
                               Fax: 818-623-6390
                               www.summitview.org
                               nnrosenfelt@thehelpgroup.org
Nancy Rosenfelt, Director
Keri Borzello, Head of School
Anne Studer, Coordinator
Serving students with specific learning disabilities.

3112 **Summit View School: Los Angeles**
12101 W Washington Blvd
Los Angeles, CA 90066   310-751-1100
                               Fax: 310-397-4417
                               www.summitview.org
                               nnrosenfelt@thehelpgroup.org
Nancy Rosenfelt, Director
Keri Borzello, Head of School
Anne Studer, Coordinator
Serving students with specific learning disabilities.

3113 **Tobinworld School: Glendale**
920 E Broadway
Glendale, CA 91205-1204   818-247-7474
                                 Fax: 818-247-6516
                                 www.tobinworld.org
                                 judyw@tobinworld.org
Charles Conrad, Principal
A non-profit school for children and young adults with behavior problems. Typically students have been classified as
severely emotionally disabled, autistic or developmentally
disabled.

3114 **Turning Point School**
8780 National Blvd
Culver City, CA 90232   310-841-2505
                               Fax: 310-841-5420
                               www.turningpointschool.com
                               info@turningpointschool.org
Nancy Von Wald, Director
Deborah Richman, Head of the School
A private, non profit school providing education for those
with specific learning disabilities, Dyslexia.

3115 **University of California: Irvine**
Office for Disability Services
Building 313
100 Disability Services
Irvine, CA 92697-5130   949-824-7494
                               Fax: 949-824-3083
                               TDD: 949-824-6272
                               www.disability.uci.edu
                               dsc@uci.edu
Jan Serrantino EdD, Director
Lori Palmerton, Assistant Director
David Andrade, Senior Disability Specialist
Our mission is to provide effective and reasonable academic
accommodations and related disability services to UCI students, Extension and Summer Session students, and other
program participants. Consults with and educates faculty
about reasonable academic accommodations. Strives to improve access to UCI programs, activities, and facilities for
students with disabilities. Advises and educates academic
and administrative departments about access issues to
programs or facilities.

3116 **University of Redlands**
1200 E Colton Ave
PO Box 3080
Redlands, CA 92373-0999   909-793-2121
                                 Fax: 909-793-2029
                                 www.redlands.edu
                                 amy.wilms@redlands.edu
Amy Wilms ller, Asst Dean of Academics
Bradley N. Adams, Board Member
Jamison J. Ashby, Board Member
Small, private 4-year, residential, liberal arts university.

3117 **Valley Oaks School: Turlock**
Fountain Court Plaza 1001 Tower Way
Suite 250
Bakersfield, CA 93309   661-323-1233
                               Fax: 661-323-8090
                               www.aspiranet.org
Vernon McFarland Brown, Chief Executive Officer
John Reiber, Chief Financial Officer
Holly Thauwald, Director of Human Resources

Focuses on specific learning techniques designed for students with learning disabilities and/or emotional disturbance.

3118 Ventura College
Mainstream Computer Program
4667 Telegraph Rd
Ventura, CA 93003-3899 805-289-6000
Fax: 805-648-8947
www.venturacollege.edu

Robin Calote, Coordinator
Implemented assistive technology for students with disabilities through the Mainstream Computer Program.

3119 Westmark School
After School Learning Center
5461 Louise Ave
Encino, CA 91316-2540 818-986-5045
Fax: 818-986-2605
www.westmarkschool.org
dseaman@westmarkschool.org

Rae Sanchini Tobey, Chair
Chip Robertson, Vice Chair
Andrea Mack, Secretary
Provides a caring environment where motivated students with learning differences discover their unique paths to personal and academic excellence in preparation for a successful college experience.

3120 Westview School
12101 W. Washignton Blvd.
Los Angeles, CA 90066 310-478-5544
Fax: 310-397-4417
www.westviewschool.com
info@westviewschool.com

Jackie Strumwasser MA, Executive Director
A private, non-profit day school in Los Angeles for students with learning, attentional and/or mild emotional concerns in grades six through twelve.

Colorado

3121 Denver Academy
4400 E Iliff Ave
Denver, CO 80222-6019 303-777-5870
Fax: 303-777-5893
www.denveracademy.org
info@denveracademy.org

Ed Callahan, President
Nicky Gittelman, Vice President
Lisa Patterson, Secretary
The only co-ed 1st-12th grade independent school in the Denver-metro area dedicated to teaching students with learning differences and unique learning profiles.

3122 Havern School
4000 S Wadsworth Blvd
Littleton, CO 80123-1308 303-986-4587
Fax: 303-986-0590
www.haverncenter.org

Cathy Pasquariello, Executive Director
Christoph P Koupal, Chairman
Cathy Pasquariello, Head of School
Provides a specialized education program for elementary and middle school students with learning disabilities.

3123 Lamar Community College
2401 South Main Street
Lamar, CO 81052-3999 719-336-2248
800-968-6920
Fax: 719-336-5626
www.lamarcc.edu
admissions@lamarcc.edu

John Marrin, President
Angela Woodward, Director Admissions
Becky Young, Special Populations Coordinator

Offers a variety of services to students with disabilities including notetakers, extended testing time, counseling services, and special accommodations.

3124 Regis University
Disability Services
3333 Regis Blvd
Denver, CO 80221-1099 303-458-4100
800-388-2366
Fax: 303-964-5498
TTY: 800-388-266
www.regis.edu
mbwillia@regis.edu

Michael J Sheeran, Director
Father JohnP Fitzgibbons, President
A four-year private university with 110 students recieving disability services out of 1,600.

3125 University of Colorado: Boulder
Academic Resource Team (ART)
107 CU-Boulder
Boulder, CO 80309-0107 303-492-8671
Fax: 303-492-5601
TDD: 303-492-8671
TTY: 303-492-6106
http://disabilityservices.colorado.edu
dsinfo@colorado.edu

John Meister, Director
Carla Hoskins, Assistant Director
Pramila Patel, Program Manager
Provides a variety of services to individuals with nonvisible disabilities, including individualized strategy sessions with a disability specialist, an assistive technology lab, and a career program for students with disabilities. Disability specialists also assist with obtaining reasonable accommodations if documentation meets disability services requirements and supports the need for them.

3126 University of Colorado: Denver
Autism and Developmental Disabilities Clinic
13121 E 17th Ave
C234
Aurora, CO 80045-2535 303-724-5266
Fax: 303-724-7664
www.ucdenver.edu
bev.murdock@uchsc.edu

Cordelia Robinson, Director
The Autism and Developmental Disorders Clinic has provided a fall range of outpatient clinical services to individuals with autism spectrum disorders or other development disorders, and their families. Services are organized around consumer and family goals, Clinical activities available to clients include disciplinary and interdisciplinary evaluations for purposes of diagnostic clarification and for provision of recommendations for treatment.

3127 University of Denver
Learning Effectiveness Program
2199 S. University Blvd.
Denver, CO 80208 303-871-4333
Fax: 303-871-3939
www.du.edu
tmay@du.edu

Ted May, Director
Gregg Kvistad, Interim Chancellor
Peg Bradley-Doppes, Vice Chancellor
A fee for service program offering comprehensive, individualized services to University of Denver Students with learning disabilities and or ADHD. The LEP is part of a larger organization called University Disability Services.

Connecticut

3128 Ben Bronz Academy
Learning Incentive
141 North Main Street
P.O. Box 370065
West Hartford, CT 06107-1264   860-236-5807
Fax: 860-233-9945
www.benbronzacademy.org
tli@tli.com

Aileen Stan-Spence, Director
Ben Bronz Acadamy is a day school for bright disabled students. Guides 60 students through an intensive school day that includes writing, mathematics, literature, science and social studies. Oral language is developed and stressed in all classes.

3129 Connecticut College
Office of Disability Services
270 Mohegan Ave
New London, CT 06320-4150   860-447-1911
Fax: 860-439-5065
www.conncoll.edu
slduq@conncoll.edu

Leo Higdon, Director
Lee Coffin, Admissions Director
Offers a variety of services to students with disabilities including notetakers, extended testing time, counseling services, and special accommodations.

3130 Eagle Hill School
45 Glenville Rd
Greenwich, CT 06831-5392   203-622-9240
Fax: 203-622-0914
www.eaglehillschool.org
info411@eaglehill.com

Marjorie E. Castro, Head of School
Jeremy Henderson, Board Chair
A language based remedial program committed to educating children with learning disabilities.

3131 Forman School
12 Norfolk Rd
P.O. Box 80
Litchfield, CT 06759-2537   860-567-8712
Fax: 860-567-8317
www.formanschool.org
admissions@formanschool.org

Louise Hoppe Finnerty, President
Thomas G. Sorell, Vice-President
John Forman, Founder
Forman offers students with learning differences the opportunity to achieve academic excellence in a traditional college preparatory setting. A coeducational boarding school of 180 students, we maintain a 3:1 student:teacher ratio. Daily remedial instruction balanced with course offerings rich in content provide each student with a flexible program that is tailored to his or her unique learning style and needs.

3132 Marvelwood
Marvelwood School
476 Skiff Mountain Rd
PO Box 3001
Kent, CT 06757-3001   860-927-0047
800-440-9107
Fax: 860-927-0021
www.marvelwood.org
summer@marvelwood.org

Craig Ough, Director
Arthur F. Goodearl, Jr., Head of School
A coeducational boarding and day school enrolling 150 students in grades 9-12. Provides an environment in which young people of varying abilities and learning needs can prepare for success in college and in life. In a nurturing, structured community, students who have not thrived academically in traditional settings are guided and motivated to reach and exceed their personal potential.

3133 Mitchell College
Learning Resource Center
437 Pequot Avenue
New London, CT 06320-4498   860-701-5000
800-443-2811
Fax: 860-701-5090
www.mitchell.edu
love_p@mitchell.edu

Elizabeth Ivey, Chair
Daniel Spring, Vice Chair
Janet Steinmayer, President
Small private college with comprehensive subject program for student with Learning Disabilities and/or ADHD.

3134 St. Joseph College
Academic Resource Center
60 College Avenue
West Hartford, CT 06117-2791   860-231-5399
866-442-8752
Fax: 860-232-4757
www.sjc.edu
judyarzt@sjc.edu

Judy Arzt, Director
Pamela Trotman Reid, Ph.D, President
Offers a variety of services to students with disabilities including notetakers, extended testing time, counseling services, and special accommodations.

3135 The Glenholme School Devereux Connecticut
81 Sabbaday Lane
Washington, CT 06793   860-868-7377
Fax: 860-868-7413
www.theglenholmeschool.org
admissions@theglenholmeschool.org

Julie Smallwood, Director of External Affairs
David Dunleavy, Director of Admissions
Denise Watson, Director of Public Relations
The Glenholme School is a therapeutic boarding school for students, ages 10-21, with high-functioning autism spectrum disorders, ADHD, OCD, Tourette's, depression, anxiety and various learning differences. Our comprehensive educational environment, which includes a rigorous curriculum and a rich selection of extracurricular activities, supports development in academic and social competence for students.

3136 University of Hartford
Learning Plus Program
200 Bloomfield Ave
West Hartford, CT 06117-1599   860-768-4100
Fax: 860-768-4183
www.hartford.edu
uofhart@hartford.edu

Lynne Golden, Director
Walter Harrison, President
Arosha Jayawickrema, Vice President for Finance
Provides academic support to students with specific learning disabilities and/or attention deficit disorder. The support consists of one 45 minute appointment a week with an adult Learning Plus specialist presenting applicable learning strategies.

3137 Vocational and Life Skills Center
1356 Old Clinton Rd
Westbrook, CT 06498-1858   860-399-8080
Fax: 860-399-3103
www.vistavocational.org
hbosch@vistavocational.org

Robert B. Ostroff, M.D, President
Barbara Segen Gould, Vice President & Treasurer
Helen K. Bosch, B.S., M.S, Executive Director
Building self-esteem and confidence in the lives of adults with disabilities through work, independence and friendship. Offers a post-secondary program for young adults with learning disabilities providing individualized training and support in career development, independent living skills, social skills development and community involvement.

3138 Woodhall School
58 Harrison Lane
PO Box 550
Bethlehem, CT 06751-550 203-266-7788
Fax: 203-266-5896
www.woodhallschool.org
woodhallschool@woodhallschool.org
Patricia R. Burns, President
Sharon L. Poole, Vice-President
Andrew Hess, Secretary /Treasurer
Offers an opportunity to experience success for young men of above average intellectual ability in grades 9 -12 who have not achieved at a level commensurate with their ability in traditional school programs.

Delaware

3139 Centreville School
6201 Kennett Pike
Centreville, DE 19807-1017 302-571-0230
Fax: 302-571-0270
www.centrevilleschool.org
centreville@centrevilleschool.org
Denise Orenstein, Head of School
Provides an educational program that produces academic success and social development for children with learning disabilities.

District of Columbia

3140 American University
Learning Services Program, Academic Support Center
4400 Massachusetts Ave NW
Washington, DC 20016-8200 202-885-3360
Fax: 202-885-1042
www.american.edu/asc
asc@american.edu
Nancy Sydnor-Greenberg, Coordinator
Focuses on assisting students with their transition from high school to college during their freshman year. It is a small, mainstream program offering weekly individual meetings with the coordinator of the Learning Services Program throughout the student's first year. For additional information, see www.american.edu/asc.

3141 Catholic University of America
Disability Support Services
620 Michigan Ave
Washington, DC 20064 202-319-5000
Fax: 202-319-5126
TTY: 202-319-5211
http://dss.cua.edu
cua-disabilityservices@cua.edu
Emily Lucio, Director
Ian Kunkes, Learning Disability Coordinator
Julia Aldrich, Administrative Assistant
Four-year college that has support services for students with learning disabilities.

3142 Georgetown University
Disability Support Services/Learning Services
37th & O St NW
Washington, DC 20057 202-687-0100
Fax: 202-687-8992
www.georgetown.edu
help@georgetown.edu
Paul Tagliabue, Chair
William R. Berkley, Vice Chair
John J. DeGioia, Ph.D., President
A four-year private university with a total enrollment of 6,418.

3143 Saint Coletta: Greater Washington
1901 Independence Ave SE
Washington, DC 20003-1733 202-350-8680
Fax: 202-350-8699
TTY: 202-350-8695
www.stcoletta.org
Sharon B Raimo, Executive Director
Carl Nelson, Treasurer
Joseph Watkins, Board Member
Is a non-sectarian, non-profit organization that operates school and adult day programs for children and adults with mental retardation and autism.

3144 The Lab School of Washington
4759 Reservoir Rd NW
Washington, DC 20007-1921 202-965-6600
TTY: 202-350-8695
www.labschool.org
katherine.schantz@labschool.org
Katherine Schantz, Head Of School
Diana Meltzer, Associate Head
Bob Lane, Director of Admissions
An innovative, rigorous, arts-based program for intelligent students with moderate to severe learning disabilities.

Florida

3145 Barry University
Center for Advanced Learning
11300 NE 2nd Ave
Miami Shores, FL 33161-6695 305-899-3000
800-756-6000
Fax: 305-899-3679
www.barry.edu
webmaster@barry.edu
Linda Bevilacqua, President
William J. Heffernan, Chairperson
Christopher Gruchacz, Vice President
A comprehensive support program for students with learning disabilities and attention deficit disorders.

3146 Beacon College
105 E Main St
Leesburg, FL 34748-5162 352-787-9731
855-220-5374
Fax: 800-889-2319
www.beaconcollege.edu
admissions@beaconcollege.edu
Brenda Meli, Director of Admisssions
Stephanie Knight, Asst. Director of Admissions
Andrew Marvin, Admissions Counselor
Offer academic degree programs to students with learning disabilities.

3147 Center Academy
341 North Orlando Avenue
Maitland, FL 32751 407-772-8727
Fax: 407-772-8747
www.centeracademy.com
infomait@centeracademy.com
Mack R. Hicks, Founder and Chairman
Andrew P. Hicks, CEO, Clinical Director
Eric V. Larson, President, COO
Private school, college prep, AD/HD, SLD, small classes, SACS & NIPSA accredited.

3148 DePaul School for Dyslexia
2747 Sunset Point Rd
Clearwater, FL 33759-1504 727-796-7679
Fax: 727-796-7927
www.thedepaulschool.org
admin@thedepaulschool.org
Vicki Howell, Head of School
Provides an alternative educational experience for students K-8th grade with dyslexia, ADHD, ADD and other learning disabilities and attention deficits.

3149 Florida Community College: Jacksonville
Independent Living for Adult Blind
601 State St W
Jacksonville, FL 32202-4774   904-633-8498
                                     Fax: 904-633-5979
                                     www.fscj.edu

Carol Spadling, President
Carolyn Krall, LD Specialist
An instructional program for adults who have vision loss to a
degree that they experience some difficulty in their daily activities. Through guidance and specialized training offered
through the ILAB program, individuals learn necessary
skills for work and independence in their home and
community.

**3150 Jericho School for Children with Autism and Other De-
velopmental Delays**
1351 Sprinkle Dr
Jacksonville, FL 32211-5448   904-744-5110
                                     Fax: 904-744-3443
                                     www.thejerichoschool.org
                                     jerichoschool@yahoo.com
Angelo Martinez, Executive Director
Provides comprehensive, individualized science-based education not otherwise available in the community. Believes
that those children with autism and other developmental delays deserve the opportunity to reach their full potential.

3151 Lynn University
Institute for Achievement and Learning
3601 N Military Trl
Boca Raton, FL 33431-5598   561-237-7000
                                    800-888-5966
                                    www.lynn.edu
                                    dkendrick@lynn.edu
Kevin Ross, President
Christine E. Lynn, Chairman
Stephen F. Snyder, Vice Chairman
Provides a series of support services to students with learn-
ing differences through a series of programs designed to help
the students to succeed in their academic endeavors.

3152 Morning Star School
4661 80th Ave
Pinellas Park, FL 33781-2496   727-544-6036
                                    Fax: 727-546-9058
                                    www.morningstarschool.org
                                    sue.conza@morningstarschool.org
Mary Lou Giacobbe, Principal
Students with special educational requirements need more
care and attention than is offered in a traditional school
setting.

3153 PACE-Brantley Hall School
3221 Sand Lake Rd
Longwood, FL 32779-5850   407-869-8882
                                    Fax: 407-869-8717
                                    www.mypbhs.org
                                    info@pacebrantley.org
Richard Dunn, D.D.S, Chairman
Kathy Ilkka, Secretary
Pam Ohab, Treasurer
Specializes in teaching learning disabled children. Children
that have been diagnosed with ADD, ADHD, and Dyslexia
attend PACE.

3154 Paladin Academy
1250 Dykes Rd
Sunrise, FL 33326-1901   954-920-2008
                                    Fax: 954-921-4657
Beth Cleary, Manager

3155 Tampa Bay Academy
Educational Program
12012 Boyette Rd
Riverview, FL 33569-5631   813-445-3125
                                    800-678-3838
                                    Fax: 813-671-3145
                                    www.tampabay-academy.com
                                    info@tampa.yfcs.com
Ed Hoefle, Executive Director
John Tracy, Founder
The curriculum is designed with academic goals that encom-
pass both special and vocational education. Individual Edu-
cational Plans are developed to address the goals and
learning styles of students.

3156 Tampa Day School
12606 Henderson Rd
Tampa, FL 33625-6548   813-269-2100
                                    Fax: 813-490-2554
                                    www.tampadayschool.com
Lois Delaney, Head of School
Patricia Soloski, Learning Solutions Director
Pat Missak, Business Manager
To provide a learning environment that promotes that individual feeling of success for each child, and to find the
unique key that opens the door to optimize his/her learning
potential. The purpose of our school is to meet each child's
needs.

3157 The Vanguard School
22000 Hwy 27
Lake Wales, FL 33859-6858   863-676-6091
                                    Fax: 863-676-8297
                                    www.vanguardschool.org
                                    info@vanguardschool.org
Cathy Wooley-Brown, President
Derri Park, Principal
Maria Hewitt, Business Manager
The Vanguard School is a fully accredited (SCAS and FCIS)
coeducational boarding school and day school educating
students in grades 5-12 with learning differences such as at-
tention issues, challenging reading disorder, dyslexia, and
Asperger's Syndrome.

3158 Victory School
PO Box 630266
Miami, FL 33163-0266   305-466-1142
                                    Fax: 305-466-1143
                                    www.thevictoryschool.org
                                    office@thevictoryschool.org
Pat Rosen, Executive Director
Richard Shan, Chairman
A Florida, non-secretarian, not-for-profit corporation that
provides children with autism and smiliar disorders compre-
hensive individualized treatment with a 1:1 student/teacher
ratio, in a classroom setting that is unique in Southeast
Florida.

3159 Woodland Hall Academy
Dyslexia Research Institute
5246 Centerville Rd
Tallahassee, FL 32309-2893   850-893-2216
                                    Fax: 850-893-2440
                                    www.woodlandhallacademy.org
                                    dri@talstar.com
Pat Hardman, Founder, CEO
Amber Mitchell, Principal
Robyn Rennick, Program Director
Designed to remediate and prevent the learning and behavior
problems associated with the dyslexic and ADD/ADHD
student.

Georgia

3160 Andrew College
FOCUS Program
501 College St
Cuthbert, GA 39840-5599

229-732-5908
800-664-9250
Fax: 229-732-5905
www.andrewcollege.edu
development@andrewcollege.edu

David Seyle, President
George Flowers, Chair
Andy Brubaker, VP Administration
The FOCUS program offers an intensive level of academic support designed for and limited to documented learning disabilities or attention deficit disorder. While FOCUS supplements and complements the tutorial and advising to all students, the program also provides an additional level of professional assistance and mentoring. Those accepted into FOCUS are charged regular tuition andd fees, plus a FOCUS laboratory fee.

3161 Brandon Hall School
1701 Brandon Hall Dr
Atlanta, GA 30350-3799

770-394-8177
Fax: 770-804-8821
www.brandonhall.org
jsingleton@brandonhall.org

Dr John L Singleton, President/Headmaster
Johnny Graham, Associate Head
Merridee Ann Michelsen, Assistant Head
College preparatory, co-ed day and boys' boarding school for students in grades 4-12. Designed for academic under-achievers and students with minor learning disabilities, attention deficit disorders and dyslexia.

3162 Cottage School
700 Grimes Bridge Rd
Roswell, GA 30075-4615

770-641-8688
Fax: 770-641-9026
www.cottageschool.org
tcs@cottageschool.org

Jacque Digieso, Executive Director
Stephanie Johnson, Executive Assistant
Tracy Ballot, Director of Advancement
Building a sense of self for students with special learning needs through academic and experiential programming, The Cottage School prepares individuals for fulfillment of their true potential as confident, productive, and independent adults.

3163 Fort Valley State University
Differently Abled Services Center
1005 State University Dr
Fort Valley, GA 31030-3298

478-827-3878
Fax: 478-825-6266
www.fvsu.edu
smitht0@fvsu.edu

Larry E Rivers, Director
Ivelaw Lloyd Griffith, President
Our mission is to increase retention for students with learning disorders by ensuring equal treatment, opportunity, and access for persons with impairments and/or disorders.

3164 Gables Academy
811 Gordon St
Stone Mountain, GA 30083-3533

770-465-7500
877-465-7500
Fax: 770-465-7700
www.gablesacademy.com
info@gablesacademy.com

James Meffen, Headmaster
A fully accredited non-profit learning center providing a full spectrum of educational services for students in the special needs population ages 9-18.

3165 Georgia State University
Margaret A Staton Office of Disability Services
P.O. Box 3965
Atlanta, GA 30302-3965

404-413-2000
Fax: 404-413-1563
www.gsu.edu
disrep@langate.gsu.edu

Mark P. Becker, President
Risa Palm, SVP Academic Affairs and Provost
Works with any student who has a disability to ensure meaningful access to the goods and services offered by GSU. To achieve this goal, academic accommodations are often made on behalf of the student.

3166 Howard School
1192 Foster St NW
Atlanta, GA 30318-4329

404-377-7436
Fax: 404-377-0884
www.howardschool.org
info@howardschool.org

Marifred Cilella, Head of School
Anne Beisel, Admissions Director
Educates students with language learning disabilitiesand learning differences. Instruction is personalized to complement individual learning styles, to address student needs and to help each student understand his or her learning process. The curriculum focuses on depth of understanding in order to make learning meaningful and therefore, maximize educational success.

3167 Mill Springs Academy
13660 New Providence Rd
Alpharetta, GA 30004-3413

770-360-1336
Fax: 770-360-1341
www.millsprings.org
rmoore@millsprings.org

Robert Moore, President
Angel Murr, Chairperson
Bruce Bowers, Board Member
Committed to a comprehensive, holistic program design that is multifaceted to meet the needs of the 'total child'.

3168 Schenck School
282 Mount Paran Rd NW
Atlanta, GA 30327-4698

404-252-2591
Fax: 404-252-7615
www.schenck.org
office@schenck.org

Gena Calloway, Head of School
Janet Brown, Associate Head
Vicki Ahnrud, Administration and Staff
Offers a unique learning environment for children with dyslexia, as well as several auxiliary programs

3169 St. Francis School
9375 Willeo Rd
Roswell, GA 30075-4743

770-641-8257
Fax: 770-641-0283
www.saintfrancisschools.com

Drew Buccellato, Headmaster
Linda Crawford, Associate Headmaster
Jay Wilson, Elementary Receptionist
Providing an educational program of the highest quality that can meet the needs of students with diverse abilities who would profit from a smaller teacher-pupil ratio than is available in most public or private schools.

3170 Toccoa Falls College
107 Kincaid Dr.
Toccoa Falls, GA 30598-13

706-886-6831
888-785-5624
Fax: 706-886-0210
www.tfc.edu
wgardner@tfc.edu

Robert M. Myers, President
Ken Gassiot, VP Student Affairs
Dan Griffin, VP Enrollment

Four-year college that provides services to the learning disabled.

3171 Wardlaw School
Atlanta Speech School
3160 Northside Pkwy NW
Atlanta, GA 30327-1598   404-233-5332
                                Fax: 404-266-2175
                                www.atlantaspeechschool.org

Russ Richards, Chairman
Glenn D. Warren, Vice Chairman
Kathryn B. Miller, Secretary
For children ages 5 to 12 years old with average to very superior intelligence and mild to moderate language-based learning disabilities. The types of learning disabilities that are served include written language disorders, mathematical disabilities, ADD, dyslexia, and difficulty understanding and/or using spoken language.

Hawaii

3172 University of Hawaii: Manoa
Center on Disability Services
1776 University Ave
Honolulu, HI 96822-2447   808-956-9199
                                Fax: 808-956-7878
                                www.cds.hawaii.edu
                                stodden@hawaii.edu

Robert Stodden, Director
Dedicated to supporting the quality of life, inclusion, and empowerment of all persons with disabilities and their families through partnerships in training, service, evaluation, research, dissemination, and technical assistance. Nurtures, sustains, and expands promising practices for people with disabilities.

Idaho

3173 Community High School
PO Box 2118
Sunvalley, ID 83353   208-622-3955
                                Fax: 208-622-3962
                                www.communityschool.org
                                info@communityschool.org

Jay Hagenbuch, Chair
Guy Cherp, Treasurer
Ellen S. Gillespie, Secretary
Complete college prep HS program for LD/ADD adolescent grades 9-12.

3174 University of Idaho
Center on Disabilities and Human Development
875 Perimeter Drive MS 4061
Moscow, ID 83844-4061   208-885-6000
                                800-393-7290
                                Fax: 208-885-6145
                                TTY: 800-432-8324
                                www.idahocdhd.org
                                idahocdhd@uidaho.edu

Julie Fodor, Director
Currently operates a variety of independent grant programs and carries out training, services, technical assistance, research and dissemination activities across the state and nation.

Illinois

3175 Acacia Academy
6425 Willow Springs Rd
La Grange Highlands, IL 60525-4468   708-579-9040
                                        Fax: 708-579-5872
                                        www.acaciaacademy.com
                                        info@acaciaacademy.com

Kathryn Fouks, Principal
Eileen Petzold, Asst. Principal
Jim Shoemaker-Saif, Head of High School
A school for grades K-12 for children with learning disabilities. NCA accredited and approved for out of district students in special education in the state of Illinois.

3176 Brehm Preparatory School
950 S. Brehm Lane
Carbondale, IL 62901-3603   618-457-0371
                                Fax: 618-529-1248
                                www.brehm.org
                                admissionsinfo@brehm.org

Stacy Brehm Tate, President
Gerry Schermerhorn, Ph.D., Vice-President
Rita Dodd, Secretary
A coeducational boarding school for students with learning differences. Services are provided for students in grades 6-12. A post-secondary program, OPTIONS, is also available.

3177 College of Dupage
Vocational Skills Program
425 Fawell Blvd
Glen Ellyn, IL 60137-6599   630-942-2800
                                Fax: 630-942-2800
                                TDD: 630-858-9692
                                www.cod.edu
                                mullan@cdnet.cod.edu

Erin Birt, Chairman
Kathy Hamilton, Vice Chairman
Allison O'Donnell, Secretary
Offers courses to students challenged with mild to moderate cognitive impairment. The courses are developmental-level, non-transferable credit courses designed to develop vocational skills that can lead to competitive, entry-level employment and enhance everyday living skills.

3178 Cove School
350 Lee Rd
Northbrook, IL 60062-1521   847-562-2100
                                Fax: 847-562-2112
                                www.coveschool.org
                                ssover@coveschool.org

Sally Sover, Executive Director
John Stieper, Director of Education
Robin S. Johnstone, Clinical Director
For children and young adults in grades K-12 who are coping with a wide range of learning disabilities. The Cove School creates an exceptional environment for the children where they develop the emotional and social skills needed to reach their fullest potential.

3179 DePaul University
PLuS Program
1 E. Jackson Blvd.
Chicago, IL 60604   312-362-8000
                                www.depaul.edu

Patricia O'Donoghue, Interim President
Robert L. Kozoman, CPA, Executive Vice President
Edward R. Udovic, Secretary
PLuS is a comprehensive program designed to assist students with specific learning disabilities and/or attention deficit disorders in experiencing academic success at DePaul University. Please visit PLuS' website for a description of services and application forms.

3180 Hamel Elementary School
P.O Box 250
Edwardsville, IL 62025   618-656-1182
                                Fax: 618-692-7423
                                www.ecusd7.org
                                bhutton@ecusd7.org

Jill Bertels, President
Brad Hewitt, Board Member
Monica Laurent, Board Member
Offer programs for students with learning disabilities, ADD and/or emotional difficulties.

3181 Kaskaskia College
27210 College Rd
Centralia, IL 62801-7878
618-545-3000
800-642-0859
Fax: 618-545-3029
www.kaskaskia.edu
cquick@kaskaskia.edu
James Underwood, President's Office
Cathy Quick, Executive Assistant to President
Cheryl Boehne, Admissions/Records
Offers a variety of services to students with disabilities including note takers, extended testing time, counseling services, and special accommodations.

3182 Lewis and Clark Community College
College Life Program
5800 Godfrey Rd
Godfrey, IL 62035-2466
618-466-7000
Fax: 618-466-4044
TTY: 618-466-4100
www.lc.cc.il.us
khaberer@lc.edu
Robert Watson, Chairman
Brenda Walker McCain, Vice Chairman
Walter S. Ahlemeyer, Secretary
For those students with disabilities who have had few inclusive experiences in high school, the College for Life Program provides courses that continue the educational experience and also provides social growth opportunities on a college campus.

3183 Roosevelt University
Learning and Support Services Program
430 S Michigan Ave
Chicago, IL 60605-1394
312-341-3500
Fax: 312-341-2003
www.roosevelt.edu
Charles R. Middleton, President
Brett Batterson, Executive Director
Douglas Knerr, Executive Vice President
The Disabled Student Services office serves all students with special needs. The use of services is voluntary and confidential. This office is a resource for students and faculty. The goal of this office is to ensure educational opportunity for all students with special needs by providing access to full participation in all aspects of campus life and increase awareness of disability issues on campus.

3184 Saint Xavier University
Student Success Program
3700 W 103rd St
Chicago, IL 60655-3105
773-298-3000
Fax: 773-779-9061
www.sxu.edu
fuller@sxu.edu
Josiah Fuller, Director
Christine M. Wiseman, J.D., President
Offers a variety of services to students with disabilities including notetakers, extended testing time, counseling services, and special accommodations.

3185 Southern Illinois University: Carbondale
Clinical Center Achieve Program
1263 Lincoln Drive
Carbondale, IL 62901-6899
618-453-2121
Fax: 618-453-6126
www.siu.edu
lukidawg@siu.edu
Sally DeDecker, Coordinator
The Achieve Program is a comprehensive academic support service for students with LD and/or ADHD. Students must apply to both Achieve and the University.

3186 University of Illinois: Chicago
Institute on Disability and Human Development
1640 W Roosevelt Rd
Chicago, IL 60608-1316
312-413-1647
Fax: 312-413-1630
TTY: 361-241-0453
www.uic.edu
idhd@uic.edu
Tamar Heller, Director
James Schmidt, Director of Athletics
Paula Allen-Meares, Chancellor
Dedicated to promoting the independence, productivity and inclusion of people with disabilities into all aspects of society.

3187 University of Illinois: Urbana
Disability Resources and Educational Services
1207 S Oak St
Champaign, IL 61820-6901
217-333-1970
Fax: 217-244-0014
TDD: 217-333-4603
www.disability.illinois.edu
disability@illinois.edu
Karen Wold, Learning Disabilities Specialist
Mylinda Granger, Coordinator
Marlene Hedrick, Clerk
Provides comprehensive disability services to University of Illinois students with disabilities, including disabilities.

Indiana

3188 Ball State University
Disabled Student Development
2000 W University Ave
Muncie, IN 47306
765-289-1241
800-382-8540
Fax: 765-285-4003
http://cms.bsu.edu
Rick Hall, Chair
Frank Hancock, Vice Chair
Thomas C. Bracken, Secretary
Offers a variety of services to students with disabilities including note takers, extended testing time, counseling services, and special accommodations.

3189 Cathedral High School
5225 E 56th St
Indianapolis, IN 46226-1487
317-542-1481
Fax: 317-543-5050
www.cathedral-irish.org
smatteson@cathedral-irish.org
Dave Worland, President
Provides, to a diverse group of students, opportunities for spiritual, intellectual, social, emotional and physical growth through service and academic excellence.

3190 Indiana Wesleyan University
TRIO Scholars Program
4201 S Washington St
Marion, IN 46953-4974
866-468-6498
Fax: 765-677-2499
www.indwes.edu
aldersgatecenter@indwes.edu
Henry L Smith, Coordinator
David Wright, President
To help students realize their full potential in relation to their academic pursuits at Indiana Wesleyan University. Benefits to TRIO Scholars include academic and cultural enrichment, disability services, mentoring, personal counseling, tutorial support, and the opportunity to apply for grant aid.

3191 Ivy Tech Community College
3501 N 1st Ave
Evansville, IN 47710-3398   812-426-2865
                                              888-489-5463
                                   Fax: 812-429-0591
                                   TDD: 812-429-9803
                                   www.ivytech.edu
                                   Evansville-finaid@ivytech.edu
Thomas J. Snyder, President
Jeff Terp, Executive Vice President, COO
Pat Bauer, VP External Partnerships
Provides reasonable and effective accommodations to qualified students with learning disabilities.

3192 Manchester College
Academic Development & Programming for Transition
604 E College Ave
North Manchester, IN 46962-1232   260-982-5000
                                   Fax: 260-982-5042
                                   www.manchester.edu
                                   bsoconnell@manchester.edu
Jo Young Switzer, Director
A specially designed academic advising program for students with disabilities.

3193 Pinnacle School
2182 W Industrial Park Dr
Bloomington, IN 47404   812-339-8141
                                   Fax: 812-339-8390
                                   www.pinnacleschool.org
                                   info@pinnacleschool.org
Stephanie Robertson-Powers, President
Ronna Papesh, Secretary and Treasurer
Denise Lessow, Executive Director
Provides an independent, full-time specialized elementary (K-8) curriculum for children with dyslexia and other related specific learning disabilities.

3194 Saint Mary-of-the-Woods College
1 St Mary of Woods Coll
Saint Mary of the Woods, IN 47876-1099 812-535-5151
                                   Fax: 812-535-5169
                                   www.smwc.edu
                                   smwc@smwc.edu
David Behrs, Vice President
Joan Lescinski, President
Offers a variety of services to students with disabilities including note takers, extended testing time, counseling services, and special accommodations.

3195 University of Indianapolis
BUILD Program
1400 E Hanna Ave
Indianapolis, IN 46227-3697   317-788-3368
                                              800-232-8634
                                   Fax: 317-788-6152
                                   www.uindy.edu
                                   mcavanaugh@uindy.edu
Debbie Spinney, Exec Director Student Dev
Connie Dunn, Administrative Assistant
Is a full support program at the University of Indianapolis designed to help the college students with specific learning disability earn an associate or baccalureate degree.

3196 Worthmore Academy
3535 Kessler Boulevard East Dr
Indianapolis, IN 46220-5154   317-251-6516
                                   Fax: 317-251-6516
                                   www.worthmoreacademy.org
Brenda Jackson, Director
A place where children with learning differences may come and receive individualized instruction to help remediate his or her learning differences.

3197 Clinton High School
1401 12th Ave. N.
Clinton, IA 52732-5698   563-243-9600
                                   Fax: 563-243-2415
                                   www.clinton.k12.ia.us
                                   ktharaldson@clintonia.org
Karinne Tharaldson, Principal
Provide services for individuals with special needs to achieve high levels of learning through equitable access to quality education for each student in an environment of mutual respect, trust, enthusiasm and cooperation.

3198 Des Moines Area Community College
2006 S Ankeny Blvd
Ankeny, IA 50023-3993   515-964-6200
                                              800-362-2127
                                   Fax: 515-965-7316
                                   TDD: 964-381-1551
                                   TTY: 515-964-6809
                                   http://go.dmacc.edu/Pages/welcome.aspx
                                   webmaster@dmacc.cc.ia.us
Robert Denson, President
DMACC is committed to providing an accessible environment that supports students with disabilities in reaching their full potential. Support services are available for students with disabilities to ensure equal access to educational opportunities.

3199 Iowa Central Community College
One Triton Circle
Fort Dodge, IA 50501-5739   515-576-7201
                                              800-362-2793
                                   Fax: 515-576-7206
                                   www.iccc.cc.ia.us
                                   lundeen@triton.iccc.cc.ia.us
Mark R. Crimmins, Board Member
Thomas O. Chelesvig, Board Member
Darrell Determann, Board Member
A public two-year college with approximately 50 special needs students out of a total of 3,003.

3200 Iowa Lakes Community College: Emmetsburg
Project Learning
3200 College Dr
Emmetsburg, IA 50536-1055   712-852-3554
                                              800-242-5108
                                   Fax: 712-852-2152
                                   www.iowalakes.edu
                                   info@iowalakes.edu
Tom Brotherton, Executive Dean
Colleen Peltz, Developmental Studies Professor
Developmentally disabled students learn basic independent living skills, which allow them to be integrated into the community. This program is conducted in conjunction with the local work activity center.

3201 Iowa Western Community College: Council Bluffs
Bridges for Learning in Applied Science & Tech
2700 College Rd
Council Bluffs, IA 51503-1057   712-325-3418
                                              800-432-5852
                                   Fax: 712-325-3424
                                   www.iwcc.cc.ia.us
                                   hirwin@iwcc.edu
Dan Kinney, President
Erin Stopak, Administrative Asst to President
Kristin Buscher, Associate Dean
The services are to assist studnts in participating in the vocational/technical training programs at IWCC by providing special education support and instructional services. This provides students with disabilities an opportunity to develop career or occupationally specific skills.

3202   Loras College
Office of Disability Services
1450 Alta Vista St
Dubuque, IA 52001-4399   563-588-7100
                                        Fax: 563-588-7964
                                          www.loras.edu
                                          ods@loras.edu

James Collins, Director
The Enhanced Program is a comprehensive program designed to provide additional support for students with a primary disability of learning disability or attention deficit disorder, however students with other disabilities will be considered. A fee is charged for the Enhanced Program.

3203   North Iowa Area Community College
On Track: Time Management Program
500 College Dr
Mason City, IA 50401-7299   641-423-1264
                                        Fax: 641-423-1711
                                           www.niacc.edu
                                        vancelis@niacc.edu

Debra Derr, Coordinator
Dr. Steven Schulz, President
Our On Track Program is meant for students with disabilities who have realized they need a little extra help keeping track of assignments, due dates, and a busy schedule of activities. Balancing all these demands can be overwhelming, but you don't have to do it alone.

3204   SAVE Program
Iowa Lakes Community College: Emmetsburg
3200 College Dr
Emmetsburg, IA 50536-1055   712-362-2604
                                             800-521-5024
                                        Fax: 712-852-2152
                                        www.iowalakes.edu

Ann Petersen, Director
Provide special education secondary students with an option where they will receive, based on their IEP goals, further education in the areas of life skills training, vocational/employability skills training, and transitional/self advocacy skills training.

3205   Simpson College
Hawley Academic Resource Center
701 N C St
Indianola, IA 50125-1202   515-961-6251
                                             800-362-2454
                                        Fax: 515-961-1363
                                     www.simpson.edu/hawley
                                         little@simpson.edu

John Byrd, Director
Dr. Jay Simmons, President
Simpson College is a private, four-year liberal arts college located south of Des Moines, Iowa. The Hawley Center offers services to students with disabilities including academic accommodations and other support services.

3206   University of Iowa
Realizing Educational and Career Hopes Program
N297 Lindquist Ctr
Iowa City, IA 52242-1529   319-335-5359
                                        Fax: 319-384-2167
                                        TTY: 800-735-2942
                                     www.education.uiowa.edu
                                         reach@uiowa.edu

Nicholas Colangelo, Ph.D., Dean
Specifically designed to meet the needs of young adults with multiple learning and cognitive disabilities.

3207   Wartburg College
100 Wartburg Blvd
Waverly, IA 50677   319-352-8260
                                             800-772-2085
                                        Fax: 319-352-8568
                                          www.wartburg.edu
                                      deb.lovers@wartburg.edu

Darrel Colson, President
Deborah Loers, VP Student Life
Scott Leisinger, VP Advancement
Four year private, residential college

Kansas

3208   Baker University
Learning Resource Center
PO Box 65
Baldwin City, KS 66006-65   785-594-6451
                                             800-955-7747
                                          www.bakeru.edu
                                   marian@harvey.bakeru.edu

Kathy Marian, Director
Paige Illum, Admissions Director
Daniel Lambert, President
A private four-year college with a total of 923 students.

3209   Fort Scott Community College
2108 Horton St
Fort Scott, KS 66701-3141   620-223-2700
                                             800-874-3722
                                         www.fortscott.edu
                                  beckyw@ftscott.cc.ks.us

Robert Nelson, Chair
Dick Hedges, President
Mark McCoy, Vice Chair
A public two-year college with 34 special education students out of a total of 1,928.

3210   Horizon Academy
4901 Reinhardt Drive
Roeland Park, KS 66205   913-789-9443
                                        Fax: 913-789-8180
                                    www.horizon-academy.org
                                  info@horizon-academy.com

Ann Cooling, President
Sharyl Kennedy, Executive Director
Private school for children with learning disabilities. Students learn word decoding skills in reading, oral and written language comprehension and/or expression, math skills, organizational and social skills.

3211   Newman University
3100 W McCormick St
Wichita, KS 67213-2008   316-942-4291
                                        Fax: 316-942-4483
                                         www.newmanu.edu
                                      niedensr@newmanu.edu

Noreen Carrocci, President
Mark Dresselhaus, Vice President
Offers a variety of services to students with disabilities including notetakers, extended testing time, counseling services, and special accommodations.

Kentucky

3212   Brescia University
717 Frederica St
Owensboro, KY 42301-3019   270-685-3131
                                             877-273-7242
                                        Fax: 270-684-2507
                                          www.brescia.edu
                                     chris.houk@brescia.edu

Chris Houk, M.B.A., Executive Director
Christy Rohner, Director of Admissions
Terri Higdon, Assistant Director of Admissions
Provides the following for students with learning disabilities: developmental courses (English, mathematics and study skills); individual tutoring for all areas; and academic and career counseling.

3213 DePaul School
1925 Duker Ave
Louisville, KY 40205-1099
502-459-6131
Fax: 502-458-0827
www.depaulschool.org
dpinfo@depaulschool.org

Tony Kemper, Head of School
Lisa Stepp, Principal
Pam Grayson, Dean of Students
We teach a lot of bright kids who learn differently. And we teach them the way they actually learn.

3214 Eastern Kentucky University
Project SUCCESS
521 Lancaster Ave
Richmond, KY 40475-3102
859-622-2933
Fax: 859-622-6794
www.disabilities.eku.edu
disserv@eku.edu

Teresa L. Belluscio, Director
Crystal Gail Brookshire, Senior Office Associate
Sandra Michelle Douglas, Disabilities Analyst
Offers a comprehensive support program for college students with learning disabilities, attention deficit disorder and other cognitive disorders. Upon admittance, Project SUCCESS develops an individualized program of services which serve to enhance the academic success of each student.

Louisiana

3215 Louisiana College
Program to Assist Student Success
1140 College Dr
PO Box 545
Pineville, LA 71359-0001
318-487-7629
Fax: 318-487-7285
www.lacollege.edu
himel@lacollege.edu

Dr. Joe Aguillard, President
Mr. Randall Hargis, VP Business Affairs, CFO
Dr. Travis Wright, VP Academic Affairs
This highly individualized program for students who have disabilities, provides support services and personal attention to students who may need special academic guidance, tutoring, and/or classroom assistance.

3216 Louisiana State University: Alexandria
8100 Highway 71 S
Alexandria, LA 71302-9119
318-445-3672
888-473-6417
Fax: 318-473-6480
www.lsua.edu

David P Manuel, Director Student Services
Donna Roberts, Administrative Assistant
Robert Cavanaugh, Manager
Offers a variety of services to students with disabilities including extended testing time, counseling services, and special accommodations.

3217 Louisiana State University: Eunice
2048 Johnson Hwy
Eunice, LA 70535-6726
337-457-7311
888-367-5783
Fax: 337-546-6620
www.lsue.edu

William Nunez, President
A public two-year college with 31 special education students out of a total of 2,595.

3218 Nicholls State University
Office of Disability
PO Box 2087
Thibodaux, LA 70310
985-448-4430
Fax: 985-449-7009
www.nicholls.edu
stacey.guidry@nicholls.edu

Stacey Guidry, Director
The Center provides assessments and remediation to students with Dyslexia and related learning disabilities. Programs are offered for college students as well as K-12 students.

3219 Northwestern State University
Learning Disabilities Association of Louisiana
Room 104-J
Teacher Education Center
Natchitoches, LA 71497
318-357-6011
Fax: 318-357-3275
www.lacec.org
duchardt@nsula.edu

Barbara Duchard MD, Associate Professor
Randy Webb, President
Northwestern State University is continuing the process of switching to new software to handle academic and financial records. On August 3, Northwestern State began implementation of student accounts receivable in the new software. By this fall, the university will be fully transitioned to the new software, and the migration will enhance services for students which include but are not limited to: extended hours for system access via the web for the purpose of applying for admission, registerin

3220 Southeastern Louisiana University
Slu 10496
Hammond, LA 70402
985-549-2185
800-222-7358
Fax: 985-549-2771
www.southeastern.edu

Dr. John Crain, President
Dr. Marvin Yates, VP Student Affairs
Sam Domiano, VP Administration, Finance
Four-year college that offers programs for students whom are disabled.

Maine

3221 University of Maine
Disability Support Services
Onward Building
Orono, ME 04469
207-581-1865
1-877-486-23
Fax: 207-581-2969
www.umaine.edu
ann.smith@umit.maine.edu

Susan J. Hunter, President
Judy Ryan, VP Administration and Finance
Karlton Creech, Director of Athletics
The primary goal of the University of Maine Disability Support Services is to create educational access for students with disabilities at UMaine by providing a point of coordination, information and education for those students and the campus community.

3222 University of New England: University Campus
Disability Services
11 Hills Beach Rd
Biddeford, ME 04005-9599
207-602-2306
Fax: 207-602-5971
www.une.edu
hnass@une.edu

Danielle Ripich, President
Holly Hammond Nass, Executive Assistant to President
William J. Bola, Vice President for Operations
Disability Services exists to ensure that the University fulfills the part of its mission that seeks to promote respect for individual differences and to ensure that no person who meets the academic and technical standards requisite for admission to, and continued enrollment at, the University is denied benefits or subjected to discrimination at UNE solely by reason of his or her disability.

Maryland

3223 Chelsea School
2970 Belcrest Center Drive
Suite 300
Hyattsville, MD 20782
301-585-1430
Fax: 301-585-9621
www.chelseaschool.edu
information@chelseaschool.edu
Katherine Fedalen, Head of School
Kristal Weems-Bradner, Dean of Students
Frank Mills, Director of Education
To prepare students with language based learning disabilities for higher education by providing a world-class school which embeds literacy remediation and technology into all aspects of the curriculum.

3224 Greenwood School
6525 Belcrest Road
Suites G-80 & G-90
Hyattsville, MD 20782-8965
301-458-4860
Fax: 802-387-5396
TDD: 301-277-6877
http://greenwoodschoolmd.org
greenwoodschoolmd@verizon.net
Stewart Miller, Headmaster
Laurie Meltzer Klinovsky, Director
A boarding school dedicated to taking bright and talented boys with learning differences and learning disabilities (LD) such as dyslexia, attentional difficulties (ADD / ADHD), or executive functioning deficits and empowering them with the skills and strategies necessary to bridge the gap between their outstanding promise and present abilities.

3225 Harbour School
1277 Green Holly Drive
Annapolis, MD 21409
410-974-4248
Fax: 410-757-3722
www.harbourschool.org
info@harbourschool.org
Linda J Jacobs EdD, Executive Director
Our mission is to provide a supportive, caring and individualized education to students with learning disabilities, autism, speech language impairments, and other disabilities like ADD/ADHD in grades one through twelve by assisting each child to attain academic and personal achievement and success commensurate with the child's abilities. Personal achievement includes success in social, physical and vocational skills

3226 Highlands School
2409 Creswell Rd
Bel Air, MD 21015-6507
410-836-1415
Fax: 410-412-1098
www.highlandsschool.net
info@highlandsschool.net
Patricia Bonney, Executive Director
Richard Molinaro, President
Rowan C. Glidden, Viice-President
Offering a full academic program for students in grades k-8 with dyslexia, ADHD, and laguage based learning differences.

3227 Ivymont School
Autism Program
11614 Seven Locks Rd
Rockville, MD 20854-3261
301-469-0223
Fax: 301-469-0778
www.ivymount.org
lgladstone@ivymount.org
Rick Weintraub, President
Molly Meegan, Vice President
Provides a non-diploma functional life skills program for students ages 6-21 diagnosed with autism and offers a proactive generalization program which ensures student progress is generalized to their community and home.

3228 James E Duckworth School
11201 Evans Trl
Beltsville, MD 20705-3903
301-572-0620
Fax: 301-572-0628
www.1.pgcps.org
jedworth@pgcps.org
Lisa M. Wenzel, Principal
Is a public school in the Prince George's County Public School System., And serves students with moderate to severe disabilities ages 5 through 21.

3229 Jemicy School
11 Celadon Rd
Owings Mills, MD 21117-3099
410-653-2700
Fax: 410-653-1972
www.jemicyschool.org
mmcgowan@jemicyschool.org
Ben Shifrin, Head of School
Empowers students with dyslexia and language-based learning differences to realize their intellectual and social potential through a proven, multisensory curriculum.

3230 Jemicy School: Towson
11 Celadon Rd
Owings Mills, MD 21117-3099
410-653-2700
Fax: 410-653-1972
www.jemicyschool.org
mmcgowan@jemicyschool.org
Ben Shifrin, Head of School
Empowers students with dyslexia / language-based learning differences to realize their intellectual and social potential through a proven, multisensory curriculum.

3231 Margaret Brent School
5816 Lamont Ter
New Carrollton, MD 20784-3541
301-918-8780
Fax: 301-918-8771
www.1.pgcps.org
Lisa M. Wenzel, Principal
Offers a language-based curriculum which infuses both language and literacy skills throughout the curriculum, utilizing 'picture communication symbols'.

3232 McDaniel College
Student Academic Support Services
2 College Hl
Westminster, MD 21157-4303
410-848-7000
800-638-5005
Fax: 410-386-4617
www.mcdaniel.edu
sass@mcdaniel.edu
Roger N. Casey, Ph.D., President
Florence W. Hines, M.B.A., Dean of Admissions
Ethan A. Seidel, Ph.D., VP, Administration and Finance
Is an optional service that is primarily for students with learning disabilities, ADD/HD, but there may be other students with disabilities who have a documented need for this service.

3233 Model Asperger Program
Ivymont School
11614 Seven Locks Rd
Rockville, MD 20854-3261
301-469-0223
Fax: 301-469-0778
www.ivymount.org
aspergerinfo@ivymont.org
Lennie Gladstone, Director
Students in this program have average to gifted cognitive abilities but struggle in mainstream learning environments due to difficulties with social skills, executive functioning, flexible thinking and self-regulation.

3234 Odyssey School
3257 Bridle Rdg
Stevenson, MD 21153-2034
410-580-5551
Fax: 410-580-5352
www.theodysseyschool.org
msweeney@theodysseyschool.org

Patrick C. Crain, Chair
Christopher Pope, Vice-Chair
Roger J. Bennett, Board Member
Provides a warm and creative environment that balances a stimulating hands-on curriculum with a personalized approach to meet the needs of the individual child. Early intervention program, daily tutoring, visual arts/music/dance, leading edge technology, sports, character education and clubs.

3235 Summit School
Academic Program
664 Central Ave E
Edgewater, MD 21037-3429 410-798-0005
Fax: 410-798-0008
www.thesummitschool.org
jane.snider@thesummitschool.org
Joan A. Mele-McCarthy, Executive Director
Joe Budge, Chairman
Kathy Heefner, M.Ed., Director of Admissions
Committed to providing a mainstream academic program that challenges intelligent young minds while addressing students with dyslexia and other learning differences.

3236 The Forbush School at Hunt Valley
Sheppard Pratt Health System
6501 N. Charles Street
Baltimore, MD 21285-6815 410-938-3000
Fax: 410-527-0329
www.sheppardpratt.org
info@sheppardpratt.org
Steven S. Sharfstein, M.D., President, CEO
Robert Roca, M.D., Vice President, Medical Affairs
Gerald A. Noll, Vice President, CFO
Special education classes for children and young adults ages 5-21 with autism, developmental delays, pervasive developmental disorder and multiple learning problems. Programs include motor skill development and sensory integration strategies, natural aided language stimulation, positive behavioral support and vocational programming.

3237 The Forbush Therapeutic Preschool at Towson
Sheppard Pratt Health System
6501 N. Charles Street
Baltimore, MD 21285-6815 410-938-3000
Fax: 410-938-4412
www.sheppardpratt.org
info@sheppardpratt.org
Steven S. Sharfstein, M.D., President, CEO
Robert Roca, M.D., Vice President, Medical Affairs
Gerald A. Noll, Vice President, CFO
Provides special education and related services to children ages 3-7 with autism, pervasive developmental disorder, developmental delays, emotional and severe behavioral problems. Programs are designed to meet each students specific needs.

3238 Towson University
8000 York Rd
Towson, MD 21252 410-828-0622
800-225-5878
Fax: 410-830-3030
TDD: 410-704-2000
www.towson.edu
swillemin@towson.edu
Maravene S. Loeschke, President
Debra Moriarty, VP Student Affairs
Tim Leonard, Director of Athletics
With more than 20,000 students, Towson University is the second largest public university in Maryland. Founded in 1866, the University offers more than 100 bachelor's, master's and doctoral degree programs in the liberal arts and sciences, and applied professional fields. Approximately 1,200 students are registered with the Disability Support Services office on campus.

Massachusetts

3239 American International College
Supportive Learning Services Program
1000 State St
Springfield, MA 01109-3155 413-737-7000
800-242-3142
Fax: 413-205-3051
www.aic.edu
inquiry@www.aic.edu
Peter J. Bittel, Chair
A. Craig Brown, Treasurer
Vincent Maniaci, President
An independent four-year college with 95 special education students out of a total of 1,433. There is an additional fee for the special education program.

3240 Berkshire Center
40 Main St
Suite 3
Lee, MA 01238-1702 413-243-2576
877-566-9247
Fax: 413-243-3351
http://cipworldwide.org/cip-berkshire/berkshire
admissions@cipworldwide.org
Lucy Gosselin, MSBM, Program Director
George Greiner. Ed.D., Program Quality Assistant
Travis McArthur, M.A., Admissions Coordinator
Provides individualized social, academic, career & life skills instruction to young adults 18-26 with Aspergers, ADD and other learning differences. With our support and direction, students learn to realize & develop their potential.

3241 Berkshire Meadows
249 N Plain Rd
Housatonic, MA 01236-9736 413-528-2523
Fax: 413-528-0293
www.jri.org/berkshiremeadows
lkelly@jri.org
Kathy Green, Director
Programs based on the philosophy that all people, no matter how severe their disabilities, should be given the opportunity to achieve their maximum potential.

3242 Boston College
One Silber Way
Boston, MA 02215 617-353-9550
Fax: 617-353-7030
www.bc.edu
ibernier@bu.edu
Robert A. Brown, President
Douglas Sears, VP, Chief of Staff
Gary W. Nicksa, SVP Operations
An independent four-year college with 195 special education students out of a total of 14,230. There is an additional fee for the special education program in addition to the regular tuition.

3243 Boston University
Office of Disability Services
One Silber Way
Boston, MA 02215 617-353-9550
Fax: 617-353-7030
www.bu.edu
ibernier@bu.edu
Robert A. Brown, President
Douglas Sears, VP, Chief of Staff
Gary W. Nicksa, SVP Operations
Provides basic support services such as test taking accommodations, note taking assistance, etc. Provides comprehensive services that include learning strategies instruction for an additional fee. LDSS offers a six-week summer program, The Summer Transition Program, for high school graduates.

3244 Bridgewater State College
Pre-College Workshop for Students with Disabilitie
131 Summit Street
Bridgewater, MA 02325
508-531-1000
Fax: 508-531-1725
TTY: 508-531-6113
www.bridgew.edu
p1connolly@bridgew.edu

Dana Mohler-Faria, President
A two-day program for new students with disabilities. Gives new students with disabilities an opportunity to talk about what BSC offers with upper-class students with disabilities.

3245 Bristol Community College
Program for Academic Support and Success
777 Elsbree Street
Fall River, MA 02720-7399
508-678-2811
Fax: 508-674-4315
www.bristolcc.edu
president@bristolcc.edu

Joseph A. Marshall, FRC, Chair
John J. Sbrega, Ph.D., President
Max Volterra, Esq., Secretary
Provides an integrated program of early academic and career guidance for students with physical and/or learning disabilities.

3246 Carroll School
25 Baker Bridge Road
Lincoln, MA 01773-3199
781-259-8342
Fax: 781-259-8842
www.carrollschool.org
admissions@carrollschool.org

Sam Foster, Chair
Josh Levy, Vice Chairman
Steve Wilkins, Head of School
A dynamic independent day school for elementary and middle school students who have been diagnosed with specific learning disabilities in reading and writing, such as dyslexia.

3247 Cotting School
453 Concord Avenue
Lexington, MA 02421-8088
781-862-7323
Fax: 781-861-1179
www.cotting.org
info@cotting.org

David Cushing, CFA, Chairman
David W. Manzo, M. Ed., President
Michael Durkin,, CEO
Day school for children with a broad spectrum of learning and communication disabilities, physical challenges, and complex medical conditions.

3248 Curry College
Program for Advancement of Learning
1071 Blue Hill Ave
Milton, MA 02186-2395
617-333-0500
Fax: 617-333-2114
www.curry.edu
pal@curry.edu

Kenneth K Quigley Jr, President
Adkins Nathan, Assisstant Director
Aiello Melanie, Prof Development Instructor
PAL is a program within Curry College, a co-educational, four-year liberal arts institution serving 2,000 students and located in the Boston suburb of Milton, Massachusetts. For over 25 years, PAL has both shaped and been shaped by Curry's distinctive philosophy of education. Serves college age students with specific learning disabilities.

3249 Dearborn Academy
34 Winter St
Arlington, MA 02474-6920
781-641-5992
Fax: 781-641-5997
www.dearbornacademy.org
hrossman@dearbornacademy.org

Dr. Howard Rossman, Director
Carol Cole, Director
Mark Dix, Director

A program of psycho-educational day schools serving children in elementary, middle, and high school with emotional, behavioral, and learning difficulties. Students struggling to learn find a secure environment in which to thrive.

3250 Eagle Hill School
242 Old Petersham Road
PO Box 116
Hardwick, MA 01037-0016
413-477-6000
Fax: 413-477-6837
www.ehs1.org
admission@ehs1.org

Jim Richardson, Chairman
Marilyn Waller, President
Alden Bianchi, Vice President
Co-educational, college preparatory boarding and day school for students in grades 8-12 diagnosed with learning disabilities and ADD.

3251 Evergreen Center
Educational Programs and Services
345 Fortune Blvd
Milford, MA 01757-1723
508-478-2631
Fax: 508-634-3251
www.evergreenctr.org
services@evergreenctr.org

Robert Littleton Jr, Executive Director
Is a residential school serving children and adolescents with severe developmental disabilities.

3252 Harvard School of Public Health
Harvard University
677 Huntington Ave
Rm G29
Boston, MA 02115-6096
617-495-1000
Fax: 617-432-3879
www.hsph.harvard.edu
aeisenma@hsph.harvard.edu

Julio Frenk, Dean
Andrew Eisenmann, Student Affairs Director
An independent four-year college with 45 special education students out of a total of 6,621. Disabled students are encouraged to take advantage of opportunities available to help them achieve their educational goals.

3253 Hillside School
404 Robin Hill Road
Marlborough, MA 01752-1099
508-485-2824
Fax: 508-485-4420
www.hillsideschool.net
admissions@hillsideschool.net

David Beecher, Headmaster
William Bullard, Director of Communications
Frances Cincotta, Assistant to the Headmaster
Hillside School is an independent boarding and day school for boys, grades 5-9. Hillside provides educational and residential services to boys needing to develop their academic and social skills while building self-confidence and maturity. The 200-acre school is located in a rural section of Marlborough and includes a working farm. Hillside accommodates both traditional learners who want a more personalized education, and those boys with learning difficulties and/or attention problems.

3254 Landmark Elementary and Middle School Program
Landmark School
429 Hale Street
P O Box 227
Prides Crossing, MA 01965
978-236-3010
Fax: 978-927-7268
www.landmarkschool.org
admission@landmarkschool.org

Moira James, Chairman
Martin P. Slark, Vice Chairman
Robert J. Broudo, President and Headmaster

Our mission is to enable and empower students with language-based learning disabilities to realize their educational and social potential through an exemplary school program complemented by outreach and training, diagnosis, and research.

3255   Landmark High School Program
Landmark School
429 Hale Street
P.O. Box 227
Prides Crossing, MA 01965
978-236-3010
Fax: 978-927-7268
www.landmarkschool.org
admission@landmarkschool.orgkschool.org
Moira James, Chairman
Martin P. Slark, Vice Chairman
Robert J. Broudo, President and Headmaster
Our mission is to transform lives by helping students with language-based learning disabilities realize their educational and social potential.

3256   Landmark School Outreach Program
Landmark School
429 Hale Street
P.O. Box 227
Prides Crossing, MA 01965-0227
978-236-3216
Fax: 978-927-7268
www.landmarkoutreach.org
outreach@landmarkschool.org
Dan Ahearn, Director
Deborah Blanchard, Academic Dean
Robert Broudo, Head of School
Seeks to empower children with language-based learning disabilities by offering their teachers an exemplary program of applied research and professional development.

3257   Lesley University
Threshold Program
29 Everett Street
Cambridge, MA 02138-2702
617-868-9600
800-999-1959
Fax: 617-349-8544
www.lesley.edu
admissions@lesley.edu
Deborah Schwartz Raizes, Chair
Hans D. Strauch, Vice Chair
Joe Moore, President
The Threshold Program is a comprehensive, nondegree campus-based program at Lesley University for highly motivated young adults with diverse learning disabilities and other special needs.

3258   Linden Hill School
154 S Mountain Rd
Northfield, MA 01360-9701
413-498-2906
Fax: 413-498-2908
www.lindenhs.org
office@lindenhs.org
James Mc Daniel, Headmaster
A middle school dedicated to helping boys with dyslexia or language-learning differences realize their full potential.

3259   Middlesex Community College
Transition Program
591 Springs Road
Bedford, MA 01730
978-656-3370
800-818-3434
www.middlesex.mass.edu
middlesex@middlesex.mass.edu
Royall M. Mack Sr., Chairman
Robert A. Barton, Board Member
William J. Chemelli, Board Member
Designed expressly for students with significant learning disabilities. This two-year certificate program teaches consumer and business skills, independent living, and personal and social development.

3260   Northeastern University
Learning Disabilities Program
360 Huntington Ave.
Boston, MA 02115
617-373-2000
Fax: 617-373-3758
TTY: 617-373-3768
www.northeastern.edu
m.barrows@neu.edu
Jim O'Shaughnessy, Director
Susie Guszcza, Executive Assistant to President
Susan Cromwell, Assistant to President
Offers a variety of services to students with disabilities including note takers, extended testing time, counseling services, and special accommodations.

3261   Riverview School
551 Route 6a
East Sandwich, MA 02537-1494
508-888-0489
Fax: 508-833-7001
www.riverviewschool.org
admissions@riverviewschool.org
Deborah Cowan, Chair
Justin Gray, Vice Chair
James Shallcross, Treasurer
An independent, residential school of international reputation and service enrolling 183 male and female students in its secondary and post-secondary programs. Students share a common history of lifelong difficulty with academic achievement and the development of friendships. On measures of intellectual ability, most students score within the 70-100 range and have a primary diagnosis of learning disability and/or complex language or learning disorder.

3262   Smith College
College Hall 104
Northampton, MA 01063-0001
413-584-2700
Fax: 413-585-4498
TTY: 413-585-2071
www.smith.edu
lrausche@email.smith.edu
Laura Rauscher, Director
Support services office for students, staff and faculty with disabilities.

3263   Springfield Technical Community College
PO Box 9000
Springfield, MA 01102-9000
413-781-7822
Fax: 413-755-6306
www.stcc.edu
Christopher Johnson, Chairman
Jeffrey E. Poindexter, Secretary
Trevor Eliason, Student Trustee
Springfield Technical Community College, a leader in technology and instructional innovation, transforms lives through educational opportunities that promote personal and professional success.

3264   The Kolburne School, Inc.
343 NM Southfield Rd
New Marlborough, MA 01230-2035
413-229-8787
Fax: 413-229-4165
www.kolburne.net
info@kolburne.net
Jeane K Weinstein, Executive Director
A family operated residential treatment center located in the Berkshire Hills of Massachusetts. Through integrated treatment services, effective behavioral management, recreational programming, and positive staff relationships, our students develop the emotional stability, interpersonal skills and academic/vocational background necessary to return home with success.

3265   White Oake School
533 North Rd
Westfield, MA 01085
413-562-9500
Fax: 413-562-9010
www.whiteoakschool.org
admissions@whiteoakschool.org

David Drake, Headmaster
Betty Knapik, Administrative Assistant
Nancy Coleman, Dean of Studies
Offer programs for students with learning disabilities, ADD and/or emotional difficulties.

3266 Willow Hill School
98 Haynes Rd
Sudbury, MA 01776
978-443-2581
Fax: 978-443-7560
www.willowhillschool.org
rtaft-farrell@willowhillschool.org
Marilyn G. Reid, Head of School
Shamus Brady, Director of Education
Tina Kaplan, Director
Offers secondary level students with learning challenges opportunities to acquire academic and social skills needed to shape their own future. Ensuring that our students fulfill their potential is our priority. We are dedicated to attainment of academic excellence and a wide range of personal talents.

Michigan

3267 Andrews University
Old Us 31
Berrien Springs, MI 49104
269-471-7771
800-253-2874
Fax: 269-471-6293
www.andrews.edu
enroll@andrews.edu
Niels-Erik Andreasen, President
Andrea Luxton, Provost
Lorena Bidwell, Chief Information Officer
Offers a variety of services to students with disabilities including notetakers, extended testing time, counseling services, and special accommodations.

3268 Aquinas College
1607 Robinson Rd SE
Grand Rapids, MI 49506-1799
616-632-8900
800-678-9593
Fax: 616-459-2563
www.aquinas.edu
admissions@aquinas.edu
Juan Olivarez, Ph.D., President
Gilda Gely, Ph.D., EVP, Provost & Dean of Faculty
Leonard V. Kogut, Jr., Ph.D., VP for Finance
An independent four-year college with 32 special education students out of a total of 2,300 students.

3269 Coaching Program
Calvin College
1845 Knollcrest Cir SE
Grand Rapids, MI 49546-4436
616-526-6113
800-618-0122
Fax: 616-526-7066
www.calvin.edu
acadservices@calvin.edu
Todd Dornbos, Director
Provides the coaching program for students with learning disabilities, attention deficit disorders and other students who benefit from help with time management and study skills.

3270 Eastern Michigan University
Students with Disabilities Office
Suite 240
Student Center
Ypsilanti, MI 48197
734-487-1849
Fax: 734-487-5784
www.emich.edu
cbracke1@emich.edu
Susan M. Martin, Ph.D., President
Kim Schatzel, Ph.D., Provost/EVP of Student Affairs
John Lumm, CFO
Four year college that offers students with learning disabilities support and services.

3271 Eton Academy
Academic Program
1755 E Melton Rd
Birmingham, MI 48009
248-642-1150
Fax: 248-642-3670
www.etonacademy.org
Pete Pullen, Head of School
Our primary focus is to help students who learn differently achieve their fullest potential for academic excellence. Eton Academy offers a comprehensive curriculum that integrates the best available multi-sensory, hands-on and experiential learning methods to meet the individual needs of its students.

3272 Lake Michigan Academy
2428 Burton St SE
Grand Rapids, MI 49546
616-464-3330
Fax: 616-285-1935
www.mylma.org/
info@mylma.org
Robert Woodhouse, Chairman
Phil Wood, Vice Chairman
Ben Pitcher, Treasurer
Lake Michigan academy provides academic excellence for students with specific learning disabilities and/or attention deficit disorder in grades 1-12

3273 Michigan Technological University
1400 Townsend Dr
Houghton, MI 49931-1295
906-487-1885
Fax: 906-487-3589
www.mtu.edu
gbmelton@mtu.edu
Glenn D. Mroz, President
Max Seel, Provost/VP for Academic Affairs
Ellen S. Horsch, VP, administration
A public undergraduate and graduate university with programs in engineering, sciences, business, technology, forestry, social sciences, and humanities. In 2005/06, there were requests for services from 70 individuals with physical or learning disabilities. Services include extended testing time, books on tape, and counseling. Total student enrollment 6,510.

3274 Montcalm Community College
2800 College Dr
Sidney, MI 48885
989-328-2111
Fax: 989-328-2950
www.montcalm.edu
info@montcalm.edu
Karen Carbonelli, Chairman
Robert Marston, Vice Chairman
Robert C. Ferrentino, J.D., President
Offers a variety of services to students with disabilities including note takers, extended testing time, counseling services, and special accommodations.

3275 Northwestern Michigan College
1701 E Front St
Traverse City, MI 49686
231-995-1000
800-748-0566
Fax: 231-995-1253
www.nmc.edu/tss
admissions@nmc.edu
Douglas S. Bishop, Chairman
William D. Myers, Vice Chairman
Kennard R. Weaver, Treasurer
Community college in Northern Michigan.

Minnesota

3276 Alexandria Technical and Community College
1601 Jefferson St
Alexandria, MN 56308   320-762-0221
                                     888-234-1222
                                     Fax: 320-762-4501
                                     www.alextech.edu
                                     marya@alextech.edu

Jon Hall, President
Rose Shorma, Vice President
Kathy Pfeffer Nohre, Executive Director
Educational Institution

3277 Augsburg College
Center for Learning and Adaptive Student Services
2211 Riverside Ave
Minneapolis, MN 55454   612-330-1000
                                     Fax: 612-330-1443
                                     TDD: 612-330-1748
                                     TTY: 612-330-1748
                                     www.augsburg.edu
                                     admissions@augsburg.edu

Paul Pribbenow, President
Karen L. Kaivola, Provost & Chief Academic Officer
Leif Anderson, VP & Chief Information Officer
The Center for Learning and Adaptive Student Services co-
ordinates academics accommodations and services for stu-
dents with learning, attentional and psychiatric disabilities.

3278 College of Saint Scholastica
1200 Kenwood Ave
Duluth, MN 55811-4199   218-723-6000
                                     800-249-6412
                                     Fax: 218-723-6290
                                     www.css.edu
                                     admissions@css.edu

Larry Goodwin, President
Beth Domholdt, VP for Academic Affairs
Patrick Flattery, VP for Finance
Offers a variety of services to students with disabilities in-
cluding note takers, extended testing time, counseling ser-
vices, and special accommodations.

3279 Groves Academy
3200 Highway 100 South
Saint Louis Park, MN 55416   952-920-6377
                                     Fax: 952-920-2068
                                     www.grovesacademy.org
                                     alexanderj@grovesacademy.org

Mark Donahoe, Chairman
TBD TBD, Vice Chairman
John Alexander, Head of School
A private, independent, day school for adults with langauge,
learning and attentional disabilities.

3280 Institute on Community Integration
University of Minnesota
109 Pattee Hall
150 Pillsbury Dr SE
Minneapolis, MN 55455   612-624-4512
                                     Fax: 612-624-9344
                                     http://ici.umn.edu
                                     icipub@umn.edu

David R Johnson PhD, Director
A federally designated University Center for Excellence in
Developmental Disabilities, has over 400 print and electronic resources on topics relating to community living for
persons with intellectual and developmental disabilities
across the lifespan.

3281 Minnesota Life College
7501 Logan Ave S
STE 2A
Richfield, MN 55423   612-869-4008
                                     Fax: 612-869-0443
                                     www.minnesotalifecollege.org
                                     info@minnesotalifecollege.org

Jennifer Greene, Chairman
Michael Zalk, Vice Chairman
Amy Gudmestad, Executive Director
Minnesota Life College is a not-for-profit, vocational and
life skills training program for young adults with learning
disabilities.

**3282 Minnesota State Community and Technical College:
Moorhead**
1900 28th Ave S
Moorhead, MN 56560   218-299-6500
                                     877-450-3322
                                     Fax: 218-299-6810
                                     TTY: 800-627-2539
                                     www.minnesota.edu
                                     jerome.migler@minnesota.edu

Dr. Peggy D. Kennedy, President
Pat Nordick, CFO
Kathleen Brock, Chief Academic Officer
Offers a variety of services to students with disabilities in-
cluding notetakers, extended testing time, counseling ser-
vices, and special accommodations.

3283 Northwest Technical College
1900 28th Ave S
Moorhead, MN 56560-4899   218-299-6500
                                     877-450-3322
                                     Fax: 218-299-6810
                                     TTY: 800-627-3529
                                     www.minnesota.edu
                                     jerome.migler@minnesota.edu

Tom Julsrud, President
Marlis Ziegler, Secretary
Richard Smestad, Vice President
Offers a variety of services to students with disabilities in-
cluding notetakers, extended testing time, counseling ser-
vices, and special accommodations.

3284 Student Disability Services
St. Cloud State University
720 4th Ave S
Saint Cloud, MN 56301-4498   320-308-4080
                                     Fax: 320-308-5100
                                     www.stcloudstate.edu/sds
                                     sds@stcloudstate.edu

Earl H. Potter III, President
Owen Zimpel, Disability Services Director
Joyce Koshiol, Office Manager
A public comprehensive university that provides services
for students with learning disabilities and other needs: alternative testing, note taking, referrals to campus resources and
advocacy/support.

3285 University of Minnesota: Morris
Student Disability Services
600 E 4th St
Morris, MN 56267   320-589-6035
                                     888-866-3382
                                     Fax: 320-589-6035
                                     TDD: 320-589-6178
                                     www.morris.umn.edu
                                     freyc@morris.umn.edu

Jacqueline Johnson, Coordinator
Offers a variety of services to students with disabilities including note takers, extended testing time, counseling services, and special accommodations.

Mississippi

3286 Mississippi State University
Adaptive Driving Program
PO Box 9736
Mississippi State, MS 39762   662-325-2323
                                     Fax: 662-325-0896
                                     TTY: 662-325-0520
                                     www.msstate.edu
                                     jcirlotnew@tkmartin.msstate.edu

Mark E. Keenum, President
Jerome A. Gilbert, Provost & EVP
Don Zant, VP, Budget and Planning
Specializes in the evaluation and training of persons with disabilities who wish to consider driving. Services may result in a recommendation for driving or further training, and when appropriate, will include specific recommendations regarding vehicle modifications and adaptive driving equipment. Also offers evaluation and training services for driving candidates using bioptic lenses.

3287 Project Art
Mississippi State University
PO Box 9736
Mississippi State, MS 39762   662-325-2323
                                     Fax: 662-325-0896
                                     TTY: 662-325-0520
                                     www.msstate.edu
                          jcirlotnew@tkmartin.msstate.edu
Mark E. Keenum, President
Jerome A. Gilbert, Provost & EVP
Don Zant, VP, Budget and Planning
Provides recreational activities for students with and without disabilities in grades K-12. With the use of assistive technology and evnironmental adaptation, the program makes available recreational activities that have not traditionally been an option for children with disabilities.

3288 University of Southern Mississippi
118 College Drive
Hattiesburg, MS 39406-1   601-266-1000
                                  Fax: 601-266-5756
                                  TDD: 601-266-6837
                                  www.usm.edu
                          latouisha.wilson@usm.edu
Rodney D. Bennett, President
Dr. Denis Wiesenburg, Provost
Douglas H. Vinzant, VP-Finance& Administration
Four year college that provides students with support and resources whom are disabled.

Missouri

3289 Central Missouri State University
Office of Accessibility Services
PO Box 800
Warrensburg, MO 64093   660-543-4111
                                Fax: 660-543-4658
                                TDD: 660-543-4421
                                www.ucmo.edu
                                admit@ucmo.edu
John Merrigan, VP, Finance/ COO
Dorothy Salsman, Budget and Planning Director
Sharon Brinton, Administrative Assistant
Provider of equal opportunity to education for students with disabilities through notetakers, extended testing time, interpreters and other accommodations.

3290 Churchill Center and School for Learning Disabilities
1021 Municipal Center Dr
Town & Country, MO 63131   314-997-4343
                                   Fax: 314-997-2760
                                   www.churchillstl.org
                                   info@churchillstl.org
Sandra Gilligan, Director
Beth Brookshier, Business Manager
Deborah Wardon, Assistant Director Operations
Our mission is to give high potential children with learning disabilities the finest, individualized, remedial education and the support they need to achieve and return to a traditional classroom .

3291 Longivew Community College
ABLE Program
3200 Broadway
Kansas City, MO 64111   816-604-1000
                                Fax: 816-672-2025
                                www.mcckc.edu

Carolyn Watley, Chair
Jason Stuart Dalen, Vice Chair
Mark James, Chancellor
The program teaches students with neurological disabilities including, but not limited to, learning disabilities or brain injuries how to become independent learners.

3292 Missouri State University
Learning Diagnostic Clinic
901 South National Avenue
Springfield, MO 65897   417-836-6841
                                Fax: 417-836-8330
                          www.psychology.missouristate.edu
                          stevecapps@missouristate.edu
Steven C. Capps, Director
Timothy A. Bender, Professor
Tracie D. Burt, Sr Instructor
Project Success is an academic support program for college students with a learning disability, ADHD, or other diagnosis who desire more comprehensive services. Those enrolled in Project Success will be offered a wide variety of services tailored for students with learning disabilities.

3293 North Central Missouri College
1301 Main St
Trenton, MO 64683   660-359-3948
                            Fax: 660-359-2211
                            www.ncmissouri.edu/
Dr Neil Nuttall, President
Offers a variety of services to students with disabilities including note takers, extended testing time, counseling services, and special accommodations.

3294 St Louis Community College: Forest Park
5600 Oakland Ave
Saint Louis, MO 63110   314-644-9100
                                Fax: 314-644-9752
                                www.stlcc.edu
Dennis F. Michaelis, Ph.D, Interim Chancellor
Donna Dare, Vice Chancellor
Pam McIntyre, President, Meramec campus
St. Louis Community College expands minds and changes lives every day. We create accessible, dynamic learning environments focused on the needs of our diverse communities.

3295 St Louis Community College: Meramec
11333 Big Bend Rd
Saint Louis, MO 63122   314-984-7500
                                Fax: 314-984-7166
                                www.stlcc.edu
Dennis F. Michaelis, Ph.D, Interim Chancellor
Donna Dare, Vice Chancellor
Pam McIntyre, President, Meramec campus
St. Louis Community College expands minds and changes lives every day. We create accessible, dynamic learning environments focused on the needs of our diverse communities.

3296 University of Missouri: Kansas City
Department of Disability Services
5100 Rockhill Rd
Kansas City, MO 64110   816-235-1000
                                Fax: 816-235-6363
                                www.umkc.edu
                                disability@umkc.edu
Murray Blackwelder, President
Leo Morton, Chancellor
Curt Crespino, Vice Chancellor
Offers a variety of services to students with disabilities including note takers, extended testing time, counseling services, and special accommodations.

Montana

3297 Western Montana College
710 S Atlantic St
Dillon, MT 59725   406-683-7331
                          877-683-7331
                          www.umwestern.edu
Estee Aiken, Assistant Professor
Matt Allen, Program Coordinator
Kelly Allen, Program Coordinator
A public four-year college with 6 special education students
out of a total of 1,100.

Nebraska

3298 Midland Lutheran College
Academic Support Services
900 N Clarkson
Fremont, NE 68025   402-941-6501
                          800-642-8382
                          Fax: 402-941-6513
                          www.midlandu.edu
                          info@midlandu.edu
Dr. Benjamin Sasse, President
Lindsay Adams, Director of External Relations
Jocelyn Allen, Admissions Counselor
Four-year college that provides academic support for stu-
dents who have a learning disability.

3299 Southeast Community College: Beatrice Campus
Career and Advising Program
4771 W Scott Rd
Beatrice, NE 68310-7042   402-228-3468
                          800-233-5027
                          Fax: 402-228-2218
                          www.southeast.edu
Kathy Boellstorff, Chair
Dale Kruse, Vice Chair
Helen E. Griffin, Treasurer
The Beatrice Campus offers the Academic Transfer program
providing first and second year college coursees for students
who wish to transfer credits to a four-year college.

3300 University of Nebraska: Omaha
6001 Dodge St
Omaha, NE 68182   402-554-2800
                          800-858-8648
                          Fax: 402-554-3777
                          www.unomaha.edu
John Christensen, Chancellor
Lee Denker, President/CEO Alumni Association
Lori Byrne, VP & UNO Director
Offers a variety of services to students with disabilities in-
cluding notetakers, extended testing time, counseling ser-
vices, and special accommodations.

New Hampshire

3301 Dartmouth College
Student Accessibility Services
301 Collis Ctr
Hanover, NH 03755   603-646-1110
                          Fax: 603-646-1629
                          TDD: 603-646-1564
                          http://dartmouth.edu/
                          contact@dartmouth.edu
Carl Thum, Ph.D, Direcror

The Student Accessibility Services (SAS) Office works with
students, faculty and staff to ensure that the programs and
activities of Dartmouth College are accessible, and students
with disabilities receive reasonable accommodations in
their curricular and co-curricular pursuits. Over 350
Dartmouth students are registered with SAS including students with learning disabilities, attentional or psychiatric
disorders, and mobility, visual, hearing or chronic health
conditions.

3302 Hampshire Country School
28 Patey Circle
Rindge, NH 03461-5950   603-899-3325
                          Fax: 603-899-6521
                          www.hampshirecountryschool.org
                          admissions@hampshirecountryschool.net
Ellen Bingham, Administrative Assistant
Thomas Ciglar, Dean of Students
William Dickerman, Director of Admissions
Hampshire Country School is a boarding school for middle
school boys with very high ability who need an unusual
amount of adult attention and support, including boys with
Asperger's, nonverbal learning disabilities and ADHD.

3303 Hunter School
PO Box 600
Rumney, NH 03266   603-786-9427
                          Fax: 603-786-2221
                          www.hunterschool.org
                          info@hunterschool.org
Tim Tyler, Director
A small, non-profit school where young boys and girls with
Attention Deficit Disorder (ADD), Attention Deficit/Hyper-
activity Disorder (ADHD) or Asperger's Syndrome are nur-
tured, educated and celebrated. Offers both a residential
program and a day school.

3304 Keene State College
229 Main St
Keene, NH 03435   603-352-1909
                          800-KSC-1909
                          Fax: 603-358-2257
                          www.keene.edu
Anne E. Huot, Ph.D., President
Patricia Francis, Chief of Staff
Amy Proctor, Sr Administrative Assistant
A public four-year college with 105 special education stu-
dents out of a total of 3,800.

3305 Learning Skills Academy
1247 Washington Rd
Rye, NH 03870   603-964-4903
                          Fax: 603-964-3838
                          www.learningskillsacademy.org/
                          lsa@learningskillsacademy.org
Barbara Gregg, Chair
Bill Carpenter, Asst. Chair
Gary Rohr, Co-Treasurer
Our purpose is to ignite every potential in our students and
since 1985 they have been successful both academically and
socially. We prepare them for success in life by helping them
to understand their learning profile: advocate for their
needs; interact appropriately in scholastic and social situations; and bring their academic work to a level that matches
their potential. When students reach these goals, our staff
works with the student, parents and LEA to support
successful transitions.

3306 New England College
98 Bridge St
Henniker, NH 03242   603-428-2000
                          Fax: 603-428-7230
                          www.nec.edu
Michelle D. Perkins, President
Paula A. Amato, VP, Finance & Administration
Tia M. Hooper, Asst. to the President
An independent four-year college with 140 students with
learning differences out of a total undergraduate
enrollment of 750.

3307 New Hampshire Vocational Technical College
379 Belmont Rd
Laconia, NH 03246-1364

603-524-3207
800-357-2992
Fax: 603-524-8084
TDD: 603-524-3207
www.laconia.nactc.edu
laconow@nactc.edu

Maureen Baldwin-Lamper, Special Services
Don Morrissey, Vice President
Offers a variety of services to students with disabilities including notetakers, extended testing time, counseling services, and special accommodations.

3308 Rivier College
420 S Main St
Nashua, NH 03060

603-888-1311
800-44-RIVIE
Fax: 603-897-8883
TDD: 800-735-2964
www.rivier.edu
kricci@rivier.edu

Paula Marie Buley, President
Karen Cooper, VP, University Advancement
Kurt Stimeling, VP, Student Affairs
An independent four-year college with 17 special education students out of a total of 1,651.

3309 Southern New Hampshire University
Office of Disability Services
2500 N River Rd
Manchester, NH 03106

603-626-9100
800-688-1249
Fax: 603-626-9100
TTY: 603-645-4671
www.snhu.edu
info@snhu.edu

Paul Leblanc, President
Karen D. Anbbott, General Counsel
Johnson Au-Yeung, Chief Information Officer
Offers services to students with disabilities based on recommendations from documentaion supporting a disability. Accommodations are made for specific needs.

3310 University of New Hampshire
118 Memorial Union Building
Durham, NH 03824

603-862-1234
Fax: 603-862-4043
TTY: 603-862-2607
www.unh.edu/disabilityservices
disability.office@unh.edu

Kathy Berger, M.S., Director
Becky Michaud, Disability Specialist
Rebecca McMillan, M.Ed, Assistive Technology Specialist
Disability Services for Students provides services to students with documented disabilities to ensure that University activities and programs are accessible. It also promotes the development of student self-reliance and the personal independence necessary to succeed in a university climate.

New Jersey

3311 Banyan School
12 Hollywood Ave
Fairfield, NJ 07004

973-439-1919
Fax: 973-439-1396
www.banyanschool.com
msaunders@banyanschool.com

Dee Herrman, Admin. Asst./Guidance
Yael Kamara, Occupational Therapist
Susan Gorden, Secretary

3312 Caldwell College
Office of Disability Services
120 Bloomfield Avenue
Caldwell, NJ 07006

973-618-3000
Fax: 973-618-3358
www.caldwell.edu
abenowitz@caldwell.edu

Marilyn Bastardi, Chair
Nancy Costello Miller, Vice Chair
Nancy Blattner, President
Four-year college that provides disability services to those students who are learnig disabled.

3313 Camden County College
PO Box 200
College Drive
Blackwood, NJ 08012-200

856-227-7200
Fax: 856-374-4975
www.camdencc.edu
jkinzy@camdencc.edu

Raymond Yannuzzi, President
Margaret Hamilton Ph.D., RN, VP, Academic Affairs
Helen Erskine, Administrative Assistant
A two-year college that provides services to the learning disabled.

3314 Centenary College
Office of Disabilities Services
400 Jefferson St
Hackettstown, NJ 07840

908-852-1400
800-236-8679
Fax: 908-852-5410
www.centenarycollege.edu
dso@centenarycollege.edu

Tiffany Zappulla, Director of Career
Jeffery Wolthoff, Corporate Realtions
Ginna Oksienik, Career Center/Internship Coor
Offers two programs specifically designed to support students with mild emotional and learning disabilities: Project Able and Step Ahead. The goals of these programs are to provide a bridge between the structured and sometimes modified secondary-school setting to the predominantly self-directed college environment.

3315 Children's Center of Monmouth County
1115 Green Grove Rd
Neptune, NJ 07753

732-922-0228
Fax: 732-922-8133
www.ccprograms.com

George Scheer, Director
Offers educational services, training in adaptive living and pre-vocational skills for students, ages 3 to 21, with multiple disabilities or a diagnosis of autism and pervasive developmental delays.

3316 College of New Jersey
Office of Differing Disabilities
2000 Pennington Road
Ewing, NJ 08628-718

609-771-2571
Fax: 609-637-5131
http://tcnj.pages.tcnj.edu/
degennar@tcnj.edu

Christopher Gibson, Chair
R. Barbara Gitenstein, President
Jacqueline Taylor, Provost/Vice President
Four-year college provides services to students with disabilities.

3317 College of Saint Elizabeth
2 Convent Rd
Morristown, NJ 07960-6989

973-290-4000
www.cse.edu

Rosemary Moynihan, Chair
Helen J. Streubert, President/ Treasurer
Patricia Butler, Secretary
Offers a variety of services to students with disabilities including notetakers, extended testing time, counseling services, and special accommodations.

3318 Community School
PO Box 2118
Sunvalley, ID 83353

208-622-3955
Fax: 208-622-3962
www.communityschool.org
info@communityschool.org

Jay Hagenbuch, Chair
Guy Cherp, Treasurer
Ellen S. Gillespie, Secretary
Comprehensive academic program for LD/ADD children grades K-8; NY and NJ funding available.

3319 Craig School
10 Tower Hill Rd
Mountain Lakes, NJ 07046

973-334-1295
Fax: 973-334-1299
www.craigschool.org
info@craigschool.org

Christopher Coates, Chairman
Norman Lobins, Vice Chairman
Grant L. Jacks, Head of School
A school for children with learning differences such as dyslexia, auditory processing issues and ADD.

3320 Cumberland County College
Project Assist
PO Box 1500
College Drive
Vineland, NJ 08362-1500

856-691-8600
Fax: 856-690-0059
www.cccnj.net
ssherd@cccnj.edu

Keith C. Figgs, Ed.D, Chairman
Ginger Chase, Vice Chairman
Donna M Perez, Secretary
A two-year college that offers services to its learning disabled students.

3321 Fairleigh Dickinson University: Metropolitan Campus
1000 River Rd
Teaneck, NJ 07666

201-692-2000
800-338-8803
Fax: 201-692-2030
www.fdu.edu

Patrick J. Zenner, Chair
Sheldon Drucker, President
Karin Hamilton, Exec Asst to the President
Comprehensive support services to students with language based LD.

3322 Forum School
107 Wyckoff Ave
Waldwick, NJ 07463

201-444-5882
Fax: 201-444-4003
www.theforumschool.com
info@theforumschool.com

Steven Krapes, Executive Director
Linda Oliver, Office Manager
Day school for children through age 16 who have neurologically based developmental disabilities, including autism, ADHD, LD, and asperger syndrome. Services include extended year, speech, adaptive physical education, music, art therapy, and parent program.

3323 Georgian Court University
The Learning Center (TLC)
900 Lakewood Ave
Lakewood, NJ 08701

732-987-2700
800-458-8422
Fax: 732-987-2026
www.georgian.edu
admissions@georgian.edu

Patricia A. Cohen, MSW, MA, Director
Luana Fahr, Deputy Director

The Learning Center is an assistance program designed to provide an environment for students with mild to moderate learning disabilities who desire a college education. The program is not one of remediation, but it is an individualized support program to assist candidates in becoming successful college students. Emphasis is placed on developing self-help strategies, study techniques, content tutoring, time management, organization skills, and social skills all taught by a certified professional.

3324 Gloucester County College
1400 Tanyard Rd
Sewell, NJ 08080

856-468-5000
Fax: 856-468-9462
TDD: 856-468-8452
www.gccnj.edu
dcook@gccnj.edu

???Gene J. Concordia, Chairperson
Yolette C Ross, Vice Chairperson
Frederick Keating, President
The Office of Special Needs Services addresses supportive needs toward academic achievement for those students with documented disabilties such as learning disabled, visually impaired, hard of hearing and mobility impaired individuals.

3325 Hudson County Community College
70 Sip Avenue
Jersey City, NJ 07306

201-714-7100
201-714-7100
Fax: 201-963-0789
www.hudson.cc.nj.us

William J. Netchert, Esq., Chairperson
Bakari Gerard Lee, Esq., Vice Chairperson
Dr. Glen Gabert, President
Offers a variety of services to students with disabilities including note takers, extended testing time, counseling services, and special accommodations.

3326 Jersey City State College
2039 Kennedy Boulevard
Jersey City, NJ 07305-1597

201-200-2000
888-441-NJCU
www.njcu.edu

T. Steven Chang, Chair
Sue Henderson, Ph.D., President
Daniel J. Julius, Provost
Offers a variety of services to students with disabilities including notetakers, extended testing time, counseling services, and special accommodations.

3327 Kean University
Community Disabilities Services
1000 Morris Ave
Union, NJ 07083

908-737-5326
Fax: 908-737-5235
TDD: 908-737-5156
www.kean.edu
webmaster@kean.edu

Ada Morell, Chair
Donald J Soreiro, Vice Chair
Audrey M. Kelly, Executive Director
Provides services to disabled students.

3328 Middlesex County College
Project Connections
2600 Woodbridge Avenue
Edison, NJ 08818-3050

732-548-6000
Fax: 732-906-7767
http://www2.middlesexcc.edu/
elizabeth_lowe@middlesex.edu

Dorothy K. Power, Chair
Thomas Tighe, Vice Chair
Robert P. Sica, Secretary
Project Connections is a comprehensive academic and counseling service for students with learning disabilities who are enrolled in mainstream programs at Middlesex County College.

3329 Morristown-Beard School
70 Whippany Rd
Morristown, NJ 07960 973-539-3032
Fax: 973-539-1590
www.mobeard.org

Michael Ranger, President
John Eagen, Vice President
Peter J. Caldwell, Headmaster
Offer programs for students with learning disabilities, ADD and/or emotional difficulties.

3330 New Jersey City University
2039 Kennedy Boulevard
Jersey City, NJ 07305-1597 201-200-2000
888-441-NJCU
Fax: 201-200-2044
www.njcu.edu

T. Steven Chang, Chair
Sue Henderson, Ph.D., President
Daniel J. Julius, Provost
Provides students with learning disabilities a mentor, a teacher, advisor or a faculty member.

3331 Ocean County College
College Dr
Toms River, NJ 08754-2001 732-255-0400
Fax: 732-255-0444
TDD: 732-255-0424
www.ocean.edu
mreustle@ocean.edu

Carl V. Thulin, Chair
Linda L. Novak, Vice Chair
Jon H. Larson, Ph.D., President
A regional resource center and comprehensive support center for college students with learning disabilities, offering a range of services including psycho-educational assessments, faculty/staff in-service training, program development assistance and consultation, and technical support. Individual and/or small group counseling is available, and vocational/career counseling on transition issues is also offered.

3332 Princeton University
303 W College
Princeton, NJ 08544 609-258-3000
Fax: 609-258-1020
www.princeton.edu

Christopher Eisgruber, President
David S. Lee, Provost
Deborah Prentice, Dean
Offers a variety of services to students with disabilities including note takers, extended testing time, counseling services, and special accommodations.

3333 Ramapo College of New Jersey
Office of Specialized Services
505 Ramapo Valley Rd
Mahwah, NJ 07430 201-684-7500
Fax: 201-684-7004
www.ramapo.edu/
oss@ramapo.edu

George C. Ruotolo, Jr., Chair
William F. Dator, Vice Chair
David G. Schlussel, Secretary
Ramapo College demostated a strong commitment to providing equal access to all students through the removal of architectural and attitudinal barriers. Integration of qualified students with disabilities into college community has been the Ramapo way since the College opened in 1971.

3334 Raritan Valley Community College
118 Lamington Road
Branchburg, NJ 08876 908-526-1200
Fax: 908-429-8589
www.raritanval.edu

Paul J. Hirsch, Chair
Robert P. Wise, Vice Chair
Tracy DiFrancesco Zaikov, Vice Chair

A public two-year college with 250 students with disabilities of a total of 6,000 per semster.

3335 Richard Stockton College of New Jersey
101 Vera King Farris Drive
Galloway, NJ 08205-9441 609-652-1776
Fax: 609-626-5550
http://www2.stockton.edu
webmaster@stockton.edu

Dr. Richard Bjork, President
David Pinto, Manager
Offers a variety of services to students with disabilities including note takers, extended testing time, counseling services, and special accommodations.

3336 Rider University
2083 Lawrenceville Rd
Lawrenceville, NJ 08648 609-896-5000
800-257-9026
Fax: 609-895-6645
www.rider.edu
serv4dstu@rider.edu

Michael B. Kennedy, Chair
Ernestine Lazenby Gast, Vice Chair
Mordechai Rozanski, President
Four-year college that provides resources, programs and support for students with learning disabilities through their SSD (Services for Students with Disabilities) center.

3337 Robert Wood Johnson Medical School
Elizabeth M Boggs Center on Dev. Disabilities
335 George Street
New Brunswick, NJ 08901 732-235-9300
Fax: 732-235-9330
www.rwjms.umdnj.edu/boggscenter

Brian L. Strom, MD, MPH, Chancellor
Robert Prodoehl, Executive Director
Patricia M. Hansen, MA, Director
The Elizabeth M. Boggs Center, as a University Center for Excellence in Developmental Disabilities, values uniqueness and individuality and promotes the self-determination and full participation of people with disabilities and their families in all aspects of community life. The Boggs Center prepares students through interdisciplinary programs, provides community training and technical assistance, conducts research, and disseminates information and educational materials.

3338 Rutgers Center for Cognitive Science
152 Frelinghuysen Rd
Piscataway, NJ 08854-8020 848-445-1625
Fax: 732-445-6715
http://ruccs.rutgers.edu/
admin@ruccs.rutgers.edu

Sue Cosentino, Business Manager
JoAnn Meli, Administrative Assistant
Hristiyan Kourtev, Scientific Programmer
A public four-year college with 2 special education students out of a total of 437.

3339 Salem Community College
460 Hollywood Ave
Carneys Point, NJ 08069-2799 856-299-2100
Fax: 856-351-2634
www.salemcc.org
SCCinfo@salemcc.org

Peter Contini, President
Offers a variety of services to students with disabilities including extended testing time, counseling services, and special accommodations.

3340 Seton Hall University
400 S Orange Ave
South Orange, NJ 07079 973-761-9000
Fax: 973-761-7494
www.shu.edu
fraziera@shu.edu

John J. Myers, Chair
TBD TBD, Vice Chair
Pamela M. Swartzberg, Esq., Secretary
Student Support Services is an academic program that addresses the needs of students with disabilities.

3341 Trenton State College
2000 Pennington Rd
Ewing, NJ 08628-718
609-771-3080
Fax: 609-637-5161
www.tcnj.edu
webmaster@tcnj.edu

Christopher Gibson, Esq, Chair
R. Barbara Gitenstein, President
Jacqueline Taylor, Provost/Vice President
A public four-year college with 24 special education students out of a total of 6,118.

3342 William Paterson College of New Jersey
Special Education Services
300 Pompton Rd
Wayne, NJ 07470
973-720-2000
Fax: 973-720-2090
www.wpunj.edu
BOONES@wpunj.edu

Kathleen Woldrone, President
Warren Sandmann, Provost/SVP for Academic Affairs
Stephen Bolyai, VP for Administration & Finance
Offers a variety of services to students with disabilities including notetakers, extended testing time, counseling services, and special accommodations.

New Mexico

3343 Albuquerque Technical Vocational Institute
Special Services
525 Buena Vista Dr SE
Albuquerque, NM 87106
505-224-3000
Fax: 505-224-4684
TDD: 505-224-3262
www.cnm.edu
pauls@cnm.edu

Michael D. DeWitte, Chair
Mark Armijo, Vice Chair
Pauline J. Garcia, Board Member
Provides or coordinates services for students with all disabilities. For students with learning disabilities can arrange for special testing situations, notetaker/scribes, tape recorders, use of wordprocessors or other accommodations based on individual needs.

3344 College of Santa Fe
6401 Richards Ave.
Santa Fe, NM 87508
505-428-1000
Fax: 505-428-1204
www.sfcc.edu
theresa.garcia2@sfcc.edu

Linda Siegle, Chair
Martha Romero, Vice Chair
Janet Wise, Executive Director, Mark and PR
Provides services to the learning disabled.

3345 Eastern New Mexico University
Special Programs and Services
1500 S Ave K
Portales, NM 88130
575-562-1011
800-FOR-ENMU
www.enmu.edu
webmaster@enmu.edu

Brett Leach, Vice President
Jane Christensen, Vice President
Chad Lydick, Secretary/Treasurer
Four year college that provides programs for the learning disabled.

3346 Eastern New Mexico University: Roswell
PO Box 6000
Roswell, NM 88202-6000
575-624-7000
800-243-6687
Fax: 505-624-7350
www.roswell.enmu.edu
denise.mcghee@roswell.enmu.edu

Brett Leach, President
Jane Christensen, Vice President
Chase Sturdevant, Secretary/Treasurer
A public two-year college with a total of 2500 students. Has a one year certificate program designed to teach vocational and life skills to individuals with significant cognitive impairments.

3347 Institute of American Indian Arts
83 Avan Nu Po Rd
Santa Fe, NM 87508
505-424-2300
Fax: 505-988-6446
www.iaia.edu

Loren Kieve, Chairman
Brenda L. Kingery, Vice Chair
Dr. Robert Martin, President
A public two-year college with 8 special education students out of a total of 237.

3348 New Mexico Institute of Mining and Technology
801 Leroy Pl
Socorro, NM 87801
575-835-5434
800-428-8324
Fax: 575-835-5655
www.nmt.edu

Daniel H. Lopez, President
Mary Dezember, Vice President
Van Romero, Vice President
A public four-year college with 5 special education students out of a total of 1,128.

3349 New Mexico Junior College
1 Thunderbird Circle
Hobbs, NM 88240
575-392-4510
800-657-6260
Fax: 505-392-3668
www.nmjc.edu

Pat Chappelle, Chair
Ron Black, Secretary
Travis Glenn, Board Member
A public two-year college with 170 special education students out of a total of 2,438.

3350 New Mexico State University
PO Box 30001
Las Cruces, NM 88003
575-646-2432
800-662-6678
Fax: 575-646-7855
www.nmsu.edu
boffice@nmsu.edu

Angela Throneberry, SVP for Administration & Finance
Anna Price, Assoc. VP/Controller
Glen Haubold, Assoc. VP, Facilities & Services
A public four-year college with 230 registered students with disabilities out of a total of 12,922.

3351 Northern New Mexico Community College
921 N. Paseo de Oñate
Espanola, NM 87532
505-747-2100
Fax: 505-747-2180
www.nnmc.edu

Riosario Garcia, President
Alfred J. Herrera, Vice President
Dr. Pedro L Martinez, Provost/VP for Academic Affairs
If you have a learning disability, support services include: reading class, readers of tests, notetakers, taped texts, tutoring, math class, recorders for classroom use, library assistance, extra time for tests, self-esteem counseling, resume assistance and kurzweil reading computers.

3352 San Juan College
4601 College Blvd
Farmington, NM 87402
505-326-3311
Fax: 505-566-3790
www.sanjuancollege.edu
Toni Hopper Pendergrass, President
Dave Eppich, VP, Student Services
Barbara Ake, VP, Learning
A public two-year college with 28 special education students out of a total of 3,654.

3353 University of New Mexico
Main Campus
Albuquerque, NM 87131
505-277-0111
Fax: 505-277-7224
www.unm.edu
lssunm@unm.edu
Thomas A. Aguirre, Dean of Students
Kayla Russo, Administrative Assistant
Leonel A. Diaz, Jr., Special Projects Coordinator
Offers a variety of services to students with disabilities including notetakers, extended testing time, counseling services, and special accommodations.

3354 University of New Mexico/School of Medicine
Center for Development and Disability
The University of New Mexico
Albuquerque, NM 87131
505-277-0111
800-Call UNM
Fax: 505-272-5280
TDD: 505-272-0321
www.cdd.unm.edu
cdd@unm.edu
Cate McClain, Director
Melody Smith, Assistant Director
Elena Aguirre, Executive Director
The mission of the CDD is the full inclusion of people with disabilities and their families in their community by: engaging individuals in making life choices; partnering with communities to build resources; and improving systems of care.

3355 University of New Mexico: Los Alamos Branch
4000 University Dr
Los Alamos, NM 87544
505-662-5919
800-894-5919
Fax: 505-662-0344
www.la.unm.edu
Stephen T. Boerigter, Sc.D., Chair
Lisa Wismer, Campus Resources Director
Gayle Burns, Manager, Business Services
Offers a variety of services to students with disabilities including notetakers, extended testing time, counseling services, and special accommodations.

3356 University of New Mexico: Valencia Campus
280 La Entrada Rd
Los Lunas, NM 87131
505-925-8500
Fax: 505-925-8501
www.unm.edu/~unmvc/
Paul Luna, Chair
Alice Letteney, Executive Director
Robert G. Frank, President
A public two-year college with 57 special services students out of a total of 1,400.

3357 Western New Mexico University
PO Box 680
Silver City, NM 88062
575-538-6336
800-872-9668
Fax: 575-538-6278
www.wnmu.edu
Janice Baca-Argabright, President
Jack Crocker, Provost/VP for Academic Affairs
Sherri Bays, VP for Business Affairs
Offers a variety of services to students with disabilities including notetakers, extended testing time, counseling services, and special accommodations.

New York

3358 Academic Resource Program
Long Island University/C.W. Post Campus
720 Northern Blvd
Brookville, NY 11548
516-299-2000
Fax: 516-299-2126
www.liu.edu/CWPost/StudentLife/Services/
susan.rock@liu.edu
Beth Carson, Registratr
Ronald Edwards, Human Resources Officer
Patricia Demarest, Customer Relations Manager
A comprehensive, structured, fee-for-service, support program designed to teach undergraduate students with learning disabilities and/or ADHD skill and strategies that will help then achiece their academic potential in a university setting.

3359 Adelphi University
Disability Support Services
PO Box 701
1 South Ave
Garden City, NY 11530-701
516-877-3145
800-233-5744
Fax: 516-877-3139
TTY: 516-877-3138
www.adelphi.edu/
admissions@adelphi.edu
Robert B. Willumstad, Chair
Thomas F. Motamed, Vice Chair
Robert A. Scott, President
The Bridges to Adelphi Project is designed to enhance college life for students with nonverbal learning disabilities by providing help with organizational skills, time management, independent living skills and social skills training.

3360 Adirondack Community College
640 Bay Rd
Queensbury, NY 12804
518-743-2200
888-SUNY-ADK
Fax: 518-745-1433
www.sunyacc.edu/
admission@sunyacc.edu
Kristine Duffy, Ed.D., President
Sue Trumpick, Chief Information Officer
Kim Thomas, Administrative Assistant
A two-year community college that provides services to the learning disabled.

3361 Albert Einstein College of Medicine
1300 Morris Park Ave
Bronx, NY 10461
718-430-2000
Fax: 718-430-3989
www.einstein.yu.edu
helpdesk@yu.edu
Edward R. Burns, Executive Dean
Stephen G. Baum, Senior Associate Dean
Arlene Reisman, Executive Assistant
Provides evaluation and psychoeducational treatment to children and adults of normal intelligence, 21 years or older, who have serious reading difficulties.

3362 Bank Street College: Graduate School of Education
610 W 1112th St
New York, NY 10025-1898
212-875-4400
Fax: 212-875-4759
http://bankstreet.edu/graduate-school/
GradCourses@bnkst.edu
Yolanda Ferrell-Brown, Chair
Sue Kaplan, Vice Chair
Jeffrey I Sussman, Vice Chair
For learning disabled college students who are highly motivated to become teachers of children and youth with learning problems and who wish to earn a masters degree in Special Education.

3363 Binghamton University
4400 Vestal Parkway East
Binghamton, NY 13902   607-777-2000
                              Fax: 607-777-6893
                              TDD: 607-777-2686
                              www.binghamton.edu/
                              info@binghamton.edu
Harvey G. Stenger, President
Andrea Snyder, LD Specialist
Provides assistance to BU students with physical, learning
or other disabilities.

3364 Bramson Ort Technical Institute
69-30 Austin St
Forest Hills, NY 11375   718-261-5800
                              Fax: 718-575-5118
                              www.bramsonort.org
                  admissions_queens@bramsonort.edu
David Kanani, Ph.D. EECS, President
Robert Adelberg, Academic Dean
Angelina Marra, Financial Aid/Marketing Coor
Offers a variety of services to students with disabilities in-
cluding notetakers, extended testing time, counseling ser-
vices, and special accommodations.

3365 CUNY Queensborough Community College
222-05 56th Ave
Bayside, NY 11364   718-631-6262
                              Fax: 718-631-8539
                              www.qcc.cuny.edu
                          Admissions@qcc.cuny.edu
Dr. Diane Bova Call, President & Chair
Oluwadamisi Atanda, Vice Chairperson
Ellen F. Hartigan, Secretary
The Office of Services for Students with Disabilities (Science Building, Room 132) offers special assistance and
counseling to students with specific needs. The services offered include academic, vocational, psychological and rehabilitation counseling, as well as liasion with community
social agencies.

3366 Canisius College
Disability Support Service
2001 Main St
Buffalo, NY 14208-1098   716-883-7000
                              Fax: 716-888-2525
                              TDD: 716-888-3748
                              www.canisius.edu
                              info@canisius.edu
Edward Burke Carey, Chair
Ben K. Wells, MBA, Vice Chair
John J. Hurley, President
Four-year college offering services to students with physical
and cognitive disabilities.

3367 Cazenovia College
22 Sullivan St
Cazenovia, NY 13035-1085   315-655-3210
                              800-654-3210
                              Fax: 315-655-4000
                              www.cazenovia.edu
                          cazenovia@cazenovia.edu
Mark J Tierno, Special Services
Jesse Lott, Director
An independent college with a significant number of special
education students.

3368 Center for Spectrum Services: Ellenville
4 Yankee Pl
Ellenville, NY 12428   845-647-6464
                              Fax: 845-647-3456
                  www.centerforspectrumservices.org
                  mwerher@centerforspectrumservices.org
Marjorie S. Rovereto, President
Rick Regan, Vice President
Robert S. Casey, Treasurer

This center-based program is a school for preschool and
school-age children who are 3 through 8 eight years old and
have the educational classification of preschooler with a disability, autism, emotional disability or multiple disabilities.

3369 Center for the Advancement of Post Secondary Studies
Maplebrook School
5142 Route 22
Amenia, NY 12501   845-373-9511
                              Fax: 845-373-7029
                              www.maplebrookschool.org
                          admin@maplebrookschool.org
Mark J. Metzger, Chairman
Robert Audia, Vice Chair
Donna Konkolics, Head of School
A program based on students successfully completing the
goals and objectives designed to prepare them for integra-
tion into today's world. Through small group and individual-
ized instruction, the student will be assisted in reaching
his/her academic, social, vocational, and physical potential.

3370 Churchill School and Center
Programs for Children
301 E 29th St
New York, NY 10016   212-722-0610
                              Fax: 212-722-1387
                              www.churchillschool.com
                          wfederico@churchillschool.com
Cynthia Wainwrigh, President
Lauri Kien Kotcher, Vice President
Maryl Hosking, Secretary
Offers educational programs, professional development in
the field of learning disabilities, and advisory and referral
services to students, parents, teachers of general and special
education, and related service provides.

3371 Colgate University
Office Disabilities Services
13 Oak Dr
Hamilton, NY 13346   315-228-7000
                              Fax: 315-228-7831
                              www.colgate.edu
                          admission@mail.colgate.edu
Denis F. Cronin, Chair
Robert A. Kindler, Vice Chair
Jeffrey Herbst, President
Provides for a small body of liberal arts education that will
expand individual potential and ability to particpate effec-
tively in the society.

3372 College of New Rochelle: New Resources Division
Student Services
29 Castle Pl
New Rochelle, NY 10805   914-654-5000
                              800-933-5923
                              Fax: 914-654-5554
                              www.cnr.edu
                              info@cnr.edu
Elizabeth LeVaca, Chair
Judith Huntington, President
Gwen Adolph, Board Member
Offers a variety of services to students with disabilities in-
cluding notetakers, extended testing time, counseling ser-
vices, and special accommodations.

3373 College of Saint Rose
432 Western Ave
Albany, NY 12203   518-454-5111
                              800-637-8556
                              Fax: 518-438-3293
                              TDD: 1-800-637-85
                              www.strose.edu
                              hermannk@strose.edu
Carolyn J. Stefanco, President
Marcus Buckley, Coordinator Supported Education
Debra Liberatore-LeBlanc, Asst. to the President
Four year college that provides disabled students with ser-
vices and support.

3374 **College of Staten Island of the City University of New York**
2800 Victory Blvd
Staten Island, NY 10314   718-982-2000
Fax: 718-982-4002
TDD: 718-982-2515
www.csi.cuny.edu
venditti@postbox.csi.cuny.edu
William J. Fritz,PhD., President
Fred Naider,PhD, SVP for Academic Affairs/Provost
Susan L. Holak,PhD, Dean of the School of Business
A public four-year college with 33 special education students out of a total of 11,136. Priority registration, test accommodations and tutoring.

3375 **Columbia College**
Disability Services
116th Street and Broadway
New York, NY 10027   212-854-1754
Fax: 212-854-3448
www.columbia.edu
disability@columbia.edu
Jonathan D. Schiller, Chair
A'Lelia Bundles, Vice Chair
Lee C. Bollinger, President
Four-year college that offers disability services to its students.

3376 **Columbia-Greene Community College**
4400 State Route 23
Hudson, NY 12534   518-828-4181
Fax: 518-822-2015
www.sunycgcc.edu
Richard Brooks, Chair
Martin Smith, Vice Chair
James R. Campion, President
A public two-year college in upstate New York with an enrollment of about 1,800. Services available to students with a documented learning disability include various academic accommodations, peer tutoring and academic counselling. Six developmental courses are offered in reading, math, English, and study skills.

3377 **Concordia College: New York**
Connections
171 White Plains Rd
Bronxville, NY 10708   914-337-9300
Fax: 914-395-4500
www.concordia-ny.edu
ghg@concordia-ny.edu
Jean Hanson, Esq., Chair
John M. Pietruski, Jr., Vice Chair
Viji George, Ed.D., President

3378 **Cornell University**
Student Disability Services
420 C Cc Garden Avenue Ext
Ithaca, NY 14853   607-245-4636
Fax: 607-255-1562
TDD: 607-255-7665
www.cornell.edu
info@cornell.edu
Robert Harrison, Chair
Kent Fuchs, Provost
David J. Skorton, President
Cornell University is committed to ensuring that students with disabilities have equal access to all university programs and activities. Policy and procedures have been developed to provide students with as much independence as possible, to preserve confidentiality, and to provide students with disabilities the same exceptional opportunities available to all Cornell students.

3379 **Corning Community College**
1 Academic Dr
Corning, NY 14830   607-962-9222
800-358-7171
Fax: 607-962-9485
TDD: 607-962-9459
TTY: 607-962-9459
www.corning-cc.edu
northop@corning-cc.edu
Dr. Neil J. Milliken III, Chair
Carl H. Blowers, Vice Chair
Katherine P. Douglas, President
A public two-year community college. There are approximately 100 LD students out of a student body of 4,500. A variety of services are available to students with LD, including specialized advising and registration, individualized tutoring, academic advisoring, and accommodations. Also on campus: Kurzweil reading machines, voice activated word processing, etc.

3380 **Dowling College**
Program for Potentially Gifted
150 Idle Hour Blvd
Oakdale, NY 11769   631-244-3000
800-369-5464
Fax: 631-563-7831
www.dowling.edu
strached@dowling.edu
Michael P. Puorro, Chair
Gerald J. Curtin, Vice Chairman
Dr Norman R Smith, President
Academic program to help college students with LD develop strategies for success. They work one-on-one with graduate students.

3381 **Dutchess Community College**
53 Pendell Rd
Poughkeepsie, NY 12601-1595   845-431-8000
800-378-9707
Fax: 845-431-8981
www.sunydutchess.edu
webmaster@sunydutchess.edu
Thomas E. LeGrand, Chair
Vincent J. DiMaso, Vice Chair
Dr. Pamela Edington, President
A public two-year college with 45 special education students out of a total of 7,511.

3382 **Erie Community College: South Campus**
Special Education Department
4041 Southwestern Blvd
Orchard Park, NY 14127   716-851-1003
Fax: 716-851-1629
TDD: 716-851-1831
www.ecc.edu
adamsjm@ecc.edu
Jack Quinn, Counselor
William Reuter, CEO
A public two-year college with 200 special education students out of a total of 3,455.

3383 **Farmingdale State University**
2350 Broadhollow Rd
Farmingdale, NY 11735-1021   631-420-2000
Fax: 631-420-2689
TDD: 631-420-2623
www.farmingdale.edu
doo@farmingdale.edu
W Hubert Keen, Director
Kim Birnholz CRC, Counselor
Jonathan Gibralter, President
Our services are designed to meet the unique educational needs of currently enrolled students with documented permanent or temporary disabilities. The Office of Support Services is dedicated to the principle that equal opportunity be afforded each student to realize his/her fullest potential.

3384 Finger Lakes Community College
3325 Marvin Sands Drive
Canandaigua, NY 14424
585-394-3500
Fax: 585-394-5005
www.fingerlakes.edu
admissions@flcc.edu

Joan Geise, Chair
Donna Mihalik, Vice Chair
Barbara Risser, President
Provides services such as pre-admission counseling, academic advisement, tutorials, computer assistance, workshops, peer counseling and support groups. The college does not offer a formal program but aids students in arranging appropriate accommodations.

3385 Fordham University
Disabled Student Services
Room 201
Keating Hall
Bronx, NY 10458
718-817-1000
Fax: 718-367-7598
TDD: 718-817-0655
www.fordham.edu
disabilityservices@fordham.edu

Stephen Freedman, Ph.D., Provost
Jonathan Crystal, Associate Vice President
Diane Cuomo, Executive Admin Assistant
The Office of Disability Services collaborates with students, faculty and staff to ensure appropriate services for students with disabilities. The University will make reasonable acccommodations, and provide appropriate aids.

3386 Fulton-Montgomery Community College
2805 State Highway 67
Johnstown, NY 12095
518-736-3622
Fax: 518-762-4334
www.fmcc.suny.edu
efosmire@fmcc.suny.edu

Michael Pepe, Chair
Edmund C. Jasewicz, Vice Chairman
Dustin Swanger, Ed.D, President
A public two-year college with 76 special education students out of a total of 1,748.

3387 Gateway School of New York
Fl 6
211 W 61st St
New York, NY 10023
212-777-5966
Fax: 212-777-5794
www.gatewayschool.org
info@gatewayschool.org

Warren H. Feder, Chair
Kieran Claffey, Secretary
Hilary Woods Giuliano, Secretary
An ungraded lower school dedicated to helping children with learning disabilities develop the academic skills, learning strategies, social competence and self-confidence necessary to succeed.

3388 Genesee Community College
SUNY (State University of New York) Systems
1 College Rd
Batavia, NY 14020
585-343-0055
Fax: 585-343-4541
www.genesee.edu/
admissions@genesee.suny.edu

Maureen T. Marshall, Chairwoman
Diane Torcello, Vice Chairwoman
Dr. James Sunser, President
A public two-year college with 78 special education students out of a total of 3,212.

3389 Hamilton College
198 College Hill Rd
Clinton, NY 13323-1295
315-859-4011
Fax: 315-859-4083
TDD: 315-859-4294
www.hamilton.edu
rbellmay@hamilton.edu

Joan Stewart, President
Karen Leach, VP, Administration and Finance
Jan Risel, Secretary to the VP
Four year college that offfers services for learning disabled students.

3390 Harmony Heights
PO Box 569
Oyster Bay, NY 11771
516-922-4060
Fax: 516-922-6126
www.harmonyheights.org
eb@harmonyheightsschool.com

Denis Garbo, President
Peter Roach, Vice President
Ellen Benson ACSW PD, Executive Director
A therapeutic residential and day school serving girls with emotional needs that cannot be adequately served in the standard high school setting.

3391 Herkimer County Community College
100 Reservoir Rd
Herkimer, NY 13350
315-866-0300
888-GO-4-HCC
Fax: 315-866-7253
TDD: 888-GO4HCCC
www.hccc.ntcnet.com
coylemf@hcc.suny.edu

Isabella S. Crandall, Vice Chairperson
Ann Marie Murray, President
Mary Ellen Clark, Secretary
A public two-year college with approximately 200 documented disabled students. Tuition and fees: $2,450 (annual basis); overall enrollment 95-96: $2,445 (1,857 full time/588 part-time).

3392 Hofstra University
Program for Academic Learning Skills
212 Memorial Hall
Hempstead, NY 11549-1000
516-463-6600
Fax: 516-463-7070
www.hofstra.edu
pals@hofstra.edu

Janis M. Meyer, Chair
James E. Quinn, Vice Chair
Stuart Rabinowitz, President
Provides auxillary aids and compensatory services to certified learning disabled students who have been accepted to the University through regular admissions. These services are provided free of charge.

3393 Houghton College
Student Academic Services
1 Willard Ave
Houghton, NY 14744
585-567-9200
800-777-2556
Fax: 585-567-9572
www.houghton.edu
admission@houghton.edu

Bobbie Strand, Chair
Terry Slye, Vice Chair
Shirley Mullen, President
Four year college that provides academic support to disabled students.

3394 Hudson Valley Community College
Disabilities Resource Center
80 Vandenburgh Ave
Troy, NY 12180
518-629-4822
877-325-4822
Fax: 518-629-7586
TDD: 518-629-7596
TTY: 1 8-7 3-5 48
www.hvcc.edu
editor@hvcc.edu

Conrad H. Lang, Jr., Chairman
Neil J. Kelleher, Vice Chairman
Drew Matonak, President
A public two-year college with 28 special education students out of a total of 10,106.

3395 **Hunter College of the City University of New York**
Office for Students with Disabilities
695 Park Ave
New York, NY 10065   212-772-4000
Fax: 212-650-3456
TTY: 212-650-3230
www.hunter.cuny.edu
icitdir@hunter.cuny.edu
Jennifer J. Raab, President
Vita Rabinowitz, Provost and Vice President
Eija Ayravainen, VP
Provides services to over 250 students with learning disabilities. A learning disability is a disorder in one or more of the basic psychological processes involved in understanding or in using spoken or written language.

3396 **Iona College**
College Assistance Program
715 North Ave
New Rochelle, NY 10801   914-633-2077
800-231-IONA
Fax: 914-633-2642
www.iona.edu
lrobertello@iona.edu
Joseph E. Nyre, PhD, President
Maryellen Callaghan, Senior Policy Advisor
Charles J. Carlson, Vice Provost for Student Life
Offers a comprehensive support program for students with learning disabilities. CAP is designed to encourage success by providing instruction tailored to individual strenghts and needs.

3397 **Ithaca College**
110 Towers Concourse
953 Danby Road
Ithaca, NY 14850   607-274-1005
Fax: 607-274-3957
www.ithaca.edu/sds
sas@ithaca.edu
Thomas H. Grape, Chair
David A. Lebow, Vice Chair
Thomas R. Rochon, President

3398 **Ithaca College: Speech and Hearing Clinic**
953 Danby Road
Ithaca, NY 14850   607-274-3011
Fax: 607-274-3237
www.ithaca.edu
webmaster@ithaca.edu
Thomas H. Grape, Chair
David A. Lebow, Vice Chair
Thomas R. Rochon, President
Offers a variety of services to students with disabilities including notetakers, extended testing time, counseling services, and special accommodations.

3399 **Jamestown Community College**
State University of New York Systems
PO Box 20
525 Falconer Street
Jamestown, NY 14702-20   716-665-1000
800-388-8557
Fax: 716-665-9110
www.sunyjcc.edu
admissions@mail.sunyjcc.edu
Wally Huckno, Chair
Dale Robbins, Esq., Vice Chair
Dr. Cory Duckworth, President
A public two-year college with 41 special education students out of a total of 4,541.

3400 **Jefferson Community College**
Jefferson Community College
1220 Coffeen St
Watertown, NY 13601   315-786-2200
888-435-6522
Fax: 315-786-0158
www.sunyjefferson.edu
webmaster@sunyjefferson.edu
Michael W. Crowley, Chairman
James P. Scordo, Vice Chair
Carol Mc Coy, President
A public two-year college whose focus is teaching and learning. Through educational excellence, innovative services and community partnerships. Jefferson advances the quality of life of our students and community.

3401 **John Jay College of Criminal Justice of the City University of New York**
524 W 59th St
New York, NY 10019   212-237-8000
Fax: 212-237-8901
TDD: 212-237-8233
www.jjay.cuny.edu
admiss@jjay.cuny.edu
Benno C. Schmidt, Chair
Philip Alfonso Berry, Vice Chair
Jeremy Teravis, President
An independent two-year college with 67 special education students out of a total of 7,912.

3402 **Kildonan School**
425 Morse Hill Rd
Amenia, NY 12501   845-373-8111
Fax: 845-373-9793
www.kildonan.org
admissions@kildonan.org
Christina Lang, Chair
Richard S. Berg, Vice Chair
Kevin Pendergast, Headmaster
Offers a fully accredited College Preparatory curriculum. The school is co-educational, enrolling boarding students in Grades 6-Postgraduate and day students in Grade 2-Postgraduate. Provides daily one-on-one Orton-Gillingham tutoring to build skills in reading, writing, and spelling. Daily independent reading and writing work reinforces skills and improves study habits. Interscholastic sports, horseback riding, clubs and community service enhance self-confidence.

3403 **Learning Disabilities Program**
ADELPHI UNIVERSITY
PO Box 701
Garden City, NY 11530-701   516-877-4710
800-ADELPHI
Fax: 516-877-4711
http://academics.adelphi.edu/ldprog
lrp@adelphi.edu
Susan Spencer Farinacci, Assistant Dean/Director
Janet Cohen, Assistant Director
The programs professional staff, all with advanced degrees, provide individual tutoring and counseling to learning disabled students who are completely mainstream in the University.

3404 **Manhattan College: Specialized Resource Center**
4513 Manhattan College Parkway
Riverdale, NY 10471   718-862-8000
800-MC2-XCEL
Fax: 718-862-7808
www.manhattan.edu
Kenneth A. Rathgeber, Chairman
Dennis Malloy, Vice Chair
Brennan O'Donnell, Ph.D, President
The Specialized Resource Center serves all students with special needs including individuals with temporary disabilities, such as those resulting from injury or surgery. The mission of the center is to ensure educational opportunity for all students with special needs by providing access to full participation in all aspects of the campus life.

3405 **Maplebrook School**
Academic Program
5142 Route 22
Amenia, NY 12501   845-373-9511
Fax: 845-373-7029
www.maplebrookschool.org
admin@maplebrookschool.org

Mark J. Metzger, Chairman
Robert Audia, Vice Chair
Donna Konkolics, Head of School
The school offers several levels of academic achievement toward which a student may strive. Our curriculum follows the New York State guidelines, the teachers are trained in a multi-sensory approach and provide a small, nurturing classroom in which each student can reach their full potential.

3406 Maria College
700 New Scotland Ave
Albany, NY 12208

518-482-3111
Fax: 518-438-7170
www.mariacollege.edu
laurieg@mariacollege.edu

Frederic M. Stutzman, Chairman
Jerry Jennings, Vice Chair
Dr. Lea Johnson, President
An independent two-year college with 13 special education students out of a total of 875.

3407 Marist College
Learning Disabilities Support Program
3399 North Rd
Poughkeepsie, NY 12601

845-575-3000
Fax: 845-471-6213
www.marist.edu
specserv@marist.edu

Ellen M. Hancock, Chair
Ross A. Mauri, Vice Chair
Dennis J. Murray, President
Provides a comprehensive range of academic support services and accommodations which promote the full integration of students with disabilities into the mainstream college environment.

3408 Marymount Manhattan College
Academic Access and Learning Disabilities Program
221 E 71st St
New York, NY 10021

212-517-0400
Fax: 212-517-0567
www.mmm.edu
jbonomo@mmm.edu

Hope Knight, Chair
Judson R. Shaver, President
Ronald J. Yoo, Secretary
The College's program for students with learning disabilities is designed to provide a structure that fosters academic success.

3409 Medaille College
Disability Services Department
18 Agassiz Cir
Buffalo, NY 14214-2695

716-880-2000
800-292-1582
Fax: 716-884-0291
www.medaille.edu
sageadmissions@medaille.edu

Charles E. Morgan, Chair
Michael J. Moley, Vice Chair
Richard T. Jurasek, President
Offers a variety of services to students with disabilities including notetakers, extended testing time, counseling services, and special accommodations.

3410 Mercy College
Star Program
555 Broadway
Dobbs Ferry, NY 10522

914-674-7200
877-MERCY-GO
Fax: 914-674-7395
www.mercy.edu/
admissions@merlin.mercynet.edu

Gary W. Brown, Chair
Joseph Gantz, Vice Chair
Timothy L. Hall, President
Helps people with learning disabilities.

3411 Mohawk Valley Community College
1101 Sherman Dr
Utica, NY 13501

315-792-5400
Fax: 315-731-5858
TDD: 315-792-5413
www.mvcc.edu
dowsland@mvcc.edu

David Mathis, Chair
William S. Calli, Vice Chair
Randall J. VanWagoner, President
MVCC'S LD program is staffed by a half time LD specialist. Service provided to students with learning disabilities include advocacy, information and referral to on and off campus services, testing accommodations, taped materials, loaner tape recorders and note takers.

3412 Molloy College
1000 Hempstead Avenue
Kellenberg Hall
Rockville Centre, NY 11571-5002

516-678-5000
888-4-MOLLOY
Fax: 516-678-2284
www.molloy.edu
info@molloy.edu

Daniel T. Henry, Chair
Laura A. Cassell, Vice Chair
Drew Bogner, President
STEEP (Success Through Expanded Education), is a program specifically designed to assist students with learning disabilities and enable them to become successful students. The program offers the student the opportunities to learn techniques which alleviate some of their problems. Special emphasis is directed toward the development of positive self-esteem.

3413 Nassau Community College
Disabled Support Department
1 Education Dr
Garden City, NY 11530-6793

516-572-7501
Fax: 516-572-9874
TTY: 513-572-7617
www.ncc.edu
schimsj@ncc.edu

Jorge Gardyn, Chair
Kathy Weiss, Vice Chair
Dr. Kenneth Saunders, President
Our goal is to help students achieve success while they are attending Nassau Community College by learning to become their own advocates through talking with their professors about their disability and the accommodations they need for the course.

3414 Nazareth College of Rochester
Disability Support Services
4245 East Ave
Rochester, NY 14618

585-389-2525
Fax: 716-586-2452
www.naz.edu
web@naz.edu

James Constanza, Chair
Sergio Esteban, Vice Chair
Daan Braveman, President
Four-year college that offers students with a learning disablility support and services.

3415 New York City College of Technology
Student Support Services Program
300 Jay St
Brooklyn, NY 11201

718-260-5500
Fax: 718-260-5631
TTY: 718-260-5443
www.citytech.cuny.edu/
connect@citytech.cuny.edu

Russell K. Hotzler,Phd, President
Bonne August, Ph.D., Provost/VP for Academic Affairs
Miguel F. Cairol, VP for Admin and Finance

The Student Support Services Program, located in A-237, provides comprehensive services to students with disabilities. The array of interventions includes counseling, tutorials, workshops, use of computer lab with adaptive software, testing accommodations, sign-language interpreters, captioning, and implementation of accommodations as per documentation.

3416 New York Institute of Technology: Old Westbury
Northern Boulevard
PO Box 8000
Old Westbury, NY 11568-8000

516-686-1000
800-345-NYIT
Fax: 516-686-7789
www.nyit.edu
eguillano@nyit.edu

Linda Davila, Chair
Bharat B. Bhatt, Vice chair
Edward Guiliano, President & CEO
Offers the Vocational Independence Progran for students who have significant learning disabilities.

3417 New York University
Henry and Lucy Moses Center
70,WashingtonSquare South
New York, NY 10012

212-998-2500
Fax: 212-995-4114
www.nyu.edu/csd
lc83@nyu.edu

Martin Lipton, Chair
Laurence D. Fink, Vice Chair
John Sexton, President
The Henry and Lucy Moses Center for Students with Disabilities (CSD) functions to determine qualified disability status and to assist students in obtaining appropriate accommodations and services. CSD operates according to the Independent Living Philosophy, and thus strives in its policies and practices to empower each student to become an independent as possible. Our services are designed to encourage independence, backed by a strong system of supports.

3418 New York University Medical Center
Learning Diagnostic Program
550 First Avenue
New York, NY 10016

212-263-7300
Fax: 212-263-7721
www.med.nyu.edu

Kenneth G. Langone, Chair
Laurence D. Fink, Vice Chair
John Sexton, President
Assessment team, neurology, neuro-psychology, psychiatry services are offered.

3419 Niagara County Community College
3111 Saunders Settlement Rd
Sanborn, NY 14132

716-614-6222
Fax: 716-614-5954
www.niagaracc.suny.edu

Dr. James P. Klyczek, President
The College provides reasonable accommodations for students with disabilties, including those with specific learning disabilities. Students with learning disabilities must provide documentation by a qualified professional that proves thry are eligible for accommodations.

3420 Niagara University
Disability Services
1st Floor
Seton Hall
Niagara University, NY 14109

716-285-1212
800-462-2111
Fax: 716-286-8063
www.niagara.edu
kadams@niagara.edu

Jeffery R. Holzschuh, Chair
Michael J. Carroll, Vice Chair
James J. Maher, President

Reasonable accommodations are provided to students with disabilities based on documentation of disability. Depending on how the disability impacts the individual, reasonable accommodations may include extended time on tests taken in a separate location with appropriate assistance, notetakes or use of a tape recorder in class, interpreter, textbooks and course materials in alternative format, as well as other academic and non-academic accommodations.

3421 Norman Howard School
Education Enterprise of New York
275 Pinnacle Rd
Rochester, NY 14623

585-334-8010
Fax: 585-334-8073
www.normanhoward.org
info@normanhoward.org

Rosemary Hodges, Co-Head of School
Linda Lawrence, Co-Head of School
Joe Martino, Executive Director & CEO
An independent co-educational day school for students with learning disabilities in grades 5-12. An approved special education program by the New York State Education Department and accredited by the New York Association of Independent Schools. Program supports many youngsters with various types of learning disabilities, including dyslexia, non-verbal LD, Asperger's Syndrome, anxiety and ADHD.

3422 North Country Community College
State University of New York
23 Santanoni Ave
PO Box 89
Saranac Lake, NY 12983

518-891-2915
888-879-6222
Fax: 518-891-2915
www.nccc.edu
admissions@nccc.edu

Fred Smith, Learning Lab/Malone
Scott Lambert, Enrollment/Financial Aid Counsel
Dr. Steve Tyrell, President
Located in the Adirondack Olympic Region of northern New York, NCCC is committed to providing a challenging and supportive environment where the aspirations of all can be realized. The college provides a variety of services for students with special needs which includes: specialized advisement, tutors and supplemental instruction, specialized accommodations, technology and equipment to accommodate learning disabilities and other resources.

3423 Onondaga Community College
Disability Services Office
4585 W Seneca Turnpike
Syracuse, NY 13215

315-498-2622
Fax: 315-498-2977
www.sunyocc.edu
occinfo@sunyocc.edu

Margaret M. O'Connell, Chair
Allen J. Naples, Vice Chair
Casey Crabill, President
A public two-year college with 650 students with disabilities.

3424 Orange County Community College
115 South St
Middletown, NY 10940-6437

845-341-4444
Fax: 845-341-4998
www.sunyorange.edu

Joan H. Wolfe, Chair
Helen G. Ullrich, Vice Chair
Dr. William Richards, President
The Office of Special Services for the Disabled provides support services to meet the individual needs of students with disabilities. Such accommodations include oral testing, extended time testing, tape recorded textbooks, writing lab, note-takers and others. Pre-admission counseling ensures accessibility for the qualified student.

3425 Purchase College State University of New York
Special Services Office
735 Anderson Hill Rd
Purchase, NY 10577   914-251-6020
                            Fax: 914-251-6019
                            www.purchase.edu

Thomas J. Schwarz, President
Donna Siegmann, Coordinator Supported Education
Offers a variety of services to students with disabilities including note takers, extended testing time, counseling services, and special accommodations.

3426 Queens College City University of New York
Special Services Office
65-30 Kissena Blvd
Flushing, NY 11367   718-997-5000
                            Fax: 718-997-5895
                            TDD: 718-997-5870
                            www.qc.cuny.edu/
                            christopher_rosa@qc.edu

Evangelos Gizis, Interim President
Elizabeth Hendrey, Provost/VP for Academic Affairs
William Keller, VP for Finance & Administration
Services include tutoring and notetaking, accommodating testing alternatives, counseling, academic and vocational advisement, as well as diagnostic assessments in order to pinpoint specific deficits.

3427 Readiness Program
New York Institute for Special Education
999 Pelham Pkwy
Bronx, NY 10469   718-519-7000
                            Fax: 718-231-9314
                            www.nyise.org
                            bkappen@nyise.org

Bernadette M Kappen PhD, Executive Director
A pre-school that helps children who are developmentally delayed from ages 3 to 5. They have disabilities that include speech impairment, mild orthopedic impairment, or a learning or emotional disability. By providing specialized instruction, intensive therapies and early intervention many are able to be mainstreamed or are placed in a least restrictive educational environment when they reach the age of five.

3428 Rensselaer Polytechnic Institute
110 8th St
Troy, NY 12180-3590   518-276-6000
                            800-448-6562
                            Fax: 518-276-4072
                            www.rpi.edu
                            hamild@rpi.edu

Shirley Ann Jackson, Disabled Student Services
Claude Rounds, VP, Administration Division
An independent four-year college with 53 learning disabled students out of a total of 6,000.

3429 Rochester Business Institute
1630 Portland Ave
Rochester, NY 14621   585-266-0430
                            888-741-4271
                            Fax: 585-266-8243
                            www.rochester-institute.com
                            dpfluke@cci.edu

Carl Silvio, President
Jim Rodriguez, Admissions Representative
An independent two-year college with 12 special education students out of a total of 528.

3430 Rochester Institute of Technology
Structured Monitoring Program
1 Lomb Memorial Drive
Rochester, NY 14623-5603   585-475-2411
                            Fax: 585-475-2215
                            www.rit.edu
                            smacst@rit.edu

Lisa Fraser, Chair Leraning Support Services
Pamela Lloyd, Disability Services Coordinator
Albert Simone, President

An independent four-year college offers a wide variety of accommodations and support services to students with documented disabilities.

3431 Rockland Community College
145 College Rd
Suffern, NY 10901   845-574-4000
                            Fax: 845-574-4424
                            www.sunyrockland.edu

Dr. Cliff L. Wood, President
Joseph Marra, Assoc. VP, Finance/Controller
Dr. Nayyer Hussain, VP for Admin & Finance
A public two-year college with 300 special education students out of a total of 5,500. The office of Disability Services provides a variety of support services tailored to meet the individual needs and learning styles of students with documented learning disabilities.

3432 Rose F Kennedy Center
Albert Einstein College of Medicine
1410 Pelham Pkwy S
Bronx, NY 10461-1116   718-430-8522
                            Fax: 718-904-1162
                            www.einstein.yu.edu.com

Robert Marion, Director
Mission is to help children with disabilities reach their full potential and to support parents in their efforts to get the best care, education, and treatment for their children.

3433 Ryken Educational Center
Xaverian High School
7100 Shore Rd
Brooklyn, NY 11209   718-836-7100
                            www.xaverian.org
                            ctrasborg@xaverian.org

Lawrence Harvey, Chair
Daniel E. Skala, Vice chair
Robert B. Alesi, President
Provides programs and services for high school students of average, or above-average intelligence who have specific learning disabilities. Its mission is to challenge and support learning disabled young men so that they achieve academically at their intellectual level. Our goal is to turn them into effective life-long learners who will go on to college.

3434 SUNY Canton
34 Cornell Dr
Campus Center 233
Canton, NY 13617-1098   315-386-7011
                            800-388-7123
                            Fax: 315-379-3877
                            TDD: 315-386-7943
                            www.canton.edu
                            leev@canton.edu

Zvi Szafran, President
Karen Spellacy, Provost/VP Academic Affairs
Courtney Bish, Dean of Students
Four year state college that provides resources and services to learning disabled students.

3435 SUNY Cobleskill
142 Schenectady Ave
State Route 7
Cobleskill, NY 12043   518-255-5011
                            800-295-8988
                            Fax: 518-255-6430
                            TDD: 518-255-5454
                            TTY: 518-255-6500
                            www.cobleskill.edu/
                            dss@cobleskill.edu

Dr. Debra H. Thatcher, President
Carol Bishop, VP for Business & Finance
Bonnie Martin, VP for Operations
A public two-year college with a Bachelor of Technology component in agriculture. Approximately 170 students identify themselves as having a learning disability out of the 2,000 total population. Tuition $3,500 in state/$8,300 out of state. Academic support services and accommodations for documented LD students.

3436   SUNY Institute of Technology: Utica/Rome
100 Seymour Road
Utica, NY 13502

315-792-7500
866-278-6948
Fax: 315-792-7837
www.sunyit.edu
admissions@sunyit.edu

Robert E. Geer, President
William W. Durgin, Provost
Upper division bachelor's degree in a variety of professional and technical majors; masters degree and continuing educational coursework is also available.

3437   Sage College
140 New Scotland Ave
Albany, NY 12208

518-244-2000
Fax: 578-292-1910
www.sage.edu
chowed@sage.edu

Dr. Susan Scrimshaw, President
Terry S. Weiner, Provost
Kevin R. Stoner, Associate Provost
Four year college that offers services to students with a learning disability.

3438   Schenectady County Community College
Disability Services Department
78 Washington Ave
Schenectady, NY 12305

518-381-1200
Fax: 518-346-0379
www.sunysccc.edu

Ann Fleming Brown, Chair
Dr. William Levering, Vice Chair
Martha Asselin, Ph.D., President
Access for All program is designed to make programs and facilities accessible to all students in pursuit of their academic goals. Disabled Student Services seeks to ensure accessible educational opportunities in accordance with individual needs. Offers general support services and program services such as: exam assistance, special scheduling, adaptive equipment, readers, taping assistance and more.

3439   Schermerhorn Program
New York Institute for Special Education
999 Pelham Pkwy N
Bronx, NY 10469-4905

718-519-7000
Fax: 718-231-9314
www.nyise.org
bkappen@nyise.org

Bernadette M Kappen PhD, Executive Director
It offers diverse educational services to meet the needs of children who are legally blind, from the ages of 5 to 21. Students participate in individually designed academic and modified academic programs that emphasize independence.

3440   Siena College
515 Loudon Rd
Loudonville, NY 12211

518-785-6537
888-AT-SIENA
Fax: 518-783-4293
www.siena.edu
jpellegrini@siena.edu

Howard S. Foote, Chair
John F. Murray, Vice Chair
Fr. Kevin Mullen, President
Four year college that offers programs for the learning disabled.

3441   St. Bonaventure University
Teaching & Learning Center
3261 West State Road
St Bonaventure, NY 14778

716-375-2000
800-462-5050
Fax: 716-375-2072
www.sbu.edu
nmatthew@sbu.edu

Raymond C. Dee, Chair
Robert J. Daughtery, Vice Chair
Margaret Carney, President

Catholic University in the Franciscan tradition. Independent coeducational institution offering programs through its schools of arts and sciences, business administration, education and journalism and mass communication. 2500 students, tuition $16,210, room and board $6,190.

3442   St. Lawrence University
23 Romoda Dr
Canton, NY 13617

800-285-1856
Fax: 315-229-5502
www.stlawu.edu
jmeagher@mail.stlawu.edu

William L. Fox, President
Liv Regosin, Director of Advising
The Office of Special Needs is here to ensure that all students with disabilities can freely and actively participate in all facets of University life, to coordinate support services and programs that enable students with disabilities to reach their educational potential, and to increase the level of awareness among all members of the University so that students with disabilites are able to perform at a level limited only by their abilities, not their disabilities.

3443   St. Thomas Aquinas College
Pathways
125 Route 340
Sparkill, NY 10976

845-398-4000
Fax: 845-359-8136
www.stac.edu
pathways@stac.edu

Lanny S. Cohen, Chair
Joseph McSweeny, Vice Chair
Margaret Fitzpatrick, President
Comprehensive support program for selected college students with learning disabilites and/or ADHD. Services include individual professional mentoring, study groups, academic counseling, priority registration, assistive technology, and a specialized summer program prior to the first semester.

3444   State University of New York College Technology at Delhi
2 Main St
Delhi, NY 13753

607-746-4000
800-96-DELHI
Fax: 607-746-4004
www.delhi.edu
weinbell@delhi.edu

Dr. Candace Vancko, President
Carol Bishop, VP Business and Finance
Dr. John Nader, Provost
Provide services for students with disabilities. Alternate test-taking arrangements, adapted equipment, assistive technology, accessibility information, note taking services, reading services, tutorial assistance, interpreting services, accessble parking and elevators, sounseling, guidance and support, refferral information and advocacy services, workshops and support groups.

3445   State University of New York College at Brockport
State University of New York
350 New Campus Dr
Brockport, NY 14420

585-395-5409
800-382-8447
Fax: 585-395-5291
TDD: 585-395-5409
www.brockport.edu
osdoffic@brockport.edu

John R. Halstead, PhD, President
Mary Ellen Zuckerman, Provost/VP Academic Affairs
James Willis, VP Administration and Finance
Provides support and assistance to students with medical, physical, emotional or learning disabilities, specially those experiencing problems in areas such as academic environment.

3446 State University of New York College of Agriculture and Technology
State Route 7
Cobleskill, NY 12043
518-255-5011
800-295-8988
Fax: 518-255-6430
TDD: 518-255-5454
TTY: 518-255-5454
www.cobleskill.edu
labarno@cobleskill.edu

Dr. Debra H. Thatcher, President
Carol Bishop, VP for Business& Finance
Bonnie Martin, VP for Operations
The primary objective is to develop and maintain a supportive campus environment that promotes academic achievement and personal growth for students with disabilities. Services provide by the office are based on each student's documentation and are tailored to each student's unique individual needs.

3447 State University of New York: Albany
1400 Washington Ave
Albany, NY 12222
518-442-3300
Fax: 518-442-5400
TDD: 518-442-3366
www.albany.edu

Robert Jones, President
Susan D. Phillips, Provost/VP Academic Affairs
Leanne Wirkkula, Chief of Staff
4-year public University.

3448 State University of New York: Buffalo
Special Services Department
1300 Elmwood Ave
Buffalo, NY 14222
716-878-4000
Fax: 716-645-3473
TTY: 716-645-2616
www.buffalostate.edu
savinomr@buffalostate.edu

Katherine Conway-Turner, President
Denise K. Ponton, Provost
Bonita R. Durand, Chief of Staff
The Office of Disability Services (ODS) is the University at Buffalo's center for coordinating services and accommodations to ensure accessiblity and usability of all programs, services and activities of UB by people with disabilities, and is a resource for information and advocacy toward their full participation in all aspects of campus life.

3449 State University of New York: Geneseo College
1 College Cir
Geneseo, NY 14454
585-245-5000
Fax: 585-245-5032
http://disability.geneseo.edu
web@geneseo.edu

Carol S. Long, President
Dr. Savi Iyer, Dean of Curriculum
To provide qualified students with disabilities, whether temporary or permanent, equal and comprehensive access to college-wide programs, services, and campus facilities by offering academic support, advisement, and removal of architectural and attitudinal barriers.

3450 State University of New York: Oswego
Disability Services Office
7060 Route 104
Oswego, NY 13126-3599
315-312-2500
Fax: 315-312-2943
www.oswego.edu
dss@oswego.edu

Deborah F. Stanley, President
Lorrie Clemo, VP for Academic Affairs/Provost
Nicholas Lyons, VP for Administration & Finance
A public four-year college of arts and sciences currently serving 140 students identified with disabling conditions. Total enrollment is approximately 8,000. Full time coordinator of academic support services for students with disabilities works with students on an individual basis.

3451 State University of New York: Plattsburgh
Student Support Services
101 Broad St
Plattsburgh, NY 12901
518-564-2000
Fax: 518-564-2807
www.plattsburgh.edu
michele.carpentier@plattsburgh.edu

John Ettling, President
Keith Tyo, Executive Assistant
Dawn Short, Secretary
Academic support program funded by the United States Department of Education. Staffed by caring and commited professional whose mission is to provide services for students with disabilities.

3452 State University of New York: Potsdam
44 Pierrepont Avenue
Potsdam, NY 13676
315-267-2000
Fax: 315-267-3268
TDD: 315-267-2071
TTY: 315-267-2071
www.potsdam.edu
housese@potsdam.edu

H.Carl McCall, Chair
Samuel L. Stanley, President
Nancy L. Zimpher, Chancellor
A public four-year college with approximately 200 students with disabilities out of a total of 4,000.

3453 Stony Brook University
Disability Support Services
128 Educational Communications Ctr
Stony Brook, NY 11794
631-632-6000
Fax: 631-632-6747
TTY: 631-632-6748
www.sunysb.edu
dss@notes.cc.sunysb.edu

H.Carl McCall, Chair
Samuel L. Stanley, President
Nancy L. Zimpher, Chancellor
The Office of Disability Support Services provides assistance for both students and employees. It coordinates advocacy and support services for students with disabilities in their academic and student life activities. Assuring campus accessibility, assisting with academic accommodations and providing assistive devices are important components of the programs.

3454 Suffolk County Community College: Ammerman
Special Services
533 College Rd
Selden, NY 11784-2899
631-451-4045
Fax: 631-451-4473
TTY: 631-451-4041
www.sunysuffolk.edu

Dafny Irizarry, Chair
Dr. Shaun L. McKay, President
Bryan Lilly, Secretary
Office of services for students with disabilities.

3455 Suffolk County Community College: Eastern Campus
Speonk-Riverhead Rd
Riverhead, NY 11901
631-548-2500
Fax: 631-369-2641
www.sunysuffolk.edu

Dafny Irizarry, Chair
Dr. Shaun L. McKay, President
Bryan Lilly, Secretary
The Eastern Campus is an accessible, open admissions institution. Services are provided to learning disabled students to allow them the same or equivalent educational experiences as nondisabled students.

3456 Suffolk County Community College: Western Campus
Crooked Hill Rd
Brentwood, NY 11717
631-851-6700
Fax: 631-851-6509
www.sunysuffolk.edu

Dafny Irizarry, Chair
Dr. Shaun L. McKay, President
Bryan Lilly, Secretary
The goal of Suffolk Community College with regard to students with disabilities is to equalize educational opportunities by minimizing physical, psychological and learning barriers. We attempt to provide as typical a college experience as is possible, encouraging students to achieve academically through the provision of special services, auxillary aids, or reasonable program modifications.

3457 Sullivan County Community College
Learning & Student Development Services
112 College Rd
Loch Sheldrake, NY 12759   845-434-5750
                                         800-577-5243
                                         Fax: 845-434-4806
                                         www.sullivan.suny.edu

Russ Heyman, Chair
Lyman Holmes, Vice Chair
Patricia Adams, Trustee
SCCC is fully committed to institutions accessability for individuals with disabilities. Students who wish to obtain particular services or accommodations should communicate their needs and concerns as early as possible. These may include, but are not limited to, extended time for tests, oral examinations, reader and notetaker services, campus maps, and elevator privileges. Books on tape may be ordered through recordings for the blind. Appropriate documentation needed.

3458 Syracuse University
Services For Students with Disabilities
900 South Crouse Ave
Syracuse, NY 13244   315-443-1870
                                         Fax: 315-443-4410
                                         TDD: 315-443-1312
                                         www.syracuse.edu
                                         dtwillia@syr.edu

Richard L. Thompson, Chair
Joanne F. Alper, Vice Chair
James D. Kuhn, Vice Chair
The office of disability services provides and coordinates services for students with documented disabilities. Students must provide current documentation of their disability in order to receive disability services and reasonable accommodations.

3459 The Gow School
2491 Emery Road
P.O. Box 85
South Wales, NY 14139-0085   716-652-3450
                                         Fax: 716-652-3457
                                         www.gow.org

M. Bradley Rogers, Jr., Headmaster
Boarding school for boys, grades 7-12, with dyslexia and other language based learning disabilities.

3460 Trocaire College
360 Choate Ave
Buffalo, NY 14220-2094   716-826-1200
                                         Fax: 716-828-6107
                                         www.trocaire.edu

Paul Hurley, President
An independent two-year college with 3 special education students out of a total of 1,056.

3461 Ulster County Community College
Student Support Services
491 Cottekill Rd
Stone Ridge, NY 12484   845-687-5000
                                         800-724-0833
                                         Fax: 845-687-5292
                                         www.sunyulster.edu

William L. Spearman, Chair
Timothy J. Sweeney, Vice Chair
Dr. Donald C Katt, President

The Student Support Services program promotes student success for students who are academically disadvantaged, economically disadvantaged, first-generation college students, and or students with disabilities. The goals of the program are to increase the retention, graduation, and transfer rates of those enrolled.

3462 University of Albany
1400 Washington Ave.
Albany, NY 12222   518-442-3300
                                         Fax: 518-442-3583
                                         TDD: 518-442-3366
                                         www.albany.edu
                                         cmalloch@uamail.albany.edu

Robert J. Jones, President
Leanne Wirkkula, Chief of Staff
Susan Supple, Senior Assistant to President
Offers a full time Learning Disability Specialist to work with students that have learning disabilities and or attention deficit disorder. The specialist offers individual appointments to develop study and advocacy skills.

3463 Utica College
1600 Burrstone Rd
Utica, NY 13502   315-792-3111
                                         Fax: 315-223-2504
                                         www.utica.edu
                                         admiss@utica.edu

Kateri Henkel, Learning Services Director
Provides students with disabilities individualized learning accommodations designed to meet the academic needs of the student. Counseling support and the development of new strategies for the learning challenges posed by college level work are an integral part of the services offered through Academic Support Services.

3464 Van Cleve Program
The New York Institute for Special Education
999 Pelham Pkwy
Bronx, NY 10469   718-519-7000
                                         Fax: 718-231-9314
                                         www.nyise.org

Bernadette M Kappen PhD, Executive Director
Thomas Bergett, Ph.D, Assistant Executive Director
The children of this program have emotional or learning difficulties. Our goal is to reduce the behavioral and learning deficits of students by providing academic and social skills necessary to enter less restrictive programs.

3465 Vassar College
124 Raymond Ave
Box 9
Poughkeepsie, NY 12604-9   845-437-7400
                                         Fax: 845-437-7187
                                         TTY: 845-437-5458
                                         www.vassar.edu
                                         info@vassar.edu

Frances D Fergusson, Director
Milbrey Rennie Taylor, President
Matthew Vassar, Founder
Offers a variety of services to students with disabilities including note takers, extended testing time, counseling services, and special accommodations.

3466 Wagner College
1 Campus Rd
Staten Island, NY 10301   718-390-3100
                                         800-221-1010
                                         Fax: 718-390-3467
                                         www.wagner.edu

Dr. Richard Guarasci, President
Pat Fitzpatrick, Assistant to the President
An independent four-year college with 25 special education students out of a total of 1,272. There is an additional fee for the special education program in addition to the regular tuition.

3467   Westchester Community College
75 Grasslands Rd
Valhalla, NY 10595   914-606-6600
                                   Fax: 914-785-6540
                                   www.sunywcc.edu

Joseph N. Hankin, President
Gloria Leon, Director
Students with Disabilities parallels the mission of WCC to
be accessable, community centered, comprehensive, adaptable and dedicated to lifelong learning for all students. Full
participation for students with disabilities is encouraged.

3468   Xaverian High School
Legacy Program
7100 Shore Rd
Brooklyn, NY 11209   718-836-7100
                                   www.xaverian.org
                                   ctrasborg@xaverian.org

Lawrence Harvey, Chair
Daniel E. Skala, Vice Chair
Robert B. Alesi, President
Our mission is to challenge and support learning disabled
young men so that they achieve academically at their intellectual level. Our goal is to turn them into effective life-long
learners who will go on to college.

North Carolina

3469   Appalachian State University
Learning Disability Program
ASU Box 32158
Boone, NC 28608   828-262-3056
                                   Fax: 828-262-7904
                                   www.ods.appstate.edu
                                   ods@appstate.edu

Maranda R. Maxey, Director Disability Services
Courtney K. McWhorter, Assistant Director
The Office of Disability Services (ODS) assists students
with indentified disabilities by providing the support they
need to become successful college graduates. ODS provides
academic advising, alternative testing, assistance with technology, tutoring, practical solutions to learning problems,
counseling, self-concept building and career exploration.

3470   Bennett College
900 E Washington St
Greensboro, NC 27401   336-571-2100
                                   800-413-5323
                                   Fax: 336-517-2228
                                   www.bennett.edu

Charles Barrentine, Chair
Deborah W. Foster, Vice Chair
Dr. Rosalind Fuse-Hall, President
An independent four-year college with 10 special education
students out of a total of 568.

3471   Brevard College
Office for Students with Special Needs & Disab
1 Brevard College Dr
Brevard, NC 28712   828-883-8292
                                   800-527-9090
                                   Fax: 828-884-3790
                                   www.brevard.edu
                                   admissions@brevard.edu

David C. Joyce, President
Four year college provides services to special needs students.

3472   Caldwell Community College and Technical Institute
Basic Skills Department
2855 Hickory Blvd
Hudson, NC 28638   828-726-2200
                                   Fax: 828-726-2216
                                   www.cccti.edu
                                   ccrump@cccti.edu

Kenneth A. Boham, President
Cindy Richards, Administrative Assistant

A public two-year college with 18 special education students out of a total of 2,744.

3473   Catawba College
Learning Disability Department
2300 W Innes St
Salisbury, NC 28144   704-637-4259
                                   800-CATAWBA
                                   Fax: 704-637-4401
                                   www.catawba.edu
                                   ekgross@catawba.edu

Brien Lewis, President
Jim Stringfield, Dean
Steve McKinzie, Director
An independent four-year liberal arts college with an enroll-
ment of 1,400.

3474   Catawba Valley Community College
Student Services Office
2550 Us Highway 70 SE
Hickory, NC 28602-8302   828-327-7000
                                   Fax: 828-327-7276
                                   www.cvcc.edu
                                   dulin@cvcc.edu

Charles R. Preston, Chair
Larry Aiello, Vice Chair
Garrett D. Hinshaw, President
The following is a partial list of accommodations provided
by the college: counseling services, tutors, note-takers and
carbonless duplication paper, recorded textbooks, tape recorders for taping lecture classes, interpeters, computer with
voice software, and extended time for texts. Catawba Valley
Community College provides services for students with
disabilities.

3475   Central Carolina Community College
1105 Kelly Dr
Sanford, NC 27330-9840   919-775-5401
                                   Fax: 919-718-7380
                                   www.ccc.edu

Paula Wolff, Chair
Ellen Alberding, Vice Chair
Larry R. Rogers, Secretary
Adopted to guide its delivery of services to students with disabilities that states that no otherwise qualified individual
shall by reason of disability be excluded from the participation in, be denied benefits of, or be subjected to discrimination under any program at Central Carolina Community
College. The college will make program modification adjustments in instructional delivery and provide
supplemental services.

3476   Central Piedmont Community College
Learning Disability Department
PO Box 35009
Charlotte, NC 28235-5009   704-542-0470
                                   Fax: 704-330-4020
                                   TDD: 704-330-5000
                                   TTY: 704-330-4223
                                   www.cpcc.edu/
                                   patricia.adams@cpcc.edu

Edwin A. Dalrymple, Chair
Judith A. Allison, Vice Chair
P. Anthony Zeiss, President
A public two-year college with 300 special education stu-
dents out of a total of 60,000.

3477   Davidson County Community College
PO Box 1287
Lexington, NC 27293-1287   336-249-8186
                                   Fax: 336-249-0088
                                   www.davidsoncc.edu
                                   emorse@davidsoncc.edu

Ed Morse MD, Dean
Mary Rittling, President
Offers a variety of services to students with disabilities including notetakers, extended testing time, counseling services, and special accommodations.

3478 Dore Academy
5146 Parkway Plaza Blvd.
Charlotte, NC 28217
704-365-5490
Fax: 704-365-3240
http://johncroslandschool.org/
info@johncroslandschool.org
Sean Preston, Head of School
Portia Eley, Admissions Director
Faye Lakey, Director of Finance & Operations
Dore Academy is Charlotte's oldest college-prep school for students with learning differences. A private, non-profit, independent day school for students in grades 1-12, it is approved by the state of North Carolina, Division of Exceptional children. All teachers are certified by the state and trained in the theory and treatment of dyslexia and attention disorders. With a maximum of 10 students per class (5 in reading classes), the teacher student ratio is 1 to 7.

3479 East Carolina University
Project STEPP
E 5th Street
Greenville, NC 27858-4353
252-328-6131
www.ecu.edu
williamssar@ecu.edu
Dr. Marilyn Sheerer, Provost
Chris Locklear, Chief of Staff
The program offers comprehensive academic, social, and life-skills support to a select number of students with identified Specific Learning Disabilities who have shown the potential to succeed in college.

3480 Evergreen Valley College
Disabilities Support Programs
East Fifth Street
Greenville, NC 27858-4353
252-328-6131
Fax: 408-223-6341
TDD: 408-238-8722
www.euc.edu
bonnie.clark@euc.edu
David W Coon, LD Specialist
John D. Messick, President
A public two-year college with 82 learning disabled students out of a total of 9,000.

3481 Fletcher Academy
400 Cedarview Ct
Raleigh, NC 27609
919-782-5082
Fax: 919-782-5980
www.thefletcheracademy.com
info@thefletcheracademy.com
Paul Atkinson, Headmaster
Tiffany Gregory, Dean of Admissions
Nancy Steinauer, Business Manager/ IT Specialist
A coeducational, independent day school serving students from grades 1-12 with learning differences.

3482 Gardner-Webb University
Noel Program
PO Box 997
110 South Main Street
Boiling Springs, NC 28017
704-406-4000
Fax: 704-406-3524
www.gardner-webb.edu
cpotter@gardner-webb.edu
Dr. A Frank Bonner, President
Dr. Ben Leslie, Provost
Four year college that provides a program for disabled students.

3483 Guilford Technical Community College
PO Box 309
601 E. Main Street
Jamestown, NC 27282
336-334-4822
Fax: 336-841-2158
TTY: 336-841-2158
www.gtcc.cc.nc.us
dcameron@gtcc.cc.nc.us
Dr. Randy Parker, President
Sonny White, Vice President

The purpose of disability access services is to provide equal access and comprehensive, quality services to all students who experience barriers toacademic, personal and social success.

3484 Hill Center
3200 Pickett Rd
Durham, NC 27705
919-489-7464
Fax: 919-489-7466
www.hillcenter.org
info@hillcenter.org
David Riddle, Chair
Nancy Farmer, Vice Chair
Beth Anderson, President
Half day school and teacher training facility, established for students with LD/ADHD.
1977

3485 Isothermal Community College
Department of Disability Services
PO Box 804
286 ICC Loop Road
Spindale, NC 28160
828-286-3636
Fax: 828-286-8109
TDD: 828-286-3636
TTY: 828-288-9844
www.isothermal.edu/
kharris@isothermal.cc.nc.us
John Condrey, Chair
Bobby England, Vice Chair
Buck Petty, Trustee
Isothermal Community College, in compliance with the Americans with Disabilities Act, makes every effort to provide accommodations for students with disabilities. It is our goal to integrate students with disabilities into the college and help them participate and benefit from programs and activities enjoyed by all students. We at Isothermal are committed to improving life through learning.

3486 Johnson C Smith University
Disability Support Services Department
100 Beatties Ford Rd
Charlotte, NC 28216
704-378-1010
Fax: 704-372-1242
www.jcsu.edu
admissions@jcsu.edu
Ronald L. Carter, President
James Saunders, Director
Four year college that provides support to those who are disabled.

3487 Key Learning Center
Carolina Day School
1345 Hendersonville Rd
Asheville, NC 28803
828-274-0757
Fax: 828-274-0116
www.cdschool.org
bsgro@cdschool.org
Jeff Baker, Chair
Marie-Louise Murphy, President
Kirk Duncan, Head of School
Provides students with learning differences the educational opportunity to overcome their differences and to achieve their maximum potential in school and life.

3488 Lenoir-Rhyne College
PO Box 7470
Hickory, NC 28603-7470
828-328-7315
Fax: 828-328-7329
www.lr.edu
kirbydr@lrc.edu
Donavon Kirby, Coordinator
Wayne Powell, President
Four year college that provides services for those students that are learning disabled.

3489 Mariposa School for Children with Autism
203 Gregson Dr
Cary, NC 27511-6495 919-461-0600
Fax: 919-461-0566
www.mariposaschool.org
info@mariposaschool.org

Dane Shears, Chairman
Palma Fouratt, Vice Chair
Jacinta Johnson, Executive Director
Provides year round one-on-one instruction to children with autism, using innovative teaching techniques targeting multiple developmental areas in a single integrated setting. A school of excellence choice for children with autism to maximize developemtn of their communication, social and academic skills.

3490 Mars Hill College
100 Atletic Street
PO Box 370
Mars Hill, NC 28754 866-642-4968
800-543-1514
Fax: 828-689-1478
www.mhu.edu/
ccain@mhc.edu

J. Dixon Free, Chairman
Cheryl B. Pappas, Vice Chair
Dan Lunsford, President
An independent four-year college with 15 special education students out of a total of 1,321.

3491 Mayland Community College
Support Options for Achievement and Retention
PO Box 547
Spruce Pine, NC 28777 828-766-1200
800-462-9526
www.mayland.edu
dcagle@mayland.edu

Charles Ronald Kates, Chairman
Edwina Sluder, Vice Chair
Dr. John C. Boyd, President
Offers a variety of services to students with disabilities including notetakers, extended testing time, counseling services, and special accommodations.

3492 McDowell Technical Community College
Student Enrichment Center
54 College Dr
Marion, NC 28752 828-652-6021
Fax: 828-652-1014
www.mcdowelltech.edu
donnashort@cc.nc.us

Darren Waugh, Chairman
Joy Shuford, Vice Chair
Dr. Bryan W Wilson, President
A public two-year college with 15 special education students out of a total of 857. Free auxiliary services for LD students include: tutors, books on tape, unlimited testing, oral testing, notetakers and counseling. All faculty are trained in working with the LD student.

3493 Montgomery Community College: North Carolina
1011 Page St
Troy, NC 27371-8387 910-576-6222
Fax: 910-576-2176
www.montgomery.edu

Mary Kirk, President
Offers a variety of services to students with disabilities including note takers, extended testing time, counseling services, and special accommodations.

3494 North Carolina State University
Campus Box 7509
Raleigh, NC 27695 919-515-2011
Fax: 919-513-2840
TDD: 919-515-8830
TTY: 919-515-8830
www.ncsu.edu/dso
cheryl_branker@ncsu.edu

Cheryl Branker, Director

Academic accommodations and services are provided for students at the university who have documented learning disabilities. Admission to the university is based on academic qualifications and learning disabled students are considered in the same manner as any other student. Special assistance is available to accommodate the needs of these students, including courses in accessible locations when appropiate.

3495 North Carolina Wesleyan College
3400 N Wesleyan Blvd
Rocky Mount, NC 27804 252-985-5100
800-488-6292
Fax: 252-985-5284
www.ncwc.edu
albunn.infowc@edu

Will H. Lassiter III, Chairman
Michael Hancock, Vice Chair
Dr. Dewey G. Clark, President
The Center provides support to students interested in achieving academic success. The staff works to provide you with information about academic matters and serves as an advocate for you. Services focus on pre-major advising, tutoring, mentoring, skills enrichment, disabilities assistance, self-assessment and retention.

3496 Piedmont International University
420 S Broad St
Winston Salem, NC 27101-5025 336-725-8344
800-937-5097
Fax: 336-725-5522
www.pbc.edu

Dr. Charles Petitt, President
Dr. Beth Ashburn, Provost
Dr. Barkev Trachian, VP Graduate Studies
Prepares men and women for Christian ministries, both lay and professional, through a rigorous program of biblical, general and professional studies.

3497 Randolph Community College
629 Industrial Park Ave
Asheboro, NC 27205 336-626-0200
Fax: 336-629-4695
www.randolph.edu/
jbranch@randolf.edu

F. Mac Sherrill, Chairman
Fred E. Meredith, Vice Chair
Robert S. Shackleford Jr, President
A public two-year college with 23 special education students out of a total of 1,487. Applicants with disabilities who wish to request accommodations in compliance with the ADA must identify themselves to the admissions counselor before placement testing.

3498 Rockingham Community College
215 Wrenn Memorial Road
Hwy. 65
Wentworth, NC 27375 336-342-4261
Fax: 336-349-9986
TDD: 336-634-0132
www.rockinghamcc.edu
rkeys@rcc.cc.nc.us

William C Aiken, President
Suzanne Rohrbaugh, Vice President, Academic Affairs
Steve Woodruff, VP Administrative Services
Offers a variety of services to students with disabilities including notetakers, extended testing time, counseling services, and special accommodations.

3499 Salem College
S Church Street
Winston-Salem, NC 27108 336-721-2600
Fax: 336-917-5339
www.salem.edu
smith@salem.edu

Stephen G. Jennings, Chair
Leigh Flippin Krause, Vice Chair
Lorraine Sterritt, President

Offers a variety of services to students with disabilities including notetakers, extended testing time, counseling services, and special accommodations.

3500 Sandhills Community College
3395 Airport Rd
Pinehurst, NC 28374 · · · · · · · · · · · · 910-692-6185
800-338-3944
Fax: 910-695-1823
www.sandhills.edu

George Little, Chair
Robert Hayter, Vice Chair
John R Dempsey, President
Offers a variety of services to students with disabilities including notetakers, extended testing time, counseling services, and special accommodations.

3501 Southwestern Community College: North Carolina
447 College Dr
Sylva, NC 28779 · · · · · · · · · · · · · · · 828-339-4000
800-447-4091
Fax: 828-339-4613
www.southwesterncc.edu
cheryl@southwest.cc.nc.us

Terry Bell, Chair
W. Paul Holt, Vice Chair
Don Tomas, Ed.D., President
Southwestern Community College provides equal access to education for persons with disabilities. It is the responsibility of the student to make their disability known and to request academic adjustments. Requests should be made in a timely manner and submitted to the Director of Student Support Services. Every reasonable effort will be made to provide service, however, not requesting services prior to registration may delay implementation.

3502 St Andrews Presbyterian College
1700 Dogwood Mile
Laurinburg, NC 28352 · · · · · · · · · · · · 910-277-5555
800-763-0198
Fax: 910-277-5020
www.sapc.edu
info@sapc.edu

Paul Baldasare, President
Glenn Batten, VP Administration
Erin Cooper Balduf, Admissions Counselor
Four year college that supports and provides services to the learning disabled students.

3503 Stone Mountain School
126 Camp Elliott Rd
Black Mountain, NC 28711-9003 · · · · · · 888-631-5994
Fax: 828-669-2521
www.stonemountainschool.org
smoore@stonemountainschool.com

Sam Moore, Executive Director
Paige Thomas, Admissions Director

3504 Surry Community College
630 S Main St
Dobson, NC 27017 · · · · · · · · · · · · · · 336-386-8121
Fax: 336-386-8951
www.surry.edu
riggsj@surry.edu

Dr. Ann Vaughn, Chair
George L. Anderson, Vice Chair
Tony Martin, Vice President, Finance
Offers a variety of services to students with disabilities including notetakers, extended testing time, counseling services, and special accommodations.

3505 University of North Carolina Wilmington
Disability Resource Center
601 S College Rd
Wilmington, NC 28403 · · · · · · · · · · · · 910-962-3000
Fax: 910-962-7556
TDD: 800-735-2962
TTY: 800-735-2962
www.uncw.edu/disability
waybrantj@uncw.edu

Wendy F. Murphy, Chair
Britt A. Preyer, Vice Chair
Bill Sederburg, Chancellor
Offer accommodative services, consultation, counseling and advocacy for students with disabilities enrolled at UNCW.

3506 University of North Carolina: Chapel Hill
450 Ridge Rd
Ste 2109
Chapel Hill, NC 27599-5135 · · · · · · · · 919-962-3782
Fax: 919-962-7797
http://learningcenter.unc.edu
learning_center@unc.edu

Kim Abels, Director
Robin Blanton, Academic Coach
Billie Shambley, Program Manager
Promotes learning by providing academic support to meet the individual needs of students diagnosed with specific learning disabilities. Strives to ensure the independence of participating students so that they may succeed during and beyond their university years.

3507 University of North Carolina: Charlotte
Special Education Department
9201 University Blvd
Charlotte, NC 28223-1 · · · · · · · · · · · · 704-687-8622
Fax: 704-547-3239
www.uncc.edu
abennett@email.uncc.edu

Karen A. Popp, Chair
Joe L. Price, Vice Chair
Philip L. Dubois, Chancellor
Introduction to Students with Special Needs. Characteristics of students with special learning needs, including those who are gifted and those who experience academic, social, emotional, physical and developmental disabilities. Legal, historical and philosophical foudations of special education and current issues in providing appropriate educational services to students with special needs.

3508 University of North Carolina: Greensboro
Disability Services
910 Raleigh Rd.
PO Box 2688
Chapel Hill, NC 27514 · · · · · · · · · · · · 919-962-1000
Fax: 336-334-4412
www.uncg.edu
ods@uncg.edu

John C. Fennebresque, Chair
W. Louis Bissette, Vice Chair
Thomas W. Ross, President
A public four-year university with over 300 students with disabilities out of a total of 12,000.

3509 Wake Forest University
1834 Wake Forest Road
Winston Salem, NC 27106 · · · · · · · · · · 336-758-5000
Fax: 336-758-6074
www.wfu.edu

Donald E. Flow, Chair
Donna A. Boswell, Vice Chair
Bobby R. Burchfield, Vice Chair
Offers a variety of services to students with disabilities including notetakers, extended testing time, counseling services, and special accommodations.

3510 Wake Technical Community College
Disabilities Support Department
9101 Fayetteville Rd
Raleigh, NC 27603

919-866-5000
Fax: 919-779-3360
TDD: 919-779-0668
www.waketech.edu
jtkillen@waketech.edu

Stephen C Scott, Director
Elaine Sardi, Coordinator
If you are a person with a documented disability who requires accommodations to achieve equal access to Wake Tech facilities, academic programs or other activities, you may request reasonable accommodations.

3511 Western Carolina University
Student Support Services
137 Killian Anx
Cullowhee, NC 28723

828-227-7211
Fax: 828-227-7078
www.wcu.edu
mellen@wcu.edu

Teresa Wiiliams, Chair
F. Edward Broadwell, Vice Chair
David O. Belcher, Chancellor
Students with a documented disability may be provided with appropriate academic accommodations such as, note takers, testing accomadations, books on tape, readers/scribes, use of adaptive equipment and priority registration.

3512 Wilkes Community College
Student Support Services
PO Box 120
1328 S.Collegiate Dr.
Wilkesboro, NC 28697

336-838-6100
Fax: 336-838-6277
www.wilkescc.edu
nancy.sizemore@wilkescc.edu

Kim Faw, Director
Nancy Sizemore, Disability Coordinator
A public two-year community college. Special services include: testing and individualized education plans; oral and extended time testing; individual and small group tutoring; study skills; readers and proctors and specialized equipment.

3513 Wilson County Technical College
North Carolina Community College
PO Box 4305
902 Herring Avenue
Wilson, NC 27893

252-291-1195
Fax: 252-243-7148
TDD: 252-246-1362
www.wilsoncc.edu

Dr. Rusty Stephens, President
Lynn Moore, Director
Jane S. Elliott, Grant Assistant
Offers a variety of services to students with disabilities including notetakers, extended testing time, counseling services, and special accommodations.

3514 Wingate University
Disability Services Department
220 N. Camden St.
Wingate, NC 28174

704-233-8000
800-755-5550
Fax: 704-233-8014
www.wingate.edu
admit@wingate.edu

Dr. Jerry McGee, President
Peter Frank, Associate Professor of Economics
Joe Graham, Professor of Accounting
An independent four-year college with 50 special education students out of a total of 1,372. There is an additional fee for the special education program in addition to the regular tuition.

3515 Winston-Salem State University
601 S. Martin Luther King Jr. Drive
Winston Salem, NC 27110

336-750-2000
Fax: 336-750-2392
www.wssu.edu/

Brenda A. Allen, Provost
Donald J. Reaves, Ph.D, Chancellor
Dr. Carolyn Berry, Associate Provost
Offers a variety of services to students with disabilities including notetakers, extended testing time, counseling services, and special accommodations.

North Dakota

3516 Anne Carlsen Center for Children
701 3rd St NW
P.O. Box 8000
Jamestown, ND 58402

701-252-3850
800-568-5175
Fax: 701-952-5154
www.annecenter.org

Bruce Iserman, Chair
Harvey Huber, Vice Chair
Eric Monson, COO
Provides students a safe, secure and loving atmosphere to learn and grow. The program is filled with an array of sensory and literary enriched experiences and materials that allow each student to become an independent, freethinking being.

3517 Bismarck State College
1500 Edwards Ave
PO Box 5587
Bismarck, ND 58506

701-224-5400
800-445-5073
Fax: 701-224-5550
www.bsc.nodak.edu
Ischlafm@gwmail.nodak.edu

Patrick J. Bjork, Web Manager
Zachery Allen, Project Manager
Dusty Anderson, Production Coordiator
Offers a variety of services to students with disabilities including notetakers, extended testing time, counseling services, and special accommodations.

3518 Dakota College at Bottineau
105 Simrall Blvd
Bottineau, ND 58318

701-228-5488
800-542-6866
Fax: 701-228-5499
www.dakotacollege.edu
jan.nahinurk@dakotacollege.edu

David Fuller, President
Dr. Ken Grosz, Dean
Karen Bowen, Director of Business Affairs
Dakota College at Bottineau offers a variety of services to students with disabilities including note takers, extended testing time, academic advising, and special accommodations.

3519 Dickinson State University
Student Support Services
291 Campus Dr
Dickinson, ND 58601

701-483-2507
800-279-HAWK
Fax: 701-483-2006
www.dickinsonstate.edu/
dsu.hawk@dickinsonstate.edu

D. C. Coston, President
Dr. Cynthia Pemberton, Provost/ VP for Academic Afairs
Mark Lowe, VP for Finance & Administration
Four year college offers support services to learning disabled students.

3520 Fort Berthold Community College
PO Box 490
280 8th Ave. N.
New Town, ND 58763   701-627-4378
                                  Fax: 701-627-3609
                                  www.fortbertholdcc.edu/
                                  lgwin@spcc.bia.edu
Patrick J. Packineau, President
Phillip Lewis, CFO/ VP, Support Services
Keith Smith, Facilties Manager
An independent two-year college with 3 special education
students out of a total of 279.

3521 Mayville State University
Learning Disabilities Department
330 3rd St NE
Mayville, ND 58257   701-788-2301
                                       800-437-4104
                                  Fax: 701-788-4748
                                  www.mayvillestate.edu
                                  kyllo@mayvillestate.edu
Charlotte Anderson, Office Manager
Karen A. Amundson, Business Office
Jessica P. Amb, Administrative Coordinator
Offers a variety of services to students with disabilities in-
cluding notetakers, extended testing time, counseling ser-
vices, and special accommodations.

3522 Minot State University
North Dakota Center for Persons with Disabilities
500 University Ave W
Minot, ND 58707   701-858-3371
                                       800-777-0750
                                  Fax: 701-858-3686
                                  TDD: 701-858-3580
                                  www.minotstateu.edu
                                  ndcpd@minotstateu.edu
Leslie Coughlin, Chair
Steven W. Shirley, President
Brian Foisy, VP for Finance & Administration
NDCPD works with the disability community, university,
faculty and researchers, policy makers and service providers
to identify emerging needs in the disability community and
how to obtain resources to address them.

3523 North Dakota State College of Science
Disability Support Services (DSS) Office
800 6th St N
Wahpeton, ND 58076   701-671-2401
                                       800-342-4325
                                  Fax: 701-671-2499
                                  joy.eichhorn@ndscs.nodak.edu
                                  www.ndscs.nodak.edu
Gregory Anderson, Chair
John Richman, President
Christine Ahlsten, Director
A public two-year comprehensive college with a student
population of 2400. Students with disabilites comprise
seven percent of the population. Tuition $2025.

3524 North Dakota State University
Disability Services
Post Office Box 6050
Fargo, ND 58108-6050   701-231-8011
                                  Fax: 701-231-6318
                                  TDD: 800-366-6888
                                  www.ndsu.edu
                                  bunnie.johnson-messelt@ndsu.edu
Dean L. Bresciani, President
Bruce Bollinger, VP for Finance & Administration
Timothy Alvarez, VP for Student Affairs

Students with permanent physical, psychological or learning disabilities may obtain accommodations. The Disability
Services (DS) staff meet with the student to determine eligibility and identify reasonable accomodations.
Accomodations are based on the functional limitations of the
disability. DS staff assist in the implementation of approved
accommodations. Referrals for disability diagnosis and for
other support services such as tutoring are also provided by
staff.

3525 Standing Rock College
9299 Hwy 24
Fort Yates, ND 58538   701-854-8000
                                  Fax: 701-854-3403
                                  www.sittingbull.edu
                                  info@sbci.edu
Sharon Two Bears, Chair
Joe L. McNeil, Vice Chair
Dr.Laurel Vermillion, President
Offers a variety of services to students with disabilities in-
cluding notetakers, extended testing time, counseling ser-
vices, and special accommodations.

Ohio

3526 Art Academy of Cincinnati
1212 Jackson St
Cincinnati, OH 45202   513-562-6262
                                       800-323-5692
                                  Fax: 513-562-8778
                                  www.artacademy.edu/
Mark Grote, Chair
Susan Crabtree, Vice Chair
John M. Sullivan, President
Offers a variety of services to students with disabilities in-
cluding notetakers, extended testing time, counseling ser-
vices, and special accommodations.

3527 Baldwin-Wallace College
275 Eastland Rd
Berea, OH 44017-2088   440-826-2900
                                  Fax: 440-826-3777
                                  www.bw.edu
                                  info@bw.edu
Paul H. Carleton, Chair
Robert C. Helmer, President
Stephen D. Stahl, Provost
Offers a variety of services to students with disabilities in-
cluding notetakers, extended testing time, counseling ser-
vices, and special accommodations.

3528 Bluffton College
Special Student Services
1 University Dr.
Bluffton, OH 45817-2104   419-358-3000
                                       800-488-3257
                                  Fax: 419-358-3323
                                  www.bluffton.edu
                                  bergerd@bluffton.edu
James H. Harder, President
Four year college offers special programs to learninig dis-
abled students.

3529 Bowling Green State University
413 S Hall
Bowling Green, OH 43403-1   419-372-2531
                                  Fax: 419-372-8496
                                  www.bgsu.edu
                                  dss@bgsu.edu
Mary Ellen Mazey, President
Dr. Rodney Rogers, SVP for Academic Affairs/Provost
Jill Carr, VP for Student Affairs

The Disability Services Office is evidence of Bowling Green State University's commitment to provide a support system which assists in conquering obstacles that persons with disabilities may encounter as they pursue their educational goals and activities. Our hope is to facilitate mainstream mobility and recognize the diverse talents that persons with disabilities have to offer to our university and our community.

3530   Brown Mackie College: Akron
2791 Mogadore Rd
Akron, OH 44320   330-896-3600
                                Fax: 330-733-5853
                                www.brownmackie.edu
Jannette Mason, Administrative Assistant
Fred Baldwin, Dean of Academic Services
Offers a variety of services to students with disabilities including notetakers, extended testing time, counseling services, and special accommodations.

3531   Case Western Reserve University
10900 Euclid Ave
Cleveland, OH 44106   216-368-2000
                                Fax: 216-368-8826
                                www.cwru.edu
Barbara R. Snyder, President
W.A. Bud Baeslack III, EVP & Provost
Robert Clark Brown, Treasurer
While all students will have preferences for learning, students with physical or learning disabilities have different actual needs as well. Students with physical disabilities such as visual impairments, hearing impairments, or temporary or permanent motor impairments may need guide dogs, interpeters, note-takers, wheelchair accessible rooms, or other types of assistance to help them attend and participate in class. Also available, extra time or a separate room for exams, tutoring and more.

3532   Central Ohio Technical College
Developmental Education
1179 University Dr
Newark, OH 43055   740-366-9494
                                     800-963-9275
                                Fax: 740-366-5047
                                www.cotc.edu
Cheryl Snyder, Chair
John Hinderer, Vice Chair
Bonnie Coe, President
Learning Assitance Center and Disability Services (LAC/DS) is the academic support unit in Student Support Services. LAC/DS provides FREE programs and services designed to help students sharpen skills necessary to succeed in college.

3533   Central State University
Office of Disability Services
1400 Brush Row Rd
PO Box 1004
Wilberforce, OH 45384   937-376-6011
                                     800-388-2781
                                Fax: 937-376-6245
                                www.centralstate.edu
                                publicrelations@centralstate.edu
Curtis Pettis, Executive Director
Daarel E. Burnette, VP for Adminstration & CFO
Charles Wesley Ford, Provost
Four year college that provides services for the learning disabled students.

3534   Cincinnati State Technical and Community College
3520 Central Pkwy
Cincinnati, OH 45223   513-569-1500
                                Fax: 513-569-1719
                                TDD: 877-569-0115
                                www.cincinnatistate.edu
                                dcover@cinstate.cc.oh.us
Cathy T. Crain, Chair
Mark D. Walton, Vice Chair
O'Dell M. Owens, M.D., M.P.H, President

Services include assistance and support services for students with permanent and temporary disabilities, test proctoring, readers/scribes, taping, tape recording loan, reading machines, assistance with locating interpeters, mediating between student and faculty to overcome specific disability issues; also offers braille access.

3535   Clark State Community College
Disability Retention Center
570 East Leffel Lane
Springfield, OH 45505-4795   937-325-0691
                                Fax: 937-328-6133
                                www.clarkstate.edu
Jo Alice Blondin, Ph.D., President
James N. Doyle, Chair
Peggy Noonan, Vice Chair
In accordance with the Americans with Disabilities Act, it is the policy of Clark State Community College to provide reasonable accommodations to persons with disabilities. The office of disability services offers a variety of services to Clark State students who have documented physical, mental or learning disabilities.

3536   Cleveland Institute of Art
Academic Services
11141 East Boulevard
Cleveland, OH 44106-1700   216-421-7450
                                     800-223-4700
                                Fax: 216-421-7438
                                www.cia.edu
                                cinema@cia.edu
Michael Schwartz, Board Chair
Grafton Nunes, President and CEO
Almut Zvosec, VP Business AffairS/CFO
No student should be discouraged from attending CIA because of a learning disability. A student working on their BFA degree at the Institute of Art can get academic support from the tutoring director in the Office of Academic Services. Services include books-on-tape, one-on-one tutoring, alternative curriculum advising, notetaking services, alternative test taking and assignment arrangements. Services outside the scope of the program can be arranged at the student's expense.

3537   Cleveland State University
2121 Euclid Avenue
Cleveland, OH 44115-2214   216-687-2000
                                     888-278-6446
                                Fax: 216-687-9366
                                www.csuohio.edu
                                m.zuccaro@csuohio.edu
Ronald M. Berkman, President
Michael Artbauer, Chief of Staff
Barbara E. Smith, Director Special Events
CSU aims to provide equal opportunity to all of its students. Services are available to those who might need some extra help because of a physical disability, communication impairment or learning disability. This program is designed to address the personal and academic issues of the physically handicapped students as they become oriented to campus. A full range of services is offered.

3538   College of Mount Saint Joseph
Project EXCEL
5701 Delhi Road
Cincinnati, OH 45233-1670   513-244-4200
                                     800-654-9314
                                Fax: 513-244-4601
                                www.msj.edu
                                debra_mato@mail.msj.edu
Tony Aretz, Ph.D., President
Kenneth W. Stecher, Chairperson
Jason P. Niehaus, Vice Chairperson
Project EXCEL is a nationally recognized, comprehensive academic support system for students with specific learning disabilities and/or Attention Deficit/Attention Deficit Hyperactivity Disorder. Project EXCEL is a fee-for-service program. Students must be admitted to the College of Mount St. Joseph before applying for Project EXCEL.

3539 College of Wooster
1189 Beall Ave
Wooster, OH 44691-2363   330-263-2000
Fax: 330-263-2427
www.wooster.edu

Grant H. Cornwell, President
David H. Gunning, Chairman
Douglas F. Brush, Vice Chairman
Offers a variety of services to students with disabilities including notetakers, extended testing time, counseling services, and special accommodations.

3540 Columbus State Community College Disability Services
550 East Spring St
Columbus, OH 43215-1722   614-287-5353
800-621-6407
Fax: 614-287-3645
TDD: 614-287-2570
TTY: 614-287-2570
www.cscc.edu
information@cscc.edu

David T. Harrison, Ph.D., President
Richard D. Rosen, Chair
Michael E. Flowers, Vice-Chair
A public two-year college serving qualified students with disabilities, including learning disabilities. Support services are provided based on disability documentation and can include, books, tapes, alternative testing, notetaking, counseling, equipment use, reader, scribe, and peer tutoring.

3541 Cuyahoga Community College: Eastern Campus
4250 Richmond Road
Highland Hills, OH 44122-6195   800-954-8742
866-933-5175
Fax: 216-987-2054
TDD: 866-933-5175
www.tri-c.edu
Maryann.Syarto@tri-c.cc.oh.us

Jerry L. Kelsheimer, Chairman
Nadine H. Feighan, Vice Chairperson
Alex Johnson, Ph.D., President
The ACCESS Programs strive to assist Tri-C students with disabilities to realize their learning potential, bring them into the mainstream of the College community, enhance their self-sufficiency, and enable them to achieve academic success. Services include tuoring, test proctoring, interpreters, adaptive equipment, readers and/or scribes for exams, alternative test taking arrangements, alternative format for printed materials and textbooks on tape.

3542 Cuyahoga Community College: Western Campus
1000 West Pleasant Valley Rd
Parma, OH 44130   216-987-5077
800-954-8742
Fax: 516-987-5050
TDD: 216-987-5117
www.tri-c.edu
rose.kolovrat@tri-c.edu

Jerry L. Kelsheimer, Chairman
Nadine H. Feighan, Vice Chairperson
Alex Johnson, Ph.D., President
The ACCESS programs strive to assist Tri-C students with disabilities to realize their learning potential, bring them into the mainstream of the College community, enhance their self-suffciency and enable them to achieve academic success. Services provided include tutoring, test proctoring, interpeters, adaptive equipment, readers/scribes for exams, alternative testing arrangements, alternative format for printed material and textbooks on tape.

3543 Defiance College
701 N Clinton St
Defiance, OH 43512-1695   419-784-4010
800-520-4632
Fax: 419-784-0426
www.defiance.edu
admissions@defiance.edu

Mark C. Gordon, President
Lois McCullough, VP for Finance and Management
Michael Suzo, VP for Enrollment Management
Offers a variety of services to students with disabilities including notetakers, extended testing time, counseling services, and special accommodations.

3544 Denison University
100 West College Street
Granville, OH 43023   740-587-6666
800-336-4766
Fax: 740-587-5629
www.denison.edu
vestal@denison.edu

Thomas E. Hoaglin, B.A., M.B.A., Chair
Dana Hart, B.A., M.A., Vice Chair
Adam Weinberg, President
The Office of Academic Support (OAS) offers a wide range of services for students with disabilities. In supporting our students as they move forward toward graduation and the world of work beyond, we strongly encourage and promote self advocacy regarding disability related issues.

3545 FOCUS Program
Program for Students with Learning Disabilities
2550 Lander Road
Pepper Pike, OH 44124-4318   440-449-4200
888 URSULINE
Fax: 440-684-6138
www.ursuline.edu
info@ursuline.edu

Eileen Delaney Kohut, Director
John M. Newman, Jr., Chair
Sister Diana Stano, President
A voluntary, comprehensive, fee-paid program for students with learning disabilities and ADHD. The goals of the FOCUS Program include providing a smooth transition for college life, helping students learn to apply the most appropriate learning strategies in college courses, and teaching students self-advocacy skills.

3546 Franklin University
201 S Grant Ave
Columbus, OH 43215-5399   614-797-4700
877-341-6300
Fax: 614-224-8027
www.franklin.edu
admissions@franklin.edu

Dr. David Decker, President
Gary L. Flynn, Chairman of the Board
Mary Laird Duchi, Vice Chairman
Students who have disabilities may notify the University of their status by checking the appropriate space on the registration form each trimester. Then the Coordinator of Disability Services will help them file proper documentation so that accommodations can be made for their learning needs.

3547 Hiram College
11715 Garfield Road
Hiram, OH 44234-67   330-569-3211
800-705-5050
Fax: 330-569-5398
www.hiram.edu
alumnirel@hiram.edu

Lori E. Varlotta, President
Brittney Braydich, Director of Major Gifts
Patrick Roberts, VP Dev & Alumni Relations
Offers a variety of services to students with disabilities including notetakers, extended testing time, counseling services, and special accommodations.

3548 Hocking College
3301 Hocking Parkway
Nelsonville, OH 45764-9588   740-753-3591
877-462-5464
Fax: 740-753-7065
www.hocking.edu
admissions@hocking.edu

John Light, President
Rosie Smith, Director
The Access Center Office of Disability Support Services is dedicated to serving the various needs of individuals with disabilities and promoting their participation in college life.

3549   ITT Technical Institute
1030 North Meridian Road
Youngstown, OH 44509-4098

330-270-1600
800-832-5001
Fax: 330-270-8333
www.itt-tech.edu

Frank Quartini, Manager
Offers a variety of services to students with disabilities including note takers, extended testing time, counseling services, and special accommodations.

3550   Julie Billiart School
4982 Clubside Rd
Lyndhurst, OH 44124-2596

216-381-1191
Fax: 216-381-2216
www.juliebilliartschool.org
jjohnston@jbschool.org

Agnesmarie Loporto, SND, President
Jodi Johnston M Ed, Principal
William D. Glubiak, Chairman
Rooted in the educational vision of the Sisters of Notre Dame, Julie Billiart School is a Catholic, alternative K-8 school, which educates children of all faith traditions who experience special learning needs.

3551   Lorain County Community College
1005 N Abbe Road
Elyria, OH 44035-1691

440-366-4100
800-955-5222
Fax: 440-365-6519
www.lorainccc.edu
info@lorainccc.edu

Roy Church, President
Lawrence Goodman, Chairman
Benjamin Fligner, Vice Chairman
LCCC serves over 80 learning disabled students per year out of a total student population of over 7,000. Services include readers/testers, scribes, notetaking accommodations, assistive technology, advocacy training and personal counseling. Free tutoring is available to all students at the college. No diagnostic testing is available.

3552   Malone University
2600 Cleveland Ave NW
Canton, OH 44709-3308

330-471-8100
800-521-1146
Fax: 330-471-8149
TDD: 330-471-8496
www.malone.edu
ameadows@malone.edu

Anna Meadows, Student Access Services Director
Dr Wil Friesen, President
David P. Murray, Chair?
An independent four-year college with about 40 special education students out of a total of almost 2,000.

3553   Marburn Academy
1860 Walden Drive
Columbus, OH 43229-3627

614-433-0822
Fax: 614-433-0812
www.marburnacademy.org
marburnadmission@marburnacademy.org

Earl B Oremus, Headmaster
A not-for-profit, independent, day school devoted to serving the educational needs of bright students with learning differences such as dyslexia and ADHD. The school programs are designed to help the student's learn strong work habits, teach values of persistance and courage in overcoming challenges and to build effective social interaction and problem solving patterns.

3554   Marietta College
Marietta College
215 Fifth Street
Marietta, OH 45750-4047

740-376-4786
800-331-7896
Fax: 740-376-4530
www.marietta.edu
higgisd@marietta.edu

Walter Miller, Director
Jean Scott, President
An Independent four-year college that offers a variety of servies to students with disabilities including note takers, extended testing time, counseling services, and special accommodations. There is no separate fee for these services.

3555   Marion Technical College
1467 Mount Vernon Ave
Marion, OH 43302-5694

740-389-4636
Fax: 740-389-6136
www.mtc.edu
enroll@mtc.edu

J Richard Bryson,Ph.D., President
Jeff Nutter, VP/CFO
Brenda Feasel, Director of Human Resources
The Student Resource Center also houses the Office of Disabilities. The SRC director will advocate on student's behalf for resonable accommodations for those with physical, mental and or emotional disabilities.

3556   Miami University Rinella Learning Center
Room 14
501 E. High St.
Oxford, OH 45056-2481

513-529-1809
www.muohio.edu

David C. Hodge, President
Ray Gorman, Interim Provost and EVP
J. Peter Natale, VP Information Technology
A public four-year college.

3557   Miami University: Middletown Campus
4200 N University Blvd
Middletown, OH 45042-3458

513-727-3200
86-MIAMI-MID
Fax: 513-727-3451
TDD: 513-727-3308
TTY: 513-727-3431
www.mid.muohio.edu
nferguson@mid.muohio.edu

Kelly Cowan, Executive Director
Margir Perkins, Academic Services
Offers a variety of services to students with disabilities including notetakers, extended testing time, counseling services, and special accommodations.

3558   Mount Vernon Nazarene College
800 Martinsburg Rd
Mount Vernon, OH 43050-9500

740-392-6868
866-462-6868
Fax: 740-393-0511
www.mvnu.edu
admissions@mvnu.edu

Dr. Henry Spaulding, II, President
Dr. Robert Hamill, VP for Finances & CFO
Dr. Lanette Sessink, VP for Student Life
Four year college that provides programs for learning diabled students.

3559   Muskingum College
Center for Advancement of Learning
163 Stormont Street
New Concord, OH 43762

740-826-8137
800-752-6082
Fax: 740-826-8100
www.muskingum.edu
adminfo@muskingum.edu

Beth DaLonzo, Senior Director of Admission
Jake Burnett, Associate Director of Admission
Gary Atkins, Assistant Director of Admission

The PLUS Program provides students identified as learning-disabled with individual and group learning strategies instruction embedded within course content.

3560   Oberlin College
Academic Support for Students with Disabilities
101 N. Professor St.
Oberlin, OH 44074
440-775-8411
800-622-6243
Fax: 440-775-6905
www.oberlin.edu
college.admissions@oberlin.edu

Marvin Krislov, President
Debra Chermonte, VP/Dean of Admissions
Tom Abeyta, Senior Associate Director
An independent four-year college with small percentage of education students.

3561   Ohio State University Agricultural Technical Institute
1328 Dover Road
Wooster, OH 44691-4000
330-287-1330
800-647-8283
Fax: 330-287-1333
http://ati.osu.edu
ati@osu.edu

Rhonda Billman, Assistant Director
Jim Kinder, Ph.D., Interim Director
Gail Miller, Director - Upward Bound
A public two-year college with nearly 10% special education students. There is no fee for the special education program in addition to the regular tuition.

3562   Ohio State University: Lima Campus
Disability Services
4240 Campus Dr
Lima, OH 45804-3576
419-995-8600
Fax: 419-995-8483
www.lima.ohio-state.edu
meyer.193@osu.edu

Deborah Ellis, Chair
Susan Hubbell, Vice Chair
Lori Schleeter, Secretary
A public four-year college providing services to learning disabled students including extended test time, counseling, notetakers and other special accommodations.

3563   Ohio State University: Mansfield Campus
Disability Services
1760 University Drive
Mansfield, OH 44906-1547
419-755-4011
Fax: 419-755-4241
http://mansfield.osu.edu
abedon.1@osu.edu

Stephen M. Gavazzi, Ph.D., Dean and Director
Christ J. Ticoras, Chair
Patrick A. Heydinger, Vice-Chair
A public four-year college providing services to learning disabled students including peer tutoring, extended test time, quiet rooms and other special accommodations.

3564   Ohio State University: Marion Campus
1465 Mount Vernon Avenue
Marion, OH 43302-5628
740-389-6786
Fax: 740-725-6258
www.osumarion.osu.edu

Matt Moreau, Director
Kathleen Clemons, Counselor
Holly Jacobson, Coordinator of Admission
A public four-year college providing a full range of services for students with disabilities.

3565   Ohio State University: Newark Campus
1179 University Drive
Founders Hall
Newark, OH 43055-1797
740-366-9333
800-963-9275
Fax: 740-364-9645
www.newark.osu.edu

William L. Mac Donald, Dean/Director
Anne Federlein, President
Ann Donahue, Director of Admissions
A public four-year college providing services to learning disabled students including peer tutoring, extended test time, quiet rooms and other special accommodations. There is no separate fee for these services.

3566   Ohio State University: Nisonger Center
1581 Dodd Drive
Columbus, OH 43210-1257
614-685-3192
855-983-9955
Fax: 614-366-6373
TDD: 614-688-8040
www.nisonger.osu.edu
nisongeradmin@osumc.edu

Marc J. Tasse, Director
Jane Case-Smith, President
Paula Rabidoux, Associate Director
The Ohio State University Nisonger Center for Mental Retardation and Developmental Disabilities provides interdisciplinary training, research and exemplary services pertaining to people with developmental disabilities. The center, which is a part of a national network of activities called University Afffiliated Programs, was founded in 1968. Training is provided in medicine (pediatrics and psychiatry), dentistry, education, physical therapy, psychology and other relevant disciplines.

3567   Ohio University
Ohio University
101 University Drive
P.O. Box 629
Chillicothe, OH 45601
740-774-7200
Fax: 740-593-2708
www.ohiou.edu
chillicothe@ohio.edu

David Brightbill, Chair
David A. Wolfort, Vice Chair
Rodrick J. McDavis, President
A public four-year college with a small percentage of special education students.

3568   Ohio University Chillicothe
101 University Drive
Chillicothe, OH 45601-629
740-774-7200
877-462-6824
Fax: 740-774-7290
www.ohiou.edu/~childept
diekroge@ohio.edu

Diane Diekroger MD, Student Support Coordinator
Richard Bebee, Manager
Offers a variety of services to students with disabilities including note takers, extended testing time, counseling services, and special accommodations.

3569   Otterbein College
1 S. Grove St.
Westerville, OH 43081-2006
614-823-1618
800-488-8144
Fax: 614-823-1983
www.otterbein.edu
lmonaghan@otterbein.edu

Rebecca D. Vazquez-Skillings, VP for Business Affairs
Kathy Krendl, President
Alec Wightman, Secretary
An independent four-year college with a small percentage of special education students.

3570   Owens Community College
Disability Resources Department
PO Box 10000
Toledo, OH 43699-1947
567-661-7000
800-466-9367
Fax: 419-661-7607
www.owens.edu
bscheffert@owens.cc.oh.us

Thomas P Perin, Associate Vice President
Dr. Mike Bower, Ph.D., President
Renay M Scott, Vice President/Provost
A comprehensive Community College that offers educational programs in over 50 technical areas of study leading to the Associate of Applied Science, Associate of Applied Business or Associate of Technical Studies degree. Provides programs designed for college transfer and leads to the Associate of Arts or Associate of Science degree. Finally, a number of certificate programs as well as short term credit and non-credit programs are available.

3571 Shawnee State University

940 Second Street
Portsmouth, OH 45662-4347

740-351-4778
800-959-2778
Fax: 740-351-3470
TTY: 740-351-3159
www.shawnee.edu
jmoore@shawnee.edu

Rita Rice-Morris, President
Elinda C. Boyles, Ph.D, VP of Finance & Administration
Elizabeth Blevins, M.S., Director of Communications
Offers a variety of services to students with disabilities including notetakers, extended testing time, counseling services, and special accommodations.

3572 Sinclair Community College

Learning Disability Support Services
Rm 11342
444 West Third Street
Dayton, OH 45402-1453

937-512-2855
800-315-3000
Fax: 937-512-4564
TDD: 937-512-3096
www.sinclair.edu

Jeff Boudouris, Vice President
Dr. Dave Collins, Provost
Steven L. Johnson, Ph.D., President and CEO
Funded by the Federal Department of Education, Student Support Services is an organization devoted to helping students meet the challenges of college life. Our goals are to help students stay in school, then eventually graduate and/or transfer to a four-year college or university. We strive to develop new ways of helping students achieve their educational, career and professional goals.

3573 Southern State Community College

100 Hobart Drive
Hillsboro, OH 45133-9406

937-393-3431
Fax: 937-393-9831
www.sscc.edu

Robin Lashley, Exe Assistant to the President
Dr Kevin Boys, President
James Bland, Vice President
Offers a variety of services to students with disabilities including notetakers, extended testing time, counseling services, and special accommodations.

3574 Terra State Community College

Special Education Services
2830 Napoleon Road
Fremont, OH 43420-9600

419-559-2349
866-288-3772
Fax: 419-334-3667
www.terra.cc.us/terra2.html
admissions@terra.edu

Jerome Webster, President
Jack Fatica, VP, Academic Affairs
Jeffery Huffman, Director
Provides quality learning experiences which are accessible and affordable. Terra is actively committed to excellence in learning and offers associate degrees in various technologies as well as in arts and sciences, applied business, and applied science. Our office of student support services works with students with learning disabilities and other disabilities.

3575 University of Cincinnati: Raymond Walters General and Technical College

9555 Plainfield Road
Blue Ash, OH 45236-1007

513-745-5600
Fax: 513-745-5780
TDD: 513-745-8300
www.ucblueash.edu
questions@ucblueash.edu

Cady Short-Thompson, Dean
Raymond Walters, President
Meredith Delaney, Director of Development
Offers a variety of services to students with disabilities including notetakers, extended testing time, counseling services, and special accommodations.

3576 University of Findlay

Disability Services Office
1000 N. Main St.
Findlay, OH 45840-3653

419-422-8313
800-472-9502
Fax: 419-434-4822
TDD: 419-434-5532
www.findlay.edu
campuscompact@findlay.edu

Debow Freed, Ph.D., President Emeritus
Katherine Fell, President
William D. Miller, Director of Christian Ministry
An independent four-year college with a small percentage of special needs students.

3577 University of Toledo

Libbey Hall
Mail Stop 524
Toledo, OH 43606-3390

419-530-8888
Fax: 419-530-4505
www.utoledo.edu
enroll@utoledo.edu

Patricia M. Mowery, B.A., Interim Director
Julianne Bonitati, Administrative Assistant
Nagi Naganathan, PhD, President
A public four-year college whose mission is to provide the support services and accommodations necessary for all students to succeed.

3578 Urbana University

Student Affairs Office
597 College Way
Urbana, OH 43078

937-772-9200
Fax: 937-484-1322
www.urbana.edu
webmaster@urbana.edu

Dr. David Decker, President
J. Steven Polsley, Chairman
Jim Wehrman, Vice Chair
An independent four-year college with a small percentage of special education students.

3579 Walsh University

2020 East Maple Street
North Canton, OH 44720-3336

330-490-7090
800-362-9846
Fax: 330-499-7165
www.walsh.edu
bfreshour@walsh.edu

Richard Jusseaume, President
Nancy Blackford, Vice President
Derrick Wyman, Director
An independent four-year college. The Office of Student Support Services maintains an early warning system for students in academic, financial, social and/or emtional difficulty. The Office proudly communicates regularly with students regarding their general well being, and assists in the students' academic and financial concerns with referals to appropriate offices.

3580 Washington State Community College
710 Colegate Drive
Marietta, OH 45750-9225
740-374-8716
Fax: 740-376-0257
www.wscc.com

Bradley J. Ebersole, Ph.D, President
Gary Williams, Executive Director
Jess N. Raines, CPA, CFO/Treasurer
A public two-year college with a small percentage of special education students.

3581 Wilmington College of Ohio
1870 Quaker Way
Wilmington, OH 45177-2499
937-382-6661
800-341-9318
Fax: 937-382-7077
www.wilmington.edu

Jim Renoylds, President
Robert Touchton, Chair
Sandra W. Neville, Vice Chair
Offers a variety of services to students with disabilities including notetakers, extended testing time, counseling services, and special accommodations.

Oklahoma

3582 Bacone College
2299 Old Bacone Rd
Muskogee, OK 74403-1568
918-683-4581
888-682-5514
Fax: 918-682-5514
www.bacone.edu
stewarta@bacone.edu

Dr. Robert K Brown, Executive Vice President
Ann Stewart, Coordinator
Frank K. Willis, President
Offers a variety of services to students with disabilities including notetakers, extended testing time, counseling services, and special accommodations.

3583 Cascade College
PO Box 11000
2501 E.Memorial Road
Edmond, OK 73013-1100
405-425-5000
800-877-5010
Fax: 503-257-1222
www.cascade.edu
info@oc.edu

John DeSteiguer, President
Dr. Bill Goad, Executive Vice President
Scott LaMascus, VP Academic Affairs
Offers a variety of services to students with disabilities including note takers, extended testing time, counseling services, and special accommodations.

3584 East Central University
1100 E 14th St
Ada, OK 74820-6999
580-332-8000
Fax: 580-310-5654
www.ecok.edu/

Duane C. Anderson, Provost and Vice President
Jessica A. Boles, VP, Administration and Finance
John R. Hargrave, President
A public four-year college with a small percentage of special education of students.

3585 Moore-Norman Technology Center
PO Box 4701
Norman, OK 73070-4701
405-364-5763
Fax: 405-360-9989
www.mntechnology.com
sjohnson@mntechnology.com

Jane Bowen, Superintendent
Barbara Rice, Disability Coordinator
Roger Adair, Director, Finance

Offers a variety of services to students with disabilities including notetakers, extended testing time, counseling services, and special accommodations.

3586 Northeastern State University
600 N Grand Ave
Tahlequah, OK 74464-2301
918-456-5511
800-722-9614
Fax: 918-458-2363
www.nsuok.edu
offices.nsuok.edu/publicsafety

Dr. Laura D Boren, Vice President Student Affairs
Ben Hardcastle, Executive Director
Dr. Steve Turner, President
Four year college that offers programs and services to disabled students.

3587 Oklahoma City Community College
Department of Student Support Services
7777 South May Avenue
Oklahoma City, OK 73159-4444
405-682-1611
Fax: 405-682-7585
TDD: 405-682-7520
TTY: 405-682-7529
www.occc.edu
webmaster@occc.edu

Teresa Moisant, Chair
Devery Youngblood, Vice-Chair
Dr. Paul W. Sechrist, President
Comprehensive community college with individualized services and accommodations for students with disabilities arranged by the Office of Student Support Services. Services include Deaf Program, and accommodations as described by section 504 & ADA. Five tutoring labs are available on campus and assistive technology including voice synthesizers and voice recognition for computer based word processing.

3588 Oklahoma Panhandle State University
PO Box 430
Goodwell, OK 73939-430
580-349-2611
800-664-OPSU
Fax: 580-349-2302
TDD: 580-349-1559
www.opsu.edu
opsu@opsu.edu

David A. Bryan, President
Lynna Brakhage, Director
Apryl Burleson, Financial Aid Conselor
Four year college that offers programs to the learning disabled.

3589 Oklahoma State University: Oklahoma City Technical School
900 N Portland Ave
Oklahoma City, OK 73107-6195
405-947-4421
800-580-4099
Fax: 405-945-3289
www.osuokc.edu
emilytc@osuokc.edu

Natalie Shirley, President
Shane Crawford, Assoc. Vice President
Rachel Rittenhouse, Secretary
Offers access to students with disabilities based upon the diagnostic documentation which is provided by the student and the functional impact of the disability.

3590 Oklahoma State University: Okmulgee Technical School
1801 E 4th Street
Okmulgee, OK 74447-3901
918-293-4678
800-722-4447
Fax: 918-293-4643
www.osuit.edu
osuit.admissions@okstate.edu

Claudette Butcher, Exe Assistant to the President
Bill R. Path, President
Dr. Linda Avant, Executive Vice President
Offers a variety of services to students with disabilities including notetakers, extended testing time, counseling services, and special accommodations.

3591 Oral Roberts University
7777 South Lewis Avenue
Tulsa, OK 74171

918-495-6161
Fax: 918-495-7229
www.oru.edu
droberson@oru.edu

William M. Wilson, President
Reverend Robert Hoskins, Board Chair
Mart Green, Vice Chair
Four year college that offers resources to students with a learning disability.

3592 Rogers State University
1701 W Will Rogers Blvd
Claremore, OK 74017-3259

918-343-7777
800-256-7511
Fax: 918-343-7712
www.rsu.edu
msith@rsu.edu

Misty Smith, Acting VP for Student Affairs
Richard A. Beck, VP for Academic Affairs
Thomas M. Volturo, EVP Administration and Finance
A public four-year university with several special education students out of a total of approximately 3,300.

3593 Rose State College
Academic Support Department
6420 SE 15th Street
Midwest City, OK 73110-2704

405-733-7673
866-621-0987
Fax: 405-733-7399
TDD: 405-736-7308
www.rose.edu
rjones@rose.edu

Dr. Jeanie Webb, President
Dr. Jeff Caldwell, Vice President
Betty J.C Wright, Chairman
Services and facilities include academic advisement, referal and liaison with other community agencies, recorded textbooks and individual testing for qualified students.

3594 Southeastern Oklahoma State University
1405 North 4th Ave
Durant, OK 74701-609

580-745-2000
800-435-1327
Fax: 580-745-2515
TDD: 580-745-2704
www.se.edu
sdodson@sosu.edu

Dr. Doug McMillan, VP for Academic Affairs
Sean Burrage, President
Michele Campbell, Executive Assistant
Four year college that provides services to the learning disabled students.

3595 Southwestern Oklahoma State University
100 Campus Drive
Weatherford, OK 73096-3098

580-774-3063
Fax: 580-774-3795
www.swosu.edu
cindy.dougherty@swosu.edu

John Hays, President
Offers a variety of services to students with disabilities including notetakers, extended testing time, counseling services, and special accommodations.

3596 St. Gregory's University
Partners in Learning
1900 W. MacArthur St.
Shawnee, OK 74804-2403

405-878-5100
Fax: 405-878-5198
TDD: 405-878-5103
www.stgregorys.edu
info@stgregorys.edu

D. Gregory Main, President
Donald Wolf, Board Chair
Michael Scaperlanda, Vice Chair
Four-year college offering assistive programs for students with learning disabilities.

3597 Tulsa Community College
Disabled Student Resource Center
909 South Boston Avenue
Tulsa, OK 74119-2095

918-595-7000
800-331-3050
Fax: 918-595-7179
TDD: 918-595-7287
admission@utulsa.edu

Roger N. Blais, Provost/VP for Academic Affairs
Kevan C. Buck, EVP/Treasurer
Dr. Steadman Upham, President
Offers a variety of services to students with disabilities including note takers, extended testing time, counseling services, and special accommodations.

3598 Tulsa University
Center for Student Academic Support
800 South Tucker Drive
Tulsa, OK 74104-9700

918-631-2000
Fax: 918-631-5003
TDD: 918-631-3329
www.utulsa.edu
jcorso@utulsa.edu

Jane Corso PhD, Director
Ruby Wile, Assistant Director
Dr. Steadman Upham, President
The Center offers a comprehensive range of support services and accommodations for students with disabilities.

3599 University of Oklahoma
660 Parrington Oval
Norman, OK 73019-0390

405-325-0311
800-522-0772
Fax: 405-325-7605
TDD: 405-325-4173
www.ou.edu/
sdyer@ou.edu

Suzette Dyer, Disability Services Director
Caryn Pacheco, Director, Financial Aid
David L. Boren, President
A public doctoral degree-granting research university. The University of Oklahoma is an equal opportunity institution.

Oregon

3600 Central Oregon Community College
2600 NW College Way
Bend, OR 97701-5933

541-383-7700
Fax: 541-383-7506
www.cocc.edu

James E. Middleton, President
Julie Smith, Executive Assistant
Jeff Stuermer, Board Chair
Central Oregon Community College will be a leader in regionally and globally responsive adult, lifelong, postsecondary education for Central Oregon.

3601 Clackamas Community College
Disability Resource Center
19600 Molalla Avenue
Oregon City, OR 97045

503-594-6100
Fax: 503-722-5865
TDD: 503-650-6649
www.clackamas.edu
admissions@clackamas.edu

Joanne Truesdell, President
Lisabeth Pacheco, Disability Coordinator
A public two-year college. Special education services are designed to support student success by creating full access and providing appropriate accommodations for all students with disabilities.

3602 Corban College
5000 Deer Park Drive SE
Salem, OR 97317-9392
503-581-8600
Fax: 503-585-4316
www.corban.edu
visit@corban.edu

Heidi Stowman, Director of Admissions
Reno Hoff, President
Chris Vetter, Associate Provost
Private four year Christian college offering assistance for learning disabled students.

3603 George Fox University
Disability Services Office
414 N Meridian St
Newberg, OR 97132-2697
503-538-8383
800-765-4369
Fax: 503-554-3880
http://ds.georgefox.edu
webmaster@georgefox.edu

Rick Muthiah, Associate Director
Missy Terry, Executive Assistant
Robin Baker, President
An independent faith-based four-year college with a small percentagge of students with disabilities.

3604 Lane Community College
4000 East 30th Ave.
Eugene, OR 97405-640
541-463-3100
Fax: 541-463-5201
TDD: 541-463-3079
www.lanecc.edu
webmaster@lanecc.edu

Mary Spilde, President
Sonya Christian, Vice-President
Anna Kate Malliris, Assistant to the Vice President
We provide accommodations, technology, advising, support systems, training and education.

3605 Linfield College
900 SE Baker St
McMinnville, OR 97128-6894
503-883-2200
Fax: 503-883-2472
TDD: 503-883-2396
TTY: 503-883-2396
www.linfield.edu
admission@linfield.edu

Susan Agre-Kippenhan, VP for Academic Affairs
Thomas L. Hellie, President
Susan Hopp, Vice President
An independent four-year college. Services include tutoring, extended time for testing, assistance with advising and counseling. Student needs are considered in customizing individual programs of support for documented special needs.

3606 Linn-Benton Community College Office of Disability Services
6500 Pacific Blvd. SW
Albany, OR 97321
541-917-4999
Fax: 541-917-4328
TDD: 541-917-4703
www.linnbenton.edu/go/ds
ods@linnbenton.edu

Carol Raymundo, Coordinator
Greg Hamann, President
Dave Henderson, Vice President
A public two-year college. LBCC provides a number of services and programs for students with disabilities including classes, supportive services and aids.

3607 Mount Bachelor Academy
33051 NE Ochoco Hwy
Prineville, OR 97754-7990
541-462-3404
800-462-3404
Fax: 541-462-3430
www.mtba.com/

Sharon Bitz, Executive Director
Matthew Lovell, Program Director
Kelli Hoffman, Admissions Director
Aspen Education Group is recognized nationwide as the leading provider of education programs for struggling or underachieving young people. As the largest and most comprehensive network of therapeutic schools and programs, Aspen offers professionals and families the opportunity to choose a setting that best meets a student's unique academic and emotional needs.

3608 Mt. Hood Community College Disability Services Department
Learning Disabilities Department
26000 SE Stark St
Gresham, OR 97030-3300
503-491-6422
Fax: 503-491-7670
www.mhcc.edu
dsoweb@mhcc.edu

Richard Doughty, VP Administrative Services
Pam Benjamin, Executive Assistant
Debbie Derr, Ed.D, President
A commitment to providing educational opportunities for all students forms the foundation of the disability services program. If you are a student with a disability, disability services will help you overcome potential obstacles so that you may be successful in your area of study. Disability services gives you the needed support to help you meet your goals without separating you and other students with disabilities from existing programs.

3609 Oregon Institute of Technology
Oregon State University Systems
3201 Campus Drive
Klamath Falls, OR 97601-8801
541-885-1000
800-422-2017
Fax: 541-885-1777
TDD: 541-885-1072
TTY: 541-885-1072
www.oit.edu
access@oit.edu

Christopher Maples, President
MaryAnn Zemke, VP Finance & Administration
Bradley Burda, Provost/VP For Academic Affairs
A public four-year college enrolling about 3,000 students. Accommodations are tailored to the needs of individual students on a case-by-case basis for those self-identified as having learning disabilities.

3610 Oregon State University
Services for Students with Disabilities
A202 Kerr Administration Building
1500 SW Jefferson Avenue
Corvallis, OR 97331-2133
541-737-4098
Fax: 541-737-7354
TDD: 541-737-3666
www.oregonstate.edu
disabilty.services@oregonstate.edu

Martha Smith, Director
Dr. Edward Ray, President
Elizabeth Grubb, Executive Secretary
A public four-year college with a small percentage of students.

3611 Portland Community College
PO Box 19000
Portland, OR 97280-990
503-244-6111
866-922-1010
Fax: 503-977-4882
TTY: 503-246-4072
www.pcc.edu

Deanna Palm, Vice Chair
Dr. Jeremy Brown, President
Denise Frisbee, Chair
Our team includes rehabilitation guidance counselors, learning disability specialists, sign language interpreters, a technology specialist, vocational progarm and special needs coordinatiors.

3612 Reed College
3203 SE Woodstock Boulevard
Portland, OR 97202-8199   503-771-1112
                                            800-547-4750
                                       Fax: 503-777-7769
                                            www.reed.edu
                                   admissions@reed.edu

John R. Kroger, President
Lorraine Arvin, Vice President & Treasurer
Dawn Thompson, Executive Assistant
Offers a variety of services to students with disabilities including notetakers, extended testing time, counseling services, and special accommodations.

3613 Southwestern Oregon Community College
1988 Newmark Ave
Coos Bay, OR 97420-2911   541-888-2525
                                            800-962-2838
                                       Fax: 541-888-7285
                                            www.socc.edu

Patty M. Scott,Ed. D., President
Marcia Jensen, Chair
David Bridgham, Vice-Chair
The college will provide reasonable accommodation for students with learning disabilities. Some instructors in academic skills have special training in working with learning disabled students.

3614 Treasure Valley Community College
650 College Blvd
Ontario, OR 97914-3423   541-881-8822
                                       Fax: 541-881-2717
                                            www.tvcc.cc.or.us

Dana M. Young, President
Randy Griffin, VP Administrative Services
Dr. Rachel Anderson, VP Academic Affairs
Offers a variety of services to students with disabilities including notetakers, extended testing time, counseling services, and special accommodations.

3615 Umpqua Community College
PO Box 967
1140 Umpqua College Rd
Roseburg, OR 97470-226   541-440-4622
                                       Fax: 541-440-4666
                                            www.umpqua.edu

Elin Miller, Board Chair
David Beyer, Administrator
Dr. Joe Olson, UCC President
A public two-year college with a small percentage of special education students.

3616 University of Oregon
5278 University of Oregon
164 Oregon Hall
Eugene, OR 97403-5278   541-346-1155
                                       Fax: 541-346-6013
                                       TTY: 541-346-1155
                                            www.ds.uoregon.edu
                                   uoaec@uoregon.edu

Michele Gottfredson, President
Yvette Marie Alex-Assensoh, VP Equity and Inclusion
Scott Coltrane, SVP/Provost
A public four-year college with about 5% of students with disabilities.

3617 Warner Pacific College
2219 SE 68th Ave
Portland, OR 97215-4099   503-517-1142
                                            800-582-7885
                                       Fax: 503-517-1350
                                            www.warnerpacific.edu
                                   webmaster@warnerpacific.edu
Andrea P. Cook, Ph.D., President
Steve Anderson, Chair
Steve Robertson, Vice-Chair

Offers a variety of services to students with disabilities including notetakers, extended testing time, counseling services, and special accommodations.

3618 Western Oregon University
345 N. Monmouth Avenue
Monmouth, OR 97361-1371   503-838-8000
                                            877-877-1593
                                       Fax: 503-838-8399
                                            www.wou.edu
                                   webmaster@wou.edu

Louann Brant, Program Assistant
Mark D. Weiss, President
Malissa Larson, Director
A public four-year college. Strives to provide and promote a supportive, accessible, non-discriminatory learning and working environment for students, faculty, staff and community members with disabilities. These goals are realized through the provision of individualized support services, advocacy and the identification of current technology and information.

3619 Willamette University
Learning Disabilities Department
900 State Street
Salem, OR 97301-3930   503-370-6300
                                       Fax: 503-370-6148
                                       TDD: 503-375-5383
                      www.willamette.edu/dept/disability/main.
                                   jhill@willamette.edu

Kristen Grainger, VP
Marlene Moore, VP Academic Affairs
Stephen E. Thorsett, President
Offers a variety of services to students with disabilities including notetakers, extended testing time, counseling services, and special accommodations. Provides services for all students on campus, including graduate schools.

Pennsylvania

3620 Albright College
13th & Bern Streets
P.O. Box 15234
Reading, PA 19612-5234   610-921-2381
                                       Fax: 610-921-7530
                                            www.albright.edu
                                   albright@alb.edu

Kathleen C. Hittner, M.D, Vice Chair
Lex O. McMillan III, Ph.D., President
Jeffrey J. Joyce, Chair
An independent four-year college with a small percentage of special education students. There is an additional fee for the education program in addition to the regular tuition.

3621 Bloomsburg University
400 E. Second St.
Bloomsburg, PA 17815-1301   570-389-4000
                                       Fax: 570-389-3700
                                            www.bloomu.edu
                                   buadmiss@bloomu.edu

MAry Vasta, Vice Chairperson
David L. Soltz, President
Patrick Wilson, Chairperson
Offers a variety of services to students with disabilities including notetakers, extended testing time, counseling services, and special accommodations.

3622 Bryn Mawr College
Educational Support Services
101 North Merion Avenue
Bryn Mawr, PA 19010-2899   610-526-5000
                                       Fax: 610-526-6525
                                            www.brynmawr.edu
                                   info@brynmawr.edu

Kim Cassidy, President
Marge Garber, Vice President
Jerry Berenson, Chief Administrative Officer

Bryn Mawr is a private liberal arts college located in Bryn Mawr, Pennsylvania not far from Philadelphia. The College provides support services for qualified students with documented learning, physical, and psychological disabilities. For additional information visit www.brynmawr.edu/access_services .

3623 Cabrini College
Disability Support Services
610 King of Prussia Rd
Radnor, PA 19087-3698   610-902-8100
                                     Fax: 610-902-8204
                                     TDD: 610-902-8582
                                     www.cabrini.edu
                                     ama722@cabrini.edu
Thomas P. Nerney, Chair
Frank R. Emmerich Jr., Vice Chair
Donald B. Taylor, Ph.D., President
Offers support services and appropriate accommodations to students with documented learning disabilities.

3624 Carnegie Mellon University
Equal Opportunity Services, Disability Resources
143 North Craig Street
Whitfield Hall
Pittsburgh, PA 15213   412-268-3386
                                     Fax: 412-268-1524
          www.cmu.edu/hr/eos/disability/index.html
                                     hrhelp@andrew.cmu.edu
Larry Powell, Manager, Disability Resources
Daniel McNulty, Interim Associate Vice President
Haley Lantz, Senior Administrative
Four year college that offers its students services for the learning disabled.

3625 College Misericordia
Alternative Learners Project
301 Lake St
Dallas, PA 18612-1090   570-674-6400
                                          800-262-6363
                                     Fax: 570-675-2441
                                     www.misericordia.edu
                                     info@misericordia.edu
Thomas J. Botzman, Ph.D, President
John Metz, Chair
Christopher Borton, Vice Chair
An independent four-year college with about 5% special education students.

3626 Community College of Allegheny County: College Center, North Campus
Learning Disabilities Services
8701 Perry Highway
Pittsburgh, PA 15237-5353   412-366-7000
                                     Fax: 412-366-7000
                                     TDD: 412-369-4110
                                     TTY: 412-369-4110
                                     www.ccac.edu
                                     kwhite@ccac.edu
Amy M. Kuntz, Chair
Quintin B. Bullock, President
Mary Frances Archey, VP Student Success & Completion
Support services for students with disabilities are provided according to individual needs. Services include assistance with testing, advisement, registration, classroom accommodations, professor and agency contact.

3627 Community College of Allegheny County: Boyce Campus
595 Beatty Road
Monroeville, PA 15146-1396   724-327-1327
                                     Fax: 724-325-6733
                                     TTY: 724-325-6733
                                     www.ccac.edu
                                     mailto:Pflorent@ccac.edu
Amy M. Kuntz, Chair
Quintin B. Bullock, President
Mary Frances Archey, VP Student Success & Completion

A 2 year community college campus in a suburban setting. Offers a variety of services to students with disabilities including notetakers, extended testing time, counseling services, and special accommodations.

3628 Community College of Philadelphia
Center on Disability
1700 Spring Garden Street
Philadelphia, PA 19130-3991   215-751-8010
                                     Fax: 215-751-8762
                                     www.ccp.edu
                                     fdirosa@ccp.edu
Dr. Donald Generals, President
Matthew Bergheiser, Chair
Suzanne Biemiller, Vice Chair
With more than 70 associate's degree, certification and continuing education programs, a lively campus near Center City, and a supportive, top-flight faculty,Community College of Philadelphia is your path to possibilities.

3629 Delaware County Community College
901 S. Media Line Road
Media, PA 19063-1027   610-359-5000
                                     Fax: 610-359-5055
                                     TDD: 610-359-5020
                                     TTY: 610-359-5020
                                     www.dccc.edu
                                     abinder@dccc.edu
Donald L. Heller, Vice-Chair
Jerome S. Parker, President
Michael L. Ranck, Chair
Delaware County Community College, the ninth largest college in the Philadelphia metropolitan area, is a public, two year institution offering more than 60 programs of study. Its open-door policy, and affordable tuition make it accessible to all. Services to physically and learning disabled students include counseling services, tutoring, extended testing, tape recorded lectures, spelling allowances, assistive equipment, notes copied and study skills workshops.

3630 Delaware Valley College of Science and Agriculture
700 East Butler Ave
Doylestown, PA 18901-2698   215-345-1500
                                     Fax: 215-230-2968
                                     www.delval.edu
                                     Admitme@delval.edu
Frances Flood, Transfer Coordinator
Bashar W. Hanna, VP Academic Affairs
Thomas O'Connor, Associate Director of Admission
Offers a variety of services to students with disabilities including notetakers, extended testing time, counseling services, and special accommodations.

3631 Delaware Valley Friends School
19 E Central Avenue
Paoli, PA 19301-1345   610-640-4150
                                     Fax: 610-296-9970
                                     www.dvfs.org
Pritchard Garrett, Head of School
Rick Mosenkis, President and CEO
Robert Turner, Chairman
Our mission is to prepare students with learning differences for future work and study.

3632 Dickinson College
Services for Students with Disabilities
Post Office Box 1773
Carlisle, PA 17013-2896   717-243-5121
                                          800-644-1773
                                     Fax: 717-245-1080
                                     TTY: 717-245-1134
                                     www.dickenson.edu
                                     admissions@dickinson.edu
Bronte Jones, VP Finance and Administration
Nancy A. Roseman, President
Joyce Bylander, VP, Student Development

The Office of Counseling and Disability Services is dedicated to the enhancement of healthy student development. Professional and paraprofessional staff offer confidential individual and group counseling sessions and outreach services which help students with both general developmental issues and with specific personal or interpersonal difficulties.

3633 Drexel University
Office of Disability Services
3141 Chestnut Street
Main Building, Room 212, 2nd Floor
Philadelphia, PA 19104-2875
215-895-2000
Fax: 215-895-1414
www.drexel.edu

John A. Fry, President
Mark L. Greenberg, PhD, Provost and SVP
Susan C. Aldridge, PhD, Senior Vice President
Drexel University's mission is to serve their students and society through comprehensive integrated academic offerings enhanced by technology, co-operative education, and clinical practice in an urban setting, with global outreach embracing research, scholarly activities, and community initiatives.

3634 East Stroudsburg University of Pennsylvania
200 Prospect St
East Stroudsburg, PA 18301-2999
570-422-3211
877-230-5547
Fax: 570-422-3777
TDD: 570-422-3543
www.esu.edu
emiller@po-box.esu.edu

Marcia G. Welsh, Ph.D., President
L. Patrick Ross, Chair
Nancy V. Perretta, Vice Chair
Four year college that offers services to disabled students.

3635 Gannon University
Program for Students with Learning Disabilities
109 University Square
Erie, PA 16541
814-871-7000
814-426-6668
Fax: 814-871-7338
www.gannon.edu
theisen001@gannon.edu

Thomas C. Guelcher, Vice Chairperson
Keith Taylor, Ph.D., President
Lawrence T. Persico, Chairperson
Special Support Services are provided for students who have a diagnosed learning disability and choose to enroll in PSLO. Charge of $300.00 per semester special services include individual sessions with Educational Specialists, Kurzweil Reader, Copying Services, Advocacy Seminar Courses I and II, Reading Efficiency sessions, testing accommodations, etc.

3636 Gettysburg College
300 N Washington Street
Gettysburg, PA 17325-1483
717-337-6100
800-431-0803
Fax: 717-337-6145
www.gettysburg.edu
admiss@gettysburg.edu

Janet Morgan Riggs, President
Gail Sweezey, Director of Admissions
Darryl Jones, Senior Associate Director
Offers a variety of services to students with disabilities including notetakers, extended testing time, counseling services, and special accommodations.

3637 Gwynedd: Mercy College
PO Box 901
1325 Sumneytown Pike
Gwynedd Valley, PA 19437-901
215-646-7300
800-342-5462
Fax: 215-641-5598
www.gmc.edu
guido.r@gmc.edu

Dr. Frank E. Scully, Jr., VP for Academic Affairs
Kathleen Owens, PhD, President
Kevin O'Flaherty, VP Finance and Administration
Recognizing the diversity of our student population and the challenges and needs this brings to the educational enterprise, Gwynedd-Mercy College, within the bounds of its resources, intends to provide reasonable accommodations for students with disabilities so that all students accepted into a program of study have equal access and subsequent opportunity to reach their academic and personal goals. Requests for specific accommodations are processed on an individual basis.

3638 Harcum Junior College
750 Montgomery Ave
Bryn Mawr, PA 19010-3476
610-525-4100
Fax: 610-526-6086
www.harcum.edu

Denise Beauchamp, Executive Director
Susan E. Barrett, Ed.D., Vice President
Jon Jay DeTemple, PhD, President
An independent two-year college. There is an additional fee for the special education program in addition to the regular tuition.

3639 Harrisburg Area Community College
Disability Services Office
One Hacc Drive
Harrisburg, PA 17110-2999
717-780-2538
800-222-4222
Fax: 717-780-2551
www.hacc.edu
bookstor@hacc.edu

Edna V Baehre, Affairs/Enrollment Management
Carol Keeper, Director
John J. Sygielski, President
A public two-year college with a small percentage of special needs students.

3640 Hill Top Preparatory School
737 S Ithan Ave
Rosemont, PA 19010-1197
610-527-3230
Fax: 610-527-7683
www.hilltopprep.org

Tom Needham, Headmaster
Bud Haly, President
Sissy Wickes, Chairman of the Board
Prepares students in grades 6-12 with diagnosed learning differences for higher education and successful futures. The school is d co-educational day school that offers an individually structures, rigorous curriculum that is complemented by a dynamic counseling support and menotoring program.

3641 Indiana University of Pennsylvania
1011 South Dr ive
Indiana, PA 15705-1098
724-357-2100
800-442-6830
Fax: 724-357-6281
TDD: 724-357-4067
www.iup.edu/advisingtesting
admissions_inquiry@iup.edu

Michael A. Driscoll, President
Susan S. Delaney, Chair
Jonathan B. Mack, Vice Chair
Disability Support Services is a component of the Advising and Testing Center. The mission of DSS is to ensure that students with disabilities who attend Indiana University of Pennsylvainia receive an integrated, quality education.

3642 Keystone Junior College
P.O .Box 50
One College Green
La Plume, PA 18440-0200
570-945-8000
877-4college
Fax: 570-945-8962
www.keystone.edu
admissions@keystone.edu

Dr. David Coppola, President
Cheryl Guse, Executive Assistant
Nancy Allan, Secretary to the President
Offers a variety of services to students with disabilities including notetakers, extended testing time, counseling services, and special accommodations.

3643 King's College
Academic Skills Center
133 N River Street
Wilkes Barre, PA 18711-801
570-208-5900
Fax: 570-208-5967
www.kings.edu
admissions@kings.edu

John Ryan, C.S.C., Ph.D., President
Thomas R. Smith, Chairman
Mark DeCesaris, Vice Chairman
First Year Academic Studies Program (FASP) - A proactive program to facilitate transition to college with intensive first-year programming with indivdual support in subsequent years. Students are enrolled as full-time students completing general education and major course requirements. Support includes regular meetings with a learning disability specialist, faculty tutorials/study groups, priority advisement, and development of self-advocacy skills. A fee charged for the first year.

3644 Kutztown University of Pennsylvania
15200 Kutztown Road
Kutztown, PA 19530
610-683-4000
Fax: 610-683-1520
TDD: 610-683-4499
www.kutztown.edu
sutherla@kutztown.edu

Jesus Pena, Esq, Associate Vice President
Dr. Carlos Vargas-Aburto, Acting President
Gerald Silberman, VP Administration and Finance
Kutztown University of Pennsylvania, a member of the Pennsylvania State System of Higher Education, was founded in 1856 as Keystone Normal School, and achieved University status in 1983. Today Kutztown University is a modern, comprehensive University. There are approximately 7,900 full and part time undergraduate and graduate students.

3645 Lebanon Valley College
101 N College Avenue
Annville, PA 17003-1400
717-867-6275
Fax: 717-867-6124
www.lvc.edu
perry@lvc.edu

Dr. Lewis Evitts Thayne, President
Shawn P. Curtin, VP Finance and Administration
Karen M. Feather, Executive Assistantt
Four year college that offers learning disabled students support and services.

3646 Lehigh Carbon Community College
4525 Education Park Drive
Schnecksville, PA 18078-2598
610-799-2121
Fax: 610-799-1527
TTY: 610-799-1792
www.lccc.edu
mmitchell@lccc.edu or lkelly@lccc.edu

Thomas C. Leamer, President
Brian Kahler, VP Finance and Facilities
Audrey L. Larvey, Chair
Disability Support Services provides learning support to qualified students with disabilities in compliance with section 504 of the Rehabilitation Act and Americans with Disabilities Act, 1990. Requests for access and/or academic accommodations are reviewed on a case by case basis. Additional learning support is available through Educational Support Services.

3647 Lock Haven University of Pennsylvania
Learning Disabilities Office
401 N Fairview St
Lock Haven, PA 17745-2390
570-893-2011
800-332-8900
Fax: 570-893-2432
www.lhup.edu
admissions@lhup.edu

Dr. Michael Fiorentino, Jr., President
Dr. Donna Wilson, Provost/SVP
William Hanelly, VP Finance and Administration
A public four-year college with a small percentage of students with disabilities.

3648 Lycoming College
700 College Place
Williamsport, PA 17701
570-321-4000
800-345-3920
Fax: 570-321-4337
www.lycoming.edu
webmaster@lycoming.edu

Peter R. Lynn, Chair of the Board
Kent Trachte, Ph.D., President
Jeff Bennett, VP Finance and Administration
An independent four-year college with a small percentage of special education students.

3649 Manor Junior College
700 Fox Chase Road
Jenkintown, PA 19046-3399
215-885-2360
Fax: 215-576-6564
www.manor.edu
ftadmiss@manor.edu

Sister Mary Cecilia Jurasinski, President
Sally Mydlowec, Executive Vice President
Jeffrey Levine, M.Ed., Director of Admissions
Offers a variety of services to students with disabilities including notetakers, extended testing time, counseling services, and special accommodations.

3650 Mansfield University of Pennsylvania
Services for Students with Learning Disabilities
31 South Academy St.
Ste. 1
Mansfield, PA 16933
570-662-4000
800-577-6826
Fax: 570-662-4995
www.mansfield.edu
wchabala@mansfield.edu

Steven M. Crawford, Vice Chairman
Francis L. Hendricks, President
Ralph H. Meyer, Chairman
Offers a variety of services to students with disabilities including, extended testing time, counseling services, and special accommodations.

3651 Marywood University
Special Education Department
2300 Adams Avenue
Scranton, PA 18509-1598
570-348-6211
866-279-9663
Fax: 570-961-4739
www.marywood.edu

Anne Munley, I.H.M., Ph.D., President
Alan M. Levine, Ph.D., Vice President
Marion Munley, Chair
Marywood challenges students to broaden their understanding of globale issues and to make decisions based on spiritual, ethical, and religious values.

3652 Mercyhurst College
Learning Differences Program
501 East 38th Street
Erie, PA 16546
814-824-2000
800-825-1926
Fax: 814-824-2438
www.mercyhurst.edu
drogers@mercyhurst.edu

Thomas J. Gamble, Ph.D., President
Marlene D Mosco, Chair of the Board
Richard A. Lanzillo, Vice Chair
Mercyhurst provides a comprehensive program of academic accommodations and support services to students with documented learning disabilities. Accommodations may include audiotaped textbooks, extended time for tests, a test reader and use of a computer to complete essay tests.

3653 Messiah College
One College Avenue
Suite 3059
Mechanicsburg, PA 17055-9800   717-796-5382
                                                800-233-4220
                                           Fax: 717-796-5217
                                               www.messiah.edu
                                disabilityservices@messiah.edu
Kim S. Phipps, Ph.D., President
Anne Barnes, Executive Assistant
Carol Wickey, Special Assistant
Private Christian college.

3654 Millersville University of Pennsylvania
Disability and Learning Services
1 South George St
P.O. Box 1002
Millersville, PA 17551-302   717-872-3011
                                           Fax: 717-871-2129
                                               www.millersv.edu
                             admissions@millersville.edu
John M. Anderson, Ph.D., President
Dr. Aminta Hawkins Breaux, Vice President
Michael G. Warfel, Chairman
Four year college that provides services to learning disabled students.

3655 Moravian College
1200 Main Street
Bethlehem, PA 18018   610-861-1320
                                                800-441-3191
                                           Fax: 610-861-1577
                                               www.moravian.edu
                                memld02@moravian.edu
Robert J. Schoenen, Jr., Vice Chair
Bryon L. Grigsby, President
Kenneth J. Rampolla, Chair
Four year college that offers programs for the learning disabled.

3656 Northampton Community College
Disability Support Services
3835 Green Pond Rd
Bethlehem, PA 18020-7599   610-861-5300
                                           Fax: 610-861-5373
                                           TDD: 610-861-5351
                          www.northampton.edu/disabilityservices
                               LDemshock@northampton.edu
Robert R. Fehnel, Vice Chairman
Dr. Mark H. Erickson, President
Karl A. Stackhouse, Chairman
Encourages academically qualified students with disabilities to take advantage of educational programs. Services and accommodations are offered to facilitate accessiblity to both college programs and facilities. Services provided to students with disabilities are based upon each student individual needs.

3657 Pace School
2432 Greensburg Pike
Pittsburgh, PA 15221-3611   412-244-1900
                                           Fax: 412-244-0100
                                               www.paceschool.org
                                     pace@paceschool.org
Gerri L. Sperling, President
Robert Gold, Vice President
Brian P. Fagan, Secretary
A placement option for school districts in Allegheny and surrounding counties that serves kids, K-9, with emotional challenges or Autism.

3658 Pathway School
162 Egypt Rd
Jeffersonville, PA 19403-3090   610-277-0660
                                           Fax: 610-539-1973
                                               www.pathwayschool.org
David J Schultheis, President/CEO
Louise Robertson, M.Ed., Vice President for Development
Hadley Williams, Ph.D., Chair
Provides a comprehensive program of services for children between the ages of 9 and 21 for whom mainstream public and private school education is insufficient to meet their needs. These youngsters display severe neuropsychiatric disorders and complex learning issues necessitating focused learning environments.

3659 Pennsylvania Institute of Technology
800 Manchester Ave
Media, PA 19063-4089   610-892-1000
                                                800-422-0025
                                           Fax: 610-892-1510
                                               www.pit.edu
                                               info@pit.edu
Walter R. Garrison, President
Gerard C. Gambs Jr., Program Manager
Raymond P. Altieri, Chair
Offers a variety of services to students with disabilities including notetakers, extended testing time, counseling services, and special accommodations.

3660 Pennsylvania State University
Support Services for Students with Learning Disab
116 Boucke Building
University Park, PA 16802-5902   814-863-1807
                                           Fax: 814-863-3217
                                           TDD: 814-863-1807
                                        www.equity.psu.edu/ods
                           william.welsh@equity.psu.edu/ods
Eric J. Barron, President
Keith Masser, Chairman
Janine S. Andrews, Director
Penn State provides academic accommodations and support services to students with documented learning disabilities. Accommodations may include audiotaped textbooks, extended time for tests, a test reader and use of a computer to complete essay tests.

3661 Pennsylvania State University: Mont Alto
1 Campus Dr
Mont Alto, PA 17237-9799   717-749-6000
                                           Fax: 717-749-6116
                                               www.ma.psu.edu
                                               nmhz@psu.edu
Derk S. Barnett, Assistant Director of Admissions
Dr. Francis Achampong, Chancellor
Dr. Michael Doncheski, Director of Academic Affairs
It is the intention of Penn State University to provide equal access to students with disabilities as mandated by the Americans with Disabilities Act, and the Rehabilitiation Act. Students with disabilities are encouraged to take advantage of the support services provided to help them successfully meet the high academic standards of the university.

3662 Pennsylvania State University: Schuylkill Campus
Disability Services
200 University Drive
Schuylkill Haven, PA 17972-2202   570-385-6000
                                           Fax: 570-385-3672
                                               www.sl.psu.edu
Allen E. Kiefer, President
Charles M. Miller, 1st Vice President
Dr. Jack T. Dolbin, 2nd Vice President
Offers a variety of services to students with disabilities including notetakers, extended testing time, counseling services, and special accommodations.

3663 Pennsylvania State University: Shenango Valley Campus
Office for Disability Services
147 Shenango Avenue
Sharon Hall 207
Sharon, PA 16146-5902
724-983-2803
Fax: 724-983-2820
TDD: 814-863-1807
TTY: 814-863-1807
www.equity.psu.edu/ods
william.welsh@equity.psu.edu/ods
Thomas Burich, President
Sam Bernstine, Vice President
Fredric M. Leeds, Secretary
Penn State encourages academically qualified students with disabilities to take advantage of its educational programs. To be eligible for disability related accommodations, individuals must have a documented disability as defined by the Americans with Disabilities Act. A disability is defined by the physical or mental impairment that substantially limits a major life function. Individuals seeking accommodations are required to provided documentation.

3664 Pennsylvania State University: Worthington Scranton Campus
120 Ridgeview Drive
Dunmore, PA 18512-1699
570-963-2500
Fax: 570-963-2535
www.sn.psu.edu
Dean L. Butler, Chair
Darlene Dunay D.O., Vice Chair
Dr. Alan Peslak, President
Penn State encourages academically qualified students with disabilities to take advantage of its educational programs. It is the policy of the university not to discriminate against persons with disabilities in its admissions policies or procedures or its educational programs, services and activities.

3665 Point Park College
Program for Academic Success
201 Wood Street
Pittsburgh, PA 15222-1984
412-391-4100
800-321-0129
Fax: 412-392-3998
www.pointpark.edu
pboykin@pointpark.edu
Dr. Karen S. McIntyre, SVP, Academics
Dr. Paul Hennigan, President
Anne Lewis, Chair
Provides appropriate, reasonable accommodations for students who are disabled in accordance with the Americans with Disabilities Act. All campus accommodations are coordinated through the Program for Academic Success (PAS).

3666 Reading Area Community College
10 South Second Street
Reading, PA 19603-1706
610-372-4721
800-626-1665
Fax: 610-607-6264
www.racc.edu
Dr. Anna Weitz, President
Edwin L. Stock, Chair
Zylkia R. Rivera, Vice Chair
A public two-year college with a small percentage of special education students.

3667 Seton Hill University
One Seton Hill Drive
Greensburg, PA 15601
724-834-2200
800-826-6234
Fax: 724-834-2752
TTY: 724-830-1151
www.setonhill.edu
bassi@setonhill.edu
Michele Ridge, Chair
David Myron, Vice President for Finance, CFO
Mary C. Finger, President
Offers programs to those who are eligible and learning disabled.

3668 Shippensburg University of Pennsylvania
1871 Old Main Drive
Shippensburg, PA 17257-2299
717-477-1301
Fax: 717-477-1273
www.ship.edu
lawate@wharf.ship.edu
Dr. Jody Harpster, President
Robin Maun, Executive Assistant
Joy Arnold, Secretary to the President
Four year college that offers services to the learning disabled students.

3669 Solebury School
Learning Skills Program
6832 Phillips Mill Road
New Hope, PA 18938-9682
215-862-5261
Fax: 215-862-3366
www.solebury.org
admissions@solebury.org
Tom Wilschutz, Head of School
Scott Eckstein, Director of Admission
Janice Poinsett, Associate Director of Admission
A special program for bright students who are hampered by specific learning differences. It is ideally suited for students who require specialized instruction to assist them in unlocking their potential.

3670 Stratford Friends School
2 Bishop Hollow Road
Newtown Square, PA 19073-5319
610-355-9580
Fax: 610-355-9585
www.stratfordfriends.org
info@stratfordfriends.org
Tim Madigan, Ph.D., Head of School
Offer programs for students with language-based learning disabilities who have had difficulty learning in a traditional classroom.

3671 Summer Matters
1777 North Valley Rd
PO Box 730
Paoli, PA 19301
610-296-6725
Fax: 610-640-0132
www.summermatters.org
info@summermatters.org
James Kirkpatrick, Chief Financial Officer
Scott Wheeler, Chair
Mark Oebbecke, Vice-Chair
Represents a continuum of innovative summer enrichment and remedial experiences for youth and young adults. Offers 3 separate and unique programs for learning and fun.

3672 Temple University
1301 Cecil B Moore Avenue
100 Ritter Annex
Philadelphia, PA 19122
215-204-1280
Fax: 215-204-6794
TTY: 215-204-1786
www.temple.edu/disability
drs@temple.edu
Vanessa Dash, Student Services Coordinator
Reene Kirby, Assistant Director
Aaron Spector, Associate Director
Offers a variety of services to students with disabilities including proctoring, interpreting and academic accommodations.

3673 Thaddeus Stevens College of Technology
750 East King Street
Lancaster, PA 17602-3198
717-299-7701
800-842-3832
Fax: 717-391-6929
www.stevenscollege.edu
admissions@stevenscollege.edu
Ronald E. Ford, Vice Chair
William E. Griscom, ED.D., President
Donna Kreiser, Chairperson

A 2-year trade and technical college primarily serving socially and economically under-resourced students.

3674 Thiel College
Office of Special Needs
75 College Ave
Greenville, PA 16125-2181

724-589-2000
800-248-4435
Fax: 724-589-2850
www.thiel.edu
scowan@thiel.edu

Mark Benninghoff, Chair
Lynn Franken, Ph.D., VP Academic Affairs
Troy D. VanAken, Ph.D., President
Four year college that provides an Office of Special Needs for those students with disabilities.

3675 University of Pennsylvania
3101 Walnut Street
Philadelphia, PA 19104

215-898-5000
Fax: 215-898-5756
www.upenn.edu
lrcmail@pobox.upenn.edu

Valerie Dorsey Allen, Director
Gregory S. Rost, Vice President/Chief of Staff
Dr. Amy Gutmann, President
Services for People with Disabilities coordinates academic support services for students with disabilities; services include readers, notetakers, library research assistants, tutors or transcribers.

3676 University of Pittsburgh: Bradford
Learning Development Department
300 Campus Drive
Bradford, PA 16701-2898

814-362-7500
800-872-1787
Fax: 814-362-7684
www.upb.pitt.edu

William C. Conrad, Executive Director
Thomas R. Bromeley, Chairman and CEO
Dr. Livingst Alexander, President
Offers a variety of services to students with disabilities including extended testing time, counseling services, and special accommodations.

3677 University of Pittsburgh: Greensburg
Disabilities Services Office
150 Finoli Drive
Greensburg, PA 15601

724-837-7040
Fax: 724-836-7134
www.pitt.edu/~upg
upgadmit@pitt.edu

Rick A. Fogle, Dean of Student Services
J. Wesley Jamison, VP Academic Affairs
Sharon P. Smith, PhD, President
The Learning Resources Center is an important place for students with disabilities at Pitt Greensburg. Students are encouraged to register with Lou Ann Sears to recieve any accommodations they are entitled to.

3678 University of Scranton
Memorial Hall
800 Linden Street
Scranton, PA 18510-4699

570-941-7400
Fax: 570-941-7899
http://matrix.scranton.edu
addmissions@scranton.edu

Donald R. Boomgaarden, Ph.D., Provost/Senior Vice President
Kevin P. Quinn, S.J., President
Gary R. Olsen, Vice President
Four year college that offers programs for learning disabled students.

3679 University of the Arts
320 S Broad St
Philadelphia, PA 19102-4994

215-717-6030
800-616-2787
Fax: 215-717-6045
www.uarts.edu

Sean T. Buffington, President
Thomas H. Carnwath, VP
Megan Storti, Executive Assistant
Within this community of artists, the process of learning engages, refines, and articulates all of our creative capabilities; the Office of Educational Accessibility is here to assist students with disabilities in the pursuit of their personal, creative, artisitic and educational objectives.

3680 Ursinus College
PO Box 1000
Collegeville, PA 19426-1000

610-409-3000
Fax: 610-489-0627
www.ursinus.edu
admissions@ursinus.edu

Jonathan Ivec, VP for Finance & Administration
Bobby Fong, President
Terry Winegar, Dean of the College
Offers a variety of services to students with disabilities including notetakers, extended testing time, counseling services, and special accommodations.

3681 Valley Forge Educational Services
1777 North Valley Road
PO Box 730
Paoli, PA 19301

610-296-6725
Fax: 610-640-0132
www.vfes.net
info@vfes.net

Tim Krushinski, Director of The Vanguard School
Janet McDwell, Admin Assistant for Director
Lynne Sansone, Administrative Assistant
Offers a wide variety of educational services focused on guiding 21st century learners to independence. Provides premier educational optoins for young children, adolescents and pre-21 adults ranging from school-based and summer programs to career planning to clinical and consulting services.

3682 Vanguard School
PO Box 730
1777 North Valley Road
Paoli, PA 19301-0730

610-296-6700
Fax: 610-640-0132
www.vanguardschool-pa.org
info@vanguardschool-pa.org

Tim Krushinski, Director of The Vanguard School
Janet McDwell, Admin Assistant for Director
Lynne Sansone, Administrative Assistant
Serves students whose exceptionalities include austism spectrum disorders, mild emotional disturbance and cognitive disabilities.

3683 Washington and Jefferson College
60 South Lincoln Street
Washington, PA 15301-4801

724-229-5139
888-926-3529
Fax: 724-503-1049
www.washjeff.edu
SAIL@washjeff.edu

Tori Haring-Smith, President
Denny Trelka, Dean
John Zimmerman, VP Academic Affairs
An independent four-year college with a small percentage of special education students.

3684   Westmoreland County Community College
145 Pavilion Lane
Youngwood, PA 15697   724-925-4000
                                    800-262-2103
                               Fax: 724-925-3823
                               TDD: 724-925-4297
                                    www.wccc.edu
                                    beresm@wccc-pa.edu

Kevin Pahach, Vice Chairman
Larry J. Larese, Chairman
Tuesday Stanley, President
Offers a variety of services to students with disabilities including notetakers, extended testing time, counseling services, and special accommodations. All services are based on a review of a current evaluation presented by the student. Appropriate services are then arranged by the student support service counselor.

3685   Widener University
Disabilities Services
One University Place
Chester, PA 19013-5792   610-499-4000
                               Fax: 610-499-4386
                                    www.widener.edu
                                    csimonds@mail.widener.edu

James T Harris III, President
Linda S. Durant, MEd, SVP for University Advancement
Nicholas P. Trainer, Chair
An independent four-year college with comprehensive support services, including disabilities services, academic coaching, tutoring services, a math center and writing center.

Rhode Island

3686   Brown University, Disability Support Services
20 Benevolent St
Box 1876
Providence, RI 02912-9012   401-863-2378
                               Fax: 401-863-9300
                               TDD: 401-863-9588
                                    www.brown.edu
                                    dss@brown.edu

Kimberly Roskiewicz, Assistant To The President
Christina H. Paxson, President
Elizabeth Huidekoper, EVP Administration and Finance
Brown University has as its primary aim the education of a highly qualified and diverse student body and respects each student's dignity, capacity to contribute, and desire for personal growth and accomplishment. Brown's commitment to students with disabilities is based on awareness of what students require for success. The University desires to foster both intellectual and physical independence to the greatest extent possible in all of its students.

3687   Bryant College
Academic Services
1150 Douglas Pike
Smithfield, RI 02917-1287   401-232-6000
                               Fax: 401-232-6319
                                    www.bryant.edu
                                    lhazard@bryant.edu

Ronald K. Machtley, President
James Damron, VP for University Advancement
James Patti, M.B.A., Executive Assistant
An independent four-year Business and Liberal Arts College. A learning specialist is on campus to provide services for students with learning disabilities.

3688   Community College of Rhode Island: Knight Campus
400 East Ave
Warwick, RI 02886-1807   401-825-1000
                               Fax: 401-825-2365
                                    www.ccri.edu
                                    webservices@ccri.edu

Deb Zielinski, Assistant to the President
Ray M. Di Pasquale, President
Greg Lamontagne, VP Academic Affairs
Academic accommodations are available to students with disabilities who demonstrate a documented need for the requested accommodation. Accommodations include but are not limited to adapted equipment, alternative testing, course accommodations, sign language interpreters, reader/audio taping services, scribes and peer note-takers.

3689   Disability Services for Students
University of Rhode Island
302 Memorial Union
Kingston, RI 02881   401-874-2098
                               Fax: 401-874-5574
                               TTY: 800-745-5555
                                    www.uri.edu
                                    dss@etal.uri.edu

Dr. David M. Dooley, President
Dr. Gerald Sonnendeld, VP Research & Economic Dev
Naomi R. Thompson, AVP Community
Disability Service for Students fosters a barrier free environment to individuals with disabilities through education that focuses on inclusion, awareness, and knowledge of ADA/504 compliance. Our mission is two fold: 1. To encourage a sense of empowerment for students with disabilities by providing a process that involves the student. 2. To be an information resource to the University faculty and staff regarding disability awareness and academic services.

3690   Johnson & Wales University
8 Abbott Park Place
Providence, RI 02903-3775   401-598-1000
                                    800-343-2565
                               Fax: 401-598-2880
                                    www.jwc.edu
                                    mberstein@jwu.edu

Mim Runey, President
Marie Bernardo-Sousa, SVP Administration
Diane H. D'Ambra, VP Human Resources
An independent four-year university servicing about 5% special education students. Accommodations are individualized to students presenting documentation and may include extended time testing, tape recorders in class, notetaking assistance, reduced course load, preferential scheduling and tutorial assistance.

3691   Providence College
Disability Support Services
1 Cunningham Square
Providence, RI 02918   401-865-1000
                               Fax: 401-865-2057
                               TDD: 401-865-2494
                                    www.providence.edu/oas
                                    oas@providence.edu

Nancy Kelley, Executive Assis to the President
Brian J. Shanley, President
Kenneth Sicard, O.P., Executive Vice President
Offers a variety of services to students with disabilities including note takers, extended testing time, counseling services, and special accommodations.

3692   Rhode Island College
Paul V Sherlock Center on Disabilities
600 Mount Pleasant Ave
Providence, RI 02908-1991   401-456-8072
                               Fax: 401-456-8150
                               TDD: 401-456-8773
                                    www.sherlockcenter.org
                                    aantosh@ric.edu

Michael Ducharme, Director
Patricia Nolin, Special Assistant
Nancy Carriuolo, President
The University Affiliated Program (UAP) of Rhode Island is a member of a national network of UAPs. The UAP is charged with four core functions: 1. Providing pre-service training to prepare quality service providers. 2. Providing community outreach training and technical assistance. 3. Disseminating information about research and exemplary practice. 4. Research.

3693 **Roger Williams University**
One Old Ferry Road
Bristol, RI 02809
401-253-1040
800-458-7144
Fax: 401-254-3185
www.rwu.edu
admit@rwu.edu

Donald J. Farish, Ph.D., J.D., President
Robert H. Avery, Esq., General Counsel/SVP
Catherine C. Capolupo, VP Enrollment Management
An independent comprehensive four-year university with about 5% special education students.

South Carolina

3694 **Aiken Technical College**
Student Services
PO Drawer 696
2276 J. Davis Highway
Graniteville, SC 29829
803-593-9231
Fax: 803-593-9231
www.atc.edu
weldon@atc.edu

Richard Weldon, Counselor
Jennifer Pinckney, Manager
Winsor Susan, President
A public two-year college offering services to the learning disabled.

3695 **Camperdown Academy**
501 Howell Rd
Greenville, SC 29615-2028
864-244-8899
Fax: 864-244-8936
www.camperdown.org

Dan Blanch, Head of School
Our mission is to enable students with average to above average intelligence, who also experience learning difficulties in the areas of reading, organization, language processing, and written expression, to reach their maximum academic potential.

3696 **Citadel-Military College of South Carolina**
171 Moultrie St
Charleston, SC 29409
843-953-5230
Fax: 843-953-7036
www.citadel.edu
admissions@citadel.edu

John W. Rosa, President
Thomas J. Elzey, Vice President
John W. Powell Jr., Director
Offers a variety of services to students with disabilities including notetakers, extended testing time, counseling services, and special accommodations.

3697 **Clemson University**
Student Development Services
707 University Under
Clemson, SC 29634
864-656-3311
Fax: 864-656-0514
www.clemson.edu
bmartin@clemson.edu

David H. Wilkins, Chairman
James P. Clements, President
Nadim M. Aziz, Vice President
Four-year college offers services to learning disabled students.

3698 **Coastal Carolina University**
Disability Services Department
PO Box 261954
Conway, SC 29528-6054
843-347-3161
Fax: 843-349-2990
www.coastal.edu

D. Wyatt Henderson, Chairman
William S. Biggs, Vice Chair
David A. DeCenzo, President

Coastal Carolina University provides a program of assistance to students with disabilities. Upon acceptance to the University, students will become eligible for support services by providing documentation of their disability. Accommodations include academic labs, tutorial referral, study skills, counseling, auxillary aids, coordination with other agencies and classroom accommodations.

3699 **Erskine College**
2 Washington St
P.O. Box 338
Due West, SC 29639
864-359-4358
888-359-4358
Fax: 864-379-2167
www.erskine.edu

Dr. Paul D. Kooistra, President
W.S. Cain, Chairman
N. Bradley Christie, SVP Academic Affairs
Offers a variety of services to students with disabilities including notetakers, extended testing time, counseling services, and special accommodations.

3700 **Francis Marion University**
PO Box 100547
Florence, SC 29502-547
843-661-1310
800-368-7551
Fax: 843-661-1202
www.fmarion.edu

Luther F Carter, President
George C. McIntyre, Chair
L. Franklin Elmore, Vice Chair
A public four-year college with services for special education students.

3701 **Glenforest School**
1041 Harbor Drive
West Columbia, SC 29169-3609
803-796-7622
Fax: 803-796-1603
www.glenforest.org
info@glenforest.org

Cheri Riddell, Principal
Daphne Perugini, Vice-Principal
Ina Fournier, Superintendent
A K-12 independent, SACS accredited, non-profit day school dedicated to educationg students who learn differently. Dedicated to serving children with learning differences and attention issues including: ADD/ADHD, Dyslexia, Dysgraphia and Autism Spectrum Disorders.

3702 **Greenville Technical College**
PO Box 5616
506 S. Pleasantburg Drive
Greenville, SC 29606-5616
864-250-8000
800-922-1183
Fax: 864-250-8580
www.greenvilletech.com

Susan M. Jones, Associate VP of Human Resources
Jacqueline DiMaggio, Vice President for Finance
Dr. Keith Miller, President
Committed to providing equal access for all students and assisting students in making their college experience successful in accordance with ADA/504 and the Rehabilitation Act. The Office of Special Needs for Students with Disabilities has counselors available to assist in the planning and implementation of appropriate accommodations.

3703 **Limestone College**
Program for Alternative Learning Styles
1115 College Dr
Gaffney, SC 29340-3799
864-489-7151
800-795-7151
Fax: 864-487-8706
www.limestone.edu
kkearse@limestone.edu

Dr. Walt Griffin, President
Dr. Karen Gainey, VP Academic Affairs & Exe. VP
Dr. William Baker, Special Assistant

Independent four-year college with a program designed to serve students with learning disabilities. There is an additional fee for the first year in the program in addition to the regular tuition. However, that additional cost is reduced by 50% after the freshman year depending on the grade point average.

3704   Midlands Technical College

PO Box 2408
Columbia, SC 29202-2408   803-738-8324
                                         800-922-8038
                                    Fax: 803-790-7524
                                    TDD: 803-822-3401
                                    www.midlandstech.edu
                                    askmtc@midlandstech.edu

Dr. Marshall White, Jr., President
Gina Mounsield, Vice President
Derrah Cassidy, Director of Admissions
Services to Students with Disabilities counselors support and assist students with disabilities in meeting their personal, educational and career goals. Services include academic and career planning, faculty/student liasion, assistive technology, readers, writers, interpeters, closed circuit television in libraries, TDD, testing services, orientation sessions and a support group.

3705   North Greenville College

Learning Disabilities Services
7801 N. Tigerville Rd
P. O. Box 1892
Tigerville, SC 29688-1892   864-977-7000
                                         800-468-6642
                                    Fax: 864-977-7021
                                    www.ngc.edu
                                    nisgett@ngc.edu

Nancy Isgett, Learning Disabilities Liaison
Dr. James B. Epting, President
Offers a variety of services to students with disabilities including notetakers, extended testing time, counseling services, and special accommodations.

3706   South Carolina State University

300 College Street NE
Orangeburg, SC 29117   864-587-4000
                                          800-772-7286
                                     Fax: 864-587-4355
                                     www.scsu.edu
                                     gouveia@scsu.edu

W. Franklin Evans, VP for Academic Affairs
Andrew Hugine, President
Dr. William Small, Jr., Chair
Four-year college that provides information and resources for the learning disabled.

3707   Spartanburg Methodist College

1000 Powell Mill Road
Spartanburg, SC 29301   864-587-4000
                                          800-772-7286
                                     Fax: 864-587-4355
                                     www.smcsc.edu
                                     admiss@smcsc.edu

Dr. Phinnize Fisher, Chair
Dr. Colleen Perry Keith, President
James Fletcher Thompson, Vice Chair
2-year educational institution, Junior College

3708   Technical College of Lowcountry: Beaufort

921 Ribaut Road
Beaufort, SC 29901-1288   843-525-8211
                                     Fax: 843-525-8285
                                     www.tcl.edu

Rodney Adams, Dean of Students
Richard J. Gough, President
Offers a variety of services to students with disabilities including note takers, extended testing time, counseling services, and special accommodations.

3709   Trident Academy

1455 Wakendaw Rd
Mount Pleasant, SC 29464-9767   843-884-7046
                                     Fax: 843-881-8320
                                     www.tridentacademy.com
                                     admissions@tridentacademy.com

Kathy M. Cook, Ph.D., Headmaster
Mike Jeresaty, President
Sandi Clerici, Vice President
An independent learning disabilities school for students in grades K-12 who have Dyslexia, Dysgraphia, Dyscalculia, Non-verbal Learning Disabilities, ADHD, CAPD and other learning differences.

3710   Trident Technical College

PO Box 118067
Charleston, SC 29423-8067   843-574-6111
                                         877-349-7184
                                    Fax: 843-574-6682
                                    www.tridenttec.edu

Mary Thornley, President
Patricia J. Robertson, Vice President For Academic Aff
Patrice Mitchell, Vice President For Student Ser
Recognizes its responsibility to identify and maintain the standards (academic, admissions, scores, etc.) that are necessary to provide quality academic programs while ensuring the rights of students with disabilities.

3711   University of South Carolina

Disability Services
902 Sumter Street Access/Lieber Col
Columbia, SC 29208   803-777-7000
                                          800-868-5872
                                     Fax: 803-777-0101
                                     TDD: 803-777-6744
                                     www.sc.edu
                                     kpettus@sc.edu

Harris Pastides, President
Eugene P Warr, Jr., Chairman
John C. von Lehe, Jr., Vice Chairman
The Office of Disability Services provides accommodations for students with documented physical, emotional, and learning disabilities. The professionally trained staff works toward accessiblity for all university programs, services, and activities in compliance with ADA/504. Services include orientation, priority registration, library access, classroom adaptions, interpeters, and access to adapted housing.

3712   University of South Carolina: Aiken

471 University Parkway
Aiken, SC 29801   803-648-6851
                                     Fax: 803-641-3362
                                     www.usca.edu
                                     kayb@aiken.sc.edu

Ernest R. Allen, Chairman
Teresa Haas, Vice Chairman
Sandra Jordan, Chancellor
The mission of Disability Services (DS) is to facilitate the transition of students with disabilities into the University enviroment and to provide appropriate accommodations for each student's special needs in order to ensure equal access to all programs, activities and services at USCA.

3713   University of South Carolina: Beaufort

801 Carteret Street
Beaufort, SC 29902-4601   843-521-4100
                                     Fax: 843-521-4194
                                     www.oc.edu/beaufort

Joan Lemoine MD, Associate Dean
Jane T. Upshaw, Chancellor
A public two-year college with services for special education students.

3714 University of South Carolina: Lancaster
Admissions Office
PO Box 889
101 N. Main Street
Lancaster, SC 29721-889
803-285-1565
Fax: 803-313-7106
www.lancaster.sc.edu
ksaile@gwm.sc.edu

Debbie Horne, Administrator
Hal Hiott, Director
Carrie W. Helms, Treasurer
Offers a variety of services to students with disabilities including notetakers, extended testing time, counseling services, and special accommodations.

3715 Voorhees College
PO Box 678
Denmark, SC 29042-678
803-780-1234
866-685-9904
Fax: 866-685-9904
www.voorhees.edu
info@voorhees.edu

Cleveland L. Dr. Cleveland L., President and CEO
Dr. Lugenia Rochelle, Interim EVP, Academic Affairs
St. Clair P. Guess, III, Chair
Four-year college that offers programs to learning disabled students.

3716 Winthrop University
Student Disabilities Department
701 Oakland Ave
Rock Hill, SC 29733-7001
803-323-2211
Fax: 803-323-4861
TDD: 803-323-2233
www.winthrop.edu
smithg@winthrop.edu

Anthony Digiorio, Director
Rosanne Wallace, Administrator
DebraC. Boyd, Ph.D., Provost/VP Academic Affairs
Since each student has a unique set of special needs, the Counselor for Students with Disabilities makes every effort to provide the student with full access to programs and services. Reasonable accommodations are provided based on needs assessed through proper documentation and an intake interview with the couselor. The majority of buildings on campus are accessible.

South Dakota

3717 Black Hills State College
1200 University St
Unit 9502
Spearfish, SD 57799-9502
605-642-6343
800-255-2478
Fax: 605-642-6099
www.bhsu.edu
admissions@bhsu.edu

Beth Oaks, Director of Admissions
Tom Jackson Jr., President
Joe Rainboth, Assistant Director of Admissions
Provide the comprehensive supports necessary in meeting the individual needs of students with disabilities.

3718 Children's Care Hospital and School
Educational Program
2501 West 26th Street
Sioux Falls, SD 57105-2498
605-444-9500
800-584-9294
Fax: 605-336-0277
www.cchs.org

Jessica Wells, Foundation President
Dave Timpe, Interim CEO
Angie Brown, V.P. Strategic Initiatives
Provides a variety of innovative educational services based on the individual learning, medical, and therapeutic needs of the child.

3719 Northern State University
1200 S Jay St
Aberdeen, SD 57401-7198
605-626-3011
800-678-5330
Fax: 605-626-2587
www.northern.edu
admissions@northern.edu

Laurie Nichols, Director
James Smith, President
Four-year college that provides services to students with a learning disability.

3720 South Dakota School of Mines & Technology
501 East Saint Joseph Street
Rapid City, SD 57701-3995
605-394-2511
800-544-8162
Fax: 605-394-6131
www.sdsmt.edu
fcampone@sdsmt.edu

Heather Wilson,Dphil, President
Duane C Hrncir, Provost/VP, Academic Affairs
Patricia G Mahon, VP, Student Affairs
Four-year college that offers support services to those students whom are disabled.

3721 South Dakota State University
PO Box 2201
Brookings, SD 57007
605-688-4121
800-952-3541
Fax: 605-688-6891
TDD: 605-688-4394
www.sdstate.edu
SDSU_Admissions@sdstate.edu

Robert Otterson, Executive Assis to the President
David L. Chicoine, Ph.D., President
Laurie Nichols, Provost/VP Academic Affairs
Committed to providing equal opportunities for higher education for learning disabled students.

3722 Yankton College
PO Box 133
Yankton, SD 57078-133
605-665-3661
866-665-3661
Fax: 605-665-3662
www.yanktoncollege.org
nfo@yanktoncollege.org

Charles Kaufman, President
Joan Neubauer, Chair
Joseph Ward, Vice-Chair
Offers a variety of services to students with disabilities including note takers, extended testing time, counseling services, and special accommodations.

Tennessee

3723 Austin Peay State University
Office of Disability Services
PO Box 4578
Clarksville, TN 37044
931-221-6230
Fax: 931-221-7102
TDD: 931-221-6278
TTY: 931-221-6278
www.apsu.edu/disability
acadaffairs@apsu.edu

Amy Deaton, Director of Admissions
Tracy Comer, Assistant Director
Megan Mitchell, Associate Director
The Office of Disability Services is dedicated to providing academic assistance for students with disabilities enrolled at Austin Peay State University. We provide information to students, faculty, staff and administrators about the needs of students with disabilities. We ensure the accessiblity of programs, services, and activities to students having a disability. We are a resource of information pertaining to disability issues and advocate participation in campus life.

3724   Bryan College: Dayton
721 Bryan Drive
Dayton, TN 37321-7000   423-775-2041
                                        800-277-9522
                                        Fax: 423-775-7300
                                        www.bryan.edu
                                        info@bryan.edu
John Haynes, Chairman
Kevin Clauson, J.D., Vice President of Academics
Stephen D. Livesay , Ph.D., President
Committed to providing quality education for those who
meet admission standards but learn differently from others.
Modifications are made in the learning environment to enable LD students to succeed. Some of the modifications
made require documentation of the specific disability while
other adaptations do not. In addition to modifications the
small teacher-student ratio allows the school to provide
much individual attention to those with learning difficulties.

3725   Carson-Newman College
2130 Branner Ave.
Jefferson City, TN 37760-2232   865-471-2000
                                        800-678-9061
                                        Fax: 865-471-3502
                                        www.cn.edu
                                        ckey@cn.edu
J Randall O'Brien, President
Tom Harmon, Chairman
Janet Hayes, Vice Chairman
An independent four-year college with support services for
special education students.

3726   East Tennessee State University
1276 Gilbreath Dr.
Box 70300
Johnson City, TN 37614-1700   423-439-1000
                                        Fax: 903-886-5702
                                        www.etsu.edu
                                        go2etsu@etsu.edu
Cecilia McIntosh, PhD, Dean of Graduate Studies
Scott Kirkby, PhD, Assistant Dean
Karin Bartoszuk, PhD, Associate Dean of Grad. Studies
Offers a variety of services to students with disabilities in-
cluding note takers, extended testing time, counseling ser-
vices, and special accommodations.

3727   Knoxville Business College
1000 Volunteer Boulevard
Knoxville, TN 37996-4160   865-974-5001
                                        Fax: 865-974-4989
                                        www.kbcollege.edu
                                        execed@utk.edu
Stephen L. Mangum, Dean
Kate Atchley, Executive Director
Tom Cervone, Managing Director
Offers a variety of services to students with disabilities in-
cluding notetakers, extended testing time, counseling ser-
vices, and special accommodations.

3728   Middle Tennessee State University
1301 East Main Street
Murfreesboro, TN 37132-1   615-898-2300
                                        Fax: 615-898-5444
                                        www.mtsu.edu
                                        dssemail@mtsu.edu
Sidney McPhee, President
John Morgan, Chancellor
Dale Sims, Vice Chancellor
We offer a wide variety of services to students with disabili-
ties including testing accommodations, providing access to
adaptive computer technologies and acting as a liaison to
University departments.

3729   Motlow State Community College
PO Box 8500
Lynchburg, TN 37352-8500   931-393-1500
                                        800-654-4877
                                        Fax: 931-393-1764
                                        www.mscc.edu
                                        asimmons@mscc.cc.tn.us
A. Simmons, Dean Student Development
Billy Soloman, Owner
MaryLou Apple, President
A public two-year college with support services for special
education students.

3730   Northeast State Community College
PO Box 246
2425 Highway 75
Blountville, TN 37617-0246   423-323-3191
                                        800-836-7822
                                        Fax: 423-279-7649
                                        TDD: 423-279-7640
                                        TTY: 423-279-4649
                                        www.northeaststate.edu
                                        memask@northeaststate.edu
A. Lee Shillito, Chair
Dr. Allana Hamilton, VP, Academic Affairs
Matt DeLozier, Interim VP of Student Affairs
To assure equal educational opportunities for individuals
with disabilities.

3731   Pellissippi State Technical Community College
PO Box 22990
10915 Hardin Valley Road
Knoxville, TN 37933-990   865-694-6400
                                        Fax: 865-539-7217
                                        www.pstcc.edu
                                        admissions@pstcc.edu
Joanne Monhollen, Executive Secretary
Rebecca Ashford, Vice President
Dr.Anthony Wise, President
Services for Students with Disabilities develops individual
educational support plans, provides prioriy registration and
advisement, furnishes volunteer notetakers, provides readers, scribes, tutor bank, provides interpeter services and publishes a newsletter. The office acts as a liaison, and assists
students in location of resources appropriate to their needs.

3732   Shelby State Community College
P.O. Box 780
Memphis, TN 38101-0780   901-333-5000
                                        877-717-7822
                                        Fax: 901-333-5711
                                        www.sscc.cc.tn.us
Sherman Greer, Executive Assis to the President
Ron Parr, VP Fnancial & Admin Services
Dr. Nathan Essex, President
A two-year college providing information and resources to
disabled students.

3733   Southern Adventist University
Academic Support
5010 University Drive
P.O. Box 370
Collegedale, TN 37315-370   423-236-2000
                                        800-768-8437
                                        Fax: 423-236-1000
                                        www.ldpsych.southern.edu
                                        adossant@southern.edu
Ron Smith, Chairman
Marc Grundy, Vice President
Gordon Bietz, President
A private university offering undergraduate degrees in education designed for K-8, 1-8, 7-12, and K-12 certification
plus graduate degrees designed for inclusion (special needs
in the regular classroom), multiage/multigrade teaching,
outdoor education, and psychology and counseling of exceptional individuals. College age students with special needs
and those desiring to teach students with special needs are
welcome to apply.

3734 Southwest Tennessee Community College
5983 Macon Cove
P.O. Box 780
Memphis, TN 38101-780   901-333-5000
                                       877-717-7822
                                  Fax: 901-333-4788
                                  www.southwest.tn.edu
                                  vesails@southwest.tn.edu
Dr.Anthony Wise, President
Sherman Greer, Executive Assistant
Ron Parr, VP Fnancial & Admin Services
Offers a variety of services to students with disabilities in-
cluding note takers, extended testing time, counseling ser-
vices, and special accommodations.

3735 Tennessee State University
Office of Disabled Student Services
3500 John a Merritt Blvd
P. O. Box 9609
Nashville, TN 37209-1561   615-963-5000
                                       888-463-6878
                                  Fax: 615-963-2930
                                  TDD: 615-963-7440
                                  www.tnstate.edu
                                  pscudder@tnstate.edu
Dr. Glenda Baskin Glover, President
Monique Mitchell, Administrative Assistant ll
Steven McCrary, Coordinator
Four year college offers services for learning disabled stu-
dents.

3736 University of Memphis
110 Wilder Tower N
Memphis, TN 38152   901-678-2911
                                  Fax: 901-678-5023
                                  TDD: 901-678-2880
                                  www.saweb.memphis.edu
                                  sds@memphis.edu
Susan TePaske, Director
Jennifer Murchison, Asst Director
Phil Minyard, Coordinator
Emphasizes individual responsibility for learning by offering a developmentally oriented program of college survival
skills, learning strategies, and individualized planning and
counseling based on the student's strengths and weaknesses.
The program also coordinates comprehensive support services, including test accommodations, tutoring and learning
strategies, alternate format tests and assistive technology.
The program serves 400 to 500 students with learning
disabilities and ADHD per year.

3737 University of Tennessee
Boling Center for Developmental Disabilities
711 Jefferson Ave
Memphis, TN 38105-5003   901-448-6512
                                       888-572-2249
                                  Fax: 901-448-7097
                                  TDD: 901-448-4677
                                  www.utmem.edu
Jimmy G. Cheek, Chancellor
Susan Martin, Provost
Kennard Brown, Executive Vice Chancellor/COO
Interdisciplinary or focused evaluation of learning, behav-
ioral and developmental problems in infants, toddlers, chil-
dren and young adults. Treatment of some conditions
offered.

3738 University of Tennessee: Knoxville
Disability Services Office
2227 Dunford Hall
915 Volunteer Blvd
Knoxville, TN 37996-0001   865-974-6087
                                  Fax: 865-974-9552
                                  TDD: 865-974-6087
                                  www.ods.utk.edu
                                  ods@utk.edu
Jimmy G. Cheek, Chancellor
Susan Martin, Provost
Kennard Brown, Executive Vice Chancellor/COO

The mission of the Office of Disability Services is to provide
each individual an equal opportunity to participate in the
University of Tennessee's programs and activities.

3739 University of Tennessee: Martin
554 University Street
Martin, TN 38238-0001   731-881-7000
                                  Fax: 731-881-1886
                                  www.utm.edu
                                  success@utm.edu
Edie B. Gibson, Executive Assis to Chancellor
Dr. Margaret Toston, Vice Chancellor
Tom Rakes, Chancellor
A four-year independent college that offers a program called
Program Access for College Enhancement for students with
learning disabilities.

3740 Vanderbilt University
Vanderbilt University
2301 Vanderbilt Place
Nashville, TN 37235   615-322-7311
                                  Fax: 615-322-3762
                                  TDD: 615-322-4705
                                  www.vanderbilt.edu
                                  melissa.a.smith@vanderbilt.edu
Jackson W. Moore, Vice Chairman
Nicholas S. Zeppos, Chancellor
Mark Dalton, Chairman
An independent four-year college with support services for
special education students.

3741 William Jennings Bryan College
HEATH Resource Center
721 Bryan Drive
2121 K St NW
Dayton, TN 20202-2524   423-775-2041
                                       800-544-3284
                                  Fax: 202-973-0908
                                  www.heath.gwu.edu
                                  nfo@bryan.edu
Stephen D. Livesay , Ph.D., President
Kevin Clauson, J.D., Interim Vice President
John Haynes, Chairman
A public four-year college. The HEALTH Resource Center
operates the national clearinghouse on postsecondary edu-
cation for individuals with disabilities.

Texas

3742 Alvin Community College
Alvin Community College
3110 Mustang Road
Alvin, TX 77511-4807   281-756-3500
                                  Fax: 281-756-3858
                                  www.alvincollege.edu
                                  info@alvincollege.edu
Christal M. Albrecht, President
Alyssa Reeves, Admission Specialist
Jim Crumm, Vice President
A public two-year college with support services for special
education students.

3743 Angelina College
Student Services Office
PO Box 1768
3500 S 1st St
Lufkin, TX 75901-1768   936-639-1301
                                  Fax: 936-639-4299
                                  www.angelina.edu
                                  jtwohig@angelina.edu
Patricia M. McKenzie, Ed.D., VP/Dean of Instruction
Larry M. Phillips, President
Tim Stacy, Secretary
A public community college that offers two-year degrees in
the arts and sciences designed to transfer to four-year col-
leges and universities as well as one and two year programs
in technical and occupational fields.

3744 Brookhaven College
Special Services Office
3939 Valley View Ln
Farmers Branch, TX 75244-4997

972-860-4700
Fax: 972-860-4897
www.dcccd.edu.bhc
bhcInfo@dcccd.edu

Sharon Blackman, Grants Manager
Thom D. Chesney, Ph.D., President
Rodger Bennett, Vice President
Physically challenged and learning disabled special services office offers advisement, additional diagnostic evaluations, mobility assistance, note taking, textbook taping, interpreters for the deaf and assistance in test taking.

3745 Cedar Valley College
3030 N Dallas Ave
Lancaster, TX 75134-3799

972-860-8201
www.cedarvalleycollege.edu

Dr Jennifer Wimbish, President
Dr. Nancy Cure, Vice President of Instruction
Dr. Mickey Best, Executive Dean of Liberal Arts
The mission of Cedar Valley College is to provide quality learning that prepares students for success in a dynamic world.

3746 Central Texas College
PO Box 1800
Killeen, TX 76540-1800

254-526-7161
800-792-3348
Fax: 254-526-1700
TDD: 254-526-1378
www.ctcd.edu

Thomas Klincar, Chancellor
Rex Weaver, Chair
Jimmy Towers, Vice Chair
Offers a variety of services to students with disabilities including extended testing time, counseling services, and assistive technology.

3747 Cisco College
101 College Heights
Cisco, TX 76437

254-442-5000
Fax: 254-442-5100
www.cisco.edu

Bobby Smith, President
Jerry Dodson, Ed.D., VP Student Services
Carol Dupree, Ph.D., Provost
Provides affordable, accessible education to more than 4,200 students through its two locations in Cisco and Abilene. Offers a variety of career and technical education programs and academic transfer options as well as many student support services like tutoring, academic intervention and counseling to ensure student success.

3748 College of the Mainland
Student Support Services
1200 Amburn Rd
Texas City, TX 77591-2499

409-938-1211
888-258-8859
Fax: 409-938-1306
www.com.edu
kkimbark@com.edu

Dr. Beth Lewis, President
Roney G. McCrary, Chair
Wayne H. Miles, Vice Chair
Offers a variety of services to students with disabilities including notetakers, extended testing time, counseling services, and special accommodations. The mission of services for students with disabilities is to provide each student with the resources needed to register, enroll and complete their course work and/or degree plan.

3749 Collin County Community College
2200 W University Drive
McKinney, TX 75071-2999

972-548-6790
Fax: 972-548-6716
www.collin.edu

Cary A. Israel, President
Mac Hendricks, Chair
Dr. Sherry Schumann, VP/Provost
A public two-year college. ACCESS provides resonable accommodations, individual attention and support for students with disabilities who need assistance with any aspect of their campus experience such as accessibility, academics and testing.

3750 Dallas Academy
950 Tiffany Way
Dallas, TX 75218-2743

214-324-1481
Fax: 214-327-8537
www.dallas-academy.com
mail@dallas-academy.com

Jim Richardson, Headmaster
Troy Sturrock, Chair
Terrence S. Welch, Vice Chair
Offers a variety of services to students with disabilities including notetakers, extended testing time, counseling services, and special accommodations.

3751 Dallas Academy: Coed High School
950 Tiffany Way
Dallas, TX 75218-2743

214-324-1481
Fax: 214-327-8537
www.dallas-academy.com
mail@dallas-academy.com

Troy Sturrock, Chair
Terrence S. Welch, Vice Chair
Jim Richardson, Headmaster
Coed Day School for bright children grades 7-12 with diagnosed learning differences. Curriculum includes sports, art, music, and photography programs.

3752 Dallas County Community College
701 Elm St.
Dallas, TX 75202-2033

214-860-2283
Fax: 972-860-7227
www.dcccd.edu/
5HCRC@dcccd.edu

Charletta Rogers Compton, Chair
Dr. Joe May, Chancellor
Susan Hall, Executive Director
Offers a variety of services to students with disabilities including note takers, extended testing time, counseling services, and special accommodations.

3753 East Texas Baptist University
One Tiger Drive
Marshall, TX 75670-1498

903-935-7963
800-804-3828
Fax: 903-938-7798
www.etbu.edu
Admissions@etbu.edu

Dr. Lawrence Ressler, Interim President
Offers a variety of services to students with disabilities including notetakers, extended testing time, counseling services, and special accommodations.

3754 Eastfield College
3737 Motley Drive
Mesquite, TX 75150-2099

972-860-7100
Fax: 972-860-7622
www.eastfieldcollege.edu
efcdso@dcccd.edu

Dr Jean Conway, President
Sharon Cook, Assistant to the President
Dr. Adrian Douglas, VP Business Services
Offers a variety of support services for students with disabilities and/or special requirements. Services are coordinated to fit the individual needs of the student and may include sign language interpreters, computer aided real-time translation services, notetaking services, tutoring referral, textbook taping, testing accomodations, and use of adaptive technology. Academic counseling, priority registration, and referral information are also available.

3755 El Centro College
801 Main Street
Dallas, TX 75202   214-860-2000
                                Fax: 214-860-2440
                              www.elcentrocollege.edu
Norman Howden, Executive Dean
Karin Reed, Disability Services Coordinator
Paul McCarthy, President
A public two-year college with support services for special
education students.

3756 Fairhill School
16150 Preston Road
Dallas, TX 75248-3558   972-233-1026
                                Fax: 972-233-8205
                                   www.fairhill.org
Carla Stanford, Executive Director
Deborah Atchley, Head of Lower School
Carla Hilts, Administrative Assistant
A private, non-profit college preparatory school serving stu-
dents in grades one through twelve. Fairhill's primary pur-
pose is to provide a superior education for students of
average and above intelligence who have been diagnosed
with a learning difference such as Dyslexia, Dysgraphia,
Dyscalculia, Auditory Processing Disorder, or Attention
Deficit/Hyperactivity Disorder.

3757 Frank Phillips College
Special Populations Department
PO Box 5118
1301 W. Roosevelt St.
Borger, TX 79008-5118   806-457-4200
                                   800-687-2056
                                Fax: 806-457-4225
                                     www.fpctx.edu
Jarel Whitehead, Chairperson
Charlotte Hale, Vice Chairperson
Lew K Hunnicutt, Ph.D., VP Extended Services
Offers a variety of services to students with disabilities in-
cluding notetakers, extended testing time, counseling ser-
vices, and special accommodations.

3758 Galveston College
4015 Avenue Q
Galveston, TX 77550-7496   409-944-4242
                                Fax: 409-944-1500
                                TDD: 866-483-4242
                                         www.gc.edu
W. Myles Shelton EdD, President
Armin Cantini, Chairperson
Raymond Lewis, Jr., Vice Chairperson
A public two-year college. A variety of services and pro-
grams are available to assist students with disabilities, those
who are academically and/or economically disadvantaged
and those with limited English proficiency.

3759 Great Lakes Academy
6000 Custer Road
Building 7
Plano, TX 75023-5100   972-517-7498
                                Fax: 972-517-0133
                           www.greatlakesacademy.com
                       admissions@greatlakesacademy.com
Marjolein J. Borsten, Executive Director
Jolene Wofford, Director
Jason Campbell, Assistant Director
A full day non-profit private school that provides 1st-12th
grade students with average to above-average intelligence,
diagnosed with various Learning Differences, Asperger's
Syndrome, ADD or AD/HD a stimulating environment and
favorable atmosphere which affords each student opportuni-
ties to develop both socially and academically.

3760 Hill School
4817 Odessa Ave
Fort Worth, TX 76133-1640   817-923-9482
                                Fax: 817-923-4894
                                   www.hillschool.org
                              hillschool@hillschool.org
Whit Perryman, President
David G. Bucher, Senior Vice President
Tim Carter, Chairman of the Board
Hill School is a college preparatory, full-service school for
bright students who learn differently. Our exceptional faculty emphasize intensive small-group instruction in core
subject areas to ensure that all students have an opportunity
to reach their full academic potential. Our students explore
interests and affinities through athletics, fine arts (drama, visual arts, music, band) and a wide variety of community involvement activities. Also located in SW Ft. Worth and
Grapevine.

3761 Jarvis Christian College
PO Box 1470
Hawkins, TX 75765-1470   903-769-5700
                                   800-292-9517
                                Fax: 903-769-5005
                                      www.jarvis.edu
                            florine_white@jarvis.edu
Florine White MD, Student Support Services Dir.
Lester C. Newman, President
Stephanie Brown, Administrative Staff
Student Support Services is a federally funded program
whose purpose is to improve the retention and graduate rate
of program participants. Eligible program participants include low income, first generation college students and students with learning and physical disabilities. A variety of
support services are provided.

3762 Lamar State College - Port Arthur
PO Box 310
1500 Procter Street
Port Arthur, TX 77640-0310   409-983-4921
                                   800-477-5872
                                Fax: 409-984-6056
                                TDD: 409-984-6242
                                  www.pa.lamar.edu
                           andrea.munoz@lamarpa.edu
Mary Wickland, Vice President for Finance
Dr. Charles Gongre, Dean of Academic Programs
W. Sam Monroe, President
A public two-year college with support services for special
education students.

3763 Laredo Community College
Special Populations Office
West End Washington Street
Laredo, TX 78040   956-721-5109
                                Fax: 956-721-5367
                                     www.laredo.edu
                            sylviat@laredo.cc.tx.us
Eleazar Gonzalez, Chief Administrative Officer/CFO
Dr. Juan L. Maldonado, President
Vincent R. Solis, VP
Offers a variety of services to students with disabilities in-
cluding notetakers, extended testing time, counseling ser-
vices, and special accommodations.

3764 Lon Morris College
Disability Services: Cole Learning Enrichment Ctr
600 College Avenue
Jacksonville, TX 75766   903-589-4000
                                   800-259-5733
                                Fax: 903-589-4001
                                 www.beabearcat.com
Sandra White, Director, Enrichment Center
Angela Jones, Assistant
Dasvid Russ, Advisor

A two-year liberal arts college that offers a learning support program (the Cole Learning Enrichment Center) for students with learning disabilities. Students work collaboratively with the director of the center to develop and achieve realistic career and education goals, determine educational needs based on testing data, and foster independence while developing and demonstrating their full potential and abilities.

3765 Lubbock Christian University

5601 19th Street
Lubbock, TX 79407-2099

806-796-8800
800-933-7601
Fax: 806-720-7255
www.lcu.edu
admissions@lcu.edu

L. Timothy Perrin, President
Dr. Brian Starr, Vice President
Monica Lopez Barnard, General Counsel
Offers a variety of services to students with disabilities including notetakers, extended testing time, counseling services, and special accommodations.

3766 McLennen Community College

1400 College Drive
Waco, TX 76708-1499

254-299-8622
Fax: 254-299-8654
www.mclennan.edu
helpdesk@mclennan.edu

Dr. Johnette McKown, President
Mickey Reyes, Desktop Publishing Technician
Harry Harelik, Executive Director
A public two-year college with support services for special education students.

3767 Midwestern State University

Disability Counseling Office
3410 Taft Boulevard
Wichita Falls, TX 76308-2096

940-397-4352
800-842-1922
Fax: 940-397-4780
TDD: 940-397-4515
www.mwsu.edu
counselling@mwsu.edu

Jesse W Rogers, President
Dr. Marilyn Fowle, Vice President
Dr. Keith Lamb, VP
A public four-year college with support services for special education students.

3768 North Lake College

Disabilities Services Office
Rm A438
5001 N Macarthur Blvd
Irving, TX 75038-3899

972-273-3000
Fax: 972-273-3431
TDD: 972-273-3169
www.dcccd.edu

Debbie Eberla, Assistant to the President
Martha Hughes, VP Academic Affairs
Christa Slejko, President
A public two-year college. Our mission is to provide a variety of support services to empower students, foster independence, promote achievement of realistic career and educational goals and assist students in discovering, developing and demonstrating full potential and abilities.

3769 Notre Dame School

2018 Allen Street
Dallas, TX 75204-2604

214-720-3911
Fax: 214-720-3913
www.notredameschool.org
tfrancis@notredameschool.org

Theresa Francis, Principal
Bruce Newsome, Vice President
Randy Bacon, President
Providing a quality education to children with developmental disabilities ages 6 to 21 and facilitating their intergration into society.

3770 Odyssey School

4407 Red River St
Austin, TX 78751-4039

512-472-2262
Fax: 512-236-9385
www.odysseyschool.com
info@odysseyschool.com

Nancy Wolf, Head of School
Paul R. Teich, Vice President
F. Scott McCown, President
Committed to the development of academic excellence and self-acceptance for students with learning and attentional differences. We believe all children can be successful in their intellectual, creative and social development. Our goal is to help each student discover his or her individual potential for greatness.

3771 Pan American University

Office of Disability Services
1201 W University Drive
Edinburg, TX 78539-2999

956-381-3306
Fax: 956-381-5196
TDD: 956-316-7092
www.panam.edu

Brinda V. Torres, Assistant toVP
Magdalena Hinojosa, Senior Associate VP
Robert S. Nelsen, President
Offers a variety of services to students with disabilities including note takers, extended testing time, counseling services, and special accommodations.

3772 Rawson-Saunders School

Soaring Eagles Program
2614-A Exposition Boulevard
Austin, TX 78703-1702

512-476-8382
Fax: 512-476-1132
www.rawson-saunders.org
info@rawson-saunders.org

Laura Steinbach, Head of School
Samer Zabaneh, Legal Counsel
Kaye Knox, Chair
Developed to help learning disabled students, grades 1 to 8, maintain their language arts and math skills while increasing their self-esteem. Students participate in small group, hands-on activities in math, language arts, organized games/movement, keyboarding, sign language, and science or creative problem solving.

3773 Richland College

12800 Abrams Rd
Dallas, TX 75243-2199

972-238-6100
Fax: 972-238-6346
www.rlc.dcccd.edu

Steve Mittelstet, President
Finney Varghese, Associate Vice President
Richland College's mission is teaching, learning, and community building.

3774 Sam Houston State University

1806 Avenue J
Huntsville, TX 77340

936-294-1111
Fax: 936-294-3794
TDD: 936-294-3786
www.shsu.edu
disability@shsu.edu

Dana G. Hoyt, President
Jaimie Hebert, Provost and Vice President
Al Hooten, VP Finance and Operation
Offers a variety of services to students with disabilities including note takers, extended testing time, counseling services, and special accommodations.

3775 San Jacinto College: Central Campus

P.O.Box 2007
8060 Spencer Hwy.
Pasadena, TX 77505-2007

281-998-6150
Fax: 281-476-1892
www.sjcd.cc.tx.us

Van Wigginton, Provost
Laurel Williamson, Deputy Chancellor/SJCD President
Joanna Zimmermann, Interim VP, Student Services
Offers a variety of services to students with disabilities including notetakers, extended testing time, counseling services, and special accommodations such as test readers and writers.

3776 San Jacinto College: South Campus
San Jacinto College: South Campus
13735 Beamer Rd
Houston, TX 77089-6099
281-998-6150
Fax: 281-922-3401
www.sjcd.edu
eeverett@sjcd.edu
Laurel Williamson, Deputy Chancellor/SJCD President
Joanna Zimmermann, Interim VP of Student Services
Brenda Jones, Provost
A public two-year college with support services for special education students.

3777 Schreiner University
2100 Memorial Blvd
Kerrville, TX 78028-5697
830-792-7217
800-343-4919
Fax: 830-282-4638
www.schreiner.edu
jgallik@schreiner.edu
Tim Summerlin, President
Bill Muse, VP for Administration & Finance
Mike Pate, Chairman of the Board
Comprehensive support program for students with diagnosed specific learning disabilities with demonstrated potential for success at the college level.

3778 Shelton School
15720 Hillcrest Road
Dallas, TX 75248-4161
972-774-1772
Fax: 972-991-3977
www.shelton.org
Suzanne Stell, Executive Director
Gary Webb, Chairman
Paul Neubach, M.D., Vice Chairman
Primary emphasis is providing learning-different children (average or above intelligence) with full, effective curriculum through individualized, structured multisensory programs. Learning differences include dyslexia, attention deficit disorder (ADD), attention deficit hyperactivity disorder (ADHD), speech and language disorders.

3779 South Plains College
1401 College Ave
Levelland, TX 79336-6595
806-894-9611
Fax: 806-897-2800
www.spc.cc.tx.us
Kelvin W. Sharp, Ed.D., President
Jim Walker, M.P.A., Vice President for Academic Aff
Cathy Mitchell, M.Ed., Vice President for Student Aff
Offers a variety of services to students with disabilities including notetakers, extended testing time, counseling services, and special accommodations.

3780 Southern Methodist University
Disability Accommodations & Success Strategies
PO Box 750201
Dallas, TX 75275-100
214-768-2000
Fax: 214-768-1225
www.smu.edu/alec/dass.asp
ugadmission@smu.edu
Michael M. Boone, Chair
R. Gerald Turner, President
Thomas E. Barry, Vice President
Provides access and accomodations to all SMU students with a disability. Also offers academic waching to undergraduates with learning and attention disorders.

3781 Southwestern Assemblies of God University
1200 Sycamore St
Waxahachie, TX 75165-2397
972-937-4010
888-YES-SAGU
Fax: 972-923-0488
www.sagu.edu
sagu@sagu.edu
Kermit S Bridges, President
Paul Brooks, Vice President for Academics
Katie White, Administrative Academic
Offers a variety of services to students with disabilities including notetakers, extended testing time, counseling services, and special accommodations.

3782 St. Edwards University
Learning Disabilities Services
3001 South Congress Avenue
Austin, TX 78704-6489
512-448-8400
855-468-6738
Fax: 512-448-8492
www.stedwards.edu
seu.admit@stedwards.edu
George E. Martin, President
Donna Jurick, SND, Executive Vice President
Christie Campbell, Associate Vice President
An independent four-year college. Students with disabilities meet with a counselor from academic planning and support and they work together to ensure equal access to all academic services.

3783 St. Mary's University of San Antonio
1 Camino Santa Maria St
San Antonio, TX 78228-8500
210-436-3011
Fax: 210-436-3782
www.stmarytx.edu
Thomas Mengler, J.D., President
Charles T. Barrett Jr., Chairman of the Board
Andre Hampton, Provost and VP
Offers a variety of services to students with disabilities including tutoring, extended testing time, and academic counseling services.

3784 Stephen F Austin State University
Office of Disability Services
2008 Alumni Drive
Rusk Building, Room 206
Nacogdoches, TX 75962-3940
936-468-2504
Fax: 936-468-3849
www.sfasu.edu
admissions@sfasu.edu
Richard Berry, Provost/VP for Academic Affairs
Tito Guerrero, President
Mr. James H. Dickerson, Secretary
Offers a variety of services to students with disabilities including note takers, extended testing time, counseling services, and special accommodations.

3785 Tarleton State University
Box T-0001
1333 W. Washington
Stephenville, TX 76402
254-968-9000
Fax: 254-968-9703
www.tarleton.edu
Joe Standridge, Jr. P.E., Associate Vice President
Angie Brown, Assistant Vice President
F Dominic Dottavid, President
Four year college that provides students with learning disabilities support and services.

3786 Tarrant County College
Disability Support Services
1500 Houston Street
Fort Worth, TX 76102
817-515-5100
Fax: 817-515-6112
TDD: 817-515-6812
www.tccd.edu
judy.kelly@tccd.edu

Larry Darlage, President, Northeast Campus
O.K. Carter, Secretary
Gary Smith, M.S., VP Academic Affairs
Offers a variety of support services to students with disabilities including notetakers, testing accommodations, as well as special accommodations, tutoring.

3787 Texas A&M University
0200 TAMU
750 Agronomy Road, Suite 1601
College Station, TX 77843-200   979-845-3313
                                       Fax: 979-845-2647
                                       www.tamu.edu
                                       anne@stulife2.tamu.edu
Dr. Brett Giroir, Executive Vice President and CEO
Dr. Karan L. Watson, Provost/EVP for Academic Affairs
Mark A. Hussey, President
A public four-year college with support services for special education students.

3788 Texas A&M University: Commerce
PO Box 3011
Commerce, TX 75429-3011   903-886-5835
                                 888-868-2682
                                 Fax: 903-468-3220
                                 www.tamu-commerce.edu
                                 frank_perez@tamu-commerce.edu
Linda King, Executive Asst. to the President
Dan R. Jones, Ph.D., President & CEO
Sharon Johnson, Vice President
Four-year college that provides student support services and programs to those students who are learning disabled.

3789 Texas A&M University: Kingsville
1210 Retama Dr
Kingsville, TX 78363   361-592-4762
                             Fax: 361-593-2006
                             www.tamuk.edu
                             kacjaol@tamuk.edu
Jeanie Alexander, Coordinator Disability Svcs
Dr. Steven Tallant, President
Four-year college that provides an academic support center for students who are disabled.

3790 Texas Southern University
3100 Cleburne St
Houston, TX 77004-4597   713-313-7011
                                Fax: 713-313-7851
                                www.tsu.edu
Janis J. Newman, Chief of Staf
Dr. John M. Rudley, President
Wendy H. Adair, VP, University Advancement
A public four-year college with support services for special education students.

3791 Texas State Technical Institute: Sweetwater Campus
300 Homer K Taylor Drive
Sweetwater, TX 79556-4108   325-235-7300
                                   www.sweetwater.tstc.edu
Kyle Smith, Interim President
Mike Reeser, MBA, Chancellor
Dixon Bailey, Vice President
Offers a variety of services to students with disabilities including notetakers, extended testing time, counseling services, and special accommodations.

3792 Texas Tech University
AccessTECH & TECHniques Center
2500 Broadway
Lubbock, TX 79409   806-742-2011
                           Fax: 806-742-4837
                           TDD: 806-742-2092
                           TTY: 806-742-4837
                           www.accesstech.dsa.ttu.edu
                           webmaster@ttu.edu
M. Duane Nellis, Ph.D., President
Lawrence Schovanec, Provost/Senior Vice President
Robert V. Duncan, Vice President for Research

AccessTECH & TECHniques Center offer TTU students every opportunity to succeed in independence and education.

3793 Texas Woman's University
Disability Support Services
PO Box 425966
Denton, TX 76204-5966   940-898-3835
                               Fax: 940-898-3965
                               TDD: 940-898-3830
                               www.twu.edu
                               dss@twu.edu
A public four-year college with support services for special education students.

3794 Tri-County Community College
1500 Houston Street
Fort Worth, TX 76102   817-515-8223
                              Fax: 828-837-3266
                              TDD: 724-228-4028
                              www.tccd.edu
Louise Appleman, President
Kristin Vandergriff, Vice President
Erma Johnson Hadley, Chancellor
Offers a variety of services to students with disabilities including notetakers, extended testing time, counseling services, and special accommodations.

3795 Tyler Junior College
PO Box 9020
Tyler, TX 75711-9020   903-510-2200
                              800-687-5680
                              Fax: 903-510-2434
                              www.tyler.cc.tx.us
Vickie Geisel, Special Services
Aubry Sharp, Manager
L. Michael Metke, President
Offers a variety of services to students with disabilities including note takers, extended testing time, counseling services, and special accommodations.

3796 University of Austin Texas
Texas Center for Disability Studies
1 University Station C1200
Austin, TX 78712   512-471-3434
                          800-828-7839
                          Fax: 512-232-0761
                          www.utexas.edu
                          txcds@uttcds.org
Patricia L. Clubb, VP for University Operations
Brad Englert, AVP/CIO
William Powers Jr, President
The mission of the Texas Center for Disability Studies (TCDS) is to serve as a catalyst so that people with developmental and other disabilities are fully included in all levels of their communities and in control of their lives.

3797 University of Houston
Disability Support Services
4800 Calhoun Road
Houston, TX 77004   713-743-2255
                           Fax: 713-743-5396
                           TDD: 713-749-1527
                           TTY: 713-749-1527
                           www.uh.edu
                           wscrain@mail.uhe.edu
Eli D. Cipriano, Associate Vice President
Lisa Holdeman, Assistant Vice President
Renu Khator, President
A public four-year college with support services for students with disabilities.

3798 **University of North Texas**
Office of Disability Accommodation
PO Box 310770
1155 Union Circle #311277
Denton, TX 76203-5017 940-565-4323
Fax: 940-369-7969
TDD: 940-369-8652
www.unt.edu/oda
branding@unt.edu
Dr. Warren Burggren, Provost/VP for Academic Affairs
Neal J. Smatresk, President
Elizabeth With, VP Student Affairs
The mission of the ODA is to provide reasonable accommodations to students and to apply appropriate adjustments to the classroom and associated learning environments. In order to facilitate this process, the ODA maintains all student diability-related medical and psychological documentation and the corresponding accommodation request records.

3799 **University of Texas at Dallas**
PO Box 830688
800 West Campbell Road
Richardson, TX 75083-3021 972-883-2111
Fax: 972-883-2098
www.utdallas.edu
Kerry Tate, Asst Director Disability Service
David E. Daniel, President
Judy Snellings, Executive Associate
Offers a variety of services to students with disabilities including notetakers, extended testing time, counseling services, and special accommodations.

3800 **University of Texas: Pan American**
1201 W University Drive
Edinburg, TX 78539-2999 956-381-2011
866-441-UTPA
Fax: 956-381-2150
www.panam.edu
Dr. Havidan Rodriguez, Provost/VP for Academic Affairs
Martin V. Baylor, VP, Business Affairs
Robert S. Nelsen, President
Offers a variety of services to students with disabilities including notetakers, extended testing time, counseling services, and special accommodations.

3801 **University of the Incarnate Word**
4301 Broadway St
CPO #285
San Antonio, TX 78209-6318 210-829-6000
800-749-WORD
Fax: 210-829-3847
www.uiw.edu
uiwhr@universe.uiwtx.edu
Louis J Agnese Jr, President
Kathleen Coughlin, VP, Institutional Adv.
Dr. Denise Doyle, Chancellor
Four year college that provides services to learning disabled students.

3802 **Wharton County Junior College**
911 E Boling Hwy
Wharton, TX 77488-3298 781-583-7561
800-561-9252
Fax: 888- 898-620
www.wcjc.cc.tx.us/
Gary P. Trochta, Vice Chair
Betty A. McCrohan, President
P. D. Gertson, III, Chair
Offers a variety of services to students with disabilities including note takers, extended testing time, counseling services, and special accommodations.

3803 **Wiley College**
711 Wiley Ave
Marshall, TX 75670-5151 903-927-3300
800-658-6889
Fax: 903-938-8100
www.wilec.edu
vdavis@wileyc.edu
Haywood L Strickland, President and CEO
Dr. Glenda Carter, Executive Vice President
Dr. Ernest Plata, VP for Academic Affairs
Offers a variety of services to students with disabilities including notetakers, extended testing time, counseling services, and special accommodations.

3804 **Winston School**
5707 Royal Lane
Dallas, TX 75229-5500 214-691-6950
Fax: 214-691-1509
www.winston-school.org
info@winston-school.org
Pamela K. Murfin, Head of School
Paula Tuffin, President
Scott Becchi, 1st Vice President
Our mission is to realize the extraordinary potential of bright students who learn differently through individualized learning strategies, and to aid in preparing graduates for college level work.

Utah

3805 **College of Eastern Utah**
451 East 400 North
Price, UT 84501-2699 435-613-5000
888-202-8783
Fax: 435-613-5112
www.ceu.edu
Michael King, DRC Director
John Shattuck, President
The DRC at CEU provides academic accommodations for the learning disabled.

3806 **Latter-Day Saints Business College**
95 North 300 West
Salt Lake City, UT 84101-1302 801-524-8100
Fax: 801-524-1900
www.ldsbc.edu
Thomas S Monson, Chairman
J. Lawrence Richards, President
Bob H. Wiser, VP Finance and Controller
Offers a variety of services to students with disabilities including notetakers, extended testing time, counseling services, and special accommodations.

3807 **Salt Lake Community College**
Disability Resource Center
4600 South Redwood Road
Salt Lake City, UT 84123-3197 801-957-4111
Fax: 801-957-4440
TDD: 801-957-4646
TTY: 801-957-4646
www.slcc.edu
linda.bennett@slcc.edu
Deneece Huftalin, Ph.D., President
Gail Miller, Chair
Nancy Singer, Ph.D., Vice President
A program to assist students with disabilities in obtaining equal access to college facilities and programs. The resource center serves all disabilities and provides services and accommodations such as testing, adaptive equipment, text on tape, readers, scribes, note takers, and interpreters for the deaf.

3808 **Snow College**
150 College Ave
Ephraim, UT 84627-1299

435-283-7000
800-848-3399
Fax: 435-283-5259
www.snow.edu

Gary Carlston, President
Theressa Alder, Chair
Spencer Hill, Vice President of Finance
A public two-year college with support services for special education students.

3809 **Southern Utah University**
351 West University Boulevard
Cedar City, UT 84720-2470

435-586-7700
Fax: 435-865-8223
www.suu.edu
thompson@suu.edu

Michael T Benson, Executive Director
Scott Wyatt, President
Stuart Jones, Vice President
A public four-year University with support services for special education students.

3810 **University Accessibility Center**
Brigham Young University
800 West, University Parkway
MS 190
Orem, UT 84058-5999

801-863-8747
Fax: 801-863-8377
TTY: 801-221-0908
www.uac.byu.edu
uac@byu.edu

Sandy Parsons, Chair
Gretchen Tousey, President
Dani Anguiano, VP University Affairs
REACH was established to assist students with disabilities to reach their full potential. It is our goal to provide an environment where the pursuit of excellence is expected, and students are strongly encouraged to make a contribution toward their own success.

3811 **University of Utah**
201 Presidents Cir
Room 201
Salt Lake City, UT 84112-9049

801-581-7200
800-444-8638
Fax: 801-585-5257
TDD: 801-581-5020
www.utah.edu
onadeau@saun.saff.utah.edu

Bryon Buchmiller, Chair
Patti Carpenter, Secretary / Treasurer
Paul Larsen, President
A public four-year college. Services include admissions requirements modification, testing accommodations, priority registration, advisement on course selection and number, adaptive technology, support group. Documentation of learning disability is required.

3812 **Utah State University**
0160 Old Main Hill
Rm 102
Logan, UT 84322-0160

435-797-1079
800-488-8108
Fax: 435-797-0130
TDD: 435-797-0740
www.usu.edu
diane.baum@usu.edu

Katie Nielsen, Director of Admissions
Tagg Archibald, Assistant Director
Jeff Sorensen, Associate Director of Admissions
A public four-year college with support services for students with learning disabilities.

3813 **Utah Valley State College**
Accessibility Services Department
800 W University Pkwy
Orem, UT 84058

801-863-8105
Fax: 801-863-7265
www.uvu.edu
info@uvsc.edu

Jono Andrews, Associate VP, Academic Programs
Brian Brich, VP, Development & Alumni
Matthew Holland, President
The mission for Accessibility Services at Utah Valley State College is to ensure, in compliance with federal and state laws, that no qualified individual with a disability be excluded from participation in or be denied the benefits of a quality education at UVSC or be subjected to discrimination by the college or its personnel. UVSC offers a large variety of support services, accommodative services and assistive technology for individuals with learning disabilities.

3814 **Weber State University**
Disabilities Support Office
3848 Harrison Blvd.
Ogden, UT 84408

801-626-6000
Fax: 801-626-6744
TDD: 801-626-7283
www.weber.edu
recruit1@weber.edu

Charles A. Wight, President
Bret R. Ellis, VP Information Technology
Alan E. Hall, Chair
Offers a variety of services to students with disabilities including notetakers, extended testing time, counseling services, and special accommodations.

3815 **Westminster College of Salt Lake City**
Learning Disability Program
1840 South 1300 East
Salt Lake City, UT 84105-3697

801-484-7651
800-748-4753
Fax: 801-468-0916
TDD: 801-832-2286
www.westminstercollege.edu
gdewitt@westminstercollege.edu

Thomas A. Ellison, ESQ, Chair
William Orchow, Vice Chair
Dr.Brian Levin-Stankevich, President
Offers a variety of services to students with disabilities including notetakers, extended testing time, counseling services, and special accommodations.

Vermont

3816 **Burlington College**
351 North Avenue
Burlington, VT 05401-2998

802-862-9616
800-862-9616
Fax: 802-660-4331
www.burlington.edu
jsanders@burlcol.edu

Christine Plunkett, President
Yves Bradley, Chair
Stephen St. Onge, Vice President for Academic
Education process vs test and grades. Small classes. Learning specialist available.

3817 **Champlain College**
Support Services
251 South Willard St.
Burlington, VT 05401-3950

802-860-2700
800-570-5858
Fax: 802-860-2750
www.champlain.edu
peterson@champlain.edu

Robert D. Botjer, Chairman
Donald J. Laackman, President
RJ Sweeney, Vice President
Four year college that supports students with a learning disability.

3818 College of St. Joseph
71 Clement Rd
Rutland, VT 05701-3899
802-773-5900
877-270-9998
Fax: 802-773-5900
www.csj.edu
admissions@csj.edu

Richard Lloyd, President
Judy Morgan, Assistant to the President
James Lambert, Director of Communications
Offers a variety of services to students with disabilities including note takers, extended testing time, counseling services, and special accommodations.

3819 Community College of Vermont
Student Services Office
PO Box 489
660 Elm Street
Montpelier, VT 05602-489
802-828-2800
800-228-6686
Fax: 802-828-2805
www.ccv.vsc.edu
ccvinfo@ccv.vsc.edu

Joyce Judy, President
Lisa Yaeger, Director of Human Resources
Tapp Barnhill, Executive Director
A public two-year college offering courses, certificates and associate degrees.

3820 Green Mountain College
Calhoun Learning Center
1 Brennan Cir
Poultney, VT 05764-1078
800-776-6675
Fax: 802-287-8099
www.greenmtn.edu
admiss@greenmtn.edu

Robert C. Allen, Chair
Matthew Menner, SVP Sales and Alliance
Paul J. Fonteyn, President
Four-year college that offers support through the school's Calhoun Learning center to students with disabilities.

3821 Landmark College
19 River Road South
Putney, VT 05346
802-387-4767
Fax: 802-387-6880
www.landmark.edu
institute@landmark.edu

Peter Eden, President
Gregory Matthews, VP Enrollment Management
Carroll Pare, Senior Director
Our programs are specially designed for a particular audience. designed exclusively for students with dyslexia, attention deficit hyperactivity disorder (AD/HD), or other specific learning disabilities.

3822 Norwich University
Learning Support Center
158 Harmon Dr
Northfield, VT 05663-1035
802-485-2000
800-468-6679
Fax: 802-485-2032
www.norwich.edu
gills@norwich.edu

Richard W Schneider, President
Dr. Guiyou Huang, Senior Vice President
Gordon R. Sullivan, Chairman
The Learning Center offers an opportunity for individualized assistance with many aspects of academic life in a supportive, personalized atmosphere. Students may voluntarily choose from a wide variety of service options.

3823 Pine Ridge School
101 Thorpe circle
Pine Ridge, SD 57770-9598
802-434-2161
Fax: 802-434-5512
www.pineridgeschool.com
dkb3131@yahoo.com

Dana Blackhurst, Head of School
Mona Miyasato, Principal
Dora Gwein, Assistant Principal
An educational community that is committed to empowering students with dyslexia and other language based learning disabilities, to define and achieve success throughout their lives.

3824 University of Vermont
ACCESS
A170 Living Learning Center
Burlington, VT 05405
802-656-7753
Fax: 802-656-0739
TDD: 802-656-3865
TTY: 802-656-7753
www.uvm.edu/access
access@uvm.edu

Jean Haverstick, Learning Specialist
Nick Ogrizovich, Information Specialist
Diana Williams, M.A., M.S., Learning Specialist
Provides accommodation, consultation, collaboration and educational support services as a means to foster opportunities for students with disabilities to participate in a barrier free learning environment.

3825 Vermont Technical College
PO Box 500
124 Admin Drive
Randolph Center, VT 05061
802-728-1000
800-442-8821
Fax: 802-728-1321
TDD: 802-728-1278
www.vtc.vsc.edu
rgoodall@vtc.edu

Pamela Ankuda, Director of Human Resources
Jim Smith, Chief Technology Officer
Dan Smith, Interim President
Offers a variety of services to students with disabilities including individualized accommodations, counseling services, academic counseling.

Virginia

3826 Averett College
Support Services for Students
420 West Main St.
Danville, VA 24541
434-791-5600
Fax: 804-791-4392
www.averett.edu
priedel@averett.edu

Pamela Riedel MD, Support Services Coordinator
Bill Bradford, Assistant Professor of Aviation
Dr. Tiffany McKillip Franks, President
Four-year college that offers services for the learning disabled.

3827 College of William and Mary
PO Box 8795
Williamsburg, VA 23187-8795
757-221-4000
TDD: 757-221-1154
www.wm.edu

Terry Driscoll, Director
Taylor Reveley, President
Anna Martin, VP Administration
Offers a variety of services to students with disabilities including notetakers, extended testing time, counseling services, and special accommodations.

3828 Eastern Mennonite University
Academic Support Center - Student Disability Svcs.
1200 Park Rd
Harrisonburg, VA 22802-2462
540-432-4000
800-368-2665
Fax: 540-432-4444
TDD: 540-432-4631
TTY: 540-432-4599
www.emu.edu
hedrickj@emu.edu

Loren E Swartzendruber, Coordinator
Dr. Loren Swartzendruber, President
EMU is committed to working out reasonable accommodations for students with documented disabilities to ensure equal access to the University and its related programs.

3829 Emory & Henry College
PO Box 947
Emory, VA 24327-0947

276-944-4121
800-848-5493
Fax: 276-944-6180
www.ehc.edu
helpdesk@ehc.edu

Jake Schrum, President
David Haney, Vice President/Dean of Faculty
Pam Gourley, Vice President/Dean of Students
A private four-year liberal arts college located in the foothills of southwest Virginia. Student enrollment of appox. 1,000, almost equally divided between men and women. The Paul Adrian Powell III resource center offers a variety of services to students with disabilities including extended testing time, counseling services, and special accommodations, as well as tutorial services.

3830 Ferrum College
PO Box 1000
Ferrum, VA 24088-9001

540-365-2121
800-868-9797
Fax: 540-365-4203
TDD: 540-365-4614
www.ferrum.edu

Jennifer L Braaten, President
Dr. Gail Summer, VP Academic Affairs
Samuel L. Lionberger, Jr.m, Chairman
An independent four-year college with support services for special education students.

3831 GW Community School
9001 Braddock Road
Suite 111
Springfield, VA 22151-1002

703-978-7208
Fax: 703-978-7226
www.gwcommunityschool.com
SchoolInfo@GWCommunitySchool.com

Alexa Warden, Director
Richard Goldie, Assistant Director
Cassie Sinichko, Administrative Director
The GW Community School is owned and operated by teachers who understand the learning process and the students' needs, and who genuinely enjoy teaching adolesents. They work closely with students and their families to maximize learning. The GW School for Divergent Learners embodies a vision shared by teachers, parents, and students. A school committed to developing and optimizing the giftedness and intelligence of each student and fostering a sense of social awareness and civic responsibility

3832 Hampden-Sydney College
1 College Road
Hampden Sydney, VA 23943-685

434-223-6000
Fax: 434-223-6346
www.hsc.edu

Keary Mariannino, Executive Secretary to President
DR. Christop Howard, President
Dale Jones,Ph.D., VP Administration
Offers a variety of services to students with disabilities including note takers, extended testing time, counseling services, and special accommodations

3833 James Madison University
Office of Disabilities Services
738 S Mason St
Student Success Center, Suite 1202
Harrisonburg, VA 22807

540-568-6705
Fax: 540-568-7099
TDD: 540-568-6705
TTY: 540-568-6705
www.jmu.edu/ods
disability-svcs@jmu.edu

Jonathan R. Alger, President
Dr. A. Jerry Benson, Provost/Senior Vice President
Maggie Burkhart Evans, Executive Assistant
Offers Learning Strategies Instruction and Strategic Learning Course. Learning Resource Centers in writing, communication, math, science, and critical thinking. Assistive technology lab with various software and hardware include scanners, Kurzweil, etc. High speed scanner support alternate text accommodations. Students with learning disabilities of ADHD may participate in Learning Leaders program.

3834 John Tyler Community College
Office of Disability Services
13101 Jefferson Davis Hwy
Chester, VA 23831-5316

804-796-4000
800-552-3490
Fax: 804-796-4362
TDD: 804-796-4197
www.jtcc.edu

Mara Hilliar, Executive Secretary to President
Dr. Edward Raspiller, President
Dr. L. Ray Drinkwater, VP Student Affairs
A public two-year college with support services for special education students.

3835 Liberty University
Office of Academic Disability Support
1971 University Boulevard
Lynchburg, VA 24515-2213

434-582-2000
Fax: 434-582-2976
TDD: 434-522-0420
www.liberty.edu
wdmchane@liberty.edu

Lee Beaumont, SVP for Auxiliary Service
Jerry Falwell, President
Neal A. Askew, SVP Special Project
Religiously oriented, private, coeducational, comprehensive four year institution. Students who have documented learning disabilities are eligible to receive support services. These would include academic advising, priority class registration, tutoring and testing accommodations.

3836 Little Keswick School
PO Box 24
Keswick, VA 22947-0024

434-295-0457
Fax: 434-977-1892
www.littlekeswickschool.net
lksinfo@littlekeswickschool.net

Terry Columbus, M.Ed., Director of Admissions
Marc J. Columbus. M.Ed., Headmaster
Mark Kindler, Ed..D., Academic Coordinator
A therapeutic boarding school for 34 boys who have learning, emotional and behavioral difficulties.
1963

3837 Longwood College
201 High Street
Graham Hall
Farmville, VA 23909

434-395-2391
800-281-4677
Fax: 434-395-2434
www.longwood.edu/disability
disabilityresources@longwood.edu

Lindsay F. Farrar M.S., CRC, Director
Dana Kieran M.S., Assistant Director
Cameron D. Patterson, Program Coordinator
A public four-year college with support services for special education students.

3838 Lord Fairfax Community College
173 Skirmisher Lane
Middletown, VA 22645-1745

540-868-7000
800-906-5322
Fax: 540-868-7100
TDD: 540-868-7218
www.lfcc.edu

Mary E. Greene, Chair
Dr. Cheryl Thompson-Stacy, President
Chris Boies, Vice President

A public two-year college. Students are encouraged to identify special needs during the admissions process and to request support services, such as individualized placement testing, developmental studies, learning assistance programs, and study skills. A 504 faculty team recommends accommodations to academic programs, and communicates with area service providers.

3839 Mary Washington College
University of Mary Washington Disability Services
1301 College Ave
Fredericksburg, VA 22401-5300

540-654-1000
Fax: 540-654-1073
TDD: 540-654-1102
www.umw.edu
jhample@umw.edu

Jeffrey W. Rountree, Executive Director and CEO
Salvatore M. Meringolo, Vice President
Richard V. Hurley, President
A public four-year college with support services for special education students.

3840 New Community School
4211 Hermitage Road
Richmond, VA 23227-3718

804-266-2494
Fax: 804-264-3281
www.tncs.org
info@tncs.org

Nancy L. Foy, Head of School
H. Pettus LeCompted, President
Janet Deskevich, VP for Development
Provides a program of college preparation for dyslexic (specific language learning disabled) students, grades 6-12. The program includes both remediation of language skills and academic challenge appropriate for students of average to above-average intellectual potential.

3841 New River Community College
PO Box 1127
5251 College Drive
Dublin, VA 24084-1127

540-674-3600
866-462-6722
Fax: 540-674-3644
TDD: 540-674-3619
www.nr.edu
nrdixoj@nr.ca.cc.va.us

Pat Huber, Vice President for Instruction
F. Brad Denardo, Chair
Jack Lewis, President
A public two-year college with support services for special education students.

3842 Norfolk State University
700 Park Avenue
Norfolk, VA 23504-8090

757-823-8396
800-274-1821
Fax: 757-823-2078
www.nsu.edu
admissions@nsu.edu

Paula Paula, Assistant to the President
Eddie N. Moore Jr., President
Clementine Cone, Executive Assistant
Four year university that offers programs for the students with learning disabilities.

3843 Northern Virginia Community College
Disability Support Department
8333 Little River Turnpike
Annandale, VA 22003-3796

703-323-7000
Fax: 703-323-3559
www.nvcc.edu

Robert G Templon Jr, President
John T Denver, Executive Vice President
Pat Gary, Chair
A public two-year college.

3844 Oakwood School
7210 Braddock Rd
Annandale, VA 22003-6068

703-941-5788
Fax: 703-941-4186
www.oakwoodschool.com
oakwood@oakwoodschool.com

Robert Mc Intyre, Chairman
A private, non-profit, co-educational day school for elementary and middle school students with mild to moderate learning differences.

3845 Old Dominion University
5115 Hampton Boulevard
Norfolk, VA 23529-0001

757-683-4655
Fax: 757-683-3000
TDD: 757-683-5356
www.studentaffairs.odu.edu/disability
disabilityservices@odu.edu

Velvet Grant, Assistant to the President/CEO
John R Broderick, President
Bob Fenning, VP Administration & Finance
Providing accomodations for students admitted to Old Dominion University that have a documented disability.

3846 Patrick Henry Community College
Patrick Henry Community College
645 Patriot Avenue
Martinsville, VA 24112-5311

276-638-8777
800-232-7997
Fax: 276-656-0327
TDD: 276-638-2433
www.ph.vccs.edu
klandrum@patrickhenry.edu

Angeline D. Godwin, Ph.D., J.D., President
Christopher Parker, PhD., VP Institutional Advancement
Debbie Bryant, Financial Assistant
Offers a variety of services to students with disabilities including note takers, adaptive testing, counseling services, peer tutoring and adaptive equipment, and accessible transportation.

3847 Paul D Camp Community College
PO Box 737
100 North College Drive
Franklin, VA 23851-737

757-569-6700
Fax: 757-569-6773
TDD: 757-569-7946
www.pdc.edu/
info@pdc.edu

Richard Brooks, Chair
Paul W. Conco, President
Randy Betz, VP Workforce Development
A public two-year institution with two campuses. Students with learning disabilities are eligible for special services provided by the Student Support Service Program. Learning-disabled students may take advantage of tutors (outside of class time and during class labs), notetakers, and taped textbooks. A counselor serves as student advocate and helps students arrange for classroom accommodations with instructors.

3848 Piedmont Virginia Community College
501 College Dr
Charlottesville, VA 22902-7589

434-977-3900
Fax: 434-971-8232
www.pvcc.edu
admissions@pvcc.edu

Frank Friedman, President
John R. Donnelly, Vice President
Corinne Lauer, Administrative Assistant
A two-year comprehensive community college dedicated to the belief that individuals should have equal opportunity to develop and extend their skills and knowledge. Consistent with this philosophy and in compliance with the Americans with Disabilities Act, we encourage persons with disabilities to apply.

3849 Randolph-Macon Woman's College
2500 Rivermont Ave
Lynchburg, VA 24503-1526   434-947-8000
                                   800-745-RMWC
                                   Fax: 434-947-8139
                                   TDD: 434-947-8608
                                   www.randolphcollege.edu
                                   admissions@randolphcollege.edu
Bradley W. Bateman, Ph.D., President
Rebecca Morrison Dunn, Chair
Wesley R. Fugate, Ph. D., Vice President
An independent four-year college with support services for
students with disabilities.

3850 Rappahannock Community College
12745 College Drive
Glenns, VA 23149-2616   804-758-6700
                                  800-836-9381
                                  Fax: 804-758-3852
                                  www.rcc.vccs.edu
                                  mcralle@rappahannock.edu
Elizabeth Hinton Crowther, President
D. Kim McManus, Vice President, Finance & Admin
Cherie N. Carl, Director of College Advancement
Offers a variety of services to students with disabilities in-
cluding notetakers, extended testing time, counseling ser-
vices, and special accommodations.

3851 Riverside School
2110 McRae Road
North Chesterfield, VA 23235-7533   804-320-3465
                                      Fax: 804-320-6146
                                      www.riversideschool.org
                                      info@riversideschool.org
Julia D Wingfield, Head of School
Elizabeth F. Edwards, President
Kathleen Miller, Vice President
Provide remediation of the language skills of each of the
at-risk students with dyslexia in grades 1-8, so that they can
return to mainstream education fully prepared to realize
their highest potential.

3852 Saint Coletta: Alexandria
Adult Programs
207 S Peyton Street
Alexandria, VA 22314-2812   571-438-6940
                                 Fax: 571-438-6949
                                 TTY: 202-350-8695
                                 www.stcoletta.org
Sharon B. Raimo, Chief Executive Officer
John Shank, VP Federal Legislative Affairs
David Pryor, Jr., President
Offer adults age 18 and older opportunities to participate in
vocational and pre-vocational training, life skills training,
and community integration in order to achieve greater
independence.

3853 Southern Virginia College
One University Hill Drive
Buena Vista, VA 24416-3038   540-261-8400
                                 800-229-8420
                                 Fax: 540-266-3806
                                 http://svu.edu/
                                 student.finances@svu.edu
Paul K. Sybrowsky, President
Robert E. Huch, Vice President of Finance
Glade M. Knight, Chair
Offers a variety of services to students with disabilities in-
cluding note takers, extended testing time, counseling ser-
vices, and special accommodations.

3854 Southside Virginia Community College
109 Campus Drive
Alberta, VA 23821-2930   434-949-1000
                                 www.sv.vccs.edu
                                 rhina.jones@southside.edu

John J Cavan, President
Dorcas Helfant-Browning, Chair
Idalia Fernandez, Vice Chair
Offers a variety of services to students with disabilities in-
cluding notetakers, extended testing time, counseling ser-
vices, and special accommodations.

3855 Southwest Virginia Community College
PO Box SVCC
Richlands, VA 24641   276-964-2555
                                 Fax: 276-964-9307
                                 TDD: 276-964-7235
                                 www.sw.edu
                                 admissions@sw.edu
Dr. J. Mark Estepp, President
Michael Bales, Business Manager
Peggy Barber, Director
Offers a variety of services to students with disabilities in-
cluding note takers, extended testing time, counseling ser-
vices, and special accommodations.

3856 Thomas Nelson Community College
99 Thomas Nelson Dr
Hampton, VA 23666   757-825-2700
                                 Fax: 757-825-2763
                                 www.tncc.edu
                                 info@TNCC.edu
Thomas Kellen, Admissions Advisor
Dr. John.T Dever, President
Howard Taylor, Administrator
A public two-year college with support services for students
with disabilities.

3857 Tidewater Community College
350 Granby Street
Norfolk, VA 23510   757-822-1110
                                 TTY: 757-822-1248
                                 www.tcc.edu
                                 tcharro@tcc.edu
Edna Baehre-Kolovani, Ph.D., President
Mr. Franklin Dunn, Executive Vice President
Valary Lejman, Administrative Assistant
This public two-year college offers transfer and occupa-
tional/technical degrees on four campuses and a visual arts
center in the Hampton Roads area of Virginia. TCC offers
students evaluations, all reasonable accommodations, and a
wide array of assistive technology.

3858 University of Virginia
Learning Needs & Evaluation Cetner
400 Brandon Avenue
PO Box 800760
Charlottesville, VA 22908-760   434-924-5362
                                 Fax: 434-982-3956
                                 www.virginia.edu/studenthealth/
                                 studenthealth@virginia.edu
Chris P. Holstege, M.D., Executive Director
James.C Turner, Director
Full range of support services for students admitted to any of
the ten schools of the university, including graduate/profes-
sional schools. Including, but not limited to, alternate texts,
exam accommodations, peer-notetakers, TTY and interpreters, assistive devices and housing and transportation
accommodations.

3859 Virginia Commonwealth University
Services for Students with Disabilities
901 W Franklin St
Richmond, VA 23284-9066   804-828-0100
                                 800-841-3638
                                 Fax: 804-828-1899
                                 www.vcu.edu
                                 vcuhsinternet@mcvh-vcu.edu
Michael Rao, Ph.D., President
Marti K. S. Heil, Vice president for Development
Mark E. Rubin, Executive Director
Offers a variety of services to students with disabilities in-
cluding note takers, extended testing time, counseling ser-
vices, and special accommodations.

3860 **Virginia Highlands Community College**
PO Box 828
100 VHCC Drive
Abingdon, VA 24212-828
276-739-2400
877-739-6115
Fax: 276-739-2590
www.vhcc.edu
helpdesk@vhcc.edu

James F. Rector, Jr., Chair
Virgil C. Wimmer, Vice-Chair
Gene C. Couch, Jr., President
A public two-year college. Strives to assist students with disabilities in successfully responding to challenges of academic study and job training.

3861 **Virginia Intermont College**
1013 Moore Street
Bristol, VA 24201-4298
276-669-6101
800-451-1842
Fax: 276-466-7963
www.vic.edu
bholbroo@vic.edu

E. Clorisa Phillips, Ph.D., President
Kathleen W. O'Brien, Chair
Linda C. Morgan, SVP for Administration
Virginia Intermont College is a private, four-year Baptist affiliated liberal arts college located near the Appalachian Mountains of Southwest Virginia. Intermont has an enrollment of 850 men and women students. Accommodations, such as notetakers, extended time on tests, transcribers, oral testing, tutors and other services, are provided based on documentation of disabilities.

3862 **Virginia Polytechnic Institute and State University**
430 Old Turner Street
Blacksburg, VA 24061
540-231-3788
Fax: 540-231-3232
TTY: 540-231-0853
www.ssd.vt.edu
ssd@vt.edu

Susan Angle MD, Director For Disability Services
Charles Steger, President
Robyn Hudson, Assistant Director
A public four-year college with support services for special education students.

3863 **Virginia Wesleyan College**
Disabilities Services Office
1584 Wesleyan Dr
Norfolk, VA 23502-5599
757-455-3200
800-737-8684
Fax: 757-466-8526
www.vwc.edu
fpearson@vwc.edu

William T Greer Jr, President
Mr. Bruce Vaughan, Vice President of Operations
Gary D. Bonnewell, Chairman
Four year college that offers support to students with a learning disability.

3864 **Virginia Western Community College**
PO Box 14007
Roanoke, VA 24038-4007
540-857-7231
Fax: 540-857-6102
TDD: 540-857-6351
www.virginiawestern.edu
helpdesk@virginiawestern.edu

Michael Henderson, Special Services
Dana Asciolla, Admissions Staff
Robert Sandel, President
A public two-year college with support services for special education students.

Washington

3865 **Bellevue Community College**
3000 Landerholm Cir SE
Bellevue, WA 98007-6484
425-564-1000
Fax: 425-649-3173
TTY: 425-564-4110
www.bcc.ctc.edu
admissions@bellevuecollege.edu

Dave Rule, President
Carol Jones-Watkins, Coordinator
Disability Support Services provides accommodations for people with disabilities to make their academic careers a success. There is no separate fee for these services.

3866 **Center for Disability Services**
Central Washington University
400 E University Way
Ellensburg, WA 98926-7431
509-963-2171
Fax: 509-963-3235
www.cwu.edu
DS@cwu.edu

James L. Gaudino, President
Rob Harden, Director
Pamela Wilson, Associate Director
A public four-year college with disability support services for students with disabilities.

3867 **Centralia College**
600 Centralia College Blvd
Centralia, WA 98531-4099
360-736-9391
Fax: 360-330-7501
TTY: 360-807-6227
www.centralia.edu
demerson@centralia.ctc.edu

Robert A. Frost, President
Donna Emerson, Secretary Lead
Michael Grubiak, Vice President
The Special Services Office offers a variety of services to students with disabilities including notetakers, extended testing time, counseling services, and special accommodations.

3868 **Children's Institute for Learning**
4030 86th Ave SE
Mercer Island, WA 98040-4198
206-232-8680
Fax: 206-232-9377
www.childrensinstitute.com
shannonr@childrensInstitute.com

Carrie Fannin, Executive Director
Cathy DeLeon, OTR/L, Director of Clinical Services
Dominic Jimenez, Director of Education
A full-day academic and therapeutic program for children ages 3 to 17. Provides social, emotional, developmental and neurological strategies for children with challenging learning differences and behavior disorders.

3869 **Clark College**
1933 Fort Vancouver Way
Vancouver, WA 98663-3598
360-992-2314
Fax: 360-992-2879
www.clark.edu/dss
tjacobs@clark.edu

Robert K. Knight, President
Bob Williamson, Vice President
Dr. Tim Cook, Vice President
Offers a variety of services to students with disabilities including note takers, extended testing time, counseling services, and special accommodations.

3870 **Columbia Basin College, Resource Center Program**
2600 N 20th Ave
Pasco, WA 99301-4108
509-547-0511
Fax: 509-546-0401
TDD: 509-547-0400
www.columbiabasin.edu
pbuchmiller@columbiabasin.edu

Richard W. Cummins PhD, President
Peggy Buchmiller, Assistant Dean & Director
Pat Wright, Associate Director
Provides advocacy and Auxillary aids and services to students with a disability.

3871   Cornish College of the Arts
1000 Lenora St
Seattle, WA 98121-2718   800-726-ARTS
                                   www.cornish.edu
                                   hello@cornish.edu
Dr. Nancy Uscher, President
Lois Harris, Ph.D., Provost and Vice President
Virginia Anderson, Chair
Through the Student Affairs Office, appropriate accommodations are provided for students with learning disabilities.

3872   Dartmoor School
2340 130th Avenue NE
Suite 110
Bellevue, WA 98005-2322   425-649-8976
                                  Fax: 425-603-0038
                                  www.dartmoorschool.org
Doris.J Bower, Founder and Executive Director
Andrew Wahl, President
Denise Leiby, Director of Special Education
A school where intellectual development and interest creates a mentorship between teacher and student, where students call teachers by their first name, and where staff invest actively in student achievement.

3873   Eastern Washington University
124 Tawanka
Cheney, WA 99004   509-359-6871
                                  Fax: 509-359-7458
                                  www.ewu.edu
                                  dsss@ewu.edu
Dr. Mary Cullinan, President
Paul Tanaka, Chair
Michael Finley, Trustee
Although the University does not offer a specialized program specifically for learning disabled students, the disability support services office works with students on a case by case basis.

3874   Edmonds Community College
20000 68th Ave W
Lynnwood, WA 98036-5999   425-640-1459
                                  Fax: 425-640-1622
                                  TDD: 425-354-3113
                                  TTY: 425-774-8669
                                  www.edcc.edu/ssd
                                  ssdmail@edcc.edu
Dee Olson, Director
Kaleb Cameron, Assistant Director
Ruben Alatorre, Coordinator-Sign Language
Offers a variety of services to students with disabilities including notetakers, extended testing time, and special accommodations.

3875   Epiphany School
3611 East Denny Way
Seattle, WA 98122-3471   206-323-9011
                                  Fax: 206-324-2127
                                  www.epiphanyschool.org
                                  office@epiphanyschool.org
Laurie Lootens Chyz, President
Hunter Wessells, VP
Belinda Buscher, Secretary
Now, with 233 students served by 43 faculty and staff, Epiphany School and the Board of Trustees turn their attention to a new educational vision, examining the student needs in a changing world, while staying true to the strengths that have served them well for over 53 years. Epiphany has proudly served more than 1,000 students, many of whom return to the School and increasingly bring their own children to be educated here.

3876   Everett Community College
Center for Disabilities Services
2000 Tower St
Everett, WA 98201-1390   425-388-9100
                                  Fax: 425-388-9129
                                  TDD: 425-388-9438
                                  www.everettcc.edu
                                  cds@everettcc.edu
Jerod Grant, Director
Esther Moss, Program Coordinator
Abraham Rodriguez-Hernandez, Program Manager
Offers a variety of services to students with disabilities including notetakers, extended testing time, adaptive software and individual accommodations.

3877   Evergreen State College
2700 Evergreen Pkwy NW
Olympia, WA 98505-5   360-867-6000
                                  Fax: 360-867-6577
                                  www.evergreen.edu
Thomas L Purce, President
Evergreen's mission is to sustain a vibrant academic community and to offer students an education that will help them excel in their intellectual, creative, professional and community service goals.

3878   Green River Community College
12401 SE 320th St
Room 126
Auburn, WA 98092-3622   253-833-9111
                                  TDD: 253-288-3359
                                  www.greenriver.edu
                                  rblosser@greenriver.edu
Dr. Eileen Ely, President
Jennifer Nelson, Program Assistant
Tom Campbell, Chair
Support services for students with disabilities to ensure that our programs and facilities are accessible. Our campus is organized to provide reasonable accommodations, including core services, to qualified students with dissabilities.

3879   Heritage Christian Academy
19527 104thAvenue NE
Bothell, WA 98011-2930   425-485-2585
                                  Fax: 425-486-2895
                                  www.hcabothell.org
                                  Info@hcabothell.org
Jack Middlebrooks, Chair
Cindy Bushnell, Parent Representative
Wendy Chappell, Preschool Director
Heritage Christian Academy has had the opportunity to educate thousands of children in the Puget Sound region. The school is well known throughout the region for its quality academic program and it is becoming known for its unwavering dedication in equipping students with a Kingdom Education that enables them to stand against a world view in opposition to Christian values.

3880   Highline Community College
PO Box 98000
Des Moines, WA 98198-9800   206-878-3710
                                  Fax: 206-870-3773
                                  TTY: 206-870-4853
                                  www.highline.edu
                                  cjones@highline.edu
Jini Allen, Human Resources Staff
Jack Bermingham, President
Debrena Jackson Gandy, Chair
Offers a variety of services to students with disabilities including note takers, extended testing time, counseling services, and special accommodations.

3881   Morningside Academy
901 Lenora Street
Seattle, WA 98109-5217   206-709-9500
                                  Fax: 206-709-4611
                                  www.morningsideacademy.org
                                  info@morningsideacademy.org

391

Aine O'Connor, Director of Operations
Dr. Kent Johnson, Executive Director
Tim Smith, Director
Morningside Academy's school helps both elementary and middle school students to catch up and get ahead. Its students have not previously reached their potential; many have learning disabilities or ADD/ADHD diagnoses; all have average to well above average intelligence. Morningside is not a school for children with significant emotional problems, behavioral problems, or developmental delays.

3882 New Heights School
Children's Institute for Learning Differences
4030 86th Ave SE
Mercer Island, WA 98040-4198   206-232-8680
Fax: 206-232-9377
www.childrensinstitute.com
micheleg@childrensinstitute.com
Carrie Fannin, Executive Director
Cathy DeLeon, OTR/L, Director of Clinical Services
Dominic Jimenez, Director of Education
A Pre k-12 school based program serving children ages 3-18.

3883 North Seattle Community College
Educational Access Center
9600 College Way N
Seattle, WA 98103-3599   206-527-3600
Fax: 206-527-3606
http://northseattle.edu
Mary Ellen O'Keeffe, Interim President
Orestes Monterecy, Administrative Services
Jennie Dulas, Office of Advancement
The Educational Access Center offers a variety of services to students with disabilities including notetakers, extended testing time, counseling services, and special accommodations.

3884 Northwest School
1415 Summit Ave
Seattle, WA 98122-3619   206-682-7309
Fax: 206-467-7353
www.northwestschool.org
admissions@northwestschool.org
Cory Carlson, President
Lisa Anderson, Vice President
Mike McGill, Head of School
The Northwest School is set in an urban campus that is housed in a historic landmark cared for by our students, we provide a curriculum for grades 6-12 that offers an international perspective and encourages independent and creative thinking in every class. They educate and shape their students into global citizens who will one day shape the community, nation, and world.

3885 Pacific Learning Solutions
314 N Olympic Ave
Arlington, WA 98223-9541   360-403-8885
Fax: 360-403-7607
http://pacificlearningsolutions.com
pacificlearningsolutions@gmail.com
Nola Smith, President
Leslie Platt, Tutor
Rebecca Wesson, Tutor
Tutoring for dyslexia; therapy for processing, memory recall and learning difficulties; LiFT (Listening is Fitness Training), Teacher consultant with Academy Northwest Private school helping home school families.

3886 Pierce Community College
9401 Farwest Dr SW
Lakewood, WA 98498-1999   253-964-6500
Fax: 253-964-6599
www.pierce.ctc.edu
mharris@pierce.ctc.edu
Angie Roarty, Chair
Steve Smith, Vice Chair
Brett Willis, Trustee

A federally funded TRIO progrm providing academic support services to low income students, first generation college students and students with disabilities in order to improve their retention, academic proformance, graduation and transfer to four-year institutions.

3887 Seattle Academy of Arts and Sciences
1201 E Union St
Seattle, WA 98122-3925   206-323-6600
Fax: 206-323-6618
http://seattleacademy.org
admissions@seattleacademy.org
Jean Orvis, Administrator
Barbara Burk, Administrative Assistant
Joe Puggelli, Head of School
Seattle Academy prepares students to participate effectively in modern society. They seek a diversified student body and faculty.

3888 Seattle Central Community College
Seattle Community College District
1701 Broadway
Seattle, WA 98122-2400   206-587-3800
Fax: 206-344-4390
TDD: 206-934-5450
www.seattlecentral.org
SCCCWCC@sccd.ctc.edu
Paul T. Killpatrick, Ph.D., President
Warren Brown, EVP
Adam Nance, Executive Director
Offers a variety of services to students with disabilities including notetakers, extended testing time, counseling services, and special accommodations.

3889 Seattle Christian Schools
18301 Military Rd S
Seatac, WA 98188-4684   206-246-8241
Fax: 206-246-9066
www.seattlechristian.com
ghunter@seattlechristian.org
Gloria Hunter, Superintendent
Bryan Peterson, Principal
Dave Steele, Administrator
Independent, interdenominational Christian Day School established in 1946, serving 750+ students.

3890 Seattle Pacific University
3307 3rd Ave W
Ste 214
Seattle, WA 98119-1997   206-281-2000
Fax: 206-286-7348
TDD: 206-281-2475
TTY: 206-281-2224
www.spu.edu
centerforlearning3@spu.edu
Daniel J. Martin, President
Don Mortenson, VP
Jeff Jordan, VP
Offers a variety of services to students with disabilities including notetakers, extended testing time, books on tape, interpreters and special accommodations.

3891 Shoreline Christian School
2400 NE 147th St
Shoreline, WA 98155-7395   206-364-7777
Fax: 206-364-0349
www.shorelinechristian.org
admin@shorelinechristian.org
Timothy Visser, Administrator
Rhonda Rasor, Office Staff
Laurie Dykstra, Director of Development
Shoreline Christian School educates students in preschool through

grade 12, challenging them to grow academically, socially and spiritually.

3892 Snohomish County Christian
17931 64th Ave W
Lynnwood, WA 98037-7106   425-742-9518
                                        Fax: 425-745-9306
www.cpcsschools.com/lynnwood
Dr. Clinton Behrends, District Superintendent
Jan Isakson, School Administrator
Mary Riley, Preschool/Childcare Director
The Lynnwood Campus is focused on a Christ-centered education that prepares their students to authentically live for God while serving Him and others.

3893 South Puget Sound Community College
2011 Mottman Rd SW
Olympia, WA 98512-6292   360-754-7711
                                        Fax: 360-664-0780
www.spscc.ctc.edu
advising@spscc.ctc.edu
Gerald Pumphrey, Disability Support Coordinator
Kenneth Minnaert, President
Marilyn Adair, Nursing/Director
Offers a variety of services to students with disabilities including notetakers, extended testing time, books on tape, readers, scribes, interpreters, assistance with registration.

3894 South Seattle Community College
6000 16th Ave SW
Seattle, WA 98106-1499   206-764-5300
                                        Fax: 206-764-5393
                                        TDD: 800-833-6388
www.southseattle.edu
rtillman@sccd.ctc.edu
Jill Wakefield, President
Albert Shen, Chair
Courtney Gregoire, Vice Chair
Offers a variety of services to students with disabilities including notetakers, extended testing time, counseling services and special accommodations.

3895 Spokane Community College
1810 N Greene St
Spokane, WA 99217-5399   509-533-7000
                                             800-248-5644
                                        TDD: 509-533-7482
www.scc.spokane.edu
shanson@scc.spokane.edu
Christine Johnson, Chancellor
Scott Morgan, President
Ben Wolfe, Director
Offers a variety of services to students with disabilities including notetakers, extended testing time, counseling services, and special accommodations.

3896 Spokane Falls Community College
3410 W Fort George Wright Dr
Spokane, WA 99224-5288   509-533-3500
                                             888-509-7944
                                        Fax: 509-533-3237
                                        TDD: 509-533-3838
                                        TTY: 509-533-3838
www.spokanefalls.edu
Christine Johnson, Chancellor
Scott Morgan, President
Ben Wolfe, Director
Offers a variety of services to students with disabilities including notetakers, extended testing time, counseling services, and special accommodations.

3897 St. Alphonsus
5816 15th Ave NW
Seattle, WA 98107-3096   206-782-4563
                                        Fax: 206-789-5709
www.stalphonsus-sea.org
Fr. Shane McKee, SOLT, Pastor
Matt Eisenhauer, Principal
Charleen Sweet, Administrative Assistant

The Society has assigned priests to serve the local Seattle area out of the parish rectory. The excellent relationship between the Archdiocese and the SOLT community has also afforded the assignment of dozens of SOLT sisters and novices to the convent located on St. Alphonsus parish grounds.

3898 St. Matthew's
1240 NE 127th St
Seattle, WA 98125-4021   206-363-6767
                                        Fax: 206-362-4863
http://stmatthewseattle.org
parishoffice@stmatthewseattle.org
Fr. Jerry Burns, Priest
Jean Cooney, Administrative Assistant
Jon Rowley, Facilities Manager
St. Matthews believe in Jesus Christ and welcome all who seek God's Grace. Their compassionate community embraces many cultures. Through prayer, liturgy, our ministries and service to others, they cultivate a lifelong journey of faith.

3899 St. Thomas School
8300 NE 12th Street
Medina, WA 98039-124   425-454-5880
                                        Fax: 425-454-1921
www.stthomasschool.org
info@stthomasschool.org
Kirk Wheeler, Ed.D., Head of School
Lyn-Felice Calvin, Director
Bill Palmer, Acting Director
St Thomas School aims to develop responsible citizens of a global society. In partnership with parents, they inspire and motivate intellectually curious students. Their small, nurturing environment supports the acquisition of a broad academic foundation with an emphasis on critical thinking, leadership skills, and the development of strong character and spiritual awareness.

3900 University Preparatory Academy
8000 25th Ave NE
Seattle, WA 98115-4600   206-525-2714
                                        Fax: 206-525-9659
www.universityprep.org
Matt Levinson, Head of School
Susan Lansverk, CFO
Lora Kolmer, Director of Communications
An independent school serving grades six through twelve, they offer an outstanding academic program guided by our mission statement:University Prep is committed to developing each student's potential to become an intellectually courageous, socially responsible citizen of the world. Their innovative teachers offer a collaborative journey of learning in a diverse community of talented students and involved families.

3901 University of Puget Sound
University of Puget Sound
1500 N Warner St
Tacoma, WA 98416-5   253-879-3211
                                        Fax: 253-879-3500
                                        TDD: 253-879-3399
                                        TTY: 800-833-6388
www.pugetsound.edu
admission@pugetsound.edu
Ronald R. Thomas, President
Linda Norwell King, Executive Assistant
Patti Turner, Residence Manager
Support services and accommodations are individually tailored depending upon a student's disability, its severity, the students academic environment and courses, housing situation, activities, etc. Accommodations include instruction in study strategies, free tutoring, assistance in note taking, sign language and additional academic advising.

3902   University of Washington Disability Resources for Students
011 Mary Gates
Box 352808
Seattle, WA 98195-2808   206-543-8924
                                   Fax: 206-616-8379
                                   TDD: 206-543-8925
                        http://depts.washington.edu/uwdrs
                        uwdss@u.washington.edu
Provides services and academic accommodations to students with documented permanent and temporary disabilities to ensure equal access to the university's educational programs and facilities. Services may include but are not limited to exam accommodations, notetaking, audio-taped class texts/materials, sign language interpreters, auxilary aids (assistive listening devices, and accessible furniture).

3903   University of Washington: Center on Human Development and Disability
PO Box 357920
Seattle, WA 98195-7920   206-543-7701
                                   Fax: 206-543-3417
                        www.depts.washington.edu/chdd
                        chdd@uw.edu
Michael Guralnick, Director
Richard Masse, M.P.H., Director of Administration
Elizabeth Aylward, Ph.D., Associate Director
The Center on Human Development and Disability (CHDD) at the University of Washington makes important contributions to the lives of people with developmental disabilities and their families, through a comprehensive array of research, clinical services, training, community outreach and dissemination activities.

3904   Walla Walla Community College
500 Tausick Way
Walla Walla, WA 99362-9267   509-522-2500
                                       877-992-9922
                                   Fax: 509-527-4480
                                   TDD: 509-527-4412
                                   www.wwcc.edu
Darcey Fugman-Small, Chair
Don McQuary, Vice Chair
Kris Klaveano, Trustee
The Special Services Office offers a variety of services to students with disabilities including notetakers, extended testing time, counseling services, and special accommodations.

3905   Washington State University
Disability Resource Center
217 Washington Building
PO Box 642
Pullman, WA 99164-2322   509-335-3417
                                   Fax: 509-335-8511
                                   www.drc.wsu.edu
                        drc.frontdesk@ad.wsu.edu
Meredyth Goodwin, Director
Juli Anderson, Access Advisor
Kay Smith, Proctoring Coordinator
Provide leadership in the development of an inclusive environment at WSU by eliminating barriers, whether they are physical, attitudinal, informational, or programmatic.

3906   Western Washington University
516 High St
Old Main 120
Bellingham, WA 98225-9019   360-650-3083
                                   Fax: 360-650-3715
                        www.wwu.edu/depts/drs
                        drs@wwu.edu
David Brunnemer, Director
Anna Talvi-Blick, Assistant Director
Kim Thiessen, Coordinator
disAbility Resources for Students (DRS) offers a variety of services to students with disabilities including note takers, extended testing time, counseling services and special accommodations.

3907   Whatcom Community College
237 W Kellogg Rd
Bellingham, WA 98226-8003   360-383-3000
                                   Fax: 360-676-2171
                                   www.whatcom.ctc.edu
                        advise@whatcom.ctc.edu
Dr. Kathi Hiyane-Brown, President
Anne Bowen, Executive Director
Patricia Onion, Vice President
A public two-year college with support services for special education students.

3908   Whitworth College
300 W Hawthorne Rd
Spokane, WA 99251   509-777-1000
                                   Fax: 509-777-3725
                                   www.whitworth.edu
                        mhansen@whitworth.edu
Marianne Hanson, Director of Admissions
Aaron McMurray, Director
Garrett Riddle, Associate Director
Offers a variety of services to students with disabilities including note takers, extended testing time, counseling services, and special accommodations.

3909   Yakima Valley Community College
S.16th Ave & Nob Hill Blvd.
Yakima, WA 98907-2520   509-574-4600
                                   TDD: 509-574-4600
                                   www.yvcc.edu
Robert Ozuna, Vice Chair
Paul McDonald, Trustee
Rosalinda Mendoza, Trustee
Offers a variety of services to students with disabilities including notetakers, extended testing time, counseling services, and special accommodations.

3910   Yellow Wood Academy
9655 SE 36th St
Suite 101
Mercer Island, WA 98040-3798   206-236-1095
                                   Fax: 206-236-0998
                        www.yellowwoodacademy.org
                        info@ywacademy.org
Ruth Hayes-Short, Executive Director
Tina Kennedy, CFO
Susan Small, Director of Student Services
Assessment, referral, tutorial, courses for credit, advocacy, dissertation, adults and students that are school age.

West Virginia

3911   Bethany College West Virginia
Special Advising Program
Room 4
Morlan Hall
Bethany, WV 26032   304-829-7000
                                   Fax: 304-829-7580
                                   www.bethanywv.edu
                        alumni@bethanywv.edu
Dr. Scott D. Miller, President
Dr. Darin E. Fields, Vice President
William R. Kiefer, Executive Vice President
Bethany College is an academic community founded on the close interaction between students and faculty in the educational process. Bethany College values intellectual rigor and freedom, diversity of thought and lifestyle, personal growth within a community context, and responsible engagement with public issues.

3912 Davis & Elkins College
Learning Disability Program
100 Campus Dr
Elkins, WV 26241-3996
304-637-1900
800-624-3157
Fax: 304-637-1413
www.dewv.edu
mccaulj@dne.wvnet.edu
Dr. Michael P. Mihalyo, Jr., President
June B. Myles, Chair
Richard C. Seybolt, Vice Chair
Offers a program to provide individual support to college students with specific learning disabilities. This comprehensive program includes regular sessions with one of the three full-time learning disabilities instructors and specialized assistance and technology not available elsewhere on campus.

3913 Fairmont State University
Student Disabilities Services
1201 Locust Ave
Fairmont, WV 26554-2470
304-367-4892
800-641-5678
Fax: 304-367-1803
TDD: 304-367-4200
www.fairmontstate.edu
admit@FairmontState.edu
Maria C. Bennett Rose, President
Ron Tucker, Chairman
Dixie Yann, Vice Chair
Four year college provides services to learning disabled students.

3914 Glenville State College
Student Disability Services
200 High St
Glenville, WV 26351-1200
304-462-7361
800-924-2010
Fax: 304-462-4407
TDD: 304-462-4136
www.glenville.edu
cottrill@GLENVILLE.WVNET.EDU
Peter B Barr, President
Rich Heffelfinger, Chair
Greg Smith, Vice Chair
Glenville State College, often referred to as the Lighthouse on the Hill, is West Virginia's only centrally located public college. With an enrollment of approximately 1,400 students, the college has a student to faculty ratio of 19 to 1. The college's enrollment is made up of many first generation students with approximately 90% of the students coming from West Virginia counties.

3915 Higher Education for Learning Problems (HELP)
Marshall University
Myers Hall
520 - 18th St
Huntington, WV 25703
304-696-6252
800-642-3463
Fax: 304-696-3231
www.marshall.edu/help
help@marshall.edu
Debbie Painter, Director
Missi Fisher, Assistant Director
K. Renna Moore, Administrative Assistant
Offers the following services: individual tutoring to assist with coursework, studying for tests, administration of oral tests when appropriate; assistance with improvement of memory, assistance with note taking; assistance to determine presence of learning problems.

3916 Salem International University
233 W Main St
Salem, WV 26426-1226
888-235-5024
Fax: 304-326-1246
TDD: 304-782-5011
www.salemu.edu
admissions@salemiu.edu
John Reynolds, President

Student Support Services grant program funded by the US Dept of Education for 125 college students who are identified as disadvantaged and/or disabled. On staff are a counselor, a learning disabled specialist in math and science and a learning specialist in reading and writing.

3917 Southern West Virginia Community and Technical College
PO Box 2900
Mount Gay, WV 25637-2900
304-896-7432
Fax: 304-792-7113
TTY: 304-792-7054
www.southernwv.edu
darrellt@southernwvnet.edu
Darrell Taylor, Dean of Student Development
Higher education

3918 West Virginia Northern Community College
1704 Market St
Wheeling, WV 26003-3643
304-233-5900
Fax: 304-233-0272
www.wvncc.edu
Martin Olshinsky, President
Dr. Darrell Cummings, Chair
Mary K. DeGarmo, Vice Chair
A public two-year college with support services for special education students.

3919 West Virginia State College
PO Box 1000
Institute, WV 25112-1000
304-766-3000
800-987-2112
Fax: 304-766-4100
www.wvstateu.edu
Kellie Dunlap, Disability Services
Dr.Brian.O Hemphill, President
Melvin Jones, Vice President
A public four-year college. Accommodations are individualized to meet student's needs.

3920 West Virginia University
Speech Pathology and Audiology
802 Allen Hall
PO Box 6122
Morgantown, WV 26506-6122
304-293-4241
Fax: 304-293-2905
www.wvu.edu/~speechpa
jack.aylor@mail.wvu.edu
Lynn Schrum, Dean
Cheryl Ridgway, Administrative Assistant
Jack Aylor, Director of Development
Provides high-quality programs of instruction at the undergraduate, graduate, and prefessional level; to stimulate and foster both basic and applied research and scholarship; to engage in and encourage other creative and artistic work; and to bring the resources of the University to all segments of society through continuing education, extension, and public activities.

3921 West Virginia University at Parkersburg
300 Campus Dr
Parkersburg, WV 26104-8647
304-424-8378
Fax: 304-424-8372
TDD: 304-424-8337
www.wvup.edu
wvup_disabilitysv@mail.wvu.edu
Christine Post, Dean Enrollment Management
John Gorrell, Assistant Dean/Director
Alice Harris, VP of Finance and Administration
Provides disability accomodations to qualified students based on appropriate documentation.

3922 **West Virginia Wesleyan College**
Mentor Advantage Program
59 College Ave
Buckhannon, WV 26201-2699

304-473-8000
800-722-9933
Fax: 304-472-2571
www.wvwc.edu
kuba_s@wvwc.edu

Pamela Balch, President
The mentoring program, developed from research on the transition and persistence of postsecondary students with learning disabilities and from self-regulated learning theory, is designed to create a bridge to academic regulation in the college environment.

Wisconsin

3923 **Alverno College**
3400 S 43rd St
Milwaukee, WI 53234-3922

414-382-6026
800-933-3401
Fax: 414-382-6354
www.alverno.edu
colleen.barnett@alverno.edu

Mary J Meehan, Ph.D., President
Mary Beth Berkes, Chair
Howard Jacob, Ph.D., Vice Chair
An independent liberal arts college with 2,000 students in its weekday and weekend degree programs. Support services for students with learning disabilities include appropriate classroom accommodations, assistance in developing self advocacy skills, instructor assistance, peer tutoring, study groups, study strategies workshops, a communication resource center and math resource center.

3924 **Beloit College**
700 College St
Beloit, WI 53511-5595

608-363-2000
Fax: 608-363-2717
www.beloit.edu

Scott Bierman, President
Dan Schooff, Chief of Staff and Secretary
Louise Denk, Executive Secretary
Offers a variety of services to students with disabilities such as self advocacy training, study skills and time management guidance, couseling services, and special accommodations.

3925 **Blackhawk Technical College**
6004 S County Road G
Janesville, WI 53546-9458

608-758-6900
800-498-1282
Fax: 608-757-7740
TDD: 608-743-4422
www.blackhawk.edu
OfficeofthePresident@blackhawk.edu

Dr Thomas Eckert, President
Dr. Diane Nyhammer, Vice President
Brian Gohlke, Vice President
A public two-year college with support services for special education students.

3926 **Cardinal Stritch University**
Academic Support
6801 N Yates Rd
Milwaukee, WI 53217-3985

414-410-4166
800-347-8822
Fax: 414-410-4239
www.stritch.edu

James P. Loftus, President
Robert J. Buckla, Ed.D, Vice President
Allan D Mitchler, M.A., Vice President
An independent four-year college with support services for special education students.

3927 **Carthage College**
Academic Support Program
2001 Alford Park Dr
Kenosha, WI 53140-1994

262-551-8500
Fax: 262-551-6208
www.carthage.edu

Gregory Woodward, President
William Abt, Senior Vice President
Dean Clark, Vice President
An independent four-year college with support services for special education students.

3928 **Chippewa Valley Technical College**
Chippewa Valley Technical College
620 W Clairemont Ave
Eau Claire, WI 54701-6162

715-833-6200
800-547-2882
Fax: 715-833-6470
www.cvtc.edu
infocenter@cvtc.edu

Bruce Barker, President
Joe Hegge, Vice President
Ronald Edwards, Manager
A public two-year college with support services for special education students.

3929 **Edgewood College**
1000 Edgewood College Dr
Madison, WI 53711-1997

608-663-4861
800-444-4861
Fax: 608-663-3291
www.edgewood.edu
admissions@edgewood.edu

Scott Flanagan, Ed.D., President
Michael Guns, VP Business and Finance
Christine Benedict, VP Enrollment Management
An independent four-year college with support services for students with learning disabilities.

3930 **Fox Valley Technical College**
1825 N. Bluemound Drive
PO Box 227
Appleton, WI 54912-2277

920-735-5600
800-735-3882
Fax: 920-831-4396
www.fvtc.edu
helpdesk@fvtc.edu

Dr. Patricia Robinson, Executive Dean
Dr. Susan A. May, President
Jill McEwen, V.P. Administrative Services
A public two-year college with support services for special education students.

3931 **Gateway Technical College**
3520 30th Ave
Kenosha, WI 53144-1690

262-564-2200
Fax: 262-564-2201
TTY: 262-564-2206
www.gtc.edu

Bryan D Albrecht, President
In accordance with Section 504 of the Vocational Rehabilitation Act, Gateway provides a wide range of services that assist special needs students in developing independence and sel-reliance within the Gateway campus community. Reasonable accommodations will be made for students with learning disabilities or physical limitations.

3932 **Lakeshore Technical College**
Office For Special Needs
1290 North Ave
Cleveland, WI 53015-1414

920-693-1000
888-GOT-OLTC
Fax: 920-693-1363
TTY: 920-693-8956
www.gotoltc.edu
rivi.hatt@qotoltc.edu

Michael A. Lanser, Ed.D., President
Allison Weber, Executive Assistant
Rivi Hatt, Director Student Central

A two-year college that provides comprehensive programs to students with learning disablities.

3933 Lawrence University
711 E. Boldt Way
Appleton, WI 54911
920-832-7000
Fax: 920-832-6884
www.lawrence.edu
excel@lawrence.edu
Rudi Pakendorf, Associate Director, Development
Laura Zuege, Director, Off-Campus Programs
Sandy Isselmann, Director, Human Resources
Four year college that offers services to the learning disabled.

3934 Maranatha Baptist Bible College
745 W Main St
Watertown, WI 53094-7600
920-261-9300
800-622-2947
Fax: 920-261-9109
www.mbbc.edu
cmidcalf@mbbc.edu
Larry R Oats, Director
S. Marty Marriott, President
Matthew J Davis, Chair
Four year college that offers programs for the learning disabled.

3935 Marian College of Fond Du Lac
45 S National Ave
Fond Du Lac, WI 54935-4699
920-923-7600
800-2-MARIAN
Fax: 920-923-7154
www.marianuniversity.edu
admission@marianuniversity.edu
Eric P. Stone, Chairperson
Terri L. Emanuel, Vice Chairperson
Anthony J. Ahern, Treasurer
Offers a variety of services to students with disabilities including note takers, extended testing time, counseling services, and special accommodations.

3936 Marquette University
Disability Services Department
1250 W. Wisconsin Ave.
Milwaukee, WI 53233
414-288-7250
800-222-6544
Fax: 414-288-3764
www.marquette.edu
patriciaalmon@marquette.edu
Michael R. Lovell, President
Arthur F. Scheuber, Vice President
Dr. Mary DiStanislao, Executive Vice President
An independent four-year university with support services for students with learning disabilities.

3937 Mid-State Technical College
500 32nd St N
Wisconsin Rapids, WI 54494-5512
715-422-5300
888-575-MSTC
Fax: 715-422-5345
www.mstc.edu
webmaster@midstate.tec.wi.us
Robert Beaver, Director
Patrick Costello, Director
Terry Reynolds, Director
Offers a variety of services to students with disabilities including notetakers, extended testing time, counseling services, and special accommodations.

3938 Milwaukee Area Technical College
700 W State St
Milwaukee, WI 53233-1419
414-297-MATC
Fax: 414-297-7990
www.matc.edu
info@matc.edu
Dr. Vicki J. Martin, President
A public two-year college with support services for disabled students.

3939 Nicolet Area Technical College
Disability Support Service
5364 College Dr
Rhinelander, WI 54501-0518
715-365-4410
800-544-3039
Fax: 715-365-4445
www.nicoletcollege.edu
inquire@nicoletcollege.edu
Ron Zimmerman, Chair
Thomas Umlauf, Treasurer
Robert Martini, Vice Chair
In support of the Nicolet Area Technical College Student services mission, the Special Needs Support Program provides appropriate accommodations empowering students with disabilities to identify and develop abilities for successful educational and life experiences.

3940 Northcentral Technical College
1000 W Campus Dr
Wausau, WI 54401-1899
715-675-3331
888-682-7144
Fax: 715-675-9776
www.ntc.edu
admissions@ntc.edu
Tom Felch, Trustee
Paul C. Proulx, Trustee
Kristine Gilmore, Trustee
Offers a variety of services to students with disabilities including notetakers, extended testing time, counseling services, and special accommodations.

3941 Northeast Wisconsin Technical College
Special Services Program
2740 W Mason St
PO Box 19042
Green Bay, WI 54307-9042
920-498-5400
800-422-6982
Fax: 920-498-6260
TTY: 920-498-6901
www.nwtc.edu
more.info@nwtc.edu
H. Jeffrey Rafn, Ph.D., President
Jim Blumreich, CFO
Jennifer Canavera, Procurement Manager
The Special Needs Office of NWTC offers assistance to individuals with disabilities when choosing educational and vocational goals, building self-steem and increasing their occupational potential. We offer a wide range of support services and accommodations which increases the potential of individuals with exceptional education needs to successfully complete Associate Degree and Technical Diploma programs.

3942 Northland College
Northland College
1411 Ellis Ave
Ashland, WI 54806-3999
715-682-1699
Fax: 715-682-1308
www.northland.edu
admit@northland.edu
Michael A. Miller, President
Margot Carroll Zelenz, Vice President
Robert Jackson, Vice President
Four year college that provides students with learning disabilities with support and services.

3943 Oconomowoc Developmental Training Center
36100 Genesee Lake Rd
Oconomowoc, WI 53066-9202
262-569-5515
Fax: 262-569-6337
www.odtc-wi.com
Christie Ducklow, Director
Our mission is to provide comprehensive residential treatment, educational and vocational services to children, adolescents, and young adults with dually-diagnosed emotional disturbances and developmental disabilities.

3944 Ripon College
Student Support Services
300 Seward Street
PO Box 248
Ripon, WI 54971-248

920-748-8107
800-947-4766
www.ripon.edu
adminfo@ripon.edu

Zach Messitte, President
Student Support Services (SSS) is a federally funded United
States Department of Education TRIO program and provides
a network of academic, personal and career services to hundreds of students on the Ripon campus who are first generation, lower income or physically or learning disabled.

3945 St. Norbert College
Academic Support Services
100 Grant St
De Pere, WI 54115-2099

920-337-3181
800-236-4878
Fax: 920-403-4008
www.snc.edu
karen.goode-bartholomew@snc.edu

Thomas Kunkel, President
Raechelle Clemmons, Chief Information Officer & VP
Dr. Jeffrey Frick, Dean of the College, Academic VP
Provides reasonable accommodations for documented dis-
abilities.

**3946 University of Wisconsin Center: Marshfield Wood
County**
2000 W 5th St
Marshfield, WI 54449-3310

715-389-6530
www.marshfield.uwc.edu
kimberly.kolstad@uwc.edu

Michelle Boernke, Assistant Dean Admin & Finance
Kimberly Kolstad, Academic Advisor
Matthew Lemmerman, Program Associate
A public two-year college with support services for special
education students.

3947 University of Wisconsin-Madison
Waisman Center
1500 Highland Ave
Madison, WI 53705-2280

608-263-1656
Fax: 608-263-0529
TDD: 608-263-0802
www.waisman.wisc.edu
webmaster@waisman.wisc.edu

Marsha Mailick Seltzer, PhD, Director
Qiang Chang, PhD, Faculty Core Co-Director
Joe Egan, MPA, Associate Director
To advance knowledge about human development, develop-
mental disabilities, and neurodegenerative diseases.

3948 University of Wisconsin: Eau Claire
105 Garfield Ave
P.O Box 4004
Eau Claire, WI 54702-4004

715-836-4636
Fax: 715-836-3712
www.uwec.edu
hansonbj@uwec.edu

James C. Schmidt, Chancellor
Martin Hanifin, Vice Chancellor
Dorothy Nelson, Associate Budget Director
Offers a variety of services to students with disabilities in-
cluding note takers, extended testing time, counseling ser-
vices, and special accommodations.

3949 University of Wisconsin: La Crosse
1725 State St
La Crosse, WI 54601-3742

608-785-8000
Fax: 608-785-6868
TDD: 608-785-6900
www.uwlax.edu
reinert.june@uwlax.edu

Joe Gow, Chancellor
Bob Hetzel, Vice Chancellor
Paula Knudson, Vice Chancellor

Offers a variety of services to students with disabilities including note takers, extended testing time, counseling services, and special accommodations.

3950 University of Wisconsin: Madison
McBurney Disability Resource Center
702 W. Johnson Street
Suite 2104
Madison, WI 53715

608-263-2741
Fax: 608-265-2998
TDD: 608-263-6393
TTY: 608-263-6393
www.mcburney.wisc.edu
mcburney@studentlife.wisc.edu

Cathleen Trueba, Director
B.A. Scheuers, Assistant Director
Barbara Lafferty, Office Manager
Offers a variety of services to students with disabilities in-
cluding notetakers, extended testing time, counseling ser-
vices, and special accommodations.

3951 University of Wisconsin: Milwaukee
Exceptional Education Department
PO Box 413
Milwaukee, WI 53201-413

414-229-4721
Fax: 414-229-4705
www.exed.soe.uwm.edu
oas@uwm.edu

Amy Otis Wilborn, Chairperson
Paul Ross, Director
Carol L. Colbeck, Dean
A public four-year college with support services for special
education students.

3952 University of Wisconsin: Oshkosh
Project SUCCESS
800 Algoma Blvd
Oshkosh, WI 54901-8610

920-424-1234
TTY: 920-424-1319
www.uwosh.edu
wegner@uwosh.edu

Tim Merrill, Facilities Manager
Richard H. Wells, Chancellor
A remedial program for students with language-based learn-
ing disabilities attending the University of Wisconsin
Oshkosh.

3953 University of Wisconsin: Platteville
1 University Plaza
Platteville, WI 53818-3099

608-342-1491
800-362-5515
Fax: 608-342-1122
www.uwplatte.edu
wilsonj@uwplatt.edu

Dennis J. Shields, Chancellor
Mittie N. Den Herder, Provost and Vice Chancellor
Robert Cramer, Vice Chancellor
Coordinates academic accommodations, provides an advo-
cacy resource center for students with disabilities.

3954 University of Wisconsin: River Falls
410 S. 3rd Street
River Falls, WI 54022

715-425-3911
Fax: 715-425-3277
www.uwrf.edu
dots@uwrf.edu

Dean Van Galen, Chancellor
Fernando Delgado, Provost and Vice Chancellor
Elizabeth Frueh, Assistant Chancellor
Offers a variety of services to students with disabilities in-
cluding note takers, extended testing time, counseling ser-
vices, and special accommodations.

3955 University of Wisconsin: Whitewater
Project ASSIST
800 W. Main Street
Whitewater, WI 53190-1790

262-472-1234
Fax: 262-472-1518
www.uww.edu
amachern@uww.edu

Richard J. Telfer, Chancellor
Rebecca Reichert, Assistant to the Chancellor
Elizabeth Woolever, Program Assistant Confidential
The program is based on the philosophy that students with learning disabilities can learn specific strategies that will enable them to become independent learners who can be successful in a college setting.

3956 Viterbo University
900 Viterbo Dr
La Crosse, WI 54601-8804

608-796-3000
800-VITERBO
Fax: 608-796-3050
www.viterbo.edu
communication@Viterbo.edu

Dr. Richard Artman, President
Barbara Gayle, Vice President
Todd Ericson, Vice President
An independent four-year college with special services for special education students.

3957 Walbridge School
7035 Old Sauk Rd
Madison, WI 53717-1010

608-833-1338
Fax: 608-833-1338
www.walbridgeschool.com
info@walbridgeschool.com

Steve Lien, Interim Head of School
Nancy Donahue, Director
Kristina Jasmine, Office Manager
Offers an alternative and comprehensive full day elementary through middle school program emphasizing multi-sensory teaching and individualization to address the learning differences of children. Specialized and personalized instruction is geared to children with learning disabilities including dyslexia and ADHD.

3958 Waukesha County Technical College
Special Services Department
800 Main St
Pewaukee, WI 53072-4696

262-691-5566
877-892-9282
Fax: 262-691-5593
www.wctc.edu
djilbert@wctc.edu

Barbara A. Prindiville, Ph.D., President
Caroline Tindall, Executive Assistant to President
Karen Krause, Office Assistant
Offers technical and associate degree programs. Services for students with a documented disability may include academic support services, transition services, assistance with the admissions process, testing accommodations, interpreting services, note taking and assistance with RFB&D.

3959 Western Wisconsin Technical College
400 Seventh Street North
La Crosse, WI 54601

608-785-9200
800-322-9982
www.westerntc.edu

Daniel P. Hanson, Chair
David Laehn, Vice Chair
Edward J. Lukasek, Secretary
Offers a variety of services to students with disabilities including notetakers, extended testing time, counseling services, and special accommodations.

3960 Wisconsin Indianhead Tech College: Ashland Campus
505 Pine Ridge Drive
Shell Lake, WI 54871-8727

715-468-2815
800-243-WITC
Fax: 715-468-2819
www.witc.edu

Bob Meyer, President
Morrie Veilleux, Chair
James Beistle, Treasurer
A public two-year college with support services for special education students.

3961 Wisconsin Indianhead Technical College: Rice Lake Campus
1900 College Drive
Rice Lake, WI 54868

715-234-7082
800-243-WITC
Fax: 715-234-5172
TTY: 888-261-8578
www.witc.edu

Bob Meyer, President
Morrie Veilleux, Chair
James Beistle, Treasurer
A public two-year college with support services for students with disabilities.

Wyoming

3962 Child Development Services of Wyoming (CDSWY)
PO Box 62
Story, WY 82842

307-752-0687
www.cdswy.org
sue@mediationwest.com

Sue Sharp, Executive Director
An organization of the Developmental Preschools Programs serving the state, CDSWY provides therapeutic and educational services to preschool children with developmental disabilities.
1972

3963 Laramie County Community College: Disability Support Services
1400 E. College Drive
Education & Enrichment Cntr, Room 222
Cheyenne, WY 82007-3295

307-778-1359
800-522-2993
Fax: 307-778-1262
TTY: 307-778-1266
http://lccc.wy.edu/services/disability
tkeney@lccc.wy.edu

Dr. Joe Schaffer, President
Vicki Boreing, Assistant to the President
Bill Dubois, Trustee
Disability Support Services provides comprehensive, confidential services for LCCC students with documented disabilities. Services and adaptive equipment to reduce mobility, sensory and perceptual problems are available through the DRC, and all services are provided free of charge to LCCC students.

3964 University of Wyoming
1000 E. University Avenue
Laramie, WY 82071

307-766-1121
www.uwyo.edu

An independent four-year college with support services for special education students.

3965 Wyoming Institute For Disabilities
University Of Wyoming
1000 E University Ave.
Department 4298
Laramie, WY 82071

307-766-2761
888-898-9463
www.uwyo.edu
wind.uw@uwyo.edu

Karen Williams, Executive Director WIND
Assists individuals with developmental disabilities and their families through early intervention, education, training and community services.

Alabama

3966 Good Will Easter Seals
2448 Gordon Smith Drive
Mobile, AL 36617
251-471-1581
800-411-0068
Fax: 251-476-4303
www.alabama.easterseals.com
John Ives, Chairman
Randy Thomas, Chairman Elect
Frank Harkins, Administrator
Children and adults with disabilities and special needs find highest-quality services designed to meet their individual needs.

3967 Sequel TSI
Sequel Youth And Family Services
1131 Eagletree Lane
Huntsville, AL 35801
256-880-3339
888-758-4356
Fax: 256-880-7026
www.threesprings.com
jripley@sequelyouthservices.com
John Ripley, Founder, Co-Chairman
Adam Shapiro, Founder, Co-Chairman
Mandy Moses, Executive VP, CPO
Formally known as Three Springs, Sequel TSI is a nationally recognized leader in youth services, founded in 1985 to provide therapy and education to adolescents experiencing emotional, behavioral and learning problems.

3968 Wiregrass Rehabilitation Center
WRC, Inc.
795 Ross Clark Circle
Dothan, AL 36303
334-792-0022
800-395-7044
Fax: 216-521-9460
www.wrcjobs.com
info@wrcjobs.com
Cliff Mendheim, Chairman
Denise Hattaway, Vice Chairman
Blaine Stewart, Treasurer
Trains individuals to become employable and helps in assisting them to find jobs within their communities.

3969 Workshops
4244 3rd Avenue South
Birmingham, AL 35222
205-592-9683
888-805-9683
Fax: 205-592-9687
www.workshopsinc.org
email@workshopsinc.org
Susan C Crow, Executive Director
Dana Chang, Director of Programs
Kathy Dunn, Director of Operations
Work adjustment and job development services for people with disabilities.

Alaska

3970 Center for Community
600 Telephone Ave.
Anchorage, AK 99503
907-747-6960
855-907-7005
Fax: 907-747-4868
www.ptialaska.net
Connie Sipe, Executive Director
A state-wide provider of home and community-based services for people with disabilities, the elderly and others who experience barriers to community living in Alaska.

3971 Gateway School and Learning Center
900 W. Fireweed Lane
P.O. Box 113149
Anchorage, AK 99511-3149
907-522-2240
Fax: 907-344-0304
www.gatewayschoolak.com
learning@gatewayschoolak.com
Beverly Lau, Principal
Provides specialized educational services for students grades 1-12 with dyslexia and other language-processing disorders.

Arizona

3972 Arizona Center Comprehensive Education and Lifeskills
3310 W. Cheryl Dr.
Phoenix, AZ 85051
602-997-2331
Fax: 602-995-2636
www.accel.org
Cheryl Key, VP, Operations
Rae Ann Brevig, VP, Finance / CFO
Connie F. Laird, Executive Director
A private, non-profit, special education school providing therapeutic, educational, and behavioral services to over 200 students, ages 3-21, with cognitive, emotional, orthopedic, and/or behavioral disabilities.

3973 Devereux Arizona Treatment Network
11000 N Scottsdale Road
Suite 260
Scottsdale, AZ 85254
480-998-2920
Fax: 480-443-5587
www.devereux.org
Robert Q. Kreider, President, CEO
Margaret McGill, SVP, COO
Lane Barker, Executive Director
Provides a wide array of behavioral health and social welfare services for persons with emotional and behavioral disorders or who are victims of physical or sexual abuse and neglect.

3974 Life Development Institute (LDI)
18001 North 79th Avenue
Building E-71
Glendale, AZ 85308
623-773-2774
866-736-7811
Fax: 623-773-2788
www.life-development-inst.org
info@life-development-inst.org
Robert Crawford, M.Ed, Co-Founder, CEO
Veronica Lieb, M.A., President, Crawford
Shirley Schroeder, Director, Finance
Provides a supportive residential community that gives individuals the education, skills and training they need to live independently. By offering these programs in a residential environment, the students are given a chance to learn independence, and instill in them a desire to succeed.

3975 Raising Special Kids
5025 E. Washington Street
St. #204
Phoenix, AZ 85034
602-242-4366
800-237-3007
Fax: 602-242-4306
www.raisingspecialkids.org
info@raisingspecialkids.org
Joyce Millard Hoie, Executive Director
Vickie French, Assistant Executive Director
Janna Murrell, Director, Education
A parent training and information center providing information, resources and support to families of children with disabilities and special needs in Arizona. Services are offered free of charge.

Arkansas

3976 Arkansas Disability Coalition

1501 N. University Avenue
Suite 268
Little Rock, AR 72207

501-614-7020
800-223-1330
Fax: 501-614-9082
TTY: 800-223-1330
www.adcpti.org
adcoalition@earthlink.net

Wanda Horton, Executive Director
Bryan Cozart, Director, Family-2-Family
Frances Johnson, Minority Outreach Specialist
Arkansas Disability Coalition's mission is to work for equal rights and opportunities for Arkansans with disabilities through public policy change, cross-disability collaboration, and empowerment of people with disabilities and their families.

California

3977 Almansor Transition & Adult Services

211 Pasadena Avenue
South Pasadena, CA 91030

323-341-5632
877-837-4332
Fax: 323-341-5644
www.redesignlearning.org
info@resdesignlearning.org

Nancy Lavelle, Ph.D, Executive Director
Nita Moore, MPA, Program Director
A multi-service, community-based education and training facility for at-risk youth. Offering a range of professional services and support to the students and their parents.

3978 Ann Martin Children's Center

1375 55th Street
Emeryville, CA 94608

510-655-7880
Fax: 510-655-3379
www.annmartin.org

Mojgan Vijeh, Chief Financial Officer
David S. Theis, DMH, Executive Director
Lynn Peralta, MSW, Development Director
A non-profit community agency, providing psychotherapy, educational therapy and diagnostic testing for children, adults and families. Also offer a monthly lecture series for educators and child mental health professionals.

3979 Brislain Learning Center

2545 Ceanothus Avenue
Suite 130
Chico, CA 95973

530-342-2567
800-791-6031
Fax: 530-342-2573
www.brislainlearningcenter.com
info@brislainlearningcenter.com

Dr. Judy Brislain, Ed.D., Clinical Director
P. David Graham, M.A., Diagnostic Coordinator
Bob Wright, B.A., Clinician, Education Coordinator
Assists children of all ages who have learning disabilities. Offers a diagnostic program and tutoring program for ADD and learning disabilities. Provides counseling and support groups for children and adults.

3980 Center for Adaptive Learning

3227 Clayton Rd
Concord, CA 94519-2818

925-827-3863
Fax: 925-827-4080
www.centerforadaptivelearning.org
info@centerforadaptivelearning.org

Genevieve Stolarz, President
The center provides a comprehsive program that is designed to address many needs; physical, social, emotional and vocational. To empower adults with a developmental neurological disability to realize their own potential.

3981 Charles Armstrong School

1405 Solana Drive
Belmont, CA 94002

650-592-7570
Fax: 650-591-3114
www.charlesarmstrong.org
information@charlesarmstrong.org

David Evans, Chairman
David Obershaw, President
Audrey Fox, VP
The mission of the school is to serve the dyslexic learner by providing an appropriate educational experience which not only enables the students to acquire language skills, but also instills a joy of learning, enhances self-worth, and allows each the right to identify, understand and fulfill personal potential.

3982 Devereux California

P.O.Box 6784
Santa Barbara, CA 93160

805-968-2525
Fax: 805-968-3247
www.devereux.org
info@devereux.org

Robert Q. Kreider, President, CEO
Margaret McGill, SVP, COO
Lane Barker, Executive Director
A treatment facility offering residential, educational and adult vocational or day activity programs to individuals ages 8-85 with multiple diagnoses such as; autistic spectrum disorders, emotional and/or behavioral disorders, mental retardation, developmental disabilities, and medical conditions.

3983 Dyslexia Awareness and Resource Center

928 Carpinteria St.
Suite 2
Santa Barbara, CA 93103-3477

805-963-7339
Fax: 805-963-6581
www.dyslexiacenter.org
info@dyslexiacenter.org

Joan Esposito, Executive Director
Joan T. Esposito, Program Director
Sid Smith, Chairman
The center provides direct one-on-one services to adults and children affected with dyslexia, attention disorders and other learning disabilities. In addition the center conducts outreach and training seminars for public and private schools, for the juvenile court systems, for drug and alcohol programs, for family and social service programs, for literacy programs, and for homeless and mission programs.

3984 EDU-Therapeutics

14401 Roland Canyon Road
Salinas, CA 93908

831-484-0994
Fax: 861-484-0998
www.edu-therapeutics.com
terry@EDU-Therapeutics.com

Terry McHenry, President
Dr. Joan Smith, Program Director
Martin Donald, Specialist
EDU-Therapeutics is a unique learning system that offers effective solutions for overcoming dyslexia, attention deficit, learning disabilities and reading challenges. It succeeds because it changes how an individual uses his or her brain to learn. It is unique because it identifies the underlying cause of the learning inefficiency and eliminates the symptoms.

3985 Frostig Center

971 N. Altadena Dr.
Pasadena, CA 91107

626-791-1255
Fax: 626-798-1801
www.frostig.org
center@frostig.org

Phyllis Kochavi, Chair
Norm Solomon, Esq., Vice-Chair
Dean Conklin, Ed.D., Executive Director
A non profit organization that specializes in helping children who have learning disabilities. Offers parent training, consulting, school and tutoring services to learning disabled children.

3986 Full Circle Programs
70 Skyview Terrace
San Rafael, CA 94903-1845 415-499-3320
Fax: 415-499-1542
www.marin.org
Full Circle has been actively caring for children and their families in need. Full Circle offers a continuum of care ranging from residential treatment for several emotionally disturbed boys, to outpatient counseling for children and their families.

3987 Help for Brain Injured Children
Cleta Harder Developmental School
981 N. Euclid St.
La Habra, CA 90631 562-694-5655
Fax: 562-694-5657
www.hbic.org
jcecil@hbic.org
Cleta Harder, Executive Director
Help for brain-injured children. Long-term, low cost home rehabilitation programs. School programs, rehabilitation, academic, speech and physical therapy, as needed. Offer an after-school program for youngsters in regular school who are experiencing difficulties.

3988 Institute for the Redesign of Learning
1955 Fremont Avenue
South Pasadena, CA 91030 323-257-3006
Fax: 323-341-5642
www.redesignlearning.org
Al Hernandez, EdD, Education Director
Lori Andrews, Med, Education Director
A multi-service, community-based education and training facility for at-risk youth. Offering a range of professional services and support to the students and their parents.

3989 Kayne Eras Center
Exceptional Children's Foundation
5350 Machado Road
Culver City, CA 90230 310-737-9393
Fax: 310-737-9344
www.ecf.net/programs/kayne-eras-center
mjackson@kayneeras.org
Dwight Counsel, Principal
Kayne-Eras accomplishes its mission by offering educational resources, direct service, and a professional training center. Kayne-ERAS provides personalized programming to children and young adults from at risk conditions and those challenged by emotional, learning, developmental and/or chronic neurological and/or medical disabilities.

3990 Marina Psychological Services
4640 Admiralty Way
Marina Del Rey, CA 90292-6621 310-822-0109
Fax: 310-822-1240
http://wendyjsalz.com
wendy@wendyjsalz.com
Stuart Shaffer PhD, Psychologist
Comprehensive psychological services for children and adults with learning disabilities and attention deficit disorders. Private, individualized assessment and treatment.

3991 Nawa Academy
17351 Trinity Mountain Rd
French Gulch, CA 96033-9709 530-359-2215
800-358-6292
Fax: 530-359-2229
www.nawaacademy.org
info@nawaacademy.org
David W Hull, Head of School
Jason Hull, Admissions Director
A boarding school located in a remote valley of the Trinity Alps that provides individual curriculum, theory and structure for 7-9 grade students, many of who have learning disabilities. ÆServices include individual counseling, small academic classes, and numerous after school activities.

3992 New Vistas Christian School
68 Morello Ave.
Martinez, CA 94553-3042 925-370-7767
Fax: 925-370-6395
www.newvistaschristian.com
info@newvistaschristian.com
Correne Romeo, Director
A non-profit 1st-12th grade school for students of average or above average intelligence with learning disabilities offering a non-traditional approach to multiple learning styles.

3993 Newport Audiology Center
Newport Health Network
5990 Greenwood Plaza Blvd.
Suite 120
Greenwood Village, CO 80111 720-385-3700
www.newportaudiology.com
The aim is to enhance the quality of people's lives by improving their ability to communicate. We provide the highest level of audiological services possible, through our highly efficient staff, informative education programs, community services, high quality products, and true spirit of customer service.

3994 One To One Reading & Educational Tutoring
11971 Salem Dr.
Granada Hills, CA 91344-2348 818-368-1801
Fax: 818-368-9345
drpakmanrains@aol.com
Paul Klinger, Director
Specialize in reading and math; reading grades 1-6, math through pre-algebra.

3995 Park Century School
3939 Landmark Street
Culver City, CA 90232 310-840-0500
Fax: 310-840-0590
www.parkcenturyschool.org
nbley@parkcenturyschool.org
Douglas E. Phelps, Head of School
Justin Hunt, Board Member
Paul Jennings, Board Member
An independent school for average and above average intellect children with learning disabilities. The program emphasizes developing the skills and strategies necessary to return to a traditional program. With a 2:1 student-staff ratio.

3996 Pine Hill School
1325 Bouret Dr.
San Jose, CA 95118 408-979-8210
Fax: 408-979-8219
www.pinehillschool.com
gregz@secondstart.org
L.E. Boydston, Executive Director
Dr. Seamus Eddy, Ed.D., Principal
Greg Zieman, BA, Director of Educational Programs
A private school that provides special education and alternative services to students with a wide range of learning and behavior disabilities.

3997 Prentice School
Prentice School
18341 Lassen Drive
Santa Ana, CA 92705 714-538-4511
800-479-4711
Fax: 714-538-5004
www.prentice.org
amaciel@prentice.org
Alicia Z. Maciel, Executive Director
Greg Endelman, Principal
Jayne Hall, Accounting & Operations Manager
The Prentice School is an independent, nonprofit, coeducational day school for children pre-k through 8th grade with language learning differences.

3998 Providence Speech and Hearing Center
1301 Providence Avenue
Orange, CA 92868
714-923-1521
855-901-7742
Fax: 714-639-2593
www.pshc.org
pshc@pshc.org

Lewis Jaffe, President
Bret Rathwick, VP, Finance
Linda Smith, CEO
Comprehensive services for testing and treatment of all speech, language and hearing problems. Individual and group therapy beginning with parent/infant programs.

3999 Raskob Learning Institute and Day School
3520 Mountain Blvd.
Oakland, CA 94619
510-436-1275
Fax: 510-436-1106
www.raskobinstitute.org
raskobinstitute@hnu.edu

Edith Ben Ari, Executive Director
Jessica Baiocchi, Director, Admissions
Polly Meyer, Clinic Director
A co-educational school for students from diverse cultural and economic backgrounds with language-based learning disabilities. Raskob seeks to recognize and nurture the talents and strengths of each student while remediating areas of academic weakness.

4000 Reading Center of Bruno
Ste 243
4952 Warner Ave
Huntington Beach, CA 92649-4423
714-377-7910
Fax: 562-436-4428
www.readingcenter.info
readingct.@aol.com

Walt Waid, Director
Working with children, teens and adults with dyslexia, auditory and visual perceptual confusions through our specialized training program. Diagnostic testing is available, as well.

4001 Sandhills School
650 Clark Way
Palo Alto, CA 94304
650-688-3605
http://sandhillschool.org
info@sandhillschool.org

Anne Vickers, Head of School
Erika Senneseth, Assistant Head of School
A private, nonprofit school for children with learning disabilities. Serves students from grades 1-8 and also offers diagnostic evaluations, summer school and educational therapy for all ages. Boarding with local families is also available.

4002 Santa Cruz Learning Center
2560 Soquel Avenue
Suite 200
Santa Cruz, CA 95062
831-331-5611
www.santacruzlearningcenter.com
malika@santacruzlearningcenter.com

Malika Bell, MS, Owner
Eleanor Stitt, Director
Lissa Downey, Middle School
Individualized one-to-one tutoring for individuals aged 5 to adult. Specializes in dyslexia, learning difficulties and gifted persons. Includes test preparation, math, reading, self confidence, study skills, time organization and related services.

4003 Special Education Day School Program
Inst. for the Redesign of Learning/Almansor Center
1317 Huntington Drive
South Pasadena, CA 91030
323-622-0720
Fax: 626-240-0080
www.redesignlearning.org
info@resdesignlearning.org

Nancy Lavelle, Ph.D., President
Jason D. Rubin, LCSW, Managing Director
Rachel Southard, MBA, Development Associate
Providing basic education and related services to children with language, learning, behavioral, developmental and emotional needs.

4004 Speech and Language Development Center
8699 Holder St.
Buena Park, CA 90620
714-821-3620
Fax: 714-821-5683
TDD: 714-821-3628
www.sldc.net
info@sldc.net

Aleen Agranowitz, Co-Founder
Dawn O'Connor, M.Ed., CEO, Program Director
Steve Fifield, CPA, CFO
A school and therapy center for children and young adults with language, learning, and behavior disorders (many have multiple handicapping conditions), resulting in complex educational needs.

4005 Stockdale Learning Center
Ste 104
1701 Westwind Dr
Bakersfield, CA 93301-3045
661-326-8084
Fax: 661-327-4752
www.stockdale-learning-center.com
slc@igalaxy.net

Andrew J Barling, Executive Director
A professional State Certified Educational Therapy clinic designed to collaboratively diagnose and assess individuals 5 years of age through adult who have learning disabilities. Offering extensive services for dyslexia, ADD/HD, and other specific learning disabilities.

4006 Stowell Learning Center
15192 Central Ave
Chino, CA 91710
909-598-2482
Fax: 909-598-3442
www.learningdisability.com
info@learningdisability.com

Jill Stowell, President
A diagnostic and teaching center for learning and attention disorders. Specializes in instruction for dyslexic or learning disabled children and adults. Our services include diagnostic evaluation, developmental evaluation, cognitive and educational therapy which is provided on a one-to-one basis, and a full day class for elementary age students with reading disabilities.

4007 Switzer Learning Center
2201 Amapola Court
Torrance, CA 90501-1431
310-328-3611
Fax: 310-328-5648
www.switzercenter.org
drfoo@switzercenter.org

Rebecca Foo, Ph.D., Executive Director
Len Hernandez, Principal
Wendy White, Psy.D., Programs Manager
Provides a personalized academic program in a therapeutic environment. Has one elementary, one middle school and six high school classrooms, plus two classrooms for middle and high school students with a moderate to severe autistic spectrum disorder.

4008 Team of Advocates for Special Kids
100 W. Cerritos Ave.
Anaheim, CA 92805
714-533-8275
866-828-8275
Fax: 714-533-2533
www.taskca.org
task@taskca.org

Marta Anchondo, Executive Director
A parent training and information center that parents and professionals can turn to for assistance in seeking and obtaining needed early intervention and educational, medical or therapeutic support service for children.

403

4009 **The Almansor Center**
Institute for the Redesign of Learning
1317 Huntington Drive
South Pasadena, CA 91030   323-622-0720
Fax: 626-240-0080
www.redesignlearning.org
info@resdesignlearning.org
Nancy Lavelle Ph.D., President
Jason D. Rubin, LCSW, Managing Director
Rachel Southard, MBA, Development Associate
A multi-service, community-based education and training
facility for at-risk youth. Offering a range of professional
services and support to the students and their parents.

4010 **The Center For Educational Therapy**
2816 Northview Ave
Arroyo Grande, CA 93420   805-801-9467
Fax: 805-546-8700
www.center4edu-therapy.com
Dr. Dianne Olvera, M.A., Ph.D, Director
Provides educational assessment to determine learning style
and document learning disabilities. Also provided are
one-to-one remedial or tutorial services for individuals specializing in dyslexia.

4011 **Turning Point School**
8780 National Blvd.
Culver City, CA 90232   310-841-2505
Fax: 310-841-5420
www.turningpointschool.org
info@turningpointschool.org
Deborah Richman, Head Of School
Stephen Plum, President
Dana Kitaj, VP
A private, nonprofit school for children with dyslexia, attention deficit disorder and learning disabilities who have difficulties in reading, writing, spelling and math. Also offers
camping, after-school classes and daycare.

4012 **Vision Care Clinic**
General, Preventive and Developmental Optometry
2730 Union Avenue
Suite A
San Jose, CA 95124   408-377-1150
Fax: 408-377-1152
www.visiondiva.com
Dr. V Liane Rice, Director
Diagnostic and training for those with visual disabilities.

Colorado

4013 **Developmental Disabilities Resource Center**
11177 West 8th Avenue
Lakewood, CO 80215   303-233-3363
800-649-8815
Fax: 303-233-4622
TDD: 303-462-6606
www.ddrcco.com
ahogling@ddrcco.com
Beverly Winters, M.S.W., Executive Director
Rob DeHerrera, CPA, Deputy Director, CFO
Gena Colbert, CPA, Director, Finance
The mission is to provide leading-edge services that create
opportunities for people with developmental disabilities and
their families to participate fully in the community.

4014 **Havern School**
4000 S. Wadsworth Blvd.
Littleton, CO 80123   303-986-4587
Fax: 303-986-0590
www.haverncenter.org
Cathleen Pasquariello, Head of School
Nancy Mann, Director, Admissions
Susan Powell, Director, Development
School for children with learning disabilities. Educational
programs, special language programs and occupational ther-
apy is available.

Connecticut

4015 **American School for the Deaf**
139 North Main Street
West Hartford, CT 06107   860-570-2300
TTY: 860-570-2222
www.asd-1817.org
information@asd-1817.org
Tom Wood, CFO
Jeff Bravin, Assistant Executive Director/COO
Ed Peltier, Executive Director
A residential/day program operating as a state-aided private
school and governed by a board of directors. It is the oldest
permanent school for the deaf in America, offering a comprehensive educational program for the deaf and hard of
hearing students, infants, preschoolers, primary, elementary, junior high school, high school, and post-secondary
students.

4016 **Boys and Girls Village, Inc.**
528 Wheelers Farms Rd
Milford, CT 06461-1847   203-877-0300
Fax: 203-876-0076
www.boysvill.org
fellenbaumk@boysvill.org
Steven Joffe, MSW, CEO
Catherine Murphy-Brooks, Director Of Education
The clients of Boys & Girls Village are children in crisis or
children with learning difficulties who have experienced re-
jection, failure or abuse. Through the years, the agency has
evolved into a leading therapeutic and learning facility offering residential shelter, clinical, after-school, counseling,
special educational, foster & adoptive recruitment and training, family support services, and day programs for children
and their families.

4017 **Child Care Programs**
Easter Seals Connecticut
733 Summer Street
Suite 104
Stamford, CT 06901   203-388-2192
Fax: 203-388-2196
www.ct.easterseals.com
Dr. Roslyn Burton-Robertson Ph.D, Executive Director
Kelley M. Ward-Welly, Development Manager
Chelsea Weeast, Development Associate
Meeting a growing need for high-quality child care for more
than 20 million young children and their working parents,
Easter Seals offers child care for children ages 6 months to 5
years. Young children are welcomed to a unique environ-
ment where children of all abilities learn together.

4018 **Connecticut Institute for the Blind**
The Oak Hill Cntr For Individual & Family Supports
120 Holcomb Street
Hartford, CT 06112   860-242-2274
TTY: 860-286-3113
www.ciboakhill.org
info@ciboakhill.org
Frank Szliagyi, Esq., Chairman
Patrick Johnson, Director
Gayle Wintjen, Esq., Secretary
Largest private nonprofit community provider of services
for people with disabilities in Connecticut.

4019 **Eagle Hill School**
45 Glenville Road
Greenwich, CT 06831   203-622-9240
Fax: 203-622-0914
www.eaglehillschool.org
info411@eaglehill.org
Marjorie E. Castro, Head Of School
Wendy G. Salisbury, B.A., M.A., Director, Education
Tom Cone, B.A. M.A., Director, Admissions
Eagle Hill is a languaged-based, remedial program committed to educating children with learning disabilities. The curriculum is individualized, interdisciplinary, and transitional
in nature.

4020 Focus Alternative Learning Center
P.O.Box 452
Canton, CT 06019-0452
860-693-8809
Fax: 860-693-0141
http://focuscenterforautism.org
info@focus-alternative.org
Donna Swanson, MSN, CS, APRN, Executive Director
Fred Evans, BA, MA, Associate Director
Nancy Reed-Nevin, BS, Finance and HR Director
FOCUS Alternative Learning Center is a private, licensed, non-profit, year-found clinical program committed to the treatment of children ages 6-18 diagnosed with Autism Spectrum disorders, attention and anxiety disorders, or who have processing and/or learning problems. Our Integral Model of Care™ focuses on the social, emotional and academic obstacles that impede a child's growth and success in school, at home and in the community.

4021 Forman School
Forman School
12 Norfolk Road
P.O. Box 80
Litchfield, CT 06759
860-567-8712
Fax: 860-567-8317
www.formanschool.org
firstname.lastname@formanschool.org
Louise Hoppe Finnerty, President of the Board
Thomas G. Sorell, VP
Adam Man, Principal
Forman offers students with learning differences the opportunity to achieve academic excellence in a traditional college preparatory setting. A coeducational boarding school of 180 students, we maintain a 3:1 student:teacher ratio. Daily remedial instruction balanced with course offerings rich in content provide each student with a flexible program that is tailored to his or her unique learning style and needs.

4022 Founder's Cottage
Star, Lighting The Way
182 Wolfpit Avenue
Norwalk, CT 06851
203-846-9581
Fax: 203-847-0545
www.starinc-lightingtheway.org
Katie Banzhaf, Executive Director
Bill Casale, Director of Operations
William Saguta, Director of Financial Services
Facility-based respite care is provided by STAR at Founders Cottage. A lovely home, is co-ed, and can accomodate four individuals at a time. It is for people with development disabilities who are 16 years or older and who reside within the Southwest Region. All persons must be registered with the Connecticut Department of Mental Retardation and have a DMR number assigned.

4023 Intensive Education Academy
840 North Main Street
West Hartford, CT 06117
860-236-2049
Fax: 860-231-2843
www.intensiveeducationacademy.org
iea_education@comcast.net
Jill O'Donnell, Head of School, Director - Edu.
Tracy Barbour, Assistant Director of Education
A state approved, non-profit, non sectarian special education facility for children 6 to 21 years with different learning styles. Individualized program with a 5:1 student teacher ratio. Program strives to help each student reach their potential by gaining confidence, recognizing their strengths and limitations, setting realistic goals and attaining satisfaction by achieving these goals. State approved. Full-day curriculum is offered.

4024 Klingberg Family Centers
370 Linwood Street
New Britain, CT 06052
860-224-9113
Fax: 860-832-8221
www.klingberg.org
lynner@klingberg.org

Mark H. Johnson, M.A., CFRE, Vice President
Lynne V. Roe, Director Of Intake
Jane Morris, Director, Education
Provides structured programs for residential, day treatment and day school students in a therapeutic environment. We are a private, nonprofit organization serving children and families from across Connecticut.

4025 Learning Center
Children's Home
60 Hicksville Rd
Cromwell, CT 06416
860-635-6010
Fax: 860-635-3708
www.adelbrook.org
info@adelbrook.org
Garrell Mullaney, President, CEO
Tony Gibson, LMFT, Chief Operating Officer
David Maibaum, CFO, Facilities Manager
A private special education facility serving adolescents between the ages of 10 and 21. The flexibility of the program provides students with an opportunity to meet their academic needs. Technology is an important component of the program in addition to academics and an opportunity to participate in a vocational component.

4026 Lorraine D. Foster Day School
1861 Whitney Avenue
Hamden, CT 06517
203-230-4877
Fax: 203-288-5749
www.ldfds.com
ldfds@snet.net
Dominique S. Fontaine, Executive Director
Christine Kirschenbaum, Assistant Director
Julie Hunt, Classroom Teacher
Teaches elementary grade children with special needs who have experienced difficulty learning in typical school settings.

4027 Mount Saint John
135 Kirtland Street
Deep River, CT 06417
860-343-1300
Fax: 860-343-1392
www.mtstjohn.org
mccormacke@mtstjohn.org
Douglas J. DeCerbo, Executive Director
Lee Farland, CPA, Director of Finance
Kathy White, Chief Admin & Edu. Director
This is a residential treatment program that provides comprehensive and integrated treatment services to adolescent boys and young men who are not able to function in their home community due to combinations of behavioral, emotional, family and educational problems. The staff and Board of Mount Saint John are committed to providing a treatment program to meet the evolving and changing needs of the times and of the boys who come into our care.

4028 Natchaug Hospital School Program
189 Storrs Road
Mansfield Center, CT 06250-0260
860-456-1311
800-426-7792
Fax: 860-423-6114
www.natchaug.org
Stephen Larcen, President
Deborah Weidner, M.D., MBA, Chief Medical Officer
Jonathan Chasen, M.D., Associate Medical Director
Natchaug Hospital operates three state approved K-12 special education programs for socially, emotionally disturbed youth. Natchaug Hospital also provides in patient and partial hospital programs at 9 Eastern Connecticut locations.

4029 Natchaug's Network of Care
Natchaug Hospital
189 Storrs Rd
Mansfield Center, CT 06250-0260
860-456-1311
800-426-7792
Fax: 860-423-6114
www.natchaug.org

Stephen Larcen, President
Deborah Weidner, M.D., MBA, Chief Medical Officer
Jonathan Chasen, M.D., Associate Medical Director
The hospital's 54-bed facility in Mansfield Center, provides inpatient care for seriously emotionally disturbed children and adolescents as well as adults in crisis each year.

4030 Oak Hill Center
The Oak Hill Center for Individual/Family Support
120 Holcomb Street
Hartford, CT 06112   860-242-2274
                                      TTY: 860-286-3113
                                      www.ciboakhill.org
                                      info@ciboakhill.org

Frank Szliagyi, Esq., Chairman
Patrick Johnson, Director
Gayle Wintjen, Esq., Secretary
Offers many programs and services for children and adults with developmental, intellectual, physical disabilities and visual impairements.

4031 Saint Francis Home for Children, Inc.
651 Prospect St
New Haven, CT 06511   203-777-5513
                                      Fax: 203-777-0644
                                      www.stfrancishome.com
                                      info@stfrancishome.com

Paula Moody, Executive Director
Ivan Tate, Director
A psychological treatment facility for emotionally disturbed children. Clinical Services are provided by a full and part time theraputic staff. Each child receives weekly individual, small and large group therapy as well as weekly family therapy. Children attend St. Francis School, staffed by professional special ed teachers.

4032 Saint Francis Home for Children: Highland
651 Prospect St
New Haven, CT 06511   203-777-5513
                                      Fax: 203-777-0644
                                      www.stfrancishome.com
                                      info@stfrancishome.com

Paula Moody, Executive Director

4033 St. Vincent's Special Needs Center
St. Vincent's Medical Center
95 Merritt Boulevard
Trumbull, CT 06611   203-375-6400
                                      Fax: 203-380-1190
                                      www.stvincentsspecialneeds.org
                                      feroleto.child.dev@snet.net

Raymond G. Baldwin, Jr., President, CEO
Harry Schaeffer, Chief Operating Officer
Beth Jezierny, Director, Adult Services
Began as therapy treatment program for children with cerebral palsy, and have evolved into a provider of specialized lifelong education and therapeutic programs for children and adults with multiple developmental disabilities and special health care needs.

4034 The Children's Program
Connecticut College
270 Mohegan Avenue
New London, CT 06320   860-447-1911
                                      Fax: 860-439-5317
                                      www.conncoll.edu
                                      shrad@conncoll.edu

Katherine Bergeron, President
Lee Hisle, Program Director
The mission of the Connecticut College Children's Program is to provide, within a community context, a model child and family-focused early childhood program for infants and young children of diverse backgroungs and abilities in Southeastern Connecticut.

4035 The Foundation School
719 Derby Milford Rd.
Orange, CT 06477   203-795-6075
                                      Fax: 203-799-4797
                                      www.foundationschool.org/Site/Home.html

Walter J Bell, Director
For students ages 3-21 with developmental needs, learning deficits, behavioral challenges and autism spectrum disorder. Basic developmental skills address speech/language and perceptual/motor areas. Academic skills are reading, writing and arithmetic with social studies, science and career studies.

4036 The Glenholme School - Devereux Connecticut
81 Sabbaday Lane
Washington, CT 06793   860-868-7377
                                      Fax: 860-868-7413
                                      www.theglenholmeschool.org
                                      admissions@theglenholmeschool.org

Julie Smallwood, Director of Admissions
Denise Watson, Director of Public Relations
The Glenholme School is a therapeutic boarding school that provides a supportive program and exceptional learning environment to address varying levels of academic, social and emotional development in boys and girls, ages 10-21, with high functioning autism spectrum disorders, ADHD, PDD, OCD, Tourette's, depression, anxiety and various learning differences. The goal of our program is to prepare our graduates for post-secondary college and career opportunities.

4037 The Learning Clinic
P.O.Box 324
Brooklyn, CT 06234-0324   860-774-5619
                                      Fax: 860-774-1037
                                      www.thelearningclinic.org
                                      admissions@thelearningclinic.org

Raymond W. Du Charme, Ph.D., Executive Director
A private, nonprofit educational program that provides day and residential school focused on ADHD and learning and emotional issues. The program is coeducational and serves seventy students. The aim is to assist students in meeting their academic goals and prepare for future experiences in educational, vocational, and community settings.

4038 VISTA Vocational & Life Skills Center
1356 Old Clinton Road
Westbrook, CT 06498   860-399-8080
                                      Fax: 860-399-3103
                                      www.vistavocational.org
                                      humanresources@vistavocational.org

Helen Bosch, President
Helen K. Bosch, B.S., M.S., Executive Director
Tracey Celentano, Director, Finance
Educational and support services for young adults with autism spectrum, ADD, learning disabilities, traumatic brain injuries, and developmental delays.

4039 Villa Maria Education Center
Villa Maria School
161 Sky Meadow Drive
Stamford, CT 06903-3400   203-322-5886
                                      Fax: 203-322-0228
                                      www.villamariaedu.org
                                      info@villamariaedu.org

Sister Carol Ann, Principal, Executive Director
Eileen Cassidy, Education Director
Mary Ann Tynan, Admissions Director
Dedicated to developing the full potential of students who are learning disabled, and does this by providing an education that will help children who learn differently acquire knowledge, develop skills, and increase the self-acceptance and self-esteem necessary to become responsible adults.

4040 Vocational Center for People who are Blind or Visually Impaired
Oak Hill Center
120 Holcomb Street
Hartford, CT 06112

860-242-2274
Fax: 860-242-3103
TTY: 860-286-3113
www.ciboakhill.org
info@ciboakhill.org

Frank Szliagyi, Esq., Chairman
Patrick Johnson, Director
Gayle Wintjen, Esq., Secretary
Providing children and adults with disabilities the opportunity to live, learn and work in the community.

4041 Waterford Country Schools
78 Hunts Brook Road
P.O. Box 408
Quaker Hill, CT 06375

860-442-9454
Fax: 860-442-2228
www.waterfordcountryschool.org
info@waterfordcs.org

William Martin, Executive Director
Bill Martin, Exe. Director, Administration
Sharon Butcher, Program Dir, Education/Principal
The school offers academic, prevocational, behavior management and life skills programs for children and young adults ages 8-18.

4042 Wheeler Clinic, Inc.
91 Northwest Drive
Plainville, CT 06062

888-793-3500
800-793-3588
Fax: 860-793-3520
www.wheelerclinic.org
dberkowitz@wheelerclinic.org

Susan Walkama, LCSW, President, CEO
John R. Sponauer, MBA, VP, Communications
Patricia Speicher Werbner, VP, Human Resources
A provider of behavioral health services for children, adolescents, adults and families that include mental health, substance abuse, special education, early childhood development, prevention, an employee assistance program and community education.

4043 Wilderness School
State of Connecticut Dept of Children & Families
240 N Hollow Rd
East Hartland, CT 06027-1002

860-653-8059
800-273-2293
Fax: 860-653-8120
www.ct.gov
dave.czaja@ct.gov

Nancy Wyman, Lieutenant Governor
Dannel P. Malloy, Governor
David Czaja, M.H.S.A., Director
A prevention, intervention, and transition program for troubled youth from Connecticut. The school offers high impact wilderness programs intended to foster positive youth development.

Delaware

4044 AdvoServ
4185 Kirkwood-St. Georges Road
Bear, DE 19701

302-834-7018
800-593-4959
Fax: 302-836-2516
www.advoserv.com
dusseaum@advoserv.com

Judith E. Favell, PhD, BCBA-D, Executive Chairwoman
Kelly McCrann, MBA, CEO
Kathy Shea, MBA, Chief Financial Officer

Provides services to individuals whose challenges have defied all previous attempts at treatment. Through proven, positive and comprehensive strategies that teach individuals how to live problem-free, AdvoSer can help overcome the burdens and barriers associated with severe and intractable problems.

4045 Centreville School
6201 Kennett Pike
Centreville, DE 19807

302-571-0230
Fax: 302-571-0270
www.centrevilleschool.org
centreville@centrevilleschool.org

Barton Reese, Former Head of School
Denise Orenstein, Director
Motivated by two fundamental goals; to provide learning disabled children a vibrant and challenging curriculum comparable to those found at any primary or intermediate level school, and to offer each student the specialized and focused support he or she needs.

4046 Parent Information Center of Delaware
404 Larch Circle
Larch Corporate Center
Wilmington, DE 19804

302-999-7394
888-547-4412
Fax: 302-999-7637
www.picofdel.org

Marie-Anne Aghazadian, Executive Director
Hazel Cole, Parent Consultant
Suzi Harris, Associate Director
Assists individuals with disabilities and special needs and those who serve them; also provides information and referral to other agencies.

4047 Pilot School
100 Garden of Eden Road
Wilmington, DE 19803

302-478-1740
Fax: 302-478-1746
www.pilotschool.org
info@pilotschool.org

Kathleen B. Craven, Director
John Harrison, Finance Director
Colleen Shivone, Development Director
Pilot School provides a creative, nurturing environment for children with special learning needs. The schools works with each child to give them the specific developmental tools, guidance and attention needed to learn and achieve in order to feel comfortable and successful.

District of Columbia

4048 Kingsbury Center
5000 14th Street, N.W.
Washington, DC 20011

202-722-5555
Fax: 202-722-5531
www.kingsbury.org
center@kingsbury.org

Peri-Anne Chobot, CEO/Head of School
Anne Hedman, Chief Operating Officer
Holly Cherico, Director, Mark & Comm
DC's oldest non public school for children with learning disabilities.

4049 Paul Robeson School
Washington Department Of Mental Health
3700 10th St N W
Washington, DC 20010-1445

202-576-5151
Fax: 202-576-8804
www.mental.disorder.net

Harriet Crawley, Principal

The Department of Mental Health offers therapy and treatment at special education centers, such as The Paul Robeson School. The school offers individual, group and/or family psychotherapy or art therapy, play therapy, speech therapy, and recreational principles. They also provide physical education, adaptive physical education, and occupational therapy, if needed.

4050 The Lab School of Washington
4759 Reservoir Road, NW
Washington, DC 20007-1921   202-965-6600
                    www.labschool.org
          katherine.schantz@labschool.org
Mimi W. Dawson, Chair
Mac Bernstein, Vice-Chair
Bill Tennis, Treasurer
The Lab School is internationally recognized for its innovative programs for children and adults with learning disabilities. The Lab School offers individualized instruction to students in kindergarten through 12 grade.

Florida

4051 Academic Achievement Center
313 Pruett Rd
Seffner, FL 33584-3116   813-654-4198
                    Fax: 813-871-7468
                    www.iser.com
                    ALSofAAC@aol.com
Lillian M Stark, Ph.D., Director
Arnold L. Stark, Ph.D., Educational Director
A private program for bright and gifted children with LD and/or ADD, offering multisensory-based instruction, remediation of basic skills, academic challenge in science, social science, and literature, plus award-winning art and drama, and curriculum-enhancing field trips and travel. Maximum student body is 22 and it is coeducational. After school tutoring and phonelogical awareness training are also available.

4052 Achievement Academy
716 E. Bella Vista Street
Lakeland, FL 33805   863-683-6504
                    Fax: 863-688-9292
          www.achievementacademy.com
          information@achievementacademy.com
John Burton, Executive Director
Laura Beard, Teacher
Kathy Box, Teacher
Serves children up to age 6 with autism, cerebral palsy, speech delays and down syndrome. The Birth to Three program offers services to children up to three years of age who may be at risk for developmental delays.

4053 Atlantis Academy
Educational Services of America
1950 Prairie Road
West Palm Beach, FL 33406   561-642-3100
                    Fax: 561-969-1950
          www.atlantisacademy.com
Dennis Kelley, Director
A small, private, highly individualized program, Pre K-12, for children with attention disorders, dyslexia and other academic learning problems. Day students only.

4054 Baudhuin Preschool
Nova SE University's Mailman Segal Institute
3301 College Avenue
Fort Lauderdale-Davie, FL 33314-7796   954-262-7100
                    800-541-6682
                    Fax: 954-262-3936
                    www.nova.edu
                    baudhuin@nova.edu
George L. Hanbury II, President, CEO
Jacqueline A Travisano, EVP, Chief Operating Officer
Marsabine Unzaga, Administrative Assistant

For autistic children, the program supports the qualities and capabilities of each child. This therapeutic program focuses on cognitive, social-emotional, adaptive, behavioral, motor, and communication skill development within a relationship-based environment. Providing each child with choices, challenges, and opportunities that nurture feelings of competence, promote intellectual growth, and enable each child to achieve his or her potential.

4055 Children's Center for Development and Behavior
440 Sawgrass Corporate Parkway
Suite 106
Sunrise, FL 33325   954-745-1112
                    866-290-6468
                    Fax: 954-745-1120
                    www.childpsych.org
          administrative@childpsych.org
Shana Williams, Psy.D., Director - Psychological Service
David Lubin, Ph.D., BCBA-D, Vice President - Clinical Affair
Debbie White-Maynes, Ms. Ed,, Director of Academic Services
Dedicated to supporting the social, physical, emotional, intellectual and creative development in children with speech delays, general developmental disorders, Autism, and Down's Syndrome. Some of the programs include speech language pathology, behavior management, music therapy, occupational therapy and sibling support groups.

4056 Exceptional Student Education: Assistive Technology
Orange County Public School
445 W Amelia St
Orlando, FL 32801-1220   407-317-3504
                    Fax: 407-317-3526
                    ruthie.rieder@ocps.net
Ruthie Rieder, Director
Services are provided for students who are mentally handicapped, emotionally handicapped, specific learning disabled, sensory impaired, speech and language impaired, physically impaired, hospital/homebound, autistic, gifted, and developmentally delayed. Services such as occupational/ physical therapy, assistive technology, and assistance for ESE bilingual students are also available.

4057 Kurtz Center
Complete Learning Center
1201 Louisiana Avenue
Suite C
Winter Park, FL 32789-2340   407-740-5678
                    Fax: 407-629-6886
          www.completelearningcenter.com
          ld-request@learningdisabilities.com
Sandy Dieringer, Director
A treatment facility and professional development provider, using scientifically based researched approaches in the treatment of those in need and in training other professionals, paraprofessionals and parents to use these approaches. Developed individualized programs for all ages that conquer all forms of learning disabilities/difficulties, including the various dyslexias and attention focus problems.

4058 McGlannan School
10770 S.W. 84 Street
Miami, FL 33173   305-274-2208
                    Fax: 305-274-0337
                    TDD: 305-274-2208
                    www.mcglannanschool.com
Frances K Mc Glannan, Founder, Director
A school that provides one-to-one learning for children with dyslexia and other learning disabilities. Diagnostic, multidisciplinary, prescriptive, research-based and individualized to reach the whole child.

4059 **Morning Star School**
Morning Star School
210 E. Linebaugh Avenue
Tampa, FL 33612 813-935-0232
Fax: 813-932-2321
www.morningstartampa.org
EDaly@morningstartampa.org
Eileen Daly, Principal
Paul Reed, Administrative Coordinator
Patricia Gramer, Administrative Assistant
A non-profit school for elementary and junior-high age children with learning disabilities and related learning differences.

4060 **PACE-Brantley Hall School**
3221 Sand Lake Road
Longwood, FL 32779 407-869-8882
Fax: 407-869-8717
www.mypbhs.org
bw@mypbhs.org
Pamela Tapley, Executive Director
Pamela Bellet, MA, LMHC, Assistant Director
Garry Chisley, Dean of Students
An independent, nonprofit school for children with learning differences. The PACE program has been specifically designed for students who have been diagnosed with learning disabilities, attention deficit disorder, dyslexia and similar challenges.

4061 **Reading Clinic**
Tampa Day School
12606 Henderson Road
Tampa, FL 33625 813-269-2100
Fax: 813-490-2554
www.tampadayschool.com
Lois Delaney, Head of School
Andrea Mowatt, Head of Lower School
Crystal Haralambou, Director, Performing Arts
Provides a learning environment that promotes that individual feeling of success for each child and to meet each child's needs. The Reading Clinic has been helping children become better readers for over 30 years. Once the problem is targeted, and provide the kind of help a child needs, the gains are immediate and long lasting.

4062 **Renaissance Learning Center**
5800 Corporate Way
West Palm Beach, FL 33407 561-640-0270
Fax: 561-640-0272
www.rlc2000.com
renaissance@rlc2000.com
Debra Johnson, Principal/Director
Lisa Hauser, President
Dr. Jack Scott, VP
Develops and provides effective education and treatment programs for children ages 3-14 with autism.

4063 **Summer Camp Program**
Tampa Day School
12606 Henderson Road
Tampa, FL 33625 813-269-2100
Fax: 813-490-2554
www.tampadayschool.com
Lois Delaney, Head of School
Andrea Mowatt, Head of Lower School
Crystal Haralambou, Director, Performing Arts
Summer camp program for children in grades K-8. Camp is held in the Citrus Park area and children are encouraged to learn, play and grow while enjoying such activies as arts and crafts, sports, field trips and more.

4064 **Susan Maynard Counseling**
7096 SW 48 Lane
Miami, FL 33155 305-667-5011
www.susanmaynardphd.com
info@susanmaynardphd.com
Susan Maynard, Ph.D., School Psychologist

Serices include testing, evaluations and consultations for children who are exhibiting learning/behavior problems or physical and motor difficulties.

4065 **Vanguard School**
22000 US Highway 27
Lake Wales, FL 33859 863-676-6091
Fax: 863-676-8297
www.vanguardschool.org
vanadmin@vanguardschool.org
Dr. Cathy Wooley-Brown, President
Derri Park, Principal, Administration
George FitzGerald, Director of Technology
The Vanguard School program is designed for students age 10 through high school who are experiencing academic difficulties due to learning disability such as dyslexia or dyscalculia or an attention deficit.

Georgia

4066 **Atlanta Speech School**
3160 Northside Parkway NW.
Atlanta, GA 30327 404-233-5332
Fax: 404-266-2175
www.atlantaspeechschool.org
cyates@atlspsch.org
Jack Zimmermann, CFO
Comer Yates, Executive Director
Iris Goodson, Director, Human Resources
The Atlanta Speech School is one of the Southeast's oldest therapeutic educational centers for children and adults with hearing, speech, language, or learning disabilities. We help children and adults with communication disorders realize their full potential.

4067 **Bedford School**
5665 Milam Road
Fairburn, GA 30213 770-774-8001
Fax: 770-774-8005
www.thebedfordschool.org
bbox@thebedfordschool.org
Betsy Box, Executive Director
Jeff James, Headmaster/LS Principal
Allison Day, Assis Headmaster/MS Principal
Serves children in grades 1-9 with learning disabilities. Students are grouped by skill levels in classes of 8-12. Students receive the proper academic remediation, as well as specific remedial help with physical skills, peer interaction and self-esteem.

4068 **Brandon Hall School**
1701 Brandon Hall Drive
Atlanta, GA 30350 770-394-8177
Fax: 770-804-8821
www.brandonhall.org
jsingleton@brandonhall.org
Dr. John L. Singleton, Ed.D., President/Head of School
Terry D. Lufkin, CFO
Scott Boice, LPC, Director of Counseling
Provides both one-on-one and small group college preparatory classes for students who, for a variety of reasons, have not been achieving their potential or who otherwise need a more intensive educational setting.

4069 **Chatham Academy**
4 Oglethorpe Professional Blvd
Savannah, GA 31406 912-354-4047
Fax: 912-354-4633
www.chathamacademy.com
channaford@chathamacademy.com
Carolyn Hannaford, Principal
Providing a specialized curriculum and individualized instruction for students with diagnosed learning disabilities and/or attention deficit disorder. Chatham's goal is to improve students' functioning to levels commensurate with their potential in all areas so that they may return to and succeed in regular educational programs.

4070 Creative Community Services
4487 Park Drive
Suite A
Norcross, GA 30093
770-469-6226
866-618-2823
Fax: 770-469-6210
www.ccsgeorgia.org
info@ccsgeorgia.org

Nicolette Lee, Board President
Michelle Roberts, Board Member
Sally Buchanan, Executive Director
Therapeutic foster care services for children and home-based support for developmental disabled adults. CCS gives both kids and adults hope by encouraging independent living resulting in involved, engaged citizens and community members.

4071 Horizons School
1900 Dekalb Ave NE
Atlanta, GA 30307
404-378-2219
800-822-6242
Fax: 404-378-8946
www.horizonsschool.com
HorizonsSchool@horizonschool.com

Les Garber, Director, Administrator
John Jones, Staff
Kate Cotter Reilly, Staff
The intent is to develop in students those values and skills which assure maximum opportunities. Students learn real-life skills through active participation in the classroom, as well as in other aspects of the school. They learn responsibility, decision-making, and problem-solving skills through active involvement in the management of the community. Such a leadership role empowers students, giving them the knowledge that they have control of personal decisions and interpersonal interactions.

4072 Jacob's Ladder Neurodevelopmental School & Therapy Center
407 Hardscrabble Road
Roswell, GA 30075
770-998-1017
Fax: 770-998-3258
www.jacobsladdercenter.com
jaclynr@jacobsladderschool.net

Amy O'Dell, M.Ed., LPC,TRS, Founder, Executive Director
Jaclyn Rhodes, Director of HR & Admissions
Karla Brigiotta, Director, Clinical Services
A neurodevelopmental school and therapy center established to provide the child with Autism, PDD, ADD/ADHD, Asperger's, learning differences, Down Syndrome or any other neurological delay, the services they need in order to realize their full potential. Come SEE and FEEL where HOPE resides!

4073 Mill Springs Academy
13660 New Providence Road
Alpharetta, GA 30004
770-360-1336
Fax: 770-360-1341
www.millsprings.org

Robert W. Moore, Headmaster
Angel Murr, Chairperson, Board
Ed Coco, Board Member
A value-based educational community dedicated to the academic, physical and social growth of those students who have not realized their full potential in traditional classroom settings. Learning strategies are generated from psycho-educational evaluations, previous school records, diagnostic skills assessment, observations and communication with other professionals involved with the student.

4074 Reading Success Plus, Inc.
4205 Columbia Rd
Martinez, GA 30907-1429
706-863-8173
800-997-3237
Fax: 706-863-4523
www.readingsuccess.com
readingsuccess@bellsouth.net

Roberta Hoehle, Director
Reading Success, Inc. is a locally owned and operated program, serving the CSRA for over 30 years and providing professional help to students with all kinds of learning problems. Our guarantee is; if one year of improvement has not been made in the 48 lessons, the student receives instruction free of charge for 18 lessons.

4075 The Howard School
1192 Foster Street NW
Atlanta, GA 30318
404-377-7436
Fax: 404-377-0884
www.howardschool.org
fwalsh@howardschool.org

Marifred Cilella, Head of School
Frances Walsh, Athletic Director
Will Long, Assistant Athletic Director
The Howard School is an independent school for children ages K-12th grade who have learning differences and language learning disabilities. Instruction is personalized to complement individual learning styles, to address student needs and to help each student understand his or her learning process. The curriculum focuses on depth of understanding in order to make learning meaningful and therefore, maximize educational success.

4076 Wardlaw School
Atlanta Speech School
3160 Northside Parkway NW.
Atlanta, GA 30327
404-233-5332
Fax: 404-266-2175
www.atlantaspeechschool.org
cyates@atlspsch.org

Jack Zimmermann, CFO
Comer Yates, Executive Director
Iris Goodson, Director, Human Resources
Dedicated to serving children with average to very superior intelligence and mild to moderate learning disabilities. Children served in the Wardlaw School typically exhibit underlying auditory and/or visual processing problems that make it difficult for them to learn in their present educational setting.

Hawaii

4077 Center on Disability Studies
University of Hawaii at Manoa
1776 University Ave, UA4-6
Honolulu, HI 96822-2447
808-956-9142
Fax: 808-956-5713
www.cds.hawaii.edu
Robert.Stodden@cds.hawaii.edu

David Leake, Chair
Eric Folk, Vice-Chair
Robert Stodden, Director/Professor
The Center for Disability Studies is a Hawaii Unviersity Affiliated Program at the University of Hawaii at Manoa. The mission of the CDS is to support the quality of life, community inclusion, and self-determination of all persons with disabilities and their families.

4078 Learning Disabilities Association of Hawaii
245 N. Kukui Street
Suite 205
Honolulu, HI 96817
808-536-9684
800-533-9684
Fax: 808-537-6780
www.ldahawaii.org
ldah@ldahawaiii.org

Michael Moore, Executive Director
Rosie Rowe, Education & Training Coordinator
Marge Neilson, Administrative Assistant

Serving families with children with learning disabilities and other special needs that interfere with learning by providing education advocacy, training and support in order to remove barriers and promote awareness and full educational opportunity. LDAH has several special projects that helps fulfill the mission of removing barriers and promoting awareness and full educational opportunity. The Parent Training and Information Center is one of these special projects that is offered.

4079 Variety School of Hawaii

710 Palekaua Street
Honolulu, HI 96816

808-732-2835
Fax: 808-732-4334
www.varietyschool.org
info@varietyschool.org

Duane Yee, Executive Director
To identify and educate children with learning disabilities, to assist in achieving their maximum potential, through a multi-disciplinary approach.

Idaho

4080 Idaho Parents Unlimited, Inc.

500 S 8th Street
P.O. Box 50126
Boise, ID 83702

208-342-5884
800-242-4785
Fax: 208-342-1408
www.ipulidaho.org
parents@ipulidaho.org

Angela Lindig, Executive Director
Jennifer Zielinski, Program & Parent Edu. Coord
Amy Ireland, Parent Education Coordinator
A statewide organization founded to provide support, information and technical assistance to parents of children and youth with disabilities.

Illinois

4081 Acacia Academy

6425 Willow Springs Road
La Grange Highlands, IL 60525

708-579-9040
Fax: 708-579-5872
www.acaciaacademy.com

Kathryn Fouks, Principal, Director
Eileen Petzold, Assistant Principal & Director
Jim Shoemaker Saif, Head of High School
Offering personalized and exceptional educational instruction to each individual student in the development of his/her intellectual and academic potential.

4082 Allendale Association

P.O.Box 1088
Lake Villa, IL 60046

847-245-6242
888-255-3631
Fax: 847-356-0289
www.allendale4kids.org
cborucki@allendale4kids.org

Mary Shahbazian, President
Connie Borucki, SVP, HR & Support Services
Sue Gaddy, Associate VP, Communications
A private, not-for-profit organization serving children and adolescents with moderate to profound emotional and behavioral disabilities. Allendaleis dedicated to excellence and innovation in the care, education, treatment and advocacy for troubled children, youth and their families.

4083 Associated Talmud Torahs of Chicago

2828 West Pratt
Chicago, IL 60645

773-973-2828
Fax: 773-973-6666
www.att.org
webmaster@att.org

Rabbi Mordechai Raizman, Executive Director, Operations
Rabbi Schwartzman, Executive Director Emeritus
Rabbi Yehuda Polstein, Principal of MIE Torah High
Offers mainstreaming, independent skills, therapeutic swim classes and psychological services.

4084 Brehm Preparatory School

950 S. Brehm Lane
Carbondale, IL 62901

618-457-0371
Fax: 618-529-1248
www.brehm.org
admissionsinfo@brehm.org

Brian Brown, Ph.D., Executive Director
Richard G. Collins, Ph.D., Director
Donna E. Collins, B.A., Director, Admissions
A boarding school specifically designed to meet the needs of students with complex learning disabilities and attention deficit disorder issues.

4085 Center for Speech and Language Disorders

310-D S. Main St.
Lombard, IL 60148

630-652-0200
Fax: 630-652-0300
www.csld.org
info@csld.org

Lynn Scheuer Kozak M.A., Executive Director
Mary Catherine Brady, Operations Manager
Jori , Intake, Billing Issues
The mission is to help children with speech and language disorders reach their full potential. CSLD is an internationally recognized leader in the diagnosis and treatment of hyperlexia and other language disorders.

4086 Children's Center for Behavioral Development

353 N 88th St
East Saint Louis, IL 62203-2705

618-398-1152
Fax: 618-398-6977

C P Birth, Executive Director
Special education programs for children and adults who are learning disabled, emotionally distubed or have behavioral disorders. Some of the programs include vocational education classes, computer classes, art, and physical education.

4087 Cove School

350 Lee Road
Northbrook, IL 60062

847-562-2100
Fax: 847-562-2112
www.coveschool.org
ssover@coveschool.org

Dr. Sally L. Sover, Executive Director
John Stieper, Director of Education
Stacy Post, Director, Finance & Admin.
The Cove School was established in 1947, to educate students with learning disabilities and to facilitate their return to their neighborhood schools in the shortest possible time. The heart of Cove's educational philosophy is to design a program that pulls out the child's skills.

4088 Educational Services of Glen Ellyn

364 Pennsylvania Ave
Glen Ellyn, IL 60137

630-469-1479
Fax: 630-469-1265
www.esgetutoring.com
educationalservices@juno.com

Megan Burke, Owner
Tutoring for all ages in all subject areas. Diagnostic testing, specializing in learning disabilities and career counseling for learning disabled adults.

4089 Elim Christian Services

13020 S Central Ave
Palos Heights, IL 60463

708-389-0555
877-9-ELIMCS
Fax: 708-389-0671
www.elimcs.org
info@elimcs.org

Dr. David DeJong, Chairman
Frederick Wezeman, Vice-Chairman
William Lodewyk, President
Elim Christian Services is a non-profit corporation that seeks to equip persons with special needs to achieve to their highest God-given potential.

4090   Esperanza Community Services
Esperanza School
520 N Marshfield Ave
Chicago, IL 60622   312-243-6097
                                 Fax: 312-243-2076
                                 TDD: 800-526-0844
                    www.esperanzacommunityservices.org
                          info@esperanzacommunity.org
Cindy Dombkowski, Principal
Melanie Mannerino, Director, Programs
Chivon Niziolek, Director, Adult Programs
Accredited by the Rehabilitation Accreditation Commission; Esperanza School is a private, therapeutic school serving students ages 5 to 21 with Autism, mild/moderate/severe cognitive disabilites, traumatic brain injuries and other health impairements.

4091   Family Resource Center on Disabilities
11 E. Adams St.
Suite 1002
Chicago, IL 60603   312-939-3513
                                      800-952-4199
                                 Fax: 312-854-8980
                                 TDD: 312-939-3519
                                      www.frcd.org
                                      info@frcd.org
Charlotte Des Jardins, Executive Director
FRCD was organized by parents, professionals, and volunteers who seek to improve services for all children with disabilities.

4092   Illinois Center for Autism
548 S Ruby Ln
Fairview Heights, IL 62208   618-398-7500
                                 Fax: 618-632-9094
                       www.illinoiscenterforautism.org
                       info@illinoiscenterforautism.org
Hardy Ware, Chairperson
Thomas E. Berry, Vice Chairperson
Susan Szekely, Executive Director
A not-for-profit, community based, mental health treatment, and educational agency dedicated to serving people with autism. Referrals for possible student placement are made through local school districts, hospitals, regional special education centers, and doctors.

4093   Joseph Academy
1100 North 22nd Avenue
Melrose Park, IL 60160   708-345-4500
                                 Fax: 708-345-4516
                             www.josephacademy.org
                          sbijak@josephacademy.org
Stasia Bijak, Principal
Jesus Garcia, Transportation Coordinator
Diane Malek, Administrative Assistant
Founded in 1983, Joseph Academy provides a nurturing and challenging environment for young people. Our mission is to serve children and adolescents with behavioral, emotional and learning disorders by helping them develop the social, academic and vocational skills they need to function in society.

4094   Northwestern University Learning Clinic
2240 Campus Drive
Evanston, IL 60208-0895   847-491-3184
                                 Fax: 847-467-1464
                      www.communication.northwestern.edu
                          dialogue@northwestern.edu
Frank Van Santen, Clinic Director
Rick Morris, Associate Dean, Administration
Jane Rankin, Associate Dean, Research

A teaching clinic that provides diagnostic evaluations for children and adults, remediation for children, and theory-based coursework for graduate steudents interested in teaching people with learning disabilities.

4095   Professional Assistance Center for Education (PACE)
National-Louis University
5202 Old Orchard Road
Skokie, IL 60077   224-233-2670
                                    www.nl.edu/pace
                                 paceprogram@nl.edu
Carol Burns, Director
Barb Kite, Assistant Director
Founded in 1986, PACE is a two-year, noncredit postsecondary certificate program located on the campus of National-Louis University. The PACE program is designed especially to meet the transitional needs of students with multiple learning disabilities in a university setting.

4096   South Central Community Services
8316 South Ellis Avenue
Chicago, IL 60619   773-483-0900
                                 Fax: 773-483-8090
                                    www.sccsinc.org
Anna Maria Kowalik, Chairperson
Bonnie Deshong, 1st Vice Chairperson
Felicia Y Blasingame, President, CEO
A comprehensive human service agency committed to improving the quality of life for individuals and families by providing mental health, educational, socio-economic, and recreational programs and services throughout the State of Illinois.

4097   Special Education Day School
Catholic Children's Home
1400 State Street
Alton, IL 62002   618-465-3594
                                 Fax: 618-465-1083
                       www.catholicchildrenshome.com
                       info@catholicchildrenshome.com
Candace Hovey, Administrator
Steven Roach, Executive Director
Michael Shelton-Montez, Associate Administrator
For children with learning disabilities, developmental and behavioral disorders and through its comprehensive residential services for children in crisis. Providing year-round educational and theraputic services to students who, due to a variety of social, emotional and/or educational difficulties, have been unsuccessful in public school programs.

4098   Summit School, Inc.
333 West River Road
Elgin, IL 60123   847-468-0490
                                 www.summitinc.org
                           jwhite@summitelgin.org
M. Ruth Tofanelli, Co-Founder, Executive Director
James R. Williams, Co-Founder
Johanna F. White, President, CEO
The Summit School offeres an array of services to children and young adults with learning difficulties. The school provides the necessary academic and interpersonal skills needed so that the students can live productive and meaningful lives.

4099   The Baby Fold
Hammit School
108 E Willow St
Normal, IL 61761   309-451-7202
                                 Fax: 309-452-0115
                                  www.thebabyfold.org
                               info@thebabyfold.org
Dale S. Strassheim, President, CEO
Karen Rousey, VP, Programs
Veronica Manzella, VP, Human Resources

A multi-service agency that provides Residential, Special Education, Child Welfare, and Family Support Services to children and families in central Illinois. Educational services are held at the Hammitt Elementary school and the Hammitt Junior-Senior High School for children and adolescents with behavioral, learning, emotional and pervasive developmental disabilities.

4100   The Early Achievement Center
Acacia Academy
6425 Willow Springs Road
La Grange Highlands, IL 60525   708-579-9040
Fax: 708-579-5872
www.acaciaacademy.com
info@acaciaacademy.com
Kathryn Fouks, Principal, Director
Eileen Petzold, Assistant Principal & Director
Jim Shoemaker Saif, Head of High School
The Early Achievement Center Program encourages growth of the total child in social, intellectual, physical, and emotional abilities.

4101   The Hope School Learning Center
The Hope Institute for Children and Families
50 East Hazel Dell Lane
Springfield, IL 62712   217-585-5437
Fax: 217-786-3356
TDD: 217-585-5105
www.thehopeschool.org
info@thehopeschool.org
Joseph Nyre, President
The Hope School is a private, not-for-profit eduational and residential center that has been serving children with multiple disabilities and their families since 1957.

Indiana

4102   Clearinghouse on Reading, English and Communications
Indiana University of Bloomington
201 N. Rose Avenue
Bloomington, IN 47405-1006   812-856-8500
www.indiana.edu/~reading
iuadmit@indiana.edu
Carl B. Smith, Director
Offers information on reading, English and communication skills, preschool through college.

4103   IN*SOURCE
Indiana Resource Cntr -Families with Special Needs
1703 South Ironwood Drive
South Bend, IN 46613   574-234-7101
800-332-4433
Fax: 574-234-7279
www.insource.org
insource@insource.org
Richard Burden, Executive Director
Scott Carson, Assistant Director
Dory Lawrence, Project Director
The mission of IN*SOURCE is to provide parents, families and service providers in Indiana the information and training necessary to assure effective educational programs and appropriate services for children and young adults with disabilities.

Kansas

4104   Families Together
5611 Southwest Barrington Court Sou
Suite 120
Topeka, KS 66614-2489   785-233-4777
800-264-6343
Fax: 785-233-4787
TTY: 316-945-7747
www.familiestogetherinc.org
topeka@familiestogetherinc.org

Brandelyn Nichols, Chairperson
Linda Peterson, Vice Chairperson
Lesli Girard, Center Director
Families Together is a statewide non-profit organization assisting Kansas families which include sons and/or daughters who have any form of disability.

4105   Heartspring School
8700 East 29th St. North
Wichita, KS 67226   316-634-8700
800-835-1043
Fax: 316-634-0555
www.heartspring.org
Gary W. Singleton, Ph.D., President, CEO
Paul Faber, EVP, Operations
David Dorf, CPA, CFO
Heartspring School has earned an international reputation for improving the lives of children. Heartspring is a not-for-profit private residential school that serves children 5-21. We serve children with disabilities such as autism, asperger's, communication disorders, developmental disabilities, dual diagnosed, behavoir disorders, hearing or vision impaired.

Kentucky

4106   KY-SPIN, Inc.
Kentucky Special Parent Involvement Network, Inc.
10301-B Deering Rd.
Louisville, KY 40272   502-937-6894
800-525-7746
Fax: 502-937-6464
TDD: 502-937-6894
www.kyspin.com
spininc@kyspin.com
Paulette Logsdon, Executive Director
Francis Edwards, Executive Assistant
Provides training, information and support to people with disabilities, their parents and families, and information on all types of disabilities and topics for all age groups.

4107   Meredith-Dunn School
3023 Melbourne Avenue
Louisville, KY 40220   502-456-5819
Fax: 502-456-5953
http://meredithdunnschool.org
cbunnell@meredith-dunn-school.org
Kathy Beam, Principal, Head of School
Anne Eddins, Admission Director
Ashley Ward, Director of Curriculum
Meredith-Dunn School's instruction is designed to empower students with average or above-average abilities who learn differently in becoming accomplished learners and resilient indiviiduals. At Meredith-Dunn, labels no longer define our students; we honor the uniqueness of all learners, emphasizing their talents while addressing their difficulties. Grades 1-8.

4108   Shedd Academy
P.O.Box 493
Mayfield, KY 42066-0030   270-247-8007
Fax: 270-247-0637
www.sheddacademy.org
judy.brindley@sheddacademy.org
Paul Thompson, Executive Director
The mission of the Shedd Academy is to prepare dyslexia and ADD students for college or vocational training and for their future by helping them to understand their unique learning styles; fulfill their intellectual, academic, physical, artistic, creative, social, spiritual, and emotional potential; develop a sense of self responsibility; assume a value system so that they can become contributing members of society and increase their skills to ensure they are armed with a variety of abilities.

4109 The de Paul School
1925 Duker Avenue
Louisville, KY 40205

502-459-6131
Fax: 502-458-0827
www.depaulschool.org

Tony Kemper, Head of School
Lisa Stepp, Principal
Kurt Moser, Director, Technology
Teaches students with specific learning differences how to: learn, be independent, and be successful. Co-ed, grades 1-8.

Louisiana

4110 Project PROMPT
Families Helping Families
201 Evans Road
Building 1, Suite 100
Harahan, LA 70123-5230

504-888-9111
800-766-7736
Fax: 504-888-0246
www.projectprompt.com
info@projectprompt.com

Rose Gilbert, Executive Director
Parent Training and Information Program views parents as full partners in the educational process and a significant source of support and assistance to each other. Funded by the Division of Personnel Preparation, Office of Special Education Programs, these programs provide training and information to parents to enable such individuals to participate more effectively with professionals in meeting the educational needs of disabled children.

Maine

4111 Learning Resource Center
Unity College
90 Quaker Hill Road
Unity, ME 04988

207-509-7100
800-624-1024
Fax: 207-948-6277
www.unity.edu
admissions@unity.edu

Bruce Nickerson, Chair
Stephen Mulkey, President
Dr. Melik Peter Khoury, EVP
The Learning Resource Center provides instruction and supportive services to students with learning disabilities. A staff learning disabilites specialist works with students who have specific cognitive disabilites that interfers with learning.

Maryland

4112 Academic Resource Center
Gunston Day School
P.O.Box 200
Centreville, MD 21617

410-758-0620
Fax: 410-758-0628
www.gunstondayschool.org
info@gunstondayschool.org

Susan Dillon, Chair
James D. Wright, Vice-Chair
Robert Fredland, Director, Technology
Founded in 1911, the school provides tutoring for individuals K through adult. Also offers limited and brief educational testing.

4113 Chelsea School
2970 Belcrest Center Drive
Suite 300
Hyattsville, MD 20782

301-585-1430
Fax: 301-585-9621
www.chelseaschool.edu
information@chelseaschool.edu

Katherine Fedalen, Head Of School
Frank Mills, Director, Education
Debbie Lourie, Director, Admissions
Committed to providing superior education to children with language-based learning disabilities.

4114 Children's Developmental Clinic
Prince George's Community College
301 Largo Rd
Largo, MD 20774-2199

301-336-6000
Fax: 301-322-0519
TDD: 301-322-0122
TTY: 301-322-0838
www.pgcc.edu
advising@pgcc.edu

Charlene M. Dukes, President
Thomas E. Knapp, VP, Administrative Services
Sandra F. Dunnington, VP, Academic Affairs
The Children's Development Clinic is a continuing education program conducted in cooperation with the Department of Health and Human Performance at Prince George's Community College. The clinic provides special services to children, birth and up, who are experiencing various development difficulties such as learning problems, developmental delays, physical fitness and coordination problems, brain injury, mental retardation, emotional problems, or orthopedic challenges.

4115 Frost Center
4915 Aspen Hill Rd
Rockville, MD 20853-3709

301-933-3452
Fax: 301-933-0350
www.frostcenter.com
chobbes@frostcenter.com

Sean McLaughlin, Director
The Frost school's programs and therapeutic day programs serve emotionally troubled and autistic children and adolescents and their families.

4116 Gengras Center
Saint Joseph College
60 College Avenue
Annapolis, MD 21401

410-263-2371
Fax: 860-231-6795
www.sjc.edu
Annapolis.Admissions@sjc.edu

Christopher Nelson, President
Barbara Goyette, VP, Advancement
Pamela Kraus, Dean
This state approved, private special education facility, provides a highly structured, intensive, self-contained special education program for elementary, middle and high school students. The program focuses on skill development in the core academic areas, functional application of skills, community life skills, work readiness skills, job training, social development and independent living skills. Special attention is given to the behavioral challenges of individual students.

4117 High Road School Of Baltimore County
7707 German Hill Road
Baltimore, MD 21222

410-282-8500
Fax: 410-282-1047
www.kids1inc.com
kids1@kids1inc.com

Ellyn Lerner PhD, President
Offers programs serving the educational, social and emotional needs of children with specific learning disabilities, communication disorders and/or behavioral difficulties.

4118 Kennedy Krieger Institute
University Affiliated Program
707 North Broadway
Baltimore, MD 21205

443-923-9200
888-554-2080
Fax: 443-923-2645
TTY: 443-923-2645
www.kennedykrieger.org
info@kennedykrieger.org

Gary W Goldstein, President
Joshua Ewen, M.D., Director, Clinical Laboratory
Jennifer Accardo, M.D., Director, Sleep Disorders Clinic
Internationally recognized for improving the lives of children and young adults with disorders of the brain, spinal cord and musculoskeletal system. Serves more than 14,000 individuals each year through inpatient and ouapatient clinics; homes and community services; and school-based programs.

4119   Nora School
955 Sligo Avenue
Silver Spring, MD 20910
301-495-6672
Fax: 301-495-7829
www.nora-school.org
marcia@nora-school.org
David Mullen, Head of School
Marcia Miller, Director, Admissions
Norman Maynard, Business
A small, progressive, college preparatory high school that nurtures and empowers bright students who have been frustrated in larger, more traditional school settings.

4120   Phillips Programs for Children and Families
7010 Braddock Road
Annandale, VA 22003
703-941-8810
Fax: 703-658-2378
www.phillipsprograms.org
piper.phillips@phillipsprograms.org
Piper Phillips Caswell, President/CEO
Trixie Herbert, Chief Operating Officer
Marbeth Ingle Levy, Director, HR
Phillips is a non-profit, private organization serving the needs of individuals with emotional and behavioral problems and their families through education, family support services, community education and advocacy.

4121   Ridge School of Montgomery County
Adventis Behavioral Health
14901 Broschart Road
Rockville, MD 20850
301-251-4500
800-204-8600
Fax: 301-251-4588
www.adventisthealthcare.com
Terry Forde, President, CEO
Susan L. Grover, SVP, Chief Quality Officer
James G. Lee, EVP, CFO
The school provides both a special education program and a general education program to meet the needs of the students who have difficulty learning in a traditional school environment.

4122   The Forbush School at Glyndon
Sheppard Pratt Health System
407 Central Avenue
Reisterstown, MD 21136
410-517-5400
Fax: 410-517-5600
www.sheppardpratt.org
jking@sheppardpratt.org
Steven S. Sharfstein, M.D., President/CEO
Catherine Doughty, VP, Human Resources
Jodi King, Director
Provides educational and therapeutic services for children and young adults through 12th grade who have learning disabilities. Curriculum is designed to help the growth of each student in emotional and cognitive areas, and each student follows a program that is designed to meet their needs.

4123   The Parents' Place of Maryland
801 Cromwell Park Drive
Suite 103
Glen Burnie, MD 21061
410-768-9100
Fax: 410-768-0830
TDD: 410-768-9100
www.ppmd.org
info@ppmd.org
Josie Thomas, Executive Director
Suzie Shannon, Administration
Melissa Alexander, Parent Educator

Serving the parents of children with disabilities throughout Maryland, regardless of the nature of their child's disability or the age of their child. The staff helps families obtain the appropriate information on education, health care and services for their childs disabilities.

Massachusetts

4124   Adult Center at PAL: Program for Advancement of Learning
1071 Blue Hill Avenue
Milton, MA 02186
617-333-0500
800-668-0686
Fax: 617-333-2114
TDD: 617-333-2250
www.curry.edu/pal
acoulter0811@curry.edu
Nancy Winbury PhD, Program Coordinator
Adam Coulter, Social Media Specialist
Elizabeth Deren, Associate Director
The Adult Center at PAL (Program for Advancement of Learning) is the first program to offer academic and socio-emotional services to adults with LD/ADHD/Dyslexia in a college setting in the New England area. The ACD offers one-to-one academic tutorials; small support groups that meet weekly; and Saturday Seminars that explore issues that impact the lives of adults with LD/ADHD.

4125   Berkshire Meadows
249 North Plain Road
Housatonic, MA 01236
413-528-2523
Fax: 413-528-0293
www.berkshiremeadows.org
lkelly@jri.org
Kathy Green, Director
Liisa Kelly, Program Director
Berkshire Meadows is a year-round residential school that helps children and young adults with severe cognitive disabilities, autism and challenging behaviors.

4126   CAST
40 Harvard Mills Square
Suite 3
Wakefield, MA 01880-3233
781-245-2212
888-858-9994
Fax: 781-245-5212
TDD: 781-245-9320
www.cast.org
cast@cast.org
Anne Meyer, Founder
David H. Rose, Founder
Lisa Poller, Co-President
A nonprofit organization that works to expand learning opportunities for all individuals, especially those with disabilities, through the research and development of innovative, technology-based educational resources and strategies.

4127   College Internship Program
The Berkshire Center
18 Park Street
Lee, MA 01238-1702
413-243-2576
Fax: 413-243-3351
www.berkshirecenter.org
admissions@berkshirecenter.org
Michael Mc Manmon, Executive Director
Lucy Gosselin, Program Director
Karen Noel, MSW, Admissions Coordinator
The College Internship Program provides individualized, post-secondary academic, internship and independent living experiences for young adults with learning differences. With the support and direction, students learn to realize and develop their potential.

4128 Commonwealth Learning Center

220 Reservoir Street
Suite 6
Needham, MA 02494-3133

781-444-5193
800-461-6671
Fax: 781-444-6916
www.commlearn.com
info@commlearn.com

Cecile Selwyn, M.Ed Ed.S, Director
Offers individualized one-to-one instruction specializing in multisensory methodologies such as Orton-Gillingham. Work with students of all ages in academic support, organizational and study skills, and test preparation.

4129 Cotting School

453 Concord Avenue
Lexington, MA 02421

781-862-7323
Fax: 781-861-1179
www.cotting.org.
info@cotting.org

David W. Manzo, M.Ed., President
Krista Macari, M.S., CCC-SLP, Chief Academic Officer
Bridget Irish, COO
Cotting School is for students with moderate to severe learning disabilities requiring assessment of learning style, remediation techniques and one-to-one instruction.

4130 Devereux Massachusetts

60 Miles Road
P.O. Box 219
Rutland, MA 01543-0219

508-886-4746
Fax: 508-886-4773
www.devereux.org

Robert Q. Kreider, President, CEO
Margaret McGill, SVP, COO
Lane Barker, Executive Director
A residential program for children, adolescents and young adults who have emotional, behavioral and substance abuse programs with developmental and learning disabilities.

4131 Educational Options

5 Suburban Road
605
Worcester, MA 01602

508-304-9672
Fax: 508-304-9257
www.optionsined.com
info@optionsined.com

Renee Goldberg, Director
Neil Kalt, Ph.D., Staff
Gay Jackson, R.N., BS, Staff
Full-service educational consulting practice dedicated to assisting students plan their future. Work with students to identify their strengths and match these qualities with an academic setting that meets their educational, cultural and social and social aspirations.

4132 Evergreen Center

345 Fortune Boulevard
Milford, MA 01757

508-478-2631
Fax: 508-634-3251
www.evergreenctr.org
services@evergreenctr.org

Robert Littleton Jr, Executive Director
The Evergreen Center is a residential school serving children and adolescents with severe developmental disabilities.

4133 F.L. Chamberlain School

Frederick L. Chamberlain Center, Inc.
1 Pleasant Street
P.O. Box 778
Middleboro, MA 02346

508-947-7825
Fax: 508-947-1593
www.chamberlainschool.org
rvonohlsen@chamberlainschool.org

William Doherty, Co-Founder, Executive Director
Jeanne Edwards, Co-Founder, COO
Lucille Mutty, Program Director

The F. L. Chamberlain School offers a highly structured program for students ages 11-20 who having difficulties that effect learning and behavior. Students may either live on campus or attend day classes and academic programming is tailored to meet the specific needs of each student.

4134 John Dewey Academy

389 Main Street
Great Barrington, MA 01230

413-528-9800
www.jda.org
info@jda.org

Kenneth Steiner, Head of School
Andrea Nathans, Executive Director, Admissions
Eric Krawczyk, Dean of Students
Provides an individualized and comprehensive education in a non-traditional therapeutic boarding school setting. Students are bright, troubled adolescents with a history of self-defeating or self-destructive choices. The peer-based approach leads students to high levels of achievement and inspires them to develop in ways that promote self-respect, maturity and respect for others.

4135 Landmark School Outreach Program

Landmark School
429 Hale Street
P.O. Box 227
Prides Crossing, MA 01965

978-236-3216
Fax: 978-927-7268
www.landmarkoutreach.org
outreach@landmarkschool.org

Robert Broudo, Headmaster
Dan Ahearn, Director
Rebecca Carson, Teacher
The Outreach Program provides professional development programs and publications that offer practical and effective strategies to help children learn. These strategies are based on Landmark's Six Teaching Principles and reflect Landmark's innovative instruction of students with language-based learning disabilites.

4136 Landmark School and Summer Programs

Landmark School
429 Hale Street
P.O. Box 227
Prides Crossing, MA 01965

978-236-3216
Fax: 978-927-7268
www.landmarkoutreach.org
outreach@landmarkschool.org

Robert Broudo, Headmaster
Dan Ahearn, Director
Rebecca Carson, Teacher
Landmark is a coeducational boarding and day school for emotionally healthy students who have been diagnosed with a language based learning disability. We individualize instruction for each of our students, providing an intensive program emphasizing the development of language and learning skills within a highly structured environment. We also offer an intensive six-week summer program for students who wish to explore the benefits of short-term, skill-based learning.

4137 League School of Greater Boston

300 Boston Providence Turnpike
Walpole, MA 02032

508-850-3900
Fax: 508-660-2442
www.leagueschool.com
info@leagueschool.com

Joseph DiGiantommaso, CFO
Jean Leahy, Principal
Frank Gagliardi, Executive Director
Providing social, academic, and vocational programs for children with Autism/Asperger Spectrum Disorders who need a specialized alternative to public school, preparing them to transfer into an environment offering greater independence.

4138 **Linden Hill School**
154 S Mountain Rd
Northfield, MA 01360-9701   413-498-2906
                                          866-498-2906
                                     Fax: 413-498-2908
                                          www.lindenhs.org
                                          office@lindenhs.org
James Mc Daniel, Headmaster
Gerald Shields, Principal
The Linden Hill School is a middle school for boys who
come from around the world who have dyslexia or other language learning difficulties. Classes students attend are
based on academic needs and the curriculum is designed to
allow students to progress at their own pace.

4139 **Living Independently Forever, Inc.**
550 Lincoln Road Extension
Hyannis, MA 02601   508-790-3600
                                     Fax: 508-778-4919
                                          www.lifecapecod.org
                                          diane@lifecapecod.org
William G. McKelvey, Chairperson
JoAnn Simons, Vice-Chairperson
Diane Enochs, Executive Director
Living Independently Forever, Inc. is dedicated to serving
the life-long needs of adults with significant learning disabilities within our residential communities. LIFE is committed to providing these men and women with the adult
education and the opportunities to develop their personal
and vocational / occupational skills to their maximum potential, and to supporting them appropriately in independent
and group living.

4140 **May Institute**
41 Pacella Park Drive
Randolph, MA 02368   781-440-0400
                                          800-778-7601
                                     Fax: 781-440-0401
                                     TDD: 781-440-0461
                                     TTY: 781-440-0461
                                          www.mayinstitute.org
                                          info@mayinstitute.org
Lauren C. Solotar, Ph.D., ABPP, President, CEO
Jerry Hand, SVP, Facilities
Eileen G. Pollack, M.A., SVP, Development
The May Institute provides educational and rehabilitative
services for individuals with autism, developmental disabil-
ities, neurological disorders and mental illness.

4141 **Melmark New England**
461 River Road
Andover, MA 01810   978-654-4300
                                     Fax: 978-654-4315
                                          www.melmarkne.org
                                          newstudents@melmarkne.org
Joanne Gillis-Donovan, Ph.D., President and CEO
George P. Linke, Jr., Psy.D., EVP
Delyn M. Byerly, MBA, Chief Financial Officer
Serves children and adolescents within the autism spectrum
disorders, and works to develop and enhance their abilities
and confidence in a safe and nuturing environment.

4142 **Riverbrook Residence**
4 Ice Glen Road
P.O. Box 478
Stockbridge, MA 01262   413-298-4926
                                     Fax: 413-298-5166
                                          www.riverbrook.org
                                          info@riverbrook.org
Deborah Francome, Executive Director
Rebecca Amuso, Program Director
Dawn S. Giftos, Director, Development
A residence in western Massachusetts, providing supported
living to developmentally disabled women, with therapy and
treatment focused on the arts.

4143 **Riverview School**
551 Route 6A East Sandwich
Cape Cod, MA 02537   508-888-0489
                                     Fax: 508-833-7001
                                          www.riverviewschool.org
                                          admissions@riverviewschool.org
Maureen B. Brenner, Principal, Head of School
Maria Cashdollar, Director, Education
Meghan Hammond, Director of Special Services
Riverview School is a coeducational residential school for
adolescents and young adults with complex language, learn-
ing and cognitive disabilities.

4144 **Seven Hills Academy at Groton**
Seven Hills Foundation
81 Hope Avenue
Worcester, MA 01603   508-755-2340
                                     Fax: 508-849-3882
                                     TTY: 508-890-5584
                                          www.sevenhills.org
David A. Jordan, DHA, President, CEO
Kathleen A. Jordan, DHA, SVP & Chief Program Officer
Joseph L. Tosches, DBA, EVP & Chief Operations Officer
Special education day programs for children and young
adults with complex developmental and medical disabili-
ties. Summer programs are also available.

4145 **Son-Rise Program®**
Autism Treatment Center of America
2080 Undermountain Rd
Sheffield, MA 01257-9643   413-229-2100
                                          877-766-7473
                                     Fax: 413-229-3202
                                          www.autismtreatment.com
                                          autism@option.org
Barry Kaufman, Founder
Raun Kaufman, Director of Global Education
Since 1983, the Autism Treatment Center of America has
provided innovative training programs and workshops for
parents and professionals caring for children challenged by
Autism, Autism Spectrum Disorders, Pervasive Developmental Disorder (PDD) and other developmental
difficulties.
1983

4146 **The Learning Center School**
The Protestant Guild for Human Services
411 Waverley Oaks Road
Suite 104
Waltham, MA 02452   781-893-6000
                                     Fax: 781-893-1171
                                          www.theguildschool.org
                                          development@theguildschool.org
William Sowyrda, Chief Financial Officer
Dr. Julie A. Armentrout, Chief Quality Assurance Officer
Sharon DiGrigoli, Chief Education Officer
A private, 365-day community-based, educational program
serving difficult to place students with a primary diagnosis
of mild to severe mental retardation, autism, or other developmental disability. In addition, students may carry secondary diagnosis of hearing impairments and other
communication disorders, traumatic brain injury, seizure
disorders, Tourette's syndrome and emotional and
psychiatric disorders.

4147 **The New England Center for Children**
33 Turnpike Road
Southborough, MA 01772-2108   508-481-1015
                                     Fax: 508-485-3421
                                          www.necc.org
                                          info@necc.org
Vincent Strully, Jr., Founder, CEO
Michael S. Downey, CPA, MBA, CFO
Katherine E. Foster, MEd., COO
The New England Center for Children is a private, nonprofit
organization serving children with autism and other related
disabilities.

4148 The Perkins Day Treatment Program
Perkins
971 Main Street
Lancaster, MA 01523   978-365-7376
Fax: 978-368-8861
TTY: 978-368-6437
www.perkinsprograms.org
admissions@perkinschool.org
Douglas J. Reid, M.B.A., CFO
Charles P. Conroy, Ed.D., Executive Director
David A. Cook, M.Ed., Director of Education
The program offers comprehensive educational and clinical programs for children and adolescents with ADD, bi-polar disorder, depression, post traumatic stress disorder, asperger syndrom and thought disorders. Some of the academic programs are speech and language therapy, math, reading, arts, music and swimming.

4149 Willow Hill School
98 Haynes Road
Sudbury, MA 01776   978-443-2581
Fax: 978-443-7560
www.willowhillschool.org
mgreid@willowhillschool.org
Marilyn G. Reid, Head of School
Shamus Brady, Director of Education
Ann Marie Reen, Director of Admissions
Willow Hill School provides supportive and individualized educational programs for middle and high school students grades 6-12 who are capable of advancing along a strong academic curriculum, but have experienced frustration in earlier school settings.

Michigan

4150 Eton Academy
1755 Melton Road
Birmingham, MI 48009   248-642-1150
Fax: 248-642-3670
www.etonacademy.org
contact@etonacademy.org
Pete Pullen, Principal
The Eton Academy is a co-educational private day school dedicated to educating students with learning differences. The mission is to educate students who will understand their learning styles and practice strategies that will prepare them for responsible independence, life-long learning and participation in school, family and in their community.

4151 Lake Michigan Academy
2428 Burton St SE
Grand Rapids, MI 49546-4806   616-464-3330
Fax: 616-285-1935
www.wmldf.org
abarto@wmldf.org
Andrea Goetz, Executive Director
Lake Michigan Academy is a state-certified, non-profit school for learning disabled children in grades 1 through 12 with average or above average intelligence. The learning disabilities of the children here vary. Some are dyslexic and have difficulty with decoding or comprehending written language. Some are dyscalculic and experience difficulty with mathematical computations and concepts. Many are dysgraphic and exhibit difficulties with writing skills. Our mission is to build self esteem.

4152 Specialized Language Development Center
2650 Horizon DR SE
Suite 230
Grand Rapids, MI 49546   616-361-1182
888-271-8881
Fax: 616-361-3648
www.sldcenter.org
info@sldcenter.org
Maura Race, Co-Executive Director
Carol McGlinn, Co-Executive Director
Amy Barto, Community Outreach Director

A community resources of W Michigan committed to bringing the power of reading, writing, and spelling to all individuals with dyslexia or other learning styles, enabling them to reach their full potential.

Minnesota

4153 Groves Academy
3200 Highway 100 South
Saint Louis Park, MN 55416   952-920-6377
Fax: 952-920-2068
www.grovesacademy.org
alexanderj@grovesadacemy.org
Mark Donahoe, Chairman
John Alexander, Head Of School
Kathy Boone, Director Of Education
A day school for children who because of their learning disabilities have not been successful in a traditional school setting.

4154 LDA Learning Center
LDA Minnesota
6100 Golden Valley Road
Golden Valley, MN 55422   952-582-6000
Fax: 952-582-6031
www.ldaminnesota.org
info@ldaminnesota.org
Martha Moriarty, Executive Director
Jill Pearson Wood, Resource Development Director
Mary Beth Kelley, Special Educator/Program Dev
Maximizes the potential of children, youths, adults and families, especially those with learning disabilities and other learning difficulties so that they can lead more productive and fulfilled lives. Provides consultations, tutoring, assessments, parent workshops, training and outreach on sliding fee scale.

Mississippi

4155 Heritage School
St. Columbus Episcopal Church
550 Sunnybrook Rd
Ridgeland, MS 39157   601-853-0205
Fax: 601-853-0389
www.stcolumbs.org
stcolumb@stcolumbs.org
Sammie Butler, Sexton
Michael Hrivnak, Director of Spiritual Formation
Abram Jones, Director of Youth Ministry
Heritage School was established in 1971 to provide an alternative learning environment for children with learning difficulties. A private, non-profit specialized school accredited through the State Department of Education to offer instruction for learning disabled and ADD/ADHD students from first through eighth grade.

Missouri

4156 Churchill Center & School for Learning Disabilities
1021 Municipal Center Drive
Town & Country, MO 63131   314-997-4343
Fax: 314-997-2760
www.churchillstl.org
info@churchillstl.org
Sandra Gilligan, Director
Anne Evers, Director, Admissions
Deborah Warden, Assistant Director - Operations
The Churchill School is a private, not-for-profit, coeducational day school. It is designed to serve children between the ages of 8-16 with diagnosed learning disabilities. The goal is to help each child reach his or her full potential and prepare for a successful return to a traditional classroom in as short a period of time as possible.

4157 Gillis Center

8150 Wornall Road
Kansas City, MO 64114   816-508-3500
                                  Fax: 816-508-3535
                                      www.gillis.org
                          Stephen.O'neill@gillis.org
Stephen O'Neill, President, CEO
Michelle Graff, VP, Administration
Pam Sanders, Director, Education
Gillis Center's mission is to help at-risk children and their families become contributing members of the community through education, counseling and social services.

4158 MPACT - Missouri Parents Act

8301 State Line Road
Suite 204
Kansas City, MO 64114   800-743-7634
                                  Fax: 816-531-4777
                                  TTY: 800-743-7634
                                    www.ptimpact.org
                                   info@ptimpact.org
Diana Biere, Interim Executive Director
Sandra Hamilton, MultiCultural Coordinator
Debby Loveall Stewart, Program Coordinator
MPACT assists parents to effectively advocate for their children's educational rights and services. MPACT is a statewide parent training and information center serving all disabilities. Our mission is to ensure that all children with special needs receive an education that allows them to achieve their personal goals.

4159 Miriam School

501 Bacon Avenue
Saint Louis, MO 63119-1512   314-968-3893
                                  Fax: 314-968-7338
                                  www.miriamschool.org
Joan Holland, M.Ed., Head of School
Megan Gibson, Director of Admissions
Mary Bless, Director of Media Services
A nonprofit day school for children between four and twelve years of age who are learning disabled and/or behaviorally disabled. Speech and language services and occupational therapy are integral components of the program. The focus of all the activities is to increase children's self-esteem and help them acquire the coping skills needed to successfully meet future challenges.

Montana

4160 Parents Let's Unite for Kids

516 N 32nd St
Billings, MT 59101-6003   406-255-0540
                                      800-222-7585
                                  Fax: 406-255-0523
                                      www.pluk.org
                                     info@pluk.org
Roger Holt, Executive Director
PLUK is a private, nonprofit organization formed in 1984 by parents and children with disabilities and chronic illnesses in the state of Montana for the purpose of information, support, training and assistance to aid their children at home, school and as adults.

Nebraska

4161 Nebraska Parents Training and Information Center

PTI (Parent Training & Information) Nebraska
2564 Leavenworth St
Suite 202
Omaha, NE 68105   402-346-0525
                                      800-284-8520
                                  Fax: 402-934-1479
                                  TDD: 800-284-8520
                                  www.pti-nebraska.org
                                  info@pti-nebraska.org

Paula Latham, President
Lyris Peak, Vice President
Glenda Davis, Executive Director
Parent Training and Information Program views parents as full partners in the educational process and a significant source of support and assistance to each other. Funded by the Division of Personnel Preparation, Office of Special Education Programs, these programs provide training and information to parents to enable such individuals to participate more effectively with professionals in meeting the educational needs of disabled children.

New Hampshire

4162 Becket Family of Services

61 Locust Street
Suite 317
Dover, NH 03820-3753   603-343-4440
                                  Fax: 603-343-5084
                                      www.becket.org
Jeffrey Caron, M.Ed.,CAGS, President
Eric Scharf, BS, CEO
Susan Beck, MSW, Executive Director
Becket guides and inspires adolescents having difficulties at home, in school or in the community.

4163 Center for Children with Disabilities

91 Maple Avenue
Keene, NH 03431   603-358-3384
                                  Fax: 603-358-6485
                                  www.cedarcrest4kids.org
                          cgray@cedarcrest4kids.org
Cathy Gray, MA, NHA, President, CEO
Scott Adams, MBA, CFO
Michael O'Hara, Director, Special Education
provides long-term and short-term residential care, special education and therapy services for children with complex medical and developmental needs.

4164 Hampshire Country School

28 Patey Circle
Rindge, NH 03461   603-899-3325
                                  Fax: 603-899-6521
                          www.hampshirecountryschool.org
                        office@hampshirecountyschool.net
William Dickerman, Director of Admissions
Bernd Focking, Headmaster
Katherine Focking, Summer Camp Director
Hampshire Country School is a small boarding school for middle-school students with Asperger's Syndrome, Nonverbal Learning Disabilities and Attention Deficit Hyperactivity Disorder. Faculty to student ratio is 2:3.

4165 Parent Information Center

151-A Manchester Street
Concord, NH 03301   603-224-7005
                                      800-947-7005
                                  Fax: 603-224-4365
                                  TDD: 800-947-7005
                          www.parentinformationcenter.org
                        picinfo@parentinformationcenter.org
Michelle Lewis, PIC Executive Director
Sylvia Abbott, Administrative Supervisor
Jennifer Cunha, Project Coordinator
Parent Training and Information Program views parents as full partners in the educational process and a significant source of support and assistance to each other. Funded by the Division of Personnel Preparation, Office of Special Education Programs, these programs provide training and information to parents to enable such individuals to participate more effectively with professionals in meeting the educational needs of children with disabilities.

New Jersey

4166 Bancroft
425 Kings Highway East
P.O. Box 20
Haddonfield, NJ 08033-0018

856-429-0010
800-774-5516
Fax: 856-429-1613
TTY: 856-428-2697
www.bancroft.org
lynn.tomaio@bancroft.org

Toni Pergolin, President
Nonprofit organization offering educational/vocational programs, therapeutic support services and full range of community living opportunities for children and adults with brain injury in Maine, New Jersey, Delaware, and Louisiana. Residential options include community living supervised apartments, specialized supervised apartments, group homes and supported living models.

4167 ECLC of New Jersey
Ho-Ho-Kus Campus
302 North Franklin Turnpike
Ho-Ho-Kus, NJ 07423-1040

201-670-7880
Fax: 201-670-6675
www.eclcofnj.org
vlindorff@eclofnj.org

Vicki Lindorff, Principal
A private school for individuals with disabilities between the ages of 5-21. Our mission is to help disabled students discover how they fit into the world and guide them towards becoming independent and employed adults.

4168 Eden Autism Services
One Eden Way
Princeton, NJ 08540-5711

609-987-0099
Fax: 609-987-0243
www.edenservices.org

Tom Mc Cool, President
Nonprofit organization founded in 1975 to provide a comprehensive continuum of lifespan services for individuals with autism and their families.

4169 Family Resource Associates, Inc.
35 Haddon Ave
Shrewsbury, NJ 07702-4007

732-747-5310
Fax: 732-747-1896
www.frainc.org
info@frainc.org

Nancy Phalanukorn, Executive Director
Michael Bell, President
Bill Sheeser, Vice President
A New Jersey non-profit agency dedicated to helping individuals with disabilities and their families.

4170 Forum School
107 Wyckoff Ave
Waldwick, NJ 07463-1795

201-444-5882
Fax: 201-444-4003
www.theforumschool.com
info@theforumschool.com

Brian Detlefsen, Director
Linda Oliver, Office Manager
Lourdes Wimer, Business Secretary
Special education day school for developmentally children. The Forum School offers a therapeutic education environment for children who cannot be accommodated in a public school setting.

4171 Georgian Court University
The Learning Center (TLC)
900 Lakewood Ave
Lakewood, NJ 08701-2697

732-987-2659
800-458-8422
Fax: 732-987-2026
www.georgian.edu
admissions@georgian.edu

William J. Behre, Provost
Evelyn Saul Quinn, Vice President
John McAuliffe, VP Enrollment Management
The Learning Center is an assistance program designed to provide an environment for students with mild to moderate learning disabilities who desire a college education. The program is not one of remediation, but it is an individualized support program to assist candidates in becoming successful college students. Emphasis is placed on developing self-help strategies, study techniques, content tutoring, time management, organization skills, and social skills all taught by a certified professional.

4172 Huntington Learning Centers, Inc.
496 Kinderkamack Road
Oradell, NJ 07649

201-261-8400
800-653-8400
http://raleigh.huntingtonhelps.com
franchise@hlcmail.com

Mike Gallagher, President
Huntington Learning Center helps target your child's unique needs through diagnostic testing so they could better achieve their grades.

4173 Matheny Medical and Educational Center
65 Highland Avenue
P.O. Box 339
Peapack, NJ 07977-0339

908-234-0011
Fax: 908-719-2137
www.matheny.org
info@matheny.org

Steve Proctor, President
Daniel McLaughlin, Chair
William A. Krais, Esq., Vice Chair
Matheny School and Hospital is a special educational facility and hospital for children and adults with medically complex developmental disabilities. The school provides comprehensive educational programs and functional life skills for children and young adults ages 3-21.

4174 Newgrange School
526 South Olden Avenue
Hamilton, NJ 08629-2101

609-584-1800
Fax: 609-584-6166
www.thenewgrange.org
info@thenewgrange.org

Gordon Sherman, Ph.D., Executive Director
Deardra Rosenberg, Director of Education
Ted Varias, Assistant Director
Newgrange is a non-profit organization established in 1977 to provide specialized educational programs for students with language based learning disabilities.

4175 SEARCH Day Program
73 Wickapecko Dr
Ocean, NJ 07712-4100

732-531-0454
Fax: 732-531-5934
www.searchdayprogram.com
info@searchdayprogram.com

Katherine Solana, Executive Director
SEARCH Day Program is a private, non-profit, New Jersey State certified agency serving children and adults with autism and their families.

4176 Statewide Parent Advocacy Network
Central Office
35 Halsey Street
Fourth Floor
Newark, NJ 07102-3000

973-642-8100
800-654-7726
Fax: 973-642-8080
www.spanadvocacy.org

Diane Autin, Executive Co Director
Debra Jennings, Executive Co Director

A nonprofit educational and advocacy center for parents of children from birth to 21 years of age. Assists families of infants, toddlers, children and youth with and without disabilities. Serves as a vehicle for the exchange of ideas, promoting awareness of the abilities and needs of the children and youth and improves services for children and families in the state of NJ.

4177 The Center School
2 Riverview Drive
Somerset, NJ 08873 908-253-3870
Fax: 908-685-8043
www.thecenterschool.com
John Ryan, Director
A school designed for bright students in grades 1-12 with learning and behavioral difficulties. The Center School offers counseling, speech and language, and occupational therapy. Our school is committed to helping each student become as self-sufficient and successful as possible.

4178 The Children's Institute
1 Sunset Ave
Verona, NJ 07044-5118 973-509-3050
Fax: 973-509-3060
www.tcischool.org
Bruce Ettinger, Executive Director
Michael J. Reimer, President
Richard M. Kaplan, Vice President
The Children's Institute is a private, non-profit school approved by the New Jersey State Board of Education, serving children facing learning, language and social challenges.

4179 The Craig School
10 Tower Hill Rd
Mountain Lakes, NJ 07046 973-334-1295
Fax: 973-334-1299
www.craigschool.org
info@craigschool.org
Grant L. Jacks, Head of School
Eric M. Caparulo, D.Ed., Director
Karen Meisinger, Chief Financial Officer
The Craig School is an independent, nonprofit school serving children who have difficulty succeeding in the traditional classroom environment. We specialize in a language-based curriculum for children of average or above average intelligence with such disorders as dyslexia, auditory processing and attention deficit.

4180 The Lewis School and Clinic for Educational Therapy
53 Bayard Ln
Princeton, NJ 08540-3028 609-924-8120
Fax: 609-924-5512
www.lewisschool.org
Marsha Lewis, Executive Director
The Clinic and School integrate teaching and diagnostic perspective of multisensory educational practices in the classrooms, and the perspective of clinical research into the brain's learning process.

4181 The Midland School
94 Readington Road
PO Box 5026
North Branch, NJ 08876 908-722-8222
Fax: 908-722-6203
www.midlandschool.org
info@midlandschool.org
Philip Gartlan, Executive Director
Barbara Darkan, Principal
A New Jersey approved non-profit school for children, ages 5-21 with developmental disabilities. Serving approx 210 students from public school districts throughout Northern and Central New Jersey. Midland provides a comprehensive special education program serving the individual social, emotional, academic and career education needs of its students.

4182 The Newgrange Education Center
407 Nassau Street at Cedar Lane
Princeton, NJ 08540 609-688-1280
Fax: 609-430-3030
www.thenewgrange.org
info@thenewgrange.org
Gordon Sherman, Ph.D., Executive Director
Bob Hegedus, Principal
Deardra Rosenburg, Director of Education/Supervisor
Meets the educational and specialized needs of individuals with learning disabilities and their families. The center offers tutoring, educational evaluations and professional development opportunities.

New Mexico

4183 Designs for Learning Differences Sycamore School
8600 Academy Rd NE
Albuquerque, NM 87111-1107 505-822-0476
Fax: 505-858-4427
www.dldsycamoreschool.com
dldschool1@aol.com
Linda Murray, Principal
A private, non-profit school, serving children and young adults in grades 1-12 with learning difficulties.

4184 EPICS Parent Project
Abrazos Family Support Services
P.O.Box 788
Bernalillo, NM 87004-0788 505-867-3396
Fax: 505-867-3398
www.swcr.org
info@abrazosnm.org
Martha Gorospe, Director
Norm Segel, Executive Director
Provides a variety of specialized educational programs, health, developmental and parent support programs for infants, children & adults with developmental delays or disabilities.

4185 Parents Reaching Out Network
1920 Columbia Drive Southeast
Albuquerque, NM 87106-3307 505-247-0192
800-524-5176
Fax: 505-247-1345
www.parentsreachingout.org
info@parentsreachingout.org
Sallie Van Curen, Executive Director
PRO views parents as full partners in the educational process and a significant source of support and assistance to each other. Programs provide training and information to parents to enable such individuals to participate more effectively with professionals in meeting the educational needs of disabled children.

New York

4186 Advocates for Children of New York
151 West 30th Street
5th Floor
New York, NY 10001-4197 212-947-9779
Fax: 212-947-9790
www.advocatesforchildren.org
info@advocatesforchildren.org
Kim Sweet, Executive Director
Matthew Lenaghan, Deputy Director
Melissa Atkinson, Administrative Assistant
Advocates for Children of New York, has worked in partnership with New York City's most impoverished and vulnerable families to secure quality and equal public education services. AFC works on behalf of children from infancy to age 21 who have disabilites, ethnic minorities, immigrants, homeless children, foster care children, limited English proficient children and those living in poverty.

4187 Anderson Center for Autism
4885 Route 9
P.O. Box 367
Staatsburg, NY 12580-0367
845-889-4034
Fax: 845-889-3104
www.andersoncenterforautism.org
Niel Pollack, Executive Director
Patrick D. Paul, Chief Operating Officer
Tina M. Chirico, Chief Financial Officer
The Anderson Center for Autism provides the highest quality programs for children and adults with autism and other developmental disabilities.

4188 Andrus Children's Center
1156 N Broadway
Yonkers, NY 10701-1196
914-965-3700
800-647-2301
Fax: 914-965-3883
http://andruscc.org
Mimi Clarke Corcoran, President,CEO
Bryan Murphy, Vice President and COO
Tito Del Pilar, VP Human Resources
For more than 75 years, Andrus has been a provider of programs and services for children and families with learning disabilities.

4189 Baker Victory Services
780 Ridge Rd
Lackawanna, NY 14218-1629
716-828-9500
888-287-1160
www.bakervictoryservices.org
ourladyofvictory.org
James J Casion, Executive Director
Paul J.E. Burkard, President
BVS offers a wide range of services for individuals with physical, developmental, and/or behavorial challenges. In addition, programming which supplies a lifetime of care; from infancy to late adulthood.

4190 Center for Spectrum Services
Special Education Program
4 Yankee Place
Ellenville, NY 12428-1510
845-647-6464
Fax: 845-647-3456
www.centerforspectrumservices. org
questions@centerforspectrumservices.org
Marjorie S. Rovereto, President
Rick Regan, Vice President
Robert S. Casey, Treasurer
Provides educational programs, diagnostic evaluations and clinical services to children ages 2 to 12 with autism and Asperger Syndrome.

4191 EAC Nassau Learning Center
50 Clinton Street
Suite 107
Hempstead, NY 11050-3136
516-539-0150
Fax: 516-539-0160
www.eacinc.org
Jerry Stone, Executive Director
Lance W. Elder, President/CEO
Rebecca Bell, EVP, COO
The purpose of EAC Learning Center is to help junior and senior high schools students who cannot function in a regular school environment obtain the necessary education which will make it possible for them to graduate from high school. EAC's first program, the Long Island Learning Centers have been serving learning disabled and emotionally disturbed students since 1971.

4192 Eden II Programs
150 Granite Ave
Staten Island, NY 10303-2718
718-816-1422
Fax: 718-816-1428
www.eden2.org
jgerenser@eden2.org

Donald M. Russo, Vice Chair
Gregg Iliceto, CPA, Treasurer
Jim Caldarella, Secretary
The mission of the Eden II/Genesis Programs is to provide people with autism specialized community-based programs and other opportunities, with the goal of enabling them to achieve the highest possible quality of living across life

4193 Hallen School
97 Centre Ave
New Rochelle, NY 10801-7212
914-636-6600
Fax: 914-633-4294
www.thehallenschool.net
info@thehallenschool.net
Angela Radogna, Executive Director
Hallen School is a private, special education school that serves children who exhibit learning disabilities, speech and language impairments, emotional difficulties, autistic features, and mid-health impairments.

4194 International Center for the Disabled
123 William Street
Floor 5
New York, NY 10038
212-585-6009
Fax: 212-585-6262
TTY: 212-585-6060
www.icdnyc.org
ssegal@icdrehab.org
Justin B. Wender, Chair
Dr. Richard Weber, Vice Chair
Dr. Les Halpert, President & CEO
Serving children, adolescents, adults, and seniors with disabilities and other rehabilitative and developmental needs.

4195 Julia Dyckman Andrus Memorial
Andrus Children's Center
1156 N Broadway
Yonkers, NY 10701-1108
914-965-3700
Fax: 914-965-3883
http://andruscc.org
Mimi Clarke Corcoran, President,CEO
Bryan Murphy, Vice President and COO
Tito Del Pilar, VP Human Resources
Residential treatment for youngsters who have moderate to severe emotional problems.

4196 Just Kids: Early Childhood Learning Center
35 Longwood Road
P.O. Box 12
Middle Island, NY 11953-0012
631-924-0008
Fax: 631-924-4602
www.kidsschool.com
jkiep@optonline.net
Robin Stevens, Program Director
Offers developmentally appropriate curriculum to young children, ages birth to five years of age, who are disabled and non-disabled. Offers infant/toddler programs, pre-school education programs, mental health services, speech and language therapy and physical and occupational therapy services.

4197 Karafin School
PO Box 277
Mount Kisco, NY 10549-0277
914-666-9211
Fax: 914-666-9868
www.karafinschool.com
karafin@optonline.net
Bart A Donow PhD, Direector
Private school serving students with disabilities in grades 9-12.

4198 Kildonan School
425 Morse Hill Rd
Amenia, NY 12501-5209
845-373-8111
Fax: 845-373-9793
www.kildonan.org
admissions@kildonan.org

Christina Lang, Chair
Richard S. Berg, Vice-Chair
Bruce Karsk, Treasurer
Offers a fully accredited College Preparatory curriculum. The school is co-educational, enrolling boarding students in Grades 6-Postgraduate and day students in Grade 2-Postgraduate. Provides daily one-on-one Orton-Gillingham tutoring to build skills in reading, writing, and spelling. Daily independent reading and writing work reinforces skills and improves study habits. Interscholastic sports, horseback riding, clubs and community service enhance self-confidence.

4199 Maplebrook School
5142 Route 22
Amenia, NY 12501-5357   845-373-9511
                                  Fax: 845-373-7029
                              www.maplebrookschool.org
                              admin@maplebrookschool.org
Mark J. Metzger, Chairman
Robert Audia, Vice-Chairman
George T. Whalen, Jr., Treasurer
A traditional boarding school enrolling students with learning differences and ADD. Offers strong academics and character development.

4200 Mary McDowell Friends School
20 Bergen St
Brooklyn, NY 11201-6302   718-625-3939
                                  Fax: 718-625-1456
                                www.marymcdowell.org
                              debbiez@marymcdowell.org
Debbie Zlotowitz, Executive Director
An independent friends school for children with learning disabilities ages 5-12.

4201 New Interdisciplinary School
430 Sills Rd
Yaphank, NY 11980   631-924-5583
                                  Fax: 631-924-5687
                                   www.niskids.org
                                   info@niskids.org
Jay Silverstein, Ph.D., Executive Director
Susan Cali, Director of Development
Theresa Mahoney, Director of Special Education
Offers educational and therapeutic services to children with disabilities from birth to five years of age.

4202 New York Institute for Special Education
999 Pelham Pkwy N
Bronx, NY 10469-4905   718-519-7000
                                  Fax: 718-231-9314
                                   www.nyise.org
Bernadette Kappen, Executive Director
Kim M. Benisatto, Operations Manager
Maria Grullon, Director of Fiscal Affairs
Educational facility that provides quality programs for children who are blind or visually impaired, emotionally/learning disabled or developmentally delayed. Students ages 3 to 21 attend NYISE. The school offers residential and day programs, physical, occupational and speech-language therapy, career guidance and couseling.

4203 Parent Network of WNY
1000 Main St
Buffalo, NY 14202-1102   716-332-4170
                                      866-277-4762
                                  Fax: 716-332-4171
                                www.parentnetworkwny.org
                              info@parentnetworkwny.org
Susan Barlow, Executive Director
Gary Pochatko, Business Manager
Peg Kovach, Administrative Assistant

A non-profit agency with the mission of parents helping parents and professionals enable individuals with disabilities to reach their own potential. Parent Network provides parents/caregivers of children with special needs, the tools necessary to allow them to take an active role in their child's education. this is accomplished through: information and referral services, workshops and conferences on various special education topics, library and resource materials, website & bimonthly newsletter.

4204 Program for Learning Disabled College Students: Adelphi University
1 South Ave
P.O. Box 701
Garden City, NY 11530-701   516-877-4710
                                      800-233-5744
                                  Fax: 516-877-4711
                                  TDD: 516-877-4777
                                   www.adelphi.edu
                                ldprogram@adelphi.edu
Robert A. Scott, President
Gayle D. Insler, Vice President
Timothy P. Burton, Treasurer

4205 Responsibility Increases Self-Esteem (RISE) Program
Maplebrook School
5142 Route 22
Amenia, NY 12501-5357   845-373-9511
                                  Fax: 845-373-7029
                              www.maplebrookschool.org
                              admin@maplebrookschool.org
Mark J. Metzger, Chairman
Robert Audia, Vice-Chairman
George T. Whalen, Jr., Treasurer
The RISE program provides the structure and support to awaken the learner in each student, promote responsibility and develop character, foster independence and growth and enhances social development.

4206 Robert Louis Stevenson School
24 W 74th St
New York, NY 10024-2497   212-787-6400
                                  Fax: 212-873-1872
                               www.stevenson-school.org
                              dherron@stevenson-school.org
Howard Spivak, Chair
Jonathan Bernstein, Treasurer
Dr. Billie Pivnick, Secretary
Serves students who are functioning below their potential, whether because of adjustment difficulties, problems with peers mild depression or anxiety. Some have been diagnosed as learning disabled or Attention Deficit Disordered, but the program is for bright under-achievers. A college preparatory school.

4207 St. Thomas Aquinas College Pathways
125 Route 340
Sparkill, NY 10976   845-398-4000
                                  Fax: 845-398-4229
                                    www.stac.edu
                                 pathways@stac.edu
Richard F. Heath, Director
James M. Calisi, Assistant Director
Comprehensive support program for selected college students with learning disabilities and/or ADHD.

4208 Stephen Gaynor School
148 W 90th St
New York, NY 10024-1202   212-787-7070
                                  Fax: 212-787-3312
                                www.stephengaynor.org
                              jmay@stephengaynor.org
Scott Gaynor, Head of School
Bianca Wright, Chief Financial Officer
Randi Simon, Administrative Assistant
The school offers a unique educational experience for children ages 5-14 with learning differences.

4209 **The Gow School**
2491 Emery Road
P.O. Box 85
South Wales, NY 14139-0085   716-652-3450
                                    Fax: 716-652-3457
                                    www.gow.org
                                    admissions@gow.org
Bradley Rogers, Principal
A boarding school for boys, grades 7-12, with dyslexia and
other language based learning disabilities.

4210 **The Norman Howard School**
275 Pinnacle Rd
Rochester, NY 14623-4103   585-334-8010
                                   Fax: 585-334-8073
                                   www.normanhoward.org
                                   info@normanhoward.org
Karen Baxter, Business & Facilities Manager
Carol Birdsall, Administrative Assistant
Patricia Dell, Chief Finance Officer
Norman Howard School is an independent day school for
students with disabilities in 5-12th grade.

4211 **Vocational Independence Program (VIP)**
NYIT/VIP
300 Carleton Ave
Central Islip, NY 11722   631-348-3354
                                   Fax: 631-348-3437
                                   www.nyit.edu/vip
                                   sincorva@nyit.edu
Dr Ernst VanBergeijk, Assoc. Dean, Executive Director
Sheree Incorvaia, Recruitment/Admissions Director
A 3-year certificate program that focuses on vocational, so-
cial, and independent living skills, with academics, that sup-
port these areas. Also offers those that qualify, the ability to
take credit courses towards a degree.

4212 **Windward School**
13 Windward Avenue
White Plains, NY 10605   914-949-6968
                                   Fax: 914-949-8220
                                   www.thewindwardschool.org
Thomas E. Flanagan, President
Michael R. Salzer, 1st Vice President
Mark A. Ellman, Treasurer
Independent school for language-based, learning disabled
students in grades 1-9.

North Carolina

4213 **Exceptional Children's Assistance Center**
907 Barra Row
Ste 102-103
Davidson, NC 28036-8103   704-892-1321
                                  800-962-6817
                                  Fax: 704-892-5028
                                  www.ecac-parentcenter.org
                                  ecac@ecacmail.org
Connie Hawkins, Executive Director
Mary LaCorte, Assistant Director
Judi Archer, Parent Educator
Parent Training and Information Program views parents as
full partners in the educational process and a significant
source of support and assistance to each other. Funded by the
Division of Personnel Preparation, Office of Special Education Programs, these programs provide training and information to parents to enable such individuals to participate more
effectively with professionals in meeting the educational
needs of disabled children.

4214 **Hill Center**
3200 Pickett Rd
Durham, NC 27705-6010   919-489-7464
                                  Fax: 919-489-7466
                                  www.hillcenter.org
                                  info@hillcenter.org

Dr. David Riddle, Chair
Dr. Nancy Farmer, Vice Chair
Ms. Beth Anderson, President
Offers a unique half-day program to students in grades K-12
with diagnosed learning disabilities and attention deficit
disorders. Also offers a comprehensive teacher training
program.

4215 **Manus Academy**
6203 Carmel Rd
Charlotte, NC 28226-8204   704-542-6471
                                  Fax: 704-541-2858
                                  www.manusacademy.com
Roseanne Manus, Owner and Program Developer
Lesley Taylor, M.Ed., Head of School
Susan Smith, M.B.A., Administrative Assistant
School for students with learning disabilties.

4216 **Manus Academy**
6203 Carmel Rd
Charlotte, NC 28226-8204   704-542-6471
                                  Fax: 704-541-2858
                                  www.manusacademy.com
Roseanne Manus, Owner and Program Developer
Lesley Taylor, M.Ed., Head of School
Susan Smith, M.B.A., Administrative Assistant
Manus Academy works with students from kindergarten
through college who experience learning disabilities, attention deficit disorder and other neurological and developmental difficulties. Their services include a middle and high
school accredited by the Southern Association for College
and Schools, after-school tutoring services for K-12 students who attend other schools, testing, consultation and
parent and teacher training

4217 **Parent Resource Center**
Hopewell High School
11530 Beatties Ford Rd
Huntersville, NC 28078   980-343-5988
                                  Fax: 980-343-5990
                                  http://pages.cms.k12.nc.us/hopewell
Dr Louise Jones, Principal

4218 **Piedmont School**
815 Old Mill Rd
High Point, NC 27265-9679   336-883-0992
                                  Fax: 336-883-4752
                                  www.thepiedmontschool.com
                                  info@thepiedmontschool.com
Sharyn Andrews, President
Allison Hudson, M.D., Vice President
Stephanie Migliardi, Secretary
Provides a unique, essential service to children with learning
disabilites and/or an attention deficit disorder.

North Dakota

4219 **Anne Carlsen Center for Children**
701 3rd St NW
P.O. Box 8000
Jamestown, ND 58402   701-252-3850
                                  800-568-5175
                                  Fax: 701-952-5154
                                  http://annecarlsen.org
Marcia Gums, President
Offers education, therapy, medical care and social and psy-
chological services for children and young adults with spe-
cial needs.

Ohio

4220 Bellefaire Jewish Children's Bureau
22001 Fairmount Blvd
Shaker Heights, OH 44118-4819   216-932-2800
800-879-2522
Fax: 216-932-6704
www.bellefairejcb.org
info@bellefairejcb.org
Adam Jacobs, President
Residential treatment center for adolescents, offering foster care, an adoption center, Monarch School for Children with Autism.

4221 Cincinnati Center for Developmental Disorders
Cincinnati Children's Hospital Medical Center
3333 Burnet Ave
Cincinnati, OH 45229-3026   513-636-4200
800-344-2462
TTY: 513-636-4900
www.cincinnatichildrens.org
David Schonfeld, Executive Director
Established in 1957, the center provides diagnosis, evaluation, treatment, training and education for infants, children and adolescents with a variety of developmental disorders.

4222 Cincinnati Occupational Therapy Institute for Services and Study, Inc.
4440 Carver Woods Dr
Cincinnati, OH 45242-5545   513-791-5688
Fax: 513-791-0023
www.cintiotinstitute.com
Deborah Whitcomb, Executive Director
Cincinnati Occupational Therapy Institute provides evaluation and treatment directly to children and adults with occupational therapy needs. COTI is owned and operated by therapists. The therapists are uniquely skilled at helping clients of all ages achieve or regain independence by offering creative adaptations and alternatives for carrying out daily activities, as well as remediating dysfunction through appropriate therapeutic modalities.

4223 North Coast Education Services
31300 Salon Road
Suite 1
Solon, OH 44139-2718   440-914-0200
Fax: 440-542-1504
www.northcoastcd.com
info@northcoasted.com
Carole Richards, Executive Director
Pamela Morton, Bookkeeper
Sharon Miles, BS, MA, Site Manager
Provides on-site education services to individual learners or groups. Uppermost in the delivery of these services is the development of self-esteem, expanding learner potential and utilizing problem-solving to identify strengths and weaknesses. Specializing in working with at-risk learners which include learning disabled students.

4224 Ohio Center for Autism and Low Incidence
470 Glenmont Avenue
Columbus, OH 43214   614-410-0321
866-886-2254
Fax: 614-262-1070
TTY: 614-410-1076
www.ocali.org
ocali@ocali.org
Shawn A Henry, Executive Director
Sheila Smith, Assistant Director
Heather Bridgman, Regional Consultant
Serves parents and educators of students with autism and low incidence disabilities including Autism spectrum disorders, Deaf-blindness, Deafness and hearing impairments, Multiple disabilities, Orthopedic impairments, Other health impairments, Traumatic brain injuries, and Visual impairments.

4225 Ohio Coalition for the Education of Children with Disabilities
165 W Center St
Ste 302
Marion, OH 43302-3741   740-382-5452
800-374-2806
Fax: 740-383-6421
www.ocecd.org
ocecd@ocecd.org
Margaret Burley, Executive Director
Lee Ann Derugen, Co-Director
Joy Albert, Executive Assistant
Non-profit parent training and information center serving Ohio families. Services are free.

4226 RICHARDS READ Systematic Language
North Coast Tutoring Services
31300 Solon Road
Suite 1
Solon, OH 44139   440-914-0200
800-335-7984
Fax: 440-542-1504
www.northcoasted.com
info@northcoasted.com
Carole Richards, Executive Director
Pamela Morton, Bookkeeper
Sharon Miles, BS, MA, Site Manager
North Coast Tutoring Services strives to provide on-site education services to individual learners or groups. Uppermost in the delivery of these services is the development of self-esteem, expanding learner potential and utilizing problem-solving to identify strengths and weaknesses. We specialize in working with at-risk learners which include learning disabled students. Our systematic language program is extremely successful with language learning difficulties from age 5 to adult.

4227 Springer School and Center
2121 Madison Rd
Cincinnati, OH 45208-3288   513-871-6080
Fax: 513-871-6428
www.springer-ld.org
info@springer.hccanet.org
Shelly Weisbacher, Executive Director
Carmen Mendoza, Admissions Director
Ginny Heitzman, Business Director
Springer School and Center is the only organization in the Greater Cincinnati area whose program is devoted entirely to the education of children with learning disabilities.

4228 The Children's Home Of Cincinnati
5050 Madison Road
Cincinnati, OH 45227-2784   513-272-2800
www.thechildrenshomecinti.org
Ellen Katz Johnson, President & CEO
Helps chldren with social, behavioral and learning challenges by helping them build the skills and confidence that they need in life to succeed in school, home, and the community.

Oregon

4229 Thomas A Edison High School
9020 SW Beaverton-Hillsdale Hwy
Portland, OR 97225-2436   503-297-2336
Fax: 503-297-2527
www.taedisonhs.org
thomasedison@taedisonhs.org
Patrick Maguire, Principal
A private high school in Oregon specifically designed to meet the needs of students with complex learning disabilities and attention deficit disorder issues. Thomas Edison High School empowers students with learning differences to experience academic success and personal growth, while preparing them for the future.

Pennsylvania

4230 Center for Alternative Learning
6 East Eagle Road
Havertown, PA 19083
610-446-6126
800-869-8336
www.learningdifferences.com
rcooper-ldr@comcast.net
Dr Richard Cooper, Ph.D., President
The Center for Alternative Learning was founded in 1987 to provide low cost and free educational services to individuals with learning differences, problems and disabilities.

4231 Center for Psychological Services
125 Coulter Ave
Ardmore, PA 19003-2410
610-642-4873
Fax: 610-642-4886
www.centerpsych.com
center12@verizon.net
Moss Jackson PhD, Director
Bruce V. Miller, Ph.D., Director
Charna Axelrod, Director
Individual, family and group therapy psychoeducational evaluation and school consultation.

4232 Devereux Center for Autism
Devereux New Jersey
444 Devereux Drive
Villanova, PA 19085
800-345-1292
www.devereux.org
Robert Q. Kreider, President and CEO
Margaret McGill, Senior Vice President, COO
Robert C. Dunne, Senior VP, CFO, Treasurer
Addressing the particular needs of children, adolescents and adults with Autism Spectrum Disorders, the center offers residential, educational and vocational programs. All programs are geared to reaching these individuals, helping them overcome challenging behaviors, and teaching them crucial life skills.

4233 Devereux Mapleton
Devereux Foundation
444 Devereux Drive
P.O. Box 638
Villanova, PA 19085
800-345-1292
www.devereux.org
Robert Q. Kreider, President and CEO
Margaret McGill, Senior Vice President, COO
Robert C. Dunne, Senior VP, CFO, Treasurer
Residential and in-patient program for children, adolescents and young adults with emotional disorders and learning disabilities.

4234 Dr Gertrude A Barber Center
Barber National Institute
100 Barber Place
136 East Avenue
Erie, PA 16507-1899
814-453-7661
Fax: 814-455-1132
www.barberinstitute.org
BNIerie@barberinstitute.org
John Barber, President and CEO
Maureen Barber-Carey, Ed.D., Executive Vice President
Gary Bukowski, Vice President for Advancement
Offers a complete range of educational services and support to children and adults with disabilities.

4235 Hill Top Preparatory School
737 South Ithan Avenue
Rosemont, PA 19010-1197
610-527-3230
Fax: 610-527-7683
www.hilltopprep.org
headmaster@hilltopprep.org
Tom Needham, Principal
Lex Nugent, Business Manager
Cindy Falcone, Asst. Head of Program
Preparatory School for bright students in grades five through twelve with learning disabilities.

4236 Hillside School
2697 Brookside Rd
Macungie, PA 18062-9045
610-967-3701
Fax: 610-965-7683
www.hillsideschool.org
office@hillsideschool.org
Donna Henry, Head of School
Darlene Stack, Business Manager
Jane Hottenstein, Administrative Assistant
A day school for children with learning differences. One hundred and twenty-eight children in grades K-6 attend the school. Scholarships are available.

4237 KidsPeace Orchard Hills Campus
4085 Independence Drive
Schnecksville, PA 18078
800-257-3223
www.kidspeace.org
Richard Zelko, President
Offers various programs including community residential care, specialized group homes, child and family guidance center and student assistance programs.

4238 Melmark
2600 Wayland Rd
Berwyn, PA 19312-2313
610-325-4969
888-MEL-MARK
www.melmark.org
admissions@melmark.org
Joanne Gillis-Donovan, President and CEO
H. Robert Marcus, Chairman
Eric Zee, Finance Chair
Provides residential, educational, therapeutic and recreational services for children and adults with mild to severe developmental disabilities.

4239 Parent Education Network
2107 Industrial Hwy
York, PA 17402-2223
717-600-0100
800-522-5827
Fax: 717-600-8101
TDD: 800-522-5827
TTY: 800-522-5827
www.parentednet.org
lspaar@parentednet.org
Kay Lipsitz, Director
Dawn Kauffman, Parent Support Coordinator
Rose Yingling, Fiscal/Administrative Assistant
Parent training and information center of Pennsylvania. Serves parents of all special needs children, birth to adulthood, to attain appropriate educational and support services by providing specific knowledge of state and federal laws and regulations; develops and disseminates material explaining the special education process and its relationship to other systems.

4240 Pathway School
162 Egypt Rd
Jeffersonville, PA 19403-3090
610-277-0660
Fax: 610-539-1973
www.pathwayschool.org
Bill O'Flanagan, President
Diana Phifer, Director Of Admissions
Louise Robertson, Vice President for Development
Provides day and residential programming for individuals ages 5-21, who have learning disabilities, neurological impairments and neuropsychiatric disorder. Special education, counseling, speech and language therapy, reading therapy, and other specialized services are provided in a small, warm and supportive atmosphere.

4241 Stratford Friends School
2 Bishop Hollow Road
Newtown Square, PA 19073
610-355-9580
Fax: 610-355-9585
www.stratfordfriends.org
info@stratfordfriends.org

Lydia Driscoll, Development Associate
Donna Giaquinto, School Secretary
Tim Madigan, Head
A Quaker elementary school for children with language-based learning differences who have had difficulty learning in a traditional classroom.

4242 The Children's Institute
1405 Shady Ave
Pittsburgh, PA 15217-1350   412-420-2400
                                   www.amazingkids.org

Michael J. Hannon, Chair
J. Keefe Ellis Jr., Vice Chair
Lisa C. Fagan, Secretary
Provides pediatric and adult rehabilitation services and programs.

4243 Vanguard School
1777 North Valley Road
P.O. Box 730
Paoli, PA 19355   610-296-6700
                          Fax: 610-640-0132
                          www.vfes.net

Tim Krushinski, Director
Helene Greenstein, Program Supervisor
Janet McDowell, Administrative Asst.
State licensed and approved private, non-profit, non-sectarian day school serving children from three to twenty-one years of age who have been diagnosed with neurological disorders, emotional disturbance or autism/PDD.

4244 Woods Schools
Woods Services
Route 413 & 213
P.O. Box 36
Langhorne, PA 19047-0036   215-750-4000
                                   Fax: 215-750-4591
                                   www.woods.org
                                   info@woods.org

Diana L. Ramsay, President and CEO
Peter M. Shubiak, Executive Vice President and COO
Timothy Graham, Vice President, Finance and CFO
Provides a full range of residential, special education, rehabilitation, recreation and vocational training to children and adults with Autism Spectru Disorder, Developmental Disabilities, Neurological Disorders, Traumatic Brain Injuries and Emotional Disturbances.

Rhode Island

4245 Harmony Hill School
63 Harmony Hill Rd
Chepachet, RI 02814-1429   401-949-0690
                                   Fax: 401-949-4412
                                   TDD: 401-949-4130
                                   www.harmonyhillschool.org
                                   djackson@hhs.org

Eric James, President and CEO
John Dooley, Chief Financial Officer
Jean Fallago, Treasurer
A private residential and day treatment center for behaviorally disordered and learning disabled boys, age eight through eighteen, who cannot be treated within their local educational system or community based mental health programs. Individual, group and family psychotherapy and 24-hour crisis intervention are available. Other programs include: Extended Day, Sex Offender, Diagnostic Day, Transition Programming, Summer Day, Career Education Center, and a Formalized Life Skills Program.

4246 Rhode Island Parent Information Network
1210 Pontiac Avenue
Cranston, RI 02920   401-270-0101
                             800-464-3399
                             Fax: 401-270-7049
                             TDD: 800-464-3399
                             www.ripin.org
                             info@ripin.org

Kathleen DiChiara, Chair
Ammala Douangsavanh, Vice Chair
Stephen Brunero, Executive Director
Rhode Island Parent Information Network is a statewide, nonprofit organization that provides eleven programs and services to families with children in RI, including families of children with special needs due to disabilities.

South Carolina

4247 Parents Reaching Out to Parents of South Carolina
652 Bush River Rd
Ste 203
Columbia, SC 29210-7537   803-772-5688
                                  800-759-4776
                                  Fax: 803-772-5341
                                  www.proparents.org
                                  proparents@proparents.org
Mary Eaddy, Executive Director
Private nonprofit parent oriented organization providing information, individual assistance and workshops to parents of children with disabilities ages birth-21. Services focus on enabling parents to have a better understanding of special education to participate more effectively with professionals in meeting the educational needs of disabled children. Funded by a grant from the US Department of Education and tax deductible contributions.

4248 Trident Academy
1455 Wakendaw Rd
Mt Pleasant, SC 29464-9767   843-884-7046
                                     Fax: 843-881-8320
                                     www.tridentacademy.com
                                     cnewton@tridentacademy.com
Mike Jeresaty, President
Sandi Clerici, Vice President
Eddie Street, Secretary
Trident Academy is for students with specific learning disabilities; offering an intensive, effective, multi-sensory program to remediate learning differences, tailored to each student's unique needs.

Tennessee

4249 Bodine School
2432 Yester Oaks Dr
Germantown, TN 38139-6400   901-754-1800
                                    Fax: 901-751-8595
                                    www.bodineschool.org
                                    communications@bodineschool.org
Imad Abdullah, Board Member
Allison Cates, Board Member
Douglas Dunavant, Board Member
The Bodine School has provided students with language based learning disabilities a nurturing environment and a challenging academic curriculum for the last 30 years. The Bodine School program is designed specifically for the dyslexic student and is based on current research findings on reading and reading disorders.

4250 Devereux Genesis Learning Centers
Genesis Learning Centers
430 Allied Dr
Nashville, TN 37211-3304   615-832-4222
                                   Fax: 615-832-4577
                                   www.genesislearn.org
                                   admin@genesislearn.org

Terance Adams, Executive Director
Chuck Goon, Human Resource Director
Day school and treatment programs for adolescents and young adults who have emotional disorders and learning disabilities.

4251   Genesis Learning Centers
430 Allied Dr
Nashville, TN 37211-3304
615-832-4222
Fax: 615-832-4577
www.genesislearn.org
admin@genesislearn.org
Terance Adams, Executive Director
Chuck Goon, Human Resource Director
Genesis Learning Centers offer special educational services to children and youth with distinctive needs, including emotional and behavioral disorders, learning disabilities, mental retardation, developmental delays, and short-term severe illness, physical challenges, or misconduct.

Texas

4252   Achievers' Center for Education
University United Methodist Church
5084 De Zavala Rd
San Antonio, TX 78249-2025
210-690-7359
Fax: 210-690-7307
www.achieverscenterforeducation.org
info@uchurch.tv
Roger Tetro, Chief Operating Officer
Stacey Arington, Program Assistant
Educational program for children and young adults in 6th through 8th grade who are behind academically due to dyslexia or other learning disabilities.

4253   Bridges Academy
4320 N. Stanton
El Paso, TX 79902-4506
915-532-6647
Fax: 915-532-8767
www.bridgesacademy.org
info@bridgesacademy.org
Irma Keys, Executive Director
Jesus Arreola, Assistant Director
Phillis Lane, Development Director
Private School for students with learning disabilities.

4254   Bright Students Who Learn Differently
Winston School
5707 Royal Ln
Dallas, TX 75229-5536
214-691-6950
Fax: 214-691-1509
www.winston-school.org
info@winston-school.org
Nancy W. Furney, Chair
Robert S. Hays, Treasurer
Melissa Ruman Stewart, Secretary
The environment and curriculum of The Winston School are designed for bright students who learn differently. Through Winston's Testing and Evaluation Center, students are assessed and teachers are provided with the learning profiles, training, and resources needed to respond to the needs of each student.

4255   Camelot Of Kingston
The Camelot Schools
7500 Rialto Blvd.
Suite 260
Austin, TX 78735
512-858-9900
www.cameloteducation.org
Paul Hickling, Executive Director
Tammy Kropp, Principal
Accepts children ages 4-17 who have been referred by area school systems. The campus includes a horsebarn and pasture, in ground swimming pool, playground areaas and pet therapy dogs.

4256   Camelot School: Palatine Campus
7500 Rialto Blvd. Building I
Suite 260
Austin, TX 78735
512-858-9900
Fax: 512-858-9901
www.cameloteducation.org
info@cameloteducation.org
Todd Bock, CEO & President
Joseph Carter, COO
Chris Friedrichs, CFO
Programs offered by the center are the Residential Treatment Center and the Therapeutic Day School. These programs provide effective clinical treatment, and are highly successful in transitioning children back home to their families, or home school environment.

4257   Crisman School
2455 N Eastman Rd
Longview, TX 75605-4057
903-758-9741
Fax: 903-758-9767
www.crismanschool.org
Michael Purifoy, Chair
Anthony Fail, Vice Chair
Samantha Chaikin, DO FAAP, Secretary
A private school designed to meet the needs of students with learning differences and/or Attention Deficit Disorder.

4258   Gateway School
2570 NW Green Oaks Blvd
Arlington, TX 76012-5621
817-226-6222
Fax: 817-226-6225
www.gatewayschool.com
INFO@GATEWAYSCHOOL.COM
Harriet Walber, Executive Director
Lori Glovier, Chair
Tony Romanelli, Vice-Chair
Geteway School is dedicated to providing an appropriate education in a nurturing environment to individuals with learning disorders and/or attention deficit.

4259   Overton Speech & Language Center, Inc.
4763 Barwick Drive
Suite 103
Fort Worth, TX 76132-1531
817-294-8408
Fax: 817-294-8411
www.overtonspeech.net
info@overtonspeech.net
Valerie Johnston, Director
Provides speech and language therapy.

4260   Parish School
11001 Hammerly Blvd
Houston, TX 77043-1913
713-467-4696
Fax: 713-467-8341
www.parishschool.org
Nancy Bewley, Principal
Sarah Martin, Director of Admissions
Wendy Airlie, CPA, CIA, Chief Financial Officer
Offers a multi-age, language-based, developmental curriculum for children 18 months through fifth grade. Children served have communication and learning differences, but average to above average learning potential. The Parish School utilizes a classroom based therapy program implemented by certified teachers and speech/language pathologists.

4261   Partners Resource Network
1090 Longfellow Dr
Ste B
Beaumont, TX 77706-4819
409-898-4684
800-866-4726
Fax: 409-898-4869
www.partnerstx.org
partnersresource@sbcglobal.net
Janice Meyer, Executive Director
Michael Meyer, Ph.D., Co-Director
Audrey Roy, Business Manager

Statewide network of federally funded parent training and information centers. Provides servies to parents of infants, toddlers, children & youth ages brith to 26 with all types of diabilities.

4262 Scottish Rite Learning Center of Austin, Inc.
12871 N. U.S. Highway 183
Suite 105
Austin, TX 78750 512-472-1231
Fax: 512-326-1877
www.scottishritelearningcenter.org
Linda Gladden, Director
Doris Haney, Executive Director
Focuses on the evalation and treatment of dyslexia in children. The center also provides workshops, seminars and resources for educators and parents.

4263 Shelton School and Evaluation Center
Admissions Office
15720 Hillcrest Rd
Dallas, TX 75248-4161 972-774-1772
Fax: 972-991-3977
www.shelton.org
wdeppe@shelton.org
Suzanne Stell, Executive Director
Gary Webb, Chairman
Paul Neubach, M.D, Vice Chairman
A coeducational day school serving 865 students in grades Pre-K-12. The school focuses on the development of learning disabled students of average to above average intelligence, enabling them to succeed in conventional classroom settings. Services include on-site Evaluation Center for diagnostic testing, a Speech, Language and Hearing Clinic, an Early Childhood Program, Out Reach Program, open summer school and more.

4264 Starpoint School
Texas Christian University
Bailey Bldg & Palko Hall
3000 Bellaire Drive North
Fort Worth, TX 76109-0001 817-257-7660
Fax: 817-257-7480
www.sofe.tcu.edu
coe@tcu.edu
Marilyn Tolbert, Director
Melissa Garza, Academic Advisor
Diana Woolsey, Director of Certification
Provides individualized academic programs for children with learning disabilities.

Utah

4265 Mountain Plains Regional Resource Center
1780 North Research Parkway
Suite 112
Logan, UT 84341-1940 435-797-9009
Fax: 435-797-9018
TDD: 435-797-9018
www.rrfcnetwork.org
Carol.Massanari@usu.edu
Carol Massanari, Director
Norm Ames, Associate Director
Wayne Ball, Program Specialist
The center is a United States Department of Education, Office of Special Education Programs funded project that helps build the capacity of State Education Agencies and Lead Agencies in improving programs and services for infants, toddlers, children and youth with disabilities.

4266 Reid School
2965 East 3435 South
Salt Lake City, UT 84109-3087 801-590-3548
801-335-4299
Fax: 801-590-3548
www.reidschool.com
ereid@xmission.com
Dr. Ethna R. Reid, Principal
Mervin R. Reid, President

Reid School is a private, innovative center for students who need more attention with reading, writing, speaking, and language arts education.

4267 SEPS Center for Learning
2120 S 1300 E
Ste 202
Salt Lake City, UT 84106-2828 801-467-2122
Fax: 801-467-2148
www.sepslc.com
ava.eva.seps@sepslc.com
Avajane Pickering, Director
Designs educational programs that help adults and children succeed in school and life. Specializing in one-on-one tutoring in all areas for all age levels, assessment, day school and preschool programs, computer assisted cognitive and academic therapy, reading programs, summer recreation and academic programs, consultation for schools and businesses.

4268 Utah Parent Center
230 West 200 South
Suite 1101
Salt Lake City, UT 84101 801-272-1051
800-468-1160
Fax: 801-272-8907
www.utahparentcenter.org
info@utahparentcenter.org
Helen Post, Executive Director
Utah Parent Center offers free training, information, referral and assistance to parents and professionals through the provision of information, referrals, individual assistance, workshops, presentations and displays.

Vermont

4269 Stern Center for Language and Learning
183 Talcott Road
Suite 101
Williston, VT 05495-9209 802-878-2332
Fax: 802-878-0230
www.sterncenter.org
learning@sterncenter.org
Blanche Podhajski, President
Janna Osman, M.Ed., Vice President for Programs
Michael Shapiro, M.B.A., Chief Financial Officer
Founded in 1983, the center is a nonprofit organization providing comprehensive services for children and adults with learning disabilities. The Center is also an educational resource serving all of Northern New England and Northern New York State. Programs include educational testing, individual instruction, psychotherapy, school consultation, professional training for educators and a parent/professional resource library.

Virginia

4270 Accotink Alternative Learning Center
Accotink Academy
6215 Rolling Road
Springfield, VA 22152-1508 703-451-5797
Fax: 703-451-0336
www.accotinkacademy.com
preschool@accotinkacademy.com
Lexie Winsten, Educational Director
Susan Arens, Administrative Director
Educational programs for students in grades 7-12 who have learning disabilities.

4271 BRAAC - Roanoke
Blue Ridge Autism and Achievement Center
312 Whitwell Dr
Roanoke, VA 24019-2039 540-366-7399
Fax: 540-366-5523
www.achievementcenter.org
braac.roanoke@gmail.com

Angela Leonard, Executive Director
Lisa Hensley, Business Manager
Patti Cook, Administrative Director
A private day school offering many academic and educational programs for children with Autism and learning disabilities and their families.

4272 Behavioral Directions
626 Grant St
Ste I
Herndon, VA 20170-4700   703-855-4032
                                 Fax: 571-333-0292
                        www.BehavioralDirections.com
                        info@behavioraldirections.com
Jane Barbin, Ph.D, BCBA-D, Executive Director
Kirsten Kennedy, B.A., ABA, Clinic Therapist
Lauren Ross, M.Ed., Senior ABA Clinic Therapist
A resource for applied behavior analysis and behavior disorders

4273 Chesapeake Bay Academy
821 Baker Rd
Virginia Beach, VA 23462-1004   757-497-6200
                                 Fax: 757-497-6304
                                 www.cba-va.org
                            jjankowski@cba-va.org
Stanley F. Baldwin, Chair
Donald L. Glenum, III, Vice Chair
Judy T. Jankowski, Ed.D., President & Head of School
Chesapeake Bay Academy is the only accredited independent school in Southeastern Virginia specifically dedicated to providing a strong academic program and individualized instruction for bright students with LD and ADHD. With a student/teacher ratio of 5:1 a student:computer ratio of 2:1, qualified professionals tailor their techniques to individual needs, allowing students who have difficulty learning in traditional settings to finally succed.

4274 Crawford First Education
Alternative Behavioral Services
825 Crawford Pkwy
Portsmouth, VA 23704-2301   757-391-6675
                                       877-227-7000
                                 Fax: 757-391-6651
                                 www.absfirst.com
                                 info@absfirst.com
Jeff Gray, Director
Alternative education programs that are effective, comprehensive and fiscally responsible. Dedicated and committed to addressing and improving the problems of special needs students.

4275 Grafton School
Grafton, Inc.
120 Belleview Avenue
Winchester, VA 22601-1700   540-542-0200
                                       888-955-5205
                                 Fax: 540-542-1722
                                 www.grafton.org
                            admissions@grafton.org
James G. Gaynor II, CEO/President
Kent Houchins, EVP, Behavioral Health Services
Kimberly Sanders, EVP Chief Outcomes Officer
Grafton provides individualized educational and residential services and in-community supports for children, youth and adults with severe emotional disturbance, learning disabilities, mental retardation, autistic disorder, behavioral disorders, and other complex challenges, including physical disabilities.

4276 Learning Resource Center
909 First Colonial Rd
Virginia Beach, VA 23454-3111   757-428-3367
                                 Fax: 757-428-1630
                        www.learningresourcecenter.net
            Nancy.Harris-Kroll@LearningResourceCenter.net
Nancy Harris-Kroll, Director

One-on-one remedial and tutorial sessions after school during the school year and all day and evening during the summer with specialists who have masters degrees. Advocacy services for parents of students with special needs. Psychoeducational testing is available. Special study skills and SAT courses given. Gifted, average, and learning disabled students attend.

4277 Leary School Programs
Lincolnia Educational Foundation
6349 Lincolnia Rd
Alexandria, VA 22312-1500   703-941-8150
                                 Fax: 703-941-4237
                                 www.learyschool.org
                            mail@learyschool.org
Ed Schultze, President/Executive Director
Sharon Masin, Business Manager
A private, day, co-educational, special education facility that serves 130 students with emotional, learning and behavioral problems. Along with individualized academic instruction, Leary School of Virginia offers a range of supportive and therapeutic services, including physical education, recreation therapy, group counseling, individual psychotherapy and art therapy.

4278 Little Keswick School
P.O.Box 24
Keswick, VA 22947-0024   434-295-0457
                                 Fax: 434-977-1892
                        www.littlekeswickschool.net
                        lksinfo@littlekeswickschool.net
Marc J. Columbus, M.Ed., Headmaster
Terry Columbus, M.Ed., Director Of Admissions
Mark Kindler, Ed..D., Academic Coordinator
Little Keswick School is a therapeutic boarding school for 33 learning disabled and/or emotionally disturbed boys between the ages of 10 to 15 at acceptance and served through 17. IQ range accepted is below average to superior. LKS provides a structured routine in a small, nurturing environment with services that include psychotherapy, occupational therapy, speech therapy and art therapy. Five week summer session.

4279 New Community School
4211 Hermitage Rd
Richmond, VA 23227-3718   804-266-2494
                                 Fax: 804-264-3281
                                 www.tncs.org
                                 info@tncs.org
Nancy L. Foy, Head of the School
The New Community School is an independent day school specializing in college preparatory instruction and intensive remediation for dyslexic students in grades 6-12.

4280 New Vistas School
520 Eldon St
Lynchburg, VA 24501-3604   434-846-0301
                                 Fax: 434-528-1004
                        www.newvistasschool.org
                        cmorgan@newvistasschool.org
Charlotte G. Morgan, M.Ed., M.F.A., Head Of School
Lisa J. DeJarnette, Assistant Head of School
Lara Jesser, Development Director
The New Vistas School provides individualized programs for students in grades K-12 with Attention Deficit Disorder and learning disabilities.

4281 Oakwood School
7210 Braddock Rd
Annandale, VA 22003-6068   703-941-5788
                                 Fax: 703-941-4186
                        www.oakwoodschool.com
                        oakwood@oakwoodschool.com
Robert McIntyre, Chairman of the Board
Oakwood School is a private, non-profit, co-educational day school for elementary and middle school students with mild to moderate learning disabilities. Students are of average to above average potential and exhibit a discrepancy between their potential and their current level of achievement.

4282 Riverside School

2110 McRae Rd
North Chesterfield, VA 23235-2962   804-320-3465
Fax: 804-320-6146
www.riversideschool.org
info@riversideschool.org

Patricia W. De Orio, Founding Director
Elizabeth F. Edwards, President
Kathleen Miller, Vice President
Private school for children grages 1-8 with specific language based learning disabilities and Dyslexia.

Washington

4283 Children's Institute for Learning Differences

4030 86th Ave SE
Mercer Island, WA 98040-4198   206-232-8680
Fax: 206-232-9377
www.childrensinstitute.com
info@childrensinstitute.com

Eric Nordling, President
Bo Darling, Vice President & Secretary
Carrie Fannin, Executive Director
CHILD provides two therapeutic year-round day schools, serving students who learn differently and who process information and life experiences in a unique way. On-site occupational and speech therapy, individual, group and family counseling.

4284 Glen Eden Institute

19351 8th Avenue
Suite C
Poulsbo, WA 98370-8710   360-697-0125
Fax: 360-697-4712
www.glenedeninstitute.com
director@glenedeninstitute.com

Ron Seifert, Director
Offers a unique educational alternative to meet the needs of those complex students in grades k-12 who are unable to function effectively in a school system due to medical, psychological or psychiatric causes.

4285 Hamlin Robinson School

1700 East Union Street
Seattle, WA 98122   206-763-1167
Fax: 206-763-7149
www.hamlinrobinson.org
ifno@hamlinrobinson.org

Joan Beauregard, Head Of School
A nonprofit, state approved elementary day school for children with specific language disability (dyslexia), providing a positive learning environment, meeting individual needs to nurture the whole child. Small classes use the Slingerland multi-sensory classroom approach in reading, writing, spelling and all instructional areas. It helps students discover the joy of learning, build positive self-esteem, and explore their full creative potential while preparing them for the classroom.

4286 RiteCare Of Washington

Scottish Rite Masons
157 S Howard Street
Suite 310
Spokane, WA 99201   206-324-6293
Fax: 203-365-0270
www.srccld.org

John Lunt, President
Charles Davis, Vice President
Chris Baker, Director of Dev & Comm
Provides diagnostic and therapeutic services to children whose primary disorder is a severe delay in language or speech development.

4287 STOMP Specialized Training for Military Parents

6316 South 12th Street
Tacoma, WA 98465   253-565-2266
800-5-PARENT
Fax: 253-566-8052
TDD: 283-588-1741
www.stompproject.org/
pave@wapave.org

Heather Hebdon, Founder and Director
Vicki Farnsworth, Assistant Director
Luz Adriana Martinez, Training Coordinator
STOMP (Specialized Training of Military Parents) is a federally funded center established to assist military families who have children with special education or health needs.

4288 St. Christopher Academy

Jevne Academy
4141 41st Ave SW
Seattle, WA 98116-4216   206-246-9751
Fax: 253-639-3466
www.stchristopheracademy.com
jevne@stchristopheracademy.com

Darlene Jevne, Founder and Executive Director
St. Christopher Academy is a private school for learning disabled, ADD and/or academically at-risk students.

West Virginia

4289 Parent Training and Information

1701 Hamill Ave
Clarksburg, WV 26301-1666   304-624-1436
800-281-1436
Fax: 304-624-1438
TDD: 304-624-1436
www.wvpti.org
wvpti@aol.com

Pat Haberbosch, Executive Director
Provides information to parents and to professionals who work with children with disabilities.

Wisconsin

4290 Chileda Institute

1825 Victory Street
La Crosse, WI 54601-4724   608-782-6480
Fax: 608-782-6481
www.chileda.org
inquiry@chileda.org

Ruth Wiseman, President and CEO
Serves children and young adults ages 6-21 with learning disabilities. The Institute offers on-campus day school and residential programs, on/off campus summer school, after school and weekend respite programs and individualized consulting and training programs for educators and families.

Wyoming

4291 Parent Information Center of Wyoming

500 W Lott St
Ste A
Buffalo, WY 82834-1935   307-684-2277
800-660-9742
Fax: 307-684-5314
TDD: 307-684-2277
www.wpic.org
tdawson@wpic.org

Terri Dawson, Executive Director
Juanita Bybee, Outreach Parent Liaison
Janet Kinstetter, Outreach Parent Liaison

Parent Training and Information Program views parents as full partners in the educational process and a significant source of support and assistance to each other. Funded by the Division of Personnel Preparation, Office of Special Education Programs, these programs provide training and information to parents to enable such individuals to participate more effectively with professionals in meeting the educational needs of disabled children.

Centers

4292 American College Testing Program
ACT Universal Testing
PO Box 168
Iowa City, IA 52243-168
319-337-1000
Fax: 319-339-3020
www.act.org
sandy.schlote@act.org

Jon Whitmore, CEO
Janet E. Godwin, Chief of Staff
Thomas J. Goedken, CFO/EVP
Helps individuals and organizations make informed decisions about education and work. We provide information for life's transitions.

4293 Diagnostic and Educational Resources
115 Rowell Court
Suite 2
Falls Church, VA 22046-3126
703-534-5180
Fax: 703-534-5181
www.der-online.com
aspector@DER-online.com

Annette Spector, M.S. Ed., Executive Director
Elisabeth Wester, Course Coordinator
Focuses on what the child can do and builds self-esteem. Provides a full range of psychoeducational testing, parent advocacy, case management, and tutoring services. Diagnostic testing determines individual needs, which are addressed in one-on-one tutoring sessions in the child's home or school. Staff trained in LD/ADHD methodologies remediate learning disabilities and offer practical suggestions for home programs and for working with school systems.

4294 Educational Diagnostic Center at Curry College
Curry College
1071 Blue Hill Ave
Milton, MA 02186-2302
617-333-0500
Fax: 617-333-2114
www.curry.edu
curryadm@curry.edu

Jane Fidlery, Dean Of Admission
Keith Robichaud, Director Of Admission
Kenneth K. Quigley, Jr., President
A comprehensive evaluation and testing center specializing in the learning needs of adolescents and adults. The Diagnostic Center welcomes adolescents and adults in need of learning strategies, long term educational plans, and better understanding of their learning profiles.

4295 Educational Testing Service
660 Rosedale Road
Princeton, NJ 08541-0001
609-921-9000
Fax: 609-734-5410
TDD: 800-877-2540
www.ets.org
etsinfo@ets.org

Kurt M Landgraf, President
Our mission is to help advance quality and equity in education by providing fair and valid assessments, research and related services.

4296 GED Testing Service
American Council on Education
1 Dupont Cir NW
Washington, DC 20036-1193
202-939-9300
800-626-9433
Fax: 202-293-2223
www.gedtest.org
help@GEDtestingservice.com

Randy Trask, President and CEO
The American Council on Education, founded in 1918, is the nation's coordinating higher education association. ACE is dedicated to the belief that equal educational opportunity and a strong higher education system are essential cornerstones of a democratic society.

4297 Georgetown University Center for Child and Human Development
P.O.Box 571485
Washington, DC 20057-1485
202-687-5000
Fax: 202-687-8899
TTY: 202-687-5503
http://gucchd.georgetown.edu
gucdc@georgetown.edu

Phyllis R Magrab, Executive Director
To improve the quality of life for all children and youth, especially those with, or at risk for, special needs and their families.

4298 Huntington Learning Centers, Inc.
496 Kinderkamack Rd
Oradell, NJ 07649
201-261-8400
800-226-7323
www.huntingtonlearning.com

Eileen Huntington, Founder
Helps students ages 5 to 17 achieve remarkable improvements in their grades, test scores and self esteem. Builds a personalized learning program for your child based on his or her individual strenths and needs, which is identified using their in-depth diagnostic evaluation. Helps child master a skill before moving on to more difficult tasks and mor advanced learning. Helps develop the skills to learn and solve problems independently.

4299 Munroe-Meyer Institute for Genetics and Rehabilitation
University of Nebraska Medical Center
985450 Nebraska Med Center
Omaha, NE 68198-5450
402-559-6430
800-656-3937
Fax: 402-559-5737
www.unmc.edu/mmi
munroemeyer@unmc.edu

J. Michael Leibowitz, Ph.D., Director, Munroe-Meyer Inst.
Diagnostic evaluation therapy, speech, physical, occupational, behavioral therapies, pediatrics, dentistry, nursing, psychology, social work, genetics, Media Resource Center, education, nutrition. Adult services for developmentally disabled, genetic evaluation and counseling, adaptive equipment, motion analysis laboratory, recreational therapy.

4300 National Center for Fair & Open Testing FairTest
P.O. Box 300204
Jamaica Plain, MA 02130
617-477-9792
Fax: 857-350-8209
www.fairtest.org
info@fairtest.org

Dr. Sophie Sa, Chair
Monty Neill, Ed.D, Executive Director
Robert Schaeffer, Public Education Director
Dedicated to ensuring that America's students and workers are assessed using fair, accurate, relevant and open tests.

4301 Plano Child Development Center
5401 S Wentworth Ave
Ste 14A
Chicago, IL 60609-6300
773-924-5297
Fax: 773-373-3548
www.planovision.org
pcdc59@yahoo.com

Dr. Henry R. Moore, Co-Founder
Albert Pritchett, Chairperson
Linda Ford, Vice Chairperson
A multi disciplinary, not for profit optometric service or ganization that specializes in the identification, evaluation and treatment of individuals with learning related vision skills problems.

4302 Providence Speech and Hearing Center
1301 Providence Ave
Orange, CA 92868-3892

714-923-1521
855-901-7742
Fax: 714-639-2593
TTY: 714-532-4047
www.pshc.org
pshc@pshc.org

Raul Lopez, Founder
Linda Smith, CEO
Raul Lopez, COO/Director of Finance
Comprehensive services for testing and treatment of all speech, language and hearing problems. Individual and group therapy beginning with parent/infant programs.

4303 Reading Assessment System
Harcourt Achieve
222 Berkeley Street
Boston, MA 02116

617-351-5000
800-531-5015
Fax: 800-699-9459
www.steckvaughn.com
info@steckvaughn.com

Steck-Vaughn Staff, Author
Linda K. Zecher, President, CEO & Director
Eric Shuman, Chief Financial Officer
William Bayers, EVP/General Counsel
The Reading Assessment System provides an ongoing meaure of specific student's skills and offers detailed directions for individual instruction and remediation. Up to eight reports are available. This popular program generates individual scores, class scores, school scores, and district reports.

4304 Reading Group
3011A Village Office Place
Champaign, IL 61822-7674

217-351-9144
Fax: 217-351-9149
www.readinggroup.org
jbell@readinggroup.org

Penny Porter, President
Michael Campion, Vice President
Robert Warth, Treasurer
A non-profit learning center known for its work with students who have challenging learning difficulties/differences. Individualized one-on-one instruction is offered by educational specialists in reading, writing, early childhood development, giftedness, and English as a second language.

4305 Rehabilitation Resource
University Of Wisconsin - Stout
221 10th Avenue East
Room 101A
Menomonie, WI 54751

715-232-2470
800-447-8688
Fax: 715-232-5008
http://www3.uwstout.edu.com
luij@uwstout.edu

John W. Lui, Ph.D., Executive Director
Develops, publishes, and distributes a variety of rehabilitation related materials. Also makes referrals to other sources on rehabilitation.

4306 Riley Child Development Center
Indiana University School of Medicine
702 Barnhill Dr
Room 5837
Indianapolis, IN 46202-5225

317-944-8167
Fax: 317-944-9760
www.child-dev.com
info@child-dev.com

Dr. John Rau, M.D., Director
Provides an interdisciplinary evaluation for children with behanvior, learning and other developmental disabilities.

4307 Rose F Kennedy Center
Albert Einstein College of Medicine
1410 Pelham Pkwy S
Bronx, NY 10461-1116

718-430-8600
Fax: 718-892-2296
www.einsten.yu.edu.com

Steven U. Walkley, D.V.M., Ph.D., Director
John J. Foxe, Ph.D., Associate Director
Lisa L. Guillory, M.A., Administrator
Provides comprehensive diagnostic services and intervention services for children and adults with learning disabilities. The primary mission is to improve the quality of life of persons with developmental disabilites and their families.

4308 Scholastic Testing Service
480 Meyer Rd
Bensenville, IL 60106-1617

630-766-7150
800-642-6787
Fax: 630-766-8054
www.ststesting.com
sts@ststesting.com

John Kauffman, Marketing VP
Publisher of assessment materials from birth to adulthood, ability and achievement tests for kindergarten through grade twelve. Publishes the Torrance Tests of Creative Thinking, Thinking Creatively in Action and Movement, the STS High School Placement Test and Educational Development Series.

4309 Services For Students with Disabilities
PSAT/NMSQT Students With Disabilities
P.O. Box 8060
Mt. Vernon, IL 62864-0060

212-713-8333
Fax: 866-360-0114
TTY: 609-882-4118
www.collegeboard.com/ssd
ssd@info.collegeboard.org

Provides services and reasonable accommodations that are appropriate according to the type of disability and the purpose of the exam.

4310 The Center for Learning Differences
45 North Station Plaza
Great Neck, NY 11201

646-775-6646
www.centerforlearningdifferences.org
syellin@yellincenter.com

Susan Denberg Yellin J.D., Chairman/Executive Director
Stuart Rothman, PhD
Herman Davidovicz, PhD
A not-for-profit organization dedicated to providing information to families, physicians and other professionals in the New York metropolitan area about issues they face in dealing with children and parents of children who struggle in school with the hope that others can benefit from their experiences and the information they have learned. And by sharing your experinces with them, they hope to make them available to other families who are dealing with similar issues.

Behavior & Self Esteem

4311 BASC Monitor for ADHD
Pearson Assessments
4940 Pearl East Circle
Suite 200
Boulder, CO 80301

888-977-7900
800-328-5999
Fax: 888-556-2103
www.pearsonassessments.com
info@pearsonkt.com

Randy W Kamphaus, Author
Cecil R Reynolds, Co-Author
Doug Kubach, Group President & CEO
The BASC Monitor for ADHD is a powerful new tool to help evaluate the effectiveness of ADHD treatments using teacher and parent rating scales, and database software for tracking behavior changes.

4312 Behavior Assessment System for Children
Pearson Assessments
4940 Pearl East Circle
Suite 200
Boulder, CO 80301   888-977-7900
                                             800-328-5999
                                        Fax: 888-556-2103
                                   www.pearsonassessments.com
                                        info@pearsonkt.com
Randy W Kamphaus, Author
Cecil R Reynolds, Co-Author
Doug Kubach, Group President & CEO
A powerful assessment to evaluate child and adolescent behavior. Includes a self-report form for describing the behaviors and emotions of children and adolescents. Administration time: 10 - 20 minutes (TRS & PRS) 30 - 45 minutes for SRP.

4313 Behavior Rating Profile
Pro-Ed
8700 Shoal Creek Boulevard
Austin, TX 78757-6897   512-451-3246
                                             800-897-3202
                                        Fax: 512-451-8542
                                          www.proedinc.com
                                       general@proedinc.com
Donald D Hammill, Owner
Linda Brown, Author
A global measure of behavior providing student, parent, teacher and peer scales. It helps to identify behaviors that may cause a student's learning problems. *$211.00*

4314 Child Behavior Checklist
University of Vermont
1 S Prospect St
St. Joseph's Wing (3rd Floor, Room# 3207
Burlington, VT 05401-3456   802-656-5130
                                        Fax: 802-656-5131
                                           www.aseba.org
                                           mail@aseba.org
Dr TM Achenbach, Director/Professor
Ramani Sunderaju, Operations Manager
Psychological assessments

4315 Culture-Free Self-Esteem Inventories
Pro-Ed
8700 Shoal Creek Boulevard
Austin, TX 78757-6897   512-451-3246
                                             800-897-3202
                                        Fax: 512-451-8542
                                          www.proedinc.com
                                       general@proedinc.com
Donald D Hammill, Owner
James Battle, Author
A series of self-report scales used to determine the level of self-esteem in children and adults. *$190.00*

4316 Devereux Early Childhood Assessment Program Observation Journal
Kaplan Early Learning Company
1310 Lewisville Clemmons Rd
Lewisville, NC 27023-9635   336-766-7374
                                             800-334-2014
                                        Fax: 800-452-7526
                                          www.kaplanco.com
                                        info@kaplanco.com
Hal Kaplan, President & CEO
Provides both sample and reproducible copies of suggested forms for early childhood programs to support appropriate observation and planning for individual children and the classroom. *$199.95*

4317 Disruptive Behavior Rating Scale Kit
Slosson Educational Publications, Inc.
538 Buffalo Road
East Aurora, NY 14052   716-652-0930
                                             888-756-7766
                                        Fax: 800-655-3840
                                           www.slosson.com
                                       slossonprep@gmail.com
Bradley T Erford, Author
Steven Slosson, President
John H Slosson, Vice President
Identifies common behavior problems such as attention deficit disorder, attention deficit hyperactivity disorder, oppositional disorders and anti-social conduct problems. *$186.25*

4318 Draw a Person: Screening Procedure for Emotional Disturbance
Pro-Ed
8700 Shoal Creek Boulevard
Austin, TX 78757-6897   512-451-3246
                                             800-897-3202
                                        Fax: 512-451-8542
                                          www.proedinc.com
                                       general@proedinc.com
Donald D Hammill, Owner
Jack A. Naglieri, Author
Timothy J. McNeish, Co-Author
A screening test that helps identify children and adolescents who have emotional problems and require further evaluation. *$145.00*

4319 Fundamentals of Autism
Slosson Educational Publications
538 Buffalo Road
East Aurora, NY 14052   716-652-0930
                                             888-756-7766
                                        Fax: 800-655-3840
                                           www.slosson.com
                                       slossonprep@gmail.com
Steven Slosson, President
Sue Larson, Author
Dr. Georgina Moynihan, Tech Support
The handbook and two accompanying checklists provide a quick, user-friendly approach to help in identifying and developing educationally related program objectives for the child diagnosed as Autistic. *$91.25*

4320 Multidimensional Self Concept Scale
Pro-Ed
8700 Shoal Creek Boulevard
Austin, TX 78757-6897   512-451-3246
                                             800-897-3202
                                        Fax: 512-451-8542
                                          www.proedinc.com
                                       general@proedinc.com
Donald D Hammill, Owner
Bruce Bracken, Author
A thoroughly researched, developed and standardized clinical instrument. It assesses global self-concept and six context-dependent self-concept domains that are functionally important in the social-emotional adjustment of youth and adolescents. *$114.00*

4321 Revised Behavior Problem Checklist
Psychological Assessment Resources
16204 N Florida Ave
Lutz, FL 33549-8119   813-449-4065
                                             800-899-8378
                                        Fax: 800-727-9329
                                            www.parinc.com
                                       chairman@parinc.com
Bob III, President/CEO
Kay Cunningham, Director
Cathy Smith, Vice President
Psychological test products and software designed by mental health professionals. *$195.00*

4322 SSRS: Social Skills Rating System
Pearson Assessments
4940 Pearl East Circle
Suite 200
Boulder, CO 80301
888-977-7900
800-328-5999
Fax: 888-556-2103
www.pearsonassessments.com
info@pearsonkt.com
Kevin Brueggman, President
Frank M Gresham, Author
Stephen N Elliot, Co-Author
A nationally standardized series of questionnaires that obtain information on the social behaviors of children and adolescents from teachers, parents and the students themselves. Administration time is 10-15 minutes per questionnaire.

4323 Self-Esteem Index
Pro-Ed
8700 Shoal Creek Boulevard
Austin, TX 78757-6897
512-451-3246
800-897-3202
Fax: 512-451-8542
www.proedinc.com
general@proedinc.com
Donald D Hammill, Owner
Linda Brown, Author
Jacquelyn Alexander, Co-Author
A new, multidimensional, norm-referenced measure of the way that individuals perceive and value themselves. *$132.00*

4324 Social-Emotional Dimension Scale
Pro-Ed
8700 Shoal Creek Boulevard
Austin, TX 78757-6897
512-451-3246
800-897-3202
Fax: 512-451-8542
www.proedinc.com
general@proedinc.com
Donald D Hammill, Owner
Jerry Hutton, Author
Timothy Roberts, Co-Author
A quick, well-standardized rating scale that can be used by teachers, counselors and psychologists to screen students who are at risk for conduct disorders or emotional disturbances. *$154.00*

4325 Wings for Kids
476 Meeting Street
Suite E
Charleston, SC 29403
843-442-2835
Fax: 866-562-8615
www.wingsforkids.org
hello@wingsforkids.org
Ginny Deerin, Founder
Suzan Zoukis, Chair
Alex Opoulos, Secretary
Wings for Kids is the only U.S. organization focused soley on social and emotional learning after school. Hot WINGS are social skill development activities that anyone can use to model, shape and reinforce the capabilities that equip a child to succeed. Through small lessons, you give kids the tools they need to navigate challenging situations and everyday problems. Activties include Positive Reinforcement, Cope with Anger and Stress, Express Emotions Constructively.

LD Screening

4326 ADD-H Comprehensive Teacher's Rating Scale: 2nd Edition
Slosson Educational Publications
538 Buffalo Road
East Aurora, NY 14052
716-652-0930
888-756-7766
Fax: 800-655-3840
www.slosson.com
slossonprep@gmail.com
Rina Ullmann, Robert Sprague, Author
Steven Slosson, President
John H Slosson, Vice President
Dr. Georgina Moynihan, Tech Support
This brief checklist assesses one of the most prevalent childhood behavior problems: attention-deficit disorder, with or without hyperactivity. Because this disorder manifests itself primarily in the classroom, it is best evaluated by teacher ratings. Also available in a Spanish translation; please indicate when ordering. *$62.00*

4327 Attention-Deficit/Hyperactivity Disorder Test
Slosson Educational Publications
538 Buffalo Road
East Aurora, NY 14052
716-652-0930
888-756-7766
Fax: 800-655-3840
www.slosson.com
slossonprep@gmail.com
James E Gilliam, Author
Steven Slosson, President
John H Slosson, Vice President
Dr. Georgina Moynihan, Tech Support
An effective instrument for identifying and evaluating ADHD. Contains 36 items that describe characteristic behaviors of persons with ADHD. These items comprise three subtests representing the core symptoms necessary for the diagnosis of ADHD: hyperactivity, impulsivity, and inattention. *$95.00*

4328 BRIGANCE Screens: Early Preschool
Curriculum Associates
153 Rangeway Road
North Billerica, MA 01862-901
978-667-8000
800-225-0248
Fax: 800-366-1158
www.curriculumassociates.com
info@CAinc.com
Frank E. Ferguson, Chairman
Albert Brigance, Author
Robert Waldron, Chief Executive Officer
An affordable, easy-to-administer, all-purpose solution. Accurately screen key developmental and early academic skills in just 10-15 minutes per child. Widely used in Early Head Start programs, it meets IDEA requirements and provides consistent results that support early childhood educator's observations and judgement. *$110.00*

4329 BRIGANCE Screens: Infants and Toddler
Curriculum Associates
153 Rangeway Road
North Billerica, MA 01862-901
978-667-8000
800-225-0248
Fax: 800-366-1158
www.curriculumassociates.com
info@CAinc.com
Frank E. Ferguson, Chairman
Albert Brigance, Author
Robert Waldron, Chief Executive Officer
An affordable, easy-to-administer, all-purpose solution. The Infant and Toddler Screen accurately assesses key developmental skills, and observes caregivers involvement and interactions. *$110.00*

4330 BRIGANCE Screens: K and 1
Curriculum Associates
153 Rangeway Road
North Billerica, MA 01862-901
978-667-8000
800-225-0248
Fax: 800-366-1158
www.curriculumassociates.com
info@CAinc.com
Frank E. Ferguson, Chairman
Albert Brigance, Author
Robert Waldron, Chief Executive Officer

The K and 1 Screen is an affordable, easy-to-administer, all-purpose solution. Accurately screen key developmental and early academic skills in just 10-15 mintues per child. School districts nationwide rely on BRIGANCE for screening children before entering kindergarten, grade 1, and grade 2. It meets IDEA requirements and provides consistant results that support early childhood educators observations and judgement. *$110.00*

4331 Basic School Skills Inventory: Screen and Diagnostic
Pro-Ed
8700 Shoal Creek Boulevard
Austin, TX 78757-6897   512-451-3246
                                          800-897-3202
                                     Fax: 512-451-8542
                                       www.proedinc.com
                                    general@proedinc.com
Lindy Jordaan, Marketing Coordinator
Donald D Hammill, Owner
Can be used to locate children who are high risk for school failure, who need more in-depth assessment and who should be referred for additional study. *$109.00*

4332 DABERON Screening for School Readiness
Pro-Ed
8700 Shoal Creek Boulevard
Austin, TX 78757-6897   512-451-3246
                                          800-897-3202
                                     Fax: 512-451-8542
                                       www.proedinc.com
                                    general@proedinc.com
Donald D Hammill, Owner
Virginia Danzer, Author
Theresa Lyons, Co-Author
Provides a standardized assessment of school readiness in children with learning or behavior problems. *$176.00*
Yearly

4333 Developmental Assessment for Students with Severe Disabilities
Pro-Ed
8700 Shoal Creek Boulevard
Austin, TX 78757-6897   512-451-3246
                                          800-897-3202
                                     Fax: 512-451-8542
                                       www.proedinc.com
                                    general@proedinc.com
Mary Kay Dykes & Jane Erin, Author
Donald D Hammill, Owner
Offers diagnostic and programming personnel concise information about individuals who are functioning between birth and 8 years of age developmentally. *$217.00*

4334 Educational Developmental Series
Scholastic Testing Service
480 Meyer Rd
Bensenville, IL 60106-1617   630-766-7150
                                          800-642-6787
                                     Fax: 630-766-8054
                                       www.ststesting.com/
                                       sts@ststesting.com
John Kauffman, Marketing VP
Scott Rich, J.D., Assessment Specialist
A standardized battery of ability and achievement tests. Administration time is approximately 2.5 - 5 hours, depending on grade level and subtests. The EDSERIES has the most comprehensive coverage of all the STS tests. It permits teachers, counselors and administrators to evaluate a student from the broadest possible perspective. A school may use the EDSERIES on a lease/score basis or it may purchase testing materials.

4335 Fundamentals of Autism
Slosson Educational Publications
538 Buffalo Road
East Aurora, NY 14052   716-652-0930
                                          888-756-7766
                                     Fax: 800-655-3840
                                       www.slosson.com
                                    slossonprep@gmail.com

Sue Larson, Author
Steven Slosson, President
John H Slosson, Vice President
Dr. Georgina Moynihan, Tech Support
Provides a quick, user-friendly, effective, and accurate approach to help in identifying and developing educationally related program objectives for children diagnosed as autistic.

4336 Goodenough-Harris Drawing Test
Pearson
19500 Bulverde Rd
San Antonio, TX 78259-3701   210-339-5000
                                          800-627-7271
                                     Fax: 800-232-1223
                                       www.psychcorp.com
                          clinicalcustomersupport@pearson.com
Aurelio Prifitera, President
Florence Goodenough, Author
This test focuses on mental maturity without requiring verbal skills. The fifteen-minute examination provides standard scores for children ages 3-15. *$178.00*

4337 Higher Education for Learning Problems (HELP)
Marshall University
Myers Hall
520 - 18th St
Huntington, WV 25703-1530   304-696-6252
                                     Fax: 304-696-3231
                                       www.marshall.edu/help
                                       help@marshall.edu
Debbie Painter, Director
Missi Fisher, Business Manager
K. Renna Moore, Administrative Assistant
The HELP program is committed to providing assistance through individual tutuoring, mentoring and support, as well as fair and legal access to educational opportunities for students diagnosed with learning disabilities and related disorders such as ADD/ADHD.

4338 Kaufman Assessment Battery for Children
Pearson
4940 Pearl East Circle
Suite 200
Boulder, CO 80301   888-977-7900
                                          800-328-5999
                                     Fax: 888-556-2103
                                       www.pearsonassessments.com
                                       info@pearsonkt.com
Alan Kaufman, Author
Nadeen Kaufman, Co-Author
Carol Watson, Publisher/Pres Clinical Asses
An individually administered measure of intelligence and achievement, using simultaneous and sequential mental processes.

4339 Kaufman Brief Intelligence Test
Pearson
4940 Pearl East Circle
Suite 200
Boulder, CO 80301   888-977-7900
                                          800-328-5999
                                     Fax: 888-556-2103
                                       www.pearsonassessments.com
                                       info@pearsonkt.com
Alan Kaufman, Author
Nadeen Kaufman, Co-Author
Doug Kubach, Group President & CEO
KBIT is a brief, individually administered test of verbal and non-verbal intelligence. Screens two cognitive functions quickly and easily.

4340 Peabody Individual Achievement Test
Pearson
4940 Pearl East Circle
Suite 200
Boulder, CO 80301   888-977-7900
                                       800-328-5999
                                  Fax: 888-556-2103
                            www.pearsonassessments.com
                                  info@pearsonkt.com
Frederick Markwardt Jr, Author
Matt Keller, Marketing Manager
Doug Kubach, Group President & CEO
Efficient individual measure of academic achievement.
Reading, mathematics and spelling are assessed in a simple
nonthreatning format that requires only a revised pointing
response for most items.

4341 Peabody Test-Picture Vocabulary Test
Pearson
4940 Pearl East Circle
Suite 200
Boulder, CO 80301   888-977-7900
                                       800-328-5999
                                  Fax: 888-556-2103
                            www.pearsonassessments.com
                                  info@pearsonkt.com
Lloyd Dunn, Author
Leota Dunn, Co-Author
Doug Kubach, Group President & CEO
A measure of hearing vocabulary for Standard American
English; administration time: 10-15 minutes.

4342 Restless Minds, Restless Kids
Slosson Educational Publications
538 Buffalo Road
East Aurora, NY 14052   716-652-0930
                                       888-756-7766
                                  Fax: 800-655-3840
                                  www.slosson.com
                            slossonprep@gmail.com
Rick D'Alli, Author
Steven Slosson, President
John H Slosson, Vice President
Dr. Georgina Moynihan, Tech Support
Two leading specialists in the field of childhood behavioral
disorders discuss the state-of-the-art approach to diagnosing
and testing ADHD. They are joined by four mothers of
ADHD children who share their experiences of the effects of
this disorder on the family. *$67.00*

4343 School Readiness Test
Scholastic Testing Service
480 Meyer Rd
Bensenville, IL 60106-1617   630-766-7150
                                       800-642-6787
                                  Fax: 630-766-8054
                                  www.ststesting.com
                                  sts@ststesting.com
John Kauffman, Marketing VP
Scott Rich, J.D., Assessment Specialist
An effective tool for determining the readiness of each stu-
dent for first grade. It allows a teacher to learn as much as
possible about every entering student's abilities, and about
any factors that might interfere with his or her learning.

4344 Slosson Intelligence Test
Pro-Ed
538 Buffalo Road
East Aurora, NY 14052   716-652-0930
                                       888-756-7766
                                  Fax: 800-655-3840
                                  www.slosson.com
                            slossonprep@gmail.com
Steven Slosson, President
John H Slosson, Vice President
Richard.L Slosson, Author

A widely used individual screening test for those who need
to evaluate the mental ability of individuals who are learning
disabled, mentally retarded, blind, orthopedically disabled,
normal, or gifted from ages 4 to adulthood. Revised by
Charles Nicholson and Terry Hibpshman. *$147.00*

4345 TOVA
Universal Attention Disorders
3321 Cerritos Ave
Los Alamitos, CA 90720-2105   562-594-7700
                                       800-729-2886
                                  Fax: 562-594-7770
                                  www.tovatest.com
                                  support@tovatest.com
Tammy Dupuy, Medical Director
Karen Carlson, Marketing Director
The TOVA (Tests of Variables of Attention) is a computerized, objective measure of attention and impulsivity, used in
the assessment and treatment of ADD/ADHD. It is standardized from 4 to 80 years of age. TOVA's report contains a full
analysis and interpetation of data. Variables measured include omissions, commisions, response time and response
time variability.

4346 Test of Memory and Learning (TOMAL)
Pro-Ed
8700 Shoal Creek Boulevard
Austin, TX 78757-6897   512-451-3246
                                       800-897-3202
                                  Fax: 512-451-8542
                                  www.proedinc.com
                                  general@proedinc.com
Donald D Hammill, Owner
Cecil Reynolds, Author
Judith K Voress, Co-Author
TOMAL provides ten subtests that evaluate general and spe-
cific memory functions. *$376.00*

4347 Test of Nonverbal Intelligence (TONI-3)
Pro-Ed
8700 Shoal Creek Boulevard
Austin, TX 78757-6897   512-451-3246
                                       800-897-3202
                                  Fax: 512-451-8542
                                  www.proedinc.com
                                  general@proedinc.com
Donald D Hammill, President
Linda Brown, Author
Susan Johnson, Co-Author
A language-free measure of reasoning and intelligence pres-
ents a variety of abstract problem solving tasks. *$285.00*

**4348 Vision, Perception and Cognition: Manual for Evalua-
tion & Treatment**
Therapro
225 Arlington St
Framingham, MA 01702-8773   508-872-9494
                                       800-257-5376
                                  Fax: 508-875-2062
                                  www.theraproducts.com
                                  info@theraproducts.com
Karen Conrad, Owner
Barbara Zoltan, Author
Details methods for testing perceptual, visual and cognitive
deficits, as well as procedure for evaluating test results in relation to cognitive loss. Clearly explains each deficit, provides step by step testing techniques and gives complete
treatment guidelines. Also includes information on the use
of computers in cognitive training. *$40.00*
232 pages

Math

4349
3 Steps to Math Success
Curriculum Associates
153 Rangeway Road
North Billerica, MA 01862-901
978-667-8000
800-225-0248
Fax: 800-366-1158
www.curriculumassociates.com
info@CAinc.com
Curriculum Associates, Author
Frank E. Ferguson, Chairman
Renee Foster, President and Publisher
Dave Caron, Chief Financial Officer
We developed an integrated approach to math that ensures academic success long after the final bell has rung. Together, these series create an easy-to-use system of targeted instruction designed to remedy math weakness and reinforce math strengths.

4350
AfterMath Series
Curriculum Associates
153 Rangeway Road
North Billerica, MA 01862-901
978-667-8000
800-225-0248
Fax: 800-366-1158
www.curriculumassociates.com
info@CAinc.com
Frank E. Ferguson, Chairman
Renee Foster, President and Publisher
Dave Caron, Chief Financial Officer
Galileo once said that mathematics is the alphabet in which the universe was created. This series helps students master that alphabet. As they puzzle their way through brainteasers and learn math magic, students build critical-thinking skills that are vital to comprehending and succeeding in today's world.

4351
ENRIGHT Computation Series
Curriculum Associates
153 Rangeway Road
North Billerica, MA 01862-901
978-667-8000
800-225-0248
Fax: 800-366-1158
www.curriculumassociates.com
info@CAinc.com
Frank E. Ferguson, Chairman
Renee Foster, President and Publisher
Dave Caron, Chief Financial Officer
Close the gap between expected and actual computation performance. The ENRIGHT Computation Series provides the practice necessary to master addition, subtraction, multiplication, and division of whole numbers, fractions, and decimals.

4352
Figure It Out: Thinking Like a Math Problem Solver
Curriculum Associates
153 Rangeway Road
North Billerica, MA 01862-901
978-667-8000
800-225-0248
Fax: 800-366-1158
www.curriculumassociates.com
info@CAinc.com
Frank E. Ferguson, Chairman
Renee Foster, President and Publisher
Dave Caron, Chief Financial Officer
Critical thinking is the key to unlocking the mystery of these nonroutine problems. Your students will eagerly accept the challenge! Students learn to apply eight strategies in each book including: draw a picture; use a pattern; work backwards; make a table; and guess and check.

4353
Getting Ready for Algebra
Curriculum Associates
153 Rangeway Road
North Billerica, MA 01862-901
978-667-8000
800-225-0248
Fax: 800-366-1158
www.curriculumassociates.com
info@CAinc.com
Frank E. Ferguson, Chairman
Renee Foster, President and Publisher
Dave Caron, Chief Financial Officer
NCTM encourages algebra instruction in the early grades to develop critical-thinking, communication, reasoning, and problem-solving skills. Getting Ready for Algebra exercises these skills in lessons that focus on key algebra concepts: adding and subtracting positive integers; patterns; set theory notation; open sentences; inequality and more.

4354
Learning Disability Evaluation Scale: Renormed
Hawthorne Educational Services
800 Gray Oak Dr
Columbia, MO 65201-3730
573-874-1710
800-542-1673
Fax: 800-442-9509
www.hawthorne-ed.com
info@hes-inc.com
Stephen McCarney, Author
Edina Laird, Director External Relations
Michele Jackson, Owner
The Learning Disability Evaluation Scale (LDES) is an initial screening and assessment instrument in the areas of listening, thinking, speaking, reading, writing, spelling, and mathematical calculations based on the federal definition (IDEA). The Learning Disability Intervention Manual (LDIM) is a companion to the LDES and contains goals, objectives, and intervention/instructional strategies for the learning problems identified by the LDES. *$152.00*
217 pages

4355
QUIC Tests
Scholastic Testing Service
480 Meyer Rd
Bensenville, IL 60106-1617
630-766-7150
800-642-6787
Fax: 630-766-8054
www.ststesting.com
sts@ststesting.com
John Kauffman, Marketing VP
Scott Rich, J.D., Assessment Specialist
The Quic Tests are used to determine the functional level of student comptetency in mathematics and/ or communicative arts for use in grades 2-12. Administration time is 30 minutes or less.

4356
Skills Assessments
Harcourt
222 Berkeley Street
Boston, MA 02116
617-351-5000
800-531-5015
Fax: 800-699-9459
www.hmhco.com/educators
international@harcourt.com
Linda K. Zecher, President, CEO & Director
Eric Shuman, Chief Financial Officer
William Bayers, EVP/General Counsel
This handy, all-in-one resource helps identify students strengths and weaknesses in order to determine appropriate instructional levels in each of five subjects areas: reading; language arts; math; science; and social studies. Assessments are identified by subtopics in each subject.

4357
Test of Mathematical Abilities
Pro-Ed
8700 Shoal Creek Boulevard
Austin, TX 78757-6897
512-451-3246
800-897-3202
Fax: 512-451-8542
www.proedinc.com
general@proedinc.com

Donald D Hammill, Owner
Virginia Brown, Author
Mary Cronin, Co-Author
Has been developed to provide standardized information about story problems and computation, attitude, vocabulary and general cultural application. *$95.00*

Professional Guides

4358 **Assessment Update**
Jossey-Bass
111 River St
Hoboken, NJ 07030-5774

201-748-6000
Fax: 201-748-6008
www.wiley.com
info@wiley.com

Stephen M. Smith, President/CEO
Ellis E. Cousens, EVP/COO
John Kritzmacher, EVP/CFO
Assessment Update is dedicated to covering the latest developments in the rapidly evolving area of higher education assessment. Assessment Update offers all academic leaders up-to-date information and practical advice on conducting assessments in a range of areas, including student learning and outcomes, factulty instruction, academic programs and curricula, student services, and overall institutional functioning.

4359 **Assessment of Students with Handicaps in Vocational Education**
Association for Career and Technical Education
1410 King St
Alexandria, VA 22314-2749

800-826-9972
Fax: 703-683-7424
www.acteonline.org
sheath@jeffco.k12.co.us

L Albright, Author
Sarah Heath, President
Katrina Plese, Finance Chair
Chuck Gallagher, Regional Representative
Includes teachers, supervisors, administrators and others interested in the development and improvement of career & technical and practical-arts education.

4360 **BRIGANCE Word Analysis: Strategies and Practice**
Curriculum Associates
153 Rangeway Road
North Billerica, MA 01862-901

978-667-8000
800-225-0248
Fax: 800-366-1158
www.curriculumassociates.com
info@CAinc.com

Albert Brigance, Author
Frank E. Ferguson, Chairman
Renee Foster, President and Publisher
Dave Caron, Chief Financial Officer
Our comprehensive, two-volume resource combines activities, strategies, and reference materials for teaching phonetic and structural word analysis. Two durable binders feature reproducible activity pages. Choose from more than 1,600 activities for corrective instruction or to reinforce your classroom reading program.

4361 **Career Planner's Portfolio: A School-to-Work Assessment Tool**
Curriculum Associates
153 Rangeway Road
North Billerica, MA 01862-901

978-667-8000
800-225-0248
Fax: 800-366-1158
www.curriculumassociates.com
info@CAinc.com

Robert G Forest, Author
Frank E. Ferguson, Chairman
Renee Foster, President and Publisher
Dave Caron, Chief Financial Officer

Students career plans develop and evolve over several school years. Our portfolio will help keep track of their progress.

4362 **Computer Scoring Systems for PRO-ED Tests**
Pro-Ed
8700 Shoal Creek Boulevard
Austin, TX 78757-6897

512-451-3246
800-897-3202
Fax: 512-451-8542
www.proedinc.com
general@proedinc.com

Donald D Hammill, Owner
Computer scoring systems have been developed to generate reports for many PRO-ED tests and to help examiners interpret test performance.

4363 **Goals and Objectives Writer Software**
Curriculum Associates
153 Rangeway Road
North Billerica, MA 01862-901

978-667-8000
800-225-0248
Fax: 800-366-1158
www.curriculumassociates.com
info@CAinc.com

Frank E. Ferguson, Chairman
Renee Foster, President and Publisher
Dave Caron, Chief Financial Officer
Using the Goals and Objectives program, you'll quickly and easily create, edit, and print IEPs. The CD allows you to install the program on your hard drive in order to save students data for future updates. You can easily export IEPs into any word processing program. CD-Rom for Windows and Macintosh.

4364 **Occupational Aptitude Survey and Interest Schedule**
Pro-Ed
8700 Shoal Creek Boulevard
Austin, TX 78757-6897

512-451-3246
800-897-3202
Fax: 512-451-8542
www.proedinc.com
general@proedinc.com

Donald D Hammill, Owner
Randall M Parker, Author
Consists of two related tests: the OASIS-2 Aptitude Survey and the OASIS-2 Interest Schedule. The tests were normed on the same national sample of 1,505 students from 13 states. The Aptitude Survey measures six broad aptitude factors that are directly related to skills and abilities required in over 20,000 jobs and the Interest Schedule measures 12 interest factors directly related to the occupations listed in Occupational Exploration.

4365 **Portfolio Assessment Teacher's Guide**
Harcourt
222 Berkeley Street
Boston, MA 02116

617-351-5000
800-531-5015
Fax: 800-699-9459
www.hmhco.com/educators
international@harcourt.com

Roger Farr, Author
Linda K. Zecher, President, CEO & Director
Eric Shuman, Chief Financial Officer
William Bayers, EVP/General Counsel
Start your portfolio systems with tips from the expert. Roger Farr outlines the basic steps for evaluating a portfolio, offers ideas for organizing portfolios and making the most of portfolio conferences, and provides reproducible evaluation forms for primary through intermediate grades and above. *$23.60*

4366 Teaching Test Taking Skills
Brookline Books
8 Trumbull Rd
Suite B-001
Northampton, MA 01060   603-669-7032
                               800-666-2665
                          Fax: 413-584-6184
                          www.brooklinebooks.com
                          brbooks@yahoo.com
Margo Mastropieri, Thomas Scruggs, Author
Mike Beattie, Manager
Test-wise individuals often score higher than others of equal ability who may not use test-taking skills effectively. This work teaches general concepts about the test format or other conditions of testing, not specific items on the test. *$21.95* *ISBN 0-914797-76-X*

4367 Tests, Measurement and Evaluation
American Institutes for Research
1000 Thomas Jefferson St
Washington, DC 20007-3835   202-342-5000
                               Fax: 202-403-5001
                               TTY: 877-344-3499
                                    www.air.org
                                    inquiry@air.org
David Myers, President/CEO
Marijo Ahlgrimm, EVP/CFO
Sabrina Laine, SVP/Director, Education
Our goal is to provide governments and the private sector with responsive services of the highest quality by applying and advancing the knowledge, theories, methods, and standards of the behavioral and social services to solve significant societal problems and improve the quality of life of all people.

Reading

4368 3 Steps to Reading Success: CARS, STARS, CARS II
Curriculum Associates
153 Rangeway Road
North Billerica, MA 01862-901   978-667-8000
                               800-225-0248
                          Fax: 800-366-1158
                          www.curriculumassociates.com
                          info@CAinc.com
Frank E. Ferguson, Chairman
Renee Foster, President and Publisher
Dave Caron, Chief Financial Officer
Equipping your students with the skills and strategies they need to achieve lifelong success can be a challenge. That's why we developed an integrated approach to learning that ensures academic success long after the final bell has rung.

4369 BRIGANCE Readiness: Strategies and Practice
Curriculum Associates
153 Rangeway Road
North Billerica, MA 01862-901   978-667-8000
                               800-225-0248
                          Fax: 800-366-1158
                          www.curriculumassociates.com
                          info@CAinc.com
Frank E. Ferguson, Chairman
Albert Brigance, Author
Dave Caron, Chief Financial Officer
Attend to the needs and differences of the children in your program using Readiness: Strategies and Practice. Skills are introduced, taught, and reinforced using both age-appropriate and individual appropriate activties. *$174.00*

4370 Capitalization and Punctuation
Curriculum Associates
153 Rangeway Road
North Billerica, MA 01862-901   978-667-8000
                               800-225-0248
                          Fax: 800-366-1158
                          www.curriculumassociates.com
                          info@CAinc.com
Frank E. Ferguson, Chairman
Renee Foster, President and Publisher
Dave Caron, Chief Financial Officer
Capitalization and Punctuation features structured, easy to understand lessons that are organized sequentially. Students read the rules, study sample exercises, apply the skills in practice lessons, and review the skills in maintenance lessons.

4371 Dyslexia/ADHD Institute
148 Eastern Blvd
Suite 406
Glastonbury, CT 06033   860-633-2604
                               877-342-7323
                          www.diaread.com
                          info@diaread.com
Les Fredette, Co-Operator/Co-Owner
Susan Fredette, Co-Operator/Co-Owner
Testing, diagnosis, and 1-on-1 tutoring for all ages and levels of need

4372 Extensions in Reading
Curriculum Associates
153 Rangeway Road
North Billerica, MA 01862-901   978-667-8000
                               800-225-0248
                          Fax: 800-366-1158
                          www.curriculumassociates.com
                          info@CAinc.com
Frank E. Ferguson, Chairman
Renee Foster, President and Publisher
Dave Caron, Chief Financial Officer
A unique new program teaching reading strategies and more. Extensions offers rich experiences with nonfiction and fiction. Each lesson extends to include: researching and writing; use of graphic organizers; vocabulary development; and comprehension questions with test-prep format.

4373 Gray Diagnostic Reading Tests
Pro-Ed
8700 Shoal Creek Boulevard
Austin, TX 78757-6897   512-451-3246
                               800-897-3202
                          Fax: 512-451-8542
                          www.proedinc.com
                          general@proedinc.com
Donald D Hammill, Owner
Brian Bryant, Author
Diane Bryant, Co-Author
Uses two alternate, equivalent forms to assess students who have difficulty reading continuous print and who require an evaluation of specific abilities and weaknesses. Item # 10965. *$259.00*

4374 Gray Oral Reading Tests
Pro-Ed
8700 Shoal Creek Boulevard
Austin, TX 78757-6897   512-451-3246
                               800-897-3202
                          Fax: 512-451-8542
                          www.proedinc.com
                          general@proedinc.com
Donald D Hammill, Owner
J Lee Wiederholt, Author
Brian Bryant, Co-Author
The latest revision provides an objective measure of growth in oral reading and an aid in the diagnosis of oral reading difficulties. *$233.00*

4375 Reading Assessment System
Steck-Vaughn Company
222 Berkeley Street
Boston, MA 02116   617-351-5000
                               800-289-4490
                          Fax: 800-289-3994
                          www.hmhco.com/educators
Linda K. Zecher, President, CEO & Director
Eric Shuman, Chief Financial Officer
William Bayers, EVP/General Counsel

The Reading Assessment System provides an ongoing measure of specific student's skills and offers detailed directions for individual instruction and remediation. Up to eight reports are available. This popular program generates individual scores, class scores, school scores, and district reports.

4376 Scholastic Abilities Test for Adults
Pro-Ed
8700 Shoal Creek Boulevard
Austin, TX 78757-6897
512-451-3246
800-897-3202
Fax: 512-451-8542
www.proedinc.com
general@proedinc.com

Donald D Hammill, Owner
Brian Bryant, Author
James Patton, Co-Author
Measures scholastic competence, aptitude and academic achievement for persons with learning difficulties. *$186.00*

4377 Skills Assessments
Steck-Vaughn Company
222 Berkeley Street
Boston, MA 02116
617-351-5000
800-531-5015
Fax: 800-269-5232
www.hmhco.com/educators
info@steck-vaughn.com

Linda K. Zecher, President, CEO & Director
Eric Shuman, Chief Financial Officer
William Bayers, EVP/General Counsel
This handy, all-in-one resource helps identify students strengths and weaknesses in order to determine appropriate instructional levels in each of five subjects areas: reading; language arts; math; science; and social studies. Assessments are identified by subtopics in each subject. Each book is $13.99 each. *$69.95*

4378 Standardized Reading Inventory
Pro-Ed
8700 Shoal Creek Boulevard
Austin, TX 78757-6897
512-451-3246
800-897-3202
Fax: 512-451-8542
www.proedinc.com
general@proedinc.com

Donald D Hammill, Owner
Phyllis Newcomer, Author
An instrument for evaluating students' reading ability. *$277.00*

4379 Test of Early Reading Ability
Pro-Ed
8700 Shoal Creek Boulevard
Austin, TX 78757-6897
512-451-3246
800-897-3202
Fax: 512-451-8542
www.proedinc.com
general@proedinc.com

Donald D Hammill, Owner
D Kim Reid, Author
Wayne Hresko, Co-Author
Unique test in that it measures the actual reading ability of young children. Items measure knowledge of contextual meaning, alphabet and conventions. *$274.00*

4380 Test of Reading Comprehension
Pro-Ed
8700 Shoal Creek Boulevard
Austin, TX 78757-6897
512-451-3246
800-897-3202
Fax: 512-451-8542
www.proedinc.com
general@proedinc.com

Donald D Hammill, Owner/Author
Virginia Brown, Co-Author
J Lee Wiederholt, Co-Author

A multidimensional test of silent reading comprehension for students. The test reflects current psycholinguistic theories that consider reading comprehension to be a constructive process involving both language and cognition. *$196.00*

Speech & Language Arts

4381 A Calendar of Home Activities
Curriculum Associates
153 Rangeway Road
North Billerica, MA 01862-901
978-667-8000
800-225-0248
Fax: 800-366-1158
www.curriculumassociates.com
info@CAinc.com

Frank E. Ferguson, Chairman
Donald Johnson, Author
Elaine Johnson, Co-Author
An activity-a-day: 365 activities for parents and children to share at home in just 10-15 minutes each day. Parents support their children's educational experiences in a meaningful and enjoyable way, such as cooking, playing ball, and sculpting clay.

4382 Adolescent Language Screening Test
Pro-Ed
8700 Shoal Creek Boulevard
Austin, TX 78757-6897
512-451-3246
800-897-3202
Fax: 512-451-8542
www.proedinc.com
general@proedinc.com

Donald D Hammill, Owner
Denise Morgan, Author
Arthur Guilford, Co-Author
Provides speech/language pathologists and other interested professionals with a rapid thorough method for screening adolescents' speech and language. *$145.00*

4383 Advanced Skills For School Success Series: Module 4
Curriculum Associates
153 Rangeway Road
North Billerica, MA 01862-901
978-667-8000
800-225-0248
Fax: 800-366-1158
www.curriculumassociates.com
info@CAinc.com

Anita Archer, Mary Gleason, Author
Frank E. Ferguson, Chairman
Renee Foster, President and Publisher
Dave Caron, Chief Financial Officer
Develops oral and written language abilities. Students learn valuable strategies for note-taking, brainstorming, and effectively participating in class dicussions. *$19.90*

4384 Aphasia Diagnostic Profiles
Pro-Ed
8700 Shoal Creek Boulevard
Austin, TX 78757-6897
512-451-3246
800-897-3202
Fax: 512-451-8542
www.proedinc.com
general@proedinc.com

Donald D Hammill, Owner
Nancy Helm-Estrabrooks, Author
This is a quick, efficient, and systematic assessment of language and communication impairment associated with aphasia that should be administered individually. The test can be administered in 40-45 minutes. *$175.00*

4385 BRIGANCE Assessment of Basic Skills
Curriculum Associates
153 Rangeway Road
North Billerica, MA 01862-901
978-667-8000
800-225-0248
Fax: 800-366-1158
www.curriculumassociates.com
info@CAinc.com

Frank E. Ferguson, Chairman
Albert Brigance, Author
Dave Caron, Chief Financial Officer
Critiqued and field tested by Spanish linguists and educators nationwide, the Assessment of Basic Skills meets nondiscriminatory testing requirements for Limited English Proficient students.

4386 BRIGANCE Comprehensive Inventory of Basic Skills
Curriculum Associates
153 Rangeway Road
North Billerica, MA 01862-901   978-667-8000
800-225-0248
Fax: 800-366-1158
www.curriculumassociates.com
info@CAinc.com
Frank E. Ferguson, Chairman
Albert Brigance, Author
Dave Caron, Chief Financial Officer
Designed for use in elementary and middle schools, the CIBS-R is a valuable resource for programs emphasizing individualized instruction. The Inventory is especially helpful in programs serving students with special needs, and continues to be indispensable in IEP development and program planning.

4387 BRIGANCE Employability Skills Inventory
Curriculum Associates
153 Rangeway Road
North Billerica, MA 01862-901   978-667-8000
800-225-0248
Fax: 800-366-1158
www.curriculumassociates.com
info@CAinc.com
Frank E. Ferguson, Chairman
Albert Brigance, Author
Dave Caron, Chief Financial Officer
Extensive criterion-referenced tool assesses basic skills and employability skills in the context of job-seeking or employment situations: reading grade placement; rating scales; career awareness and self-understanding; reading skills; speaking and listening; job-seeking skills and knowledge; pre-employment writing; math and concepts.

4388 BRIGANCE Life Skills Inventory
Curriculum Associates
153 Rangeway Road
North Billerica, MA 01862-901   978-667-8000
800-225-0248
Fax: 800-366-1158
www.curriculumassociates.com
info@CAinc.com
Frank E. Ferguson, Chairman
Albert Brigance, Author
Dave Caron, Chief Financial Officer
Assesses listening, speaking, reading, writing, comprehending, and computing skills in nine life-skill sections: speaking and listening; money and finance; functional writing; food; words on common signs and warning labels; clothing; health; telephone; travel and transportation.

4389 Bedside Evaluation and Screening Test
Pro-Ed
8700 Shoal Creek Boulevard
Austin, TX 78757-6897   512-451-3246
800-897-3202
Fax: 512-451-8542
www.proedinc.com
general@proedinc.com
Donald D Hammill, Owner
Joyce West, Author
Elaine Sands, Co-Author
Access and quantify language disorders in adults resulting from aphasia. *$171.00*

4390 Boone Voice Program for Adults
Pro-Ed
8700 Shoal Creek Boulevard
Austin, TX 78757-6897   512-451-3246
800-897-3202
Fax: 512-451-8542
www.proedinc.com
general@proedinc.com
Donald D Hammill, Owner
Daniel Boone, Author
Kay Wiley, Co-Author
Provides for diagnosis and remediation of adult voice disorders. This program is based on the same philosophy and therapy as The Program for Children but is presented at an adult interest level. *$153.00*

4391 Boone Voice Program for Children
Pro-Ed
8700 Shoal Creek Boulevard
Austin, TX 78757-6897   512-451-3246
800-897-3202
Fax: 512-451-8542
www.proedinc.com
general@proedinc.com
Donald D Hammill, Owner
Daniel Boone, Author
Provides a cognitive approach to voice therapy and is designed to give useful step-by-step guidelines and materials for diagnosis and remediation of voice disorders in children. *$208.00*

4392 Connecting Reading and Writing with Vocabulary
Curriculum Associates
153 Rangeway Road
North Billerica, MA 01862-901   978-667-8000
800-225-0248
Fax: 800-366-1158
www.curriculumassociates.com
info@CAinc.com
Frank E. Ferguson, Chairman
Deborah P Adcock, Author
Dave Caron, Chief Financial Officer
This vocabulary enrichment series builds successful writers and speakers by implementing strategic word techniques. Students will add 120 writing words and other word forms to their word banks. Each lesson introduces ten vocabulary words in a variety of contexts: a letter, poem, story, journal entry, classified ad, etc.

4393 Diamonds in the Rough
Slosson Educational Publications
538 Buffalo Road
East Aurora, NY 14052   716-652-0930
888-756-7766
Fax: 800-655-3840
www.slosson.com
slossonprep@gmail.com
Steven Slosson, President
Peggy Strass Dras, Author
Dr. Georgina Moynihan, Tech Support
College reference/rehabilitation guide for people with attention deficit disorder and learning disabilities. *$36.00*

4394 Easy Talker: A Fluency Workbook for School Age Children
Pro-Ed
8700 Shoal Creek Boulevard
Austin, TX 78757-6897   512-451-3246
800-897-3202
Fax: 512-451-8542
www.proedinc.com
general@proedinc.com
Donald D Hammill, Owner
Barry Guitar, Author
Julie Reville, Co-Author
A diagnostic, criterion-referenced instrument to be used with children, to determine which stutterers would benefit from early intervention. Item #4855. *$45.00*

4395 Fluharty Preschool Speech & Language Screening Test-2
Speech Bin
PO Box 1579
Appleton, WI 54912-1579 888-388-3224
Fax: 800-845-1535
www.schoolspecialty.com
orders@schoolspecialty.com
Joseph M. Yorio, President & CEO
James R. Henderson, Chairman
Patrick T. Collins, EVP, Distribution
Carefully normed on 705 children, the Fluharty yields standard scores, percentiles, and age equivalents. The form features space for speech-language pathologists to note phonological processes, voice quality, and fluency; a Teacher Questionnaire is also provided. Item number P882. *$153.00*

4396 Help for the Learning Disabled Child
Slosson Educational Publications
538 Buffalo Road
East Aurora, NY 14052 716-652-0930
888-756-7766
Fax: 800-655-3840
www.slosson.com
slossonprep@gmail.com
Steven Slosson, President
John H Slosson, Vice President
Dr. Georgina Moynihan, Tech Support
Symptoms and solutions for learning disabled children. Features issues from a medical, psychological and educational basis and illustrates learning disabilities from emotional and mental impairment. *$48.75*

4397 Learning Disability Evaluation Scale
Hawthorne Educational Services
800 Gray Oak Dr
Columbia, MO 65201-3730 573-874-1710
800-542-1673
Fax: 800-442-9509
www.hawthorne-ed.com
info@hes-inc.com
Stephen B McCarney Ed-D, Author
Tamara J Arthaud PhD, Co-Author
The Learning Disability Evaluation Scale - Renormed Second Edition (LDES-R2) was developed to enable instructional personnel to document those performance behaviors most characteristic of learning disabilities in children and youth. The LDES-R2 avoids the nature of a testing situation by relying on the performance observations of the classroom teacher or other instructional personnel. *$189.00*

4398 Oral Speech Mechanism Screening Examination
Pro-Ed
8700 Shoal Creek Boulevard
Austin, TX 78757-6897 512-451-3246
800-897-3202
Fax: 512-451-8542
www.proedinc.com
general@proedinc.com
Donald D Hammill, Owner
Kenneth St Louis, Author
Dennis Ruscello, Co-Author
Provides an efficient, quick, and reliable method to examine the oral speech mechanism of all types of speech, language, and related disorders where oral structure and function are of concern. *$105.00*

4399 Peabody Picture Vocabulary Test
4940 Pearl East Circle
Suite 200
Boulder, CO 80301 888-977-7900
800-328-5999
Fax: 888-556-2103
www.pearsonassessments.com
info@pearsonkt.com
Lloyd M Dunn, Author
Leota M Dunn, Co-Author
Doug Kubach, Group President & CEO
A wide-range measure of receptive vocabulary for standard English, and a screening test of verbal ability.

4400 Peabody Picture Vocabulary Test: Fourth Edition
Pearson Assessments
4940 Pearl East Circle
Suite 200
Boulder, CO 80301 888-977-7900
800-328-5999
Fax: 888-556-2103
www.pearsonassessments.com
info@pearsonkt.com
Karen Dahlen, Associate Director
Matt Keller, Marketing Manager
Lisa Dunttam, Development Assistant
A wide range measure of receptive vocabulary for standard English and screen of verbal ability. *$379.99*

4401 Preschool Motor Speech Evaluation & Intervention
Speech Bin
PO Box 1579
Appleton, WI 54912-1579 888-388-3224
Fax: 800-845-1535
www.schoolspecialty.com
orders@schoolspecialty.com
Joseph M. Yorio, President & CEO
James R. Henderson, Chairman
Patrick T. Collins, EVP, Distribution
This comprehensive criterion-based assessment tool differentiates motor-based speech disorders from those of phonology and determines if speech difficulties of children 18 months to six years old are characteristic of: oral nonverbal apraxia; dysarthria; developmental verbal dyspraxia; hypersensitivity; differences in tone and hyposensitivity. Item number J322. *$59.00*

4402 Receptive One-Word Picture Vocabulary Test
Speech Bin
PO Box 1579
Appleton, WI 54912-1579 888-388-3224
Fax: 800-845-1535
www.schoolspecialty.com
orders@schoolspecialty.com
Rick Brownell, Author
Joseph M. Yorio, President & CEO
James R. Henderson, Chairman
Patrick T. Collins, EVP, Distribution
This administered, untimed measure assessess the vocabulary comprehension of 0-2 through 11-18 years. New full-color test pictures are easy to recognize; many new test items have been added. It is ideal for children unable or reluctant to speak because only a gestural response is required. *$140.00*

4403 Receptive-Expressive Emergent Language Tests
Pro-Ed
8700 Shoal Creek Boulevard
Austin, TX 78757-6897 512-451-3246
800-897-3202
Fax: 512-451-8542
www.proedinc.com
general@proedinc.com
Donald D Hammill, Owner
Kenneth Bzoch, Author
Richard League, Co-Author
Designed to use with at-risk infants and toddlers to provide a multidimensional analysis of emergency language skills. *$104.00*

4404 Say and Sign Language Program
Slosson Educational Publications
538 Buffalo Road
East Aurora, NY 14052 716-652-0930
888-756-7766
Fax: 800-655-3840
www.slosson.com
slossonprep@gmail.com
Roger Hoffmann, Author
John H Slosson, Vice President
Dr. Georgina Moynihan, Tech Support

Addresses articulation skills, speech production, basic sign language skills, and finger spelling. *$71.50*

4405 Sequenced Inventory of Communication Development (SICD)
Speech Bin
PO Box 1579
Appleton, WI 54912-1579
888-388-3224
Fax: 800-845-1535
www.schoolspecialty.com
orders@schoolspecialty.com
Joseph M. Yorio, President & CEO
James R. Henderson, Chairman
Patrick T. Collins, EVP, Distribution
SICD uses appealing toys to assess communication skills of children at all levels of ability, including those with impaired hearing or vision. SICD looks at child and environment, measuring receptive and expressive language. Item number W710. *$395.00*

4406 Skills Assessments
222 Berkeley Street
Boston, MA 02116
617-351-5000
800-531-5015
Fax: 800-269-5232
www.hmhco.com/educators
info@steck-vaughn.com
Linda K. Zecher, President, CEO & Director
Eric Shuman, Chief Financial Officer
William Bayers, EVP/General Counsel
This handy, all-in-one resource helps identify students strengths and weaknesses in order to determine appropriate instructional levels in each of five subjects areas: reading; language arts; math; science; and social studies. Assessments are identified by subtopics in each subject.

4407 Slosson Intelligence Test
Slosson Educational Publications, Inc.
538 Buffalo Road
East Aurora, NY 14052
716-652-0930
888-756-7766
Fax: 800-655-3840
www.slosson.com
slossonprep@gmail.com
Steven Slosson, President
John H Slosson, Vice President
Dr. Georgina Moynihan, Tech Support
A quick and reliable individual screening test of Crystallized Verbal Intelligence. Tests include SIT-R3: Slosson Intelligence Test, Rev. - Third Edition; SORT-R3: Slosson Oral Reading Test, Rev. - Third Edition; S-VMPT: Slosson Visual Motor Performance Test; EASYOT: Educational Assessment of School Youth for Occupational Therapists. *$147.00*

4408 Slosson Intelligence Test Primary
Slosson Educational Publications
538 Buffalo Road
East Aurora, NY 14052
716-652-0930
888-756-7766
Fax: 800-655-3840
www.slosson.com
slossonprep@gmail.com
Steven Slosson, President
Bradley Erford, Author
Gary Vitali, Co-Author
Designed to facilitate the screening identification of children at risk of educational failure. Provides a quick estimate of mental ability to identify children who may be appropriate candidates for deeper testing services. *$168.00*

4409 Stuttering Severity Instrument for Children and Adults
Pro-Ed
8700 Shoal Creek Boulevard
Austin, TX 78757-6897
512-451-3246
800-897-3202
Fax: 512-451-8542
www.proedinc.com
general@proedinc.com

Donald D Hammill, Owner
Glyndon Riley, Author
With these easily administered tools you can determine whether to schedule a child for therapy using the Stuttering Prediction Instrument or to evaluate the effects of treatment using the Stuttering Severity Instrument. *$114.00*

4410 Test for Auditory Comprehension of Language: TACL-3
Speech Bin
PO Box 1579
Appleton, WI 54912-1579
888-388-3224
Fax: 800-845-1535
www.schoolspecialty.com
orders@schoolspecialty.com
Joseph M. Yorio, President & CEO
James R. Henderson, Chairman
Patrick T. Collins, EVP, Distribution
The newly revised TACL-3 evaluates the 0-3 to 9-11-year old's understanding of spoken language in three subtests: Vocabulary, Grammatical Morphemes and Elaborated Phrases and Sentences. Each test item is a word or sentence read aloud by the examiner; the child responds by pointing to one of three pictures. Item number P792. *$261.00*

4411 Test of Adolescent & Adult Language: TOAL-3
Pro-Ed
8700 Shoal Creek Boulevard
Austin, TX 78757-6897
512-451-3246
800-897-3202
Fax: 512-451-8542
www.proedinc.com
general@proedinc.com
Donald D Hammill, Owner/Author
Virginia Brown, Co-Author
Stephen Larson, Co-Author
This test is a measure of receptive and expressive language skills. In this revision easier items were added to the subtests, making them more appropriate for testing disabled students. *$202.00*

4412 Test of Auditory Reasoning & Processing Skills: TARPS
Speech Bin
PO Box 1579
Appleton, WI 54912-1579
888-388-3224
Fax: 800-845-1535
www.schoolspecialty.com
orders@schoolspecialty.com
Morrison Gardner, Author
Joseph M. Yorio, President & CEO
James R. Henderson, Chairman
Patrick T. Collins, EVP, Distribution
TARPS assesses how 5-14 year old children understand, interpret, draw conclusions, and make inferences from auditorily presented stimuli. It tests their ability to think, understand, reason, and make sense of what they hear. Item number H787. *$64.00*

4413 Test of Auditory-Perceptual Skills: Upper TAPS-UL
Speech Bin
PO Box 1579
Appleton, WI 54912-1579
888-388-3224
Fax: 800-845-1535
www.schoolspecialty.com
orders@schoolspecialty.com
Wayne Hresko, Shelley Herron, Pamela Peak, Author
Joseph M. Yorio, President & CEO
James R. Henderson, Chairman
Patrick T. Collins, EVP, Distribution
This highly respected, well-normed test evaluates a 13-18 year old's ability to perceive auditory stimuli and helps you diagnose auditory disorders in just 15-20 minutes. TAPS: UL measures the auditory perceptual skills of processing, word and sequential memory, interpretation of oral directions, and discrimination. Item number H769. *$95.00*

4414   Test of Early Language Development
Pro-Ed, Inc.
8700 Shoal Creek Boulevard
Austin, TX 78757-6897   512-451-3246
                                          800-897-3202
                                    Fax: 512-451-8542
                                    www.proedinc.com
                                    general@proedinc.com

Wayne P Hresko, Author

4415   Test of Early Language Development: TELD-3
Pro-Ed, Inc.
8700 Shoal Creek Boulevard
Austin, TX 78757-6897   512-451-3246
                                          800-897-3202
                                    Fax: 512-451-8542
                                    www.proedinc.com
                                    general@proedinc.com

Donald D Hammill, President/Author
Wayne Hresko, Co-Author
Kim Reid, Co-Author
An individually administered test of spoken language abilities. This test fills the need for a well-constructed, standardized instrument, based on a current theory, that can be used to assess spoken language skills at early ages. Now including scores for receptive language and expressive language subtests. Administration Time: 20 minutes. *$295.00*

4416   Test of Early Written Language
Pro-Ed
8700 Shoal Creek Boulevard
Austin, TX 78757-6897   512-451-3246
                                          800-897-3202
                                    Fax: 512-451-8542
                                    www.proedinc.com
                                    general@proedinc.com

Donald D Hammill, Owner
Shelley Herron, Author
Wayne Hresko, Co-Author
Measures the merging written language skills of young children and is especially useful in identifying mildy disabled students. *$197.00*

4417   Test of Written Language: TOWL-3
Pro-Ed
8700 Shoal Creek Boulevard
Austin, TX 78757-6897   512-451-3246
                                          800-897-3202
                                    Fax: 512-451-8542
                                    www.proedinc.com
                                    general@proedinc.com

Donald D Hammill, Owner/Author
Stephen Larson, Co-Author
Offers a measure of written language skills to identify students who need help improving their writing skills. Administration Time: 65 minutes. *$217.00*

4418   Test of Written Spelling
Pro-Ed
8700 Shoal Creek Boulevard
Austin, TX 78757-6897   512-451-3246
                                          800-897-3202
                                    Fax: 512-451-8542
                                    www.proedinc.com
                                    general@proedinc.com

Donald D Hammill, Owner/Author
Stephen Larsen, Co-Author
Louisa Cook Moats, Co-Author
Assesses students' ability to spell words whose spellings are readily predictable in sound-letter patterns, words whose spellings are less predictable and both types of words considered together. *$88.00*

4419   Testing & Remediating Auditory Processing (TRAP)
Speech Bin
PO Box 1579
Appleton, WI 54912-1579   888-388-3224
                                    Fax: 800-845-1535
                                    www.schoolspecialty.com
                                    orders@schoolspecialty.com

Lynn Baron Berk, Author
Joseph M. Yorio, President & CEO
James R. Henderson, Chairman
Patrick T. Collins, EVP, Distribution
TRAP gives you an easy-to-implement program to assess and treat school-age auditory processing problems. It gives you two major components: Screening Test of Auditoring Processing Skills that identifies children at risk due to auditory processing deficits; and Remediating Auditory Processing Skills that presents interactional stories, sequence pictures, and illustrated activities. Item number 1233. *$38.00*

4420   Voice Assessment Protocol for Children and Adults
Pro-Ed
8700 Shoal Creek Boulevard
Austin, TX 78757-6897   512-451-3246
                                          800-897-3202
                                    Fax: 512-451-8542
                                    www.proedinc.com
                                    general@proedinc.com

Donald D Hammill, Owner
Rebekah Pindzola, Author
Easily guides the speech pathologist through a systematic evaluation of vocal pitch, loudness, quality, breath features and rate/rhythm. *$78.00*

Visual & Motor Skills

4421   BRIGANCE Inventory of Early Development-II
Curriculum Associates
153 Rangeway Road
North Billerica, MA 01862-901   978-667-8000
                                          800-225-0248
                                    Fax: 800-366-1158
                                    www.curriculumassociates.com
                                    info@CAinc.com

Albert H Brigance, Author
Frank E. Ferguson, Chairman
Dave Caron, Chief Financial Officer
The Inventory of Early Development simplifies and combines the assessment, diagnostic, recordkeeping, and instructional planning process, and it encourages communication between teachers and parents.

4422   Benton Visual Retention Test
Pearson Assessments
4940 Pearl East Circle
Suite 200
Boulder, CO 80301   888-977-7900
                                          800-328-5999
                                    Fax: 888-556-2103
                                    www.pearsonassessments.com
                                    info@pearsonkt.com

Abigail Benton Sivan, Author
Matt Keller, Marketing Manager
Doug Kubach, Group President & CEO
Assess visual perception, memory, visoconstructive abilities. Test administration 15-20 minutes. *$199.00*

4423   Boston Diagnostic Aphasia Exam
Speech Bin
PO Box 1579
Appleton, WI 54912-1579   888-388-3224
                                    Fax: 800-845-1535
                                    www.schoolspecialty.com
                                    orders@schoolspecialty.com

Harold Goodglass, Edith Kaplan, Barbara Barresi, Author
Joseph M. Yorio, President & CEO
James R. Henderson, Chairman
Patrick T. Collins, EVP, Distribution
BDAE-3 now gives you an instructive 90-minute video plus two separate forms of the test. Item number L235. *$150.00*

4424   Developmental Test of Visual Perception (D TVP-2)
Pro-Ed
8700 Shoal Creek Boulevard
Austin, TX 78757-6897   512-451-3246
                                                 800-897-3202
                                            Fax: 512-451-8542
                                            www.proedinc.com
                                            general@proedinc.com
Donald D Hammill, Owner/Author
Nils Pearson, Co-Author
Judith Voress, Co-Author
A test that measures both visual perception and visual-motor integration skills, has eight subtests, is based on updated theories of visual perceptual development, and can be administered to individuals in 45 minutes. *$207.00*

4425   Differential Test of Conduct and Emotional Problems
Slosson Educational Publications
538 Buffalo Road
East Aurora, NY 14052   716-652-0930
                                                 888-756-7766
                                            Fax: 800-655-3840
                                            www.slosson.com
                                            slossonprep@gmail.com
Steven Slosson, President
Edward Kelly, Author
Dr. Georgina Moynihan, Tech Support
Designed to address one of the most critical challenges in education and juvenile care. Administration of test is 15-20 minutes. *$120.75*

4426   Educational Assessment of School Youth for Occupational Therapists
Slosson Educational Publications
538 Buffalo Road
East Aurora, NY 14052   716-652-0930
                                                 888-756-7766
                                            Fax: 800-655-3840
                                            www.slosson.com
                                            slossonprep@gmail.com
Sharon Kenmotsu, Author
Katy Tressler, Co-Author
Dr. Georgina Moynihan, Tech Support
The E.A.S.Y. is a school-based occupational therapy assessment tool developed by occupational therapists. *$280.00*

4427   Khan-Lewis Phonological Analysis: KLPA-2
Pro-Ed
8700 Shoal Creek Boulevard
Austin, TX 78757-6897   512-451-3246
                                                 800-897-3202
                                            Fax: 512-451-8542
                                            www.proedinc.com
                                            general@proedinc.com
Donald D Hammill, President
Linda Klan, Author
Nancy Lewis, Co-Author
An in-depth measure of phonological processes for assessment and remediation planning. Administration Time: 10-30 minutes. *$144.00*

4428   Peabody Developmental Motor Scales-2
Speech Bin
PO Box 1579
Appleton, WI 54912-1579   888-388-3224
                                            Fax: 800-845-1535
                                            www.schoolspecialty.com
                                            orders@schoolspecialty.com
Joseph M. Yorio, President & CEO
James R. Henderson, Chairman
Patrick T. Collins, EVP, Distribution

PDMS-2 gives you in-depth standardized assessment of motor skills in children birth to six years. Subtests include: fine motor object manipulation; grasping; gross motor; locomotion; reflexes; visual-motor integration and stationary. Item number P624. *$43.00*

4429   Perceptual Motor Development Series
Therapro
225 Arlington St
Framingham, MA 01702-8773   508-872-9494
                                                 800-257-5376
                                            Fax: 508-875-2062
                                            www.theraproducts.com
                                            info@theraproducts.com
Karen Conrad, Owner
Jack Capon, Author
Use these classroom tested movement education activities to assess motor strengths and weaknesses in preschool and early elementary grades or special education classes. The sequence of easily given tests and tasks requires minimal instruction time and your kids will find the activities to be interesting, challenging, and fun! Each book has 25-54 pages and costs $9.99 each. *$49.95*

4430   Phonic Reading Lessons
Academic Therapy Publications
20 Commercial Blvd
Novato, CA 94949-6120   415-883-3314
                                                 800-422-7249
                                            Fax: 888-287-9975
                                            www.academictherapy.com
                                            sales@academictherapy.com
Jim Arena, President
Joanne Urban, Manager
Samuel Kirk, Author
A step-by-step program for teaching reading to children who failed to learn by conventional methods. Consistent sound-symbol relationships are presented and reinforced using a grapho-vocal method. A two book set (Book 1: Skills; Book 2: Practice). *$140.00*
ISBN 1-571284-68-6

4431   Preschool Motor Speech Evaluation & Intervention
Speech Bin
PO Box 1579
Appleton, WI 54912-1579   888-388-3224
                                            Fax: 800-845-1535
                                            www.schoolspecialty.com
                                            orders@schoolspecialty.com
Joseph M. Yorio, President & CEO
James R. Henderson, Chairman
Patrick T. Collins, EVP, Distribution
This comprehensive criterion-based assessment tool differentiates motor-based speech disorders from those of phonology and determines if speech difficulties of children 18 months to six years old are characteristic of: oral nonverbal apraxia; dysarthria; developmental verbal dyspraxia; hypersensitivity; differences in tone and hyposensitivity. Item number J322. *$59.00*

4432   Slosson Full Range Intelligence Test Kit
Slosson Educational Publications
538 Buffalo Road
East Aurora, NY 14052   716-652-0930
                                                 888-756-7766
                                            Fax: 800-655-3840
                                            www.slosson.com
                                            slossonprep@gmail.com
Steven Slosson, President
H Robert Vance, Author
Bob Algozzine, Co-Author
Intended to supplement the use of more extensive cognitive assessment instruments. Administration of test 25-45 minutes. *$175.00*

4433 **Slosson Visual Motor Performance Test**
Slosson Educational Publications
538 Buffalo Road
East Aurora, NY 14052   716-652-0930
                                888-756-7766
                          Fax: 800-655-3840
                             www.slosson.com
                        slossonprep@gmail.com
Steven Slosson, President
Richard.L Slosson, Author
Dr. Georgina Moynihan, Tech Support
A test of visual motor integration in which individuals are asked to copy geometric figures increasing in complexity without the use of a ruler, compass or other aids. *$86.75*

4434 **Test of Gross Motor Development**
Pro-Ed
8700 Shoal Creek Boulevard
Austin, TX 78757-6897   512-451-3246
                                800-897-3202
                          Fax: 512-451-8542
                            www.proedinc.com
                        general@proedinc.com
Donald D Hammill, Owner
Dale Urlich, Author
Assists you in identifying children who are significantly behind their peers in gross motor skill development and who should be eligible for special education services in phyiscal education. *$109.00*

4435 **Test of Information Processing Skills**
Academic Therapy Publications
20 Commercial Blvd
Novato, CA 94949-6120   415-883-3314
                                800-422-7249
                          Fax: 888-287-9975
                        www.academictherapy.com
                      sales@academictherapy.com
Jim Arena, President
Joanne Urban, Manager
Raymond Webster, Author
The TIPS (formerly The Learning Efficiency Test) provides a quick and accurate measure of a child or adult's information processing abilities, sequential and nonsequential, in both visual and auditory modalities. Additional subtests include Delayed Recall and Semantic Fluency. *$140.00*
ISBN 1-571284-68-6

4436 **Visual Skills Appraisal**
Academic Therapy Publications
20 Commercial Blvd
Novato, CA 94949-6120   415-883-3314
                                800-422-7249
                          Fax: 888-287-9975
                        www.academictherapy.com
                      sales@academictherapy.com
Jim Arena, President
Regina Richards, Author
Gary Oppenheim, Co-Author
This test identifies visual problems in children ages 5-9. Can be administered by an experienced examiner. Set includes manual, stimulus cards and test forms, design completion forms, and red/green glasses. *$100.00*
ISBN 0-878794-53-0

National Programs

4437 ACT Universal Testing
ACT
500 ACT Drive
P.O. Box 168
Iowa City, IA 52243-0168

319-337-1332
Fax: 319-339-3021
TDD: 319-337-1701
www.act.org
sandy.schlote@act.org

Jon Whitmore, CEO
Janet E. Godwin, Chief of Staff
Thomas J. Goedken, CFO/EVP
To help individuals and organizations make informed decisions about education and work. We provide information for life's transitions.

4438 American College Testing Program
ACT Universal Testing
500 ACT Drive
P.O. Box 168
Iowa City, IA 52243-0168

319-337-1000
Fax: 319-339-3021
TDD: 319-337-1701
www.act.org
sandy.schlote@act.org

Jon Whitmore, CEO
Janet E. Godwin, Chief of Staff
Thomas J. Goedken, CFO/EVP
ACT provides a broad array of assessment, information, research and program management solutions pertaining to education and workforce development.

4439 Center For Accessible Technology
Alliance For Technology Access
3075 Adeline
Suite 220
Berkeley, CA 94703

510-841-3224
Fax: 510-841-7956
www.cforat.org
info@cforat.orgg

Guy Thomas, Board President
Sara Armstrong Ph.D., Board Treasurer
A national organization dedicated to providing access to technology for people with disabilities through its coalition of 39 community-based resource centers in 28 states and in the Virgin Islands. Each center provides information, awareness, and training for professionals and provides guided problem solving and technical assistance for individuals with disabilities and family members.

4440 Division on Career Development
Council for Exceptional Children
2900 Crystal Drive
Suite 1000
Arlington, VA 22202-3557

888-232-7733
Fax: 703-264-9494
TTY: 866-915-5000
www.cec.sped.org
service@ces.sped.org

Robin D. Brewer, President
James P. Heiden, President Elect
Joni L. Baldwin, Board Member
Focuses on the career development of individuals with disabilities and/or who are gifted and their transition from school to adult life. Members include professionals and others interested in career development and transition for individuals with any exception at any age. Members receive a journal twice yearly and newsletter three times per year.

4441 Independent Living Research Utilization Program
One Baylor Plaza
Houston, TX 77030

713-798-4951
Fax: 713-520-5785
TTY: 713-520-0232
www.bcm.edu

Lex Frieden, Director
Laurie Redd, Executive Director
Dr. Paul Klotman, President
A national resource center for information, training, research and technical assistance in independent living; produces and disseminates materials, develops and conducts training and publishes a monthly newsletter; provides a listing of Statewide Independent Living Councils (SILCS) in each state.

4442 Job Accommodation Network (JAN)
West Virginia University
PO Box 6080
Morgantown, WV 26506-6080

800-526-7234
Fax: 304-293-5407
TDD: 877-781-9403
http://askjan.org
jan@jan.wvu.edu

Anne Hirsh, Co-Director
Louis Orslene, Co-Director
Melanie Whetzel, Senior Consultant
Source of free, expert, and confidential guidance on workplace accomodations and disability employment issues. Working toward practical solutions that benefit both employer and employee, helps people with disabilities enhance their employability and shows employers how to capitalize on the value and talent that people with disabilities add to the workplace.

4443 National Federation of the Blind
200 E. Wells St. At Jernigan Place
Baltimore, MD 21230-4914

410-659-9314
Fax: 410-685-5653
www.nfb.org
nfb@nfb.org

Marc Maurer, President
Patricia Maurer, Community Relations Director
Provides education, information, literature and publications to the public about blindness. The National Federation of the Blind also provides programs and jobs to blind individuals, which helps them build self-confidence and self-respect.

4444 U.S. Department of Education: Office of Vocational & Adult Education
400 Maryland Avenue, SW
Lyndon Baines Johnson, Dept Ed. Bldg.
Washington, DC 20202-0001

202-401-1576
800-872-5327
http://www2.ed.gov
ovae@ed.gov

Arne Duncan, Secretary of Education
Emma Vadehra, Chief of Staff
Massie Ritsch, Acting Assistant Secretary
These agencies can provide job training, counseling, financial assistance, and employment placement to individuals who meet eligibility criteria.

Publications

4445 ADD on the Job
Taylor Publishing
7211 Circle S Road
Austin, TX 78745

512-444-0571
800-225-3687
Fax: 512-440-2160
www.balfour.com
Yearbooks@balfour.com

Lynn Weiss PhD, Author
Practical, sensitive advice for the ADD employee, his boss, and his co-workers. The book suggests advantages that the ADD worker has, how to find the right job, and how to keep it. Employers and co-workers will learn what to expect from fellow workers with ADD and the most effective ways to work with them.
232 pages Paperback
ISBN 0-878339-17-5

4446 Ability Magazine
Ability Awareness
PO Box 10878
Costa Mesa, CA 10878
949-854-8700
Fax: 949-548-5966
www.abilitymagazine.com
editorial@abilitymagazine.com
Chet Cooper, President
Brings disabilities into mainstream America. By interviewing high profile personalities such as President Clinton, Elizabeth Taylor, Mary Tyler Moore, Richard Pryor, Jane Seymour and many more, Ability Magazine is able to bring articles to the public's attention that may in the past have gone unnoticed.
80+ pages Bimonthly

4447 Current Developments in Employment and Training
National Governors Association
444 N Capitol St NW
Ste 267
Washington, DC 20001-1512
202-624-5300
Fax: 202-624-5313
www.nga.org
mjensen@nga.org
John Hickenlooper, Chair
Gary Herbert, Vice Chair
Dan Crippen, Executive Director
Highlights issues and areas of interest related to employment and training.
Bimonthly

4448 Fundamentals of Job Placement
RPM Press
737 N. Cental Avenue
Wood Dale, IL 60191
630-422-7393
888-810-1990
Fax: 630-422-7246
www.rpmpress.com
info@rpmpress.com
James Costello, Author
Paul McCray, President
Provides step-by-step guidance for educators, special counselors and vocational rehabilitation personnel on how to develop job placement opportunities for special needs students and adults.

4449 Fundamentals of Vocational Assessment
RPM Press
737 N. Cental Avenue
Wood Dale, IL 60191
630-422-7393
888-810-1990
Fax: 630-422-7246
www.rpmpress.com
info@rpmpress.com
Paul McCray, President
Provides step-by-step guidance for educators, counselors and vocational rehabilitation personnel on how to conduct professional vocational assessments of special needs students.

4450 Handbook for Developing Community Based Employment
RPM Press
737 N. Cental Avenue
Wood Dale, IL 60191
630-422-7393
888-810-1990
Fax: 630-422-7246
www.rpmpress.com
info@rpmpress.com
Paul McCray, President
Provides step-by-step guidance for educators and vocational rehabilitation personnel on how to develop community-based employment training programs for severely challenged workers.

4451 JOBS V
PESCO International
21 Paulding St
Pleasantville, NY 10570-3108
914-769-4266
800-431-2016
Fax: 914-769-2970
www.pesco.org
pesco@pesco.org
Joseph Kass, President
A software program matching people with jobs, training, employment and local employers. Provides job outlooks for the next five years.

4452 Job Access
Ability Awareness
PO Box 10878
Costa Mesa, CA 92627-4512
949-548-1986
Fax: 949-548-5966
TDD: 949-548-5966
www.jobaccess.org
custserv@jobtarget.com
Chet Cooper, President
Job Access, a program of ability awareness, is an internet driven system dedicated to employ qualified people with disabilities. Employers can list job postings and review our resume bank. People with disabilities seeking employment can also search for jobs.

4453 Job Accommodation Handbook
RPM Press
737 N. Central Avenue
Wood Dale, IL 60191
630-422-7393
888-810-1990
Fax: 630-422-7246
www.rpmpress.com
info@rpmpress.com
Paul McCray, President
Provides how-to-do-it for counselors, job placement specialists, educators and others on how to modify jobs for special needs workers.

4454 Life Centered Career Education: Assessment Batteries
Council for Exceptional Children
2900 Crystal Drive
Suite 1000
Arlington, VA 22202-3557
703-620-3660
888-232-7733
Fax: 703-264-9494
TTY: 866-915-5000
www.cec.sped.org
service@ces.sped.org
Robin D. Brewer, President
James P. Heiden, President Elect
Joni L. Baldwin, Board Member
The LCCE Batteries are curriculum-based assessment instruments designed to measure the career education knowledge and skills of regular and special education students. There are two alternative forms of a Knowledge Battery and two forms of the Performance Batteries. These assessment tools can be combined with instruction to determine the instructional goals most appropriate for a particular student.
827 pages

4455 National Governors Association Newsletter
444 N Capitol St NW
Ste 267
Washington, DC 20001-1512
202-624-5300
Fax: 202-624-5313
www.nga.org
mjensen@nga.org
John Hickenlooper, Chair
Gary Herbert, Vice Chair
Dan Crippen, Executive Director
Highlights issues and areas of interest related to employment and training.
Bimonthly

4456   PWI Profile
Goodwill Industries of America
15810 Indianola Dr
Derwood, MD 20855-2674   301-530-6500
                                       800-GOODWILL
                                       www.goodwill.org
                                       contactus@goodwill.org
David Hadani, Director
Rev. Edgar J Helms, Founder
Newsletter that deals with employment of persons with disabilities.

4457   School to Adult Life Transition Bibliography
Special Education Resource Center
25 Industrial Park Rd
Middletown, CT 06457-1516   860-632-1485
                                       Fax: 860-632-8870
                                       www.ctserc.org
                                       jlebrrun@ctserc.org
Jen Lebrun, Director
Marianne Kirner, Executive Director
A bibliography of references and resources.

4458   Self-Supervision: A Career Tool for Audiologists, Clinical Series 10
American Speech-Language-Hearing Association
2200 Research Boulevard
Rockville, MD 20850-3289   301-897-5700
                                       800-638-2255
                                       Fax: 301-897-7358
                                       TDD: 301-897-5700
                                       www.asha.org
                                       jjanota@asha.org
Elizabeth S. McCrea, President
Judith L. Page, President-Elect
Arlene A. Pietranton, Chief Executive Officer
Describes concepts of supervision, defines and presents strategies for self-supervision, discusses supervisory accountability and covers issues of self-supervision within supervisor format.

4459   Succeeding in the Workplace
4156 Library Road
Pittsburgh, PA 15234-1349   412-341-1515
                                       Fax: 412-344-0224
                                       http://ldaamerica.org
                                       lathamlaw@gmail.com
Nancie Payne, President
Ed Schlitt, First Vice President
Beth McGaw, Secretary
Comprehensive review: understanding disabilities, how to find and get the right job, how to succeed on the job, strategies, job accommodations, legal rights and personal experiences.

4460   Tales from the Workplace
Ste 707
2700 Virginia Ave NW
Washington, DC 20037-1909   202-333-1713
                                       Fax: 202-333-1735
                                       lathamlaw@gmail.com
Peter S Latham JD, Director
Patricia Horan Latham JD, Director
Easy to read. Explores through stories: What is the right job match? Should I disclose my disability? What are the signs of job trouble?

4461   Transition and Students with Learning Disabilities
Pro-Ed
8700 Shoal Creek Boulevard
Austin, TX 78757-6897   512-451-3246
                                       800-897-3202
                                       Fax: 512-451-8542
                                       www.proedinc.com
                                       general@proedinc.com
Patton Blalock, Author
Donald D Hammill, Owner
Provides important information about academic, social and vocational planning for students with learning disabilities.

4462   Vocational Training and Employment of Autistic Adolescents
Charles C Thomas
2600 S 1st St
Springfield, IL 62704-4730   217-789-8980
                                       800-258-8980
                                       Fax: 217-789-9130
                                       www.ccthomas.com
                                       books@ccthomas.com
Michael P Thomas, President
Publisher of Education and Special Education books.

4463   Workforce Investment Quarterly
National Governor's Association (NGA)
444 N Capitol St NW
Ste 267
Washington, DC 20001-1512   202-624-5300
                                       Fax: 202-624-5313
                                       www.nga.org
                                       info@nga.org
John Hickenlooper, Chair
Gary Herbert, Vice Chair
Dan Crippen, Executive Director
Highlights issues and area interests related to employment and training. Contact NGA for more information.

Alabama

4464   Achievement Center
Easter Seals Of East Central Alabama
510 W Thomason Cir
Opelika, AL 36801-5499   334-745-3501
                                       866-239-2237
                                       Fax: 334-749-5808
                                       www.achievement-center.org
                                       info@achievement-center.org
Jason Lazenby, Chairman
Kenneth Burton, Vice-Chairman
Phyllis Horace, Secretary
Provides vocational development and employment programs to developmentally and physically disabled individuals. The programs help individuals build self-esteem, self-confidence and helps to maximize their independent living skills.

4465   Easter Seals - Alabama
5960 E Shirley Ln
Montgomery, AL 36117-1963   334-395-4489
                                       800-388-7325
                                       Fax: 334-395-4492
                                       www.alabama.easter-seals.org
                                       info@al.easterseals.com
Richard W. Davidson, Chairman
Sandra L. Bouwman, 1st Vice Chairman
Lynne Stokley, CEO
Job training and employment services, senior community service employment program.

4466   Easter Seals - Camp ASCCA
PO Box 21
Jacksons Gap, AL 36861-21   256-825-9226
                                       800-843-2267
                                       Fax: 256-825-8332
                                       www.alabama.easter-seals.org
                                       matt@campascca.org
Richard W. Davidson, Chairman
Sandra L. Bouwman, 1st Vice Chairman
Lynne Stokley, CEO
Camp respite for adults and children, camperships, canoeing, day camping for adults, day camping for children, therapeutic horseback riding.

4467 Easter Seals - Capilouto Center for the Deaf
5960 E Shirley Ln
Montgomery, AL 36117-1963   334-395-4489
800-388-7325
Fax: 334-395-4492
www.alabama.easter-seals.org
info@al.easterseals.com
Richard W. Davidson, Chairman
Sandra L. Bouwman, 1st Vice Chairman
Lynne Stokley, CEO
Job training and employment services, occupational skills training, job placement/competitive-supported employment, vocational evaluation/situation assessment, work adjustment.

4468 Easter Seals - Disability Services
2448 Gordon Smith Dr
Mobile, AL 36617-2319   251-471-1581
800-411-0068
Fax: 251-476-4303
TTY: 334-872-8421
www.alabama.easterseals.org
info@al.easterseals.com
S.Lynne Stokley, CEO
Easter Seals has been helping individuals with disabilities and special needs, and their families, live better lives for more than 80 years. Whether helping someone improve physical mobility, return to work or simply gain greater independence for everyday living, Easter Seals offers a variety of services to help people with disabilities address life's challenges and achieve personal goals.

4469 Easter Seals - Opportunity Center
United Way
6300 McClellan Blvd
Anniston, AL 36206   256-820-9960
Fax: 256-820-9592
www.alabama.easter-seals.org
mikenancyoppcen@aol.com
Richard W. Davidson, Chairman
Sandra L. Bouwman, 1st Vice Chairman
Lynne Stokley, CEO
Job training and employment services, occupational skills training, job placement/competitive-supported employment, vocational evaluation/situation assessment, work adjustment.

4470 Easter Seals - Rehabilitation Center, Northwest Alabama
1450 E Avalon Ave
Muscle Shoals, AL 35661-3110   256-381-1110
Fax: 256-314-5105
www.alabama.easter-seals.org
info@al.easterseals.com
Richard W. Davidson, Chairman
Sandra L. Bouwman, 1st Vice Chairman
Lynne Stokley, CEO
Job training and employment services, occupational skills training, job placement/competitive-supported employment, vocational evaluation/situation assessment, work services.

4471 Easter Seals - West Alabama
PO Box 2817
Tuscaloosa, AL 35403   205-759-1211
800-726-1216
Fax: 205-349-1162
www.alabama.easter-seals.org
info@al.easterseals.com
Richard W. Davidson, Chairman
Sandra L. Bouwman, 1st Vice Chairman
Lynne Stokley, CEO
Job training and employment services, occupational skills training, job placement/competitive-supported employment, vocational evaluation/situation assessment, work adjustment.

4472 Good Will Easter Seals
2448 Gordon Smith Dr
Mobile, AL 36617-2319   251-471-1581
800-411-0068
Fax: 251-476-4303
TTY: 800-411-0068
www.gesgc.org
bill@gesgc.org
Frank Harkins, President/CEO
John McCain, Chief Operating Officer
Terri Bolin, VP Program Services
Job training and employment services, occupational skills training, job placement/competitive-supported employment, vocational evaluation/situation assessment, work adjustment.

4473 State Vocational Rehabilitation Agency
Alabama Dept Of Rehabilitation Services
602 South Lawrence Street
Montgomery, AL 36104   334-293-7500
800-441-7607
Fax: 334-293-7383
TDD: 334-613-2249
www.rehab.state.al.us
sshivers@rehab.state.al.us
Steve Shivers, Director
State vocational rehabilitation agencies provide direct services to persons with disabilities, including persons with learning disabilities. The services may include evaluation and diagnosis; counseling, guidance, and referral services; vocational and other training services; transportation to rehabilitation services; and assistive devices.

4474 Workforce Development Division
Alabama Dept of Economic & Community Affairs
P.O.Box 5690
Montgomery, AL 36103-5690   334-242-5100
Fax: 334-242-5099
www.adeca.state.al.us
stevew@adeca.state.al.us
Tim Alford, Executive Director
Customer focused to help Americans access the tools they need to manage their careers through information and high quality services and to help US companies find skilled workers. Alabama's Career Center System is a network of one-stop centers designed to offer these services. These centers are co-located or electronically linked to provide streamlined services.

Alaska

4475 AK Dept. of Labor and Workforce Dev.
Division of Voc. Rehab.
801 W. 10th Street
Suite A
Juneau, AK 99801-1894   907-465-2814
800-478-2815
Fax: 907-465-2856
www.labor.state.ak.us/dvr
Cheryl Walsh, Director
Assists individuals with disabilities to obtain and maintain employment.

Arizona

4476 Arizona Vocational Rehabilitation
Arizona Department of Economic Security
1717 W. Jefferson
Room 119
Phoenix, AZ 85007   602-542-4791
Fax: 602-241-7158
TTY: 602-241-1048
www.azdes.gov
Michael Scione, Program Manager
Jon Ellerston, Assistant Program Manager

Programs provide a variety of specialized services for individuals with physical or mental disabilities that create barriers to employment or independent living. RSA offers three major service programs and several specialized programs/services.

4477 Rehabilitation Services Administration
Arizona Dept Of Economic Security
1717 W. Jefferson
Room 119
Phoenix, AZ 85007   602-542-4791
                           Fax: 602-241-7158
                           TTY: 602-241-1048
                           www.azdes.gov

Katharine Levandowsky, Director
The mission of the Rehabilitation Services Administration (RSA) is to work with individuals with disabilities to achieve increased independence and/or gainful employment through the provision of comprehensive rehabilitative and employment support services in a partnership with all stakeholders.

Arkansas

4478 Arkansas Department of Career Education
Luther Hardin Building
Three Capitol Mall
Little Rock, AR 72201-1005   501-682-1500
                                    Fax: 501-682-1509
                                    http://ace.arkansas.gov

Mike Beebe, Governor
William L. Walker, Jr., Director
James H. Smith, Jr., Deputy Director
Formerly the Dept. of Workforce Education, the Arkansas Dept. of Career Education (ACE) provides many resources to serve the educational needs of Arkansas individuals living with disabilities.

4479 Arkansas Department of Health & Human Services: Division of Developmental Disabilities
425 W. Capital Avenue
Suite 1620
Little Rock, AR 72201   501-324-8900
                               www.arkansas.gov

James Green PhD, Director
The mission of the Division of Developmental Disabilities Services is to provide a variety of supports to improve the quality of life for individuals with mental retardation, autism, epilepsy, cerebral palsy or other conditions that cause a person to function as if they had a mental impairment.

4480 Arkansas Employment Security Department: Office of Employment & Training Services
425 W. Capital Avenue
Suite 1620
Little Rock, AR 72201   501-324-8900
                               www.arkansas.gov

Artee Williams, Director
Employment related services that contribute to the economic stability of Arkansa and its citizens. These services are provided to employers, the workforce and the general public.

4481 Arkansas Rehabilitation Services
Three Capitol Mall
Little Rock, AR 72201   501-682-1500
                               Fax: 501-682-1509
                               TDD: 501-686-9686
                               http://ace.arkansas.gov
                               ssholt@ars.state.ar.us

Mike Beebe, Governor
William L. Walker, Jr., Director
James H. Smith, Jr., Deputy Director
For persons who are clients of Arkansas Rehabilitation Services, individual psychological/educational evaluations and college preparatory training are provided if approved by vocational rehabilitation counselor.

4482 Department of Human Services: Division of Developmental Disabilities Services
425 W. Capital Avenue
Suite 1620
Little Rock, AR 72201   501-324-8900
                               www.state.ar.us

Dr. Charlie Fleetwood, Chairman
Angela Harrison-King, Vice Chairman
Michael Stock, Treasurer
Offers a wide range of services and supports to Arkansans with developmental disabilities and their families.

4483 Easter Seals - Adult Services Center
Easter Seals Arkansas
3920 Woodland Heights Rd
Little Rock, AR 72212-2406   501-227-3600
                                    877-221-8400
                                    Fax: 501-227-7180
                                    TTY: 501-221-8424
                                    www.ar.easter-seals.org
                                    info@easterseals.com

Rick Zilk, President
Easter Seals Arkansas helps adults with disabilities gain greater independence through vocational and independent living programs.

4484 Office For The Deaf And Hearing Impaired
Arkansas Rehabilitation Services
Three Capitol Mall
Little Rock, AR 72201   501-682-1500
                               Fax: 501-682-1509
                               TDD: 501-686-9686
                               http://ace.arkansas.gov

Mike Beebe, Governor
William L. Walker, Jr., Director
James H. Smith, Jr., Deputy Director
Providing opportunities for individuals with hearing impairment to work and have productive and independent lives.

4485 State Vocational Rehabilitation Agency of Arkansas
ARS, Vocational & Technical Education Division
Three Capitol Mall
Little Rock, AR 72201   501-682-1500
                               Fax: 501-682-1509
                               TDD: 501-686-9686
                               http://ace.arkansas.gov

William L. Walker, Jr., Director
James H. Smith, Jr., Deputy Director
Provides direct services to persons with disabilities, including persons with learning disabilities. The services may include evaluation and diagnosis, counseling, guidance, and referral services, vocational and other training services, transportation to rehabilitation services, and assistive devices. Offering opportunities for individuals with disabilities to lead productive and independent lives.

4486 Workforce Investment Board
Arkansas State Employment Board
425 W. Capital Avenue
Suite 1620
Little Rock, AR 72201   501-324-8900
                               www.arkansas.gov

Cindy Verner, Division Chief
Operates workforce centers that offer locally developed and operated services linking employers and jobseekers through a statewide delivery system. Convenient centers are designed to eliminate the need to visit different locations. The centers integrate multiple workforce development programs into a single system, making the resources much more accessible and user friendly to jobseekers as well as expanding services to employers.

California

4487 Adult Education
California Department of Education
Ste 400
1430 N St
Sacramento, CA 95814-5901
916-319-0800
Fax: 916-319-0100
www.cde.ca.gov
scheduler@cde.ca.gov

Jack O'Connell, Director
Elementary basic skills and tutor/literacy training are offered on or off site using language masters, audiocassettes, videos and computers with internet access. Workplace literacy training will also be provided, with groups of students physically coming into the Center or hooking up to the Center from their workplace by borrowing materials or going online. In the latter case, instructors will meet with students at the work site on a regular schedule for evaluation and consultation.

4488 California Department of Education
1430 N St
Sacramento, CA 95814-5901
916-319-0800
800-331-6316
TTY: 916-445-4556
www.cde.ca.gov
gedoffic@cde.ca.gov

Nancy Edmunds, Program Coordinator
Provides access to a general high school education by providing many local classes and testing services.

4489 California Department of Rehabilitation
California Health & Human Services Agency
721 Capitol Mall
P.O. Box 944222
Sacramento, CA 94244-2220
916-324-1313
Fax: 916-558-5807
www.dor.ca.gov
externalaffairs@dor.ca.gov

Catherine Campisi PhD, Executive Director
California Department of Rehabilitation works in partnership with consumers and other stakeholders to provide services and advocacy resulting in employment, independent living and equality for individuals with disabilities.

4490 California Employment Development Department
800 Capitol Mall
Sacramento, CA 95814-4807
916-654-8210
Fax: 916-657-5294
TTY: 800-815-9387
www.edd.ca.gov
phenning@edd.ca.gov

Patrick Henning, Director
The California Employment Development Department (EDD) offers a wide variety of services to millions of Californians under the Job Service, Unemployment Insurance, Disability Insurance, Workforce Investment, and Labor Market Information programs.

4491 Easter Seals - Central California, Aptos
9010 Soquel Dr
Aptos, CA 95003-4002
831-684-2166
Fax: 831-684-1018
TTY: 831-684-1054
www.centralcal.easter-seals.org
donna@es-cc.org

Tom Conway, Chief Executive Officer
June Stockbridge, Director of Human Resources
Stella Lauerman, Director of Program Services
Recreational services for adults, residential camping programs.

4492 Easter Seals - Pacoima
Eastern Seals Southern California
12510 Van Nuys Blvd
Ste 103
Pacoima, CA 91331
818-996-9902
800-996-6302
Fax: 818-975-8299
www.easterseals.com
paula.pompa-craven@essc.org

Richard W. Davidson, Chairman
Sandra L. Bouwman, 1st Vice Chairman
Joseph G. Kern, 2nd Vice Chairman
Job training and employment services, occupational skills training, job placement/competitive-support employment, vocational evaluation/situational assessment and work adjustment.

4493 Easter Seals - Redondo Beach
Ste 201
700 N Pacific Coast Hwy
Redondo Beach, CA 90277-2147
310-376-3445
800-404-3445
Fax: 310-376-5567
www.easterseals.com
dee.prescott@cssc.org

Richard W. Davidson, Chairman
Sandra L. Bouwman, 1st Vice Chairman
Joseph G. Kern, 2nd Vice Chairman
Job training and employment services, occupational skills training, job placement/competitive-support employment, vocational evaluation/situational assessment and work adjustment.

4494 Easter Seals - Southern California
1570 E 17th St
Santa Ana, CA 92705-8511
714-834-1111
Fax: 714-934-1128
www.southerncal.easterseals.com

Kimberly Michel, Chair
Andre Filip, First Vice Chair
Mark Whitley, President/CEO
Easter Seals provides job training and volunteer opportunities to those individuals with disabilities.

4495 Easter Seals - Superior California
3205 Hurley Way
Sacramento, CA 95864-3898
916-485-6711
888-887-3257
Fax: 916-485-2653
www.easterseals.com
info@easterseals-superiorca.org

Richard W. Davidson, Chairman
Sandra L. Bouwman, 1st Vice Chairman
Joseph G. Kern, 2nd Vice Chairman
Job training and employment services, occupational skills training, job placement/competitive-support employment, vocational evaluation/situational assessment and work adjustment.

4496 WorkFirst
Easter Seals Of Southern California
Ste C
11110 Artesia Blvd
Cerritos, CA 90703-2546
760-737-3990
877-855-2279
Fax: 562-860-1680
www.workfirst.us
dee.prescott@essc.org

Sandra Meredith, Executive Director
WorkFirst helps individuals with disabilities to find work and keep working in a job that is more suited to their talents. The program also helps those individuals who are looking to open a business of their own.

Colorado

4497 Colorado Department of Human Services: Division for Developmental Disabilities
1575 Sherman Street
Denver, CO 80203-3111
303-866-5700
Fax: 303-866-4047
TDD: 303-866-7471
www.cdhs.state.co.us
cdhs_communications@state.co.us.
Karen L. Beye, Executive Director
A state office that provides leadership for the direction, funding and operation of community based services to people with developmental disabilities within Colorado.

4498 Easter Seals - Colorado
5755 W Alameda Ave
Lakewood, CO 80226-3500
303-233-1666
Fax: 303-569-3857
www.co.easterseals.com
info@eastersealscolorado.org
Lynn Robinson, President/CEO
Nancy Hanson, VP, Human Resources
Job training and employment services, occupational skills training, job placement/competitive-support employment, vocational evaluation/situational assessment and work adjustment.

4499 Human Services: Division of Vocational
1575 Sherman St
4th Fl
Denver, CO 80203-1702
303-866-4150
866-870-4595
Fax: 303-866-4905
TDD: 303-866-4150
www.dvrcolorado.com
Voc.Rehab@state.co.us
Nancy Smith, Director
Assists individuals whose disabilities result in barriers to employment to succeed at work and live independently. Building partnerships to improve opportunities for safety, self-sufficiency and dignity for the people of Colorado.

Connecticut

4500 Department of Social Services: Vocational Rehabilitation Program
55 Farmington Avenue
Hartford, CT 06105
860-424-5241
800-842-1508
TDD: 800-842-4524
www.ct.gov
pgr.dss@ct.gov
John Galiette, Director
Brenda Moore, Executive Director
Provides services to people with most significant physical or mental disabilities to assist them in their effort to enter or maintain employment. The agency also oversees a statewide network of community based, consumer controlled, independent living centers that promote independence for people with disabilities.

4501 Easter Seals - Connecticut
85 Jones Street
PO Box 198
Hebron, CT 06248-0100
860-228-9496
800-874-7687
Fax: 860-228-2091
www.easterseals.com
Richard W. Davidson, Chairman
Sandra L. Bouwman, 1st Vice Chairman
Joseph G. Kern, 2nd Vice Chairman
Easter Seals Connecticut creates solutions that change the lives of children and adults with disabilities or special needs, their families and communities.

4502 Easter Seals - Employment Industries
Easter Seals Rehabilitation Center
122 Avenue of Industry
Waterbury, CT 06705-3901
203-236-0188
Fax: 203-236-0183
www.easterseals.com
eswct@eswct.com
Fran DeBlasio, CEO
Ron Bourque, Primary Contact
Job training, employment services, vocational evaluation/situational assessment and work services.

4503 Easter Seals - Fulfillment Enterprises Easter Seals Connecticut
24 Stott Ave
Norwich, CT 06360-1508
860-859-4148
Fax: 860-455-1372
www.easterseals.com
Richard W. Davidson, Chairman
Sandra L. Bouwman, 1st Vice Chairman
Joseph G. Kern, 2nd Vice Chairman
Job training, employment services, vocational evaluation/situational assessment and work services.

4504 Easter Seals - Job Training And Placement Services
Easter Seals Waterbury, Connecticut
22 Tompkins St
Waterbury, CT 06708-1496
203-754-5141
Fax: 203-757-1198
TTY: 203-754-5141
www.waterburyct.easterseals.com
Curtis Audibert, Chairman
David Segal, Vice Chairman
Francis DeBlasio, President
Offers a number of vocational rehabilitation services, application & interviewing support, individualized employment planning & supported employment, and on the job training.

Delaware

4505 Division of Vocational Rehabilitation
Delaware Department of Labor
4425 N Market St
PO Box 9969
Wilmington, DE 19809-0969
302-761-8085
Fax: 302-761-6601
TTY: 302-761-8275
www.delawareworks.com
cynthia.fairwell@state.de.us
Andrea Guest, Director
Mission is to provide information opportunities and resources to individuals with disabilities, leading to success in employment and independent living. Facebook: www.facebook.com/DE.DVR.1

4506 Easter Seals - Dover Enterprise
Easter Seals Delaware & Maryland's Eastern Shore
61 Corporate Cir
New Castle, DE 19720-2405
302-324-4444
800-677-3800
Fax: 302-324-4441
TDD: 302-324-4442
www.de.easterseals.com
Gary Cassedy, Vice President, Programs
Easter Seals offers a variety of programs and activities for children and adults with disabililties.

4507 Easter Seals Delaware & Maryland's Eastern Shore
61 Corporate Cir
New Castle, DE 19720-2405
302-324-4444
800-677-3800
Fax: 302-324-4441
TDD: 302-324-4442
www.de.easterseals.com
William Adami, President

Offers early intervention services and outpatient rehab therapies for children and adults. Also offers day programs for adults with developmental disabilties.

District of Columbia

4508 Department of Employment Services
District of Columbia
4058 Minnesota Avenue, NE
Washington, DC 20019
202-724-7000
Fax: 202-673-6993
TTY: 202-698-4817
www.does.dc.gov
does@dc.gov

Gregory Irish, Director
Helps consider career decisions and offer vocational and placement assistance at several area training locations.

4509 District of Columbia Department of Education: Vocational & Adult Education
400 Maryland Ave SW
Washington, DC 20202
202-842-0973
800-872-5327
Fax: 202-205-8748
TTY: 800-437-0833
http://www2.ed.gov
ovae@ed.gov

Arne Duncan, Secretary of Education
Emma Vadehra, Chief of Staff
Massie Ritsch, Acting Assistant Secretary
To help all people achieve the knowledge and skills to be lifelong learners, to be successful in their chosen careers, and to be effective citizens.

4510 The DC Center For Independent Living, Inc.
1400 Florida Ave NE
Washington, DC 20002-5032
202-388-0033
Fax: 202-398-3018
TDD: 202-388-0277
TTY: 202-388-0277
www.dccil.org
info@dccil.org

Richard Simms, Executive Director
Kandra Hall, Coordinator
Promotes independent life styles for persons with significant disabilities. Programs offered include advocacy/legal/information and referral services, and independent living skills training.

Florida

4511 Children's Therapy Services Center
Easter Seals Of Southwest Florida
350 Braden Ave
Sarasota, FL 34243-2001
941-355-7637
800-807-7899
Fax: 941-358-3069
www.swfl.easterseals.com

Bill Lloyd, President
Job training, employment services, vocational evaluation/situational assessment and work services.

4512 College Living Experience
6555 Nova Drive
Suite 300
Davie, FL 33317-7404
954-370-5142
800-486-5058
Fax: 954-370-1895
www.experiencecle.com
secretary@cleinc.net

Stephanie Martin, President
Amy Radochonski, Vice President
Tiffany Prior, Assistant VP

A post-secondary program for students with Autism spectrum disorders, Dyslexia, Traumatic Brain Injury, ADD/ADHD, auditory/visual processing disorders and non-verbal learning disorders. The program offers students additional support with academic, social and living skills which helps them in adulthood.

4513 Division of Vocational Rehabilitation
Florida Department of Education
2002 Old Saint Augustine Road
Building A
Tallahassee, FL 32301-4862
850-245-3399
800-451-4327
Fax: 850-245-3316
TDD: 800-451-4327
www.rehabworks.org

Bill Palmer, Director
Statewide employment resource for businesses and people with disabilities. Our mission is to enable individuals with disabilities to obtain and keep employment.

4514 Easter Seals - Florida
6050 Babcock St SE
Ste 18
Palm Bay, FL 32909-3996
321-723-4474
Fax: 321-676-3843
www.fl.easterseals.org
scaporina@fl.easterseals.com

Gail Edwards, President
Offers vocational training to adults with disabilities and special needs, giving them the opportunity to receive job and life skills training so they gain greater independence.

4515 Easter Seals - South Florida
1475 NW 14th Ave
Miami, FL 33125-1616
305-325-0470
Fax: 305-325-0578
TTY: 305-326-7351
www.southflorida.easterseals.com
lwelch@sfl.easterseals.com

Luanne K Welch, Executive President/CEO
Malerie Sloshay, VP Operations
Job training, employment services, vocational evaluation/situational assessment and work services, adult day services, outpatient medical rehabilitation.

4516 Florida Workforce Investment Act
Department of Labor & Employment Security
1580 Waldo Palmer Lane
Suite 1
Tallahassee, FL 32308
850-921-1119
Fax: 850-921-1101
http://careersourceflorida.com

Kathleen McLeskey, Director
Provides job-training services for economically disadvantaged adults and youth, dislocated workers and others who face significant employment barriers.

4517 TILES Project: Transition/Independent Living/Employment/Support
Family Network on Disabilities, Inc.
2196 Main Street
Suite K
Dunedin, FL 34698-1610
727-523-1130
800-825-5736
Fax: 727-523-8687
www.fndfl.org
fnd@fndfl.org

Tracy Stewart, President/Parliamentarian
Jennifer Morgan-Byrd, Vice President
Molly Jacobson, Secretary
Provides training information to enable individuals with disabilities and the parents, family members, guardians, advocates, or other authorized representatives to participate more effectively with professionals in meeting the vocational, independent living and rehabilitation needs of people with disabilities in Florida.

Georgia

4518 Easter Seals - East Georgia
1500 Wrightsboro Rd
PO Box 2441
Augusta, GA 30903-4079
706-667-9695
866-667-9695
Fax: 706-667-8831
www.ga-ea.easterseals.com
shthomas@esega.org
Sheila Thomas, President/CEO
Job training for disabled individuals, employment services, vocational evaluation/situational assessment and work services.

4519 Easter Seals - Middle Georgia
604 Kellam Rd
PO Box 847
Dublin, GA 31040
478-275-8850
Fax: 478-275-8852
www.easterseals.com/middlega
Wayne Peebles, President
Job training, employment services, vocational evaluation/situational assessment and work services.

4520 Easter Seals - Southern Georgia
Easter Seals Southern Georgia
1906 Palmyra Rd
Albany, GA 31701-1575
229-439-7061
800-365-4583
Fax: 229-435-6278
www.easterseals.com/southerngeorgia
benglish@swga-easterseals.org
Beth English, Executive Director
Helps individuals with disabilities and special needs by providing many services such as job training, employment services, vocational evaluation/situational assessment and work services.

4521 Vocational Rehabilitation Services
Georgia Department of Labor
10 Park Place South, SE
Suite 602
Atlanta, GA 30303-1732
404-657-2239
Fax: 404-657-4731
TTY: 404-657-2239
www.vocrehabga.org
rehab@dol.state.ga.us
Peggy Rosser, Director
Operates 5 integrated and interdependent programs that share a primary goal — to help people with disabilities to become fully productive members of society by achieving independence and meaningful employment.

Hawaii

4522 Vocational Rehabilitation and Services For The Blind Division (VRSBD)
State Of Hawaii, Department Of Human Services
1901 Bachelot Street
Honolulu, HI 96817-0339
808-586-5268
www.hawaii.gov
Lilian Poller, Director
State vocational rehabilitation agencies provide direct services to persons with disabilities, including persons with learning disabilities. The services may include evaluation and diagnosis, counseling, guidance, and referral services, vocational and other training services, transportation to rehabilitation services, and assistive devices.

Idaho

4523 Idaho Department of Commerce & Labor
State Of Idaho Department of Labor
317 W Main St
Boise, ID 83735-0001
208-332-3570
Fax: 208-334-6430
TDD: 800-377-1363
www.labor.idaho.gov
labor.idaho.gov
Roger Madsen, Director
Renee Bade, Project Coordinator
Alexis Neufeld, Administrative Assistant
Provides vocational training services for economically disadvantaged adults and youth, dislocated workers and others who face significant employment barriers.

4524 Idaho Division of Vocational Rehabilitation Administration
Idaho State Board of Education
650 W. State Street
Room 150
Boise, ID 83702-0001
208-334-3390
Fax: 208-334-5305
www.vr.idaho.gov
department.info@vr.idaho.gov
Michael Graham, Director
State vocational rehabilitation agencies provide direct services to persons with disabilities, including persons with learning disabilities. The services may include evaluation and diagnosis, counseling, guidance, and referral services, vocational and other training services, transportation to rehabilitation services, and assistive devices.

4525 State Of Idaho Department Of Labor
317 W Main St
Boise, ID 83735-0001
208-332-3570
Fax: 208-334-6430
TDD: 800-377-1363
www.labor.idaho.gov
labor.idaho.gov
Roger Madsen, Director
Renee Bade, Project Coordinator
Alexis Neufeld, Administrative Assistant
An equal opportunity employer/program with auxiliary aids and services available upon request to individuals with disabilities.

Illinois

4526 State Vocational Rehabilitation Agency
100 S Grand Ave
Springfield, IL 62762-0001
217-782-2094
800-843-6154
Fax: 217-558-4270
TDD: 217-557-2507
TTY: 888-440-8982
www.dhs.state.il.us
dhs.ors@illinois.gov
Rob Kilbury, Director
Assists people with physical, visual, and hearing disabilities in achieving their education, employment, and independent living goals, including preparing for and finding quality employment.

4527 Therapeutic School and Center For Autism Research
Easter Seals Metropolitan Chicago
1939 West 13th Street
Suite 300
Chicago, IL 60608-1226
312-491-4110
www.chicago.easterseals.com
ndavenport@eastersealschicago.org
F. Timothy Muri, President & CEO
Barbara Zawacki, CEO
Nicole Davenport, School Administrator

Campus offers educational programs that help meet the special needs of students with autism, emotional behavior disorders and severe learning disabilities. Schools are also located in Rockford, Tinley Park and Waukegan.

4528   Timber Pointe Outdoor Center
Easter Seals Of Illinois
507 East Armstrong Avenue
Peoria, IL 61603-3197   309-686-1177
www.easterseals-ci.org
info@easterseals-ci.org

Debbie England, President
Timber Pointe provides specialized camping and respite programs for individuals with disabilities or special needs and their families. For ages 7 and up. Children enjoy activities such as swimming, boating, fishing, sports, music and arts and crafts.

Indiana

4529   Easter Seals - Arc of Northeast Indiana
4919 Colwater Rd
Fort Wayne, IN 46825-5380   260-456-4534
800-234-7811
Fax: 260-745-5200
www.neindiana.easterseals.com

Steven Hinkle, President
Sue Dubay, Executive Assistant
The Easter Seals Arc of Northeast Indiana covers 16 counties and offers many services and programs to children and adults with special needs or disabilities.

4530   Easter Seals - Crossroads
4740 Kingsway Dr
Indianapolis, IN 46205-1521   317-466-1000
Fax: 317-466-2000
TTY: 317-479-3232
www.eastersealscrossroads.org

J. Patrick Sandy, President / CEO
Susan Saunders, CFO/Security Officer
Bruce Schnaith, VP Workforce Dev Services
Works with children and adults with disabilities or special needs to promote growth, dignity and independence.

4531   INdiana Camp R.O.C.K.S.
Easter Seals Crossroads
4740 Kingsway Drive
Indianapolis, IN 46205   317-466-1000
Fax: 317-466-2000
TDD: 317-479-3232
www.eastersealscrossroads.org

Anne Shupe, Director
J. Patrick Sandy, President / CEO
Susan Saunders, CFO/Security Officer
Camp for chidlren and young adults ages 10-17 who have autism.

4532   Vocational Rehabilitation Services
1452 Vaxter Ave
Clarksville, IN 47129-7721   812-288-8261
877-228-1967
Fax: 812-282-7048
TDD: 812-288-8261
www.in.gov

Delbert Hayden, Director
Purpose is to assist the community by providing services which allow individuals to maximize their potential and to participate in work, family and the community. To do this we will provide rehabilitation, education and training.

Iowa

4533   Division of Community Colleges and Workforce Preparation
Iowa Department of Education
400 E 14th St
Des Moines, IA 50319-146   515-281-5294
Fax: 515-242-5988
http://educateiowa.gov
kathy.petosa@iowa.gov

Dr. Jason Glass, Director
Kathy Petosa, Administrative Assistant
The Iowa Department of Education (the Department) works with the Iowa State Board of Education (State Board) to provide oversight, supervision, and support for the state education system that includes public elementary and secondary schools, nonpublic schools that receive state accreditation, area education agencies (AEAs), community colleges, and teacher preparation programs.

4534   Easter Seals - Iowa
401 NE 66th Ave
Des Moines, IA 50313-1200   515-289-1933
866-533-9344
Fax: 515-289-1281
TDD: 515-274-8348
TTY: 515-289-4069
www.ia.easterseals.com
info@eastersealsia.org

Sherri Nielsen, President/CEO
Krable Mentzer, Chief Development Officer
Kevin Small, Chief Financial Officer
Offers many programs and services for children and adults with disabilities or special needs.

4535   Easter Seals Center
2920 30th St
Des Moines, IA 50310-5299   515-274-1529
866-533-9344
Fax: 515-274-6434
TDD: 515-274-8348
TTY: 515-274-8348
www.easterseals.com
info@eastersealsia.org

Richard W. Davidson, Chairman
Sandra L. Bouwman, 1st Vice Chairman
Joseph G. Kern, 2nd Vice Chairman
Job training, employment services, vocational evaluation/situational assessment and work services.

4536   State Vocational Rehabilitation Agency
Iowa Division of Vocational Rehabilitation Service
510 E 12th St
Des Moines, IA 50319-9025   515-281-4211
800-532-1486
Fax: 515-281-7645
TDD: 515-281-4211
TTY: 800-532-1486
www.ivrs.iowa.gov

Stephen Wooderson, Director
We work for and with individuals with disabilities to achieve their employment, independence and economic goals. Economic independence and more and better jobs are what we are about for Iowans with disabilities.

Kansas

4537   Office of Vocational Rehabilitation
Department of Vocational Rehabilitation
915 SW Harrison St
Topeka, KS 66612-1505   888-369-4777
TTY: 785-296-1491
www.srskansas.org
cmxa@srskansas.org

Clarissa Ashdown, Director
Partnering to connect Kansans with support and services to improve lives. Vocational and transitional training.

Kentucky

4538 Easter Seals - West Kentucky
801 N 29th St
Paducah, KY 42001-3067   270-442-9687
                                 866-673-3565
                                 Fax: 270-442-4933
                                 www.easterseals.com/westkentucky
George Kennedy, President
Provides programs and services for children and adults with
disabilities and/or special needs. Provides job training, employment services, vocational evaluation/situational assessment and work services.

4539 Office of Vocational Rehabilitation
275 E Main St
Mail Drop 2EK
Frankfort, KY 40621   502-564-4440
                                 800-372-7172
                                 Fax: 502-564-6745
                                 TTY: 888-420-9874
                                 www.kydor.state.ky.us
                                 wfd.vocrehab@mail.state.ky.us
Beth Smith, Executive Director
Pam Jarboe, Program Services Director
Provides direct services to persons with disabilities, including persons with learning disabilities. The services may include evaluation and diagnosis; counseling, guidance, and
referral services, vocational and other training services,
transportation to rehabilitation services, and assistive
devices.

Maine

4540 State Vocational Rehabilitation Agency
Maine Bureau of Rehabilitation Services
150 State House Station
Augusta, ME 04333-0150   207-623-6799
                                 800-698-4440
                                 Fax: 207-287-5292
                                 www.maine.gov/rehab
Carolyn Lockwood, Executive Director
Betsy Hopkins, Director
Works to bring about full access to employment, independ-
ence and community integration for people with disabilities.
Our three service provision units are Vocational Rehabilita-
tion, Division for the Blind and Visually Impaired and
Division of Deafness.

Maryland

4541 Maryland Technology Assistance Program
Maryland Department of Disabilities
217 E. Redwood Street
Suite 1300
Baltimore, MD 21202   410-767-3660
                                 800-637-4113
                                 www.mdod.maryland.gov
Beth Lash, Director
Offers information and referrals, reduced rate loan program
for assistive technology, five regional display centers, pre-
sentations and training on request.

4542 State Vocational Rehabilitation Agency
Maryland State Dept Of Education/Div Rehab Svcs.
2301 Argonne Dr
Baltimore, MD 21218-1696   410-554-9442
                                 888-554-0334
                                 TTY: 410-554-9411
                                 www.dors.state.md.us
Robert Burns, Director
Operates more than 20 statewide offices and also operates
the Workforce and Technology Center, a comprehensive rehabilitation facility in Baltimore. Rehabilitation representatives also work in many Maryland One-Stop Career Centers.

Massachusettes

4543 Easter Seals - Massachusetts
484 Main St
Worcester, MA 01608-2629   617-226-2640
                                 800-244-2756
                                 Fax: 617-737-9875
                                 TTY: 617-226-2640
                                 www.ma.easterseals.com
Alex Cassie, President
Job training, employment services, vocational evalua-
tion/situational assessment and work services. Camp programs, assistive technology and augmentative
communication.

4544 State Vocational Rehabilitation Agency
Massachusetts Rehabilitation Commission
59 Temple Place
Suite 905
Boston, MA 02111-1619   617-357-8137
                                 800-245-6543
                                 Fax: 617-482-5576
                                 TDD: 800-223-3212
                                 TTY: 800-245-6543
                                 www.mass.gov
Elmer Bartels, Director
Provides public vocational rehabilitation, independent liv-
ing and disability determination services for residents with
disabilities in Massachusetts.

Michigan

4545 Easter Seal Michigan
2399 E. Walton Blvd.
Auburn Hills, MI 48326   248-475-6400
                                 800-757-3257
                                 TTY: 800-649-3777
                                 www.easterseals.com/michigan
Brent L. Wirth, President and CEO
Juliana Harper, Sr. Vice President
Rich Hollis, Sr. Vice President
Job training, employment services, vocational evalua-
tion/situational assessment and work services.

4546 State Vocational Rehabilitation Agency
Dept Of Labor & Economic Grwth-Rehabilitation Svcs
201 N. Washington Square, 4th Floor
P.O. Box 30010
Lansing, MI 48909-7510   517-373-4026
                                 800-605-6722
                                 Fax: 517-335-7277
                                 TDD: 888-605-6722
                                 TTY: 888-605-6722
                                 www.michigan.gov
Jaye Balthazar, Director
State vocational rehabilitation agencies provide direct services to persons with disabilities, including persons with
learning disabilities. The services may include evaluation
and diagnosis; counseling, guidance, and referral services;
vocational and other training services; transportation to rehabilitation services; and assistive devices.

Minnesota

4547 Goodwill - Easter Seals Minnesota
553 Fairview Ave N
Saint Paul, MN 55104-1708   651-379-5800
                                 Fax: 651-379-5803
                                 www.goodwilleasterseals.org
The Goodwill stores help individuals achieve their goals for
employment, education, training and independence.

4548   Minnesota Vocational Rehabilitation Agency: Rehabilitation Services Branch
Department of Employment & Economic Development
1st National Bank Building
332 Minnesota Street, Suite E-200
Saint Paul, MN 55101-1351   651-259-7114
                                            800-657-3858
                                       Fax: 651-297-5159
                                       TTY: 651-296-3900
                                       www.deed.state.mn.us
                      DEED.CustomerService@state.mn.us
Katie Clark Sieben, Commissioner
Blake Chaffee, Deputy Commissioner /COO
Robin Sternberg, Deputy Commissioner Eco Dev
Provides basic vocational rehabilitation services to consumers including vocational counseling, planning, guidance and placement, as well as certain special services based on individual circumstances.

4549   State Vocational Rehabilitation Agency: Minnesota Department of Economics Security
Rehabilitation Service Branch
1st National Bank Building
332 Minnesota Street, Suite E-200
Saint Paul, MN 55101-1351   651-259-7114
                                            800-657-3858
                                       Fax: 651-296-3900
                                       TTY: 651-296-3900
                                       www.deed.state.mn.us
                      DEED.CustomerService@state.mn.us
Katie Clark Sieben, Commissioner
Blake Chaffee, Deputy Commissioner /COO
Robin Sternberg, Deputy Commissioner Eco Dev
State vocational rehabilitation agencies provide direct services to persons with disabilities, including persons with learning disabilities. The services may include evaluation and diagnosis, counseling, guidance, and referral services, vocational and other training services, transportation to rehabilitation services, and assistive devices.

Mississippi

4550   Office Of Vocational Rehabilitation
Mississippi Dept Of Rehabilitation Services
P.O.Box 1698
Jackson, MS 39215-1698   601-853-5100
                                            800-443-1000
                                       Fax: 601-853-5158
                                       TDD: 601-351-1586
                                            www.mdrs.ms.gov
Chris Howard, Deputy Executive Director???
Anita Naik, Office Director???
Billy Taylor, Special Assistant???
Helps individuals with physical or mental disabilities to find employment, retain employment and so they feel better about themselves and can live more independently.

Missouri

4551   Rehabilitation Services for the Blind
615 E 13th St
Ste 409
Kansas City, MO 64106-2829   816-889-2677
                                            800-592-6004
                                       Fax: 816-889-2504
                      www.dss.mo.gov/fsd/rsb/index.htm
                             Rachel.M.Labrado@dss.mo.gov
Rachel Labrado, District Supervisor
Provides services to people with varing degrees of visual impairment, ranging from those who cannot read regular print to those who are totally blind. Services may include: job training, job placement, vocational rehabilitation, assistive technology, independent living skills, personal and home management, meal preparation, communications assistance, independent travel instruction, counseling and guidance, leisure activities and client assistant program.

4552   State Vocational Rehabilitation Agency Department of Elementary & Secondary Education
205 Jefferson St.
Jefferson City, MO 65109-6188   573-751-4212
                                            877-222-8963
                                       Fax: 573-751-1441
                                       TDD: 573-751-0881
                                            www.dese.mo.gov
Jeanne Loyd, Director
State vocational rehabilitation agencies provide direct services to persons with disabilities, including persons with learning disabilities. The services may include evaluation and diagnosis, counseling, guidance, and referral services, vocational and other training services, transportation to rehabilitation services, and assistive devices.

4553   United Cerebral Palsy Heartland
13975 Manchester Road
Manchester, MO 63011   636-227-6030
                                       Fax: 636-779-2270
                                            www.ucpheartland.org
Richard Forkosh, President & CEO
Kathleen Fagin, Vice President Programs
Steve Staicoff, CFO
Job training, employment services, vocational evaluation/situational assessment and work services.

Montana

4554   Easter Seals - Goodwill Career Designs Mountain
Regional Service Center
4400 Central Ave
Great Falls, MT 59405-1641   406-761-3680
                                            800-771-2153
                                       Fax: 406-761-5110
                                            www.esg.easterseals.com
                                            sharonod@esgw.org
Michelle Belknap, President
Job skill training programs for adults with developmental disabilities.

4555   Easter Seals - Goodwill Store
425 1st Ave N
Great Falls, MT 59405-1641   406-761-3680
                                            800-771-2153
                                       Fax: 406-761-5110
                                       TDD: 800-253-4093
                                       www.esgw-nrm.easterseals.com
                                            gwbillings@mcn.net
Shalene Sparling, Director
Provides vocational training sites for individuals with emotional, developmental and physical disabilities. Employees develop and improve work skills while gaining work experience.

4556   Easter Seals - Goodwill Working Partners, Great Falls
425 1st Ave N
Great Falls, MT 59405-1641   406-761-3680
                                            800-771-2153
                                       Fax: 406-761-5110
                                       TDD: 800-253-4093
                                       www.esgw-nrm.easterseals.com
                                            joelc@csgw.org
Michelle Belknap, President
Russell Plath, Board Chair
Scott Wilson, 1st Vice Chair and Treasurer
Job training, employment services, vocational evaluation/situational assessment and work services.

4557   Goodwill Staffing Services
Easter Seals Goodwill Northern Rocky Mountain
425 1st Ave. N.
Great Falls, MT 59401   406-761-3680
                                            www.easterseals.com/esgw
Marcie Bailey, Director

Temporary staffing company which provides effective solutions to businesses in Idaho by customizing staffing solutions to fit individual needs, fill orders promptly, and monitors job performance to ensure customer satisfaction.

4558 State Vocational Rehabilitation Agency
Department of Public Health & Human Services
111 North Sanders
P.O. Box 4210
Helena, MT 59604-4210   406-444-2590
877-296-1197
Fax: 406-444-3632
www.dphhs.mt.gov
Robert Wynia, Executive Director
Joe Mathews, Director
State vocational rehabilitation agencies provide direct services to persons with disabilities, including persons with learning disabilities. The services may include evaluation and diagnosis, counseling, guidance, and referral services, vocational and other training services, transportation to rehabilitation services, and assistive devices.

4559 Workforce Development Services
Easter Seals-Goodwill Northern Rocky Mountains
425 1st Ave. N.
Great Falls, MT 59401   406-761-3680
www.easterseals.com/esgw
Kim Osadchuk, Director
Job training, employment services, vocational evaluation/situational assessment and work services.

Nebraska

4560 Camp Kaleo
Easter Seals Nebraska
12565 West Center Road
Suite 100
Omaha, NE 68144-8144   402-345-2200
800-471-6425
TTY: 402-462-4721
www.ne.easterseals.com
Karen Ginder, President
Job training, employment services, vocational evaluation/situational assessment and work services.

4561 State Vocational Rehabilitation Agency: Nebraska
Nebraska Dept Of Educ. Vocational Rehabilitation
PO Box 94987
Lincoln, NE 68509-4987   402-471-3644
877-637-3422
Fax: 402-471-0788
TTY: 402-471-3659
www.vocrehab.state.ne.us
vr_stateoffice@vocrehab.state.ne.us
Cherly Ferree, Director
We help people with disabilities make career plans, learn job skills, get and keep a job. Our goal is to prepare people for jobs where they can make a living wage and have access to medical insurance.

Nevada

4562 Bureau of Services to the Blind & Visually Impaired
Nevada Dept Of Employment,Training&Rehabilitation
2800 E. St. Louis Avenue
Las Vegas, NV 89104   702-486-5230
800-326-6868
Fax: 775-684-4186
TTY: 702-486-1018
www.detr.state.nv.us
InternetHelp@nvdetr.org
Dennis A. Perea, Deputy Director/Interim Director
Services to the Blind and Visually Impaired (BSBVI) provides a variety of services to eligible individuals, whose vision is not correctable by ordinary eye care. Adaptive training, independence skills, low vision exams and aids, mobility training and vocational rehabilitation are offered.

4563 Nevada Governor's Council on Rehabilitation & Employment of People with Disabilities
2800 E. St. Louis Avenue
Carson City, NV 89713   775-684-3849
Fax: 775-684-3850
TTY: 775-687-5353
www.detr.state.nv.us
InternetHelp@nvdetr.org
Dennis A. Perea, Deputy Director/Interim Director
To help insure vocational rehabilitation programs are consumer oriented, driven and result in employment outcomes for Nevadans with disabilities. Funding for innovation and expansion grants.

4564 Rehabilitation Division Department of Employment, Training & Rehabilitation
Bureau of Services to Blind and Visually Impaired
500 East Third Street
Carson City, NV 89713   775-684-4040
Fax: 775-684-4184
TDD: 775-684-8400
TTY: 800-326-6868
www.detr.state.nv.us
InternetHelp@nvdetr.org
Dennis A. Perea, Deputy Director/Interim Director
Providing options and choices for Nevadans with disabilities to work and live independently. Our mission will be accomplished through planning, implementing and coordinating assessment, employment, independent living and training.

New Hampshire

4565 Camp Sno Mo
Easter Seals New Hampshire
Hidden Valley Reservation
260 Griswold Lane
Gilmanton Iron Works, NH 03837   603-364-5818
www.nh.easterseals.com
rkelly@eastersealsnh.org
Larry J. Gammon, President
Elin A. Treanor, COO/CFO
Robert Kelly, Camp Director
The camp gives children and young adults ages 11-21 with disabililties or special needs the chance to explore new adventures which develop confidence, gain courage and build new friendships. Some of the activities include swimming, canoeing, hiking, archery, woodcarving, and arts & crafts.

4566 Easter Seals - Keene
20 Norway Ave
Keene, NH 03431-3825   603-209-5619
800-307-2737
Fax: 603-352-1879
www.easterseals.com
Larry J. Gammon, President
Diana Castor, Primary Contact
Job training, employment services, vocational evaluation/situational assessment and work services.

4567 Easter Seals - Manchester
Joliceour School
555 Auburn St
Manchester, NH 03103-4800   603-623-8863
800-870-8728
Fax: 603-625-1148
www.nheasterseals.com
Larry J. Gammon, President
Elin A. Treanor, COO/CFO
Karen Van Der Beken, Chief Development Officer
Job training, employment services, vocational evaluation/situational assessment and work services.

4568 New Hampshire Department of Health & Human Services
129 Pleasant Street
Concord, NH 03301-3852 603-271-6200
800-322-9191
TDD: 800-735-2964
www.dhhs.nh.gov
Nick Toumpas, Director
Programs for individuals with disabilities or special needs.

4569 State Vocational Rehabilitation Agency
Department of Education
101 Pleasant Street
Concord, NH 03301-3494 603-271-3494
800-299-1647
Fax: 603-271-7095
TDD: 603-271-3471
TTY: 603-271-3471
www.education.nh.gov
Paul K Leather, Executive Director
Assisting eligible New Hampshire citizens with disabilities secure suitable employment, financial and personal independence by providing rehabilitation services.

New Jersey

4570 Assistive Technology Advocacy Center-ATAC
New Jersey Protection and Advocacy
210 South Broad Street
3rd Floor
Trenton, NJ 08608-2407 609-292-9742
800-922-7233
Fax: 609-777-0187
TTY: 609-633-7106
www.njpanda.org
advocate@drnj.com
Ellen Catanese, Director
Assists individuals in overcoming barriers in the system and making assistive technology more accessible to individuals with disabilities throughout the state.

4571 Division of Family Development: New Jersey Department of Human Services
Quakerbridge Plaza, Building 6
P.O. Box 716
Trenton, NJ 08625-0716 609-588-2000
Fax: 609-588-3051
www.state.nj.us
Jeanette Page-Hawkins, Director
Offers programs to individuals with disabilities.

4572 Eden Family of Services
Eden Services
One Eden Way
Princeton, NJ 08540-5711 609-987-0099
Fax: 609-987-0243
www.edenservices.org
info@edenservices.org
Tom Mc Cool, President
David Holmes EdD, Executive Director
Provides year round educational services, early intervention, parent training, respite care, outreach services, community based residential services and employment opportunities for individuals with autism.

4573 New Jersey Council on Developmental Disabilities
P.O. Box 700
Trenton, NJ 08625-0700 609-292-3745
800-792-8858
Fax: 609-292-7114
TDD: 609-777-3238
www.njddc.org
njddc@njddc.org
Elaine Buschbaum, Chair
Dr Allison Lozano, Executive Director
Douglas McGruher, Deputy Director

Promotes systems change, coordinates advocacy and research for 1.2 million residents with developmental and other disabilities.

4574 New Jersey State Department of Education
P.O.Box 500
Trenton, NJ 08625-0500 609-292-4469
www.state.nj.us
Lucille E Davy, Commissioner
Assists the disabled student with changes from the school environment to the working world.

4575 Programs for Children with Special Health Care Needs
NJ Department of Health
P.O. Box 360
Trenton, NJ 08625-0360 609-292-7837
800-367-6543
Fax: 609-292-9288
www.nj.gov/health/fhs/sch
Gloria Rodriguez, President
Assists families caring for children with long-term medical and developmental disabilities. Programs include early intervention and case management units

New Mexico

4576 New Mexico Department of Labor: Job Training Division
Office of Workforce Training and Development
401 Broadway NE
Albuquerque, NM 87102-3960 505-841-4000
www.dws.state.nm.us
reese.fullerton@state.nm.us
Reese Fullerton, Executive Director
Veronica Moya, Office Assistant
Helps citizens of New Mexico from all walks of life find appropriate vocational trainings, and job placement.

4577 State of New Mexico Division of Vocational Rehabilitation
491 Old Santa Fe Trail
Santa Fe, NM 87501-2753 505-827-6328
877-696-1470
TTY: 505-476-0412
www.dvrgetsjobs.com
rsmith@state.nm.us
Jim Parker, Director
Commited to improving the quality of life of those with disabilities by addressing program accessibility and economic self-sufficiency.

New York

4578 Commission for the Blind & Visually Handicapped
NYS Office Of Children & Family Services
52 Washington Street
Rensselaer, NY 12144-2796 518-473-7793
Fax: 518-486-7550
TDD: 518-473-1698
http://ocfs.ny.gov/main
Professionals and paraprofessionals are available to help those with low vision or blindness with vocational rehabilitation services.

4579 Office of Curriculum & Instructional Support
New York State Education Department
89 Washington Ave
Albany, NY 12234-1000 518-474-8892
Fax: 518-474-0319
www.p12.nysed.gov
NYSEDP12@mail.nysed.gov
Jean Stevens, Director
Works with those seeking General Educational Development diplomas and technical training.

4580 **Office of Vocational and Educational Services for Individuals with Disabilities**
New York State Department of Education
1 Commerce Plaza
Room 1624e Plz
Albany, NY 12234-0001   518-436-0008
                              800-222-5627
                         TTY: 519-486-3773
                         www.p12.nysed.gov
                    NYSEDP12@mail.nysed.gov
Harvey Rosenthal, Executive Director
Nancy Lauria, Director
Promotes educational equality and excellence for students with disabilities while ensuring that they receive the rights and protection to which they are entitled, assure appropriate continuity between the child and adult services systems, and provide the highest quality vocational rehabilitation and independent living services to all eligible people.

North Dakota

4581 **North Dakota Department of Career and Technical Education**
State Capital, 15th Floor
600 E Boulevard Ave, Dept. 270
Bismarck, ND 58505-0610   701-328-3180
                            Fax: 701-328-1255
                            www.nd.gov/cte
                                 cte@nd.gov
Wayne Kutzer, Director and Executive Officer
Dwight Crabtree, Assistant State Director
Brenda Schuler, Administrative Officer
The mission of the Board for Vocational and Technical Education is to work with others to provide all North Dakota citizens with the technical skills, knowledge, and attitudes necessary for successful performance in a globally competitive workplace.

4582 **North Dakota Workforce Development Council**
North Dakota Department of Commerce
1600 E. Century Ave.
Suite 2
Bismarck, ND 58503-2057   701-328-5000
                            Fax: 701-328-5320
                            TTY: 800-366-6888
                            www.workforce.nd.gov
                            NDWorkforce@nd.gov
James Hirsch, Director
The role of the North Dakota Workforce Development Council is to advise the Governor and the Public concerning the nature and extent of workforce development in the context of North Dakota's economic development needs, and how to meet these needs effectively while maximizing the efficient use of available resources and avoiding unnecessary duplication of effort.

4583 **Vocational Rehabilitation**
North Dakota Department of Human Services
1237 West Divide Avenue
Suite 1B
Bismarck, ND 58501-1208   701-328-8950
                              800-755-2745
                         Fax: 701-328-8969
                         TDD: 701-328-8968
                         TTY: 701-328-8802
                         www.nd.gov/dhs/dvr
                              dhsvr@nd.gov
Nancy Mc Kenzie, Director
Assists individuals with disabilities to achieve competitive employment and increased independence through rehabilitation services.

4584 **Workforce Investment Act**
Governor's Employment & Training Forum
1000 E Divide Ave
POBox 5507
Bismarck, ND 58506-5507   701-328-2836
                         Fax: 701-328-1612
                         TDD: 800-366-6888
                         www.jobnd.com
                              mdaley@nd.gov
Maren Daley, Executive Director
Job service North Dakota

Ohio

4585 **Office of Workforce Development**
Ohio Department of Job and Family Services
30 E. Broad Street 32nd Floor
Columbus, OH 43215-1618   888-296-7541
                         Fax: 614-728-8366
                         http://jfs.ohio.gov/owd
John Weber, Deputy Director
Operates several US department of labor-funded programs that focus on improving Ohio's workforce through career and job search realted services, assistance to employers, training and education.

4586 **State Vocational Rehabilitation Agency**
Ohio Dept Of Rehabilitation Services Commission
150 E. Campus View Blvd.
Columbus, OH 43235-4604   614-438-1200
                              800-282-4536
                         Fax: 614-438-1257
                         TDD: 614-438-1726
                         TTY: 614-438-1200
                         http://ood.ohio.gov
                    rsc_rir@vscnet.a1.state.oh.us
John M Connelly, Executive Director
Bill Bishilany, Assistant Executive Director
Erik Williamson, Deputy Director
State vocational rehabilitation agencies provide direct services to persons with disabilities, including persons with learning disabilities. The services may include evaluation and diagnosis, counseling, guidance, and referral services, vocational and other training services, transportation to rehabilitation services, and assistive devices.

Oklahoma

4587 **State Vocational Rehabilitation Agency: Oklahoma Department of Rehabilitation Services**
3535 NW 58th Street
Suite 500
Oklahoma City, OK 73112-4824   405-951-3400
                              800-845-8476
                         Fax: 405-951-3529
                         TTY: 405-951-3400
                         www.okrehab.org
                              info@okdrs.gov
Linda S Parker, Executive Director
State vocational rehabilitation agencies provide direct services to persons with disabilities, including persons with learning disabilities. The services may include evaluation and diagnosis counseling, guidance, and referral services, vocational and other training services, transportation to rehabilitation services and assistive devices.

4588 **Workforce Investment Act**
Oklahoma Employment Security Commission
Will Rogers Memorial Office Bldg.
2401 N. Lincoln Blvd., P.O. Box 52003
Oklahoma City, OK 73152-2003   405-557-7100
                         Fax: 405-557-7256
                         TDD: 800-722-0353
                         www.ok.gov
John Brock, Executive Director

Partnership of local goverments offering resource conservation and development and workforce development.

Oregon

4589 Oregon Employment Department
875 Union St NE
Salem, OR 97311
503-947-1470
877-345-3484
TTY: 503-947-1472
www.employment.oregon.gov
Laurie Warner, Director
Tom Fuller, Communciations Manager
Craig Spivey, Backup Manager
Supports economic stability for Oregonians and communities during times of unemployment through the payment of unemployment benefits. Serves businesses by recruiting and referring the best qualified applicants to jobs, and provides resources to diverse job seekers in support of their employment needs.

4590 Recruitment and Retention Special Education Jobs Clearinghouse
Teaching Research Institute
Western Oregon University
345 Monmouth Ave
Monmouth, OR 97361
503-838-8391
Fax: 503-838-8150
TTY: 503-838-9623
http://teachingresearchinstitute.org
samplesb@wou.edu
John Killoran, Director
A free on-line jobs clearinghouse with access to position openings in Oregon in the area of Special Education and related services. A Job Seeker Listing and resumes also sent via e-mail to districts and agencies looking for qualified individuals.

Pennsylvania

4591 State Vocational Rehabilitation Agency: Pennsylvania
Department of Labor & Industry
1521 N 6th St
Harrisburg, PA 17102-1104
717-787-5244
800-442-6351
Fax: 717-783-5221
TTY: 717-787-5244
www.portal.state.pa.us
wgannon@dli.state.pa.us
William Gannon, Executive Director
Provides individualized services to assist people with disabilities to pursue, obtain, and maintain satisfactory employment. Counselors are available for training, planning and placement services.

Rhode Island

4592 Rhode Island Vocational and Rehabilitation Agency
Rhode Island Department of Human Services
40 Fountain St
Providence, RI 02903-1898
401-421-7005
Fax: 401-421-9259
TDD: 401-421-7016
www.ors.ri.gov
ronald.racine@dhs.ri.gov
Ronald Racine, Acting Associate Director
John Microulis, Administrator
Roberta Greene-Whittemore, Assistant Administrator of VR
Assists people with disabilities to become employed and to live independently in the community. In order to achieve this goal, we work in partnership with the State Rehabilitation Council, our customers, staff and community.

4593 State Vocational Rehabilitation Agency: Rhode Island
Rhode Island Department of Human Services
40 Fountain St
Providence, RI 02903-1830
401-421-7005
Fax: 401-421-9259
TDD: 401-421-7016
www.ors.ri.gov
ronald.racine@dhs.ri.gov
Ronald Racine, Acting Associate Director
John Microulis, Administrator
Roberta Greene-Whittemore, Assistant Administrator of VR
Assists people with disabilities to become employed and to live independently in the community. In order to achieve this goal, we work in partnership with the State Rehabilitation Council, our customers, staff and community.

South Carolina

4594 Americans with Disabilities Act Assistance Line
Employment Security Commission
1550 Gadsden Street
P.O. Box 995
Columbia, SC 29202-1406
803-737-9935
800-436-8190
Fax: 803-737-0140
www.sces.org
rratterree@sces.org
Regina Ratterree, Director
Provides information, technical assistance and training on the Americans with Disabilities Act.

4595 South Carolina Vocational Rehabilitation Department
PO Box 15
West Columbia, SC 29171-0015
803-896-6500
Fax: 803-896-6529
TTY: 803-896-6500
www.scvrd.net
info@scrvd.state.sc.us
Barbara G Hollis, Commissioner
Enabling eligible South Carolinians with disabilities to prepare for, achieve and maintain competitive employment.

South Dakota

4596 South Dakota Department of Labor
700 Governors Dr
Pierre, SD 57501-2291
605-773-3165
800-952-3216
Fax: 605-773-6184
TDD: 605-773-5017
TTY: 605-773-3101
www.dss.sd.gov
Mike Ryan, Director
Job training programs provide an important framework for developing public-private sector partnerships. We help prepare South Dakotans of all ages for entry or re-entry into the labor force.

4597 South Dakota Department of Social Services
700 Governors Dr
Pierre, SD 57501-2291
605-773-3165
Fax: 605-773-4855
www.dss.sd.gov
Deborah K Bowman, Director

4598 South Dakota Rehabilitation Center forthe Blind
Department of Human Services
Ste 101
2900 W 11th St
Sioux Falls, SD 57104-2594
605-334-4491
800-658-5441
Fax: 605-367-5263
TTY: 605-367-5260
www.dss.sd.gov
dawn.backer@state.sd.us

Gaye Mattke, Director
Helping people lead a full, productive life — regardless of how much one does or does not see. Upon completion of training, individuals usually return to their community and use these new skills in their home, school or job.

4599 State Vocational Rehabilitation Agency
Division of Rehabilitation Services
East Highway 34
Hillsview Plaza
Pierre, SD 57501-5070
605-773-3195
800-265-9684
Fax: 605-773-5483
TDD: 605-773-3195
www.dhs.sd.gov/drs
steve.stewart@state.sd.us
Grady Kickul, Executive Director
Assists individuals with disabilities to obtain employment, economic self-sufficiency, personal independence and full inclusion into society.

Tennessee

4600 State Vocational Rehabilitation Agency
Tennessee Department of Human Services
Citizens Plaza State Office Buildin
2nd Floor, 400 Deaderick Street
Nashville, TN 37243-1403
615-313-4891
866-311-4288
Fax: 615-741-6508
TTY: 615-313-5695
http://tennessee.gov/humanserv/rehab/vrs.html
car.w.brown@state.tn.us
Terry Smith, Director
State vocational rehabilitation agencies provide direct services to persons with disabilities, including persons with learning disabilities. The services may include evaluation and diagnosis counseling, guidance, and referral services, vocational and other training services, transportation to rehabilitation services and assistive devices.

4601 Tennessee Department of Education
Tennessee Department of Education
710 James Robertson Parkway
Nashville, TN 37243-0382
615-741-5158
800-531-1515
www.tn.gov/education/
education.comments@tn.gov
Kevin S. Huffman, Commissioner
Kathleen Airhart, Deputy Commissioner
Hanseul Kang, Chief of Staff
Mission is to take Tennessee to the top in education. Guides administration of the state's K-12 public schools.

4602 Tennessee Department of Labor & Workforce Development: Office of Adult Education
11th Fl
500 James Robertson Pkwy
Nashville, TN 37243-1204
615-741-7054
800-531-1515
Fax: 615-532-4899
TDD: 800-848-0299
www.tn.gov/labor-wfd/AE/
Phyllis.Pardue@tn.gov
Burns Phillips, Commissioner
Dustin Swayne, Deputy Commissioner
Marva Doremus, Administrator

4603 Tennessee Services for the Blind
Tennessee Department Of Human Services
400 Deaderick Street
2nd Floor
Nashville, TN 37243-1403
615-313-4700
800-628-7818
Fax: 615-313-6617
TDD: 615-313-6601
TTY: 615-313-6601
www.state.tn.us
Human-Services.Webmaster@state.tn.us
Terry Smith, Director
Offering training and services to help blind or low-vision citizens of Tennessee become more independent at home, in the community and at work.

Texas

4604 Department of Assistive & Rehabilitative Services
Texas Department of Health & Human Services
4800 N Lamar Blvd
Austin, TX 78756-3106
512-377-0500
800-628-5115
TTY: 866-581-9328
www.dars.state.tx.us
DARS.Inquiries@dars.state.tx.us
Veronda L. Durden, Commissioner
Glenn Neal, Deputy Commissioner
Karin Hill, Director of Internal Audit
Transitional and vocational programs aid independence in the home, community and at work for Texans who are blind, deaf, or have other impairments that would benefit from assistive technology.

4605 State Vocational Rehabilitation Agency
Texas State Rehabilitation Commission
4800 N Lamar Blvd
Austin, TX 78756-3106
512-424-4000
800-628-5115
Fax: 512-424-4337
TTY: 800-628-5115
www.dars.state.tx.us
DARS.Inquiries@dars.state.tx.us
Veronda L. Durden, Commissioner
Glenn Neal, Deputy Commissioner
Karin Hill, Director of Internal Audit
State vocational rehabilitation agencies provide direct services to persons with disabilities, including persons with learning disabilities. The services may include evaluation and diagnosis, counseling, guidance, and referral services, vocational and other training services, transportation to rehabilitation services and assistive devices.

4606 Texas Department of Assistive and Rehabilitative Services
4800 N Lamar Blvd
Austin, TX 78756-3106
512-377-0500
800-628-5115
Fax: 512-424-4730
TTY: 866-581-9328
www.dars.state.tx.us
DARS.Inquiries@dars.state.tx.us
Veronda L. Durden, Commissioner
Glenn Neal, Deputy Commissioner
Karin Hill, Director of Internal Audit
A place where people with disabilities and families with children who have developmental delays enjoys independent and productive lives. The mission is to wo

4607 Texas Workforce Commission
101 E 15th St
Austin, TX 78778-0001
512-463-2294
Fax: 512-475-2321
TDD: 800-735-2989
www.twc.state.tx.us
larry.temple@twc.state.tx.us
Larry Temple, Executive Director

Provides oversight, coordination, guidance, planning, technical assistance and implementation of employment and training activities with a focus on meeting the needs of employers throughout the state of Texas.

Utah

4608 Adult Education Services
Utah State Office of Education
250 East 500 South
Salt Lake City, UT 84114-4200
801-538-7500
Fax: 801-538-7882
www.schools.utah.gov
marty.kelly@schools.utah.gov
Marty Kelly, Director
Provides oversight of state and federally funded adult education programs. Offers adult basic education, adult high school completion, English as a second language, and general education development programs.

4609 Utah State Office of Rehabilitation
250 E 500 S
Salt Lake City, UT 84111-4200
801-538-7500
Fax: 801-538-7882
www.schools.utah.gov
Russell Thelin, Director
Assisting and empowering eligible individuals. Disabled, learning disabled, blind, low vision and deaf people can prepare for and obtain employment and increase their independence through job training and assistive technology.

Vermont

4610 Adult Education & Literacy
State Department of Education
120 State St
Montpelier, VT 05602-2703
802-828-3101
Fax: 802-828-3146
http://wwww.education.vermont.gov
edinfo@education.state.vt.us
Kay Charron, Director
Provides adults with educational opportunities to acquire the essential skills and knowledge to achieve career, post-secondary and life goals.

4611 State of Vermont Department of Education: Adult Education and Literacy
120 State Street
Montpelier, VT 05602
802-828-3101
Fax: 802-828-3146
www.vermont.gov
Kay Charron, Director
Adult Education and Literacy Programs provide adults with educational opportunities to acquire the essential skills and knowledge to achieve career, post-secondary and life goals. The Department of Education supports and administers a number of programs that focus on essential literacy and academic skills as well as workplace and introductory occupational skills.

4612 Vermont Dept of Employment & Training
5 Green Mountain Drive
P.O. Box 488
Montpelier, VT 05601-0488
802-828-4000
Fax: 802-828-4022
TDD: 802-825-4203
www.labor.vermont.gov
Mike Calcagni, Director
The Disability Program Navigator Initiative provides professionals who help individuals with disabilities to find jobs, gain access to jobs, or help in re-entering the job market.

4613 Vermont Division of Vocational Rehabilitation
VocRehab Of Vermont
103 South Main Street
Weeks 1A Building
Waterbury, VT 05671-2303
866-879-6757
TTY: 802-241-1455
www.vocrehab.vermont.gov
jana.sherman@ahs.state.vt.us
Diane Dalmasse, Director of VocRehab Division
VocRehab's mission is to assist Vermonters with disabilities, find and maintain meaningful employment in their communities. VocRehab Vermont works in close partnership with the Vermont Association of Business, Industry and Rehabilitation. Contact local VocRehab office for information about services.

4614 Vermont Family Network
600 Blair Park Road
Suite 240
Williston, VT 05495-7549
802-876-5315
800-800-4005
Fax: 802-876-6291
www.vermontfamilynetwork.org
info@vtfn.org
June Heston, President/CEO
Provides educational programs for children and young adults with special educational needs.

4615 VocRehab Reach-Up Program
VocRehab Of Vermont
103 South Main Street
Weeks 1A Building
Waterbury, VT 05671-2303
802-241-1455
866-879-6757
Fax: 802-241-2830
www.vocrehabvermont.org
jana.sherman@ahs.state.vt.us
Pamela Dalley, Director
The program helps individuals with disabilities find meaningful work at a level that is appropriate for them.

Virginia

4616 Adult Education and Literacy
Virginia Department of Education
101 N 14th St, James Monroe Bldg.
P.O. Box 2120
Richmond, VA 23218
804-225-2053
Fax: 804-225-3352
www.doe.virginia.gov
gedinfo@doe.virginia.gov
Randall Stamper, Director
Distributes funds and provides leadership and services related to adult education programs in Virginia. The goal is to raise the performance levels of adult education programs, increase the number of GED credentials issued by Virginia, and provide alternatives for youth who are at risk of dropping out of school.

4617 Virginia Department of Rehabilitative Services
8004 Franklin Farms Dr
Richmond, VA 23229-5019
804-662-7000
800-552-5019
Fax: 804-662-9532
TTY: 804-662-9040
www.vadrs.org
James.Rothrock@drs.virginia.gov
James Rothrock, Commissioner
In partnership with people with disabilities and their families, the Virginia Department of Rehabilitative Services collaborates with the public and private sectors to provide and advocate for the highest quality services that empower individuals with disabilities to maximize their employment, independence and engagement in the community.

Washington

4618 **State Vocational Rehabilitation Agency: Washington Division of Vocational Rehabilitation**
Department of Social Services & Health
P.O. Box 45340
Olympia, WA 98504-5340

360-725-3636
800-637-5627
Fax: 360-438-8007
TDD: 360-438-8000
TTY: 360-438-8000
www.dshs.wa.gov
obrien@dshs.wa.gov

Michael O'Brien, Director
State vocational rehabilitation agencies provide direct services to persons with disabilities, including persons with learning disabilities. The services may include evaluation and diagnosis, counseling, guidance, and referral services, vocational and other training services, transportation to rehabilitation services, and assistive devices.

4619 **State of Washington, Division of Vocational Rehabilitation**
P.O. Box 45340
Olympia, WA 98504-5340

360-725-3636
800-637-5627
Fax: 360-438-8007
http://www1.dshs.wa.gov
ruttllm@dshs.wa.gov

Lynnea Ruttledge, Director
Provides employment-related services to individuals with disabilities who want to work but need assistance. These individuals might experience difficulty getting or keeping a job due to a physical, sensory and/or mental disability. A DVR counselor works with each individual to develop a customized plan of services designed to help the individual achieve his or her job goal.

West Virginia

4620 **West Virginia Division of Rehabilitation Services**
West Virginia Department of Education & the Arts
107 Capitol Street
PO Box 50890
Charleston, WV 25301-2609

304-766-4601
800-642-8207
Fax: 304-766-4905
TDD: 304-766-4809
www.wvdrs.org
susan.n.weinberger@wv.gov

Deborah Lovely, Director
Susan Weinberger, Supervisor, Ed. & Employment
A state agency responsible for the operation of the state and federal vocational rehabilitation program in West Virginia. Specializes in helping people with disabilities who want to find a job or maintain current employment.

Wisconsin

4621 **Wisconsin Division of Vocational Rehabilitation**
PO Box 7852
Madison, WI 53707-7852

608-261-0050
800-442-3477
Fax: 608-266-1133
TDD: 888-877-5939
http://dwd.wisconsin.gov/dvr
dwddvr@dwd.wisconsin.gov

Charlene Dwyer, Administrator
Federal and state program designed to obtain, maintain and improve employment for people with disabilities by working with vocational rehabilitation consumers, employers and other partners.

Wyoming

4622 **Wyoming Department of Workforce Services: State Vocational Rehabilitation Agency**
1510 E Pershing Blvd
Cheyenne, WY 82002-0001

307-777-3700
Fax: 307-777-5870
TTY: 307-777-7389
www.wyomingworkforce.org
jmcint@state.wy.us

Norma Whitney, Vocational Rehabilitation
Assists Wyoming citizens with disabilities to prepare for, enter into, and return to suitable employment. Individuals with a disability that prevents them from working may apply for these services as long as a physical or mental impairment which constitutes or results in a substantial impediment to employment exists, and they have the ability to benefit in terms of an employment outcome from vocational services.

Alabama

Achievement Center, 4464
Alabama Commission on Higher Education, 1926
Alabama Council for Developmental Disabili ties, 1469
Alabama Department of Industrial Relations, 1470
Alabama Disabilities Advocacy Program, 1471
Auburn University, 3030
Auburn University at Montgomery, 3031
Birmingham-Southern College, 3032
Camp ASCCA, 458
Camp Merrimack, 459
Chattahoochee Valley State Community College, 3033
Churchill Academy, 3034
Easter Seals - Alabama, 119, 4465
Easter Seals - Birmingham Area, 120
Easter Seals - Camp ASCCA, 4466
Easter Seals - Capilouto Center for the Deaf, 4467
Easter Seals - Central Alabama, 121
Easter Seals - Disability Services, 4468
Easter Seals - Opportunity Center, 4469
Easter Seals - Rehabilitation Center, Northwest Alabama, 4470
Easter Seals - West Alabama, 122, 4471
Employment Service Division: Alabama, 1472
Enterprise Ozark Community College, 3035
Good Will Easter Seals, 460, 3966, 4472, 4472
International Dyslexia Association of Alab ama, 123
Jacksonville State University, 3037
James H Faulkner State Community College, 3038
Learning Disabilities Association of Alaba ma, 124
Sequel TSI, 3967
South Baldwin Literacy Council, 1927
The Literacy Council, 1928
Troy State University Dothan, 3039
University of Alabama, 3040
University of Montevallo, 3041
University of North Alabama, 3042
University of South Alabama, 3043
Wallace Community College Selma, 3044
Wiregrass Rehabilitation Center, 3968
Workforce Development Division, 4474
Workshops, 3969

Alaska

AK Dept. of Labor and Workforce Dev., 4475
Alaska Adult Basic Education, 1929
Alaska Pacific University, 3045
Alaska State Commission for Human Rights, 1473
Anchorage Literacy Project, 1930
Assistive Technology of Alaska (ATLA), 1474
Center for Community, 1475, 3970
Center for Human Development (CHD), 125
Correctional Education Division: Alaska, 1476
Disability Law Center of Alaska, 1477
Easter Seals - Alaska, 126
Employment Security Division, 1478
Gateway School and Learning Center, 3046, 3971
Juneau Campus: University of Alaska Southeast, 3047
Ketchikan Campus: University of Alaska Southeast, 3048
Literacy Council of Alaska, 1931
State Department of Education & Early Deve lopment, 1479
State GED Administration: GED Testing Program, 1480
University of Alaska Anchorage, 3049

Arizona

Arizona Center Comprehensive Education and Lifeskills, 3972
Arizona Center for Disability Law, 127, 1481
Arizona Center for Law in the Public Inter est, 1482
Arizona Department of Economic Security, 1483
Arizona Department of Education, 1484

Arizona Governor's Committee on Employment of the Handicapped, 1485
Arizona Vocational Rehabilitation, 1476
Camp Civitan, 461
Center for Applied Studies in Education Le arning (CASE), 128
Chandler Public Library Adult Basic Educat ion, 1932
Commission on the Accreditation of Rehabilitation Facilities (CARF), 33
Devereux Arizona Treatment Network, 3973
Division of Adult Education, 1487
Fair Employment Practice Agency, 1488
GED Testing Services, 1489
Institute for Human Development: Northern Arizona University, 129
International Dyslexia Association of Ariz ona, 130
Life Development Institute (LDI), 3974
Literacy Volunteers of Maricopa County, 1933
Literacy Volunteers of Tucson A Program of Literacy Connects, 1934
National Association of Parents with Child ren in Special Education (NAPCSE), 78
New Way Learning Academy, 3050
Parent Information Network, 131
Raising Special Kids, 3975
Rehabilitation Services Administration, 4477
SALT Center, 3051
Upward Foundation, 3052
Yuma Reading Council, 1935

Arkansas

AR-CEC Annual Conference, 1001
Arkansas Adult Learning Resource Center, 1936
Arkansas Department of Career Education, 4478
Arkansas Department of Corrections, 1491
Arkansas Department of Education, 1492
Arkansas Department of Health & Human Services: Division of Developmental Disabilities, 4479
Arkansas Department of Special Education, 1493
Arkansas Department of Workforce Education, 1494
Arkansas Department of Workforce Services, 1495
Arkansas Disability Coalition, 3976
Arkansas Employment Security Department: Office of Employment & Training Services, 4480
Arkansas Governor's Developmental Disabili ties Council, 1496
Arkansas Literacy Council, 1937
Arkansas Rehabilitation Services, 4481
Client Assistance Program (CAP) Disability Rights Center of Arkansas, 1498
Department of Human Services: Division of Developmental Disabilities Services, 4482
Drew County Literacy Council, 1938
Easter Seals - Adult Services Center, 462, 4483
Easter Seals - Arkansas, 132
Faulkner County Literacy Council, 1939
Increasing Capabilities Access Network, 1499
Jones Learning Center, 3053
Learning Disabilities Association of Arkan sas (LDAA), 133
Literacy Action of Central Arkansas, 1940
Literacy Council of Arkansas County, 1941
Literacy Council of Benton County, 1942
Literacy Council of Crittenden County, 1943
Literacy Council of Garland County, 1944
Literacy Council of Grant County, 1945
Literacy Council of Hot Spring County, 1946
Literacy Council of Jefferson County, 1947
Literacy Council of Lonoke County, 1948
Literacy Council of Monroe County, 1949
Literacy Council of North Central Arkansas, 1950
Literacy Council of Western Arkansas, 1951
Literacy League of Craighead County, 1952
Office For The Deaf And Hearing Impaired, 4484
Office of the Governor, 1500
Ozark Literacy Council, 1953
Philander Smith College, 3054
Pope County Literacy Council, 1954
Southern Arkansas University, 3055

St. John's ESL Program, 1955
State Vocational Rehabilitation Agency of Arkansas, 4485
Twin Lakes Literacy Council, 1956
University of Arkansas, 3056
Van Buren County Literacy Council, 1957
Workforce Investment Board, 4486

California

ACCESS Program, 3057
Ability Magazine, 4446
Adult Education, 4487
Allan Hancock College, 3058
Almansor Transition & Adult Services, 3977
Ann Martin Children's Center, 3978
Antelope Valley College, 3059
Ants in His Pants: Absurdities and Realiti es of Special Education, 768
Aspen Education Group, 3060
Assistive Technology Training Program, 1006
Autism Research Institute, 19
Bakersfield College, 3061
Barstow Community College, 3062
Berkeley Policy Associates, 134
Bridge School, 3063
Brislain Learning Center, 3979
Butte College, 3064
Butte County Library Adult Reading Program, 1958
CSUN Conference, 1013
Cabrillo College, 3065
California Association of Private Special Education Schools, 135
California Association of Special Educatio n & Services, 1959
California Department of Education, 1960, 4488
California Department of Fair Employment and Housing, 1503
California Department of Rehabilitation, 1504, 4489
California Department of Special Education, 1505
California Employment Development Department, 4490
California Employment Development Departme nt, 1506
California Literacy, 1961
California State Board of Education, 1507
California State Council on Developmental Disabilities, 1508
California State University: East Bay, 3066
California State University: Fullerton, 3067
California State University: Long Beach- Stephen Benson Program, 3068
Camp Krem: Camping Unlimited, 463
Camp ReCreation, 464
Camp Ronald McDonald at Eagle Lake, 465
Caps, Commas and Other Things, 958
Career Assessment and Placement Center Whittier Union High School District, 1509
Center For Accessible Technology, 4439
Center for Adaptive Learning, 3980
Center on Disabilities Conference, 1014
Chaffey Community College District, 3069
Charles Armstrong School, 3070, 3981
Chartwell School: Seaside, 3071
Clearinghouse for Specialized Media, 1510
College of Alameda, 3072
College of Marin, 3073
College of the Canyons, 3074
College of the Redwoods, 3075
College of the Sequoias, 3076
College of the Siskiyous, 3077
Community Alliance for Special Education (CASE), 136
Cuesta College, 3079
DBTAC: Pacific ADA Center, 1511
Devereux California, 3982
Disability Rights California (California's Protection and Advocacy System), 1512
Disability Rights Education & Defense Fund (DREDF), 38
Disabled Students Programs & Services, 3080
Division for Early Childhood of CEC, 42

Canada

Colorado

Connecticut

Indiana

Iowa

National Federation of Families for Childr en's Mental Health, 222
National Federation of the Blind, 91, 4443
National Institute of Mental Health, 1456
National Institute of Mental Health (NIMH) Nat'l Institute of Neurological Disorders and Stroke, 362
National Rehabilitation Information Center (NARIC), 98
National Resource Center on AD/HD, 363
Nora School, 4119
PWI Profile, 4456
Ridge School of Montgomery County, 4121
Self-Supervision: A Career Tool for Audiologists, Clinical Series 10, 4458
Shelley, the Hyperactive Turtle, 426
Social Security Administration, 1466
Summit School, 3235
The Forbush School at Glyndon, 4122
The Forbush School at Hunt Valley, 3236
The Forbush Therapeutic Preschool at Towson, 3237
The Parents' Place of Maryland, 4123
Towson University, 3238
Youth for Understanding USA, 1444

Massachusetts

A Legacy for Literacy, 2110
ABC's, Numbers & Shapes, 952
ADHD Challenge Newsletter, 374
Activities Unlimited, 851
Activities for the Elementary Classroom, 656
Activities of Daily Living: A Manual of Group Activities and Written Exercises, 657
Activity Schedules for Children with Autism: Teaching Independent Behavior, 852
Adaptive Environments, 223
Adult Center at PAL, 2111
Adult Center at PAL: Program for Advancement of Learning, 4124
Alert Program with Songs for Self-Regulati on, 853
American Government Today, 886
American International College, 3239
An Introduction to How Does Your Engine Run?, 854
Analogies 1, 2 & 3, 614
Animals of the Rainforest Classroom Librar y, 767
Attack Math, 687
Autism Support Center: Northshore Arc, 1647
Autism Treatment Center of America, 21
Basic Essentials of Math: Whole Numbers, Fractions, & Decimals Workbook, 689
Beads and Baubles, 910
Beads and Pattern Cards, 911
Berkshire Center, 3240
Berkshire Meadows, 3241, 4125
Beyond the Code, 771
Big Little Pegboard Set, 912
Boston College, 3242
Boston University, 3243
Breakthroughs Manual: How to Reach Student s with Autism, 856
Bridges To Independence Programs, 514
Bridgewater State College, 3244
Bristol Community College, 3245
Building Mathematical Thinking, 690
Busy Kids Movement, 857
CAST, 4126
Callirobics: Advanced Exercises, 954
Callirobics: Exercises for Adults, 955
Callirobics: Handwriting Exercises to Music, 956
Callirobics: Prewriting Skills with Music, 957
Camp Connect, 515
Camp Discovery, 516
Camp Endeavor, 517
Camp Joy, 518
Camp Lapham, 519
Camp Ramah, 520
Camp Starfish, 521
Camp Summit, 522
Carroll School, 3246
Center for Applied Special Technology (CAS T), 30

Changes Around Us CD-ROM, 659
Claims to Fame, 773
Classroom Visual Activities, 660
Clues to Meaning, 774
Cognitive Strategy Instruction for Middle and High Schools, 661
College Internship Program, 4127
Colored Wooden Counting Cubes, 914
Commonwealth Learning Center, 4128
Cotting School, 3247, 4129
Courageous Pacers Classroom Chart, 859
Courageous Pacers Program, 860
Creative Expressions Program, 523
Crossroads for Kids, 524
Curry College, 3248
Dearborn Academy, 3249
Decimals: Concepts & Problem-Solving, 697
Department of Corrections, 1648
Devereux Massachusetts, 4130
Disc-O-Bocce, 915
Driven to Distraction: Attention Deficit Disorder from Childhood Through Adulthood, 395
Dysgraphia: Why Johnny Can't Write, 959
Dyslexia Training Program, 779
ESL Center, 2112
Early Communication Skills for Children with Down Syndrome, 620
Early Listening Skills, 621
Early Movement Skills, 755
Early Sensory Skills, 757
Early Visual Skills, 758
Easter Seals - Massachusetts, 224, 4543
Eastern Massachusetts Literacy Council, 2113
Educational Foundation for Foreign Study, 1429
Educational Options, 4131
Evergreen Center, 3251, 4132
Experiences with Writing Styles, 904
Explode the Code, 784
Explode the Code: Wall Chart, 625
Explorer Camp, 525
Explorers & Exploration: Steadwell, 894
Eye-Hand Coordination Boosters, 919
F.L. Chamberlain School, 4133
Familiar Things, 920
Federation for Children with Special Needs, 51
Fine Motor Activities Guide and Easel Acti vities Guide, 662
Finger Frolics: Fingerplays, 663
First Biographies, 895
Focus on Math, 700
Fonts 4 Teachers, 965
Fractions: Concepts & Problem-Solving, 702
From Scribbling to Writing, 966
Fun with Handwriting, 967
Fun with Language: Book 1, 627
Funsical Fitness With Silly-cise CD: Motor Development Activities, 863
GEPA Success in Language Arts Literacy and Mathematics, 703
Games we Should Play in School, 864
Geoboard Colored Plastic, 923
Geometrical Design Coloring Book, 924
Geometry for Primary Grades, 704
Get in Shape to Write, 925
Getting Ready to Write: Preschool-K, 968
Getting it Write, 969
Grade Level Math, 706
Great Series Great Rescues, 786
Guide to Summer Programs, 455
HELP for Preschoolers at Home, 759
Half 'n' Half Design and Color Book, 926
Handi Kids Camp, 526
Handprints, 787
Handwriting: Manuscript ABC Book, 971
Harvard School of Public Health, 3252
Health, 665
Higher Scores on Math Standardized Tests, 711
Hillside School Summer Program, 527
Hippotherapy Camp Program, 528
Home/School Activities Manuscript Practice, 972
Horse Camp, 529
Institute for Human Centered Design, 1909
Institute for Human Centered Design (IHCD), 56
Intermediate Geometry, 715

International Dyslexia Association of Massachusetts, 225
JOBS Program: Massachusetts Employment Services Program, 2114
Jarvis Clutch: Social Spy, 865
John Dewey Academy, 4134
Keyboarding Skills, 905
Landmark Elementary and Middle School Prog ram, 3254
Landmark High School Program, 3255
Landmark School Outreach Program, 61, 1030, 3256, 3256, 4135
Landmark School Summer Boarding Program, 530
Landmark School and Summer Programs, 4136
Landmark Summer Program: Exploration and R ecreation, 531
Landmark Summer Program: Marine Science, 532
Landmark Summer Program: Musical Theater, 533
League School of Greater Boston, 4137
Learning Disabilities Worldwide (LDW), 226
Learning in Motion, 866
Lesley University, 3257
Let's Read, 796
Let's-Do-It-Write: Writing Readiness Workbook, 974
Life Cycles Beaver, 839
Linden Hill School, 3258, 4138
Linden Hill School & Summer Program, 534
Link N' Learn Activity Book, 927
Link N' Learn Activity Cards, 928
Link N' Learn Color Rings, 929
Literacy Network of South Berkshire, 2115
Literacy Volunteers of Greater Worcester, 2116
Literacy Volunteers of Massachusetts, 2117
Literacy Volunteers of Methuen, 2118
Literacy Volunteers of the Montachusett Area, 2119
Living Independently Forever, Inc., 4139
MORE: Integrating the Mouth with Sensory & Postural Functions, 667
Magicatch Set, 930
Magnetic Fun, 931
Massachusetts Association of Approved Private Schools (MAAPS), 227
Massachusetts Commission Against Discrimin ation, 1649
Massachusetts Correctional Education: Inmate Training & Education, 2120
Massachusetts Family Literacy Consortium, 2121
Massachusetts GED Administration: Massachu setts Department of Education, 2122
Massachusetts General Education Developmen t (GED), 1650
Massachusetts Job Training Partnership Act: Department of Employment & Training, 2123
Massachusetts Office on Disability, 1651
Massachusetts Rehabilitation Commission, 1652
Mastering Math, 717
May Institute, 4140
Maze Book, 932
Measurement: Practical Applications, 718
Megawords, 798
Melmark New England, 4141
Memory Workbook, 668
Middle School Math Collection Geometry Basic Concepts, 721
Middle School Writing: Expository Writing, 977
Middlesex Community College, 3259
Mike Mulligan & His Steam Shovel, 799
Moose Hill Nature Day Camp, 535
More Primary Phonics, 800
Multiplication & Division, 724
National Center for the Study of Adult Learning & Literacy, 1919
Natural Therapies for Attention Deficit Hyperactivity Disorder, 420
New Language of Toys: Teaching Communicati on Skills to Children with Special Needs, 867
Next Stop, 802
Northeastern University, 3260
Nutritional Treatment for Attention Defici t Hyperactivity Disorder, 421
One-Handed in a Two-Handed World, 669
Opposites Game, 933

Michigan

Minnesota

Mississippi

Missouri

Camp Encourage, 552
Central Missouri State University, 3289
Churchill Center & School for Learning
  Disabilities, 4156
Churchill Center and School for Learning D
  isabilities, 3290
EEOC St. Louis District Office, 1679
Easter Seals - Heartland, 235
Friends-In-Art, 52
Gillis Center, 4157
Great Plains Disability and Business Technical
  Assistance Center (DBTAC), 1680
H.O.R.S.E., 553
Interest Driven Learning Master Class Work shop,
  1025
Joplin NALA Read, 2140
LIFT: St. Louis, 2141
Learning Disabilities Association of Misso uri, 236
Literacy Kansas City, 2142
Literacy Roundtable, 2143
Longivew Community College, 3291
MPACT - Missouri Parents Act, 4158
MVCAA Adult/Family Literacy, 2144
Miriam School, 4159
Missouri Protection & Advocacy Services, 237,
  1681
Missouri State University, 3292
North Central Missouri College, 3293
Parkway Area Adult Education and Literacy, 2145
People to People International, 1439
Rehabilitation Services for the Blind, 4551
Sertoma Inc., 105
St Louis Community College: Forest Park, 3294
St Louis Community College: Meramec, 3295
St Louis Public Schools Adult Education and
  Literacy, 2146
St. Louis Learning Disabilities Associatio n, 238
State Vocational Rehabilitation Agency
  Department of Elementary & Secondary
  Education, 4552
United Cerebral Palsy Heartland, 4553
University of Missouri: Kansas City, 3296

Montana

ACRES -American Council on Rural Special
  Education Conference, 1000
Assistive Technology Project, 1497, 1678, 1685,
  1685
Easter Seals - Goodwill Career Designs Mountain,
  4554
Easter Seals - Goodwill Store, 4555
Easter Seals - Goodwill Working Partners, Great
  Falls, 4556
Goodwill Staffing Services, 4557
LVA Richland County, 2147
Learning Disabilities Association of Monta na, 239
Montana Council on Developmental Disabilities
  (MCDD), 1687
Montana Department of Labor & Industry, 1688
Montana Literacy Resource Center, 2148
Montana Office of Public Instruction, 1689
Montana Parents, Let's Unite for Kids (PLU K),
  240
Office of Adult Basic and Literacy Educati on,
  1690
Parents Let's Unite for Kids, 4160
University of Montana's Rural Institute -
  MonTECH, 1691
Western Montana College, 3297
Workforce Development Services, 4559

Nebraska

Answers4Families: Center on Children, Families,
  Law, 2149
Answers4Families: Center on Children, Fami lies
  and the Law, 1692
Assistive Technology Partnership, 1693
Camp Kaleo, 4560
Camp Kitaki, 554

Client Assistance Program (CAP): Nebraska
  Division of Persons with Disabilities, 2150
Client Assistance Program (CAP): Nebraska
  Division of Persons with Disabilities, 1694
Easter Seals - Nebraska, 241, 555
International Dyslexia Association of Nebr aska,
  242
Learning Disabilities Association of Nebra ska, 243
Lincoln Literacy Council, 2151
Literacy Center for the Midlands, 2152
Midland Lutheran College, 3298
Nebraska Advocacy Services, 1695
Nebraska Department of Labor, 1696
Nebraska Equal Opportunity Commission, 1697
Nebraska Parents Training and Information
  Center, 4161
Platte Valley Literacy Association, 2153
Southeast Community College: Beatrice Camp us,
  3299
State GED Administration: Nebraska, 1699
State Vocational Rehabilitation Agency: Nebraska,
  4561
University of Nebraska: Omaha, 3300

Nevada

Bureau of Services to the Blind & Visually
  Impaired, 4562
Children's Cabinet, 244
Client Assistance Program (CAP): Nevada
  Division of Persons with Disability, 1702
Correctional Education and Vocational Trai ning,
  1703
Department of Employment, Training and Reh
  abilitation, 1704
Easter Seals - Nevada, 245
Learning Disabilities Association of Nevad a, 246
National Council of Juvenile and Family Court
  Judges (NCJFCJ), 87
Nevada Bureau of Disability Adjudication, 1705
Nevada Department of Adult Education, 2154
Nevada Disability and Law Center, 1706
Nevada Economic Opportunity Board: Communi ty
  Action Partnership, 2155
Nevada Equal Rights Commission, 1707
Nevada Governor's Council on Developmental
  Disabilities, 1708
Nevada Governor's Council on Rehabilitatio n &
  Employment of People with Disabilities, 4563
Nevada Literacy Coalition: State Literacy
  Resource Center, 2156
Nevada State Rehabilitation Council, 1709
Northern Nevada Literacy Council, 2157
Rehabilitation Division Department of
  Employment, Training & Rehabilitation, 4564

New Hampshire

AppleSeeds, 769
Becket Family of Services, 4162
Calliope, 887
Calumet Camp, 556
Camp Sno Mo, 4565
Center for Children with Disabilities, 4163
Crotched Mountain, 247
Dartmouth College, 3301
Disability Rights Center, 1712
Easter Seals - Keene, 4566
Easter Seals - Manchester, 4567
Easter Seals - New Hampshire, 248
Easter Seals - New Hempshire, 557
Granite State Independent Living, 1713
Hampshire Country School, 3302, 4164
Hunter School, 3303
Institute on Disability, 1714
International Dyslexia Association of New
  Hampshire, 249
Keene State College, 3304
Learning Skills Academy, 3305
NH Family Ties, 250
New England College, 3306
New Hampshire Commission for Human Rights,
  1715

New Hampshire Department of Health & Human
  Services, 4568
New Hampshire Developmental Disabilities
  Council, 1716
New Hampshire Disabilities Rights Center (DRC),
  251
New Hampshire Employment Security, 1717
New Hampshire Governor's Commission on Dis
  ability, 1718
New Hampshire Literacy Volunteers of Ameri ca,
  2158
New Hampshire Second Start Adult Education,
  2159
New Hampshire Vocational Technical College,
  3307
Parent Information Center, 1719, 4165
Rivier College, 3308
ServiceLink, 1720
Southern New Hampshire University, 3309
State Department of Education: Division of Career
  Technology & Adult Learning-Vocational
  Rehab, 1721
University of New Hampshire, 3310

New Jersey

ASPEN Asperger Syndrome Education Network,
  252
Assistive Technology Advocacy Center-ATAC,
  4570
Assistive Technology Center (ATAC), 1722
Bancroft, 4166
Banyan School, 3311
Caldwell College, 3312
Camden County College, 3313
Camp Merry Heart, 558
Camp Moore, 559
Centenary College, 3314
Center for Parent Information & Resources, 31
Children's Center of Monmouth County, 3315
College of New Jersey, 3316
College of Saint Elizabeth, 3317
Colleges for Students with Learning Disabi lities or
  ADD, 3018
Craig School, 3319
Cumberland County College, 3320
Disability Rights New Jersey, 253
Division of Family Development: New Jersey
  Department of Human Services, 4571
ECLC of New Jersey, 4167
Easter Seals - New Jersey, 254
Eden Autism Services, 48, 4168
Eden Family of Services, 1020, 4572
Fairleigh Dickinson University: Metropolit an
  Campus, 3321
Family Resource Associates, Inc., 255, 4169
Family Support Center of New Jersey, 256
Forum School, 3322, 4170
Georgian Court University, 3323, 4171
Gloucester County College, 3324
How to Reach & Teach Teenagers With ADHD,
  401
Hudson County Community College, 3325
Huntington Learning Centers, Inc., 4172
ISS Directory of International Schools, 3023
International Dyslexia Association of New Jersey,
  257
Jersey City Library Literacy Program, 2160
Jersey City State College, 3326
Kean University, 3327
Learning Ally: National Headquarters, 62
Learning Disabilities Association of New J ersey,
  258
Literacy Volunteers in Mercer County, 2161
Literacy Volunteers of America Essex/Passa ic
  County, 2162
Literacy Volunteers of Camden County, 2163
Literacy Volunteers of Cape-Atlantic, 2164
Literacy Volunteers of Englewood Library, 2165
Literacy Volunteers of Gloucester County, 2166
Literacy Volunteers of Middlesex, 2167
Literacy Volunteers of Monmouth County, 2168
Literacy Volunteers of Morris County, 2169

North Carolina

Utah

Vermont

Virginia

Washington

West Virginia

Wisconsin

A

AAC Institute, 308
AACE, 1081
Abbreviation/Expansion, 1403
ABC's of Learning Disabilities, 2735
ABC's, Numbers & Shapes, 952
ABE Career and Lifelong Learning: Vermont Department of Education, 2290
ABE:College of Southern Idaho, 2024
Abilitations Speech Bin, 622, 623, 628, 629, 630, 633, 634, 635, 780, 781, 916, 917, 1165, 1174
Ability Awareness, 4446, 4452
Ability Magazine, 4446
ABLE DATA, 1445
ABLE Program, 3291
AbleData National Institute on Disability & Rehab. Research, 1049
Ablenet, 1050
About Dyslexia: Unraveling the Myth, 2423
Abrazos Family Support Services, 4184
Absurdities of Special Education: The Best of Ants...Flying...and Logs, 2424
ACA Charlotte, 999
ACA Membership Division, 999
Acacia Academy, 3175, 4081, 4100
Academic Access and Learning Disabilities Program, 3408
Academic Achievement Center, 4051
Academic Communication Associates, 2648, 2988
Academic Development & Programming for Transition, 3192
Academic Drill Builders: Wiz Works, 1115
Academic Fun & Fitness Camp, 590
Academic Institute, 1895
Academic Program, 3235, 3271, 3405
Academic Resource Center, 4112, 3134
Academic Resource Program, 3358
Academic Resource Team (ART), 3125
Academic Services, 3536, 3687
Academic Skills Center, 3643
Academic Skills Problems Workbook, 2918
Academic Skills Problems: Direct Assessment and Intervention, 2919
Academic Software, 1051, 1123, 1129
Academic Success Press, 2649, 2569, 2997
Academic Support, 3733, 3926
Academic Support Center - Student Disability Svcs., 3828
Academic Support Department, 3593
Academic Support Program, 3927
Academic Support Services, 3298, 3945
Academic Support for Students with Disabilities, 3560
Academic Therapy Publications, 2650, 631, 788, 958, 2459, 2926, 2952, 4430, 4435, 4436
Academy of Hope, 1996
ACCESS, 3824
Access Aware: Extending Your Reach to People with Disabilities, 2425
ACCESS Program, 3057
Access Technologies, 1781
Access for All: Integrating Deaf, Hard of Hearing, and Hearing Preschoolers, 2999
Access to Math, 1230
AccessTECH & TECHniques Center, 3792
Accessibility Services Department, 3813
Accessing Parent Groups, 2573
Accessing Programs for Infants, Toddlers and Preschoolers, 2574
Accommodations in Higher Education under the Americans with Disabilities Act (ADA), 2897
Accotink Academy, 4270
Accotink Alternative Learning Center, 4270
Accurate Assessments, 1328
Achievement Academy, 4052
Achievement Center, 4464
Achievers' Center for Education, 4252
ACRES -American Council on Rural Special Education Conference, 1000
ACT, 4437
ACT Universal Testing, 4437, 4292, 4438

Active Parenting Publishers, 1003, 2651
Activities Unlimited, 851
Activities for a Diverse Classroom, 2426
Activities for the Elementary Classroom, 656
Activities of Daily Living: A Manual of Group Activities and Written Exercises, 657
Activity Schedules for Children with Autism: Teaching Independent Behavior, 852
Activity Schedules for Children with Autism: A Guide for Parents and Professionals, 2427
ADA Information Line, 1446
ADA Quiz Book, 2389
ADA Technical Assistance Programs, 1447
Adapted Physical Education, 3106
Adapted Physical Education for Students with Autism, 2920
Adapting Curriculum & Instruction in Inclusive Early Childhood Settings, 2921
Adapting to Your Child's Personality, 2741
Adaptive Device Locator System (ADLS), 1051
Adaptive Driving Program, 3286
Adaptive Environments, 223
Adaptive Physical Education Program, 1116
Adaptive Technology Tools, 1349
ADD Helpline for Help with ADD, 439
ADD Warehouse, 442
ADD and Creativity: Tapping Your Inner Muse, 367
ADD and Romance: Finding Fulfillment in Love, Sex and Relationships, 368
ADD and Success, 369
ADD in Adults, 370
ADD on the Job, 4445
ADD-H Comprehensive Teacher's Rating Scale: 2nd Edition, 4326
ADD/ADHD Behavior-Change Resource Kit: Ready-to-Use Strategies & Activities for Helping Children, 371
The ADD/ADHD Checklist, 428
ADDvance Online Newsletter, 441
ADELPHI UNIVERSITY, 3403
Adelphi University, 3359
ADHD, 2736
ADHD - What Can We Do?, 372
ADHD - What Do We Know?, 373
The ADHD Book of Lists: A Practical Guide for Helping Children and Teens With ADD, 429
ADHD Challenge Newsletter, 374
AD/HD For Dummies, 366
ADHD Report, 375
ADHD and the Nature of Self-Control, 376
ADHD in Adolescents: Diagnosis and Treatment, 2422
ADHD in Adolescents: Diagnosis and Treatment, 377
ADHD in Adults, 2737
ADHD in Adults: What the Science Says, 378
ADHD in the Classroom: Strategies for Teachers, 2738
ADHD in the Schools: Assessment and Intervention Strategies, 3012
ADHD in the Schools: Assessment and Intervention Strategies, 379
ADHD/Hyperactivity: A Consumer's Guide For Parents and Teachers, 380
ADHD: Attention Deficit Hyperactivity Disorder in Children, Adolescents, and Adults, 381
ADHD: What Can We Do?, 2739
ADHD: What Do We Know?, 2740
Adirondack Community College, 3360
Adirondack Leadership Expeditions, 563
Admissions Office, 3714, 4263
Adolescent Language Screening Test, 4447
Adolph & Rose Levis Jewish Community Center, 490
Adult Basic Education, 1888, 2130, 2024
Adult Basic Education Division of Dona Ana Community College, 2174
Adult Basic Education and Adult Literacy Program, 2057
Adult Center at PAL, 2111
Adult Center at PAL: Program for Advancement of Learning, 4124
Adult Education, 4487

Adult Education & Literacy, 4610
Adult Education Foundation of Blount County, 2260
Adult Education Services, 4608
Adult Education Team, 1634
Adult Education and Literacy, 4616
Adult Education and Literacy Program, 2257
Adult Learning Center, 2296
Adult Literacy Advocates of Baton Rouge, 2084
Adult Literacy League, 2002
Adult Literacy Program, 1973
Adult Literacy Program of Gibson County, 2052
Adult Literacy Resource Institute, 2625
Adult Literacy at People's Resource Center, 2029
Adult Programs, 3852
Adult Resource Center, 1971
Adult and Community Learning Services, 1658
Adults with Learning Problems, 2742
Advanced Skills For School Success Series: Module 4, 4383
Adventis Behavioral Health, 4121
Adventure Learning Center at Eagle Village, 540
AdvoServ, 4044
Advocacy, 1830
Advocacy Center, 1628, 1629
Advocacy Center for Persons with Disabilities, 2003
Advocacy Center of Louisiana: Lafayette, 208
Advocacy Center of Louisiana: New Orleans, 209
Advocacy Center of Louisiana: Shreveport, 210
Advocacy Services for Families of Children in Special Education, 2575
ADVOCAP Literacy Services, 2325
Advocates for Children of New York, 265, 4186, 2972
Aetna InteliHealth, 2835
Affect and Creativity, 2898
After School Learning Center, 3119
AfterMath Series, 4350
AGS, 2792
Aids and Appliances for Independent Living, 658
Aiken Technical College, 3694
AK Dept. of Labor and Workforce Dev., 4475
Akron Rotary Camp, 591
Alabama Commission on Higher Education, 1926
Alabama Council for Developmental Disabilities, 1469
Alabama Department of Industrial Relations, 1470
Alabama Dept Of Rehabilitation Services, 4473
Alabama Dept of Economic & Community Affairs, 4474
Alabama Disabilities Advocacy Program, 1471
Alaska Adult Basic Education, 1929
Alaska Department of Education, 1480
Alaska Department of Labor & Workforce Development, 1478
Alaska Pacific University, 3045
Alaska State Commission for Human Rights, 1473
Albert Einstein College of Medicine, 3361, 3432, 4307
Albright College, 3620
Albuquerque Technical Vocational Institute, 3343
Alert Program with Songs for Self-Regulation, 853
Alexander Graham Bell Association, 2613
Alexander Graham Bell Association for the Deaf and Hard of Hearing, 2652
Alexandria Literacy Project, 2131
Alexandria Technical and Community College, 3276
Algebra Stars, 686, 1231
Alien Addition: Academic Skill Builders in Math, 1232
All About Vision, 2010
All Children Learn Differently, 2743
All Kinds of Minds: Young Student's Book About Learning Disabilities & Disorders, 2344
Allan Hancock College, 3058
Allendale Association, 4082
Alliance for Technology Access, 4439
Alliance for Technology Access, 1052, 2425, 2446, 2462
Allyn & Bacon, 2960
The Almansor Center, 4009
Almansor Transition & Adult Services, 3977

Boldface indicates Publisher

Attention Deficit Disorder (ADD or ADHD), 2838

Attention Deficit Disorder Association, 18, 352, 397, 399, 438

Attention Deficit Disorder Warehouse, 383

Attention Deficit Disorder in Adults Workbook, 384

Attention Deficit Disorder: A Concise Source of Information for Parents, 385

Attention Deficit Hyperactivity Disorder: Handbook for Diagnosis & Treatment, 386

Attention Deficit/Hyperactivity Disorder Fact Sheet, 387

Attention-Deficit Disorders and Comorbidit ies in Children, Adolescents, and Adults, 388

Attention-Deficit Hyperactivity Disorder, 2433

Attention-Deficit Hyperactivity Disorder: A Handbook for Diagnosis and Treatment, 389, 2434

Attention-Deficit/Hyperactivity Disorder Test, 4327

Attention-Deficit/Hyperactivity Disorder: A Clinical Guide To Diagnosis and Treatment, 390

Attitude Magazine, 440

Atypical Cognitive Deficits in Development al Disorders: Implications for Brain Function, 2925

Auburn University, 3030

Auburn University at Montgomery, 3031

Auditory Processes, 2926

Auditory Skills, 1136

Augmentative Communication Without Limitat ions, 2749

Augsburg College, 3277

Austin Peay State University, 3723

Author's Toolkit, 953, 1404

Autism, 2750

Autism Program, 3227

Autism Research Institute, 19, 2864

Autism Research Review International, 2864

Autism Society, 20

Autism Support Center: Northshore Arc, 1647

Autism Treatment Center of America, 21, 107, 1041, 2820, 4145

Autism and Developmental Disabilities Clinic, 3126

Autism and the Family: Problems, Prospects and Coping with the Disorder, 2435

Averett College, 3826

AVKO Educational Research Foundation, 1, 642, 803, 973, 1154, 2485, 2550, 2981

Awesome Animated Monster Maker Math, 688, 1233

Awesome Animated Monster Maker Math and Mo nster Workshop, 1234

Awesome Animated Monster Maker Number Drop, 1235

B

The Baby Fold, 4099

Backyards & Butterflies: Ways to Include Children with Disabilities, 2436

Bacone College, 3582

Bailey's Book House, 1352

Baker University, 3208

Baker Victory Services, 4189

Bakersfield College, 3061

Baldwin-Wallace College, 3527

Ball State University, 3188

Ballantine Books, 2557

Ballard & Tighe, 1145, 1153

Bancroft, 4166

Bank Street College: Graduate School of Education, 3362

Bantam Partners, 2355

Banyan School, 3311

Barber National Institute, 4234

Barry University, 3145

Barstow Community College, 3062

Barton County Community College, 1613, 2070

BASC Monitor for ADHD, 4311

Basic Essentials of Math: Whole Numbers, Fractions, & Decimals Workbook, 689

Basic Facts on Study Abroad, 1426

Basic Level Workbook for Aphasia, 770

Basic Math Competency Skill Building, 1236

Basic School Skills Inventory: Screen and Diagnostic, 4331

Basic Signing Vocabulary Cards, 616

Basic Skills Department, 3472

Basic Skills Products, 1137, 1237

Basic Vocabulary: American Sign Language Basic Vocabulary: American Sign Language for Parents, 2364

Baudhuin Preschool, 4054

BBC - Autism Treatment Center of America, 2770

Beacon College, 3146

Beads and Baubles, 910

Beads and Pattern Cards, 911

Becket Family of Services, 4162

Bedford School, 4067

Bedside Evaluation and Screening Test, 4389

Beech Center on Disability, University of Kansas, 2794, 2814

Beginning Signing Primer, 2365

Behavior Assessment System for Children, 4312

Behavior Change in the Classroom: Self-Management Interventions, 3013

Behavior Rating Profile, 4313

Behavior Survival Guide for Kids, 2556

Behavior Technology Guide Book, 2437

Behavioral Directions, 4272

Behavioral Institute for Children and Adolescents, 1008

Behind the Glass Door: Hannah's Story, 2751

Bellefaire Jewish Children's Bureau, 4220

Bellevue Community College, 3865

Belmont Community Adult School, 1968

Beloit College, 3924

Ben Bronz Academy, 3128

Bennett College, 3470

Benton Visual Retention Test, 4422

Berkeley Policy Associates, 134

Berkshire Center, 3240

The Berkshire Center, 4127

Berkshire Meadows, 3241, 4125

Best Buddies International, 22

Best Practice Occupational Therapy: In Com munity Service with Children and Families, 2899

Bethany College West Virginia, 3911

Bethany House Publishers, 2659

Beyond Drill and Practice: Expanding the Computer Mainstream, 1329

Beyond the ADD Myth, 2752

Beyond the Code, 771

Bibliography of Journal Articles on Microcomputers & Special Education, 1082

Biddeford Adult Education, 2088

Big Little Pegboard Set, 912

Binghamton University, 3363

Birmingham Alliance for Technology Access Center, 1090

Birmingham Independent Living Center, 1090

Birmingham-Southern College, 3032

Birth Defect Research for Children (BDRC), 23

Bismarck State College, 3517

Black Hills State College, 3717

Blackhawk Technical College, 3925

Blackwell Publishing, 2660, 2858, 2877

Blocks in Motion, 1118

Bloomsburg University, 3621

Blue Ridge Autism and Achievement Center, 611, 4271

Blue Ridge Literacy Council, 2193

Bluegrass Technology Center, 1091

Bluffton College, 3528

Bodine School, 4249

Body and Physical Difference: Discourses of Disability, 2927

Boling Center for Developmental Disabilities, 3737

Books on Special Children, 2526

Boone Voice Program for Adults, 4390

Boone Voice Program for Children, 4391

Boston Centers for Youth & Families, 518

Boston College, 3242

Boston Diagnostic Aphasia Exam, 4423

Boston University, 3243

Bowling Green State University, 3529

Boy Scouts of America, 24

Boys and Girls Village, Inc., 4016

Bozons' Quest, 1201

BRAAC - Roanoke, 4271

Braille Keyboard Sticker Overlay Label Kit, 1053

Brain Injury Association of America, 25

BrainTrain, 1303, 1319, 1320

Bramson Ort Technical Institute, 3364

Brandon Hall School, 3161, 4068

Breakthroughs Manual: How to Reach Student s with Autism, 856

Brehm Preparatory School, 3176, 4084

Brescia University, 3212

Brevard College, 3471

The Bridge Center, 514, 515, 516, 517, 522, 523, 526, 528, 529

Bridge School, 3063

Bridgerland Literacy, 2287

Bridges Academy, 4253

Bridges To Independence Programs, 514

Bridges for Learning in Applied Science & Tech, 3201

Bridgewater State College, 3244

Brief Intervention for School Problems: Ou tcome-Informed Strategies, 2928

BRIGANCE Assessment of Basic Skills, 4385

BRIGANCE Comprehensive Inventory of Basic Skills, 4386

BRIGANCE Employability Skills Inventory, 4387

BRIGANCE Inventory of Early Development-II, 4421

BRIGANCE Life Skills Inventory, 4388

BRIGANCE Readiness: Strategies and Practice, 4369

BRIGANCE Screens: Early Preschool, 4328

BRIGANCE Screens: Infants and Toddler, 4329

BRIGANCE Screens: K and 1, 4330

BRIGANCE Word Analysis: Strategies and Practice, 4360

Brigham Young University, 3810

Bright Students Who Learn Differently, 4254

Brislain Learning Center, 3979

Bristol Community College, 3245

Brookes Publishing Company, 2661, 2457, 2492, 2497, 2498, 2501, 2504, 2505, 2510, 2520, 2731, 2736, 2752, 2806, 2931, 2942, 2946, 2956

Brookhaven College, 3744

Brookline Books, 424, 661, 2436, 2512, 2529, 2908, 2929, 2954, 2963, 2979, 2989, 3004, 3011, 4366

Brookline Books/Lumen Editions, 2662

Brown Mackie College: Akron, 3530

Brown University, 2244

Brown University, Disability Support Services, 3686

Bryan College: Dayton, 3724

Bryant College, 3687

Bryn Mawr College, 3622

Bubbleland Word Discovery, 617

BUILD Program, 3195

Building Blocks, 751

Building Mathematical Thinking, 690

Building Perspective, 691, 1238

Building Perspective Deluxe, 692, 1239

Bureau of Adult Basic & Literacy Education, 1790

Bureau of Adult Education and Training, 1539

Bureau of Child & Adolescent Health Dept of Health, 1745

Bureau of Early Intervention, 1746

Bureau of Rehabilitation Services, 1635

Bureau of Services to Blind and Visually Impaired, 4564

Bureau of Services to the Blind & Visually Impaired, 4562

Bureau of Special Education & Pupil Servic es, 1530

Burlington College, 3816

Busy Box Activity Centers, 913

Busy Kids Movement, 857

Butler Community College Adult Education, 2067

Butte College, 3064

Boldface indicates Publisher

D

Boldface indicates Publisher

Department of Correctional Education, 1857
Department of Correctional Services, 1737
Department of Corrections, 1648, 1543, 1776, 1863
Department of Corrections/Division of Institutions, 1476
Department of Corrections: Prisoner Education Prog, 1660
Department of Disability Services, 3296, 3485
Department of Economic Development, 1609
Department of Education, 1530, 1547, 1632, 1666, 1671, 1727, 1734, 1735, 1779, 1823, 2060, 4569
Department of Employment & Economic Development, 4548
Department of Employment Services, 4508
Department of Employment, Training and Rehabilitation, 1704
Department of Human Services, 1784, 1820, 4598
Department of Human Services: Division of Developmental Disabilities Services, 1825, 4482
Department of Industrial Relations, 1472
Department of Labor, 1635, 1824
Department of Labor & Employment Security, 4516
Department of Labor & Industry, 4591
Department of Personnel & Human Services, 1864
Department of Public Health & Human Services, 4558
Department of Public Instruction, 1881, 1883, 1990
Department of Public Safety, 1567
Department of Rehabilitation & Correction, 1765
Department of Social Services, 1532
Department of Social Services & Health, 4618
Department of Social Services: Vocational Rehabilitation Program, 4500
Department of Student Support Services, 3587
Department of Technical & Adult Education, 2011
Department of Technical and Adult Education, 1564
Department of VSA and Accessibility, 37
Department of Vocational Rehabilitation, 4537
Department of Workforce Services, 1844
Dept Of Labor & Economic Grwth-Rehabilitation Svcs, 4546
Dept of Administrative and Financial Services, 1640
Dept of Social Services/Bureau of Rehab Services, 1536
Des Moines Area Community College, 3198
Designs for Learning Differences Sycamore School, 4183
Developing Fine and Gross Motor Skills, 2452
Developing Minds: Parent's Pack, 2761
Developing Minds: Teacher's Pack, 2762
Developmental Assessment for Students with Severe Disabilities, 4333
Developmental Disabilities Council, 1637
Developmental Disabilities Resource Center, 4013
Developmental Education, 3532
Developmental Profile, 1334
Developmental Test of Visual Perception (D TVP-2), 4424
Developmental Variation and Learning Disorders, 2937
Devereux Arizona Treatment Network, 3973
Devereux California, 3982
Devereux Center for Autism, 4232
Devereux Early Childhood Assessment (DECA), 753
Devereux Early Childhood Assessment Program Observation Journal, 4316
Devereux Early Childhood Assessment: Clinical Version (DECA-C), 754
Devereux Foundation, 4233
Devereux Genesis Learning Centers, 4250
Devereux Mapleton, 4233
Devereux Massachusetts, 4130
Devereux New Jersey, 4232
Diagnostic and Educational Resources, 4293

Dialog Information Services, 1098
Diamonds in the Rough, 2453, 4393
Dickinson College, 3632
Dickinson State University, 3519
Dictionary of Special Education & Rehabilitation, 2454
Dictionary of Special Education and Rehabilitation, 2938
Different Way of Learning, 2806
Differential Test of Conduct and Emotional Problems, 4425
Differently Abled Services Center, 3163
Dino-Games, 1123
Directory for Exceptional Children, 2939
Directory of Organizations, 2579
Disabilities Resource Center, 3394
Disabilities Services, 3685
Disabilities Services Office, 3677, 3768, 3863
Disabilities Support Department, 3510
Disabilities Support Office, 3814
Disabilities Support Programs, 3480
Disability Accommodations & Success Strategies, 3780
Disability Compliance for Higher Education, 2867
Disability Counseling Office, 3767
Disability Law Center, 1643, 1845, 1655, 1778
Disability Law Center of Alaska, 1477
Disability Programs and Services, 3069
Disability Resource Center, 3076, 3505, 3601, 3807, 3905
Disability Resources, 2823
Disability Resources Department, 3570
Disability Resources and Educational Services, 3187
Disability Retention Center, 3535
Disability Rights - Idaho, 185
Disability Rights California (California's Protection and Advocacy System), 1512
Disability Rights Center, 1712, 1501, 1639
Disability Rights Center of Kansas, 1612
Disability Rights Center of Kansas (DRC), 203
Disability Rights Education & Defense Fund (DREDF), 38
Disability Rights Idaho, 1571
Disability Rights Network of Pennsylvania, 1792
Disability Rights New Jersey, 253, 1722
Disability Rights Oregon, 1783
Disability Rights Washington, 337, 1865
Disability Rights Wisconsin, 1882
Disability Services, 3124, 3222, 3375, 3420, 3508, 3524, 3562, 3563, 3662, 3711
Disability Services Department, 3409, 3438, 3514, 3698, 3936
Disability Services Office, 3423, 3450, 3576, 3603, 3639, 3738
Disability Services for Students, 3689
Disability Services: Cole Learning Enrichment Ctr, 3764
Disability Support Department, 3843
Disability Support Programs and Services, 3103
Disability Support Service, 3366, 3939
Disability Support Services, 214, 3037, 3141, 3221, 3359, 3414, 3453, 3623, 3656, 3691, 3786, 3793, 3797
Disability Support Services (DSS) Office, 3523
Disability Support Services Department, 3486
Disability Support Services/Learning Services, 3142
Disability and Learning Services, 3654
DisabilityInfo.gov, 2822
Disabled Faculty and Staff in a Disabling Society: Multiple Identities in Higher Education, 3019
Disabled Student Development, 3188
Disabled Student Programs, 3082
Disabled Student Programs and Services, 3055, 3061, 3062, 3064, 3065, 3074, 3075, 3083, 3085, 3086, 3088, 3090, 3091, 3092, 3094, 3095, 3096, 3097, 3102
Disabled Student Resource Center, 3597
Disabled Student Services, 3043, 3045, 3067, 3068, 3072, 3385
Disabled Student Services Program, 3059
Disabled Students Program, 3073
Disabled Students Programs & Services, 3080

Disabled Support Department, 3413
Disc-O-Bocce, 915
Discipline, 2390
Discoveries: Explore the Desert Ecosystem, 888, 1387
Discoveries: Explore the Everglades Ecosystem, 889, 1388
Discoveries: Explore the Forest Ecosystem, 890, 1389
Discovery Camp, 584
Discovery Health, 2828
Dispute Resolution Journal, 2391
Disruptive Behavior Rating Scale Kit, 4317
Distance Education Accrediting Commission (DEAC), 39
Distance Education and Training Council (DETC), 1903
District of Columbia, 4508
District of Columbia Department of Corrections, 1550
District of Columbia Department of Education: Vocational & Adult Education, 4509
District of Columbia Fair Employment Practice Agencies, 1551
District of Columbia Public Schools, 1998
Diverse Learners in the Mainstream Classroom: Strategies for Supporting ALL Students Across Areas, 2346
Division for Children's Communication Development, 1904
Division for Communicative Disabilities and Deafness (DCDD), 40
Division for Culturally & Linguistically Diverse Exceptional Learners, 41
Division for Culturally and Linguistically Diverse Learners, 1905
Division for Early Childhood of CEC, 42
Division for Research, 1906
Division of Adult Education, 1487
Division of Career Technology & Adult Learning, 1642
Division of Community Colleges and Workforce Preparation, 4533
Division of Family Development: New Jersey Department of Human Services, 4571
Division of Rehabilitation Services, 215, 4599
Division of Research, 43
Division of Technical & Adult Education Services: West Virginia, 2322
Division of Voc. Rehab., 4475
Division of Vocational Rehabilitation, 2315, 4505, 4513
Division on Career Development, 4440
Division on Career Development & Transition (DCDT), 44
Division on Visual Impairments and Deafblindness, 45
DLM Math Fluency Program: Addition Facts, 1245
DLM Math Fluency Program: Division Facts, 1246
DLM Math Fluency Program: Multiplication Facts, 1247
DLM Math Fluency Program: Subtraction Facts, 1248
Does My Child Have An Emotional Disorder, 2848
Dominican Literacy Center, 2034
Don Johnston, 1114, 1118, 1120, 1126, 1130, 1230, 1355, 1373, 1402
Don Johnston Reading, 1355
Don't Give Up Kid, 2367
Dore Academy, 3478
Dowling College, 3380
The Down & Dirty Guide to Adult ADD, 430
Dpt of Employment, Training and Rehabilitation, 1702
Dr Gertrude A Barber Center, 4234
Dr. Peet's Picture Writer, 1405
Dr. Peet's TalkWriter, 1398
Dragon Mix: Academic Skill Builders in Math, 1250
The Drama Play Connection, Inc., 538
Draw a Person: Screening Procedure for Emotional Disturbance, 4318
Drew County Literacy Council, 1938

Boldface indicates Publisher

G

Boldface indicates Publisher

H

H.O.R.S.E., 553
Hachette Book Group, 2474
Half 'n' Half Design and Color Book, 926
Hallen School, 4193
Halloween Bear, 2371
Hallowell Center, 395
Hamel Elementary School, 3180
Hamilton College, 3389
Hamlin Robinson School, 4285
Hammit School, 4099
Hampden-Sydney College, 3832
Hampshire Country School, 3302, 4164
Handbook for Developing Community Based Employment, 4450
Handbook for Implementing Workshops for Siblings of Special Needs Children, 2470
Handbook of Adaptive Switches and Augmentative Communication Devices, 3rd Ed, 1061
Handbook of Psychological and Educational Assessment of Children, 2907
Handbook of Research in Emotional and Behavioral Disorders, 2471
Handi Kids Camp, 526
Handling the Young Child with Cerebral Palsy at Home, 2472
Handmade Alphabet, 2372
Handprints, 787
Hands-On Activities for Exceptional Students, 664
Handwriting Without Tears, 970
Handwriting: Manuscript ABC Book, 971
Harbour School, 3225
Harcourt, 4356, 4365
Harcourt Achieve, 711, 827, 828, 831, 904, 4303
Harcum Junior College, 3638
Harmony Heights, 3390
Harmony Hill School, 4245
Harris Communications, 616, 1134, 2363, 2364, 2365, 2372, 2374, 2377, 2378, 2381, 2429, 2430, 2456, 2460, 2495, 2509, 2744, 2962, 2986, 2991, 2999
Harrisburg Area Community College, 3639
Hartnell College, 3086
Harvard Graduate School of Education, 1919
Harvard School of Public Health, 3252
Harvard University, 3252
Havern School, 3122, 4014
Hawaii Disability Rights Center, 1568
Hawaii Literacy, 2022
Hawaii State Council on Developmental Disabilities, 1569
Hawley Academic Resource Center, 3205
Hawthorne Educational Services, 4354, 4397
Hazelden Publishing, 2674
Health, 665
Health Answers Education, 2829
Health Science Center, 320
Health Services Building, 1624
Health Services Minneapolis, 1665
HealthCentral Network, 2831
HealthyMind.com, 2832
HearFones, 629
Heartspring School, 4105
HEATH Resource Center, 1099, 2887, 3741
HEATH Resource Directory: Clearinghouse on Postsecondary Edu for Individuals with Disabilities, 2559
Heinemann, 2346, 2348, 2349, 2351, 2352, 2358, 2361, 2362
Heinemann-Boynton/Cook, 2675
HELP Activity Guide, 2947
Help Build a Brighter Future: Children at Risk for LD in Child Care Centers, 2473
Help Me to Help My Child, 2474
Help for Brain Injured Children, 3987
HELP for Preschoolers Assessment and Curriculum Guide, 2948
HELP for Preschoolers at Home, 759
Help for the Hyperactive Child: A Good Sense Guide for Parents, 2475
Help for the Learning Disabled Child, 2476, 4396
Help! This Kid's Driving Me Crazy!, 2768

HELP...at Home, 2906
Helping Students Become Strategic Learners: Guidelines for Teaching, 2908
Helping Your Child with Attention-Deficit Hyperactivity Disorder, 2477
Helping Your Hyperactive Child, 2478
Henry and Lucy Moses Center, 3417
Heritage Christian Academy, 3879
Heritage School, 4155
Herkimer County Community College, 3391
The Hidden Disorder: A Clinician's Guide to Attention Deficit Hyperactivity Disorder in Adults, 431
Hidden Treasures of Al-Jabr, 709
Hidden Youth: Dropouts from Special Education, 2949
High Frequency Vocabulary, 1150
High Noon Books, 788, 2676
High Road School Of Baltimore County, 4117
High School Math Bundle, 710, 1308
High School Student's Guide To Study, Travel and Adventure Abroad, 1430
High Tech Center Training Unit, 1100
Higher Education Consortium for Urban Affairs, 1431
Higher Education for Learning Problems (HELP), 53, 3915, 4337
Higher Scores on Math Standardized Tests, 711
Highlands Educational Literacy Program, 2300
Highlands School, 3226
Highline Community College, 3880
Hill Center, 3484, 4214
Hill School, 3760
Hill Top Preparatory School, 3640, 4235
Hillside School, 3253, 4236
Hillside School Summer Program, 527
Hint and Hunt I & II, 1151
Hippotherapy Camp Program, 528
Hiram College, 3547
A History of Disability, 2916
HMH Supplemental Publishers, 638, 643, 644, 645, 646, 647, 648, 651, 653, 665, 767, 786, 806, 839, 841, 842, 849, 886, 894, 895, 899
Ho-Ho-Kus Campus, 4167
Hocking College, 3548
Hofstra University, 3392
Home Row Indicators, 1062
Home/School Activities Manuscript Practice, 972
Hooleon Corporation, 1053, 1062, 1066, 1067
The Hope Institute for Children and Families, 4101
The Hope School Learning Center, 4101
Hopewell High School, 4217
Horizon Academy, 3210
Horizons School, 3036, 4071
Horizons, Inc., 481
Horse Camp, 529
Hot Dog Stand: The Works, 712
Houghton College, 3393
Houghton Mifflin, 799, 805, 2506
Houghton Mifflin Achieve, 732
Houghton Mifflin Harcourt, 637, 675, 678, 683, 689, 697, 700, 702, 703, 704, 706, 715, 717, 718, 721, 724, 731, 741, 742
How Difficult Can This Be?, 2769, 2950
How Does Your Engine Run? A Leaders Guide to the Alert Program for Self Regulation, 2951
How Not to Contact Employers, 2809
How the Special Needs Brain Learns, 2479
How the West Was 1+3x4, 713
How to Get Services by Being Assertive, 2350, 2480
How to Organize Your Child and Save Your Sanity, 2481
How to Organize an Effective Parent-Advocacy Group and Move Bureaucracies, 2482
How to Own and Operate an Attention Deficit Disorder, 2483
How to Reach & Teach Teenagers With ADHD, 401
How to Write an IEP, 2952
Howard School, 3166
The Howard School, 4075

Howard University School of Continuing Education, 2106
Hudson County Community College, 3325
Hudson Valley Community College, 3394
Hui Malama Learning Center, 2023
A Human Development View of Learning Disabilities: From Theory to Practice, 2917
Human Services: Division of Vocational, 4499
Hunter College of the City University of New York, 3395
Hunter School, 3303
Huntingdon County PRIDE, 312
Huntington Learning Centers, Inc., 4172, 4298
Hutchinson Public Library: Literacy Resources, 2069
HyperStudio Stacks, 1152
Hyperactive Child Book, 402
Hyperactive Child, Adolescent and Adult, 403
Hyperactive Children Grown Up, 2484
Hyperactive Children Grown Up: ADHD in Children, Adolescents, and Adults, 404

I

I Can Read, 789
I Can Read Charts, 2373
I Can Say R, 630
I Can See the ABC's, 790
I Can Sign My ABC's, 2374
I Want My Little Boy Back, 2770
I Would if I Could: A Teenager's Guide To ADHD/Hyperactivity, 405
I'd Rather Be With a Real Mom Who Loves Me: A Story for Foster Children, 406
I'm Not Stupid, 2771
IA University Assistive Technology, 1101
Ice Cream Truck, 714, 1309
IDA Conference, 1023
Idaho Adult Education Office, 2025
Idaho Assistive Technology Project, 1572
Idaho Coalition for Adult Literacy, 2026
Idaho Department of Commerce & Labor, 4523
Idaho Department of Education, 1573
Idaho Division of Vocational Rehabilitation Administration, 4524
Idaho Division of Vocational Rehabilitation, 1574
Idaho Fair Employment Practice Agency, 1575
Idaho Human Rights Commission, 1576, 1575
Idaho Parents Unlimited, Inc., 4080
Idaho Professional Technical Education, 1577
Idaho State Board of Education, 4524
Idaho State Library, 2027
IDEA Amendments, 2587
IDEA Cat I, II and III, 1153
Identifying Learning Problems, 2772
Identifying and Treating Attention Deficit Hyperactivity Disorder: A Resource for School and Home, 407
Idiom's Delight, 631
IEP Success Video, 2953
If Your Child Stutters: A Guide for Parents, 2588
If it is to Be, It is Up to Me to Do it!, 2485
Illinois Affiliation of Private Schools for Exceptional Children, 1583
Illinois Assistive Technology, 1584
Illinois Center for Autism, 4092
Illinois Council on Developmental Disabilities, 1585
Illinois Department of Commerce and Community Affairs, 1586
Illinois Department of Corrections, 1581
Illinois Department of Employment Security, 1587
Illinois Department of Human Rights, 1588
Illinois Department of Human Services, 1590, 2041
Illinois Department of Rehabilitation Services, 1589
Illinois Library Association, 2039
Illinois Literacy Resource Development Center, 2040
Illinois Office of Rehabilitation Services, 1590, 2041

Jewish Child & Family Services Downtown Chicago - Central Office, 190
Jewish Community Center of Metropolitan Detroit, 546
JKL Communications, 2677, 2395
Job Access, 4452
Job Accommodation Handbook, 4453
Job Accommodation Network (JAN), 4442
JOBS Program: Massachusetts Employment Services Program, 2114
JOBS V, 4451
John Dewey Academy, 4134
John Jay College of Criminal Justice of the City University of New York, 3401
John Tyler Community College, 3834
John Wiley & Sons Inc, 401, 413, 425, 432, 433, 2502, 2543, 2553, 2903
Johnson & Wales University, 3690
Johnson C Smith University, 3486
Joliceour School, 4567
Jones Learning Center, 3053
Joplin NALA Read, 2140
Joseph Academy, 4093
Jossey-Bass, 4358
Journal of Learning Disabilities, 2874
Journal of Physical Education, Recreation and Dance, 2635
Journal of Postsecondary Education and Disability, 2875
Journal of Rehabilitation, 2876
Journal of School Health, 2877
Journal of Social and Clinical Psychology, 2857
Journal of Special Education Technology, 2878
Journal of Speech, Language, and Hearing Research, 2893
Joystick Games, 1297
JR Mills, MS, MEd, 2847
JTPA Programs Division, 1586
Judy Lynn Software, 1357
Julia Dyckman Andrus Memorial, 4195
Julie Billiart School, 3550
Jumpin' Johnny, 409
Jumpin' Johnny Get Back to Work: A Child's Guide to ADHD/Hyperactivity, 2375
Juneau Campus: University of Alaska Southeast, 3047
Junior League of Oklahoma City, 2222
Just Kids: Early Childhood Learning Center, 4196

K

Kaleidoscope After School Program, 473
Kaleidoscope, Exploring the Experience of Disability Through Literature and Fine Arts, 2894
Kamp A-Kom-plish, 513
Kamp Kiwanis, 577
Kansas Adult Education Association, 1613, 2070
Kansas Board of Regents, 1618
Kansas Board of Regents Adult Education, 1620
Kansas Correctional Education, 2071
Kansas Department of Corrections, 2072
Kansas Department of Labor, 1614
Kansas Department of Social & Rehabilitati on Services, 2073
Kansas Department of Social and Rehabilita tion Services, 1615
Kansas Human Rights Commission, 1616
Kansas Literacy Resource Center, 2074
Kansas State Department of Adult Education, 2075
Kansas State Department of Education, 1617
Kansas State GED Administration, 1618
Kansas State Literacy Resource Center: Kansas State Department of Education, 2076
Kaplan Early Learning Company, 753, 754, 760, 761, 762, 763, 764, 4316
Karafin School, 4197
Kaskaskia College, 3181
Katie's Farm, 1155
Kaufman Assessment Battery for Children, 4338
Kaufman Brief Intelligence Test, 4339
Kaufman Speech Praxis Test, 633
Kayne Eras Center, 3089, 3989

KC & Clyde in Fly Ball, 1126
KDES Health Curriculum Guide, 2962
Kean University, 3327
Keene State College, 3304
Keeping Ahead in School: A Students Book About Learning Disabilities & Learning Disorders, 2560
Kennedy Center for the Performing Arts, 37
Kennedy Krieger Institute, 4118
Kent County Literacy Council, 2126
Kent State University, 2212
Kentucky Adult Education, 1622
Kentucky Client Assistance Program, 1623
Kentucky Department of Corrections, 1624
Kentucky Department of Education, 1625
Kentucky Laubach Literacy Action, 2079
Kentucky Literacy Volunteers of America, 2080
Kentucky Protection and Advocacy, 1626
Kentucky Special Ed TechTraining Center, 1344
Kentucky Special Parent Involvement Network, Inc., 4106
KET Basic Skills Series, 2810
KET Foundation Series, 2811
KET, The Kentucky Network Enterprise Division, 2729, 2730, 2810, 2811, 2812, 2813
KET/GED Series, 2812
KET/GED Series Transitional Spanish Edition, 2813
Ketchikan Campus: University of Alaska Southeast, 3048
Key Concepts in Personal Development, 2496, 2713
Key Learning Center, 3487
Keyboarding Skills, 905
Keystone Junior College, 3642
Khan-Lewis Phonological Analysis: KLPA-2, 4427
Kid Pix, 1156
KidDesk, 1337
KidDesk: Family Edition, 1338
KidTECH, 1299
Kids Behind the Label: An Inside at ADHD f or Classroom Teachers, 2352
Kids Media Magic 2.0, 793, 1157, 1399
KidsPeace Orchard Hills Campus, 4237
Kildonan School, 3402, 4198
KIND News, 2615
Kind News, 2616, 2617
KIND News Jr: Kids in Nature's Defense, 2616
KIND News Primary: Kids in Nature's Defens e, 2617
KIND News Sr: Kids in Nature's Defense, 2618
Kindercomp Gold, 1298
King's College, 3643
Kingsbury Center, 4048
Kirkwood Community College, 2057
Klingberg Family Centers, 4024
Knoxville Business College, 3727
Kolburne School, 539
The Kolburne School Summer Program, 539
The Kolburne School, Inc., 3264
Kurtz Center, 4057
Kurzweil 3000, 1358
Kurzweil Educational Systems, 1358
Kutztown University of Pennsylvania, 3644
KY-SPIN, Inc., 4106

L

The Lab School of Washington, 3144, 4050
Ladders to Literacy: A Kindergarten Activity Book, 2497
Ladders to Literacy: A Preschool Activity Book, 2498
Lake County Literacy Coalition, 1962
Lake Michigan Academy, 3272, 4151
Lakeshore Technical College, 3932
Lamar Community College, 3123
Lamar State College - Port Arthur, 3762
Landmark College, 3821
Landmark Elementary and Middle School Prog ram, 3254
Landmark High School Program, 3255
Landmark Method for Teaching Arithmetic, 2996

Landmark School, 61, 530, 1030, 2499, 2541, 2987, 2995, 2996, 3254, 3255, 3256, 4135, 4136
Landmark School Outreach Program, 61, 1030, 3256, 4135
Landmark School Summer Boarding Program, 530
Landmark School and Summer Programs, 4136
Landmark School's Language-Based Teaching Guides, 2499
Landmark Summer Program: Exploration and R ecreation, 531
Landmark Summer Program: Marine Science, 532
Landmark Summer Program: Musical Theater, 533
Lane Community College, 3604
Laney College, 3080
Language Activity Resource Kit: LARK, 635
Language Arts, 2895
Language Carnival I, 1158
Language Carnival II, 1159
Language Experience Recorder Plus, 1409
Language Learning Everywhere We Go, 2988
Language Master, 1160
Language and Literacy Learning in Schools, 2500
Language-Related Learning Disabilities, 2501
LAP-D Kindergarten Screen Kit, 760
Laramie County Community College: Disabili ty Support Services, 3963
Laredo Community College, 3763
Large Print Keyboard, 1066
Large Print Lower Case Key Label Stickers, 1067
Latest Technology for Young Children, 2775
Latter-Day Saints Business College, 3806
Laureate Learning Systems, 1339, 1119, 1170, 1190, 1191, 1192, 1193, 1206, 1208, 1209, 1210, 1212, 1213, 1220, 1290, 1293, 1372
Lawrence Hall Youth Services, 1583
Lawrence Productions, 1155
Lawrence University, 3933
LD Advocate, 2645
LD Child and the ADHD Child, 410
LD News, 2646
LD OnLine, 60
LD OnLine/Learing Disabilities Resource, 1045
LD OnLine/Learning Disabilities Resource, 1044
LD Online, 448
LD Pride Online, 2840
LDA Alabama Newsletter, 2636, 2879
LDA Annual International Conference, 1027
LDA Illinois Newsletter, 2637
LDA Learning Center, 4154
LDA Life and Learning Services, 271
LDA Minnesota, 4154
LDA Minnesota Learning Disability Association, 2133
LDA Rhode Island Newsletter, 2880
LDAT Annual State Conference, 1028
LDR Workshop: What Are Learning Disabiliti es, Problems and Differences?, 1029
League School of Greater Boston, 4137
Learn About Life Science: Animals, 836, 1381
Learn About Life Science: Plants, 837, 1382
Learn About Physical Science: Simple Machi nes, 838
Learn to Match, 1161
Learn to Read, 2007
LEARN: Regional Educational Service Center, 1980
Learning & Student Development Services, 3457
Learning About Numbers, 1259
Learning Accomplishment Profile Diagnostic Normed Screens for Age 3-5, 761
Learning Accomplishment Profile (LAP-R) KI T, 762
Learning Accomplishment Profile Diagnostic Normed Assessment (LAP-D), 763
Learning Ally: Athens Recording Studio, 178
Learning Ally: Austin Recording Studio, 329
Learning Ally: Denver Recording Studio, 153
Learning Ally: Menlo Park Recording Studio, 147
Learning Ally: National Headquarters, 62
Learning Ally: New York Recording Studio, 272
Learning Ally: Orland Pk Recording Studio, 191
Learning Ally: Washington Recording Studio, 170
The Learning Camp, 476

Learning Center, 4025
The Learning Center (TLC), 3323, 4171
The Learning Center School, 4146
Learning Center for Adults and Families, 2264
The Learning Clinic, 4037
Learning Company, 1340
Learning Development Department, 3676
Learning Diagnostic Clinic, 3292
Learning Diagnostic Program, 3418
Learning Differences Program, 3652
Learning Disabilities & ADHD: A Family Gui de to Living and Learning Together, 2502
Learning Disabilities A to Z, 2503
Learning Disabilities Association, 273, 1831
Learning Disabilities Association Alabama, 2636
Learning Disabilities Association Illinois, 2637
Learning Disabilities Association of Hawaii, 212, 230, 357, 1627, 4078
Learning Disabilities Association of Alaba ma, 124
Learning Disabilities Association of Alabama, 2879
Learning Disabilities Association of Ameri ca, 63, 2679
Learning Disabilities Association of America, 357, 1027, 2357, 2386, 2408, 2467, 2473, 2475, 2477, 2481, 2483, 2494, 2582, 2771, 2882
Learning Disabilities Association of Arkan sas (LDAA), 133
Learning Disabilities Association of Calif ornia, 148
Learning Disabilities Association of Centr al New York, 274
Learning Disabilities Association of Color ado, 154
Learning Disabilities Association of Cuyah oga County, 300
Learning Disabilities Association of Flori da, 173, 2008
Learning Disabilities Association of Georg ia, 179
Learning Disabilities Association of Georgia, 411
Learning Disabilities Association of Hawai i (LDAH), 184
Learning Disabilities Association of Illin ois, 192
Learning Disabilities Association of India na, 198
Learning Disabilities Association of Iowa, 202, 1610, 2062
Learning Disabilities Association of Kansa s, 206
Learning Disabilities Association of Kentu cky, 207
Learning Disabilities Association of Louisiana, 3219
Learning Disabilities Association of Maryl and, 219
Learning Disabilities Association of Minne sota, 232
Learning Disabilities Association of Missi ssippi, 234
Learning Disabilities Association of Misso uri, 236
Learning Disabilities Association of Monta na, 239
Learning Disabilities Association of Nebra ska, 243
Learning Disabilities Association of Nevad a, 246
Learning Disabilities Association of New York City, 263, 275
Learning Disabilities Association of New J ersey, 258
Learning Disabilities Association of New M exico: Las Cruces, 264
Learning Disabilities Association of Oklah oma, 302
Learning Disabilities Association of Orego n, 305
Learning Disabilities Association of Penns ylvania, 314, 2235
Learning Disabilities Association of Rhode Island, 2880
Learning Disabilities Association of South Dakota, 319
Learning Disabilities Association of Tenne ssee, 323
Learning Disabilities Association of Texas, 330, 2889
Learning Disabilities Association of Utah, 333
Learning Disabilities Association of Washi ngton, 340

Learning Disabilities Association of Weste rn New York, 276
Learning Disabilities Department, 3521, 3608, 3619
Learning Disabilities Office, 3647
Learning Disabilities Program, 3403, 3260
Learning Disabilities Quarterly, 2881
Learning Disabilities Research & Practice, 2858
Learning Disabilities Resources, 2680, 1005, 1016, 1024, 1029, 1031, 1032, 1040, 1043, 2722, 2725, 2742, 2761, 2762, 2769, 2788
Learning Disabilities Services, 3626, 3705, 3782
Learning Disabilities Support Program, 3407
Learning Disabilities Worldwide (LDW), 226
Learning Disabilities and Discipline: Rick Lavoie's Guide to Improving Children's Behavior, 2776
Learning Disabilities and Self-Esteem, 2777
Learning Disabilities and Social Skills: Last One Picked..First One Picked On, 2778
Learning Disabilities and the Law in Highe r Education and Employment, 2395
Learning Disabilities and the World of Work Workshop, 1031
Learning Disabilities in Higher Education and Beyond: An International Perspective, 3024
Learning Disabilities: A Complex Journey, 2779
Learning Disabilities: A Multidisciplinary Journal, 2882
Learning Disabilities: Lifelong Issues, 2504
Learning Disabilities: Literacy, and Adult Education, 2505
Learning Disabilities: Theories, Diagnosis and Teaching Strategies, 2506
Learning Disability Department, 3473, 3476
Learning Disability Evaluation Scale, 4397
Learning Disability Evaluation Scale: Reno rmed, 4354
Learning Disability Program, 3469, 3815, 3912
Learning Disability Support Services, 3572
Learning Effectiveness Program, 3127
Learning Incentive, 3128
Learning Incentive/American School for the Deaf, 478
Learning Independence through Computers, 1102
Learning Lab, 2028
Learning Needs & Evaluation Cetner, 3858
Learning Outside The Lines: Two Ivy League Students with Learning Disabilities and ADHD, 2507
Learning Plus Program, 3136
Learning Problems and Adult Basic Educatio n Workshop, 1032
Learning Problems in Language, 2780
Learning Project at WETA, 2839
Learning Resource Center, 4111, 4276, 3133, 3208
Learning Resource Network, 64, 1912
Learning Services Program, Academic Support Center, 3140
Learning Skills Academy, 3305
Learning Skills Program, 3669
Learning Source, 1977
Learning Strategies Curriculum, 906
Learning Support Center, 3822
Learning Times, 411
Learning and Individual Differences, 2883
Learning and Support Services Program, 3183
Learning in Motion, 866
Leary School Programs, 4277
Least Restrictive Environment, 2396
Lebanon Valley College, 3645
Legacy Program, 3468
A Legacy for Literacy, 2110
Legacy of the Blue Heron: Living with Lear ning Disabilities, 2508, 2781
Legal Center for People with Disabilities and Older People, 1525
Legal Notes for Education, 2397
Legal Rights of Persons with Disabilities: An Analysis of Federal Law, 2398
Legal Services for Children, 149
Lehigh Carbon Community College, 3646
Lekotek of Georgia, 1068, 1073

Lekotek of Georgia Shareware, 1068
Lenoir-Rhyne College, 3488
Leo the Late Bloomer, 2376
Lesley University, 3257
Let's Find Out, 2619
Let's Go Read 1: An Island Adventure, 794
Let's Go Read 2: An Ocean Adventure, 795
Let's Learn About Deafness, 2509
Let's Read, 796
Let's Write Right: Teacher's Edition, 973
Let's-Do-It-Write: Writing Readiness Workbook, 974
Letter Sounds, 1162
Letters and First Words, 1163
Letting Go: Views on Integration, 2782
The Lewis School and Clinic for Educational Therapy, 4180
Lewis and Clark Community College, 3182
Lexia Cross-Trainer, 1359
Lexia Early Reading, 1360
Lexia Learning Systems, 1164, 1359, 1360, 1361, 1362
Lexia Phonics Based Reading, 1164
Lexia Primary Reading, 1361
Lexia Strategies for Older Students, 1362
Liberty University, 3835
Library Literacy Programs: State Library o f Iowa, 2063
Library Reproduction Service, 2681
Life After High School for Students with Moderate and Severe Disabilities, 2814
Life Beyond the Classroom: Transition Strategies for Young People with Disabilities, 2510
Life Centered Career Education: Assessment Batteries, 4454
Life Cycles Beaver, 839
Life Development Institute (LDI), 3974
Life-Centered Career Education Training, 666
LIFT: St. Louis, 2141
Lighthouse Central Florida, 1103
Lighthouse International, 797
Lighthouse Low Vision Products, 797
LILAC, 634
Lily Videos : A Longitudinel View of Lily with Down Syndrome, 2783
Limestone College, 3703
LINC, 1102
Lincoln Literacy Council, 2151
Lincolnia Educational Foundation, 4277
Lindamood Bell, 2994
Lindamood-Bell Learning Processes Professi onal Development, 1033
Linden Hill School, 3258, 4138
Linden Hill School & Summer Program, 534
Linfield College, 3605
LinguiSystems, 2682
Link N' Learn Activity Book, 927
Link N' Learn Activity Cards, 928
Link N' Learn Color Rings, 929
Link Newsletter, 2638
Linn-Benton Community College Office of Disability Services, 3606
Lion's Workshop, 1216
Lions Club International, 1434
Lisle, 1435
Literacy & Evangelism International, 2223
Literacy Action of Central Arkansas, 1940
Literacy Alliance, 2054
Literacy Austin, 2275
Literacy Center for the Midlands, 2152
Literacy Center of Marshall: Harrison Coun ty, 2276
Literacy Center of Milford, 1981
Literacy Chicago, 2042
Literacy Connection, 2043
Literacy Council, 2044
The Literacy Council, 1928
Literacy Council Of Buncombe County, 2196
Literacy Council of Alaska, 1931
Literacy Council of Arkansas County, 1941
Literacy Council of Benton County, 1942
Literacy Council of Clermont/Brown Countie s, 2209
Literacy Council of Crittenden County, 1943

Boldface indicates Publisher

Literacy Council of Frederick County, 2107
Literacy Council of Garland County, 1944
Literacy Council of Grant County, 1945
Literacy Council of Greater Waukesha, 2328
Literacy Council of Hot Spring County, 1946
Literacy Council of Jefferson County, 1947
Literacy Council of Kingsport, 2265
Literacy Council of Kitsap, 2316
Literacy Council of Lancaster/Lebanon, 2236
Literacy Council of Lonoke County, 1948
Literacy Council of Monroe County, 1949
Literacy Council of Montgomery County, 2108
Literacy Council of North Central Arkansas, 1950
Literacy Council of Northern Virginia, 2301
Literacy Council of Prince George's County, 1991
Literacy Council of Seattle, 2317
Literacy Council of Southwest Louisiana, 2085
Literacy Council of Sumner County, 2266
Literacy Council of Western Arkansas, 1951
Literacy Florida, 2009
Literacy Kansas City, 2142
Literacy League of Craighead County, 1952
Literacy Mid-South, 2267
Literacy Network, 2329
Literacy Network of South Berkshire, 2115
Literacy Program: County of Los Angeles Public Library, 1963
Literacy Roundtable, 2143
Literacy Services of Wisconsin, 2330
Literacy Source: Community Learning Center, 2318
Literacy Volunteers Centenary College, 2086
Literacy Volunteers Serving Adults: Northe rn Delaware, 1992
Literacy Volunteers in Mercer County, 2161
Literacy Volunteers of America Essex/Passa ic County, 2162
Literacy Volunteers of America: Bastrop, 2277
Literacy Volunteers of America: Bay City Matagorda County, 2278
Literacy Volunteers of America: Chippewa Valley, 2331
Literacy Volunteers of America: Dona Ana County, 2178
Literacy Volunteers of America: Eau Claire, 2332
Literacy Volunteers of America: Forsyth County, 2014
Literacy Volunteers of America: Illinois, 2045
Literacy Volunteers of America: Laredo, 2279
Literacy Volunteers of America: Las Vegas, San Miguel, 2179
Literacy Volunteers of America: Marquette County, 2333
Literacy Volunteers of America: Middletown, 2186
Literacy Volunteers of America: Montgomery County, 2280
Literacy Volunteers of America: Nelson Cou nty, 2302
Literacy Volunteers of America: New River Valley, 2303
Literacy Volunteers of America: Pitt Count y, 2197
Literacy Volunteers of America: Port Arthu r Literacy Support, 2281
Literacy Volunteers of America: Prince William, 2304
Literacy Volunteers of America: Rhode Isla nd, 2239
Literacy Volunteers of America: Shenandoah County, 2305
Literacy Volunteers of America: Socorro County, 2180
Literacy Volunteers of America: Tulsa City County Library, 2224
Literacy Volunteers of America: Willits Public Library, 1964
Literacy Volunteers of America: Wilmington Library, 1993
Literacy Volunteers of America: Wimberley Area, 2282
Literacy Volunteers of Androscoggin, 2090
Literacy Volunteers of Aroostook County, 2091
Literacy Volunteers of Atlanta, 2015
Literacy Volunteers of Bangor, 2092
Literacy Volunteers of Camden County, 2163

Literacy Volunteers of Cape-Atlantic, 2164
Literacy Volunteers of Central Connecticut, 1982
Literacy Volunteers of Charlottesville/Alb emarle, 2306
Literacy Volunteers of DuPage, 2046
Literacy Volunteers of Eastern Connecticut, 1983
Literacy Volunteers of Englewood Library, 2165
Literacy Volunteers of Fox Valley, 2047
Literacy Volunteers of Gloucester County, 2166
Literacy Volunteers of Greater Augusta, 2093
Literacy Volunteers of Greater Hartford, 1984
Literacy Volunteers of Greater New Haven, 1985
Literacy Volunteers of Greater Portland, 2094
Literacy Volunteers of Greater Saco/Biddef ord, 2095
Literacy Volunteers of Greater Sanford, 2096
Literacy Volunteers of Greater Worcester, 2116
Literacy Volunteers of Kent County, 2240
Literacy Volunteers of Lake County, 2048
Literacy Volunteers of Maine, 2097
Literacy Volunteers of Maricopa County, 1933
Literacy Volunteers of Massachusetts, 2117
Literacy Volunteers of Methuen, 2118
Literacy Volunteers of Mid-Coast Maine, 2098
Literacy Volunteers of Middlesex, 2167
Literacy Volunteers of Monmouth County, 2168
Literacy Volunteers of Morris County, 2169
Literacy Volunteers of Northern Connecticu t, 1986
Literacy Volunteers of Oswego County, 2187
Literacy Volunteers of Otsego & Delaware Counties, 2188
Literacy Volunteers of Plainfield Public Library, 2170
Literacy Volunteers of Providence County, 2241
Literacy Volunteers of Roanoke Valley, 2307
Literacy Volunteers of Santa Fe, 2181
Literacy Volunteers of Somerset County, 2171
Literacy Volunteers of South County, 2242
Literacy Volunteers of Tucson A Program of Literacy Connects, 1934
Literacy Volunteers of Union County, 2172
Literacy Volunteers of Waldo County, 2099
Literacy Volunteers of Washington County, 2243
Literacy Volunteers of Western Cook County, 2049
Literacy Volunteers of the Lowcountry, 2251
Literacy Volunteers of the Montachusett Area, 2119
Literacy Volunteers of the National Capita l Area, 1999
Literacy Volunteers-Valley Shore, 1987
Literacy Volunteers: Campbell County Publi c Library, 2308
Literacy Volunteers: Stamford/Greenwich, 1988
Literary Resources Rhode Island, 2244
Little Keswick School, 3836, 4278
Living Independently Forever, Inc., 4139
Living With Attention Deficit Disorder, 2714
Living with a Learning Disability, 2511
Lock Haven University, 1438
Lock Haven University of Pennsylvania, 3647
Lon Morris College, 3764
Long Beach City College: Liberal Arts Camp us, 3090
Long Island University/C.W. Post Campus, 3358
Longivew Community College, 3291
Longwood College, 3837
Look! Listen! & Learn Language!, 1165
Lorain County Community College, 3551
Loras College, 3202
Lord Fairfax Community College, 3838
Lorraine D. Foster Day School, 4026
Los Angeles Mission College, 3091
Los Angeles Pierce College, 3092
Los Angeles Valley College Services for Students with Disabilities (SSD), 3093
Loudoun Literacy Council, 2309
Louisiana Assistive Technology Access Network, 1631
Louisiana College, 3215
Louisiana Department of Education, 1630, 1633
Louisiana State University: Alexandria, 3216
Louisiana State University: Eunice, 3217
Love Publishing Company, 2683, 2454, 2786, 2938, 2945

LRP Publications, 2398, 2867
Lubbock Christian University, 3765
Lutheran Braille Workers, 150
LVA Richland County, 2147
Lycoming College, 3648
Lynn University, 3151

M

M-ss-ng L-nks Single Educational Software, 1166
MA Department of Elementary & Secondary Education, 1650
MA Dept of Elementary & Secondary Education, 2121
MACcessories: Guide to Peripherals, 1085
Magicatch Set, 930
Magination Press, 2684
Magnetic Fun, 931
Maine Bureau of Rehabilitation Services, 4540
Maine Department of Education, 1634
Maine Human Rights Commission, 1638
Maine Literacy Resource Center, 2100
Maine Parent Federation, 213
Mainstream Computer Program, 3118
Mainstreaming at Camp, 578
Make-a-Map 3D, 897
Making Handwriting Flow, 975
Making School Inclusion Work: A Guide to Everyday Practices, 2963
Making Sense of Sensory Integration, 2784
Making the System Work for Your Child with ADHD, 412
Making the Writing Process Work: Strategies for Composition & Self-Regulation, 2989
Making the Writing Process Work: Strategie s for Composition & Self-Regulation, 2512
Malone University, 3552
Managing Attention Deficit Hyperactivity D isorder: A Guide for Practitioners, 413
Manchester College, 3192
Manhattan College: Specialized Resource Ce nter, 3404
Manor Junior College, 3649
Mansfield University of Pennsylvania, 3650
Manus Academy, 4215
Manus Academy, 4216
Maplebrook School, 3405, 4199, 3369, 4205
Maps & Navigation, 840, 898
Maranatha Baptist Bible College, 3934
Marathon County Literacy Council, 2334
MarbleSoft, 1219, 1294, 1317
Marburn Academy, 3553
Marburn Academy Summer Programs, 602
Margaret A Staton Office of Disability Services, 3165
Margaret Brent School, 3231
Maria College, 3406
Marian College of Fond Du Lac, 3935
Marianne Frostig Center of Educational Therapy, 3084
Marietta College, 3554
Marin Literacy Program, 1965
Marina Psychological Services, 3990
Marion Technical College, 3555
Mariposa School for Children with Autism, 3489
Marist College, 3407
Marquette University, 3936
Marriott Foundation, 2842
Mars Hill College, 3490
Marsh Media, 1217, 2685, 2496, 2713, 2790
Marshall University, 53, 3915, 4337
Marshware, 1217
Marvelwood, 3132
Marvelwood School, 3132
Mary McDowell Friends School, 4200
Mary Washington College, 3839
Maryland Adult Literacy Resource Center, 2109
Maryland Association of University Centers on Disabilities, 220
Maryland Department of Disabilities, 4541
Maryland Developmental Disabilities Counci l, 1644
Maryland State Department of Education, 215

Boldface indicates Publisher

My House: Language Activities of Daily Living, 1220
My Mathematical Life, 725
My Own Bookshelf, 1172
My Signing Book of Numbers, 2378
Myofascial Release and Its Application to Neuro-Developmental Treatment, 2965
Myth of Laziness, 2353

N

NACE Journal, 2896
NAHEE, 2615, 2618
Napa Valley College, 3096
NAPSEC, 3025
Narrative Prosthesis: Disability and the Dependencies of Discourse, 2966
NASDSE, 68
Nashville Adult Literacy Council, 2268
NASP, 69
Nassau Community College, 3413
Nat'l Clearinghouse of Rehab. Training Materials, 2809
Nat'l Dissemination Center for Children Disabiliti, 450
Natchaug Hospital, 4029
Natchaug Hospital School Program, 4028
Natchaug's Network of Care, 4029
National ARD/IEP Advocates, 70
National Academies Press, 3003, 3009
National Adult Education Professional Deve lopment Consortium, 71, 1913
National Adult Literacy & Learning Disabilities Center (NALLD), 1914
National Aeronautics and Space Administration, 1112
National Alliance on Mental Illness (NAMI) Attention-Deficit/Hyperactivity Disorder Fact Sheet, 358, 419
National Association for Adults with Special Learning Needs, 1915
National Association for Adults with Speci al Learning Needs (NAASLN), 72
National Association for Child Development (NACD), 73
National Association for Community Mediati on (NAFCM), 74
National Association for Gifted Children (NAGC), 75
National Association for Humane and Enviro nmental Education, 2620
National Association for Visually Handicap ped, 2687
National Association for the Education of Young Children (NAEYC), 76
National Association of Colleges and Employers, 2896
National Association of Councils on Develo pmental Disabilities (NACDD), 77
National Association of Parents with Child ren in Special Education (NAPCSE), 78
National Association of Private Special Education Centers, 1916
National Association of Private Special Ed ucation Centers (NAPSEC), 79
National Association of Special Education Teachers (NASET), 80
National Association of the Education of African American Children with Learning Disabilities, 81
National Autism Association, 82
National Bible Association, 2688
National Business and Disability Council at The Viscardi Center, 83
National Center For Family Literacy, 1034
National Center for Fair & Open Testing FairTest, 4300
National Center for Families Literacy (NCFL), 84
National Center for Family Literacy, 1917
National Center for Gender Issues and AD/HD, 449
National Center for Learning Disabilities, 85, 359, 1918, 2644, 2645, 2646, 2647

National Center for State Courts, 1448
National Center for Youth Law, 86
National Center for the Study of Adult Learning & Literacy, 1919
National Center on Adult Literacy (NCAL), 1920
National Clearinghouse of Rehabilitation Training Materials (NCRTM), 360
National Council of Juvenile and Family Court Judges (NCJFCJ), 87
National Council of Teachers of English, 193, 2895
National Council on Disability, 1455, 2558
National Council on Rehabilitation Educati on (NCRE), 88
National Data Bank for Disabled Service, 221
National Disabilities Rights Network (NDRN), 89
National Disability Rights Network, 2003
National Dissemination Center for Children, 361, 387, 457
National Easter Seals Society, 501
National Education Association (NEA), 90, 1921
National Federation of Families for Childr en's Mental Health, 222
National Federation of the Blind, 91, 4443
National Governor's Association (NGA), 4463
National Governors Association, 4447
National Governors Association Newsletter, 4455
National Head Start Association, 1035, 2624
National Head Start Association Parent Conference, 1036
National Institute for Learning Developmen t, 92
National Institute of Art and Disabilities Art Center, 93
National Institute of Health, 1332
National Institute of Mental Health, 1456, 418
National Institute of Mental Health (NIMH) Nat'l Institute of Neurological Disorders and Stroke, 362
National Institute on Disability and Rehabilitation Research, 1457
National Institutes of Health, 1454
National Joint Committee on Learning Disab ilities, 94
National Lekotek Center, 1922
National Library Services for the Blind and Physically Handicapped, 1458
National Organization for Rare Disorders (NORD), 95
National Organization of Easter Seals, 470
National Organization on Disability, 2884
National Organization on Disability (NOD), 96
National Rehabilitation Association, 97, 2876
National Rehabilitation Information Center (NARIC), 98
National Resource Center on AD/HD, 363, 445
National Resources, 2591
National School Boards Association, 2862
National Society for Experimental Educatio n, 1437
National Techinical Information Service, 2844
National Technical Information Service: US Department of Commerce, 1459
National Toll-free Numbers, 2592
National Wildlife Foundation/Membership Services, 2621
National-Louis University, 4095
Natural Therapies for Attention Deficit Hyperactivity Disorder, 420
Navigating College College Manual for Teac hing the Portfolio, 3026
Navigating College: Strategy Manual for a Successful Voyage, 3027
Nawa Academy, 3991
Nazareth College of Rochester, 3414
NCFL Conference, 1034
ND Department of Human Services, 1762
Nebraska Advocacy Services, 1695
Nebraska Department of Education, 1694, 1699, 1700
Nebraska Department of Labor, 1696
Nebraska Dept Of Educ. Vocational Rehabilitation, 4561
Nebraska Equal Opportunity Commission, 1697

Nebraska Parents Training and Information Center, 4161
Negotiating the Special Education Maze, 2517
Nevada Bureau of Disability Adjudication, 1705
Nevada Department of Adult Education, 2154
Nevada Department of Education, 1710
Nevada Dept Of Employment,Training&Rehabilitation, 4562
Nevada Disability and Law Center, 1706
Nevada Economic Opportunity Board: Communi ty Action Partnership, 2155
Nevada Equal Rights Commission, 1707
Nevada Governor's Council on Developmental Disabilities, 1708
Nevada Governor's Council on Rehabilitatio n & Employment of People with Disabilities, 4563
Nevada Literacy Coalition: State Literacy Resource Center, 2156
Nevada Rehabilitation Division, 1709
Nevada State Rehabilitation Council, 1709
New Community School, 3840, 4279
New Directions, 2399
The New England Center for Children, 4147
New England College, 3306
New Hampshire Commission for Human Rights, 1715
New Hampshire Department of Health & Human Services, 4568
New Hampshire Developmental Disabilities Council, 1716
New Hampshire Disabilities Rights Center (DRC), 251
New Hampshire Employment Security, 1717
New Hampshire Governor's Commission on Dis ability, 1718
New Hampshire Literacy Volunteers of Ameri ca, 2158
New Hampshire Second Start Adult Education, 2159
New Hampshire Vocational Technical College, 3307
New Heights School, 3882
New Horizons Information for the Air Traveler with a Disability, 2354
New IDEA Amendments: Assistive Technology Devices and Services, 2400
New Interdisciplinary School, 4201
New Jersey City University, 3330
New Jersey Council on Developmental Disabi lities, 4573
New Jersey Department of Education, 1724, 1728
New Jersey Department of Health, 1725
New Jersey Department of Law and Public Safety, 1723
New Jersey Department of Special Education, 1724
New Jersey Division on Civil Rights, 1723
New Jersey Programs for Infants and Toddle rs with Disabilities: Early Intervention System, 1725
New Jersey Protection and Advocacy, 4570
New Jersey Self-Help Group Clearinghouse, 259
New Jersey State Department of Education, 4574
New Jersey State Elks Association, 559
New Language of Toys, 2518
New Language of Toys: Teaching Communicati on Skills to Children with Special Needs, 867
A New Look at ADHD: Inhibition, Time, and Self-Control, 365
New Mexico Coalition for Literacy, 2182
New Mexico Department of Labor: Job Traini ng Division, 4576
New Mexico Department of Workforce Solutio ns: Workforce Transition Services Division, 1730
New Mexico Human Rights Commission Educati on Bureau, 1731
New Mexico Institute of Mining and Technol ogy, 3348
New Mexico Junior College, 3349
New Mexico Public Education Department, 1732, 1733
New Mexico State GED Testing Program, 1733
New Mexico State University, 3350

New Mexico Technology-Related Assistance Program, 1734
New Orleans Corporate Office, 511
New River Community College, 3841
New Room Arrangement as a Teaching Strateg y, 2715
NEW START Adult Learning Program, 1994
New Vistas Christian School, 3992
New Vistas School, 4280
New Way Learning Academy, 3050
New York City College of Technology, 3415
New York Department of Labor: Division of Employment and Workforce Solutions, 1740
New York Institute for Special Education, 4202, 3427, 3439
The New York Institute for Special Education, 3464
New York Institute of Technology: Old Westbury, 3416
New York Literacy Assistance Center, 2189
New York Literacy Resource Center, 2190
New York Literacy Volunteers of America, 2191
New York State Commission on Quality Care and Advocacy for Persons with Disabilities (CQCAPD), 1741
New York State Department of Education, 1744, 4580
New York State Education Department, 4579
New York State Office of Vocational & Educ ational Services for Individuals with Disabilities, 1742
New York University, 3417
New York University Medical Center, 3418
The Newgrange Education Center, 4182
Newgrange School, 4174
Newman University, 3211
Newport Audiology Center, 3993
Newport Beach Public Library Literacy Services, 1969
Newport Health Network, 3993
Newton County Reads, 2016
Next Stop, 802
NH Family Ties, 250
Niagara County Community College, 3419
Niagara University, 3420
NICHCY, 2571, 2572, 2573, 2574, 2576, 2577, 2578, 2579, 2580, 2584, 2585, 2586, 2587, 2589, 2590, 2591, 2592, 2593, 2594, 2595, 2596
NICHCY News Digest, 2612
Nicholls State University, 3218
Nicolet Area Technical College, 3939
Nimble Numeracy: Fluency in Counting and Basic Arithmetic, 726
NIMH Neurological Institute, 362
NIMH-Attention Deficit-Hyperactivity Diso rder Information Fact Sheet, 418
900 W.Fireweed Lane, 3046
92ny Street Y, 565
NJ Department of Health, 260, 4575
No Barriers to Study, 1438
No Easy Answer, 2355
No One to Play with: The Social Side of Learning Disabilities, 2519
Nobody's Perfect: Living and Growing with Children who Have Special Needs, 2520
Noel Program, 3482
NOLO, 2444
Non Verbal Learning Disorders Association (NLDA), 99
Nonverbal Learning Disorders Association, 162
Nora School, 4119
Nordic Software, 1314
Norfolk State University, 3842
Normal Growth and Development: Performance Prediction, 2786
Norman Howard School, 3421
The Norman Howard School, 4210
North American Montessori Teachers' Association Conference, 1037
North Carolina Community College, 1757, 2198, 3513
North Carolina Council on Developmental Disabilities, 1752

North Carolina Division of Vocational Reha bilitation, 1753
North Carolina Division of Workforce Servi ces, 1754
North Carolina Employment Security Commission, 1755
North Carolina Literacy Resource Center, 2198
North Carolina Office of Administrative Hearings: Civil Rights Division, 1756
North Carolina State University, 3494
North Carolina Wesleyan College, 3495
North Central Missouri College, 3293
North Coast Education Services, 4223
North Coast Tutoring Services, 4226
North Country Community College, 3422
North Dakota Adult Education and Literacy Resource Center, 2200
North Dakota Association For The Disabled (NDAD), 290
North Dakota Association for Lifelong Learning (NDALL), 291
North Dakota Autism Center, 292
North Dakota Center for Persons with Disab Ilities (NDCPD), 293
North Dakota Center for Persons with Disabilities, 3522
North Dakota Department of Career and Tech nical Education, 2201, 4581
North Dakota Department of Commerce, 4582
North Dakota Department of Human Services, 1759, 4583
North Dakota Department of Human Services: Welfare & Public Assistance, 2202
North Dakota Department of Labor: Fair Employment Practice Agency, 1760
North Dakota Department of Public Instruct ion, 1761, 2203
North Dakota Protection & Advocacy Project, 294
North Dakota Reading Association, 2204
North Dakota State College of Science, 3523
North Dakota State Council on Developmenta l Disabilities, 1762
North Dakota State University, 3524
North Dakota Workforce Development Council, 2205, 4582
North Georgia Technical College Adult Educ ation, 2017
North Greenville College, 3705
North Iowa Area Community College, 3203
North Lake College, 3768
North Seattle Community College, 3883
North Texas Rehabilitation Center, 331
Northampton Community College, 3656
Northcentral Technical College, 3940
Northeast ADA Center, 277
Northeast State Community College, 3730
Northeast Wisconsin Technical College, 3941
Northeastern State University, 3586, 2217
Northeastern University, 3260
Northern Nevada Literacy Council, 2157
Northern New Mexico Community College, 3351
Northern State University, 3719
Northern Virginia Community College, 3843
Northland College, 3942
Northwest Community Action Programs - Casp er (NOWCAP), 348
Northwest Community Action Programs - Cody (NOWCAP), 349
Northwest Community Action Programs - Rock Springs (NOWCAP), 350
Northwest Media, 2689
Northwest Oklahoma Literacy Council, 2226
Northwest School, 3884
Northwest Technical College, 3283
Northwestern Michigan College, 3275
Northwestern State University, 3219
Northwestern University Learning Clinic, 4094
Norwich University, 3822
Notre Dame School, 3769
Nova SE University's Mailman Segal Institute, 4054
Now You're Talking: Extend Conversation, 2716
Number Farm, 1273
Number Meanings and Counting, 727

Number Please, 1274
Number Sense & Problem Solving CD-ROM, 728, 1315
Number Sense and Problem Solving, 1275
Number Stumper, 1276
Numbers Undercover, 729
Numbers that add up to Educational Rights for Children with Disabilities, 2401
Nutritional Treatment for Attention Defici t Hyperactivity Disorder, 421
NY Commission on Quality of Care, 1747
NY District Kiwanis Foundation, 577
NYS Commission on Quality of Care/TRAID Pr ogram, 1738
NYS Developmental Disabilities Planning Co uncil, 1739
NYS Office Of Children & Family Services, 4578

O

O'Net: Department of Labor's Occ. Information, 2824
Oak Hill Center, 4030, 4040
The Oak Hill Center for Individual/Family Support, 4030
The Oak Hill Cntr For Individual & Family Supports, 4018
Oakstone Business Publishing, 2397
Oakwood School, 3844, 4281
Oberlin College, 3560
Occupational Aptitude Survey and Interest Schedule, 4364
Occupational Outlook Quarterly, 2886
Ocean County College, 3331
Oconee Adult Education, 2252
Oconomowoc Developmental Training Center, 3943
Octameron Associates, 3015
Odyssey School, 3234, 3770
Office Disabilities Services, 3371
Office For Civil Rights, 1684
Office For Special Needs, 3932
Office For The Deaf And Hearing Impaired, 4484
Office Of Vocational Rehabilitation, 4550
Office for Civil Rights: US Department of Health and Human Services, 1460
Office for Civil Rights: US Department of Education, 1461
Office for Disability Services, 3115, 3663
Office for Students with Disabilities, 3395
Office for Students with Special Needs & Disab, 3471
Office of Academic Disability Support, 3835
Office of Accessibility Services, 3289
Office of Adult Basic Education, 1871
Office of Adult Basic and Literacy Educati on, 1690
Office of Adult Education, 1603
Office of Adult Education and Literacy, 1858, 1859, 1860
Office of Aviation Enforcement and Proceedings, 2354
Office of Civil Rights, 1526
Office of Civil Rights: California, 1516
Office of Civil Rights: District of Columb ia, 1552
Office of Civil Rights: Georgia, 1562
Office of Civil Rights: Illinois, 1592
Office of Civil Rights: Massachusetts, 1653
Office of Civil Rights: Missouri, 1682
Office of Civil Rights: New York, 1743
Office of Civil Rights: Ohio, 1766
Office of Civil Rights: Pennsylvania, 1793
Office of Civil Rights: Texas, 1832
Office of Curriculum & Instructional Suppo rt, 1744, 4579
Office of Developmental Services, 3042
Office of Differing Disabilities, 3316
Office of Disabilities Services, 3314, 3833
Office of Disability, 3218
Office of Disability Accommodation, 3798
Office of Disability Employment Policy: US Department of Labor, 1462

Boldface indicates Publisher

S

Special Education Day School Program, 4003
Special Education Department, 3382, 3507, 3651
Special Education Law Update, 2409
Special Education Program, 3052, 4190
Special Education Resource Center, 1082, 2390, 2396, 2400, 2403, 2404, 2406, 4457
Special Education Resources on the Internet, 2833
Special Education Services, 3342, 3574
Special Education and Related Services: Communicating Through Letterwriting, 2605
Special Education in Juvenile Corrections, 2410
Special Law for Special People, 2411
Special Needs Program, 673
Special Needs Project, 1084, 2379, 2384, 2413, 2443, 2470, 2486, 2487, 2545, 2853
Special Populations Department, 3757
Special Populations Office, 3763
Special Programs and Services, 3098, 3345
Special Services, 3343
Special Services Department, 3448, 3958
Special Services Office, 3425, 3426, 3744
Special Services Program, 3941
Special Student Services, 3528
Specialized Language Development Center, 4152
Specialized Program Individualizing Reading Excellence (SPIRE), 822
Spectral Speech Analysis: Software, 1397
Speech Bin, 1133, 1397, 4395, 4401, 4402, 4405, 4410, 4412, 4413, 4419, 4423, 4428, 4431
Speech Bin Abilitations, 1347
Speech Pathology and Audiology, 3920
Speech Therapy: Look Who's Not Talking, 2793
Speech and Language Development Center, 4004
Speed Drills for Arithmetic Facts, 739
Spell-a-Word, 1183
Spellagraph, 1184
Spelling Ace, 1185
Spelling Mastery, 1186
Spelling Workbook Video, 2722
Spelling: A Thematic Content-Area Approach, 648
Spider Ball, 943
Splish Splash Math, 740, 1283
Spokane Community College, 3895
Spokane Falls Community College, 3896
Springall Academy, 3107
Springall Program, 3107
Springer School and Center, 4227
Springfield Technical Community College, 3263
Squidgie Flying Disc, 944
SRA Order Services, 1115, 1121, 1122, 1125, 1131, 1132, 1141, 1151, 1158, 1159, 1189, 1198, 1199, 1200, 1203, 1211, 1232, 1245, 1246, 1247, 1248
SRA/McGraw-Hill, 1186
SSRS: Social Skills Rating System, 4322
St Andrews Presbyterian College, 3502
St Louis Community College: Forest Park, 3294
St Louis Community College: Meramec, 3295
St Louis Public Schools Adult Education and Literacy, 2146
St. Alphonsus, 3897
St. Bonaventure University, 3441
St. Christopher Academy, 4288
St. Cloud State University, 3284
St. Columbus Episcopal Church, 4155
St. Edwards University, 3782
St. Francis School, 3169
St. Gregory's University, 3596
St. James Cathedral, 2320
St. James ESL Program, 2320
St. John's ESL Program, 1955
St. John's University, Learning Styles Network, 2728
St. Joseph College, 3134
St. Lawrence University, 3442
St. Louis Learning Disabilities Association, 238
St. Martin's Press, 402
St. Mary's University of San Antonio, 3783
St. Matthew's, 3898
St. Norbert College, 3945
St. Thomas Aquinas College Pathways, 3443, 4207
St. Thomas School, 3899

St. Vincent's Medical Center, 4033
St. Vincent's Special Needs Center, 4033
Stanbridge Academy, 3108
Standardized Reading Inventory, 4378
Standing Rock College, 3525
Stanley Sticker Stories, 1187
Star Center, 1107
Star Program, 3410
Star, Lighting The Way, 4022
Starbridge, 271
Starpoint School, 4264
Start to Finish: Developmentally Sequenced Fine Motor Activities for Preschool Children, 874
StartWrite, 979
StartWrite Handwriting Software, 1416
Starting Comprehension, 823
Starting Out Right: A Guide to Promoting Children's Reading Success, 3009
Startly Technologies, 1071
State Capital, 15th Floor, 4581
State Department of Adult Basic Education, 1671
State Department of Adult Education, 1658, 1663, 1675, 1710, 1727, 1735, 1757, 1779, 1807, 1814
State Department of Education, 1529, 1564, 1602, 1632, 1646, 1676, 1698, 1711, 1772, 1799, 1826, 1859, 1877, 1892, 1749, 1773, 1780, 1876, 1893, 4610
State Department of Education & Early Development, 1479
State Department of Education: Division of Career Technology & Adult Learning-Vocational Rehab, 1721
State Department of Education: Special Education, 1578
State Education Resources Center of Connecticut, 164
State GED Administration, 1502, 1539, 1603, 1633, 1664, 1749, 1773, 1780, 1800, 1815, 1824, 1827, 1834, 1860, 1878, 1883, 1893
State GED Administration: Delaware, 1547
State GED Administration: GED Testing Program, 1480
State GED Administration: Georgia, 1565
State GED Administration: Hawaii, 1570
State GED Administration: Nebraska, 1699
State GED Administration: Office of Specialized Populations, 1728
State Literacy Resource Center, 1620
State Of Hawaii, Department Of Human Services, 4522
State Of Idaho Department Of Labor, 4525
State Of Idaho Department of Labor, 4523
State Resource Sheet, 2606
State University of New York, 2190, 3422, 3445
State University of New York College Technology at Delhi, 3444
State University of New York College at Brockport, 3445
State University of New York College of Agriculture and Technology, 3446
State University of New York Systems, 3399
State University of New York: Albany, 3447
State University of New York: Buffalo, 3448
State University of New York: Geneseo College, 3449
State University of New York: Oswego, 3450
State University of New York: Plattsburgh, 3451
State University of New York: Potsdam, 3452
State Vocational Rehabilitation Agency, 4473, 4526, 4536, 4540, 4542, 4544, 4546, 4552, 4558, 4569, 4586, 4599, 4600, 4605
State Vocational Rehabilitation Agency of Arkansas, 4485
State Vocational Rehabilitation Agency: Washington Division of Vocational Rehabilitation, 4549, 4561, 4587, 4618
State Vocational Rehabilitation Agency: Pennsylvania, 4591
State Vocational Rehabilitation Agency: Rhode Island, 4593
State of Alaska, 1479
State of Connecticut Board of Education & Services for the Blind, 1540

State of Connecticut Dept of Children & Families, 4043
State of Delaware Adult and Community Education Network, 1995
State of New Mexico Division of Vocational Rehabilitation, 4577
State of Vermont Department of Education: Adult Education and Literacy, 4611
State of Washington, Division of Vocational Rehabilitation, 4619
Statewide Parent Advocacy Network, 4176
Statutes, Regulations and Case Law, 2412
Steck-Vaughn Company, 1369, 4375, 4377
Stellar Academy for Dyslexics, 3109
STEP/Teen: Systematic Training for Effective Parenting of Teens, 2792
Stephen F Austin State University, 3784
Stephen Gaynor School, 4208
Stepwise Cookbooks, 674
Stern Center for Language and Learning, 4269, 1376, 2709, 2711, 2718, 2724
Sterne School, 3110
Steuben County Literacy Coalition, 2056
Stevens Point Area YMCA, 612
Stickybear Software, 1226, 1374
Stimulant Drugs and ADHD Basic and Clinical Neuroscience, 427
Stockdale Learning Center, 4005
STOMP Specialized Training for Military Parents, 4287
Stone Mountain School, 3503
Stone Soup, The Magazine by Young Writers & Artists, 2622
Stony Brook University, 3453
Stop, Relax and Think, 875
Stop, Relax and Think Ball, 876
Stop, Relax and Think Card Game, 877
Stop, Relax and Think Scriptbook, 878
Stop, Relax and Think Workbook, 879
Stories Behind Special Education Case Law, 2413
Stories and More: Animal Friends, 824
Stories and More: Time and Place, 649, 825
Stories from Somerville, 826
Story of the USA, 900
Stowell Learning Center, 4006
Strangest Song: One Father's Quest to Help His Daughter Find Her Voice, 2974
Strategic Planning and Leadership, 2723
Strategies for Problem-Solving, 675, 741
Strategies for Success in Mathematics, 742
Strategies for Success in Writing, 980
Strategy Challenges Collection: 1, 1321
Strategy Challenges Collection: 2, 1322
Stratford Friends School, 3670, 4241
String A Long Lacing Kit, 945
Strong Center for Developmental Disabilities, 279
Structured Monitoring Program, 3430
Student Academic Services, 3393
Student Academic Support Services, 3232
Student Accessibility Services, 3301
Student Affairs Office, 3578
Student Development Services, 3697
Student Directed Learning: Teaching Self Determination Skills, 2794
Student Disabilities Department, 3716
Student Disabilities Services, 3913
Student Disability Services, 3284, 3104, 3285, 3378, 3914
Student Enrichment Center, 3492
Student Services, 3372, 3694
Student Services Office, 3474, 3743, 3819
Student Success Program, 3184
Student Support Program (SPARK), 3054
Student Support Services, 3451, 3461, 3511, 3512, 3519, 3748, 3944
Student Support Services Program, 3415
A Student's Guide to Jobs, 2571
A Student's Guide to the IEP, 2572
Students with Disabilities Office, 3270
Students with Disabilities and Special Education, 2414
Study Abroad, 1442
Study Skills Web Site, 2841

Study Skills: A Landmark School Student Gu ide, 2385

Study Skills: A Landmark School Teaching G uide, 2541

Study Skills: How to Manage Your Time, 2795

Stuttering Foundation of America, 108, 2542, 2588

Stuttering Severity Instrument for Childre n and Adults, 4409

Stuttering and Your Child: Questions and A nswers, 2542

A Subsidiary of Visiting Nurse Association, 241

Substance Use Among Children and Adolescen ts, 2543

Succeeding in the Workplace, 4459

Success in Mind, 283

Success with Struggling Readers: The Bench mark School Approach, 2544

Successful Movement Challenges, 880

Suffolk County Community College: Ammerman, 3454

Suffolk County Community College: Eastern Campus, 3455

Suffolk County Community College: Western Campus, 3456

Sullivan County Community College, 3457

Summer Camp Program, 4063

Summer Camps for Children with Disabilitie s, 457

Summer Day Programs, 483

Summer Matters, 3671

Summer PLUS Program, 611

Summer Reading Camp at Reid Ranch, 610

Summer@Carroll, 537

Summit Camp, 561

Summit Camp & Travel Programs, 561

Summit School, 3235

Summit School, Inc., 4098

Summit View School, 3111

Summit View School: Los Angeles, 3112

Sunbuddy Math Playhouse, 743

Sunbuddy Writer, 981, 1401

Sunburst, 1348

Sunburst Technology, 615, 617, 619, 624, 626, 632, 636, 639, 640, 650, 686, 688, 691, 692, 693, 694, 695, 696, 698, 699, 701

Sunburst Visual Media, 2658

Sunken Treasure Adventure: Beginning Blend s, 650, 1188

SUNY (State University of New York) Systems, 3388

SUNY Buffalo Office of International Education, 1440

SUNY Canton, 3434

SUNY Cobleskill, 3435

SUNY Institute of Technology: Utica/Rome, 3436

Super Study Wheel: Homework Helper, 907

Support Options for Achievement and Retention, 3491

Support Services, 3817

Support Services for Students, 3826

Support Services for Students with Learning Disab, 3660

Supporting Children with Communication Difficulties In Inclusive Settings, 2545

Supportive Learning Services Program, 3239

Surry Community College, 3504

Survey of Teenage Readiness and Neurodevel opmental Status, 676

Survival Guide for Kids with ADD or ADHD, 2565

Survival Guide for Kids with LD Learning D ifferences, 2566

Survival Guide for Teenagers with LD Learn ing Differences, 2567

Susan Maynard Counseling, 4064

SUWS Wilderness Program, 497

SVE & Churchill Media, 1202, 1215

Swallow Right 2nd Edition, 677

Sweetwater State Literacy Regional Resourc e Center, 1971

Switch Accessible Trackball, 1073

Switch to Turn Kids On, 1086

Switzer Learning Center, 4007

Syllasearch I, II, III, IV, 1189

Syracuse Univ./Facilitated Communication Institute, 2766

Syracuse University, 3458

Syracuse University, Institute on Communication, 2767

T

Tactics for Improving Parenting Skills (TIPS), 2546

Take Me Home Pair-It Books, 827

Take Part Art, 2975

Taking Your Camera To...Steadwell, 828

Tales from the Workplace, 4460

Talisman Camps & Programs, 586, 584

Talisman Summer Camp, 587

Talking Fingers, 1176, 1368

Talking Fingers, California Neuropsych Services, 1415

Talking Nouns II: Sterling Edition, 1190

Talking Nouns: Sterling Edition, 1191

Talking Verbs Sterling Edition, 1192

Talking Walls, 844, 1385

Talking Walls Bundle, 901

Talking Walls: The Stories Continue, 845, 1386

Tampa Bay Academy, 3155

Tampa Day School, 3156, 4061, 4063

Target Spelling, 678

Tarleton State University, 3785

Tarrant County College, 3786

TASH Annual Conference Social Justice in the 21st Century, 1042

Taylor Associated Communications, 1079

Taylor Publishing, 367, 368, 369, 370, 384, 2347, 4445

TDLWFD/Adult Education, 1827

Teach Me Language, 2547

Teacher Support Software, 1408, 1409

Teachers Ask About Sensory Integration, 2976

Teachers of English to Speakers of Other Languages, 2641, 2642, 2643

Teaching & Learning Center, 3441

Teaching Adults with Learning Disabilities, 2724

Teaching Comprehension: Strategies for Sto ries, 829

Teaching Developmentally Disabled Children, 2548

Teaching Dressing Skills: Buttons, Bows and More, 679

Teaching Exceptional Children, 2888

Teaching Gifted Kids in the Regular Classroom CD-ROM, 2977

Teaching Gifted Kids in the Regular Classr oom, 2978

Teaching Kids with Mental Health and Learn ing Disorders in the Regular Classroom, 881

Teaching Language Deficient Children: Theory and Application of the Association Method, 2993

Teaching Math, 2725

Teaching Math Workshop, 1043

Teaching Mathematics to Students with Learning Disabilities, 2998

Teaching People with Developmental Disabilities, 2726

Teaching Phonics: Staff Development Book, 651

Teaching Reading Workshop, 1044

Teaching Reading to Children with Down Syn drome, 2549

Teaching Reading to Disabled and Handicapp ed Learners, 3010

Teaching Research Institute, 4590

Teaching Spelling Workshop, 1045

Teaching Strategies, 2715, 2932

Teaching Strategies Library: Research Based Strategies for Teachers, 2727

Teaching Students Through Their Individual Learning Styles, 2728

Teaching Students Ways to Remember: Strategies for Learning Mnemonically, 2979

Teaching Students with Learning and Behavior Problems, 2914

Teaching Test Taking Skills, 4366

Teaching Visually Impaired Children, 3rd E d., 2980

Teaching of Reading: A Continuum from Kindergarten through College, 2550

Teaching the Dyslexic Child, 2551

Team of Advocates for Special Kids, 4008

Team of Advocates for Special Kids (TASK), 109

Tech-Able, 1108

Technical Assistance Alliance for Parent C enters: PACER Center, 233

Technical College System of Georgia, 1560

Technical College of Lowcountry: Beaufort, 3708

Technology & Persons with Disabilities Con ference, 1046

Technology Access Center, 1109

Technology Access Foundation, 1110

Technology Assistance for Special Consumers, 1111

Technology Utilization Program, 1112

Technology and Media Division, 110

Technology for Language and Learning, 1113, 1140, 1146, 1150, 1152, 1161, 1297

Technology, Curriculum, and Professional Development, 2415

Teddy Barrels of Fun, 1131

Teddy Bear Press, 2700, 789, 790, 819, 820, 2366, 2370, 2371, 2373, 2380, 2383, 2387, 2563

Teenage Switch Progressions, 1227

TeleSensory, 1228, 1059, 1078

Telling Tales, 2729

Temeron Books, 385, 394, 2982

Temple University, 3672

Ten Tricky Tiles, 744

Tennessee Council on Developmental Disabil ities, 1828

Tennessee Department Of Human Services, 4603

Tennessee Department of Education, 2270, 4601

Tennessee Department of Human Services, 4600

Tennessee Department of Labor & Workforce Development: Office of Adult Education, 4602

Tennessee School-to-Work Office, 2271

Tennessee Services for the Blind, 4603

Tennessee State University, 3735

Tennessee Technology Access Project, 1829

Tenth Planet Roots, Prefixes & Suffixes, 1375

Tenth Planet: Combining & Breaking Apart Numbers, 1284

Tenth Planet: Combining and Breaking Apart Numbers, 745

Tenth Planet: Comparing with Ratios, 746, 1285

Tenth Planet: Equivalent Fractions, 747, 1286

Tenth Planet: Fraction Operations, 748, 1287

Tenth Planet: Grouping and Place Value, 749

Tenth Planet: Roots, Suffixes, Prefixes, 830

TERC, 1378

Terra State Community College, 3574

TESOL Journal, 2641

TESOL Newsletter, 2642

TESOL Quarterly, 2643

Test Practice Success: American History, 902

Test for Auditory Comprehension of Language: TACL-3, 4410

Test of Adolescent & Adult Language: TOAL- 3, 4411

Test of Auditory Reasoning & Processing Skills: TARPS, 4412

Test of Auditory-Perceptual Skills: Upper TAPS-UL, 4413

Test of Early Language Development, 652, 4414

Test of Early Language Development: TELD-3, 4415

Test of Early Reading Ability, 4379

Test of Early Written Language, 4416

Test of Gross Motor Development, 4434

Test of Information Processing Skills, 4435

Test of Mathematical Abilities, 4357

Test of Memory and Learning (TOMAL), 4346

Test of Nonverbal Intelligence (TONI-3), 4347

Test of Reading Comprehension, 4380

Test of Written Language: TOWL-3, 4417

Test of Written Spelling, 4418

Testing & Remediating Auditory Processing (TRAP), 4419

U

University of South Carolina: Beaufort, 3713
University of South Carolina: Lancaster, 3714
University of Southern Mississippi, 3288
University of St Thomas, 1665, 2136, 2137
University of Tennessee, 3737, 2261
University of Tennessee: Knoxville, 3738
University of Tennessee: Martin, 3739
University of Texas at Dallas, 3799
University of Texas: Pan American, 3800
University of Toledo, 3577
University of Utah, 3811
University of Vermont, 3824, 4314
University of Virginia, 3858
University of Washington Disability Resources for
     Students, 3902
University of Washington: Center on Human
     Development and Disability, 3903
University of Wisconsin Center: Marshfield Wood
     County, 3946
University of Wisconsin-Madison, 3947, 2826
University of Wisconsin: Eau Claire, 3948
University of Wisconsin: La Crosse, 3949
University of Wisconsin: Madison, 3950
University of Wisconsin: Milwaukee, 3951
University of Wisconsin: Oshkosh, 3952
University of Wisconsin: Platteville, 3953
University of Wisconsin: River Falls, 3954
University of Wisconsin: Whitewater, 3955
University of Wyoming, 3964
University of the Arts, 3679
University of the Incarnate Word, 3801
University of the Ozarks, 3053
Up and Running, 1077
Updown Chair, 883
Upward Foundation, 3052
Urbana University, 3578
Ursinus College, 3680
US Autism & Asperger Association, 113
US Bureau of the Census, 1467
US Department Health & Human Services, 1656
U.S. Department Of Education, 2000
U.S. Department of Education, 1049
US Department of Education, 1450, 1457, 1465,
     1516, 1517, 1552, 1562, 1592, 1653, 1682,
     1743, 1766, 1793, 1832, 1867, 1923
**U S Department of Education/Special Ed-Rehab
     Srvcs**, 407
US Department of Education: Office for Civil
     Rights, 114
U.S. Department of Education: Office of
     Vocational & Adult Education, 4444
US Department of Health & Human Services,
     1468, 1594, 1798, 1868
U.S. Department of Health & Human Services
     Administration on Developmental Disabilities,
     364
US Department of Justice, 1446, 1447
US Department of Justice: Disabilities Rig hts
     Section, 2417
US Department of Justice: Disability Right s
     Section, 2418
US Department of Labor, 1528, 1595, 1654,
     1866, 2886
US Government Printing Office, 2640
USDE National Institution on Disability/Rehab,
     1445
Utah Antidiscrimination and Labor Division, 1846
Utah Developmental Disabilities Council, 1847
Utah Labor Commission, 1846
Utah Literacy Action Center, 2289
Utah Parent Center, 4268
Utah State Office of Education, 1848, 4608
Utah State Office of Rehabilitation, 4609
Utah State University, 3812, 360, 1843
Utah Valley State College, 3813
Utica College, 3463

V

Valencia County Literacy Council, 2185
Valentine Bear, 2387
Valley Forge Educational Services, 3681
Valley Oaks School: Turlock, 3117

Valley-Shore YMCA, 485
Van Buren County Literacy Council, 1957
Van Cleve Program, 3464
Vanderbilt University, 3740
The Vanguard School, 3157
Vanguard School, 3682, 4065, 4243
Variety School of Hawaii, 4079
Vassar College, 3465
Ventura College, 3118
Verbal Images Press, 2367
Vermont Assistive Technology Project: Dept of
     Aging and Disabilities, 2293
Vermont Department of Children & Families, 1849
Vermont Department of Education, 1850, 1855
Vermont Department of Labor, 1851
Vermont Dept of Employment & Training, 4612
Vermont Developmental Disabilities Council, 1852
Vermont Division of Vocational Rehabilitation,
     2294, 4613
Vermont Family Network, 4614
Vermont Governor's Office, 1853
Vermont Literacy Resource Center: Dept of
     Education, 2295
Vermont Protection & Advocacy, 334
Vermont Protection and Advocacy Agency, 1854
Vermont Special Education, 1855
Vermont Technical College, 3825
Via West, 474
Victoria Adult Literacy, 2285
Victory Junction Gang Camp, 588
Victory School, 3158
Villa Maria Education Center, 4039
Villa Maria School, 4039
Virginia Adult Learning Resource Center, 2312
Virginia Board for People with Disabilitie s, 1861
Virginia Commonwealth University, 3859
Virginia Council of Administrators of Spec ial
     Education, 2313
Virginia Department of Education, 1858, 4616
Virginia Department of Rehabilitative Services,
     4617
Virginia Highlands Community College, 3860
Virginia Intermont College, 3861
Virginia Literacy Foundation, 2314
Virginia Office for Protection & Advocacy
     Agency, 1862
Virginia Polytechnic Institute and State University,
     3862
Virginia Wesleyan College, 3863
Virginia Western Community College, 3864
Virtual Labs: Electricity, 850
VisagraphIII Eye-Movement Recording System &
     Reading Plus, 1079
Vision Care Clinic, 4012
Vision Literacy of California, 1972
Vision, Perception and Cognition: Manual for
     Evaluation & Treatment, 4348
VISTA, 1078
VISTA Vocational & Life Skills Center, 4038
Visual Perception and Attention Workbook, 2388
Visual Skills Appraisal, 4436
Visualizing and Verbalizing for Language
     Comprehension and Thinking, 2994
VITA (Volunteer Instructors Teaching Adult s),
     2087
Viterbo University, 3956
VocRehab Of Vermont, 2294, 4613, 4615
VocRehab Reach-Up Program, 4615
Vocabulary Connections, 653
Vocational Center for People who are Blind or
     Visually Impaired, 4040
Vocational Independence Program (VIP), 4211
Vocational Rehabilitation, 1700, 4583
Vocational Rehabilitation Services, 4521, 4532
Vocational Rehabilitation and Services For The
     Blind Division (VRSBD), 4522
Vocational Skills Program, 3177
Vocational Training and Employment of Autistic
     Adolescents, 4462
Vocational and Life Skills Center, 3137
Voice Assessment Protocol for Children and
     Adults, 4420
Volta Voices, 2613

Volunteers for Literacy of Habersham Count y,
     2020
Voorhees College, 3715
Vowel Patterns, 1197
Vowels: Short & Long, 832

W

W Virginia Regional Education Services, 2323
WA State Board for Community and Technical
     Colleges, 1869
Wadsworth Publishing Company, 2705
Wagner College, 3466
Waisman Center, 3947
Wake Forest University, 3509
Wake Technical Community College, 3510
Walbridge School, 3957
Walla Walla Community College, 3904
Wallace Community College Selma, 3044
Walsh University, 3579
Walworth County Literacy Council, 2337
Wardlaw School, 3171, 4076
Warner Pacific College, 3617
Wartburg College, 3207
Washington Department Of Mental Health,
     4049
Washington Human Rights Commission, 1870
Washington Literacy Council, 2001
Washington PAVE: Specialized Training of
     Military Parents (STOMP), 115
Washington Parent Training Project: PAVE, 341
Washington State Board for Community and T
     echnical Colleges, 1871
Washington State Client Assistance Program, 1872
Washington State Community College, 3580
Washington State Developmental Disabilitie s
     Council, 1873
Washington State Governor's Committee on D
     isability Issues & Employment, 1874
Washington State University, 3905
Washington and Jefferson College, 3683
Waterford Country Schools, 4041
Waukesha County Technical College, 3958
Wayne State University Press, 654, 655, 685, 770
Web MD Health, 453, 2843
Weber State University, 3814
Weslaco Public Library, 2286
West Virginia Adult Basic Education, 1879
West Virginia Advocates, 1875
West Virginia Assistive Technology System, 1880
West Virginia Department of Education, 2324,
     1879
**West Virginia Department of Education & the
     Arts**, 4620
West Virginia Division of Rehabilitation Services,
     4620
West Virginia Northern Community College, 3918
West Virginia State College, 3919
West Virginia University, 3920, 4442
West Virginia University at Parkersburg, 3921
West Virginia Wesleyan College, 3922
Westchester Community College, 3467
Westchester Institute for Human Developmen t,
     280
Westchester Medical Center, 280
Western Carolina University, 3511
Western Illinois University: Macomb Projects,
     1085, 1086, 2775
Western Iowa Tech Community College, 2065
Western Montana College, 3297
Western New Mexico University, 3357
Western Oregon University, 3618
Western Psychological Services, 1334
Western Washington University, 3906
Western Wisconsin Technical College, 3959
Westmark School, 3119
Westminster College of Salt Lake City, 3815
Westmoreland County Community College, 3684
Westview School, 3120
**WETA-TV, Department of Educational
     Activities**, 2791
Wharton County Junior College, 3802

Boldface indicates Publisher

X

Y

Z

ADD/ADHD

Churchill Center & School for Learning Disabilities, 4156
Cincinnati Center for Developmental Disorders, 4221
Commonwealth Learning Center, 4128
Cotting School, 3247, 4129
Crisman School, 4257
DBTAC: Northeast ADA Center, 1736
Designs for Learning Differences Sycamore School, 4183
Developmental Disabilities Resource Center, 4013
EAC Nassau Learning Center, 4191
The Early Achievement Center, 4100
Educational Options, 4131
Evergreen Center, 3251, 4132
F.L. Chamberlain School, 4133
Focus Alternative Learning Center, 4020
The Forbush School at Glyndon, 4122
The Foundation School, 4035
Founder's Cottage, 4022
Frost Center, 4115
Frostig Center, 3084, 3985
Gateway School, 4258
Gillis Center, 4157
Hampshire Country School, 3302, 4164
Havern School, 3122, 4014
Heritage School, 4155
Hillside School, 3253, 4236
The Howard School, 4075
Huntington Learning Centers, Inc., 4172, 4298
Institute for the Redesign of Learning, 3087, 3988
Jacob's Ladder Neurodevelopmental School & Therapy Center, 4072
Karafin School, 4197
KidsPeace Orchard Hills Campus, 4237
League School of Greater Boston, 4137
Leary School Programs, 4277
Living with a Learning Disability, 2511
Mary McDowell Friends School, 4200
Matheny Medical and Educational Center, 4173
Meredith-Dunn School, 4107
The Midland School, 4181
Mill Springs Academy, 3167, 4073
Morning Star School, 3152, 4059
Natchaug Hospital School Program, 4028
New Community School, 3840, 4279
New Vistas School, 4280
New York Institute for Special Education, 4202
Newgrange School, 4174
Newport Audiology Center, 3993
The Norman Howard School, 4210
Office of Disability Employment Policy: US Department of Labor, 1462
Overton Speech & Language Center, Inc., 4259
Parish School, 4260
Paul Robeson School, 4049
The Perkins Day Treatment Program, 4148
Pine Hill School, 3996
Professional Assistance Center for Education (PACE), 4095
Readiness Program, 3427
Reading Success Plus, Inc., 4074
Reid School, 4266
Renaissance Learning Center, 4062
Ridge School of Montgomery County, 4121
Riley Child Development Center, 4306
Riverbrook Residence, 4142
Riverside School, 3851, 4282
Riverview School, 3261, 4143
Robert Louis Stevenson School, 4206
Saint Francis Home for Children: Highland, 4032
Schermerhorn Program, 3439
Sequel TSI, 3967
Special Education Day School Program, 4003
Starpoint School, 4264
Stratford Friends School, 3670, 4241
Summit School, Inc., 4098
Susan Maynard Counseling, 4064
Thomas A Edison High School, 4229
Trident Academy, 3709, 4248
VISTA Vocational & Life Skills Center, 4038
Van Cleve Program, 3464
Vision Care Clinic, 4012
Wilderness School, 4043

Willow Hill School, 3266, 4149
Windward School, 4212

Creative Expression

Affect and Creativity, 2898
Author's Toolkit, 953, 1404
Basic Skills Products, 1137, 1237
Create with Garfield, 1121
Create with Garfield: Deluxe Edition, 1122
Easybook Deluxe Writing Workshop: Immigration, 892, 962
Easybook Deluxe Writing Workshop: Rainforest & Astronomy, 893, 963
Once Upon a Time Volume I: Passport to Discovery, 1411
Painting the Joy of the Soul, 2357

Crisis Intervention

American Red Cross (National Headquarters), 13

Critical Thinking

Read and Solve Math Problems #3, 1280

Curriculum Guides

Print Module, 1342
Springer School and Center, 4227
Teaching Students with Learning and Behavior Problems, 2914

Daily Living

ABC's of Learning Disabilities, 2735
Aids and Appliances for Independent Living, 658
Aphasia Diagnostic Profiles, 4384
BRIGANCE Life Skills Inventory, 4388
Calendar Fun with Lollipop Dragon, 1202
A Calendar of Home Activities, 4381
Disabled Faculty and Staff in a Disabling Society: Multiple Identities in Higher Education, 3019
District of Columbia Department of Education: Vocational & Adult Education, 4509
District of Columbia Public Schools, 1998
Get Ready to Read!, 2644
Imagination Express Destination: Neighborhood, 1391
Imagination Express Destination: Pyramids, 1393
LD Advocate, 2645
LD News, 2646
Literacy Volunteers of the National Capital Area, 1999
Math Spending and Saving, 1218
Math for Everyday Living, 1265
Money Skills, 1219
Our World, 2647
Special Needs Program, 673
Succeeding in the Workplace, 4459
Travel the World with Timmy Deluxe, 684
U.S. Department Of Education, 2000
Upward Foundation, 3052
World Class Learning Materials, 1288
Zap! Around Town, 750, 1289

Databases

Dialog Information Services, 1098

Developmental Disabilities

Adirondack Leadership Expeditions, 563
Alabama Council for Developmental Disabilities, 1469
Birth Defect Research for Children (BDRC), 23
Body and Physical Difference: Discourses of Disability, 2927
California Association of Private Special Education Schools, 135
California Association of Special Education & Services, 1959

Camp ASCCA, 458
Camp Akeela, 564
Camp Bari Tov, 565
Camp Buckskin, 547
Camp Kavod, 490
Camp Lee Mar, 608
Camp Northwood, 570
Camp Sky Ranch, 583
Center for Disabilities and Development, 199
Charis Hills, 609
Client Assistance Program (CAP): New Mexico Protection and Advocacy System, 1729
Colorado Developmental Disabilities, 1523
Defects: Engendering the Modern Body, 2936
Developmental Disabilities Council, 1637
Developmental Variation and Learning Disorders, 2937
Division for Early Childhood of CEC, 42
EBL Coaching Summer Programs, 574
Easter Seals - New York, 267
Easter Seals - Southwestern Idiana, 196
FAT City, 2764
Frames of Reference for the Assessment of Learning Disabilities, 2946
Gainesville Hall County Alliance for Literacy, 2010
Illinois Council on Developmental Disabilities, 1585
Institutes for the Achievement of Human Potential (IAHP), 57
International Dyslexia Association Southwest Branch, 262
LDA Life and Learning Services, 271
LDA Minnesota Learning Disability Association, 2133
LDAT Annual State Conference, 1028
Landmark School Summer Boarding Program, 530
Learning Disabilities A to Z, 2503
Learning Disabilities Association, 1831
Learning Disabilities Association of Alabama, 124
Learning Disabilities Association of America (LDAA), 63
Learning Disabilities Association of Arkansas (LDAA), 133
Learning Disabilities Association of California, 148
Learning Disabilities Association of Colorado, 154
Learning Disabilities Association of Cuyahoga County, 300
Learning Disabilities Association of Florida, 173, 2008
Learning Disabilities Association of Iowa, 202, 1610, 2062
Learning Disabilities Association of Kansas, 206
Learning Disabilities Association of Kentucky, 1627
Learning Disabilities Association of Maine (LDA), 212
Learning Disabilities Association of Missouri, 236
Learning Disabilities Association of New Mexico: Albuquerque, 263
Learning Disabilities Association of New Mexico: Las Cruces, 264
Learning Disabilities Association of New York City, 275
Learning Disabilities Association of Oklahoma, 302
Learning Disabilities Association of Oregon, 305
Learning Disabilities Association of Pennsylvania, 314, 2235
Learning Disabilities Association of Texas, 330
Learning Disabilities Association of Washington, 340
Learning Disabilities Association of Western New York, 276
Learning Disabilities Worldwide (LDW), 226
Learning Disabilities: Theories, Diagnosis and Teaching Strategies, 2506
Lily Videos : A Longitudinel View of Lily with Down Syndrome, 2783
Living Independently Forever, Inc., 4139
Maryland Developmental Disabilities Council, 1644

Directories

Discrimination

Dispute Resolution Dyslexia

Dyscalculia

Dyslexia

ESL

Education

Team of Advocates for Special Kids, 4008
Technology, Curriculum, and Professional Development, 2415
Tennessee Department of Education, 2270, 4601
Tennessee Department of Labor & Workforce Development: Office of Adult Education, 4602
Tenth Planet: Combining & Breaking Apart Numbers, 1284
Tenth Planet: Combining and Breaking Apart Numbers, 745
Tenth Planet: Comparing with Ratios, 746, 1285
Tenth Planet: Equivalent Fractions, 747, 1286
Tenth Planet: Fraction Operations, 748, 1287
Tenth Planet: Grouping and Place Value, 749
Testing Students with Disabilities, 2416
Texas Education Agency, 1838
US Department of Education: Office for Civil Rights, 114
United Cerebral Palsy Of Georgia, 495
Vermont Department of Education, 1850
Villa Maria Education Center, 4039
Vocational Center for People who are Blind or Visually Impaired, 4040
West Virginia Department of Education, 2324
Wheeler Clinic, Inc., 4042
Wheeler Regional Family YMCA, 486
Wings for Kids, 4325
Write On! Plus: Elementary Writing Skills, 985

Elementary Education

Academic Drill Builders: Wiz Works, 1115
Activities for the Elementary Classroom, 656
EarobicsM® Step 1 Home Version, 781
Inclusive Elementary Schools, 2491, 2959
New Room Arrangement as a Teaching Strategy, 2715
Stories and More: Animal Friends, 824
Stories and More: Time and Place, 649, 825

Equality

Florida Advocacy Center for Persons with Disabilities, 171
Wisconsin Equal Rights Division, 1886

Ethics

Association of Educational Therapists, 16, 1898
Discipline, 2390
Ethical Principles of Psychologists and Code of Conduct, 2904
Ethical and Legal Issues in School Counseling, 2581
Ethical and Legal Issues in School Counseling, 2393
Key Concepts in Personal Development, 2496, 2713

Evaluations

Accommodations in Higher Education under the Americans with Disabilities Act (ADA), 2897
Adolescent Language Screening Test, 4382
Assessing Children for the Presence of a Disability, 2576
Assessment of Students with Handicaps in Vocational Education, 4359
Behavior Assessment System for Children, 4312
Behavior Rating Profile, 4313
Berkeley Policy Associates, 134
BRIGANCE Comprehensive Inventory of Basic Skills, 4386
BRIGANCE Inventory of Early Development-II, 4421
The Children's Home Of Cincinnati, 4228
Computer Scoring Systems for PRO-ED Tests, 4362
Culture-Free Self-Esteem Inventories, 4315
Developing Minds: Parent's Pack, 2761
Developing Minds: Teacher's Pack, 2762
Devereux Early Childhood Assessment Program Observation Journal, 4316

Devereux Early Childhood Assessment(DECA), 753
Devereux Early Childhood Assessment: Clinical Version (DECA-C), 754
Easter Seals - Bay Area, Lakeport, 138
Easter Seals - Eastern Pennsylvania, 309
Easter Seals - Nothern California, Novato, 142
Easter Seals - Southeastern Pennsylvania, 310
Easter Seals - Western & Central Pennsylvania, 311
Educational Diagnostic Center at Curry College, 4294
Georgetown University, 3142
Georgetown University Center for Child and Human Development, 4297
Gray Diagnostic Reading Tests, 4373
Gray Oral Reading Tests, 4374
HELP for Preschoolers Assessment and Curriculum Guide, 2948
HELP...at Home, 2906
Identifying Learning Problems, 2772
LAP-D Kindergarten Screen Kit, 760
Learning Accomplishment Profile (LAP-R) KIT, 762
Learning Accomplishment Profile Diagnostic Normed Assessment (LAP-D), 763
Learning Accomplishment Profile Diagnostic Normed Screens for Age 3-5, 761
Learning Disability Evaluation Scale, 4397
National Association for Child Development(NACD), 73
National Center for Fair & Open Testing FairTest, 4300
Partners for Learning (PFL), 764
Peabody Individual Achievement Test, 4340
Receptive One-Word Picture Vocabulary Test, 4402
SSRS: Social Skills Rating System, 4322
Saint Coletta: Greater Washington, 3143
Sandhills School, 4001
Scholastic Abilities Test for Adults, 4376
Skills Assessments, 4356, 4377, 4406
Standardized Reading Inventory, 4378
Test of Auditory Reasoning & Processing Skills: TARPS, 4412
Test of Auditory-Perceptual Skills: Upper TAPS-UL, 4413
Test of Early Reading Ability, 4379
Testing & Remediating Auditory Processing (TRAP), 4419
Tests, Measurement and Evaluation, 4367
Voice Assessment Protocol for Children and Adults, 4420
Your Child's Evaluation, 2610

Eye/Hand Coordination

Beads and Baubles, 910
Beads and Pattern Cards, 911
Geoboard Colored Plastic, 923
Half 'n' Half Design and Color Book, 926
Primer Pak, 937
String A Long Lacing Kit, 945
VisagraphIII Eye-Movement Recording System& Reading Plus, 1079
Windup Fishing Game, 950

Family Involvement

Children and Families, 2624
In Time and with Love, 2487
Innovations in Family Support for People with Learning Disabilities, 2492
KidDesk: Family Edition, 1338
Learning Disabilities & ADHD: A Family Guide to Living and Learning Together, 2502
Massachusetts Family Literacy Consortium, 2121
Matrix Parent Network & Resource Center, 65
A Miracle to Believe In, 2343, 2420
Misunderstood Child, 2516
NCFL Conference, 1034
National Center for Families Literacy(NCFL), 84
Parent Teacher Meeting, 2788

Parenting a Child with Special Needs: A Guide to Reading and Resources, 2593
Parents Guide, 2594
Practical Parent's Handbook on Teaching Children with Learning Disabilities, 2528
Questions and Answers About the IDEA News Digest, 2601
Raising Your Child to be Gifted: Successful Parents, 2529
School-Home Notes: Promoting Children's Classroom Success, 2971
Serving on Boards and Committees, 2604
Tactics for Improving Parenting Skills (TIPS), 2546
Texas Key, 2889
Understanding Learning Disabilities: A Parent Guide and Workbook, Third Edition, 2552
What Every Parent Should Know about Learning Disabilities, 2608
What to Expect: The Toddler Years, 2554

Family Resources

American Autism Association, 266
Easter Seals, 47
Exceptional Parent Magazine, 2629
Help Me to Help My Child, 2474
Learning Disabilities Association of New York State (LDANYS), 273
Maybe You Know My Kid: A Parent's Guide to Identifying ADHD, 415
Northeast ADA Center, 277
Parents Helping Parents, 102
Success in Mind, 2830d@MINOR HEADING = Financial Resources
Chronicle Financial Aid Guide, 3017
Kansas Department of Social and Rehabilitation Services, 1615
Parent's Guide to the Social Security Administration, 2402
Social Security Administration, 1466
Vermont Department of Children & Families, 1849

Fluency

DLM Math Fluency Program: Addition Facts, 1245
DLM Math Fluency Program: Division Facts, 1246
DLM Math Fluency Program: Multiplication Facts, 1247
DLM Math Fluency Program: Subtraction Facts, 1248
Educating Deaf Children Bilingually, 2456

Gameboards

Bozons' Quest, 1201
Curious George Preschool Learning Games, 752
Garfield Trivia Game, 1125
PCI Educational Publishing, 909

Gifted Education

CEC Today, 2866
Center on Disabilities Conference, 1014
Council for Exceptional Children, 2626
National Association for Gifted Children(NAGC), 75
State Resource Sheet, 2606
Teaching Gifted Kids in the Regular Classroom CD-ROM, 2977

Graphing

Data Explorer, 696, 1249
Graphers, 707

Health Care

America's Health Insurance Plans, 2
KDES Health Curriculum Guide, 2962
National Organization for Rare Disorders (NORD), 95

History

Hotlines

Human Services

Easter Seals Goodwill - Headquarters, 289
Employment Security Division, 1478
Employment Service Division: Alabama, 1472
Governor's Council on Developmental Disabilities,
1490, 1561, 1605
Granite State Independent Living, 1713
Hawaii State Council on Developmental
Disabilities, 1569
Human Services: Division of Vocational, 4499
Idaho Division of Vocational Rehabilitation, 1574
Idaho Human Rights Commission, 1576
Illinois Department of Human Rights, 1588
Increasing Capabilities Access Network, 1499
Indiana ATTAIN Project, 1598
Institute for Human Development: Northern
Arizona University, 129
Institute on Disability, 1714
Kansas Department of Labor, 1614
Kansas Human Rights Commission, 1616
Maine Human Rights Commission, 1638
Michigan Protection and Advocacy Service, 1662
Minnesota Department of Children, Families &
Learning, 1666
Minnesota Department of Human Rights, 1667
Minnesota Governor's Council on Developmental
Disabilities, 1668
NYS Developmental Disabilities Planning Council,
1739
Nevada Governor's Council on Developmental
Disabilities, 1708
New Hampshire Department of Health & Human
Services, 4568
New Mexico Human Rights Commission
Education Bureau, 1731
North Carolina Division of Vocational
Rehabilitation, 1753
North Dakota Association For The
Disabled(NDAD), 290
North Dakota Association for Lifelong Learning
(NDALL), 291
North Dakota Autism Center, 292
North Dakota Center for Persons with Disabllities
(NDCPD), 293
North Dakota Department of Human Services,
1759
North Dakota Department of Human Services:
Welfare & Public Assistance, 2202
North Dakota Protection & Advocacy Project, 294
Northwest Community Action Programs - Casper
(NOWCAP), 348
Northwest Community Action Programs -
Cody(NOWCAP), 349
Northwest Community Action Programs - Rock
Springs (NOWCAP), 350
Office of Human Rights: District of Columbia,
1553
Oregon Department of Human Resource Adult &
Family Services Division, 2230
Oregon Department of Human Services: Children,
Adults & Families Division, 1788
Pathfinder Services, 295
Pennsylvania Human Rights Commission, 1796
Pennsylvania's Initiative on Assistive Technology,
1797
Rhode Island Commission for Human Rights, 1803
Rhode Island Human Resource Investment
Council, 2245
ServiceLink, 1720
South Carolina Human Affairs Commission, 1813
South Dakota Advocacy Services, 1819
South Dakota Department of Labor, 4596
South Dakota Department of Social Services, 4597
South Dakota Division of Human Rights, 1822
Texas Workforce Commission: Civil Rights
Division, 1839
University of Oregon Center for Excellence in
Developmental Disabilities, 307
University of Washington: Center on Human
Development and Disability, 3903
Utah Developmental Disabilities Council, 1847
Vermont Family Network, 4614
Virginia Board for People with Disabilities, 1861
VocRehab Reach-Up Program, 4615
Washington Human Rights Commission, 1870

Inclusion

Andreas: Outcomes of Inclusion, 2745
Backyards & Butterflies: Ways to Include Children
with Disabilities, 2436
Devereux California, 3982
Devereux Mapleton, 4233
Devereux Massachusetts, 4130
Easter Seals - Central Alabama, 121
General Guidelines for Providers of Psychological
Services, 2905
Inclusion Series, 2773
Inclusion: An Essential Guide for the
Paraprofessional, 2958
Making School Inclusion Work: A Guide to
Everyday Practices, 2963
National Business and Disability Council at The
Viscardi Center, 83
National Organization on Disability (NOD), 96
Social-Emotional Dimension Scale, 4324
Southern Adventist University, 3733
Take Part Art, 2975
YACHAD/National Jewish Council for
Disabilities, 117

Infancy

New Jersey Programs for Infants and Toddlers with
Disabilities: Early Intervention System, 1725
Programs for Infants and Toddlers with
Disabilities, 1746

Information Resources

Ablenet, 1050
Army & Air Force Exchange Services, 1424
Bethany House Publishers, 2659
Center for Parent Information & Resources, 31
Charles C Thomas, Publisher, Ltd., 2663
How to Organize Your Child and Save Your
Sanity, 2481
A Human Development View of Learning
Disabilities: From Theory to Practice, 2917
Including Students with Severe and Multiple
Disabilities in Typical Classrooms, 2956
Institute for Human Centered Design (IHCD), 56
LD OnLine, 2591
Learning Company, 1340
National Bible Association, 2688
National Joint Committee on Learning Disabilities,
94
National Resources, 2591
Northwest Media, 2689
Reader's Digest Partners for Sight Foundation,
2694
Stuttering Foundation of America, 108
Sunburst, 1348
Tales from the Workplace, 4460
Thomas Nelson Publishers, 2702
Thorndike Press, 2703
Underachieving Gifted, 2607

Integration

Division on Career Development, 4440
Inclusion: 450 Strategies for Success, 2957
Michigan Department of Community Health, 1661
Regular Lives, 2791
South Dakota Council on Developmental
Disabilities, 1820

International Associations

American-Scandinavian Foundation, 1421
Andeo International Homestays, 1422
Association for Childhood Education International
(ACEI), 168
Council on International Educational Exchange,
1427
International Dyslexia Association of Austin, 326
International Dyslexia Association of Central Ohio,
297

International Dyslexia Association of DC Capital
Area, 218
International Dyslexia Association of Dallas, 327
International Dyslexia Association of Houston, 328
International Dyslexia Association of
Massachusetts, 225
International Dyslexia Association of New
Hampshire, 249
International Dyslexia Association of Northern
Ohio, 145, 298
International Dyslexia Association of Utah, 332
International Dyslexia Association of Virginia, 336
International Dyslexia Association of Western New
York, 270
International Dyslexia Association: Ohio Valley
Branch, 299
International Dyslexia Association: Tennessee
Branch, 322
International Reading Association Newspaper:
Reading Today, 408, 2634
Lisle, 1435
People to People International, 1439
SUNY Buffalo Office of International Education,
1440
Sister Cities International, 1441
World Experience, 1443

Intervention

Academic Skills Problems Workbook, 2918
Accessing Programs for Infants, Toddlers and
Preschoolers, 2574
The Baby Fold, 4099
Behavior Change in the Classroom:
Self-Management Interventions, 3013
Brief Intervention for School Problems:
Outcome-Informed Strategies, 2928
Child Who is Ignored: Module 6, 2757
Easy Talker: A Fluency Workbook for School Age
Children, 4394
Focus on Exceptional Children, 2945
Guidelines and Recommended Practices for
Individualized Family Service Plan, 2469
HELP Activity Guide, 2947
Intervention in School and Clinic, 2961
Just Kids: Early Childhood Learning Center, 4196
National Association for Community Mediation
(NAFCM), 74
National Disabilities Rights Network (NDRN), 89
Practitioner's Guide to Dynamic Assessment, 2911
When Slow Is Fast Enough: Educating the Delayed
Preschool Child, 3000

Job/Vocational Resources

Adult Education & Literacy, 4610
Alabama Department of Industrial Relations, 1470
Alaska State Commission for Human Rights, 1473
Arizona Governor's Committee on Employment of
the Handicapped, 1485
Arkansas Department of Workforce Services, 1495
BRIGANCE Employability Skills Inventory, 4387
California Department of Fair Employment and
Housing, 1503
California Employment Development Department,
1506
Career Planner's Portfolio: A School-to-Work
Assessment Tool, 4361
Colorado Department of Labor and Employment,
1522
DC Department of Employment Services, 1549
Department of Employment Services, 4508
Department of Employment, Training and
Rehabilitation, 1704
Department of Personnel & Human Services, 1864
Different Way of Learning, 2806
District of Columbia Fair Employment Practice
Agencies, 1551
Division of Family Development: New Jersey
Department of Human Services, 4571
Division on Career Development & Transition
(DCDT), 44
Easter Seal Michigan, 4545

Keyboards

Kits

Language Skills

Leadership

Legal Issues

Libraries

Listening Skills

Literacy

Tutorial Center, 2292
Twin Lakes Literacy Council, 1956
VITA (Volunteer Instructors Teaching Adults), 2087
Valencia County Literacy Council, 2185
Van Buren County Literacy Council, 1957
Victoria Adult Literacy, 2285
Virginia Adult Learning Resource Center, 2312
Volunteers for Literacy of Habersham County, 2020
W Virginia Regional Education Services, 2323
Walworth County Literacy Council, 2337
Washington Literacy Council, 2001
Washington State Board for Community and Technical Colleges, 1871
West Virginia Adult Basic Education, 1879
Western Iowa Tech Community College, 2065
Whatcom Literacy Council, 2321
Winchester Adult Education Center, 2083
Winnebago County Literacy Council, 2338
York County Literacy Council, 2238
Yuma Reading Council, 1935

Literature

Assessing the ERIC Resource Collection, 2577
Island Reading Journey, 632, 792
Journal of Social and Clinical Psychology, 2857
Kaleidoscope, Exploring the Experience of Disability Through Literature and Fine Arts, 2894
Learning Times, 411
Library Reproduction Service, 2681
Navigating College College Manual for Teaching the Portfolio, 3026
Navigating College: Strategy Manual for a Successful Voyage, 3027
PsycINFO Database, 1343
Stone Soup, The Magazine by Young Writers& Artists, 2622
Write On! Plus: Literature Studies, 989
Write On! Plus: Responding to Great Literature, 991

Logic

Anne Carlsen Center for Children, 3516, 4219
Autism and the Family: Problems, Prospects and Coping with the Disorder, 2435
Dyna Vox Technologies, 1056
Early Discoveries: Size and Logic, 1292
Freddy's Puzzling Adventures, 1306
Kayne Eras Center, 3089, 3989
Ladders to Literacy: A Kindergarten Activity Book, 2497
Ladders to Literacy: A Preschool Activity Book, 2498
Marina Psychological Services, 3990
Merit Software, 1312
Pathway School, 3658, 4240
Problem Solving, 1316
Revised Behavior Problem Checklist, 4321
School Psychology Quarterly, 2859
Summit Camp, 561
Switzer Learning Center, 4007
Teaching Students Through Their Individual Learning Styles, 2728
To Teach a Dyslexic, 2981

Mainstreaming

Ability Magazine, 4446
Associated Talmud Torahs of Chicago, 4083
Least Restrictive Environment, 2396
Mainstreaming at Camp, 578
New Jersey State Department of Education, 4574
Purposeful Integration: Inherently Equal, 2405

Matching

Early and Advanced Switch Games, 1295
Educational Advisory Group, 1907
Familiar Things, 920

Learn to Match, 1161
Multi-Scan, 1129
Sound Match, 1181

Mathematics

Access to Math, 1230
AfterMath Series, 4350
Colored Wooden Counting Cubes, 914
Concert Tour Entrepreneur, 694, 1242
ENRIGHT Computation Series, 4351
Fast-Track Fractions, 1255
Figure It Out: Thinking Like a Math Problem Solver, 4352
Fraction Fuel-Up, 1257
Get Up and Go!, 705, 1258
Getting Ready for Algebra, 4353
Hidden Treasures of Al-Jabr, 709
Hot Dog Stand: The Works, 712
Ice Cream Truck, 714, 1309
Introduction to Patterns, 716
Math and the Learning Disabled Student: A Practical Guide for Accommodations, 2997
Mirror Symmetry, 723
Penny Pot, 730
See Me Subtract, 820
Shape Up!, 736, 1281
Speed Drills for Arithmetic Facts, 739
Splish Splash Math, 740, 1283
Sunbuddy Math Playhouse, 743
Teaching Mathematics to Students with Learning Disabilities, 2998
Ten Tricky Tiles, 744
3 Steps to Math Success, 4349
2+2, 1229
Winning at Math: Your Guide to Learning Mathematics Through Successful Study Skills, 2569

Maturity

Goodenough-Harris Drawing Test, 4336

Memorization Skills

Memory Fun!, 719
Memory I, 1168
Memory Match, 1310
Memory: A First Step in Problem Solving, 1311
Sequencing Fun!, 735, 1178
Teaching Students Ways to Remember: Strategies for Learning Mnemonically, 2979
Test of Memory and Learning (TOMAL), 4346

Motivation

Dr. Peet's Picture Writer, 1405
Faking It: A Look into the Mind of a Creative Learner, 2348
From Disability to Possibility: The Powerof Inclusive Classrooms, 2349
Inclusion-Classroom Problem Solver; Structures and Supports to Serve ALL Learners, 2351
Kids Behind the Label: An Inside at ADHD for Classroom Teachers, 2352
A Mind of Your Own, 2734
Motivation to Learn: How Parents and Teachers Can Help, 2785
Rethinking the Education of Deaf Students: Theory and Practice from a Teacher's Perspective, 2358
What About Me? Strategies for Teaching Misunderstood Learners, 2361
You're Welcome: 30 Innovative Ideas for the Inclusive Classroom, 2362

Motor Development

Big Little Pegboard Set, 912
Children's Developmental Clinic, 4114
Early Screening Inventory: Revised, 756
Handbook of Adaptive Switches and Augmentative Communication Devices, 3rd Ed, 1061

Indy Reads: Indianapolis/Marion County Public Library, 2053
Magnetic Fun, 931
Mobility International (MIUSA), 1436
North Dakota Reading Association, 2204
Peabody Developmental Motor Scales-2, 4428
Preschool Motor Speech Evaluation & Intervention, 4401, 4431
Swallow Right 2nd Edition, 677
Test of Gross Motor Development, 4434
Wikki Stix, 949

Multicultural Education

Activities for a Diverse Classroom, 2426
TESOL Quarterly, 2643

Multisensory Education

Journal of Learning Disabilities, 2874
Specialized Program Individualizing Reading Excellence (SPIRE), 822

Music

Busy Box Activity Centers, 913
Camp New Hope, 550
Department of VSA and Accessibility, 37
Imagination Express Destination: Castle, 1390
Imagination Express Destination: Ocean, 1392
Thinkin' Things Collection: 3, 1323
Thinkin' Things: All Around Frippletown, 1324
Thinkin' Things: Collection 1, 1325
Thinkin' Things: Collection 2, 1326
Thinkin' Things: Sky Island Mysteries, 1327
Valley-Shore YMCA, 485
Whistle Kit, 948
Working with Visually Impaired Young Students: A Curriculum Guide for 3 to 5 Year-Olds, 2984

Neurological Disorders

May Institute, 4140
Menninger Clinic, 67
Vanguard School, 3682, 4065, 4243

Newsletters

Family Resource Associates, Inc., 255, 4169
Mountain Plains Regional Resource Center, 4265
NICHCY News Digest, 2612
New Directions, 2399

Occupational Therapy

American Journal of Occupational Therapy, 2861
American Occupational Therapy Association, 10
California Employment Development Department, 4490
Career College and Technology School Databook, 3016
Center for Speech and Language Disorders, 4085
Centreville School, 3139, 4045
Cincinnati Occupational Therapy Institute for Services and Study, Inc., 4222
Huntingdon County PRIDE, 312
Miriam School, 4159

Pathology

American Journal of Speech-Language Pathology: A Journal of Clinical Practice, 2891
Annals of Otology, Rhinology and Laryngology, 2863
ASHA Leader, 2890

Peer Programs

Best Buddies International, 22

Perception Skills

Building Perspective, 691, 1238
Building Perspective Deluxe, 692, 1239
Maze Book, 932
PAVE: Perceptual Accuracy/Visual Efficiency, 1222
Parquetry Blocks & Pattern Cards, 934
Shape and Color Sorter, 939
Shapes Within Shapes, 737
Spatial Relationships, 738, 1282

Pets

KIND News Sr: Kids in Nature's Defense, 2618
National Association for Humane and Environmental Education, 2620

Phonics

Chess with Butterflies, 772
Clues to Meaning, 774
Common Ground: Whole Language & Phonics Working Together, 2442
First Phonics, 626, 1148
Fishing with Balloons, 785
High Noon Books, 788, 2676
I Can See the ABC's, 790
Lexia Phonics Based Reading, 1164
Lexia Primary Reading, 1361
More Primary Phonics, 800
Phonemic Awareness: The Sounds of Reading, 804, 2789
Phonic Ear Auditory Trainers, 1070
Phonology and Reading Disability, 3002
Phonology: Software, 1174
Primary Phonics, 807
Python Path Phonics Word Families, 640, 1175
Reading Who? Reading You!, 814, 1371
Sentence Master: Level 1, 2, 3, 4, 1372
Simon Sounds It Out, 1373

Physical Education

Adapted Physical Education for Students with Autism, 2920
Boy Scouts of America, 24
ECLC of New Jersey, 4167
Journal of Physical Education, Recreation and Dance, 2635
Prentice School, 3100, 3997

Play Therapy

Children's Cabinet, 244
Flagship Carpets, 921
Link N' Learn Color Rings, 929
New Language of Toys, 2518

Program Planning

Adventure Learning Center at Eagle Village, 540
Calumet Camp, 556
Camp Frog Hollow, 1120
Camp Happiness, 594
Camp Joy, 518
Camp Kehilla, 569
Camp Lapham, 519
Camp Little Giant: Touch of Nature Environmental Center, 499
Camp Moore, 559
Camp Shriver, 477
Camp Sunshine-Camp Elan, 571
Camp Winnebago, 551
Eagle Hill Summer Program, 479
Easter Seals - Camp Hemlocks, 480
Groves Academy, 3279, 4153
Guide to ACA Accredited Camps, 454
Kamp A-Kom-plish, 513
The Kolburne School Summer Program, 539
The Kolburne School, Inc., 3264
Landmark Summer Program: Exploration and Recreation, 531

Landmark Summer Program: Marine Science, 532
Landmark Summer Program: Musical Theater, 533
Lesley University, 3257
Marburn Academy, 3553
Marburn Academy Summer Programs, 602
Marvelwood, 3132
Patriots' Trail Girl Scout Council Summer Camp, 536
Pilgrim Hills Camp, 603
Project LEARN of Summit County, 2213
Recreation Unlimited Farm and Fun, 604
School Vacation Camps: Youth with Developmental Disabilities, 581
Summer Day Programs, 483
Timber Trails Camps, 484
Wilderness Experience, 589

Public Awareness & Interest

Crotched Mountain, 247
NH Family Ties, 250
New Hampshire Governor's Commission on Disability, 1718
Public Agencies Fact Sheet, 2598
Vermont Governor's Office, 1853
Wisconsin Governor's Committee for People with Disabilities, 1887

Publishers

Academic Communication Associates, 2648
Academic Success Press, 2649
Academic Therapy Publications, 2650
Alexander Graham Bell Association for the Deaf and Hard of Hearing, 2652
At-Risk Youth Resources, 2658
Blackwell Publishing, 2660
Brookes Publishing Company, 2661
Brookline Books/Lumen Editions, 2662
Concept Phonics, 775, 2665
Corwin Press, 2666
Decoding Automaticity Materials for Reading Fluency, 778
Educators Publishing Service, 2667
Federation for Children with Special Needs, 51, 2668
Free Spirit Publishing, 2669
Gordon Systems & GSI Publications, 2671
Guilford Publications, 2673
Hazelden Publishing, 2674
Heinemann-Boynton/Cook, 2675
Love Publishing Company, 2683
Magination Press, 2684
Marsh Media, 1217, 2685
Nimble Numeracy: Fluency in Counting and Basic Arithmetic, 726
Performance Resource Press, 2691
Peytral Publications, 2692
Research Press Publisher, 2695
Riggs Institute, 2696
Scholastic, 1346, 2697
Schwab Learning, 2698
Sounds and Spelling Patterns for English, 821
Stories from Somerville, 826
Teaching Comprehension: Strategies for Stories, 829
Teddy Bear Press, 2700
Therapro, 2701
Wadsworth Publishing Company, 2705
Woodbine House, 2706

Puzzles

ADA Quiz Book, 2389
Equation Tile Teaser, 698
Equation Tile Teasers, 1252
KIND News, 2615
KIND News Jr: Kids in Nature's Defense, 2616
KIND News Primary: Kids in Nature's Defense, 2617
Mind Over Matter, 1127
Puzzle Tanks, 733
Toddler Tote, 947

Wordly Wise ABC 1-9, 835

Recognition Skills

Creating Patterns from Shapes, 695
Curious George Pre-K ABCs, 619, 1143
Mind Matters, 282

Rehabilitation

AbleData National Institute on Disability & Rehab. Research, 1049
American Rehabilitation Counseling Association (ARCA), 14
Answers4Families: Center on Children, Families and the Law, 1692
Answers4Families: Center on Children, Families, Law, 2149
Arizona Department of Economic Security, 1483
Arkansas Department of Corrections, 1491
Arkansas Rehabilitation Services, 4481
California Department of Rehabilitation, 1504, 4489
The Children's Institute, 4178, 4242
Client Assistance Program (CAP): Nebraska Division of Persons with Disabilities, 2150
Client Assistance Program (CAP): Nebraska Division of Persons with Disabilities, 1694
Cognitive Rehabilitation, 1140
Connecticut Bureau of Rehabilitation Services, 1532
Council on Rehabilitation Education (CORE), 36
Department of Assistive & Rehabilitative Services, 4604
Department of Correctional Services, 1737
Department of Social Services: Vocational Rehabilitation Program, 4500
District of Columbia Department of Corrections, 1550
Division of Rehabilitation Services, 215
Fundamentals of Job Placement, 4448
Fundamentals of Vocational Assessment, 4449
Help for Brain Injured Children, 3987
Illinois Department of Rehabilitation Services, 1589
Iowa Vocational Rehabilitation Agency, 2060
Job Accommodation Network (JAN), 4442
Journal of Rehabilitation, 2876
Kansas Correctional Education, 2071
Kansas Department of Corrections, 2072
Kansas Department of Social & Rehabilitation Services, 2073
Life After High School for Students with Moderate and Severe Disabilities, 2814
Massachusetts Correctional Education: Inmate Training & Education, 2120
Massachusetts Rehabilitation Commission, 1652
Minnesota Vocational Rehabilitation Agency: Rehabilitation Services Branch, 4548
Minnesota Vocational Rehabilitation Services, 2138
Munroe-Meyer Institute for Genetics and Rehabilitation, 4299
National Council on Rehabilitation Education (NCRE), 88
National Rehabilitation Association, 97
National Rehabilitation Information Center(NARIC), 98
North Texas Rehabilitation Center, 331
Office For The Deaf And Hearing Impaired, 4484
Office of Vocational Rehabilitation Services, 1784
Rehabilitation International (RI Global), 104
Rehabilitation Services Administration, 4477
Rhode Island Vocational and Rehabilitation Agency, 2246, 4592
Section 504 of the Rehabilitation Act, 2406
Student Directed Learning: Teaching Self Determination Skills, 2794
Texas Department of Assistive and Rehabilitative Services, 1836
Virginia Department of Rehabilitative Services, 4617
Wiregrass Rehabilitation Center, 3968

531

Remediation

Art-Centered Education & Therapy for Children with Disabilities, 2924
Auditory Skills, 1136
Boone Voice Program for Adults, 4390
Boone Voice Program for Children, 4391
Challenging Our Minds, 1138
Complete Learning Disabilities Resource Library, 2445
Cyber Launch Pad Camp, 478
Differential Test of Conduct and Emotional Problems, 4425
Help for the Learning Disabled Child, 2476, 4396
International Center for the Disabled, 4194
Khan-Lewis Phonological Analysis: KLPA-2, 4427
Lake Michigan Academy, 3272, 4151
Landmark School and Summer Programs, 4136
A Practical Parent's Handbook on Teaching Children with Learning Disabilities, 2421
Reading Problems: Consultation and Remediation, 3005
Slosson Full Range Intelligence Test Kit, 4432
Slosson Intelligence Test, 4344, 4407
Slosson Intelligence Test Primary, 4408
Slosson Visual Motor Performance Test, 4433
Teach Me Language, 2547
Wardlaw School, 3171, 4076
The de Paul School, 4109

Research

Artificial Language Laboratory, 1088
Association Book Exhibit: Brain Research, 1007
Center for Applied Studies in Education Learning (CASE), 128
Computer Retrieval of Information on Scientific Project (CRISP), 1332
Division for Research, 1906
Division of Research, 43
Easter Seals - Arkansas, 132
Hyperactive Child, Adolescent and Adult, 403
International Conference on Learning Disabilities, 1026
Learning Disabilities Research & Practice, 2858
Narrative Prosthesis: Disability and the Dependencies of Discourse, 2966
World Institute on Disability (WID), 116

Resource Centers

Alabama Commission on Higher Education, 1926
Center for Adult Learning and Literacy: University of Maine, 2089
The Center for Learning Differences, 4310
Center for Literary Studies, 2261
Complete Set of State Resource Sheets, 2578
Connecticut Literacy Resource Center, 1979
Council for Exceptional Children (CEC), 34, 354
Council for Learning Disabilities CLD, 355
Florida Literacy Resource Center, 2005
Georgia Literacy Resource Center: Office of Adult Literacy, 2013
Iowa Literacy Resource Center, 2059
Kansas Literacy Resource Center, 2074
LEARN: Regional Educational Service Center, 1980
Laureate Learning Systems, 1339
Learning Disabilities Association of Maryland, 219
Literacy Program: County of Los Angeles Public Library, 1963
Literacy Volunteers of America: Willits Public Library, 1964
Literacy Volunteers of Greater Hartford, 1984
Literary Resources Rhode Island, 2244
Maine Literacy Resource Center, 2100
Marin Literacy Program, 1965
Maryland Adult Literacy Resource Center, 2109
Merced Adult School, 1966
Metropolitan Adult Education Program, 1967
Mid City Adult Learning Center, 1968
Montana Literacy Resource Center, 2148

National Center for Learning Disabilities (NCLD), 85, 1918
National Center for Learning Disabilities(NCLD), 359
National Organization on Disability, 2884
New Hampshire Second Start Adult Education, 2159
New York Literacy Resource Center, 2190
Newport Beach Public Library Literacy Services, 1969
North Carolina Literacy Resource Center, 2198
Office of Special Education Programs, 1923
Ohio Literacy Resource Center, 2212
Oklahoma Literacy Resource Center, 2228
Parent Advocacy Coalition for Educational Rights (PACER), 100
Pennsylvania Literacy Resource Center, 2237
Pomona Public Library Literacy Services, 2340
Sacramento Public Library Literacy Service, 1970
South Carolina Literacy Resource Center, 2255
South Dakota Literacy Resource Center, 2259
Sweetwater State Literacy Regional Resource Center, 1971
Utah Literacy Action Center, 2289
Vermont Literacy Resource Center: Dept of Education, 2295
Vision Literacy of California, 1972
Wisconsin Literacy Resource Center, 2339

School Administration

CABE Journal, 2865
Journal of School Health, 2877
OT Practice, 2885
Restructuring America's Schools, 2720

Science

Discoveries: Explore the Desert Ecosystem, 888, 1387
Discoveries: Explore the Everglades Ecosystem, 889, 1388
Discoveries: Explore the Forest Ecosystem, 890, 1389
GeoSafari Wonder World USA, 922
Imagination Express Destination: Rain Forest, 1394
Learn About Life Science: Animals, 836, 1381
Learn About Life Science: Plants, 837, 1382
Learn About Physical Science: Simple Machines, 838
Make-a-Map 3D, 897
Maps & Navigation, 840, 898
Ranger Rick, 2621
Thinkin' Science, 847
Thinkin' Science ZAP!, 848

Secondary Education

Algebra Stars, 686, 1231
Dallas Academy: Coed High School, 3751
GED Testing Services, 1489
Green Globs & Graphing Equations, 708
High School Math Bundle, 710, 1308
Idaho Professional Technical Education, 1577
Journal of Postsecondary Education and Disability, 2875
KET/GED Series, 2812
Kansas State GED Administration, 1618
Massachusetts GED Administration: Massachusetts Department of Education, 2122
Massachusetts General Education Development (GED), 1650
New Mexico State GED Testing Program, 1733
Oregon GED Administrator: Office of Community College Services, 2232
Publications from HEATH, 2887
SMARTS: A Study Skills Resource Guide, 2531
State GED Administration, 1502, 1539, 1603, 1633, 1664, 1749, 1773, 1780, 1800, 1815, 1824, 1827, 1834, 1860, 1878, 1883, 1893
State GED Administration: Delaware, 1547

State GED Administration: GED Testing Program, 1480
State GED Administration: Georgia, 1565
State GED Administration: Hawaii, 1570
State GED Administration: Nebraska, 1699
State GED Administration: Office of Specialized Populations, 1728
Utah State Office of Education, 1848
WA State Board for Community and Technical Colleges, 1869
Write On! Plus: High School Writing Skills, 988

Self-Advocacy

Advocacy Center for Persons with Disabilities, 2003
Advocacy Services for Families of Children in Special Education, 2575
Arizona Center for Disability Law, 127, 1481
Client Assistance Program (CAP) C.A.R.E.S., Inc., 1636
Community Legal Aid Society, 1542
Connecticut Office of Protection and Advocacy for Persons with Disabilities, 1534
Disability Rights - Idaho, 185
Disability Rights Center, 1712
Disability Rights Center of Kansas, 1612
Disability Rights Idaho, 1571
Disability Rights Network of Pennsylvania, 1792
Disability Rights New Jersey, 253
Disability Rights Oregon, 1783
Disability Rights Washington, 337, 1865
Disability Rights Wisconsin, 1882
Equip for Equality, 2035
Equip for Equality: Carbondale, 2036
Equip for Equality: Moline, 2037
Equip for Equality: Springfield, 2038
Georgia Advocacy Office, 1559
Hawaii Disability Rights Center, 1568
How to Get Services by Being Assertive, 2350, 2480
Illinois Protection & Advocacy Agency: Equip for Equality, 188
Indiana Protection & Advocacy Services, 1601
Kentucky Protection and Advocacy, 1626
Missouri Protection & Advocacy Services, 237, 1681
Montana Parents, Let's Unite for Kids (PLUK), 240
Nevada Disability and Law Center, 1706
Protection & Advocacy Agency, 1501, 1538, 1593, 1639, 1655, 1670, 1683, 1747, 1771, 1778, 1802
Protection & Advocacy Agency (NJP&A), 1726
Protection & Advocacy Services, 1611
Protection & Advocacy System, 1891
Protection & Advocacy for People with Disabilities, 1809
Vermont Protection & Advocacy, 334
Who I Can Be Is Up To Me: Lessons in Self-Exploration and Self-Determination, 2568

Self-Esteem

Draw a Person: Screening Procedure for Emotional Disturbance, 4318
I'm Not Stupid, 2771
Learning Disabilities and Self-Esteem, 2777
Me! A Curriculum for Teaching Self-Esteem Through an Interest Center, 2514
Multidimensional Self Concept Scale, 4320
Positive Self-Talk for Children, 2527
Rosey: The Imperfect Angel, 2379
Self-Esteem Index, 4323
Someone Special, Just Like You, 2384

Sensory Integration

Adaptive Physical Education Program, 1116
New Interdisciplinary School, 4201
Sensory Integration: Theory and Practice, 2536, 2973
Visualizing and Verbalizing for Language Comprehension and Thinking, 2994

Multisensory Teaching Approach, 2990
Patterns of English Spelling, 803
Preventing Academic Failure, 2969
Raskob Learning Institute and Day School, 3101, 3999
Read, Write and Type Learning System, 1415
Read, Write and Type! Learning System, 1176
Read, Write and Type! Learning Systems, 1368
Sequential Spelling 1-7 with Student Respose Book, 642
Slingerland Multisensory Approach to Language Arts, 2992
Spell-a-Word, 1183
Spelling Ace, 1185
Spelling Mastery, 1186
Spelling Workbook Video, 2722
Teaching Reading to Children with Down Syndrome, 2549
Teaching Spelling Workshop, 1045
Test of Written Spelling, 4418
ThemeWeavers: Animals Activity Kit, 680
ThemeWeavers: Nature Activity Kit, 681, 846
Thinking and Learning Connection, 1925

Strategies

Academic Skills Problems: Direct Assessment and Intervention, 2919
ADHD in the Classroom: Strategies for Teachers, 2738
Americans with Disabilities Act (ADA) Resource Center, 1448
Auditory Processes, 2926
Ben Bronz Academy, 3128
BRIGANCE Word Analysis: Strategies and Practice, 4360
Child Who Appears Aloof: Module 5, 2753
Child Who is Rejected: Module 7, 2758
Closer Look: Perspectives & Reflections on College Students with LD, 2345
Cognitive Strategy Instruction That Really Improves Children's Performance, 2929
Cognitive Strategy Instruction for Middleand High Schools, 661
Cooperative Learning and Strategies for Inclusion, 2931
Creative Mind: Building Foundations that will Last Forever, 1018
Factory Deluxe, 699, 1254
Factory Deluxe: Grades 4 to 8, 1305
Fischer Decoding Mastery Test, 2368
From Talking to Writing: Strategies for Scaffolding Expository Expression, 2987
Handbook of Psychological and Educational Assessment of Children, 2907
Inclusion: A Practical Guide for Parents, 2489
Instructional Strategies for Learning Disabled Community College Students, 2712
Interventions for Students with Learning Disabilities, 2590
Landmark Method for Teaching Arithmetic, 2996
Landmark School's Language-Based Teaching Guides, 2499
Learning Disability Evaluation Scale: Renormed, 4354
Lexia Cross-Trainer, 1359
Lexia Early Reading, 1360
Lexia Strategies for Older Students, 1362
National Clearinghouse of Rehabilitation Training Materials (NCRTM), 360
No Easy Answer, 2355
Park Century School, 3099, 3995
Purdue University Speech-Language Clinic, 2719
Self-Supervision: A Career Tool for Audiologists, Clinical Series 10, 4458
Strategy Challenges Collection: 1, 1321
Study Skills: A Landmark School Student Guide, 2385
Study Skills: A Landmark School Teaching Guide, 2541
Survival Guide for Kids with LD Learning Differences, 2566
Teaching Strategies Library: Research Based Strategies for Teachers, 2727

United Learning, 2803
University of Illinois: Urbana, 3187
University of New England: University Campus, 3222
University of Virginia, 3858
When a Child Doesn't Play: Module 1, 2805
Writing: A Landmark School Teaching Guide, 2995

Student Workshops

AtoZap!, 615, 1135
Glen Eden Institute, 4284
A Student's Guide to the IEP, 2572
Study Skills: How to Manage Your Time, 2795

Support Groups

Accessing Parent Groups, 2573
Brain Injury Association of America, 25
Easter Seals - Camp Heron, 139
Easter Seals - Capper Foundation, 204
Easter Seals - Central California, Fresno, 141
Easter Seals - Colorado Camp Rocky Mountain Village, 152
Easter Seals - DC, MD, VA, 216
Easter Seals - Delaware & Maryland's Easten Shore, New Castle, 165
Easter Seals - Georgetown, 166
Easter Seals - Hawaii, 182
Easter Seals - Heartland, 235
Easter Seals - Maine, 211
Easter Seals - Metropolitan Chicago, 187
Easter Seals - Nevada, 245
Easter Seals - New Jersey, 254
Easter Seals - North Georgia, 175
Easter Seals - Santa Maria El Mirador, 261
Easter Seals - South Carolina, 317
Easter Seals - South Dakota, 1818
Easter Seals - Tennessee, 321
Easter Seals - UCP North Carolina & Virginia, 335
Easter Seals - Washington, 338
Easter Seals - West Virginia, 342
How to Organize an Effective Parent-Advocacy Group and Move Bureaucracies, 2482
Learning Disabilities in Higher Educationand Beyond: An International Perspective, 3024
Nevada Economic Opportunity Board: Community Action Partnership, 2155
Rockland County Association for the Learning Disabled (YAI/RCALD), 579
Rose F Kennedy Center, 3432, 4307
Team of Advocates for Special Kids (TASK), 109
Westchester Institute for Human Development, 2800d@MINOR HEADING = Surveys
Let's Learn About Deafness, 2509
Phonic Reading Lessons, 4430
Test of Information Processing Skills, 4435
US Bureau of the Census, 1467

Switches

Adaptive Device Locator System (ADLS), 1051
Tech-Able, 1108

Synthesizers

Mega Dots 2.3, 1410

Tape Recorders

Albuquerque Technical Vocational Institute, 3343
Johnson & Wales University, 3690

Technology

ABLE DATA, 1445
Abbreviation/Expansion, 1403
Accurate Assessments, 1328
Adapting Curriculum & Instruction in Inclusive Early Childhood Settings, 2921
Adaptive Environments, 223

Adaptive Technology Tools, 1349
American Foundation for the Blind, 1087
An Open Book, 1350
Assistive Technology, 1597, 1677, 1701, 1763, 1774
Assistive Technology Advocacy Center-ATAC, 4570
Assistive Technology Center, 1841
Assistive Technology Center (ATAC), 1722
Assistive Technology Office, 1621
Assistive Technology Partners, 1520
Assistive Technology Partnership, 1693
Assistive Technology Program, 1750, 1781, 1808, 1842
Assistive Technology Project, 1497, 1678, 1685
Assistive Technology System, 1856
Assistive Technology of Alaska (ATLA), 1474
Behavior Technology Guide Book, 2437
Birmingham Alliance for Technology Access Center, 1090
Bluegrass Technology Center, 1091
Center for Accessible Technology, 1093
Center for Applied Special Technology (CAST), 30
Center for Enabling Technology, 1094
Closing the Gap, 32
Closing the Gap Conference, 1015
Closing the Gap Newsletter, 1083
Communication Outlook, 2892
Communication Skills for Visually Impaired Learners, 2nd Ed., 2985
Computer Access-Computer Learning, 1084
ConnSENSE Conference, 1017
Connecticut Tech Act Project, 1536
Division of Vocational Rehabilitation, 2315, 4505, 4513
Educational Technology, 2872
Family Guide to Assistive Technology, 2461
HEATH Resource Center, 1099
Idaho Assistive Technology Project, 1572
Illinois Assistive Technology, 1584
International Society for Technology in Education (ISTE), 1336
Iowa Program for Assistive Technology, 201, 1101
Journal of Special Education Technology, 2878
Latest Technology for Young Children, 2775
Learning Independence through Computers, 1102
Lighthouse Central Florida, 1103
Louisiana Assistive Technology Access Network, 1631
Michigan Assistive Technology: Michigan Rehabilitation Services, 2127
Michigan Technological University, 3273
Microsoft Corporation, 1341
Minnesota's Assistive Technology Act Program, 1669
NYS Commission on Quality of Care/TRAID Program, 1738
New IDEA Amendments: Assistive Technology Devices and Services, 2400
New Mexico Technology-Related Assistance Program, 1734
Pennsylvania Institute of Technology, 3659
Project TECH, 1104
RESNA Technical Assistance Project, 1105
Rehabilitation Engineering and Assistive Technology Society of North America (RESNA), 103
SUNY Institute of Technology: Utica/Rome, 3436
Star Center, 1107
TASH Annual Conference Social Justice inthe 21st Century, 1042
Teaching Exceptional Children, 2888
Technical Assistance Alliance for Parent Centers: PACER Center, 233
Technology & Persons with Disabilities Conference, 1046
Technology Access Center, 1109
Technology Access Foundation, 1110
Technology Assistance for Special Consumers, 1111
Technology Utilization Program, 1112
Technology and Media Division, 110
Technology for Language and Learning, 1113
TeleSensory, 1228

Rehabilitation Division Department of Employment, Training & Rehabilitation, 4564
Rehabilitation Resource, 4305
Rehabilitation Services Administration State Vocational Program, 1465
Rehabilitation Services for the Blind, 4551
Resources for Children with Special Needs, 278, 2192
Rhode Island Parent Information Network, 4246
Rhyming Sounds Game, 938
Right from the Start: Behavioral Intervention for Young Children with Autism: A Guide, 765, 869, 2530
RiteCare Of Washington, 4286
Rocky Mountain Disability and Business Technical Assistance Center, 156
S'Cool Moves for Learning: A Program Designed to Enhance Learning Through Body-Mind, 870
STEP/Teen: Systematic Training for Effective Parenting of Teens, 2792
STOMP Specialized Training for Military Parents, 4287
School-Based Home Developmental PE Program, 2532
Scottish Rite Learning Center of Austin, Inc., 4262
Seeing Clearly, 2533
Sensory Integration and the Child: Understanding Hidden Sensory Challenges, 2535
Sensory Motor Activities for Early Development, 766
Shapes, 940
Siblings of Children with Autism: A Guide for Families, 2537
Simple Steps: Developmental Activities for Infants, Toddlers & Two Year Olds, 871, 2538
Skillstreaming Video: How to Teach Students Prosocial Skills, 2721
Snail's Pace Race Game, 941
So What Can I Do?, 672
Song Games for Sensory Integration, 873
SoundSmart, 1320
Southwest Texas Disability & Business Technical Assistance Center: Region VI, 1833
Specialized Language Development Center, 4152
Spider Ball, 943
Squidgie Flying Disc, 944
St. Vincent's Special Needs Center, 4033
Start to Finish: Developmentally Sequenced Fine Motor Activities for Preschool Children, 874
StartWrite, 979
StartWrite Handwriting Software, 1416
State Of Idaho Department Of Labor, 4525
Stepwise Cookbooks, 674
Stern Center for Language and Learning, 4269
Successful Movement Challenges, 880
Super Study Wheel: Homework Helper, 907
Teachers Ask About Sensory Integration, 2976
Teaching Dressing Skills: Buttons, Bowsand More, 679
Teenage Switch Progressions, 1227
Tennessee School-to-Work Office, 2271
Tennessee Services for the Blind, 4603
Things in My House: Picture Matching Game, 946
Time Together: Adults Supporting Play, 2797
Tool Chest: For Teachers, Parents and Students, 982
Tools for Students, 2798
Tools for Teachers, 2799
TrainerVision: Inclusion, Focus on Toddlers and Pre-K, 2800
2's Experience Fingerplays, 751
Type to Learn 3, 1194
Type to Learn Jr, 1195
Type to Learn Jr New Keys for Kids, 1196
U.S. Department of Education: Office of Vocational & Adult Education, 4444
US Department of Health & Human Services, 1468
Understanding and Managing Vision Deficits, 2983
University of Hawaii: Manoa, 3172
Utah Parent Center, 4268
Vision, Perception and Cognition: Manual for Evaluation & Treatment, 4348
Visual Skills Appraisal, 4436
Vocational Rehabilitation Services, 4521, 4532

Vocational Training and Employment of Autistic Adolescents, 4462
Vocational and Life Skills Center, 3137
Washington PAVE: Specialized Training of Military Parents (STOMP), 115
Washington Parent Training Project: PAVE, 341
Who's Teaching Our Children with Disabilities?, 2609
Wikki Stix Hands On-Learning Activity Book, 884
Wilson Language Training, 833, 1047
Winning the Study Game, 2570
Wisconsin Department of Workforce Development, 1885
Wonder Ball, 951
Woods Schools, 4244
Workforce Investment Act, 4584, 4588
Workforce Investment Board, 4486
Workforce Investment Quarterly, 4463
YAI Network, 118

Transportation

AK Dept. of Labor and Workforce Dev., 4475
Idaho Division of Vocational Rehabilitation Administration, 4524
Let's Find Out, 2619
National Technical Information Service: US Department of Commerce, 1459
New Horizons Information for the Air Traveler with a Disability, 2354
Office of Vocational Rehabilitation, 4537, 4539
Office of Vocational and Educational Services for Individuals with Disabilities, 4580
Related Services for School-Aged Children with Disabilities, 2602
South Carolina Vocational Rehabilitation Department, 4595
State Vocational Rehabilitation Agency, 4473, 4526, 4536, 4540, 4542, 4544, 4546, 4558, 4569, 4586, 4599, 4600, 4605
State Vocational Rehabilitation Agency Department of Elementary & Secondary Education, 4552
State Vocational Rehabilitation Agency of Arkansas, 4485
State Vocational Rehabilitation Agency: Minnesota Department of Economics Security, 4549
State Vocational Rehabilitation Agency: Nebraska, 4561
State Vocational Rehabilitation Agency: Oklahoma Department of Rehabilitation Services, 4587
State Vocational Rehabilitation Agency: Pennsylvania, 4591
State Vocational Rehabilitation Agency: Rhode Island, 4593
State Vocational Rehabilitation Agency: Washington Division of Vocational Rehabilitation, 4618
State of New Mexico Division of Vocational Rehabilitation, 4577
State of Washington, Division of Vocational Rehabilitation, 4619
TILES Project: Transition/Independent Living/Employment/Support, 4517
Texas Department of Assistive and Rehabilitative Services, 4606
Utah State Office of Rehabilitation, 4609
Vocational Rehabilitation, 1700, 4583
Vocational Rehabilitation and Services For The Blind Division (VRSBD), 4522
West Virginia Division of Rehabilitation Services, 4620
Wisconsin Division of Vocational Rehabilitation, 4621
Wyoming Department of Workforce Services: State Vocational Rehabilitation Agency, 4622

Treatment

ADHD in Adolescents: Diagnosis and Treatment, 2422
AdvoServ, 4044
American Psychological Association, 11, 2655

American Psychologist, 2855
Andrus Children's Center, 4188
Attention-Deficit Hyperactivity Disorder: A Handbook for Diagnosis and Treatment, 2434
BASC Monitor for ADHD, 4311
Boys and Girls Village, Inc., 4016
Camelot Of Kingston, 4255
Camelot School: Palatine Campus, 4256
Chileda Institute, 4290
Cognitive-Behavioral Therapy for Impulsive Children, 2900
Crawford First Education, 4274
Devereux Arizona Treatment Network, 3973
Devereux Genesis Learning Centers, 4250
Emergence: Labeled Autistic, 2459
Full Circle Programs, 3986
Genesis Learning Centers, 4251
Harmony Hill School, 4245
Heartspring School, 4105
Helping Your Hyperactive Child, 2478
Hyperactive Children Grown Up, 2484
Illinois Center for Autism, 4092
International Dyslexia Association, 58, 1911
International Dyslexia Association Quarterly Newsletter: Perspectives, 2631
Interventions for ADHD: Treatment in Developmental Context, 2493
Journal of Speech, Language, and Hearing Research, 2893
Julia Dyckman Andrus Memorial, 4195
Kennedy Krieger Institute, 4118
Klingberg Family Centers, 4024
Lorraine D. Foster Day School, 4026
Natchaug's Network of Care, 4029
Nawa Academy, 3991
The New England Center for Children, 4147
Providence Speech and Hearing Center, 3998, 4302
Saint Francis Home for Children, Inc., 4031
Stuttering Severity Instrument for Children and Adults, 4409
Treatment of Children's Grammatical Impairments in Naturalistic Context, 2801
Waterford Country Schools, 4041

Visual Assistive Devices

The American Printing House for the Blind, Inc., 111
Benton Visual Retention Test, 4422
Braille Keyboard Sticker Overlay Label Kit, 1053
Connecticut Institute for the Blind, 4018
Developmental Test of Visual Perception (D TVP-2), 4424
Genie Color TV, 1059
Home Row Indicators, 1062
Miami Lighthouse for the Blind and Visually Impaired, 174
National Association for Visually Handicapped, 2687
SmartDriver, 1319
Ulverscroft Large Print Books, 2704
Updown Chair, 883
VISTA, 1078
Xavier Society for the Blind, 2707

Visual Discrimination

Associated Services for the Blind, 2656
Bureau of Services to the Blind & Visually Impaired, 4562
Commission for the Blind & Visually Handicapped, 4578
Comparison Kitchen, 1203
Educating Students Who Have Visual Impairments with Other Disabilities, 2457
Gremlin Hunt, 1149
I Can Read, 789
Jewish Braille Institute of America, 2678
Lighthouse Low Vision Products, 797
Lutheran Braille Workers, 150
Same or Different, 1177
Second Sense, 194
Sliding Block, 1318

South Dakota Rehabilitation Center for the Blind, 4598

Visual Perception and Attention Workbook, 2388

Vocabulary

Analogies 1, 2 & 3, 614
Bailey's Book House, 1352
Basic Signing Vocabulary Cards, 616
Bubbleland Word Discovery, 617
Carolina Picture Vocabulary Test (CPVT): For Deaf and Hearing Impaired Children, 618
Christmas Bear, 2366
Connecting Reading and Writing with Vocabulary, 4392
Emergent Reader, 782
Explode the Code, 784
Following Directions: One and Two-Level Commands, 1213
Funny Bunny and Sunny Bunny, 2370
Halloween Bear, 2371
High Frequency Vocabulary, 1150
I Can Read Charts, 2373
Language Learning Everywhere We Go, 2988
Language Master, 1160
Learning Disabilities Resources, 2680
My Own Bookshelf, 1172
Nordic Software, 1314
Old MacDonald's Farm Deluxe, 1299
Once Upon a Time Volume II: Worlds of Enchantment, 1412
Once Upon a Time Volume III: Journey Through Time, 1413
Once Upon a Time Volume IV: Exploring Nature, 1414
Peabody Picture Vocabulary Test, 4399
Peabody Picture Vocabulary Test: Fourth Edition, 4400
Peabody Test-Picture Vocabulary Test, 4341
Reading Comprehension in Varied Subject Matter, 812
Scare Bear, 2380
Secondary Print Pack, 1225
See Me Add, 819
Signs of the Times, 2991
Snowbear, 2383
Space Academy GX-1, 843
Speaking Language Master Special Edition, 1182
Stanley Sticker Stories, 1187
Story of the USA, 900
Summer@Carroll, 537
Talking Walls, 844, 1385
Talking Walls: The Stories Continue, 845, 1386
Tenth Planet Roots, Prefixes & Suffixes, 1375
Tenth Planet: Roots, Suffixes, Prefixes, 830
Test of Mathematical Abilities, 4357
Thinkin' Science ZAP, 682
Valentine Bear, 2387
Virtual Labs: Electricity, 850
Word Wise I and II: Better Comprehension Through Vocabulary, 1200
Wordly Wise 3000 ABC 1-9, 834

Voice Output Devices

Kurzweil 3000, 1358
Oral Speech Mechanism Screening Examination, 4398

Reading Pen, 813, 1072

Volunteer

Aloha Special Technology Access Center, 180
Delaware County Literacy Council, 2234
International Cultural Youth Exchange (ICYE), 1432
International Partnership for Service-Learning and Leadership, 1433
Kentucky Literacy Volunteers of America, 2080
LDA Rhode Island Newsletter, 2880
Learning Disabilities Association of Michigan (LDA), 230
Literacy Chicago, 2042
Literacy Volunteers of America: Rhode Island, 2239
Literacy Volunteers of Massachusetts, 2117
New York Literacy Volunteers of America, 2191
People Care Center, 2173
Teaching People with Developmental Disabilities, 2726

Workshop Training

ACA Charlotte, 999
Active Parenting Publishers, 1003, 2651
Assessing Learning Problems Workshop, 1005
Boston University, 3243
Computer Access Center, 1096
Dr. Peet's TalkWriter, 1398
Easybook Deluxe Writing Workshop: Colonial Times, 891, 961
Educational Options for Students with Learning Disabilities and LD/HD, 1022
Elim Christian Services, 4089
The Fowler Center For Outdoor Learning, 545
Handbook for Implementing Workshops for Siblings of Special Needs Children, 2470
How Difficult Can This Be?, 2769, 2950
Inclusion of Learning Disabled Students in Regular Classrooms Workshop, 1024
Interest Driven Learning Master Class Workshop, 1025
International Dyslexia Association Long Island, 268
International Dyslexia Association New York, 269
International Dyslexia Association Upper Midwest Branch, 231
International Dyslexia Association of Florida, 172
International Dyslexia Association of Georgia, 177
International Dyslexia Association of Hawaii, 183
International Dyslexia Association of Indiana, 197
International Dyslexia Association of Iowa, 200
International Dyslexia Association of Los Angeles, 144
International Dyslexia Association of Michigan, 229
International Dyslexia Association of Nebraska, 242
International Dyslexia Association of Oregon, 304
International Dyslexia Association of Rhode Island, 316
International Dyslexia Association of San Diego, 146
International Dyslexia Association of South Carolina, 318

International Dyslexia Association of Wisconsin, 344
International Dyslexia Association: Philadelphia Branch Newsletter, 2633
LDA Learning Center, 4154
LDR Workshop: What Are Learning Disabilities, Problems and Differences?, 1029
Landmark School Outreach Program, 61, 1030, 3256, 4135
Learning Disabilities Association of Nebraska, 243
Learning Disabilities Association of South Dakota, 319
Learning Disabilities and the World of Work Workshop, 1031
Learning Problems and Adult Basic Education Workshop, 1032
Lindamood-Bell Learning Processes Professional Development, 1033
Lion's Workshop, 1216
National Head Start Association, 1035
National Head Start Association Parent Conference, 1036
Parents Reaching Out to Parents of South Carolina, 4247
Rocky Mountain International Dyslexia Association, 157
Social Skills Workshop, 1040
State University of New York: Albany, 3447
Stockdale Learning Center, 4005
Switch to Turn Kids On, 1086
Teaching Math Workshop, 1043
Workshops, 3969

Writing

Advanced Skills For School Success Series: Module 4, 4383
Easybook Deluxe, 960, 1406
Easybook Deluxe Writing Workshop: Whales & Oceans, 964
Goals and Objectives Writer Software, 4363
Handwriting Without Tears, 970
Imagination Express Destination: Time Trip USA, 1395
Making Handwriting Flow, 975
Making the Writing Process Work: Strategies for Composition & Self-Regulation, 2989
Making the Writing Process Work: Strategies for Composition & Self-Regulation, 2512
Media Weaver 3.5, 976, 1400
PAF Handwriting Programs for Print, Cursive (Right or Left-Handed), 978
Reading and Writing Workbook, 2564
Sunbuddy Writer, 981, 1401
Write On! Plus: Beginning Writing Skills, 984
Write On! Plus: Essential Writing, 986
Write On! Plus: Growing as a Writer, 987
Write On! Plus: Middle School Writing Skills, 990
Write On! Plus: Steps to Better Writing, 993
Write On! Plus: Writing with Picture Books, 994
Writer's Resources Library 2.0, 995
Writing Trek Grades 4-6, 996, 1417
Writing Trek Grades 8-10, 998, 1419

Grey House
Publishing

Grey House
Publishing

2016 Title List
Visit www.GreyHouse.com for Product Information, Table of Contents, and Sample Pages.

General Reference
An African Biographical Dictionary
America's College Museums
American Environmental Leaders: From Colonial Times to the Present
Encyclopedia of African-American Writing
Encyclopedia of Constitutional Amendments
Encyclopedia of Gun Control & Gun Rights
An Encyclopedia of Human Rights in the United States
Encyclopedia of Invasions & Conquests
Encyclopedia of Prisoners of War & Internment
Encyclopedia of Religion & Law in America
Encyclopedia of Rural America
Encyclopedia of the Continental Congress
Encyclopedia of the United States Cabinet, 1789-2010
Encyclopedia of War Journalism
Encyclopedia of Warrior Peoples & Fighting Groups
The Environmental Debate: A Documentary History
The Evolution Wars: A Guide to the Debates
From Suffrage to the Senate: America's Political Women
Global Terror & Political Risk Assessment
Nations of the World
Political Corruption in America
Privacy Rights in the Digital Era
The Religious Right: A Reference Handbook
Speakers of the House of Representatives, 1789-2009
This is Who We Were: 1880-1900
This is Who We Were: A Companion to the 1940 Census
This is Who We Were: In the 1910s
This is Who We Were: In the 1920s
This is Who We Were: In the 1940s
This is Who We Were: In the 1950s
This is Who We Were: In the 1960s
This is Who We Were: In the 1970s
U.S. Land & Natural Resource Policy
The Value of a Dollar 1600-1865: Colonial Era to the Civil War
The Value of a Dollar: 1860-2014
Working Americans 1770-1869 Vol. IX: Revolutionary War to the Civil War
Working Americans 1880-1999 Vol. I: The Working Class
Working Americans 1880-1999 Vol. II: The Middle Class
Working Americans 1880-1999 Vol. III: The Upper Class
Working Americans 1880-1999 Vol. IV: Their Children
Working Americans 1880-2015 Vol. V: Americans At War
Working Americans 1880-2005 Vol. VI: Women at Work
Working Americans 1880-2006 Vol. VII: Social Movements
Working Americans 1880-2007 Vol. VIII: Immigrants
Working Americans 1880-2009 Vol. X: Sports & Recreation
Working Americans 1880-2010 Vol. XI: Inventors & Entrepreneurs
Working Americans 1880-2011 Vol. XII: Our History through Music
Working Americans 1880-2012 Vol. XIII: Education & Educators
World Cultural Leaders of the 20th & 21st Centuries

Education Information
Charter School Movement
Comparative Guide to American Elementary & Secondary Schools
Complete Learning Disabilities Directory
Educators Resource Directory
Special Education: A Reference Book for Policy and Curriculum Development

Health Information
Comparative Guide to American Hospitals
Complete Directory for Pediatric Disorders
Complete Directory for People with Chronic Illness
Complete Directory for People with Disabilities
Complete Mental Health Directory
Diabetes in America: Analysis of an Epidemic
Directory of Drug & Alcohol Residential Rehab Facilities
Directory of Health Care Group Purchasing Organizations
Directory of Hospital Personnel
HMO/PPO Directory
Medical Device Register
Older Americans Information Directory

Business Information
Complete Television, Radio & Cable Industry Directory
Directory of Business Information Resources
Directory of Mail Order Catalogs
Directory of Venture Capital & Private Equity Firms
Environmental Resource Handbook
Food & Beverage Market Place
Grey House Homeland Security Directory
Grey House Performing Arts Directory
Grey House Safety & Security Directory
Grey House Transportation Security Directory
Hudson's Washington News Media Contacts Directory
New York State Directory
Rauch Market Research Guides
Sports Market Place Directory

Statistics & Demographics
American Tally
America's Top-Rated Cities
America's Top-Rated Smaller Cities
America's Top-Rated Small Towns & Cities
Ancestry & Ethnicity in America
The Asian Databook
Comparative Guide to American Suburbs
The Hispanic Databook
Profiles of America
"Profiles of" Series – State Handbooks
Weather America

Financial Ratings Series
TheStreet Ratings' Guide to Bond & Money Market Mutual Funds
TheStreet Ratings' Guide to Common Stocks
TheStreet Ratings' Guide to Exchange-Traded Funds
TheStreet Ratings' Guide to Stock Mutual Funds
TheStreet Ratings' Ultimate Guided Tour of Stock Investing
Weiss Ratings' Consumer Guides
Weiss Ratings' Guide to Banks
Weiss Ratings' Guide to Credit Unions
Weiss Ratings' Guide to Health Insurers
Weiss Ratings' Guide to Life & Annuity Insurers
Weiss Ratings' Guide to Property & Casualty Insurers

Bowker's Books In Print® Titles
American Book Publishing Record® Annual
American Book Publishing Record® Monthly
Books In Print®
Books In Print® Supplement
Books Out Loud™
Bowker's Complete Video Directory™
Children's Books In Print®
El-Hi Textbooks & Serials In Print®
Forthcoming Books®
Large Print Books & Serials™
Law Books & Serials In Print™
Medical & Health Care Books In Print™
Publishers, Distributors & Wholesalers of the US™
Subject Guide to Books In Print®
Subject Guide to Children's Books In Print®

Canadian General Reference
Associations Canada
Canadian Almanac & Directory
Canadian Environmental Resource Guide
Canadian Parliamentary Guide
Canadian Venture Capital & Private Equity Firms
Financial Post Directory of Directors
Financial Services Canada
Governments Canada
Health Guide Canada
The History of Canada
Libraries Canada
Major Canadian Cities

2016 Title List

Visit www.SalemPress.com for Product Information, Table of Contents, and Sample Pages.

Science, Careers & Mathematics

Ancient Creatures
Applied Science
Applied Science: Engineering & Mathematics
Applied Science: Science & Medicine
Applied Science: Technology
Biomes and Ecosystems
Careers in Building Construction
Careers in Business
Careers in Chemistry
Careers in Communications & Media
Careers in Environment & Conservation
Careers in Healthcare
Careers in Hospitality & Tourism
Careers in Human Services
Careers in Law, Criminal Justice & Emergency Services
Careers in Manufacturing
Careers in Physics
Careers in Sales, Insurance & Real Estate
Careers in Science & Engineering
Careers in Technology Services & Repair
Computer Technology Innovators
Contemporary Biographies in Business
Contemporary Biographies in Chemistry
Contemporary Biographies in Communications & Media
Contemporary Biographies in Environment & Conservation
Contemporary Biographies in Healthcare
Contemporary Biographies in Hospitality & Tourism
Contemporary Biographies in Law & Criminal Justice
Contemporary Biographies in Physics
Earth Science
Earth Science: Earth Materials & Resources
Earth Science: Earth's Surface and History
Earth Science: Physics & Chemistry of the Earth
Earth Science: Weather, Water & Atmosphere
Encyclopedia of Energy
Encyclopedia of Environmental Issues
Encyclopedia of Environmental Issues: Atmosphere and Air Pollution
Encyclopedia of Environmental Issues: Ecology and Ecosystems
Encyclopedia of Environmental Issues: Energy and Energy Use
Encyclopedia of Environmental Issues: Policy and Activism
Encyclopedia of Environmental Issues: Preservation/Wilderness Issues
Encyclopedia of Environmental Issues: Water and Water Pollution
Encyclopedia of Global Resources
Encyclopedia of Global Warming
Encyclopedia of Mathematics & Society
Encyclopedia of Mathematics & Society: Engineering, Tech, Medicine
Encyclopedia of Mathematics & Society: Great Mathematicians
Encyclopedia of Mathematics & Society: Math & Social Sciences
Encyclopedia of Mathematics & Society: Math Development/Concepts
Encyclopedia of Mathematics & Society: Math in Culture & Society
Encyclopedia of Mathematics & Society: Space, Science, Environment
Encyclopedia of the Ancient World
Forensic Science
Geography Basics
Internet Innovators
Inventions and Inventors
Magill's Encyclopedia of Science: Animal Life
Magill's Encyclopedia of Science: Plant life
Notable Natural Disasters
Principles of Astronomy
Principles of Chemistry
Principles of Physics
Science and Scientists
Solar System
Solar System: Great Astronomers
Solar System: Study of the Universe
Solar System: The Inner Planets
Solar System: The Moon and Other Small Bodies
Solar System: The Outer Planets
Solar System: The Sun and Other Stars
World Geography

Literature

American Ethnic Writers
Classics of Science Fiction & Fantasy Literature
Critical Insights: Authors
Critical Insights: Film
Critical Insights: Literary Collection Bundles
Critical Insights: Themes
Critical Insights: Works
Critical Survey of Drama
Critical Survey of Graphic Novels: Heroes & Super Heroes
Critical Survey of Graphic Novels: History, Theme & Technique
Critical Survey of Graphic Novels: Independents/Underground Classics
Critical Survey of Graphic Novels: Manga
Critical Survey of Long Fiction
Critical Survey of Mystery & Detective Fiction
Critical Survey of Mythology and Folklore: Heroes and Heroines
Critical Survey of Mythology and Folklore: Love, Sexuality & Desire
Critical Survey of Mythology and Folklore: World Mythology
Critical Survey of Poetry
Critical Survey of Poetry: American Poets
Critical Survey of Poetry: British, Irish & Commonwealth Poets
Critical Survey of Poetry: Cumulative Index
Critical Survey of Poetry: European Poets
Critical Survey of Poetry: Topical Essays
Critical Survey of Poetry: World Poets
Critical Survey of Shakespeare's Plays
Critical Survey of Shakespeare's Sonnets
Critical Survey of Short Fiction
Critical Survey of Short Fiction: American Writers
Critical Survey of Short Fiction: British, Irish, Commonwealth Writers
Critical Survey of Short Fiction: Cumulative Index
Critical Survey of Short Fiction: European Writers
Critical Survey of Short Fiction: Topical Essays
Critical Survey of Short Fiction: World Writers
Critical Survey of Young Adult Literature
Cyclopedia of Literary Characters
Cyclopedia of Literary Places
Holocaust Literature
Introduction to Literary Context: American Poetry of the 20th Century
Introduction to Literary Context: American Post-Modernist Novels
Introduction to Literary Context: American Short Fiction
Introduction to Literary Context: English Literature
Introduction to Literary Context: Plays
Introduction to Literary Context: World Literature
Magill's Literary Annual 2015
Magill's Survey of American Literature
Magill's Survey of World Literature
Masterplots
Masterplots II: African American Literature
Masterplots II: American Fiction Series
Masterplots II: British & Commonwealth Fiction Series
Masterplots II: Christian Literature
Masterplots II: Drama Series
Masterplots II: Juvenile & Young Adult Literature, Supplement
Masterplots II: Nonfiction Series
Masterplots II: Poetry Series
Masterplots II: Short Story Series
Masterplots II: Women's Literature Series
Notable African American Writers
Notable American Novelists
Notable Playwrights
Notable Poets
Recommended Reading: 600 Classics Reviewed
Short Story Writers

Grey House Publishing | Salem Press | H.W. Wilson | 4919 Route, 22 PO Box 56, Amenia NY 12501-0056

2016 Title List

Visit www.SalemPress.com for Product Information, Table of Contents, and Sample Pages.

History and Social Science

The 2000s in America
50 States
African American History
Agriculture in History
American First Ladies
American Heroes
American Indian Culture
American Indian History
American Indian Tribes
American Presidents
American Villains
America's Historic Sites
Ancient Greece
The Bill of Rights
The Civil Rights Movement
The Cold War
Countries, Peoples & Cultures
Countries, Peoples & Cultures: Central & South America
Countries, Peoples & Cultures: Central, South & Southeast Asia
Countries, Peoples & Cultures: East & South Africa
Countries, Peoples & Cultures: East Asia & the Pacific
Countries, Peoples & Cultures: Eastern Europe
Countries, Peoples & Cultures: Middle East & North Africa
Countries, Peoples & Cultures: North America & the Caribbean
Countries, Peoples & Cultures: West & Central Africa
Countries, Peoples & Cultures: Western Europe
Defining Documents: American Revolution
Defining Documents: Civil Rights
Defining Documents: Civil War
Defining Documents: Emergence of Modern America
Defining Documents: Exploration & Colonial America
Defining Documents: Manifest Destiny
Defining Documents: Postwar 1940s
Defining Documents: Reconstruction
Defining Documents: 1920s
Defining Documents: 1930s
Defining Documents: 1950s
Defining Documents: 1960s
Defining Documents: 1970s
Defining Documents: American West
Defining Documents: Ancient World
Defining Documents: Middle Ages
Defining Documents: Vietnam War
Defining Documents: World War I
Defining Documents: World War II
The Eighties in America
Encyclopedia of American Immigration
Encyclopedia of Flight
Encyclopedia of the Ancient World
Fashion Innovators
The Fifties in America
The Forties in America
Great Athletes
Great Athletes: Baseball
Great Athletes: Basketball
Great Athletes: Boxing & Soccer
Great Athletes: Cumulative Index
Great Athletes: Football
Great Athletes: Golf & Tennis
Great Athletes: Olympics
Great Athletes: Racing & Individual Sports
Great Events from History: 17th Century
Great Events from History: 18th Century
Great Events from History: 19th Century
Great Events from History: 20th Century (1901-1940)
Great Events from History: 20th Century (1941-1970)
Great Events from History: 20th Century (1971-2000)
Great Events from History: Ancient World
Great Events from History: Cumulative Indexes
Great Events from History: Gay, Lesbian, Bisexual, Transgender Events

Great Events from History: Middle Ages
Great Events from History: Modern Scandals
Great Events from History: Renaissance & Early Modern Era
Great Lives from History: 17th Century
Great Lives from History: 18th Century
Great Lives from History: 19th Century
Great Lives from History: 20th Century
Great Lives from History: African Americans
Great Lives from History: American Women
Great Lives from History: Ancient World
Great Lives from History: Asian & Pacific Islander Americans
Great Lives from History: Cumulative Indexes
Great Lives from History: Incredibly Wealthy
Great Lives from History: Inventors & Inventions
Great Lives from History: Jewish Americans
Great Lives from History: Latinos
Great Lives from History: Middle Ages
Great Lives from History: Notorious Lives
Great Lives from History: Renaissance & Early Modern Era
Great Lives from History: Scientists & Science
Historical Encyclopedia of American Business
Issues in U.S. Immigration
Magill's Guide to Military History
Milestone Documents in African American History
Milestone Documents in American History
Milestone Documents in World History
Milestone Documents of American Leaders
Milestone Documents of World Religions
Music Innovators
Musicians & Composers 20th Century
The Nineties in America
The Seventies in America
The Sixties in America
Survey of American Industry and Careers
The Thirties in America
The Twenties in America
United States at War
U.S.A. in Space
U.S. Court Cases
U.S. Government Leaders
U.S. Laws, Acts, and Treaties
U.S. Legal System
U.S. Supreme Court
Weapons and Warfare
World Conflicts: Asia and the Middle East
World Political Yearbook

Health

Addictions & Substance Abuse
Adolescent Health & Wellness
Cancer
Complementary & Alternative Medicine
Genetics & Inherited Conditions
Health Issues
Infectious Diseases & Conditions
Magill's Medical Guide
Psychology & Behavioral Health
Psychology Basics

Grey House Publishing | Salem Press | H.W. Wilson | 4919 Route, 22 PO Box 56, Amenia NY 12501-0056

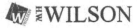
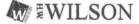

2016 Title List

Visit **www.HWWilsonInPrint.com** for Product Information, Table of Contents and Sample Pages

Current Biography
Current Biography Cumulative Index 1946-2013
Current Biography Monthly Magazine
Current Biography Yearbook: 2003
Current Biography Yearbook: 2004
Current Biography Yearbook: 2005
Current Biography Yearbook: 2006
Current Biography Yearbook: 2007
Current Biography Yearbook: 2008
Current Biography Yearbook: 2009
Current Biography Yearbook: 2010
Current Biography Yearbook: 2011
Current Biography Yearbook: 2012
Current Biography Yearbook: 2013
Current Biography Yearbook: 2014
Current Biography Yearbook: 2015

Core Collections
Children's Core Collection
Fiction Core Collection
Graphic Novels Core Collection
Middle & Junior High School Core
Public Library Core Collection: Nonfiction
Senior High Core Collection
Young Adult Fiction Core Collection

The Reference Shelf
Aging in America
American Military Presence Overseas
The Arab Spring
The Brain
The Business of Food
Campaign Trends & Election Law
Conspiracy Theories
The Digital Age
Dinosaurs
Embracing New Paradigms in Education
Faith & Science
Families: Traditional and New Structures
The Future of U.S. Economic Relations: Mexico, Cuba, and Venezuela
Global Climate Change
Graphic Novels and Comic Books
Immigration
Immigration in the U.S.
Internet Safety
Marijuana Reform
The News and its Future
The Paranormal
Politics of the Ocean
Racial Tension in a "Postracial" Age
Reality Television
Representative American Speeches: 2008-2009
Representative American Speeches: 2009-2010
Representative American Speeches: 2010-2011
Representative American Speeches: 2011-2012
Representative American Speeches: 2012-2013
Representative American Speeches: 2013-2014
Representative American Speeches: 2014-2015
Representative American Speeches: 2015-2016
Rethinking Work
Revisiting Gender
Robotics
Russia
Social Networking
Social Services for the Poor
Space Exploration & Development
Sports in America
The Supreme Court
The Transformation of American Cities

U.S. Infrastructure
U.S. National Debate Topic: Surveillance
U.S. National Debate Topic: The Ocean
U.S. National Debate Topic: Transportation Infrastructure
Whistleblowers

Readers' Guide
Abridged Readers' Guide to Periodical Literature
Readers' Guide to Periodical Literature

Indexes
Index to Legal Periodicals & Books
Short Story Index
Book Review Digest

Sears List
Sears List of Subject Headings
Sears: Lista de Encabezamientos de Materia

Facts About Series
Facts About American Immigration
Facts About China
Facts About the 20th Century
Facts About the Presidents
Facts About the World's Languages

Nobel Prize Winners
Nobel Prize Winners: 1901-1986
Nobel Prize Winners: 1987-1991
Nobel Prize Winners: 1992-1996
Nobel Prize Winners: 1997-2001

World Authors
World Authors: 1995-2000
World Authors: 2000-2005

Famous First Facts
Famous First Facts
Famous First Facts About American Politics
Famous First Facts About Sports
Famous First Facts About the Environment
Famous First Facts: International Edition

American Book of Days
The American Book of Days
The International Book of Days

Junior Authors & Illustrators
Eleventh Book of Junior Authors & Illustrations

Monographs
The Barnhart Dictionary of Etymology
Celebrate the World
Guide to the Ancient World
Indexing from A to Z
The Poetry Break
Radical Change: Books for Youth in a Digital Age

Wilson Chronology
Wilson Chronology of Asia and the Pacific
Wilson Chronology of Human Rights
Wilson Chronology of Ideas
Wilson Chronology of the Arts
Wilson Chronology of the World's Religions
Wilson Chronology of Women's Achievements

Grey House Publishing | Salem Press | H.W. Wilson | 4919 Route, 22 PO Box 56, Amenia NY 12501-0056

FOR REFERENCE

Do Not Take From This Room